Principles and Practice of
Veterinary
Technology

Principles and Practice of
Veterinary
Technology

Edited by
Paul W. Pratt, VMD

*with 339 illustrations
including 32 color plates*

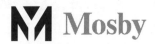

St. Louis Baltimore Boston Carlsbad Chicago Minneapolis New York Philadelphia Portland
London Milan Sydney Tokyo Toronto

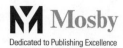

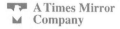

Vice President and Publisher: Don Ladig
Executive Editor: Linda Lee Duncan
Managing Editor: Janet Russell
Developmental Editor: Melba Steube
Project Manager: Mark Spann
Production Editors: Jennifer Doll, Anne Salmo
Book Design Manager: Judi Lang
Cover Design: GW Graphics
Manufacturing Supervisor: Karen Boehme

Printed in the United States of America
Composition by Mosby Electronic Production
Lithography/color film by Top Graphics
Printing/binding by The Maple-Vail Book Manufacturing Group

Mosby–Year Book, Inc.
11830 Westline Industrial Drive
St. Louis, Missouri 63146

Library of Congress Cataloging-in-Publication Data

Principles and practice of veterinary technology / edited by Paul W.
  Pratt
     p. cm.
  Includes index.
  ISBN 0-8151-7308-3
  1. Animal health technology. I. Pratt, Paul W.
SF774.4.P75 1997
636.089—dc21   97-14020
                                  CIP

98 99 00 01 02 / 9 8 7 6 5 4 3 2 1

Contributors

Ron E. Banks, DVM, Dipl ACVPM, Dipl ACLAM
Director, Office of Laboratory Animal Medicine
University of Colorado
Denver, Colorado

Susan A. Berryhill, BS, RVT
Research Veterinary Technician
Hill's Pet Nutrition, Inc.
Science and Technology Center
Topeka, Kansas

Robert L. Bill, DVM, PhD
Associate Professor of Veterinary Pharmacology
Assistant to the Director of Veterinary Technology
Purdue University School of Veterinary Medicine
West Lafayette, Indiana

James T. Blackford, DVM, MS, Dipl ACVS
Associate Professor
Department of Large Animal Surgery
University of Tennessee
College of Veterinary Medicine
Knoxville, Tennessee

Christine Bretz, RVT
Special Procedures Veterinary Technologist
Purdue University Veterinary Teaching Hospital
West Lafayette, Indiana

Linda J. Brown, AAS, CVT
Certified Veterinary Technician
College of Veterinary Medicine
University of Illinois
Urbana, Illinois

Phillip E. Cochran, MS, DVM
Department Chairman/Program Veterinarian
Veterinary Technology Program
Portland Community College
Portland, Oregon

Joann Colville, DVM
Associate Professor of Veterinary Science
Department of Veterinary and Microbiological Sciences
North Dakota State University
Fargo, North Dakota

Thomas P. Colville, DVM, MSc
Director, Veterinary Technology Program
Department of Veterinary and Microbiological Sciences
North Dakota State University
Fargo, North Dakota

Autumn P. Davidson, AHT, DVM, Dipl ACVIM
Associate Clinical Professor
Department of Medicine
University of California
School of Veterinary Medicine
Davis, California

Harold Davis, Jr., BA, RVT, VTS (Emergency & Critical Care)
Coordinator, Clinical Instruction: Hospital Practices, Veterinary Technician, Small Animal Intensive Care Unit, Veterinary Medical Teaching Hospital Charter Veterinary Technician Specialist (Emergency & Critical Care)
Academy of Veterinary Emergency & Critical Care Technicians
University of California
Veterinary Medical Teaching Hospital
Davis, California

Barbara J. Deeb, DVM, MS
Clinical Assistant Professor
Department of Comparative Medicine
University of Washington
Seattle, Washington
Private Practice, Allpet Veterinary Clinic
Shoreline, Washington

Jacqueline Ann De Jong, LVT, BS
Veterinary Technician, Large Animal
Oregon State University
College of Veterinary Medicine
Corvallis, Oregon

Gay L. De Longe, DVM
Professor of Veterinary Technology
Blue Ridge Community College
Weyers Cave, Virginia

Donald R. Dooley
Veterinary Practice Management Consultant
Los Gatos, California

Samuel M. Fassig, DVM, MA
Certified OD/Systems Design
Technical Services Veterinarian
Companion Animal Business Unit
Mallinckrodt Veterinary, Inc.
Bennett, Colorado

David J. Fisher, DVM, Dipl ACVP (Clinical Pathology)
Clinical Pathologist
CVD, Inc.
West Sacramento, California

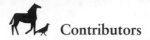
Ruth Francis-Floyd, DVM
Associate Professor
Department of Large Animal Clinical Sciences
Department of Fisheries and Aquatic Sciences
University of Florida
College of Veterinary Medicine
Gainesville, Florida

Theresa W. Fossum, DVM, MS, PhD, Dipl ACVS
Associate Professor
Department of Small Animal Medicine and Surgery
Texas A&M University
College of Veterinary Medicine
College Station, Texas

Laurie J. Gage, DVM
Director of Veterinary Services
Chief Clinical Consultant
The Marine Mammal Center
Marine World Africa USA
Vallejo, California

Franklyn B. Garry, DVM, MS, Dipl ACVIM
Associate Professor
Department of Clinical Sciences
Colorado State University
College of Veterinary Medicine and Biomedical Sciences
Fort Collins, Colorado

Peter J. Gaveras, DVM, MBA
Hospital Administrator
Animal Emergency Center
Milwaukee, Wisconsin

Madonna E. Gemus, DVM
Swine Production and Medicine Resident
Department of Large Animal Clinical Sciences
Michigan State University
College of Veterinary Medicine
East Lansing, Michigan

Richard A. Goebel, DVM
Director, Veterinary Teaching Hospital
Purdue University
School of Veterinary Medicine
West Lafayette, Indiana
Private Practice, Magrane Animal Hospital
Mishawaka, Indiana

Elizabeth A. Gorecki, LVT
Technician, Small Animal Neurology
Michigan State University
Veterinary Teaching Hospital
East Lansing, Michigan

Sheila R. Grosdidier, BS, RVT
Senior Paraveterinary Educator
Hill's Pet Nutrition, Inc.
Topeka, Kansas

Connie Han, RVT
Imaging Technologist
Purdue University
Veterinary Teaching Hospital
West Lafayette, Indiana

Christi Hayes, BS
Veterinary Assistant
Private Practice
Yorba Linda, California

Suzanne Hetts, PhD
Certified Applied Animal Behaviorist
President, Animal Behavior Associates, Inc.
Littleton, Colorado

Bruce Hopman, MS, DVM
Instructor, Veterinary Technology Program
Portland Community College
Portland, Oregon

Karen Hrapkiewicz, DVM, MS, Dipl ACLAM
Director, Veterinary Technology Program
Wayne County Community College and Wayne State University
Detroit, Michigan

Cheryl Hurd, RVT
Chief Imaging Technologist
Purdue University Teaching Hospital
West Lafayette, Indiana

Muhammed Ikram, DVM, MSc, PhD
Coordinator, Animal Health and Veterinary Medical Receptionist Technologies
Department of Animal Health Technology
Fairview College
Fairview, Alberta, Canada

Eileen M. Johnson, DVM, MS, PhD
Staff Research Associate
University of California
College of Veterinary Medicine
Veterinary Medical Teaching Hospital
Davis, California

Tina Kemper, DVM, Dipl ACVIM
Private Practice
Yorba Linda, California

Linda R. Krcatovich, LVT
Veterinary Technician
Large Animal Clinical Sciences
Michigan State University
College of Veterinary Medicine
East Lansing, Michigan

Michel Levy, DVM, Dipl ACVIM
Associate Professor of Large Animal Medicine
Purdue University
School of Veterinary Medicine
West Lafayette, Indiana

Heidi B. Lobprise, DVM, Dipl AVDC
Private Practice
Dallas Dental Service Animal Clinic
Dallas, Texas

Roger L. Lukens, DVM
Professor and Director of Veterinary Technology
Purdue University
School of Veterinary Medicine
West Lafayette, Indiana

Shawn Patrick Messonnier, DVM
Editor-in-chief, Exotic Pet Practice
Plano, Texas

Seyedmehdi Mobini, DVM, MS, Dipl ACT
Professor of Veterinary Science
Research/Extension Veterinarian
Agriculture Research Station
Fort Valley State College
Fort Valley, Georgia

Donna A. Oakley, CVT, VTS (Emergency and Critical Care)
Director of Nursing
Veterinary Hospital
University of Pennsylvania
School of Veterinary Medicine
Philadelphia, Pennsylvania

Catherine Ann Picut, VMD, JD, Dipl ACVP
Patent Attorney
Hoffmann-La Roche, Inc.
Nutley, New Jersey

Stuart L. Porter, VMD
Professor, Veterinary Technology
Blue Ridge Community College
Weyers Cave, Virginia
Vice President, National Wildlife Rehabilitators Association

Sheila M. Wing-Proctor, LVT, BS (Medical Technology), BS (Animal Science)
Large Animal Surgery
Veterinary Teaching Hospital
Michigan State University
East Lansing, Michigan

Rose Quinn, CVT, BA
Assistant Professor
Veterinary Technology
Colorado Mountain College
Glenwood Springs, Colorado

Angel M. Rivera, CVT
Animal Emergency Center
Milwaukee, Wisconsin

Bernard E. Rollin, PhD
Director of Bioethical Planning
Professor of Physiology and Philosophy
Department of Philosophy
Colorado State University
College of Veterinary Medicine and Biomedical Sciences
Fort Collins, Colorado

Cheri Barton Ross, MA
Private Practice
Montgomery Village Veterinary Clinic
Santa Rosa, California

Scott W. Rundell, DVM
Associate Professor, Veterinary Technology
Morehead State University
Morehead, Kentucky

Philip J. Seibert, Jr., CVT
Veterinary Practice Consultant
Calhoun, Tennessee

Howard B. Seim III, DVM, Dipl ACVS
Associate Professor and Chief of Small Animal Surgery
Colorado State University
College of Veterinary Medicine and Biomedical Sciences
Fort Collins, Colorado

Jane Baron-Sorensen, BSN, MA
Patient Care Manager
County of Sonoma Psychiatric Services
Santa Rosa, California

Amy E. Thiessen, DVM
Resident, Clinical Pathology
Oklahoma State University
College of Veterinary Medicine
Stillwater, Oklahoma

Mary E. Torrence, DVM, PhD, Dipl ACVPM
Epidemiologist for Epidemiology Branch
Office of Surveillance and Biometrics
Center for Devices and Radiological Health, FDA
Rockville, Maryland
Adjunct Professor
Virginia-Maryland Regional College of Veterinary Medicine
Blacksburg, Virginia

C. Lee Tyner, DVM
Coordinator, Veterinary Technology
Morehead State University
Morehead, Kentucky

Wendy E. Vaala, VMD, Dipl ACVIM
Assistant Professor of Medicine
New Bolton Center
University of Pennsylvania
Kennett Square, Pennsylvania

Steven D. Van Camp, DVM, Dipl ACT
Associate Professor
Department of Food Animal and Equine Medicine
North Carolina State University
College of Veterinary Medicine
Raleigh, North Carolina

Robert J. Van Saun, DVM, MS, PhD, Dipl ACT, Dipl ACVN
Assistant Professor of Clinical Nutrition and Theriogenology
Department of Large Animal Clinical Sciences
Oregon State University
College of Veterinary Medicine
Corvallis, Oregon

M. Randy White, DVM, PhD, Dipl ACVP
Assistant Director
Animal Disease Diagnostic Laboratory
Purdue University
School of Veterinary Medicine
West Lafayette, Indiana

Preface

The contributions of veterinary technicians and veterinary assistants to the veterinary profession and animal health industry are inestimable. These dedicated individuals typically work long hours providing nursing care for sick and injured animals. Their clinical expertise and responsibilities have steadily grown in recent years to the point where they are now an indispensable part of most veterinary practices. Many veterinary practitioners pale at the thought of attempting to operate a busy practice without their key technicians, who manage to juggle multiple clinical tasks while tactfully interacting with clients, often under harried and stressful circumstances. Veterinary technicians also play a key role in nonpractice situations, providing technical support in research laboratories, teaching hospitals, and other institutional environments. Rather than "just another pair of hands," veterinary technicians are an integral part of the animal health care team. This text is dedicated to these unheralded professionals.

In planning this book, I aimed to include all of the topics that make up a veterinary technician's duties, with space alloted in proportion to each topic's degree of import. To include an exhaustive discussion of every topic would have necessitated publishing a multivolume work costing hundreds of dollars. This text is a compromise between practicality and the ideal of comprehensive coverage. The scope of content is broad; discussions present the salient information veterinary technician students should know and entry-level technicians would find useful.

Technician students and educators will benefit from this text's useful features:

- A list of learning objectives at the beginning of each chapter
- Color plates in the section on hematology
- Numerous boxed descriptions of clinical procedures
- More than 200 review questions and answers at the end of the text

Nearly all of the contributors of this text are involved in technician education. Their clinical and pedagogic experience are evident in their discussions, which distill complex subjects down to the essentials required by students of veterinary technology. I was humbled by the breadth and depth of their knowledge and am grateful to have had this opportunity to work with them.

Paul W. Pratt, VMD

Brief Contents

Contents

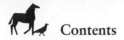

Contents   **xv**

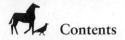

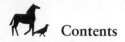

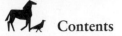

PART ONE

Introduction

CHAPTER 1

An Overview of Veterinary Technology

R.L. Lukens

Learning Objectives

After reviewing this chapter, the reader should understand the following:

Scope of a veterinary technician's duties
Nomenclature describing veterinary personnel

Education of veterinary technicians
Career opportunities, salary ranges, and organizations available to veterinary technicians
Certification and licensing procedures for veterinary technicians

Veterinary technicians are a relatively new group of professionals in veterinary medicine, similar in many respects to registered nurses in human medicine. By the American Veterinary Medical Association's (AVMA) definition, a *veterinary technician* must be a graduate of an AVMA-accredited college program in veterinary technology and work under a licensed veterinary practitioner (DVM or VMD), unless employed in a nonpractice situation.

The emergence of veterinary technicians (educated in technician training programs) as members of the veterinary team is an important development for the veterinary profession. This change was in its infancy in the 1960s, in the developmental stage in the 1970s, and in a dynamically changing stage in the 1980s. It is maturing in the 1990s. Veterinary technicians likely will play an increasingly important role in the veterinary profession, such as nurses do in human medicine.

DUTIES OF VETERINARY TECHNICIANS

Veterinary technicians often are not recognized by the public and may be misunderstood by practicing DVMs. Varying expectations and lack of standardization of employee roles allow DVMs to establish their teams by their own criteria. Before and during their veterinary medical education, veterinarians usually work in veterinary practices as unpaid volunteers, often in a practice where the DVM did not delegate many technical and/or medical tasks to staff members. This has caused many new practicing veterinarians to think of themselves as "doers" and not "delegators." Therefore, it has sometimes been difficult for recently graduated veterinary technicians to find career opportunities where delegated technical tasks are sufficient to justify a salary high enough to keep them in the veterinary technology profession.

The role of veterinary technicians in practice varies with the many different ways in which practices are organized. In years past, most DVMs trained their own helpers (on-the-job trainees) as clinical aides, and many still do today. The primary purpose of these people was to help restrain animals, to keep the premises clean, to serve as a "gopher" (go for), and to receive clients. Often one person served all of these functions, assisting a busy DVM as a closely supervised clinical aide. The licensed DVM (regulated by the state where practicing) usually practiced alone and performed the technical procedures and nursing duties him- or herself.

Veterinary technicians are now assuming a major role in practice by performing medical and surgical nursing procedures and laboratory testing, anesthesia induction, maintenance, monitoring during recovery, and other clinical procedures. A DVM's productivity is increased by delegating many income-producing procedures to veterinary technicians, allowing the doctor to concentrate on diagnosis and surgery. Table 1-1 summarizes the duties and responsibilities of veterinary technicians.

NOMENCLATURE OF VETERINARY PERSONNEL

The following definitions expand AVMA definitions to provide more complete descriptions that encompass the latest developments in the profession.

Veterinary technology The science and art of providing professional support service to veterinarians. AVMA-accredited programs that educate veterinary technicians are usually called veterinary technology programs.

Veterinary assistant Person with training, knowledge, and skills at the level of a clinical aide, but less than that required for a veterinary technician. Veterinary assistants can be compared with nurses' aides in human medicine. Generally, veterinary assistants are trained on the job, but some graduate from 6-month training programs. The duties of veterinary assistants usually include non--income-producing tasks, such as restraining, moving, feeding, and exercising patients, cleaning premises, and other clinical support tasks. These aides may also be described by other terms, combining *clinical, hospital, technician's, ward,* or *veterinary* with *aide, attendant, caretaker,* or *assistant.* They are most appropriately called *technician's assistants* or *clinical aides,* rather than *veterinary assistants.* The physician's assistant has more training and requires less supervision than a registered nurse, in contrast with the clinical aide (nurse's aide).

Veterinary technician A graduate of a 2- or 3-year, AVMA-accredited program in veterinary technology. A veterinary technician's duties are similar to, in human medicine, those of a registered nurse, nurse-anesthetist, operating room technician, dental hygienist, medical laboratory technician, or radiographic technician.

Professional nursing-related duties that produce income are delegated to a veterinary technician by a licensed DVM in a fee-for-service veterinary practice. Veterinary technicians may also work in research, educational, sales, or governmental positions.

Veterinary technologist A graduate of a 4-year, AVMA-accredited veterinary technology program who holds a baccalaureate degree from veterinary technician study; or a graduate veterinary technician with a bachelor of science (B.S.) degree in another program with studies in supervision, leadership, management, or a scientific area. Duties of veterinary technologists include veterinary technician duties, often in combination with personnel management or hospital management. They may be employed as teachers, research associates, group leaders, sales managers, or clinical technologists in a specialty practice. Their role is sometimes compared with that of the physician's assistant, except, by veterinary practice law, veterinary technologists require more direct supervision in treating patients.

Veterinarian A doctor of veterinary medicine; a graduate of a 4-year, AVMA-accredited program, such as one of the 27 American or 4 Canadian veterinary medical colleges. To practice veterinary medicine, veterinarians must pass a licensure examination in the states or provinces in which they wish to practice. Most veterinarians graduating today have 4 years of preveterinary studies, with a B.A. or B.S. degree, in addition to their 4 years of study at a veterinary college, culminating in a Doctor of Veterinary Medicine degree (DVM or VMD).

Veterinary team A combination of DVMs, professional support staff (veterinary technicians and/or veterinary technologists), and nonprofessional lay staff (veterinary assistants, technician's assistants, clinical aides, caretakers, and receptionists).

Table 1-1 on p. 5 outlines the education and roles of veterinary assistants, veterinary technicians, and veterinary technologists.

VETERINARY TECHNICIAN EDUCATION PROGRAMS

As of this writing, there are 71 AVMA-accredited veterinary technology programs in 38 states. To attain AVMA accreditation, veterinary technology education programs must meet 11 minimal requirements pertaining to facilities, faculty, admission requirements, and curricula. All programs are required to provide training in a variety of clinical tasks. They must "provide technical skill acquisition strengthened through meaningful experience to enable graduates to not only be a productive employee at entry level for veterinary technicians, but also develop the capabilities to perform satisfactorily in positions of increasing responsibility." These curricula must be designed to provide hands-on experience

TABLE 1-1 Veterinary support personnel

Category	Veterinary assistants	Veterinary technicians	Veterinary technologists
Definition	Clinical aide; generalist in animal care	Technician in technical medical skills	Specialist technologist in applied science
Knowledge and ability	Can do general tasks; does not know alternatives or why	Performs wide range of technical tasks; adaptable; knows how and why technically; normal vs abnormal focus	Knows how to organize; knows scientific basis and many specialized applications
Focus	General restraint and animal care; clinical assisting	Wide range of technical and medical nursing tasks	Plans and executes projects, supervises and/or teaches technicians
Education	OJT* experience only, entry level; correspondence or short courses	Veterinary technology program—AVMA accredited	Advanced areas of veterinary technology and science
Degree	On-the-job trained; no degree	A.A.S. degree	B.S. degree in a specialty or equivalent
College	Little or none required	2-year program required	4-year program required
Role	Clinical aide Animal caretaker/attendant Technician's assistant Veterinarian's assistant (entry-level) Orderly Janitor	Nursing technician Anesthetist Surgery tech/ORT† Radiography tech Medical lab tech Dental hygienist	Clinical specialist Working supervisor Practice manager Teaching technologist Sales representative Animal housing director
AALAS terminology	Assistant laboratory animal technician	Laboratory animal technician	Laboratory animal technologist
Regulation	None except as employee of licensed DVM	40 states regulated by VTNE‡ as registered, certified, or licensed technician	Certification developing in some specialties
Career pathway	Remain VA$ or enter technician or pre-vet program	Career as a certified veterinary technician on veterinary team	Career as technologist, supervisor, teacher, or manager on veterinary team

*On-the-job training.
†Operating room technician.
‡Veterinary Technician National Examination.
§Veterinarian's assistant.

to ensure that each student performs 200 "essential tasks" listed in the AVMA *Accreditation Policies and Procedures Manual*. It is also desirable that an additional 84 "recommended tasks" be performed by each student. Proficiency outcomes for each procedure depend on the program emphasis and the number of times the students have practiced these tasks.

In 1995 in the United States, 1,214 veterinary technician students graduated from 65 AVMA-accredited programs. There were 2,368 first-year students, 1,649 second-year students, 124 third-year students, and 105 fourth-year students enrolled in programs responding to a 1995 AVMA survey. The average rate of attrition (dropouts) was 27.1% in year one and 12.2% in year

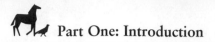

two (total of 39.3% during two years). More than 95% of veterinary technician students are female.

CAREER OPPORTUNITIES FOR VETERINARY TECHNICIANS

According to the AVMA, most (77%) career positions for veterinary technicians are in veterinary practices, with 59% employed in companion animal practices, 10% in mixed-species practices, 4% in equine practices, and about 2% each in food animal and specialty practices. The greatest demand for veterinary technicians is in companion animal practices.

Nonpractice career opportunities (22%) include diagnostic/research laboratories (13%), industry/sales (2%), veterinary technician education programs (2%), government (1%), and miscellaneous (4%). The miscellaneous category includes positions with zoos (especially in zoos with a hospital and full-time zoo veterinarians), livestock farms (animal health liaison with a consulting veterinarian), wildlife rehabilitation centers, humane shelters, the military, and colleges of veterinary medicine (clinical technicians).

SALARY RANGES FOR VETERINARY TECHNICIANS

In 1995, the AVMA reported average annual salaries for experienced veterinary technicians of about $17,000 in equine and mixed animal practices, $18,000 in food animal practices, $19,000 in companion animal and government positions, $22,000 in specialty practices, $26,000 in teaching and diagnostic/research laboratories, and $29,000 in industry sales positions. In a 1995 AVMA survey, there were 5,153 job openings on file with 54 job placement programs and only 131 recent graduates still seeking a position. Even though some employers list positions with several placement programs, the shortage of veterinary technicians remains significant in many geographic areas. How many of these potential employers were willing to delegate appropriate tasks and pay a salary sufficient to retain a veterinary technician in the profession is unknown.

ATTRITION OF VETERINARY TECHNICIANS

There is a trend toward group practices (today's average is more than two DVMs per practice in the United States, with many practices having three or more DVMs), increased client expectations of quality care, and an economic need to leverage DVM productivity.

These changes have allowed veterinary technicians to play a greater role in providing nursing care and related medical services. For decades, registered nurses have outnumbered physicians by more than 2 to 1; support staff members in human medicine have outnumbered physicians by more than 15 to 1. According to the AVMA, in 1991 there was only 1 veterinary technician for every 4 DVMs and 2.4 support staff members for every 1 DVM. These low ratios are beginning to increase, suggesting that the veterinary profession is shifting toward utilizing more support staff.

A significant number of technicians leave the profession after graduation. Issues that discourage veterinary technicians from remaining in the profession include low pay, lack of professional recognition, lack of advancement, and underutilization by veterinary employers. Of 23,900 technicians graduating in all past years from 33 veterinary technology programs, only 7,849 remained employed in 1995, which suggests an attrition rate of more than 65%.

Attrition could be reduced if DVMs would delegate more income-producing medical nursing and laboratory tasks to veterinary technicians and raise their salaries according to the additional income produced. Although most veterinary technicians are highly motivated to work as caregivers for the satisfaction of nursing patients back to health, few can afford to work for a very modest income. Veterinary technicians in this situation almost always leave the profession. Fortunately, this situation is being reversed as more DVMs are learning to delegate medical and diagnostic procedures to technicians and pay them accordingly.

CERTIFICATION AND LICENSING OF VETERINARY TECHNICIANS

Graduate veterinary technicians are licensed, certified, or registered in most states by passing an examination given by that state and the Veterinary Technician National Examination (VTNE). Results of the VTNE can be transferred to other states via the Interstate Reporting Service of the Professional Examination Service. The VTNE is validated by the Veterinary Technician Testing Committee, a committee of veterinarians and veterinary technicians appointed by various professional organizations.

Veterinary technicians are educated to follow specific ethical and legal guidelines while working under the direction and supervision of a licensed DVM. The employing veterinarian has the ultimate responsibility for using a technician in an appropriate ethical manner, consistent with state and federal laws. According to veterinary practice acts in all states, only the DVM can legally diagnose diseases and prescribe therapy, as well as perform surgery and issue a prognosis (predicted medical outcome). All of these are beyond the scope of a veterinary technician's duties (see Box 1-1). Chapter 3 presents detailed information on the laws and ethics of veterinary practice.

VETERINARY TECHNICIAN ORGANIZATIONS

There are many state and local or regional veterinary technician professional associations. The North American Veterinary Technician Association (NAVTA) represents the veterinary technician profession nationally in seeking changes that help its members and the profession as a whole. NAVTA has been very successful in many areas, including lobbying the AVMA to establish a national board examination (VTNE) validation

process. Its current emphasis is on representing its members while striving to improve utilization of veterinary technicians, thus improving career opportunities for veterinary technicians.

THE FUTURE OF VETERINARY TECHNOLOGY

If veterinary technology is to advance as a profession, veterinary technicians must join state and national organizations to advance the cause for better utilization of veterinary technicians, attain greater professional recognition, develop more effective continuing education programs, and generally represent its members in political, legal, and other related matters. Whereas an increasing number of DVMs have leveraged their productivity through full utilization of veterinary techni-

---

Box 1-1 Technical duties and responsibilities of qualified veterinary technicians*

Care of hospitalized patients

Administering medication
Applying dressings and bandages
Collecting diagnostic samples
Intensive care
Nutritional management
Physical therapy

Clinical pathology

Collecting specimens
Cytologic examination
Hematologic examination
Microbiologic examination
Parasitologic examination
Serum chemistry assays
Urinalysis

Outpatients and field service

Administering medication and vaccines
Client education
Collecting diagnostic samples
Obtaining a history
Physical examination

Radiology

Developing radiographic film
Patient preparation and positioning
Radiation safety
Radiographic technique

Anesthesiology

Administering local or general anesthetics
Patient monitoring during and after anesthesia
Preanesthetic evaluation

Dental prophylaxis

Oral and dental examination
Teeth cleaning and polishing

Surgical assisting

Assisting during surgical procedures
Instrument sterilization
Postoperative patient care
Preoperative patient preparation
Surgical suite preparation and maintenance

Hospital administration

Bookkeeping and practice management
Inventory control
Reception duties and client education
Supervision and training of staff

Biomedical research

Assist in design and implementation of research projects
Supervise maintenance of animal colonies and facilities

*Adapted from NAVTA: *Veterinary technology: a career for you in the 90s.*

cians, few have an incentive to discuss their competitive advantage with other veterinary practices. Therefore, future advances in utilization of veterinary technicians depend on the collective efforts of veterinary technicians themselves and their professional organizations.

SOURCES OF ADDITIONAL INFORMATION

North American Veterinary Technician Association (NAVTA), P.O. Box 224, Battleground, IN 47920. Posters, career brochures, technician code of ethics, newsletters, continuing education opportunities, and information on technician utilization.

Association of Veterinary Technician Educators (AVTE), Terry Teeple, DVM, Pierce College, 9401 Farwest Dr. SW, Tacoma, WA 98498. Information on educational programs.

American Veterinary Medical Association (AVMA), Suite 100, 1931 North Meacham Rd., Schaumburg, IL 60173. List of accredited veterinary technology education programs, accreditation requirements, job openings, state law summaries, career brochures, and state and local veterinary technician organizations.

AVMA Directory. Published annually by the AVMA, Suite 100, 1931 North Meacham Rd., Schaumburg, IL 60173.

RECOMMENDED READING

NAVTA Newsletter. Published monthly by NAVTA, P.O. Box 224, Battleground, IN 47920.
The Veterinary Technician. Journal published monthly by Veterinary Learning Systems, #100, 425 Phillips Blvd., Trenton, NJ 08618.

CHAPTER 2

Occupational Hazards

P.J. Seibert, Jr.

Learning Objectives

After reviewing this chapter, the reader should understand the following:

Ways in which to avoid hazards in the veterinary workplace
Hazards of handling animals
Primary zoonotic diseases that pose danger to veterinary personnel

Ways in which radiation injury can be avoided
Hazards of anesthetic and compressed gases
Methods of preventing spread of infectious disease
Information contained in and uses of Material Safety Data Sheets

As a staff member in a veterinary hospital, you are exposed to many hazards in your day-to-day routine and in the performance of nonroutine functions. Hazards can include exposure to pathogenic microorganisms, chemicals, or radiation, in addition to the obvious physical dangers. When properly identified, however, these hazards can be controlled and your risk of injury minimized.

BASIC SAFETY CONSIDERATIONS
Machinery and Moving Parts

Equipment such as fans and dryers has moving parts that can severely injure you or even sever a finger. Never operate machinery or equipment without all the proper guards in place. Long hair should be tied back or up on top of your head to prevent it from getting caught in fans or other moving objects. Avoid wearing excessive jewelry, very loose-fitting clothing, or open-toe shoes. If you become aware of an unsafe condition, report it to your supervisor immediately.

Slips and Falls

You can reduce the chances of personal injury from slips and falls by wearing slip-proof shoes and using nonslip mats or strips in wet areas. Be especially cautious when walking on uneven or wet floors. Never run inside the hospital or on uneven flooring.

Lifting

When lifting patients, supplies, or equipment, remember to keep your back straight and lift with your legs. Never bend over to lift an object. If a motorized lift table is not available, recruit some help when lifting patients who weigh more than 40 pounds. Remember to follow sound ergonomic principles when positioning or restraining, especially when working with horses or food animals.

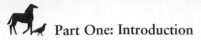

Storing Supplies

Store heavy supplies or equipment on the lower shelves to prevent unnecessary strains. Never use stairways as storage areas. Do not overload shelves or cabinets. Store liquids in containers with tight-fitting lids. When possible, store chemicals on shelves that are *at or below* eye level. Never climb onto cabinets, shelves, chairs, buckets, or similar items to reach high locations; use an appropriate ladder or step.

Toxic Substances

Eat or drink only in areas free of toxic and biologically harmful substances. Keep the staff coffee pot and utensils well away from sources of possible contamination, such as the laboratory or the treatment/bathing tub. Ensure that the cabinets above a coffee or food area contain no hazardous chemicals or supplies that could spill onto the area. Store food, drinks, condiments, and snacks in a refrigerator free from biological or chemical hazards; vaccines, drugs, and laboratory samples are all potential contamination sources.

Heating Devices

When using such equipment as autoclaves, microwave ovens, cautery irons, or other heating devices, take time to learn the rules for safe operation. Burns, especially from steam, are painful and serious and almost always can be prevented. Autoclaves also present a danger from the pressure that is used for proper sterilization. When opening the autoclave, first release the pressure with the "vent" device and let the steam rise completely before opening the door fully. Always assume cautery devices and branding irons are hot, and use the insulated handle whenever you handle them. Never place heated irons on any surface where they could overheat and start a fire or where someone could accidentally touch them.

Eye Safety

Become familiar with the locations and use of the eye wash stations. Always use safety glasses and other personal protective equipment when required. By law, this equipment must be provided by your employer; however, the primary reason it is there is for your protection. Remember, in every state and territory of the United States, an employee can be legally disciplined, including termination, for failure to follow the safety rules for the workplace.

HAZARDS OF ANIMAL HANDLING
Remaining Alert

The first rule when working around animals is to *stay alert*. Sudden noises, movements, or even light can cause an animal to react. If you are the primary restraint person, focus your attention on the animal's reactions and not on the procedure being performed. Learn the proper restraint positions for each of the species of patients you handle regularly.

Protective Gear

Make use of any available capture/restraint equipment. Wear latex examination gloves and a surgical mask when handling a stray, wild, or unvaccinated animal. Maintain an appropriate distance from the work area or animal; for example, do not place your face very close to the mouth of the animal (see also Zoonotic Hazards later in this chapter). Wear protective leather gloves when handling a fractious animal.

Barking dogs can be a threat to hearing, especially in indoor kennels. Noise levels in canine wards can reach 110 decibels (dB). Exposure to these noise levels for a short time, such as going into the kennel to retrieve a patient, poses no serious damage to your hearing, but excessive or long-term exposure can contribute to hearing loss. When working in noisy areas for extended periods (e.g., when cleaning cages), always wear personal hearing protectors rated to filter the noise by at least 20 dB. (The package label indicates the rating.)

Chutes and Enclosures

Large animals, such as horses and cattle, can severely injure or even kill you when they try to escape restraint. Never place your hand, leg, or any other part of your body between the animal and the side of the enclosure or chute; use a hook or pole to pass ropes or belts through the chute. If you must enter a stall or paddock containing a large animal, stay on the side of the animal nearer the door or gate so that you can escape if the situation becomes hazardous.

HAZARDS OF BATHING AND DIPPING
Ventilation

Always use the ventilation fan to keep fumes from shampoos and dips at a safe level.

Eye Safety

Make sure you know where the eye wash device is before you need to use it (Fig. 2-1). If you splash a chemical in your eyes, *do not rub your eyes with your hands*. Immediately call out for help. With a co-worker's assistance, go to the eye wash station and flush *both* eyes, even if only one eye is affected. Avoid using the spray attachments for tubs and sinks, because the water pressure is unregulated and the streams of water from these devices can be fine enough to lacerate the cornea.

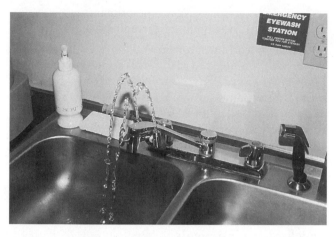

FIG. 2-1 Locate and know how to operate the eye wash devices in your hospital.

Chemical Storage

The chemicals used for bathing and dipping animals can be harmful and must be stored properly. Bottles of dips, shampoos, and parasiticides should be stored in a cabinet at or below eye level. The bottle should be properly labeled including contents and any appropriate hazard warning (see Hazards of chemicals, p. 14).

ZOONOTIC HAZARDS

When handling such specimens as fecal samples, laboratory samples, or wound exudates, wear protective gloves and *always wash your hands immediately after completing the procedure.* Contamination with these types of materials can usually be cleaned up with paper towels soaked in appropriate disinfecting solution. Latex gloves should be worn and then discarded with the cleaned-up materials.

When treating patients with potentially infectious diseases (infectious to people or other animals), wear a protective apron, latex exam gloves, and, if appropriate, eye protection. Thoroughly wash your hands with a disinfecting agent, such as chlorhexidine or povidone-iodine scrub, at the completion of treatment. Any clothing that has been contaminated should be changed immediately.

Rabies

Rabies is a very serious, usually fatal viral disease that can affect any warm-blooded animal, including people. Rabies virus is spread by contact with an infected animal's saliva. Usually a noninfected animal becomes infected through the bite of a rabid (infected) animal. The disease has also been transmitted by saliva (even the residue left on a dog's bowl after eating) that contaminates an open wound or contacts the mucous membranes.

The primary barrier to the spread of rabies from the wild animal population to humans is vaccination of pets and other domestic animals. When you must handle an unvaccinated, wild, or stray animal, *always* wear protective latex gloves and perhaps even protective gowns and goggles. A safe and effective human vaccine is available for people who work with animals. Ask your hospital administrator about the availability of this vaccine at your practice.

Bacterial Infections

Bacterial infections are certainly possible in the veterinary environment. Aside from the common bacteria that all animals harbor naturally, injury and disease in veterinary patients can expose you to such serious pathogens as *Pasteurella, E. coli,* and *Pseudomonas.* Bacteria are most commonly transferred by direct contact with the animal or its excretions, especially if you have any cuts or open sores. Some bacteria are easily aerosolized or released into the air, where they can be inhaled and absorbed through your mucous membranes. The best protection from exposure to bacteria is good personal hygiene.

Fungal Infections

Ringworm is a superficial skin infection caused by the fungus *Microsporum canis,* among others. Ringworm is very easily transmitted from animals to humans. The most effective protection from ringworm is to wear latex gloves when handling or treating animals with ringworm and to practice good personal hygiene.

Parasitism

When the eggs of common internal parasites, such as roundworms and hookworms, infect humans, they usually do not mature to adult parasites, but they can cause other problems. Roundworm larvae can migrate to virtually any organ in the body and develop into a cyst-like growth causing the condition known as *visceral larva migrans.* These "cysts" are usually not noticeable, but if they develop in a vital organ, such as the eye or brain, they can cause severe problems.

Hookworms can cause a condition known as *cutaneous larva migrans.* This condition particularly affects children who play in areas where pets defecate frequently, such as a sandbox. Unlike the visceral "cysts" caused by roundworm larvae, the lesions of cutaneous larva migrans are relatively easy to visualize. These usually appear as red, serpentine lines on the skin of the feet or lower legs.

Borreliosis or *Lyme disease,* a bacterial infection transmitted by ticks, has become a more serious concern for pets and people. When an infected deer tick bites a host (animal or person) during feeding, the bacterium *Borrelia burgdorferi* is transferred to the host.

Lyme disease in humans is characterized by joint pain, fever, and a host of other "flu-like" signs. The best defense against borreliosis is to check yourself for ticks after venturing outdoors and remove them promptly.

Mites causing *sarcoptic mange* can easily infest people. When treating animals with sarcoptic mange, always wear gloves and a protective gown, and wash your hands thoroughly with disinfecting soap immediately after the procedure.

The coccidian parasite *Toxoplasma gondii* can infect cats and people. Although it is usually not harmful to healthy humans, it can cause serious problems to the fetus of pregnant women. Toxoplasmosis is spread from cats to people usually by ingestion of the infectious oocysts in cat feces. Ideally, pregnant women should avoid cleaning cat litter pans.

Biologics

Vials containing biologics, such as vaccines and bacterins, usually are not considered hazardous unless the agent can infect humans. For example, vials containing such agents as canine distemper virus or feline calicivirus are not usually considered a danger to humans, but vials containing biologically hazardous agents, such as brucellosis bacterins, must be treated as potentially infectious during and after use.

RADIATION HAZARDS

Infrequent exposure to small amounts of radiation, such as routine thoracic or dental radiographs, poses little threat to your overall health. However, long-term exposure to small doses of radiation has been linked to genetic, cutaneous, glandular, and other disorders. Exposure to large doses of radiation can cause skin changes, cell damage, and gastrointestinal and bone marrow disorders that can be fatal.

Radiation Safety

When using radiographic equipment, never place any part of your body in the primary beam, even a hand wearing a lead-lined glove. Always wear the appropriate protective equipment, such as lead-lined aprons and gloves. Thyroid collars and lead-impregnated glasses are also recommended. Always use the collimator to restrict the primary beam to an area smaller than the size of the cassette. In other words, isolate the area to be radiographed and minimize the scatter radiation.

Portable x-ray machines, such as those used in large animal and mobile practices, can be particularly dangerous because the primary beam of these machines can be aimed in any direction. When using a portable machine, always make sure no person or human body part is in the path of the primary beam, even at a distance. Never hold a cassette, whether wearing lead-lined gloves or not; always use a cassette-holding pole. Also, wear a lead-lined apron and gloves.

Everyone involved with radiography must wear a *dosimetry badge*. This badge must always be worn during radiographic procedures to measure any scatter radiation you may receive during the procedure. Your supervisor or hospital adminstrator will regularly advise you of the readings from your personal dosimetry badge. These reports, required by law, are designed as a warning system to alert you and your supervisor if your exposure to radiation reaches a hazardous level.

Developing Chemicals

Radiographic developing chemicals (developer and fixer) can be very corrosive to materials and human tissues. Take extreme care when mixing, transferring, agitating, or transporting these chemicals, and do this only in a well-ventilated area. Always turn on the exhaust fan when you are in the darkroom. Use protective gloves and goggles when mixing or pouring the chemicals. For manual processing tanks, stir the chemicals with care and avoid splashing. After handling radiographic developing chemicals, always wash your hands.

Chapter 19 contains detailed information on radiation safety.

ANESTHETIC HAZARDS

Long-term exposure to waste anesthetic gases has been linked to congenital abnormalities in children, spontaneous abortions, and even liver and kidney damage. The Occupational Safety and Health Administration (OSHA) has set the safe exposure limit for halogenated anesthetic agents (halothane, methoxyflurane, isoflurane) at 2 parts per million.

According to some sources, as much as 90% of the anesthetic gas levels found in the surgery room during a procedure can be attributed to leaks in anesthesia machines. For this reason, always check for leaks in the hoses and anesthetic machine before use (see Box 2-1). Also, make sure to use hoses and rebreathing bags of proper size and inflate the endotracheal tube cuff before connecting the patient to the machine. Start the flow of anesthetic gas after connecting the patient to the machine. Before disconnecting the patient, continue oxygen flow until the remaining anesthesia gas has been flushed through the scavenging system.

A well-designed scavenging system captures excess gases directly at the source and transports them to a safe exhaust port, usually outside the building. This is the most effective means of reducing exposures of waste anesthetic gases in the workplace.

**Box 2-1 Procedure to check for leaks
in the anesthetic machine**

1. Assemble all hoses, canisters, valves, or tubes according to the manufacturer's instructions.
2. Turn on the oxygen supply to the machine.
3. Close the pressure-relief (pop-off) valve.
4. Use your thumb or palm to form a tight seal on the Y-piece.
5. Turn on the oxygen flow until the rebreathing bag is slightly overinflated, then close the valve.
6. Observe the pressure in the system on the manometer and watch closely for any decrease. (If your machine is not equipped with manometer, observe the size of the bag closely.) If the pressure remains constant, the machine is considered leak-free. If the pressure drops, there is a leak (or leaks) in the system. The faster the pressure drops, the larger the leak(s).
7. If there is a leak, check the rebreathing bag, hoses, and other rubber or plastic parts for evidence of cracks or deterioration. Replace any parts that are damaged. Check all connections, especially at the vaporizer inlet and outlet. Check the seals at the top and bottom of the soda lime canister and on the one-way valves (clear plastic domes). Tighten any loose connections you find.
8. After checking all connections and hoses, if there is still a leak, have the machine serviced by a qualified technician before use.
9. When the machine is leak-free, reopen the pressure-relief valve and use the machine normally.

When refilling the anesthetic machine vaporizer, move the machine to a well-ventilated area. Use a pouring funnel and avoid overfilling the vaporizer or spilling the liquid anesthetic. If you accidentally break a bottle of liquid anesthetic, immediately evacuate all people from the area. Open the window and turn on the exhaust fans. Control the liquid with a spill kit absorbent or a generous amount of kitty litter. Pick up the contaminated absorbent or kitty litter with a dust pan and place it in a plastic garbage bag.

Some procedures, such as masking or tank induction, defy collection of waste gases. In those instances, make sure that the room is well ventilated. Exhaust fans for evacuating room air to the outside are recommended. Air-handling systems that recirculate the air can expose others in the hospital. Induction chambers can be connected to the scavenging system or absorption canister to reduce levels of escaping gases.

When changing the soda lime (carbon dioxide absorbent) in anesthetic machines, wear latex gloves.

When the soda lime is wet, as it often is from humidity in the patient's breath, it can be very caustic to tissues and some metals. Place the used soda lime granules in a plastic trash bag and dispose of it in the regular trash.

If you are a woman and become pregnant, discuss the anesthetic exposure risk with your physician as soon as possible and notify your supervisor immediately.

HAZARDS OF COMPRESSED GASES

Store cylinders of compressed gas (e.g., oxygen) in a dry, cool place, away from potential heat sources, such as furnaces, water heaters, and direct sunlight. Always secure the tanks in an upright position by means of a chain or strap (including small tanks). Transportation carts and floor-mounting collars are also acceptable methods of securing compressed gas cylinders. If the cylinder is equipped with a protective cap (usually the large ones are), it must be firmly screwed in place when the cylinder is not in use. If you must move a large cylinder, do not roll or drag it; always use a hand truck or cart and strap the tank to the cart before moving. Always wear impact-resistant protective goggles when connecting or disconnecting tanks, because air escaping from tanks can cause trauma to the cornea of your eyes.

HAZARDS OF SHARP OBJECTS

The most serious hazard from sharp objects ("sharps") in a veterinary environment is from the physical trauma and possible bacterial infection caused by a puncture or laceration. To prevent accidents from punctures or lacerations, always keep needles, scalpel blades, and other sharp instruments capped or sheathed until ready for use. When practical, place the needle or sharp in a red "sharps container" immediately after use (Fig. 2-2). Do not attempt to recap the needle unless the physical danger from sticks or lacerations cannot be avoided by any other means.

When necessary, needles may be recapped using the "one-handed" method. Place the cap on a flat surface (table or counter). With one hand, "thread" the needle into the cap. The cap may then be firmly seated using both hands. The needle should not be removed from the syringe, but the entire unit should be disposed of in the red sharps containers. When full, the sharps containers must be sealed and disposed of following the hospital's prescribed policy.

Ordinary plastic milk containers are not appropriate sharps collection containers; a 22-gauge needle can easily penetrate these. The containers made for this specific purpose (usually red and labeled with a biohazard symbol) are the most effective and are usually very economical.

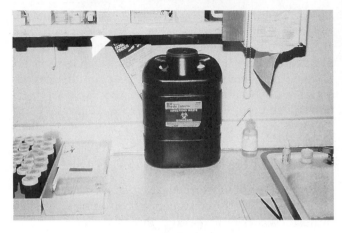

FIG. 2-2 Needles and other sharp objects must be disposed of in specially designed sharps containers.

Cutting off the end of needles before disposal increases the potential for aerosolization of the liquid involved. Collecting sharps in a smaller container and transferring them to a larger container for disposal places someone at an increased risk of exposure. Neither of these practices is recommended.

Never throw needles or other sharps directly into regular trash containers, regardless of whether or not they are capped. Never open a used sharps container. Never insert your fingers into a sharps container for any reason.

HAZARDS OF CHEMICALS

Many products you use every day can be hazardous. Every chemical, even such common ones as cleaning supplies, can cause harm. Some chemicals can contribute to health problems, whereas others may be flammable and pose a fire threat. The most common chemicals used in the veterinary workplace are insecticides, medications, and cleaning agents.

Veterinary hospitals must follow the guidelines of OSHA's Right to Know law. This law requires you to be informed of all chemicals you may be exposed to while doing your job. The Right To Know law also requires you to wear all safety equipment that is prescribed by the manufacturer when handling a chemical. The safety equipment must be provided by your employer at no cost to you. It is not optional; you must wear what is prescribed.

Hazardous Materials Plan

A key component of the Right To Know law is the *hazardous materials plan*. This plan describes the details of the practice's Material Safety Data Sheet (MSDS) filing system and the secondary container labeling system, and it lists the person responsible for ensuring that all employees have received the necessary safety training.

You have a right to review any of these materials, so ask your supervisor where your plan is located.

Part of the planning process includes knowing exactly what chemicals are present in the workplace. There must be an up-to-date list of chemicals known to be on the hospital premises. It surprises some people to learn that the average veterinary hospital has over 200 hazardous chemicals present at any one time.

Material Safety Data Sheets

More detailed information about every chemical can be found on the *Material Safety Data Sheet (MSDS)*. Ask your supervisor where your hospital's MSDS file is located and take the time to review the MSDS for chemicals you use frequently. Material Safety Data Sheets may look complicated at first glance, but the information that is important to you is easy to find.

Container Labels

When you receive a supply of chemicals from the distributor, every bottle is identified with a label containing directions and any appropriate warnings. Always read, understand, and follow these directions and warnings printed on the label. When possible, keep this label intact and readable. Sometimes it is necessary to dilute a chemical or pour it into smaller bottles for use. These smaller bottles are known as secondary containers. All secondary containers must have a label that indicates the contents and appropriate safety warnings.

Container Caps

Always remember to replace the cap on chemical bottles after use. Bottles of chemicals should always have tight-fitting, screw-on lids. Always store chemical bottles at or below eye level in a closed cabinet. Never store or use chemicals near food or beverages.

Mixing Chemicals

Be very cautious when mixing or diluting chemicals. Always wear latex gloves and protective goggles. Never mix any chemicals unless you know it is safe to do so according to the label or MSDS. Mixing often creates a new, sometimes very dangerous chemical. When making dilute solutions from a concentrate, always start with the correct quantity of water and then add the concentrate. Never add the water to the concentrate, because the chemical may splash or may not react as you would expect.

Chemical Spills

Minor spills of most chemicals can be cleaned up with paper towels or absorbent, such as kitty litter, and disposed of in the trash or sanitary sewer. However, some very dangerous chemicals, such formaldehyde or ethylene oxide, require special procedures. Before you use a chemical with which you are unfamiliar, review the MSDS and learn the procedures you must follow for cleaning up a spill. When cleaning up any spill, always wear latex gloves and any other protective equipment specified on the MSDS. Unless prohibited by the instructions on the MSDS, wash the spill site and any contaminated equipment with a detergent soap and water.

Handling Ethylene Oxide

Many hospitals use ethylene oxide gas to sterilize items that would be damaged by other sterilization procedures. Ethylene oxide is a potent human carcinogen, so special precautions must be taken:

- Carefully read the MSDS for ethylene oxide.
- Store the ethylene oxide in a safe place.
- Use only approved devices to perform ethylene oxide sterilization.
- Read, understand, and follow all written procedures and safety precautions.
- Know the emergency procedures.
- Be aware of monitoring levels.
- Keep ethylene oxide away from flames and sparks, because it is highly flammable.

Handling Formalin

Liquid or gaseous formaldehyde and formalin are serious health hazards in veterinary hospitals. Because formaldehyde is a known human carcinogen, OSHA monitors its use:

- Carefully read the MSDS for formaldehyde/formalin.
- Store formalin containers safely, including specimen jars.
- Use formalin only with good ventilation; avoid breathing the vapors.
- Wear goggles and latex gloves; avoid skin and eye contact.

Exposure to formalin can be minimized by use of premixed, premeasured vials of formalin for specimens. Veterinary hospitals that still use bulk formalin for diagnostic laboratory tests (e.g., Knott's test) should consider switching to some of the newer, less hazardous methods of testing.

HAZARDS OF ELECTRICITY

Do not remove light switch or electrical outlet covers. Always keep circuit breaker boxes closed. Only persons trained to perform maintenance duties should repair electrical outlets, switches, fixtures, or breakers. If you must use a portable dryer or other electrical equipment in a wet area, it must be properly grounded and plugged into only a ground-fault circuit interruption (GFCI) type of outlet.

Extension cords should be used only for temporary supply applications and should always be of the 3-conductor, grounded type. Never run extension cords through windows or doors that could close and damage the wires. Also, never run extension cords across aisles or floors, which creates a tripping hazard. When an extension cord is necessary, it should be adequate for the electrical load. Generally, extension cords longer than 4 feet should not be used for loads greater than 6 amps at 120 volts AC or 3 amps at 240 volts AC.

Equipment with grounded plugs must never be used with adapters or nongrounded extension cords. Never alter or remove the ground terminals on plugs. Appliances or equipment with defective ground terminals or plugs should not be used until repaired.

FIRE AND EVACUATION

Always store flammables properly; such materials as gasoline, paint thinner, and ether should never be stored inside the hospital, except in an approved storage cabinet designed for flammables. Some components of specialty dental and large animal acrylic repair kits are also very flammable. Very small amounts of these components can usually be safely stored in an area with good ventilation and free from flames or sparks.

Be alert for situations that could cause a fire. Flammable items, particularly newspapers, boxes, and cleaning chemicals, must always be stored at least 3 feet away from any ignition source, such as a water heater, furnace, or stove. Always use extra care when using portable heaters. Never leave them unattended, and always make sure they are placed no closer than 3 feet from any wall, furniture or other flammable material.

Know location of all the fire extinguishers on the premises and how to use them (Fig. 2-3). Before you decide to use a fire extinguisher, make sure the fire alarm has been sounded, everyone has left the building (or is in the process of leaving), and the fire department has been called. The National Fire Protection Association recommends that you never attempt to fight a fire if any of the following conditions apply:

- The fire is spreading beyond the immediate area where it started or has already become a large fire.
- The fire could block your escape route.
- You are unsure of the proper operation of the extinguisher.
- You doubt that the extinguisher is designed for the type of fire at hand or is large enough to suppress the fire.

Know where the designated emergency exits are. Make sure emergency exits are always unlocked and free from obstructions. If you must work in a building during non-operational hours (when security warrants that the doors are locked), make sure you have at least two clear exits from the building that can be opened without a key.

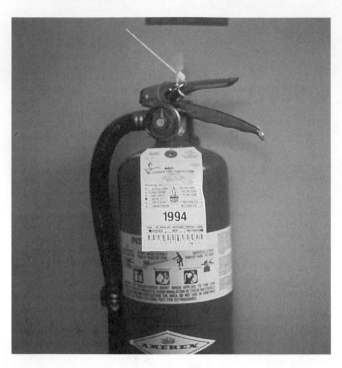

FIG. 2-3 Learn where the fire extinguishers are located and how to use them.

RECOMMENDED READING

Newman E et al: *Health hazards in veterinary practice*, ed 3, Schaumburg, Ill, 1995, American Veterinary Medical Association.

OSHA: *Employee workplace rights* (free pamphlet), 1994, US Department of Labor, OSHA, Publications Office, Room N-3101, 200 Constitution Ave, NW, Washington, DC 20210.

Renado VT, Ryan G: Technical assistance in radiology, Part 2, Basic considerations and radiation safety, *Vet Tech* 9(10):547-551, 1988.

Seibert, PJ Jr., *The complete veterinary practice regulatory manual*, ed 2, Calhoun, Tenn, 1996, Philip J. Seibert, Jr.

PERSONAL SAFETY

Workers in emergency or 24-hour practices should use the "barriers" that are usually available. Use the buzzer to control access through the front door and one-way locks on the remaining doors. (This lets you out in case of an emergency but keeps the door locked from the outside.) These personal safety techniques are almost essential in these environments.

In any practice, the potential for robbery is always present. In any situation where someone demands money or drugs while threatening your personal safety, *do not attempt to withhold the things they demand.* Cooperate with the demands, but do not go with the person, even to the parking lot. Attempt to remember every detail of the person's appearance and demeanor. This greatly increases the likelihood that the police will locate the person. As soon as safely possible, let everyone else know of the situation. Attempt to contact the police if this can be done safely without the intruder's knowledge; otherwise, do it immediately after the intruder has left the premises.

CHAPTER 3

Ethics, Animal Welfare, and Law

B.E. Rollin
C.A. Picut

Learning Objectives

After reviewing this chapter, the reader should understand the following:

Types of ethics
Ethical issues facing veterinary personnel
General categories of law

Features of the law protecting veterinary employees against physical injury, sexual harassment, and discrimination
Features of the law relating to ensuring quality veterinary service

ETHICS AND ANIMAL WELFARE

B.E. ROLLIN

AREAS OF ETHICS

There are three major areas of ethics: social ethics, personal ethics, and professional ethics. *Social ethics,* or social consensus ethics, is the consensus principles adopted by or accepted by society at large, taught to the young, and codified in laws and regulations. Laws, ranging from laws against murder and rape to laws against discrimination to local zoning ordinances that prohibit bars or pornographic bookstores in school zones, reflect (and help teach) the social ethical consensus.

Personal ethics is what is left to the discretion of the individuals by society or, more accurately, what is left to the individual's own set of principles of right and wrong. For example, such matters as whether one gives charity and to whom, how many children one has, and whether or not one adheres to a religious tradition are all left to an individual's personal ethics in our society, although not in all societies.

What, then, is *professional ethics?* Members of a profession are first and foremost members of society, and thus are bound by the consensus social ethic not to steal, murder, or commit other crimes. Democratic societies assume that professionals understand the ethical issues that they confront better than society does as a whole, and thus these societies generally leave it to professionals to set up their own rules of conduct.

ETHICS AND ANIMAL TREATMENT

Western societies are dramatically changing their consensus ethic for animal treatment. Certainly, veterinarians should be leaders in this area, because they understand the needs and interests of both those who use animals and animals themselves. Society expects veterinarians to lead; U.S. federal laws for research animals put the responsibility for proper animal care and use on the shoulders of laboratory animal veterinarians, as does British law.

Dealing with ethical issues is analogous to dealing with medical problems. Diagnosing a disease requires taking cognizance of all relevant signs. Diagnosis must come before treatment. By the same token, dealing with ethical issues requires taking cognizance of all morally relevant components of the situation. Failure to do so can lead to a very distorted view of the case and to an inappropriate moral decision.

The best way to ensure consideration of all ethical aspects of a case is to talk about it with a wide variety of people with differing perspectives. Unfortunately, many veterinarians seek counsel from other veterinarians of similar age and background, thereby minimizing the chances of getting radically new perspectives. Veterinary technicians are often helpful in this regard, because they are more often conscious of animal welfare issues than are some veterinarians who were trained during an era when animal welfare was not emphasized.

In the absence of the opportunity for dialogue, there is another way to help identify otherwise unnoticed ethical components of a veterinary situation. Examine the case in terms of each of the following five types of ethical obligations that veterinarians experience:

1. *Obligations to the client.* Obviously, veterinarians owe an obligation to clients who hire them. This obligation does not, of course, always triumph over all others, but it is usually a major component in ethical decision making.
2. *Moral obligations to peers and the profession.* These are so important that for many years they constituted the bulk of what veterinarians thought of as veterinary ethics. They include such questions as, Does one advertise? Does one criticize a colleague?
3. *Moral obligation to society in general.* These include such duties as protecting public health and being expected to lead in animal welfare matters.
4. *Moral obligations to self.* This is an extremely neglected but nonetheless significant moral consideration. Clearly, veterinarians have an obligation to themselves and their families for such things as spending time at home, allowing for recreation, and not living under constant stress.
5. *Moral obligations to the animal.* This is the most difficult and interesting branch of veterinary ethics, because social and professional ethics have, until very recently, been silent on these obligations. Thus, most veterinarians loathe euthanizing an animal merely for owner convenience, yet the consensus social ethic as embodied in law sees animals as property. Until very recently, the social ethic was silent on moral obligations to animals except for a prohibition of deliberate cruelty.

The issue of a veterinarian's obligation to the animal is clearly the most problematic aspect of veterinary ethics; traditionally, the social ethic virtually ignored that issue. In veterinarians' personal ethics, there are two possible ways veterinarians can view their obligation to the animal. At one end of the spectrum, the veterinarian could see himself or herself as analogous to a garage mechanic. If a person takes a car to a mechanic, the mechanic does strictly what the owner decrees and is morally bound to do no more. If the owner does not wish to spend money to repair a particular problem, the mechanic's responsibility ends. On the other end of the spectrum, the veterinarian may see his or her role as analogous to that of a pediatrician. If a pediatrician tells a parent, "It will cost $2,000 to cure your child," the parent cannot say, "No, we can't do that; it costs too much." The pediatrician recognizes the moral status of the child as independent of the parent's desire. Pediatricians, in fact, historically worked assiduously to raise the status of children in the social consensus ethic and in the laws mirroring it.

Most veterinarians lean more toward the pediatrician model. With society recognizing little moral status for animals, this personal ethical predilection clashed with the social ethic. Fortunately, in the last two decades, society has become increasingly concerned with elevating the moral status of animals. Further, there is evidence that society sees veterinarians as the plausible guardians and promoters of animal well-being. The aforementioned federal laboratory laws attest to this. It is to this emerging ethic and its conceptual roots we now turn.

Society has paid formal attention to limiting human behavior regarding animals for more than 2,000 years. However, such attention was restricted to prohibition of overt, intentional, extraordinary, malicious, or unnecessary cruelty, deviant sadism, or outrageous neglect, such as not providing food or water.

This minimalistic, lowest common denominator ethic was formally encapsulated in the anticruelty laws during the 19th century. These laws were designed not only to protect animals but also to ferret out sadists and psychopaths who might begin with cruelty toward animals and, if left unchecked, prey on human beings. This view of prohibiting animal cruelty can be found in Catholic theology where, although animals do not in themselves count morally, animal cruelty is forbidden for its potential consequences for people, in that people who are cruel to animals will "graduate" to abusing people.

Interestingly enough, contemporary research has buttressed this view. The traditional humane or animal welfare movement was also caught up in the categories of kindness and cruelty, and for this reason tends to simplistically categorize anyone causing animal suffering as "cruel." Hence, activists still picket medical research institutions, carrying signs that say, "Stop the cruelty."

The overwhelming majority of animal suffering at human hands is not the result of cruelty; instead, the animals suffer because of normal animal use and socially acceptable motives. Scientists may be motivated by benevolence, high ideals, and noble goals, yet far more animal suffering is occasioned by people acting in pursuit of these motives than by the actions of overt sadists. Confinement agriculturalists may be motivated by the quest for efficiency, profit, productivity, low-cost food, and other acceptable goals, yet again, their activities occasion animal suffering in magnitudes traditionally unimaginable.

Why is society suddenly concerned about the 99% of animal suffering that is not the result of deliberate cruelty? First, society has focused its concern on disenfranchised human individuals and groups, such as women, African Americans, people with disabilities, and people in developing countries. This same emphasis on moral obligation, rather than patronizing benevolence toward the powerless, has led to a new look at animal treatment. Second, the urbanization of society makes the companion animal, not the food animal, the paradigm for animals in the social mind. Third, graphic media portrayal of animal exploitation fuels social concern. Fourth, increased awareness of the magnitude of animal exploitation made possible by technologies of scale inspires massive unease among citizens. Perhaps these citizens see themselves being rendered insignificant in the face of techniques, systems, and machines that relentlessly reduce the individual, animal or human, to a replaceable quantity. Last, and by far the most important, the nature of animal use has changed significantly.

Thus, the changes both in animal use and in society foster increasing concern about all animal treatment and suffering, not just cruelty. This has in turn been reflected in increasing demands for new laws regulating many areas of animal treatment, including hunting, trapping, entertainment, and, most important, animal research. Society will demand more and more legalized protection for animals. It also sees veterinarians as the natural advocates of animals. As the status of animals rises in society, so too will that of the veterinary professionals who care for them.

RECOMMENDED READING

Tannenbaum J: *Veterinary ethics,* ed 2, St Louis, 1995, Mosby.

LAW

C.A. PICUT

In the daily practice of veterinary medicine, the veterinarian and veterinary technician are confronted with a wide variety of legal issues that affect their professional or business decisions. Bodies of law governing daily practices occurring within a veterinary clinic often overlap and fall into one of four categories: federal law, state law, local/municipal law, or common law. *State, federal, and local/municipal laws* constitute the legislative or written laws. These laws are enforced by the relevant governmental authorities and agencies, and violations of such may be punishable by fines and/or by jail sentence. In contrast, *common law* is a body of unwritten laws that has evolved from use and customs and by judge-made decisions over many years. Common law is not enforced by government authorities or agencies in the same way as legislative laws. Rather, common law is "enforced" by the judicial system when citizens who may have been injured by a "violation" of the common law file civil lawsuits against the violators.

The laws affecting a veterinary practice can be divided into two groups: (1) those directed to ensure the quality of veterinary service to patients, and (2) those directed to providing a nonhostile and safe environment for employees, clients, and the public.

LAWS ENSURING THE QUALITY OF VETERINARY SERVICE
Practice Acts

The Veterinary Practice Act of each individual state is the law prescribing which persons may practice veterinary medicine and surgery in a particular state, and under which conditions. Although the Practice Acts vary from state to state, they generally define the practice of veterinary medicine, make it illegal to practice without a license, state the qualifications for receiving a license, state the conditions under which a license can be revoked, and establish the penalties for violating the Act.

The Practice Acts generally define the practice of veterinary medicine and surgery as diagnosing, treating, prescribing, operating on, testing for the presence of animal disease, and holding oneself out as a licensed practitioner. Embryo transfer, dentistry, and alternative forms of therapy, such as acupuncture and chiropractic and holistic medicine, are generally regarded within this definition of veterinary medicine and surgery.

Allowing only licensed veterinarians to legally practice veterinary medicine may raise questions about the duties performed by veterinary technicians or veterinary assistants. After all, many of the procedures performed routinely by technicians (or assistants) fall literally within the scope of the practice of veterinary medicine and surgery, such as inserting an intravenous catheter, inducing general anesthesia, and extracting teeth. However, as long as the technician is under the direction and reasonable supervision of a licensed veterinarian and as long as the technician does not make any decisions requiring professional judgment, it is the licensed veterinarian and not the technician who is actually practicing veterinary medicine in these instances.

Whether or not a technician is under the direction and reasonable supervision of a licensed veterinarian is a subjective determination that takes into account the degree of experience and competence of the technician, the task being performed, and the risks to the animal patient involved with performing the task. For example, reasonable supervision of an untrained assistant inducing anesthesia for the first time would probably mean that the veterinarian should be standing by the assistant's side during the procedure. On the other hand, it may be reasonable for a veterinarian to, by telephone, request an experienced technician to place an intravenous catheter into an animal patient and start fluid administration. Regardless of how experienced the technician may be, the veterinarian must be on the premises or reachable by telephone or two-way radio communication during and for a reasonable time after any veterinary procedure.

Common Law Malpractice

When a veterinarian agrees to treat a client's animal, common law automatically imposes on that veterinarian a legal duty to provide medical or surgical care to that client's animal in accordance with that of a reasonably prudent veterinary practitioner of similar training under the same or similar circumstances.

A veterinarian's failure to live up to this particular duty constitutes *negligence*, which may also be referred to as *malpractice* or professional negligence. For malpractice to be subject to litigation, the plaintiff must prove three elements: the veterinarian agreed to treat that particular patient; the veterinarian failed to exercise the necessary legal obligation of skill and diligence in treating the animal (the veterinarian was negligent); and the negligence was a cause of injury to the patient.

Veterinarians can be found negligent and guilty of malpractice for the injurious actions of a technician or assistant under the common law doctrine of *respondeat superior*. For example, if a technician mistakenly gave twice the recommended dosage of anesthesia to a patient, and this doubled dose caused the death of the animal, the veterinarian may be found negligent and guilty of malpractice as if the veterinarian had given the wrong dosage.

PROVIDING A SAFE BUSINESS ENVIRONMENT FOR EMPLOYEES, CLIENTS, AND THE PUBLIC

Federal, state, and common laws exist to help ensure safe and nonhostile working conditions for employees of a veterinary practice, as well as safe conditions for the public.

Occupational Safety and Health Act

Every employer with one or more employees must operate in compliance with the *Occupational Safety and Health Act (OSHA)*.

OSHA was designed to provide a safe workplace for all persons working in any business effecting commerce. The broad judicial interpretation of "commerce" includes the business of practicing veterinary medicine and surgery. OSHA requires that all employers "furnish . . . employment and a place of employment which are free from recognized hazards that are causing or are likely to cause death or serious physical harm."

Common Law Ordinary Negligence

Common law establishes for every business owner a legal duty to provide a reasonably safe work environment for employees, as well as a reasonably safe place for clients. Failure to provide this safe environment may constitute *ordinary negligence* on the part of the veterinarian/business owner. This ordinary negligence is to be distinguished from malpractice, which is negligence associated with the rendering of professional veterinary medical services. As with malpractice, however, ordinary negligence is not subject to legal action unless it causes injury to the client or employee. For example, suppose a practice owner provided poor ventilation in a surgical suite, and an employee became drowsy from the anesthetic gases. That employee could not sue and recover damages from the veterinarian unless the employee actually experiences injury (for example, fainted and hit his or her head on the countertop) as a consequence of the poor ventilation.

A veterinarian, in meeting the obligation to provide a safe environment for employees and clients, has a common-law duty to supervise proper restraint of any animal within the veterinarian's control. When a client's animal is being examined and the client restrains the animal, it is the veterinarian and not the client who is primarily responsible for proper restraint of that animal. A veterinarian may be found guilty of ordinary negligence if he or she fails to use reasonable care to avoid foreseeable harm to the restrainer or to other people in the vicinity. The definition of reasonable care or foreseeable harm varies, depending on the experience or training of the veterinarian and the animal handler, as well as the procedure being done on the animal.

State and Local Medical Waste Management Laws

Veterinarians who own or operate a veterinary practice may be subject to the requirements of state law governing management and disposal of medical wastes. Local laws may impose additional restrictions on what types of waste transporters and disposal facilities may be acceptable. Typical waste included under these acts include discarded needles and syringes, vials containing attenuated or live vaccines, culture plates, and animal carcasses exposed or infected with pathogens infectious to humans. State and local law may extend these categories of regulated veterinary medical waste to include all carcasses, animal blood, bedding, and pathology waste.

Maintaining a Nonhostile Environment for Employees

There is a body of federal, state, and common law that restricts a veterinarian, as the owner of a business, from engaging in hiring or firing practices that wrongfully discriminate against individuals. Firing an individual for discriminatory reasons constitutes a violation of the federal or state Equal Employment Opportunity (EEO) laws and may provide a basis for the terminated employee to sue the employer under common law for wrongful termination of employment.

According to federal EEO laws, an employer of 15 or more employees may not discriminate against employees in hiring or firing practices (or in any practice, for that matter) on the basis of race, color, religion, sex, or national origin. Sexual harassment and discrimination on the basis of pregnancy or childbirth are forms of sex discrimination made illegal under federal law. Employers also cannot discriminate against individuals in hiring and firing of employees on the basis of age between 40 and 70 years or on the basis of disabilities, including AIDS and rehabilitated drug abuse.

Common law also protects employees because it prohibits an employer from terminating that employee for discriminatory reasons or other reasons violating public policy. Under the common law tort of wrongful termination, an employee can directly sue an employer for firing the employee on the basis of sex, race, or religious discrimination, or on the basis that the employee is a "whistle-blower" (i.e., has complained of sexual harrassment or other violations of the law).

RECOMMENDED READING

Brody MD: Safety in the veterinary medical workplace environment, Common issues and concerns, *Vet Clin North Am* 23(5):1071-1084, 1993.

Copeland JD: Employer-employee relations, *Vet Clin North Am* 23(5):957-974, 1993.

Stribling J, Picut C: Food and drug regulatory issues, *Vet Clin North Am* 23(5):991-1005, 1993.

Wilson JF: *Law and ethics of the veterinary profession,* Yardley, PA, 1993, Priority Press.

CHAPTER 4

Veterinary Medical Terminology

P.E. Cochran

Learning Objectives

After reviewing this chapter, the reader should understand the following:

Constituent parts of medical terms
Rules used to construct medical terms
Meanings of common prefixes and suffixes used in medical terms

Combining forms used to refer to various body parts
Terms for direction, position, and movement
Terms used for common surgical procedures, diseases, instruments, procedures, and dentistry

---

Veterinary medical terminology is the "language" of the veterinary profession. This language is used in everyday speech, recorded in medical records, and used in journal articles and published textbooks for veterinary technicians and veterinarians. One of the most important aspects of this study is to learn correct pronunciation and proper spelling of medical terms. In this chapter, the accented syllables have been printed in CAPITAL LETTERS; syllables not accented are in lowercase letters. In multisyllabic words with primary and secondary accents, the syllable with the primary (greater) accent is printed in **BOLDFACE CAPITAL LETTERS,** and the syllable with the secondary (lesser) accent is in CAPITAL LETTERS only. Unaccented syllables are printed in lowercase letters. Words of one syllable are printed in lowercase letters. Multisyllabic words, in which all syllables receive equal stress, are printed in lowercase letters.

INTRODUCTION TO MEDICAL WORD PARTS

Definitions

Prefix. A *prefix* is a syllable, group of syllables, or word joined to the beginning of another word to alter its meaning or create a new word.
Example: Pre-: meaning before, in space or in time

Root Word. A *root word* is the part of the word consisting of a syllable, group of syllables, or word that is the basis (or word base) for the meaning of the word.
Example: CARdi-: the root word (or the "root") for the heart

Combining Form. A *combining form* is a word or root word that may or may not use the connecting vowel *o* when it is used as an element in word formation. It is the combination of the root word and the combining vowel. It is generally written in the following manner: "root word"/o.

Example: CARdi/o: the combining form for the heart
CARdi = root word
/o = the combining vowel (see below)

    Combining Vowel. A *combining vowel* is the vowel, usually an *o*, used to connect a word or root word to the appropriate suffix.

    Suffix. A *suffix* is a syllable, group of syllables, or word added at the end of a word to change its meaning, give it grammatical function, or form a new word.

Example: -megaly: the enlargement of (cardiomegaly is an abnormally enlarged heart)

    Compound Word. A *compound word* is two or more words combined to make a new word.

Example: Horse and fly combine to form the following word: HORSEfly

RULES FOR WORD CONSTRUCTION
Use of the Prefix

The prefix is attached to the beginning of the root word to form the altered or new word.

Prefix	Root word	Combined	Definition
de-	horn	DEhorn	To remove the horns
semi-	PERmeable	SEMiPERmeable	Allowing only certain elements or liquids to pass through a membrane

Use of the Suffix

The suffix is attached to the end of the root word to form the altered or new word.

Root word	Suffix	Combined	Definition
TONsil	-itis	TONsilLItis	Inflammation of the tonsils
THYroid	-ectomy	THYroidECtomy	Removal of the thyroid gland

Compound Word

Two words are joined together to form the new word.

Word 1	Word 2	Combined	Definition
lock	jaw	LOCKjaw	Common name for the disease tetanus
blood	worms	BLOODworms	Worms (nematodes) that inhabit a main artery of the intestines in horses

Combining Forms

There are certain rules peculiar to the use of combining forms and the combining vowel *o*, which are as follows:

- If the suffix begins with a consonant, use the combining vowel *o* with the root word (the combining form), to which the suffix will be added.

Example: CARdi/o (combining form for heart) plus -megaly (meaning enlargement of), forms CARdioMEGaly, which means enlargement of the heart. Note the combining vowel *o* is retained.

- Do not use the combining vowel *o* when the suffix begins with a vowel.

Example: HEPat/o (combining form for liver) and -osis (meaning a condition, disease, or morbid process), combine to form HEPaTOsis, which means disease occurring in the liver. Note the combining vowel *o* is not used (otherwise there would be more than one o).

- If the suffix begins with the same vowel that the combining form ends with (minus the combining vowel *o*), do not repeat the vowel twice when forming the new word.

Example: CARdi/o minus the *o* is CARdi- plus -itis (which means inflammation of), combines to form carDItis, which means inflammation of the heart. Note, as the rule states, this word has a single *i*.

Combining form	Suffix	Combined	Definitions
cardi/o	-logy	CARdiOLogy	Study of heart diseases
mast/o	-itis	masTItis	Inflammation of the mammary glands

Use of Only the Prefix and Suffix to Form Words

In this situation, no root word is used. The prefix is added directly to the suffix.

Prefix	Suffix	Combined	Definition
dys-	-uria	dysUria	Trouble urinating
POLy-	-phagia	POLyPHAgia	Eating to excess

Use of the Prefix, Root Word, and Suffix to Form Words

Words are formed by adding both the prefix and suffix to the root word.

Prefix	Root word	Suffix	Combined	Definition
un-	sound	-ness	unSOUNDness	Some form of physical dysfunction, such as lameness
PERi-	cardi-	-al	PERiCARdial	In the area surrounding the heart

DEFINING MEDICAL TERMS USING WORD ANALYSIS

Analyzing words makes them easier to remember and teaches you to think logically. The process of word analysis is the reverse of word construction. When analyzing a word, start the end of the word (at the suffix) and work toward the prefix, analyzing the components in sequence. *Example:* oVARioHYSterECtomy = ovari/o/hyster/ectomy

$$\underset{4}{\quad}\;\underset{3}{\quad}\;\underset{2}{\quad}\;\underset{1}{\quad}$$

(1) The suffix *-ectomy* means to surgically remove. (2) The root word *hyster* refers to the uterus. (3) The *o* is the combining vowel for the previous root word. (4) The root word *ovari* refers to the ovaries. Thus, *ovariohysterectomy* means excision (surgical removal) of the uterus and ovaries. Note that steps (3) and (4) could be combined into one step, using the combining form *ovari/o,* which refers to the ovaries.

COMBINING FORMS FOR BODY PARTS

Following is a list of body parts and their respective combining forms. This is not a complete list of combining forms, but it represents some often used in veterinary terminology.

Combining Form	Body Part
abdomin/o	abdomen
adren/o, adrenal-	adrenal gland
angi/o	vessel
arteri/o	artery
arthr/o	joint
blephar/o	eyelid, eyelash
cardi/o	heart
cervic/o	cervix or neck of an organ
chol/o, chole-	bile
cholecyst/o	gallbladder
chondr/o	cartilage
col/o	colon
crani/o	cranium, skull
cyst/o	bladder
cyt/o	cell
dent/o	tooth, teeth
derm/o, dermat/o	skin
encephal/o	brain
enter/o	intestines
epididym/o	epididymis
esophag/o	esophagus
gastr/o	stomach
gloss/o	tongue
hem/o, hemat/o	blood
hepa-, hepat/o	liver
hyster/o	uterus
kerat/o	cornea or horny tissue
lapar/o	flank, abdomen
lip/o	fat
lymph/o	lymph

Combining Form (cont'd)	Body Part (cont'd)
mast/o, mamm/o	mammary glands
mening/o	meninges
metr/o	uterus (special reference to inner lining)
muscul/o, my/o, myos-	muscle
myel/o	bone marrow or spinal cord
nephr/o	kidney, nephron
neur/o	nerve
ocul/o	eye
odont/o	tooth, teeth
onych/o	claw, hoof
ophthalm/o	eye
orchi/o, orchid/o	testes
oste/o	bone
ot/o	ear
peritone/o	peritoneum
phleb/o	vein
pneum/o	lung, air, breath
proct/o	rectum
pulmo-, pulmon/o	lung
ren/o	renal (kidney)
rhin/o	nose
spondyl/o	vertebra, spinal column
thorac/o	thorax
thyr/o, thyroid-	thyroid gland
tonsill/o	tonsil
trache/o	trachea
tympan/o	tympanum (middle ear), tympanic membrane, eardrum
urethr/o	urethra
ur/o	urine
uter/o	uterus
vagin/o	vagina
ven/o	vein
ventricul/o	ventricle
vertebr/o	vertebra
vulv/o	vulva

Remember, words for some body parts have more than one combining form. Examples from the previous list are the following:

mouth = or/o, stomat/o; teeth = dent/o, odont/o

There are no general rules for when one or the other is used. This must be learned by listening and reading to be aware of how these combining forms are used. You already know some of them. For instance, you know that there is oral medication, not stomatal medication. Often, the different combining forms refer to a specific part of a structure or a specific use of the structure. *Or/o* often refers to the mouth as the first part of the digestive system, whereas *stomat/o* refers to the lining of the oral cavity or the opening to the oral cavity (e.g., stomatitis, stomatoplasty).

SUFFIXES FOR SURGICAL PROCEDURES

Following is a list of suffixes for surgical procedures. Using the rules for word construction, you can form words to describe a variety of surgical procedures on various body parts, or define these words using the word analysis technique previously described.

Suffix	Meaning	Example and definition
-ectomy	to excise or surgically remove	CHOLecys**TEC**tomy = surgical removal of the gallbladder
-tomy	to incise or cut into (making an incision	LAPa**ROT**omy = surgical incision into the abdomen
-stomy	to make a new, artificial opening in a hollow organ (to the outside of the body), *or*	coLOStomy = surgical creation of a new opening between the colon and the outside of the body
	to make a new opening between 2 hollow organs	GAStroDUode**NOS**tomy = to create a new opening between the stomach and the duodenum
-rrhaphy	to surgically repair by joining in a seam or by suturing together	HERni**ORR**haphy = surgical repair of a hernia
-pexy	fixation or suturing (a stabilizing type of repair)	**GAS**troPEXy = fixation of the stomach to the body wall
-plasty	to shape, the surgical formation of, or plastic surgery (which means to improve unction, to relieve pain, or for cosmetic reasons	**CHEI**loPLASty = plastic repair of the lips (to improve looks and function)
-centesis	to puncture, perforate, or tap, permitting withdrawal of fluid, air, etc.	abDOMinocen**TE**sis = surgical puncture of the abdomen to remove fluid from the peritoneal cavity

SUFFIXES FOR DISEASES OR CONDITIONS

The same rules and procedures used to form and analyze surgical words can be used with suffixes that refer to diseases or conditions to describe a problem affecting a particular organ or body part.

Following is a list of these suffixes:

Suffix	Meaning	Example and definition
-iasis	infestation or infection with, a condition characterized by	ACa**RI**asis = infestation with mites lith**I**asis = a condition characterized by formation of calculi
-ism	a state or condition, a fact of being, result of a process	HYper**COR**tiSONism = condition resulting from excessive cortisone
-itis	inflammation of	TONsil**LI**tis = inflammation of the tonsils
-oma	tumor	LEIomy**OM**a = tumor of smooth muscles
-osis	abnormal condition or process of degeneration	nePHROsis = degenerative disease of the kidneys

PREFIXES RELATED TO DISEASES OR CONDITIONS

Below is a list of prefixes used to create words indicating a specific problem within the body.

Prefix	Meaning	Example and definition
a-, an-	without or not having	aNEmia = not having enough red blood cells
anti-	against	ANtibi**OT**ic = drug that acts against bacteria
brady-	slow	BRAdy**CAR**dia = excessively slow heart rate
contra-	against, opposed	CONtra**IN**diCAted = something that is not indicated
de-	remove, take away, loss of	deHYdrated = excessive loss of body water
dys-	difficult, troubled	dysPHAgia = difficulty eating or swallowing
hyper-	high, excessive	HYper**THER**mia = body temperature higher than normal
hypo-	low, insufficient	HYpo**THER**mia = body temperature lower than normal
mal-	bad, poor	MALo**CCLU**sion = poor fit of upper and lower teeth when jaws close
poly-	many, much	POLy**PHA**gia = excessive eating

Prefix	Meaning	Example and definition
py/o	pus	PYo**THO**rax = pus in the thoracic cavity

Prefix	Meaning	Example and definition
tachy-	fast, rapid	TACHyCARdia = excessively fast heart rate

PLURAL ENDINGS

It is important to understand the methods for converting singular forms of medical words to their plural forms, and vice versa. Below is a list of common singular endings and their corresponding plural endings:

Singular	Plural	Example
-a	-ae	VERtebra, VERtebrae
-anx	-anges	PHAlanx, phaLANges
-en	-ina	LUmen, LUmina
-ex, -ix	-ices	Apex, Apices CERvix, CERvices
-is	-es	TEStis, TEStes
-inx	-inges	MENinx, meNINges
-ma	-mata or -mas	ENema, ENeMAta or ENemas
-um	-a	Ovum, Ova
-ur	-ora	FEMur, FEMora
-us	-i	Uterus, Uteri

SUFFIXES FOR INSTRUMENTS, PROCEDURES, AND MACHINES

Below is a list of suffixes that, when added to a combining form of a body part, form a word pertaining to an instrument, procedure, or a machine that looks into, cuts, or measures a body part.

Suffix	Meaning	Example and definition
-scope	an instrument for examining, viewing, or listening	Otoscope = instrument for looking into the ears
-scopy	act of examining or using the scope	LAPaROScopy = procedure of using a laparoscope to view the abdominal cavity
-tome	instrument for cutting, such as into smaller or thinner sections	MIcrotome = instrument for cutting tissues into microthin slices or sections
-graph	instrument or machine that writes or records	eLECtroCARdiograph = machine that records electrical impulses produced by the beating heart

Suffix	Meaning	Example and definition
-graphy	procedure of using an instrument or machine to record	eLECtroCARdiOGraphy = procedure of using an electrocardiograph to produce an electrocardiogram
-gram	the product, written record, "picture," or graph produced	eLECtroCARdiogram (ECG, EKG) = graphic tracing of the electrical currents flowing through the beating heart
-meter	instrument or machine that measures or counts	therMOmeter = instrument used to measure body temperature
-metry -IMetry	procedure of measuring	doSIMetry = act of determining the amount, rate and distribution of ionizing radiation

TERMS FOR DIRECTION, POSITION, AND MOVEMENT

Following is a list of words used to describe direction or the position of a body part relative to other body parts.

CRAnial: Pertaining to the cranium or head end of the body, or denoting a position more toward the cranium or head end of the body than some other reference point (body part) (Fig. 4-1). *Example:* The head is cranial to the tail.

CAUdal: Pertaining to the tail end of the body, or denoting a position more toward the tail or rear of the body than some other reference point (body part) (see Fig. 4-1). *Example:* The tail is caudal to the head.

ROStral: Pertaining to the nose end of the head or body, or toward the nose (see Fig. 4-1). *Example:* The nose is rostral to the eyes.

DORsal: Pertaining to the back area of a quadruped (animal with four legs), or denoting a position more toward the spine than some other reference point (body part) (see Fig. 4-1). *Example:* The vertebral column is dorsal to the abdomen.

VENtral: Pertaining to the underside of a quadruped, or denoting a position more toward the abdomen than some other reference point (body part) (see Fig. 4-1). *Example:* The intestines are ventral to the vertebral column.

MEdial: Denoting a position closer to the median plane of the body or a structure, toward the middle or median plane,

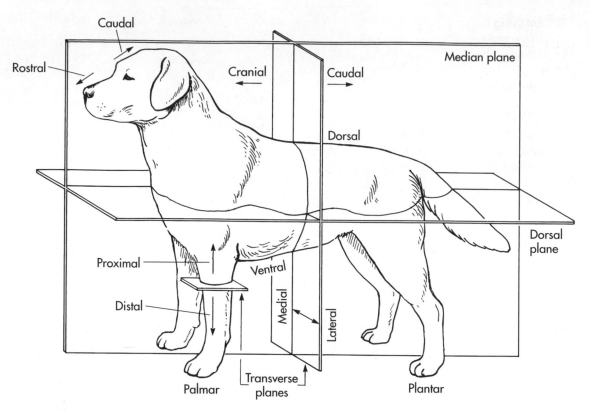

FIG. 4-1 Terms denoting position in animals. *(From McBride DF:* Learning veterinary terminology, *St Louis, 1996, Mosby.*

or pertaining to the middle or a position closer to the median plane of the body or a structure (see Fig. 4-1). *Example:* The medial surface of the leg is the "inside" surface.

LATeral: Denoting a position farther from the median plane of the body or a structure, on the side or toward the side away from the median plane, or pertaining to the side of the body or of a structure (see Fig. 4-1). *Example:* The lateral surface of the leg is the "outside" surface.

peRIPHeral: Pertaining to or situated near the periphery, the outermost part, or surface of an organ or part. *Example:* The enamel of a tooth is peripheral to the dentin and central root canal.

CENtral: Pertaining to or situated near the more proximal areas of the body or a structure; opposite of peripheral. *Example:* This spinal cord is central to the sciatic nerve.

SUperFIcial: Situated near the surface of the body or a structure; opposite of deep. *Example:* The skin is superficial to the muscles.

deep: Situated away from the surface of the body or a structure; opposite of superficial. *Example:* The muscles are deep to the skin.

adJAcent: Next to, adjoining, close. *Example:* The tongue is adjacent to the teeth.

PROXimal: Nearer to the center of the body, relative to another body part, or a location on a body part relative to another, more distant, location (see Fig. 4-1). *Example:* The humerus is proximal to the radius.

DIStal: Farther from the center of the body, relative to another body part or a location on a body part relative to another closer location (see Fig. 4-1). *Example:* The tibia is distal to the femur.

obLIQUE: At an angle, or pertaining to an angle. *Example:* The vein crosses obliquely from the dorsal left side to the ventral right side.

reCUMbent: Lying down; a modifying term is needed to describe the surface on which the animal is lying. *Example:* An animal in dorsal recumbency is lying on its dorsum (back), face up.

SUpine, SUpinNAtion: Lying face up, in dorsal recumbency. Supination is the act of turning the body or a leg so that the ventral aspect is uppermost.

prone, proNAtion: Lying face down, in ventral recumbency. Pronation is the act of turning the body or a leg so the ventral aspect is down.

PALmar: The caudal surface of the front foot distal to the antebrachiocarpal joint; also pertains to the undersurface of the front foot (see Fig. 4-1).

PLANtar: The caudal surface of the back foot distal to the tarsocrural joint; also pertains to the undersurface of the rear foot (see Fig. 4-1).

abDUCtion: Movement of a limb or part away from the median line or middle of the body (Fig. 4-2).

adDUCtion: Movement of a limb or part toward the median line or middle of the body (see Fig. 4-2).

FLEXion: The act of bending, such as a joint (Fig. 4-3).

exTENsion: The act of straightening, such as a joint; also, the act of pulling two component parts apart to lengthen the whole part (see Fig. 4-3).

DENTAL TERMINOLOGY

The teeth have their own set of positional terms listed below.

ocCLUsal: The chewing or biting surface of teeth; toward the plane between the mandibular and maxillary teeth (Fig. 4-4).

BUccal: Toward the cheek; tooth surface toward the cheek (see Fig. 4-4).

LINGual: Pertaining to the tongue; tooth surface toward the tongue (see Fig. 4-4).

CONtact: Surface of a tooth facing an adjacent or opposing tooth (see Fig. 4-4).

MEsial: Surface of a tooth closest to the midline of the dental arcade.

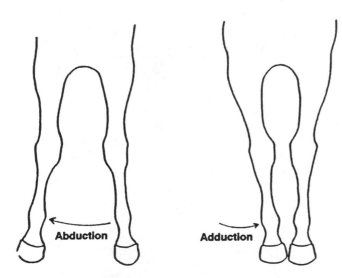

FIG. 4-2 Terms denoting limb movement: adduction and abduction. *(From Frandson RD:* Anatomy and physiology of farm animals, *ed 5, Philadelphia, 1992, Lea & Febiger.)*

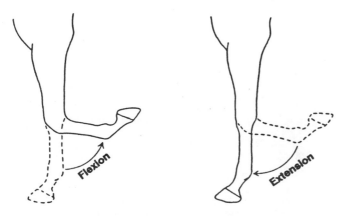

FIG. 4-3 Terms denoting limb movement: flexion and extension. *(From Frandson RD:* Anatomy and physiology of farm animals, *ed 5, Philadelphia, 1992, Lea & Febiger.)*

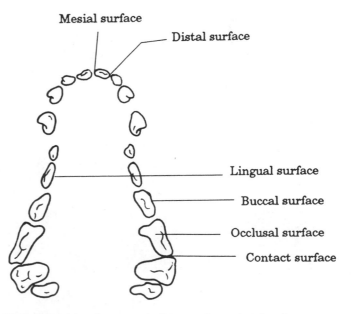

FIG. 4-4 Positional terms pertaining to the teeth. This illustrates teeth in the upper dental arcade, as seen from a ventral view. *(From Cochran PE:* Guide to veterinary medical terminology, *St Louis, 1991, Mosby.)*

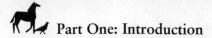

RECOMMENDED READING

Austrin G, Austrin BA: *Learning medical terminology,* ed 8, St Louis, 1995, Mosby.

Cochran PE: *Guide to veterinary medical terminology,* St Louis, 1991, Mosby.

Cohen BJ: *Medical terminology,* ed 2, Philadelphia, 1994, Lippincott.

Leonard PC: *Quick and easy medical terminology,* ed 2, Philadelphia, 1994, WB Saunders.

Mosby's Medical, Nursing & Allied Health Dictionary, ed 4, St Louis, 1994, Mosby.

PART TWO

Clinic Administration and Client Relations

CHAPTER 5

Recordkeeping, Business Transactions, and Clinic Administration

R.A. Goebel

Learning Objectives

After reviewing this chapter, the reader should understand the following:

Administrative procedures commonly used during a client's office visit and when admitting or discharging patients
Methods used in billing clients, extending credit, and collecting debts
Methods used to market veterinary services

Administrative procedures commonly used in operating a veterinary practice
Methods used in maintaining and ordering inventory and interacting with vendors
Uses of computers in veterinary practice
Procedures used for physically maintaining a veterinary facility

A successful and rewarding veterinary practice is as dependent upon practice philosophy and infrastructure as it is on the technical ability to perform medicine and surgery. This chapter's focus is on development of an infrastructure that equips the practice to meet client (and patient) needs. A "customer" focus is essential for the success of any small business, and veterinary practices are, by definition, small businesses. With proper balance and judicious application of the concepts presented in this chapter, the patient, client, staff member, and practice are all well served.

THE OFFICE VISIT

Your role, as veterinary technician, in the client visit may include several important examination room activities. After escorting the client and patient to the exam room you have an opportunity to discuss the practice's services as appropriate, to review the reason for the current visit, and to make recommendations for routine services that, by practice policy, would be timely or overdue. You can perform an initial physical examination, including measuring rectal temperature, noting gross physical abnormalities on the record, and obtaining required laboratory samples.

Some practices use a physical examination form that duplicates the information recorded in the medical record to apprise the client of the animal's health. This form should contain lay terminology and document physical examination findings as well as recommendations. This tool helps to formalize recommendations, documents information for discussion with the client's family members, and serves to refresh memories of matters discussed during the patient visit. Welcome client questions and answer them as appropriate. Veterinary technicians can play a major role in client education, as well as in patient care.

As an alternative to traditional office visits, some practices offer "drop-off" services. With this service, a client may present the patient, relate any concerns or needs, and retrieve the patient later in the day. You may record pertinent information on a standardized form to obtain an adequate history and authorization for treatment (Fig. 5-1). Obtain the client's daytime telephone number or establish some other method so that the client can be contacted following the patient's evaluation by the veterinarian. Some practices loan a paging device to clients so that they can be signaled to telephone the practice or return to pick up their pet. Alternatively, you can schedule a tentative pick-up time so that the client can be sure a technician or veterinarian will be available to discuss the case at that time.

ADMITTING A PATIENT

If the patient is scheduled for elective surgery, prepackaged folders can speed client check-in. For example, you could assemble a description of the procedure, including cost estimates, procedure authorization and consent form, home care instructions, cage card, and patient identification band, as appropriate for commonly performed elective procedures (Figs. 5-2 and 5-3).

Additional forms can facilitate the communication and authorization process. A *standard consent form* authorizes care to be provided at the practice facility (Fig. 5-4). A *boarding guest registration form* may serve as an authorization form. The boarding guest registration form lists services that should also be offered verbally by the staff member managing the admission process. Owners frequently forget or are distracted when leaving their pet and appreciate these reminders of other services that can be performed conveniently during that pet's stay in the hospital facility.

You, as technician, are frequently involved with not only performing some procedures during the patient stay but also providing patient progress reports to the client periodically during the animal's stay.

If an animal must be referred to a specialty practice, the technician can arrange for preparation of such information as referral forms, copies of medical records, laboratory reports, and radiographs. It is essential to properly label and address original radiographs that accompany referrals, as these must be returned to the primary care facility. With all other records, provide copies for the referral practice and retain originals (as legally required) in the referring practice.

Finally, the technician may arrange for patient discharge, scheduling of recheck or suture removal visits, and a telephone call to the client for a progress report 48 to 72 hours after release.

DISCHARGING A PATIENT

Complete medical and financial records before the patient is discharged from the hospital. Collect payment in full (or have payment contract signed) and make any follow-up appointment before the patient is brought to the examination room or reception area. Having the essential paperwork completed before the client and patient are reunited expedites the discharge procedure.

The final exchange with the client should always include a statement about when the patient's next visit should be. This serves as a reminder not only to the client but also to you that you expect your relationship with that client to continue. Therefore, *every* time a patient leaves the clinic, there should be some mechanism in place to reestablish contact with the client. For example, schedule an appointment for reexamination and give a reminder appointment to the client. If, for example, a blood count and chemistry profile are scheduled in 90 days, a staff member can call the client 48 hours before the appointment to remind the client of the appointment. Veterinary practices commonly send *reminder notices* to clients, suggesting an appointment for the animal's annual physical examination (Fig. 5-5). Backup methods must be in place so that staff members follow up on "no-shows" and lack of response to reminders. This maintains the cycle of clients returning to the practice.

BILLING, COLLECTION, AND CREDIT MANAGEMENT

Ideally, clients pay in full at the time services are rendered. It is usually best to provide several payment options to clients, including cash, check, credit cards (MasterCard/Visa), or medical charge cards (e.g., Care Credit and Health Cap). Medical charge cards can be useful, but common complaints include failure to approve applicant (who may be standing at your reception desk), failure to authorize needed limits of credit, or slow or cumbersome application/approval process.

Many practices extend credit to clients, although sometimes with reluctance. Good credit management procedures protect the practice and serve the clients well. To address any potential financial difficulties early, reception staff or others greeting clients and preparing records for the patient visit should simply ask, "How do you intend to pay for today's service? We offer the option of cash, check, or credit card." The client should then be honest in his or her response and indicate the method of payment (ability to pay is implied). If the client will need extension of credit by the practice, it should be apparent at this time.

The financial advantage of extending credit can be twofold. First, if credit is made available, the recom-

---

MAGRANE ANIMAL HOSPITAL (219) 259-5291

What's Wrong with Your Pet?
Please answer the following questions as thoroughly as possible.

Vomiting:
☐ food   ☐ blood   how often? _____   ☐ diet change
☐ eating foreign objects (grass, trash, etc.) _____

Diarrhea:
☐ mucus   ☐ blood   ☐ straining   how often? _____

Sneezing & Coughing:
any discharge? _____ if yes, describe _____
☐ difficulty in breathing   type of cough _____ frequency _____

Urination:
☐ painful   ☐ blood noted   ☐ straining   how often _____

Limping:
which leg(s)? _____ describe problem _____

Skin:
☐ irritation   ☐ any family members itching?   ☐ hair loss   ☐ fleas
☐ applied any shampoos, dips, etc. (explain)? _____ how long? _____

Eyes:
which one? _____ discharge (color, consistency) _____ how long? _____

Ears:
which one? _____   ☐ odor   ☐ discharge   how long? _____

Seizures:
☐ twitching   ☐ any unknown seizure activity (describe)? _____
Any additional information? _____
Any known reaction to medication or vaccinations? _____
Any other pre-existing problems (if new patient)? _____
Currently on any medication and, if so, when was the last dose given? _____
1. **At what phone number can you be reached?** _____
2. **Do you authorize us to do more than an initial exam?** _____
3. **May we start diagnostic tests or x-rays?** _____
4. **May we start treating the problem?** _____
5. **Is there a strict limit on dollars to be spent?** _____

(Unless emergency treatment is required, we intend to thoroughly discuss with you
any involved procedures and/or approximate costs before proceeding.)

Client's Name _____   Pet's Name _____
Signature _____   Date _____

FIG. 5-1   The client is asked to complete this form when dropping off an animal at the clinic for evaluation or treatment.

ANESTHESIA/SURGERY CONSENT FORM

Owner: _____   Patient: _____

Procedure: _____   Phone Number Today: _____

I hereby authorize Magrane Animal Hospital, P.C. and its designated associates to perform the above procedure(s). In addition, in the event that emergency treatment is required and I cannot be reached, I agree to any necessary diagnostic, treatment, or surgical procedures which are required.

In order to maintain a healthy, clean, hospital environment, pets must be free of parasites (fleas, ticks) and be current on vaccinations. If necessary, pets will be updated on vaccinations and treated for any fleas or ticks at an additional charge.

Additional Options/Services

Please initial if you approve any of these additional services

Blood Tests To identify potential health risks we recommend a more comprehensive blood testing to evaluate the liver and kidneys, as well as diabetes (this testing is required on all patients over 7 years of age). The cost is an additional $37.60.

Approve _____

Retained Baby Teeth Occasionally puppies and kittens will not lose their baby teeth on schedule, which results in potential dental problems. We routinely extract these unwanted teeth while the pet is anesthetized. The additional cost is $6.60-$20.20 per tooth.

Approve _____

Fecal Examination We recommend a yearly bowel movement examination for internal parasites (worms). If your pet is overdue we can obtain a sample and test it for parasites while your pet is here for a fee of $11.00.

Approve _____

Microchip Identification We are now able to permanently identify pets using a small microchip implanted beneath their skin. The benefit of microchip identification is the ability to identify missing pets. We offer a $10.00 discount when we implant a microchip during an anesthetic procedure, for a net cost of $26.00.

Approve _____

Nail Trim $6.00

Approve _____

Express Anal Sacs $6.00

Approve _____

I have read and understand this consent form, and I agree to pay for services rendered at the time my pet is discharged or when service is otherwise completed.

Owner or Agent: _____   Date: _____

Magrane Animal Hospital • 2324 Grape Road • Mishawaka, IN 46545 • (219) 259-5291

FIG. 5-2 Form used to obtain a client's consent to induce general anesthesia or perform surgery.

HOME CARE FOLLOWING SURGERY

Your pet has received a general anesthetic and, as a result, may appear more tired than normal and possibly a little uncoordinated. This is to be expected and the grogginess should disappear in the next day or so.

- To prevent vomiting due to excitement on arriving home, do not give your pet food or water for an hour after returning home. Feed the regular diet lightly today and return to normal feeding tomorrow.

- If your pet becomes listless or refuses to eat the next day, or if vomiting or diarrhea occurs, call the hospital immediately.

- Observe the incision at least twice a day for drainage, excessive swelling, redness, or pain and report any abnormalities immediately.

- Discourage excessive licking or chewing by your pet at the stitches or incision, and call us if it persists.

- Your pet's exercise should be restricted (no free running or jumping) for a week following surgery.

- If your pet is sent home with a bandage or cast, make sure it stays clean and dry. Call the hospital if it becomes wet or heavily soiled.

- If your cat was declawed, use shredded paper towels or newspaper instead of litter for the first 3-5 days at home to help prevent infection.

Future Treatment

☐ Please make an appointment for a recheck in _____ days/weeks.

☐ Please make an appointment for suture removal in _____ days.

☐ Please make an appointment in _____ days for bandage change or removal.

☐ Remove bandage at home in _____ days.

Call the hospital if you have any problems or questions.

Special Instructions

_____

_____

_____

_____

_____

_____

Magrane Animal Hospital • 2324 Grape Road • Mishawaka, IN 46545 • (219) 259-5291

FIG. 5-3 Client handout describing home care following surgery.

STANDARD CONSENT FORM

TO: Magrane Animal Hospital, P.C.; K.T. Neuhoff, DVM; R.L. Doversberger, DVM; K.M. Kline, DVM; T.J. Niemann, DVM; R.A. Goebel, DVM

OWNER'S NAME: _____   NAME OF PET: _____

ADDRESS: _____   SPECIES: _____

BREED: _____

PATIENT NUMBER: _____   SEX: _____

I am the owner or agent for the owner of the above described pet and have the authority to execute this consent.

I hereby consent to the hospitalization of the above described pet and authorize the doctor and his/her staff to administer any medication, tests, anesthetics or surgical procedures that the doctor deems necessary for the health, safety, or well-being of my pet.

I specifically request the following procedure(s) or operation(s):

_____

I understand that during the performance of the foregoing procedure(s) or operation(s), unforeseen conditions may be revealed that necessitate an extension of the foregoing procedure(s) or operation(s) or different procedure(s) or operation(s) than those set forth above. Therefore, I hereby consent to and authorize the performance of such procedure(s) or operation(s) as are necessary and desirable in the exercise of the veterinarian's professional judgement.

I also authorize the use of appropriate anesthetics and other medications, and I understand that hospital support personnel will be employed as deemed necessary by the veterinarian.

I have been advised as to the nature of the procedure(s) or operation(s) and the risks involved. I realize that results cannot be guaranteed.

I understand that all fees for professional services are due and payable at the time of discharge.

I have read and understand this authorization and consent.

ADDITIONAL INFORMATION _____

_____

_____

DATE: _____   Signature of Owner or Agent _____

Witness to Above Signature _____

FIG. 5-4   Form used to obtain a client's consent to provide veterinary care.

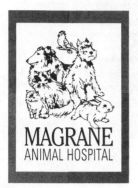

2324 Grape Road • Mishawaka, Indiana 46545 • 219/259-5291   Fax 219/259-3755

January 5, 1998

Richard Goebel
2601 Darwin Dr.
West Lafayette, IN 47906

Dear Richard,

Rudy's health is very important to us. Our records indicate that it has been more than 18 months since we have given Rudy a complete physical exam. Bringing Rudy in every year for a physical and vaccinations is a step in the right direction on the road to good health. Because dogs and cats age much more quickly than people, a yearly exam for them is the same as a doctor's visit every 6-8 years for us. A lot can change in a year.

Please call us today at 259-5291 for an appointment. We want to help you keep Rudy healthy. Remember it is far less costly to you and your pet to prevent diseases rather than treat them.

If you no longer have Rudy with you, please call to let us know. We would like to know if you have taken Rudy elsewhere for care, particularly if it is because you were dissatisfied with our service or care in any way, since we strive to provide you with the best. Please call and ask to speak with Vikky Warner.

Thank You,

Doctors and Staff of
Magrane Animal Hospital

FIG. 5-5   Letter sent to remind a client of vaccinations past due.

mended work can be performed; client and patient are well served and the practice bills additional fees. Second, many clients need more than 30 days to pay and are willing to pay interest on balances extending past 30 days from the time of billing. Some practices charge the client interest at 1.5% per month on the unpaid balance. A billing fee is also assessed to pay for bookkeeping, postage, and other costs related to extending credit. The practice collects interest, because the client has use of money owed to the practice. If accounts receivable (money owed by clients) are $24,000 for a three-doctor practice and 3/4 of the balance is more than 30 days old, $3,240 in increased revenue would be generated annually by charging interest ($24,000 × 3/4 × 1.5% = $270 per month × 12).

Each practice should clearly define criteria for extending credit so that all staff members can understand and implement the practice's policies. Box 5-1 lists sample considerations used in extending credit to clients. Box 5-2 lists factors to be considered when drawing up a payment contract.

CLIENT COMMUNICATIONS

Communication with clients is essential to learn about client/patient needs, to educate clients about animal health needs and their role in meeting those needs, and to remind clients of periodic routine visits, as well as seasonal health needs. A variety of tools can facilitate communication with clients. Examples include newslet-

---

> **Box 5-1 Sample considerations for extending credit**
>
> - Always request initial payment.
> - If the animal is ill, treat the animal and check the client's credit rating.
> - If the procedure is elective and no initial partial payment is made, reschedule the procedure for another time.
> - If the client has had a relationship with the clinic for more than 1 year and has always paid his or her bills in the past, establish a payment contract for up to $200 (not to be offered for elective services).
> - If the client has history of previous unpaid bills and the account was turned over to a collection agency, do not extend credit with or without a payment contract.
> - If credit needs exceed $200, call the clinic's designated credit manager to expedite the credit check and negotiate payment terms.

> **Box 5-2 Considerations when drawing up a payment contract**
>
> - Limit the total term of the contract to 90 days or less.
> - Be sure the client understands that interest will be applied to all unpaid balances extending beyond 30 days.
> - Be sure the person signing the payment contract is the animal owner or authorized agent and is willing to assume full financial responsibility.
> - Inspect the client's driver's license to confirm information provided (such as name, address, driver's license or Social Security number, and photo).
> - Seek agreement to pay on a weekly (or monthly) basis. Enter the specific details on the payment contract.
> - Be sure all details are provided in the credit application and payment agreement.
> - Make phone calls to verify information provided on the credit application.
> - Base your decision to extend or not to extend credit on the information provided, negotiated, and verified.

---

ters, promotions, client advisory boards, focus groups, client surveys, and posters or signs.

Newsletters

Although newsletters can be somewhat costly and time consuming to produce and distribute, they are an effective educational tool for clients. Newsletters can inform clients of health services offered by the practice and can introduce staff members. Newsletters produced in-house have the advantage of being more personal than commercially produced newsletters. Columns may include seasonal topics (e.g., heartworm or flea control or heat prostration), behavioral topics, case of the month, staff spotlight (focused on one staff member), and staff updates to introduce new staff or report on recent continuing education experiences. The newsletter may describe new or seasonal services or announce sign-up opportunities for "puppy manners" classes.

Special Promotions

Clients can be informed of special events or timely topics using various promotional methods. Examples of special events include National Pet Week, National Dental Health month, breed rescue events, and humane society projects. Clients can be informed by posters or signs in the practice facility, notices on the outside sign, and/or mailings of a special edition of the clinic's letters or postcards (Fig. 5-6). Special incentives can be used to

Pet Lines

Special Dental Health Issue

This edition of our newsletter is devoted exclusively to the topic of dental care for your pet. According to the American Veterinary Dental Society, studies show that more than 80 percent of dogs by age three and 70 percent of cats by age three show some signs of gum disease. In this issue you will find articles on the warning signs, free dental examinations, the dental procedure, and home care.

We hope you will keep this newsletter as a future reference as we help to improve your pet's dental health.

Signs Your Pet May Have Dental Problems

by TJ Niemann, DVM

- ☐ Breath odor
- ☐ Yellow or brown deposit on teeth
- ☐ Red or inflamed gums
- ☐ Gums that bleed easily
- ☐ Loose or missing teeth
- ☐ Pain on chewing

If you checked any of the above it may be time to have your pet's teeth checked.

One of the earliest signs of dental problems is the formation of dental tartar (calculus). Dental tartar is that yellow to brown deposit on the tooth surface. It is composed of bacteria, plaque and food debris literally cemented onto the tooth. If not removed it continues to accumulate, eventually migrating down between the tooth, gum, and bone that holds the tooth in place. Left untreated the tooth root can become infected, and/or the tooth falls out due to the weakened attachment between the tooth and bone - either situation is not comfortable for your pet.

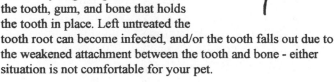

Dental Health Examinations

by Carol O'Connor, RVT

Have you looked at your pet's teeth recently? Not sure if what you see is normal? Want to learn how to provide dental care at home for your pet?

Our technicians are trained to perform oral examinations on your pets. They will explain what to look for, what is normal and abnormal, demonstrate home cleaning care, and give recommendations on additional care and tartar-fighting diets.

February is National Pet Dental Health Month. To celebrate this event our technicians will be performing free dental examinations and giving away free pet toothpaste samples and fingerbrushes during the month of February. This is a $21.23 value.

"Pets Need Dental Care, Too". Call 259-5291 to make an appointment for a dental health examination with one of our technicians.

FIG. 5-6 This special issue of a practice newsletter promotes dental care.

entice clients to participate, such as an open house during National Pet Week or free dental examinations by staff technicians during National Dental Health Month. Some practices use promotions to generate business during predictably slow times of the year. This can help keep staff fully employed and hospital revenues stable if clients respond to the campaign.

Client Surveys

Client surveys can help the practice harvest the information needed to determine the level of client satisfaction and to identify unmet client and/or patient needs. You can give surveys to clients when they visit the practice, hand them out to each client for 2 days per month, or mail them to 1 of every 10 or 20 clients within 2 weeks following a practice visit. Clients respond best if they see the results from their survey participation. Periodic reports in the practice newsletter can highlight survey findings and the action taken by the practice to meet identified needs.

Focus Groups and Advisory Boards

Veterinary practices sometimes use focus groups and advisory boards to attract desirable clients. Your favorite clients are likely to refer animal owners like themselves to the practice. It may be in your practice's best interest to cultivate these referrals by first meeting the needs of your clients and asking your favorite clients to refer the friends and family to your clinic. Always express gratitude when referrals are made. The doctors and staff should be able to quickly identify 30 to 50 top clients by any criteria (e.g., they visit the practice frequently, they always comply with instructions, or they really love their animal). Once a long client list is formed, the top 20 can be identified and invited to an evening forum, where a discussion of practice products and services takes place. These favorite clients frequently respond with enthusiasm and are eager to offer constructive criticism and suggestions for the future. Requests for pet pickup/delivery, extended hours, and puppy behavior classes are examples of new services frequently requested and appreciated. This advisory group can also give you feedback for your ideas for new products or services by letting you know if the new idea would be of value to them. Many suggestions can be implemented at little or no cost to the practice. Frequently, the group pleasantly offers affirmation that you are doing a good job meeting client needs.

Depending upon your personal practice style and how well you think this process works, you may limit these meetings to occasional use and invite a different group of clients each time. This method would be referred to as a *focus group* exercise. Box 5-3 lists some information gained from a focus group. By contrast, you may want to keep the same group of clients together and meet regularly (quarterly or semi-annually) as an

---

> **Box 5-3 Example of information gained from a focus group**
>
> Reasons for coming to your clinic:
> - "Confidence in staff (know answers or will find them)"
> - "Congeniality of staff members to each other and to clients"
> - "Compassionate veterinary care"
> - "Accommodation of special needs (early drop off, late office visits, etc.)"
> - "Staff helps ease the process of euthanasia—flowers, cards, memorial contributions are all appreciated"
> - "Excellent newsletters"
>
> Challenges/opportunities:
> - "Need improved examination room seating."
> - "Handrail at front door would be helpful."
> - "How about computerized record interface with the emergency clinic?"
> - "More evening appointments requested."
> - "Note on front page of client's record the best time to call client."

---

advisory board. Some practices have used such advisory boards to assist in putting on an open house celebration or grand opening for a new facility.

VALUE-ADDED SERVICES

Offering clients more than they expect to receive can help bond them to your practice. Ways to exceed client expectations may be referred to as *value-added* services.

Some practices have an Ask-A-Tech *telephone information "hotline,"* on which technicians answer client questions on routine, uncomplicated problems. Many clients use this hotline to ask questions they might have been reluctant to ask the doctor. Others call to obtain advice about animal care in unhurried conversation with a competent professional. Technicians must always use good judgment in advising clients. The technician should tactfully recommend an office visit or discussion with the doctor when medical judgment must be made.

Clinic tours for all new or prospective clients fosters good client relations. Tours may also be offered to 4-H, Scout, and school groups. The practice newsletter is a good place to promote tours. Clinic tours offer an opportunity to demonstrate the capability of the clinic's veterinarian(s) and staff to provide a broad range of care for animals. Most clients are surprised at the array of instruments, equipment, drugs, and supply items used to treat their animals. Tours help bond new clients to your practice and encourage others to seek services for the first time or inquire about new services to which they were exposed during the tour.

Presentations for community groups, service clubs, and school groups allow an opportunity to promote your clinic in person. A photographic tour (slides or video) of your clinic can substitute for a clinic tour for your audience. You can also highlight special patient care benefits offered by your clinic as well as seasonal animal health tips.

Puppy and kitten socialization classes can be offered free or at low cost to clients who purchase "wellness" packages of services in your practice. Surveys suggest that 30% of all former pet owners no longer own their pet because of unresolved behavioral problems.

Pet selection services are beneficial but not often used. Too many pet owners become owners of new pets as a result of an impulsive decision. Too little thought and advance planning often result in a poor match between new owner and pet. Too often, an unhappy relationship develops and is terminated when the owner puts the animal up for adoption. With some creative thought, your clinic can offer a valuable counseling service to increase the chances of a successful match between the new owner and pet. This has the potential for additional long-term client relationships for your practice. Newsletter articles and public service announcements in your local newspaper advocating important points to consider in pet selection are well received. You can encourage prospective pet owners to seek advice from the veterinarian in considering pets species and breed alternatives.

Grief counseling after an animal's death or euthanasia is essential to maintaining a good relationship with clients. Clients who are supported through this difficult time with your caring attitude, sensitive responses, and assurances on euthanasia decisions respond appropriately. They are likely to own another pet after healing from the grief associated with pet loss and are likely to bring that new pet to your clinic. Chapter 6 contains a discussion of grief counseling.

CLINIC OPERATIONS
Scheduling of Work

Scheduling of work provides the greatest opportunity for properly managing the practice's single largest investment: its people. Doctor and staff salaries typically make up 40% to 50% of a practice's expense. Managing this expense, therefore, is three times more important than managing the next largest expense: drugs and supplies (13% to 18% of practice expense). To optimize the doctor/staff salary investment, it is best to have a steady and predictable amount of work to do

on a year-round basis. Fluctuations in workload are the biggest obstacle for efficient use of staff.

If your clients tell you that evening hours are important, but so are morning hours, you face a common but difficult challenge. To avoid scheduling the entire staff for all day and the evening, some staff must work split-shifts or more part-time personnel must be employed. For most practices this is not an option but rather a necessity for financial survival.

To deal with seasonal peaks and valleys, consider how you can shift the workload from the peaks to fill the valleys. Can you recommend year-round heartworm prevention versus seasonal programs? Can you offer client incentives to purchase elective procedures during slow months, for example by promoting National Dental Health Month in February? Can you slightly reduce or expand the intervals for annual physical examinations (11 months or 13 months) instead of the usual 12 months to increase client visits during the slower months?

Scheduling challenges must consider client needs first, patients' seasonal and illness needs second, and doctor/staff preferences last. Veterinary practice is a service business. For the success of any service business, the needs of the customers must drive the priorities. With some creative thinking and planning, you may be able to make adjustments to meet the needs of clients, patients, doctors, and staff alike.

Teamwork

Clients and patients are best served by a team of professionals who are committed to responsive client service and excellent patient care. It can be challenging to assemble, maintain, and grow a successful team.

It all starts with a personnel philosophy that honors the strengths of everyone on the team and fosters mutual openness and respect. The philosophy must recognize that each person has strengths and weaknesses. It is best to focus on strengths and compensate for weaknesses. Allow people to work where they are most likely to be successful and assign to someone else tasks they do not do well. The friendly, accommodating, extroverted person may be best suited for receptionist activity; the less outgoing, meticulous perfectionist may be better suited to attend the exacting details related to patient care.

Hiring of new employees is important. The cost of hiring and training a new employee to become a dependable daily contributor to the practice can equal at least 1 year's salary. Selecting an inappropriate person means turnover and a loss of many thousands of dollars to the practice.

Staff selection must include a focus on team players. All employees who are team players readily offer help to others when they need it and are equally willing to accept help when needed. This attitude, combined with appropriate cross training, prepares the team to be responsive to peaks in client demand and patient case-load. It also prepares staff to "cover" during staff ill-nesses, vacations, and other absences.

Attitudes toward teamwork can be detected by care-fully questioning applicants about their experience working (or playing) with others. For example, has the applicant served on committees at school or with service clubs or sororities? Has the applicant played team sports? Can the applicant tell you about his or her role in group problem solving with a previous employer? Can he or she tell you about a previous experience when his or her work team came together and enjoyed success through a "crunch" time? Good team members are nei-ther too independent (lone rangers) nor too dependent (must be told everything to do). Rather, they are inter-dependent and willing to give or receive help.

Setting expectations and training is also crucial. Many new staff members are slow to succeed because expecta-tions are not clearly communicated. The "big picture" of a practice's philosophy is communicated by a mission statement and is demonstrated by having staff meetings, staff communication, and practice policies in place that drive activities that fulfill the mission statement.

Team leaders must define, teach, and periodically measure skill levels. Good performance must be recog-nized and rewarded. All staff members must have assur-ance that their jobs are important and they must per-form well in their positions to enjoy both personal and professional success. Rewards and recognition should be made as publicly as possible, such as during staff meetings, with posted announcement, or published in newsletters.

Handle reprimands or corrections in private; nothing can be gained by pointing out a person's shortcomings in public. Such embarrassment undermines trust, erodes confidence, and weakens team bonds.

Medical Records

Veterinary practice acts in most states require that med-ical records be made for each patient, litter, or herd/flock, and that these records be maintained for a minimum period, such as 3 years. As a practical matter, most practices maintain medical records for a much longer period, often for years after a client relationship is terminated or after the patient dies.

Practical reasons exist for maintaining good medical records beyond the minimal legal requirements. Quality patient care, good client communications, doc-umentation for referrals, and documentation as a legal defense are all valid reasons for maintaining good med-ical records.

Quality patient care requires tracking and accommo-dating animal's wellness and illness needs. An individual patient record should include a master sheet listing species, gender, breed, age, diet, allergies, unique behav-iors, and annual vaccination/parasite control documen-tation (Fig. 5-7). The master sheet should also include a major problem list and prescribed drug list for which refills are indicated. Follow the master sheet with lined pages on which chronologic visits, treatments, and client communications are recorded.

Make all entries in permanent ink and enter them promptly to ensure accuracy. Eliminate errors by draw-ing a single line through the erroneous entry; do not mask by "white out," using correction fluids, or "black out," using a felt-tip marker. This allows a legal observ-er to note the nature of the error and to be assured that important "evidence" has not been destroyed. Medical records should contain factual or objective information. Any subjective observations must have some basis in fact and not reflect personal opinions of doctor/staff nor judgments about the client's truthfulness, credit worthi-ness, religious or sexual orientation, or other personal characteristics. Treat all records with confidentiality. Do not discuss cases by name with clients; the privacy of owner and patient information must be respected. Clients have a right to review records kept by the prac-tice; copies must be supplied upon demand. Further, medical records can be subpoenaed for legal action and the clinic must comply. Accurate, legible, complete, and contemporaneous recordkeeping is important.

Careful documentation throughout a patient visit or hospital stay allows caregivers to review such information as previous history, diagnostic and treatment plans, and response to treatment. This review of historical informa-tion contributes to the plan for future patient care man-agement. All laboratory reports and imaging interpreta-tions must be included in a complete medical record.

You can weave client communications and summa-rized phone conversations into the medical record to document revised estimates, revised treatment plans, and important decisions dictated or declined by the client.

Use the carefully documented medical record when a patient is referred to a specialist. Photocopied medical records should accompany the patient, along with a recent, written summary of the case. Original records should always remain in the practice facility, with one exception. Radiographs are not easily duplicated and are usually sent with the patient. These must be returned to the referring clinic.

Some practices include financial documentation in the medical record. This is not a legal requirement and may not be in the practice's best interest. Many prac-tices manage financial documentation in a separate, computerized system. In the latter case, cost estimates and authorizations to treat, as well as transaction totals, may be included in the medical record, but detailed charges (visit slips or invoices) usually are not included in the medical record.

MAGRANE ANIMAL HOSPITAL

2324 Grape Rd.
Mishawaka, IN 46545
(219) 259-5291

PATIENT'S NAME		BREED		OWNER'S NAME		☐ MISS ☐ MR ☐ MRS ☐ DR ☐ MS
DATE OF BIRTH		DESCRIPTION		ADDRESS		
☐ MALE ☐ ALTERED ☐ FEMALE	DOG	CAT	OTHER	CITY	STATE	ZIP
BEHAVIOR				HOME PHONE	WORK PHONE	
ALLERGIES				SPOUSE'S NAME	OWNER'S EMPLOYER	
MEDICAL ALERT				SPOUSE'S EMPLOYER	SPOUSE'S WORK PHONE	
X-RAY NUMBER		DIET		REFERRED BY		
FORM OF PAYMENT ☐ CASH ☐ CHECK ☐ VISA/MC		CREDIT ☐ OK		OTHER PETS		

ROUTINE HEALTH MAINTENANCE

YEAR	1997	1998	1999	2000	2001	2002
DA$_2$P						
Reminder						
PARVO						
Reminder						
RABIES						
Reminder						
FVRCP						
Reminder						
FeLV						
Heartworm Test						
Result						
Reminder						
WEIGHT						
FECAL						
Result						

Date Active	Date Resolved	MASTER PROBLEMS	MEDICATION	REFILL

FIG. 5-7 The master record sheet contains a comprehensive record of an animal's medical history.

Special forms can be used to facilitate recordkeeping and enhance client communication. For example, a color-coded (by year) vaccination sheet can be developed for easy completion and ready identification within the medical record (Fig. 5-8). Another example is the anesthesia/surgery consent form (see Fig. 5-2), which is used to obtain owner authorization to perform elective procedures.

Records format. In the examples shown, the format is a paper 8½ × 11-inch record system designed to be held in a clasp-type file folder. Some clinics find a smaller paper size to be adequate. Other clinics maintain an entirely computerized medical and financial record for each client. Regardless of the format, the record must be accurate, complete, and secure. Storage and retrieval must be convenient and well organized. Various design formats are commercially available to minimize misfiling by incorporating color-coded tabs. If computerized records are used, meticulous accuracy is necessary for all data entry; incorrectly entered computer records may never be retrieved.

Standard operating procedure (SOP) can streamline medical recordkeeping detail. Although the medical record requires detailed tracking of all procedures, recording repetitious entries on record after record can become tedious. According to medical recordkeeping standards established by the American Animal Hospital Association, simply making the entry by routine procedure name, followed by "SOP," is perfectly acceptable, with one provision. For each SOP, there must be on file in the practice a description of the detailed procedures for each standardized procedure (Box 5-4).

SOP descriptions can be written for all standardized procedures used in the practice and a looseleaf binder used to store SOP sheets in a central location. Annual reviews and updates of SOP descriptions are important. Once the SOP binder is in place, you may reference all standardized procedures by "procedure name, SOP" as you complete patient medical records.

Inventory Management

The pharmacy of a veterinary clinic provides a valuable client service. If the patient needs a prescription item (e.g., an antibiotic) or an over-the-counter nonprescription item (e.g., flea spray), there are numerous advantages in dispensing the item from the clinic's pharmacy.

Client convenience is very important in the current business environment. "One-stop shopping" saves time and relieves stress for the busy client. Clients appreciate the convenience of having the clinic supply any needed products and services in one visit. Directing a busy client to the nearest feed store or human pharmacy for a needed product is neither profitable nor desirable.

Competent professional judgment is required to select the best quality and most appropriate array of pharma-

---

Box 5-4   Sample of a detailed description of the standard operating procedures for ovariohysterectomy

Procedure: Canine Ovariohysterectomy
Preoperative physical exam
Preoperative blood work: total protein & PCV
Preanesthetic medication: atropine 0.05 mg/kg
                                            acepromazine 0.1 mg/kg
Intravenous anesthetic: thiopental 20 mg/kg to effect
Intubate patient
Inhalation anesthesia: halothane 2% to effect
                                    oxygen 98%
Patient prep: clip hair, surgical scrub (SOP)
Surgical procedure:
• ventral midline incision
• expose uterus and ovaries
• double ligation of ovarian pedicles and uterine stump
• excision of ovaries and uterus
Three-layer closure:
• 2-0 chromic gut/muscle wall
• 3-0 chromic gut/subcutis
• 3-0 monofilament polypropylene/skin
Terminate inhalant anesthesia; oxygen only for 5 minutes.
Disconnect endotracheal tube from anesthetic machine.
Observe patient; extubate when swallowing reflex regained.
Return patient to housing compartment.
Continue periodic patient observation and complete the medical record.

---

ceuticals and biologicals in the practice. Each item dispensed or sold is accompanied by the professional expertise available in the practice. The veterinarian and/or veterinary technician is responsible for product selection, instruction for use, cautions about potential side effects, appropriate recordkeeping, and availability for follow-up information on patient care. The professional expertise related to the clinic's drug and supply inventory make the availability of this inventory more valuable to clients than products purchased from the pet shop, grocery store, or feed store. The veterinary practice is the best source of top-quality pharmaceuticals and biologicals for veterinary use.

Purchasing Guidelines

The veterinarian or veterinary technician must use some judgment in selecting a product to be stocked for dispensing (prescription items) or over-the-counter sale (nonprescription). Aside from drugs used for emergency use, which must be immediately available, it makes little sense to invest in inventory that will be used only

MAGRANE ANIMAL HOSPITAL
VACCINATION SHEET

DATE _____   PATIENT'S NAME _____

TIME _____   CLIENT'S NAME _____

PROCEDURES _____

<u>PUPPY</u>
DHP-M
PARVO
DHP/PARVO/CORONA
PARVO/CORONA

<u>DOG</u>
DHP/PARVO/CORONA
RABIES # _____
BORDETELLA
HW CHECK _____

<u>CAT/KITTEN</u>
FVR-CP/CHLMY
RABIES # _____
FELV
FECAL _____

<u>CANINE</u>
_____ Behavior   _____ Fecals   _____ Microchip
_____ House Brk   _____ HW
_____ Other   _____ Diet
_____ Spay   _____ Ears
_____ Castrate   _____ Nails/anal sacs
_____ Flea x   _____ Groom
_____ Dental px   _____ AEC
_____ Lepto   _____ Bordetella

<u>FELINE</u>
_____ Dental px   _____ FELV   _____ Microchip
_____ Spay   _____ Declaw
_____ Castrate   _____ Chlamydia
_____ Ear Mites   _____ Fecal
_____ Fleas   _____ Diet
_____ Inside   _____ Groom
_____ Outside   _____ AEC
_____ GIVE LITERATURE
_____ GIVE HOSPITAL TOUR

TEMP. _____
WT. _____
G.I. _____
    teeth _____
    fecal _____
    anal sacs _____
RESP. _____
    upper _____
    lower _____
EYES _____
EARS _____

C.V. _____
    m.m. _____
    heart _____
    h.w. _____
INTEG. _____
    ext. par _____
    nails _____
LYMPH _____
GEN. UR _____
MUS-SKEL _____
C.N.S. _____
ABD. PALP _____

_____
_____
_____

FIG. 5-8 Sheet summarizing vaccines given and procedures performed. These sheets are often color coded for easy location in the medical record file.

occasionally. It is better to stock only items that are used frequently and to rely on writing prescriptions or referring clients to other sources for products used only occasionally. Inactive inventory occupies valuable space and ties up capital that could be invested elsewhere. Inactive inventory represents an unnecessary and avoidable practice expense.

Economic Order Quantity. Deciding how much of an item to order is as important as deciding what product to order. If you purchase too little at one time, you risk not having the product available when needed or spending too much time and effort reordering to keep the product in stock. Maintaining excessive inventory occupies storage space and ties up capital in inventory.

A simple equation helps establish the appropriate amount to order for a clinic (Box 5-5). Use of this calculation establishes the correct *economic order quantity (EOQ)*.

$$EOQ = 2FS \div CP,$$

where F = fixed cost of placing and receiving an order, S = annual sales of an item in units, C = carrying cost (usually 25%), and P = purchase price per unit. Consider carrying cost as the cost of investing in inventory (rather than in certificates of deposit or the stock market), cost of outdated products, and the cost of products no longer used when they are replaced by new and improved products.

Use this EOQ method for all products that are frequently used on a fairly constant (nonseasonal) basis. Do not use the EOQ formula for ordering products infrequently used, such as chemotherapeutic agents, or used seasonally, such as flea products.

Inventory turnover. Use inventory turnover to measure how well you are managing your inventory. The more often a modest inventory is sold and resold

---

Box 5-5　Sample calculation of economic order quantity (EOQ)

$$EOQ = \sqrt{2FS \div CP}$$

F = fixed cost of placing/receiving/pricing/storing one order, e.g., $15
S = annual sales of the item in units, e.g., 3,000 units of vaccine
C = carrying cost, e.g., 25%
P = price per unit, e.g., $2.75 per dose
The square root of (2)(15)(3,000) ÷ (25%)(2.75) = 995 units
The 995 units should be rounded to the nearest convenient unit. Therefore 1,000 units should be ordered at one time.

(turned over) each year, the better the financial result. High inventory turnover means that minimum space and capital are tied up in inventory. An easy way to calculate inventory turnover is shown in Box 5-6.

Inventory turnover of less than 5 times per year is considered poor, whereas turnover exceeding 10 times per year is admirable. This simple tool can help monitor how well veterinary practices manage inventory.

Pricing Dispensed Products

The pharmacy operation in most practices should be quite profitable. Although some areas of a practice may be only minimally profitable (e.g., surgery or hospitalization), the pharmacy should be making a significant contribution to profitability. Without the profits generated by their pharmacy, some practices would operate at a loss.

Box 5-6　Calculating inventory turnover

$$\text{Inventory turnover} = \frac{\text{total value of product purchased annually}}{\text{average value of product in stock}}$$

The average value of product in stock can be calculated by adding the beginning physical inventory to the year-end physical inventory and dividing the total by 2.

For example:
Total expenditures = $115,000
January 1 inventory = 21,000
December 31 inventory = 19,000

$$\text{Inventory turnover} = \frac{115,000}{(21,000 + 19,000) \div 2} = \frac{115,000}{20,000} = 5.75 \text{ times}$$

Prescription Drugs. Prescription drug pricing usually considers *markup* based on drug cost and a *dispensing fee*. *Markup* is a term commonly used to price the product based on a percentage of cost, such as per tablet, per tube of ointment, or per milliliter. Markup is used to recoup the cost of the drug, the carrying cost, and the ordering cost, and also to generate profit.

A markup of 100% can be illustrated by the following example. An antibiotic purchased for 10¢ and then marked up 100% would sell for 20¢ per tablet. A markup of 50% on the same tablet would result in a selling price of 15¢ per tablet. Most practices have a standard markup established for commonly used drugs. The markup ranges from a very low 2% or 3% in a food-animal practice dispensing large quantities of vaccine in a rural setting, to markups of several hundred percent in a small animal practice where overhead and operating costs might be quite high (high labor costs, high building occupancy costs).

Standard markups may not apply to certain items, such as very inexpensive products (e.g., antihistamine tablets) and very expensive products (e.g., some chemotherapy drugs). In these cases, it is common to have a minimum per-tablet cost, such as 10¢ per tablet, even though the cost of a tablet may by only 1¢ or 2¢ (this would represent a markup of 400% to 900%). If the tablet cost is quite high (e.g., $1.50 to $2.00 per tablet, markups may be reduced to 10% or 20%. The *margin* (difference between selling price and cost per unit) is 8¢ to 9¢ in the low-cost example and 15¢ to 40¢ in the high-cost example. In these exceptional examples, very high markups on very low-cost products actually yield less revenue per unit than very low markups on high-cost products. The objective is to generate enough revenue *per unit* to cover associated costs and contribute to practice profitability.

Dispensing Fee. A dispensing fee is often assessed in addition to the markup to cover the costs of packaging, labeling, and medical and pharmacy recordkeeping. Significant responsibility and potential liability are incurred in management of the clinic's drug inventory. Potential liability issues include dispensing drugs in childproof containers; proper documentation of drug dispensing in the medical and pharmacy records; maintaining these records for the required number of years; and proper storage, dispensing, or disposing of controlled substances.

The practice should receive revenue for the cost of handling prescription drugs and also for the responsibility and potential liability (risk) associated with making these prescription drugs available to clients. The dispensing fee, which generates this revenue, might be as low as $2.50 per prescription in some practices and as high as $10 in others (Box 5-7).

Many practices also have a *minimum prescription fee* for situations when only a few low-cost tablets are dispensed.

Box 5-7 Example of prescription drug pricing

Twenty 100-mg amoxicillin tablets are to be dispensed.

Each tablet costs 10¢, the markup is 150%, and the dispensing fee is $5.

(20 tablets × 10¢/tablet) + (150% × 20 tablets × 10¢/tablet) + $5 dispensing fee = $2 + $3 + $5 = $10 total fee.

---

pensed. For example, a client might need only two tranquilizer tablets for an anxious pet's car ride. The fee to the client might be $6.50, representing a $5 dispensing fee plus a $1.50 minimum prescription fee, even though the two tablets cost the practice only 25¢.

Over-the-Counter Products. Over-the-counter (OTC) products, such as flea powder, shampoo, and pet dentifrice, carry less liability and require less labor and less recordkeeping, and therefore are commonly sold without an associated dispensing fee. These products do not require a prescription and typically arrive in prepackaged form, so the primary product and packaging liability rests with the manufacturer.

Prices of OTC products are typically marked up in a similar method as prescription drugs. For example, a pet flea spray purchased for $6 per unit and marked up 150% would sell for $15 to the client ($6 cost + $9 markup = $15). Price shopping by clients may be more common with OTC products than with prescription products, so OTC products should be priced competitively. Remember, however, that the veterinary professional has carefully selected the best-quality and the most appropriate product and has provided it for the convenience of clients. It is reasonable that a premium should be paid to recognize this value-added client benefit.

In-Hospital Items. Pricing of products used on hospitalized animals must also be considered. Common methods include charging a flat fee for injections (e.g., $10 per injection) and perhaps adding a surcharge for very expensive drugs, such as some postoperative analgesics. In-hospital tablet administration frequently is priced to include drug, labor, and recordkeeping costs, such as $3 per administration. Intravenous (IV) fluid administration frequently is priced at one large initial fee (e.g., $15) to capture revenues for setting up the IV drip and for labor related to administering the fluid. An additional per-milliliter fee is commonly assessed, such as 2¢/ml. Using these fees, for example, IV infusion of 1 L of fluids would cost

$$\$15 + (1000 \text{ ml} \times 2¢/\text{ml}) = \$35.$$

This fee would not typically include the cost of catheter placement, which should be charged separately.

CONTROLLED SUBSTANCES

Handle controlled substances in compliance with state and federal regulations. Controls must be in place so that handling of controlled drugs is careful, deliberate, precise, and secure. Access to controlled drugs by doctors and staff should not be casual. Given the stresses common today in society, temptations for abuse may be hard to resist for some practice employees. Practice decision makers must view management of controlled substances as a serious responsibility. Chapter 13 contains more information on controlled substances.

VENDOR TRANSACTIONS

You may view veterinary drug and supply company representatives either as very helpful or as a nuisance. They often appear at inconvenient times to discuss products in which you may have no interest and recommend purchase in quantities far exceeding your potential use. With prior arrangement, the representative can appear at a mutually convenient time to discuss products useful to your practice to be purchased in quantities that fit your economic order quantity and inventory turnover criteria.

A constructive and useful relationship is possible. Ask your reception staff to schedule the initial visit by a company representative for 30 to 45 minutes, during which time you can get acquainted, take the representative on a tour of the clinic, explain your supply procurement, storage, and dispensing procedures, and relate your practice philosophy. In this way, the representative can gain insight into how your practice is managed and better understand your quality and quantity priorities. The representative can then determine how to best meet your needs with the products and services his or her company has to offer.

You should reasonably expect the sales representative to provide information on the following:
- current products, including animal health and practice financial benefits
- trends in the market, such as new drugs, supplies, and equipment
- practice tips that may have application in your practice
- on-site services, such as checking for outdated products or methods of stock rotation
- special prices, such as quantity discounts, seasonal or other promotions, or delayed billing
- benefits related to carrying a "family" of products, such as a line of flea control products for use on the pet (oral and topical), in the home and in the yard
- staff and client education materials, such as on flea control, heartworm control, or vaccination programs

USING COMPUTERS

More than 90% of veterinary practices use computers in some manner for practice operations. Many vendors offer hardware and software for veterinary purchases. Operationally and financially, the decision to computerize your practice or to change computer systems can have great implications. The decision maker in your practice should proceed carefully in making this decision. Changing a practice's recordkeeping to computerized format disrupts the usual routine, but the initial inconvenience is far outweighed by the benefits of computerization.

Use of a Computer

Uses of a computer in veterinary clinics include generating the following:
- financial information (and tracking it)
- invoices for services rendered
- reminders and recall notices
- monthly statements
- client instructions linked to procedures, vaccination certificates, and prescription labels
- mailing lists for newsletter, promotional, or informational mailings
- management data, such as reports on individual and profit center production, trends related to growth or decline of income from various services (e.g., dentistry and hospitalization), cash flow, budgeting, growth or decline in client and/or patient numbers, and owner compliance with wellness recommendations.

Other computer uses that may benefit your practice include the following:
- drug and supply inventory management
- complete patient medical recordkeeping
- bookkeeping (general ledger, accounts payable, accounts receivable, payroll processing)
- medical database references
- electronic mail, network access, World Wide Web access
- word processing (letters) and desktop publishing (newsletter)

Purchasing a Computer

Purchase of a computer for a veterinary practice can be expensive and its use can have an impact on the daily work routine of many staff members. For these reasons, it may be useful for interested staff to become involved in the decision of which computer system to buy. Why not form a computer committee?

The "Computer Committee" can evaluate the benefits versus the cost before deciding to computerize or to change computer systems. Some software systems may be more appropriate for your practice than others, so develop criteria to match the computer system with your practice's size, type, and philosophy. Although you must consider initial price, price should never be the only consideration. Reliability, usefulness, new efficiencies, ease of use, user support, timely software upgrades, installation, and training are all as important as initial price. Consider computer systems from at least three vendors before any final purchase decision is made.

FACILITY MAINTENANCE

"You never get a second chance to make a first impression." This phrase is particularly pertinent in regard to maintaining the clinic's facilities. Conscientious maintenance of your facility provides many benefits, including increased client satisfaction, improved patient comfort, a pleasant work environment for staff, reduced cost of repair/replacement as a practice expense, and long-term stability of the practice in its current location.

Most clients have a limited ability to objectively judge the quality of medical and surgical care provided by your clinic. They cannot observe much of the clinic and most have inadequate knowledge to judge medical and surgical quality. The opinion clients form about your clinic is often based on nonmedical issues, such as consideration shown by staff, expressions of care for the animals, willingness and ability to answer questions, and the appearance of the practice facility.

Is the outside of your clinic appealing, readily visible, and useful in guiding people to your practice? Is your parking lot readily accessible, in good condition, and kept clean? Does your building exterior have a tasteful finish kept in good repair?

Is the air in the reception area and examination rooms odor free (free of masking deodorants as well)? Are the client reception areas and examination rooms bright, clean, and orderly? What would your clients, see, smell, and hear if you escorted them on a clinic tour right now?

An individual in the practice should be responsible for facility maintenance and repair. Various staff members can take charge of maintenance tasks to spread the workload and attain maintenance/repair goals. Properly trained staff members can complete many interior and exterior maintenance tasks. Maintenance schedules remind those responsible of daily, weekly, and monthly tasks and document completed tasks.

Skilled craftspeople must complete some repairs. Make a list of maintenance and repair personnel so that someone can be quickly summoned in case of an urgent need. This list should include the practice's plumber, electrician, carpenter, lawn service, pest controller, computer supplier, telephone company, and utility suppliers. A supplemental list might include suppliers of major pieces of equipment (e.g., x-ray machine, furnace, air conditioner, blood chemistry analyzer) or systems (telephone or computer system) and their telephone numbers.

Some practices delegate authority for repairs and maintenance to staff according to their area of responsibility. For example, the laboratory technician is responsible for all maintenance and repair of the clinic's laboratory equipment. Along with this authority goes the responsibility to keep laboratory equipment operating in good repair. Provide spending authority by way of an annual budget to maintain major pieces of equipment in addition to a small miscellaneous category. Ward staff may have the authority to manage such decisions as calling a plumber to repair or upgrade bathing fixtures or unclog a major drain obstruction. The advantage of this delegation is that the problems are resolved by the staff members they immediately affect. Repairs are usually made more quickly and appropriately when the designated employees have a vested interest in the outcome; therefore, staff members are likely to act expeditiously to solve problems in their work area.

RECOMMENDED READING

Lukens RL, Landon P: *Guide to inventory management for veterinary practices,* West Chester, Penn, 1993, SmithKline Beecham.

McCarthy JW: *Basic guide to veterinary hospital management,* ed 2, Denver, 1992, American Animal Hospital Association.

Messonnier SP: *Marketing your veterinary practice,* St Louis, 1994, Mosby.

Messonnier SP: *Marketing your veterinary practice II,* St Louis, 1997, Mosby.

Wilson JF: *Client consent forms,* Denver, 1995, American Animal Hospital Association.

CHAPTER 6

Human Interactions in the Veterinary Workplace

S.M. Fassig
D.R. Dooley
C. Barton Ross
J. Baron-Sorensen

Learning Objectives

After reviewing this chapter, the reader should understand the following:

Ways in which veterinary personnel can interact positively with each other and with clients
Ways in which personnel can meet their and their employer's professional needs
Expectations of veterinary clients
Appropriate ways to interact with clients on the telephone

Ways to interact with doctors and clients to keep the practice operating smoothly
Appropriate ways to present a bill to clients and to discuss fees
Appropriate ways to handle complaints from clients
Stages of grief
Appropriate ways in which to counsel clients on loss of a companion animal

COMMUNICATION AND HUMAN DYNAMICS

S.M. FASSIG

COMMUNICATING WITH OTHERS

Whether you are interacting with clients, supervisors, or co-workers in the workplace, the more of your senses that you use in a positive way, the more likely it is that you will inspire a positive interaction with another person. In the workplace, you can use your senses of sight, touch, hearing, and smell to create favorable surroundings, promote positive interaction, and accomplish your tasks.

Communication has several dimensions and occurs on many levels simultaneously. The more elements that are combined, the more powerful the impact. People communicate by verbal (spoken and written) and nonverbal means. Contrary to what most people think, nonverbal communication is more persuasive than verbal and is a substantial part of interactions with others.

More than 70% of communication is nonverbal. Nonverbal communication involves emotions, which alter the interpretation of the message. It also signals your social and professional position within the workplace (how you relate to supervisors, peers, and subordinates). Nonverbal communication can be likened to the way in which wolves communicate their social position within the pack, using displays of submissive or dominant behavior (e.g., posture, tail carriage, eye contact).

53

You can convey a positive attitude regarding your workplace by dressing and grooming yourself appropriately for your work environment. Maintaining eye contact and attentive facial expressions when dealing with others shows concern and displays your feelings about the content of the conversation.

In addition, creating work surroundings that are clean, uncluttered, and visually pleasing promotes a sense of "feeling good." This often reduces anxiety, making people more approachable, responsive, and engaging. It says that you have a concern for people and quality of life.

A self-initiated, firm, friendly handshake also helps to establish positive communication with clients and colleagues. A half-hearted, limp handshake is often interpreted as a lack of confidence, especially if it is without eye contact. This negative message often creates a barrier to positive interaction and a sense of uncertainty.

You can facilitate positive interactions by consciously focusing on the sound and tone of your voice, making sure your speech is consistently audible and well-paced, with the proper inflection. Combined with direct eye contact, a well-modulated voice can enhance communications with a client or co-worker and help you share information.

Consider the following scenarios:

- What are you communicating when a client tells you about her treasured cat, but you make no eye contact nor exhibit any appropriate facial expressions because you are looking down, writing the information on the chart?
- What are you communicating when you tell your supervisor that you have everything organized and are up-to-date on all work responsibilities, but your desk and work area look like they qualify for a disaster-relief program?
- What are you communicating when you tell your supervisor and co-workers how much you enjoy your job and how enthused you are to be a part of this profession, but your work clothes are usually wrinkled, soiled, torn, or generally unkempt?
- What are you communicating when you answer the telephone, "Good morning, ABC Animal Hospital. May I help you?" using a lifeless, distracted, or curt tone of voice?

To communicate well, you do not have to assume a false, nauseatingly sweet, "Pollyanna" personality. On some days you may feel upbeat and happy, and on other days you may feel more subdued. Realizing this, you can create and maintain the most positive dynamics in your workplace when you consciously put your best foot forward at any given moment. By paying special attention to your nonverbal cues and those of others, as well as verbal communication, you can help to create a productive, enjoyable workplace that is respectful of others,

allows a sense of humor and fun, and is appreciative of your role as an animal health care provider.

If you see a spill or find a mess, take the responsibility to clean it up. If you perceive that a client is uncomfortable or confused, or has misgivings about something, give him or her your full attention to explain anything not understood and answer all questions. These simple actions show your concern for the client and the patient. They also demonstrate your commitment to your team of health care providers in conveying a professional image to clients.

Once you get into the habit of consciously putting forth your best effort in communicating, you begin to feel good about doing your part in serving clients and caring for animals. That positive feeling may even lead to a firmer handshake, a bit of bounce in your step, a friendlier telephone manner, and more self-confidence. All of these communicate a positive, "can-do" attitude, which will benefit you in considerations for promotions and career development opportunities.

KEEPING NONWORK ISSUES OUT OF THE WORKPLACE

Everyone has individual circumstances but common areas of responsibilities. You can be more successful, productive, and effective as a veterinary professional if you do not carry into the workplace concerns not related to work. Personal problems related to family, relationships, finances, and health are of course very important; however, it is inappropriate to become distracted and discuss personal problems with others during work hours.

HUMAN DYNAMICS

Human dynamics are an individual's pattern of change or growth and pattern of interpersonal relationships. Human dynamics are influenced by personal, social, and professional position and motivating physical or moral forces that stimulate actions and behavior.

Although professionals should try to keep their personal lives out of the workplace, feelings of happiness or unhappiness about personal issues color attitudes about work. It is important to genuinely like what you do: to enjoy your work, your home life, and your lifestyle. It is also important to feel part of a team at work and to enjoy accomplishing something together.

Your Personal and Professional Goals. Whether you want to be a veterinary technician as a lifelong career or you view it as a step to other objectives, you should develop a *personal vision*. Just as businesses formulate a business plan and regularly revise it to guide management decisions for the company, individuals need some sense of direction, or vision, in their lives. This provides direction, familiarity with personal and professional needs, and a sense of accomplishment.

A vision is a future ideal that is more compelling than any present reality. Vision motivates people, directs allocation of resources (time and energy), and overcomes resistance and obstacles. Applied in the workplace environment, your personal vision combines personal and business (get/give) objectives. If you make your employer aware of your personal and professional goals at an appropriate time, such as during a performance review, the employer may try to accommodate some of your needs and career development plans as part of your work assignment.

What kind of work do you desire? Your aim should not be to find the "ultimate" or "perfect" job, but rather to live with the job you have (or later find) and then develop opportunities to make it "right" for you as your needs change or to negotiate and create a new position that will let you grow in accordance with your personal vision. If your vision includes career development, you will likely "outgrow" the job you start with. You do not always have to leave your employer to upgrade your position. Instead, you may be able to negotiate a better work situation, often to your advantage and the practice's.

Some of the most unhappy and unproductive people believe that their work life and personal life control them. This is in contrast to gratified people, who believe that what they can visualize, they can realize. You can determine what direction your life will take and what your rewards will be. If you define what you want to accomplish in life, you are more likely to reap considerable personal fulfillment as you work to bring your dreams to reality. You can derive energy from this sense of purpose and are less likely to feel bogged down and trapped.

Your Personal and Professional Needs. Consider your personal and professional needs, including income needed to live in the manner in which you would like. Before you accept or even apply for a position, you should tabulate the cost of housing, food, clothing, transportation, insurance (vehicle/liability, health), utilities, student loans, taxes, and sundries to find out how much income you will need to live in a specific geographic area. Accepting a position that will not provide sufficient income to meet expenses creates difficulties for you and your employer.

Just as a house is built from a set of blueprints, so should a professional life be based on a *career plan*. What do you see yourself doing a year from now? Where do you imagine you will be five years from now? What skills and talents must you have to make this happen? What additional skills must you need to acquire and how will you develop them? Setting a timetable to reach your objective will keep you on track and help

you know when you have reached your goal. You should periodically revise your career plan as new opportunities become available.

Assume you find an entry-level technician position that would meet your objectives initially. As time passes, your personal needs change as your circumstances change. Such changes include getting married or divorced, giving birth to or adopting children, upgrading your living quarters, or buying a house. New professional needs might include a more flexible work schedule, fewer or more hours, less or more overtime, and a higher salary.

Employees tend to reconsider their commitment to their employer at predictable intervals: after the "honeymoon" has ended (6 to 12 months after hire), when the original attraction of the position has waned (2 to 3 years on the job), and after significant personal investment has been made (5 to 7 years on the job). Most employers are willing to provide additional compensation to valued employees at those times. Employees tend to renegotiate their commitment at unpredictable intervals when there are significant changes in work assignments or relationships, when management personnel or culture changes, and during major life transitions.

Your Employer's Needs. At the time of the employment interview, an employer often assumes an individual has the necessary technical skills to perform in a job, based on the candidate's training, certification, licensing, advanced coursework, specialized credentials, and experience. In most employment settings, the employer assumes the new employee will receive additional training on the job, such as training in how things are done in the particular work setting. This training can be in the form of a formal program, a mentoring experience, or learning by doing ("trial by fire").

Traits that employers look for in prospective employees include the following:

- Ability to work as a team player, as both a leader and a follower
- Management and supervisory skills
- Self-confidence and a sense of humor
- Good oral and written skills: readable handwriting and ability to express a complete thought
- Ability to listen and follow instructions
- Willingness to consider other viewpoints, accept criticism, formulate constructive suggestions, take risks, and accept responsibility
- Analytical skills: critical and logical thinking, vision, and problem solving
- A positive attitude
- A good work ethic: honest, compassionate, concerned, empathetic, abides by commitments, punctual, keeps others informed, self-directed in performing duties in a timely manner, and takes

responsibility for one's self, the work area, and equipment
- Self-motivation and ability to motivate others
- Versatility and adaptability to change
- Broad background: not only in animal-related fields

Your Energy Level. You need not go home from work every day feeling tired and exhausted. You can learn to continually replace the energy expended on the job. Sleep is not the only way to restore your energy. Everyone does not require seven or eight hours of continuous sleep nightly. Time spent exercising, having fun, doing something artistic, relaxing, or meditating can revive you. A healthy balance of both work and play is needed for keeping the energy flowing. Eating the right foods at the right time is also helpful.

There is a strong link between play and energy level. Adults tend to eliminate most of their opportunities for fun, laughter, joy, physical activity, curiosity, adventure, and unrepressed emotional expression in an effort to "retain their objectivity" (be an adult) at all times. They may participate in games or sports but do so with the left brain "do your best" approach. Physical activity, the free expression of emotion, a sense of adventure and challenge, feelings of joy, anger, curiosity, fascination, surprise, apprehension, and satisfaction affect brain chemistry and/or metabolic and mental processes in a way that produces energy.

Having a strong feeling of purpose in life and feeling passionate about something will sustain your vigor and maintain your enthusiasm for life. A key to maintaining high energy levels is to feel that what you do is making the world a better place. Concerns for people and quality of life must be balanced with concerns for productivity and profit to maintain energy and vitality.

LEARNING ABOUT YOUR JOB SITUATION

Once you have been hired, start to develop an understanding of your job situation. Your job involves three basic features:

1. *Duties:* These are the things you do, things that you agree to perform.
2. *Responsibilities:* These are the functions that you agree to fulfill.
3. *Authority:* This is the empowerment to perform your duties and fulfill your responsibilities.

A *job description* is a listing of the duties, responsibilities, and results entailed in a specific job. Descriptions of job elements can be precise and exhaustive (specific), or they can be vague and incomplete (general). A written job description serves as a reference point for your performance as an employee. A job description is not a rigid set of directives—it consists of more than just guidelines.

There should be provisions so that deviations, additions, and variations are always open for discussion. The key point is that a good job description will allow you and your boss to discuss, express, and communicate expectations surrounding the position from both of your points of view. This helps to ensure a better understanding of how the job will be performed and what is to be accomplished as a result.

Your job can be an opportunity for growth, or it can become a dead end. Ultimately, the decision is yours. The job you have today is a resource for building good working relationships that may provide links to your next job, either with your current employer or with another. Try not to burn bridges behind you; instead, maintain and nurture the bonds you build in your professional relationships.

Your Boss

If you intend to be promoted or move to a better position elsewhere, you will need your supervisor's support. To understand your boss and his or her job, consider these questions:

- What does your boss want from his or her career?
- What does your boss expect from the staff?
- How can your boss be influenced to support your career growth?
- How can you serve as an ally to help your boss meet his or her goals?

Your Co-Workers

Teamwork. Effectiveness in all organizations, including veterinary practices, requires teamwork. Understanding the people with whom you work and the jobs they do will enhance your effectiveness, as well as theirs. Developing effective working relationships with co-workers and colleagues, including suppliers, clients, competitors, salespeople, and manufacturers' representatives, can also be of benefit. Your goal is to succeed and to make those around you also want to succeed.

Networking. Building a *professional network* is not limited to your immediate job situation. You should begin early in your career and network widely. Professional network building begins in school with your classmates, professors, and others encountered during your professional education. Some of these relationships will endure throughout your career. Every person in your network offers unique insights, expertise, and experience. You may have different skills, knowledge, and ideas to offer others in your network. Savor the diversity of your contacts, because that diversity offers a richness of perspectives, abilities, and opportunities.

Your Job Environment

Your *job environment* comprises the parts of the organization for which you work and the people with whom you work. Whether you work in a small veterinary practice or in a large corporation, governmental agency, or other business, how you do your job may be directly affected by how others do theirs.

Performance of Co-workers. Poor performance by co-workers can impair your effectiveness. For example, assume you are an operating room technician who prepares patients and assists during surgery in a surgery referral hospital. The office manager is responsible for ordering supplies. How well the office manager does his or her job will affect your performance on the job, especially if the appropriate gauze sponges, surgical scrub, or suture materials are not kept in stock.

In this same facility, one of the receptionist's job duties is to ensure that owners of animals undergoing orthopedic surgery are given a copy of the handout on cast and bandage care when such patients are discharged. The receptionist fails to give the owner this handout. As a result, the owner never checks the cast. The affected leg swells and the animal loses its toes because of impaired circulation. The owner thinks the surgical team did a poor job and refuses to pay the bill.

Written versus Unwritten Rules. All organizations, large or small, have written and unwritten rules concerning work procedures within the organization. In general, written rules cover routine situations and standard procedures. As a rule of thumb, the bigger the organization, the more written rules it has. *Written rules* may cover everything from conduct, job descriptions, and operating and compensation procedures to company policies and corporate actions. However, most organizations do not have the time to write a rule for every task performed.

Many tasks are not written into anyone's formal responsibility list, but these tasks must be done for work to flow smoothly. For many of the nonroutine, exceptional tasks and situations, workers develop *unwritten rules* for getting things done within the organization. These unwritten rules are often just as orderly and logical as the written ones. Sometimes, if an unwritten rule works well, it is then suggested as a change or an addition to a written policy.

For example, all outgoing mail is to be in the receptionist's outbasket by 11:30 AM. At noon, the office manager takes the mail from the receptionist's outbasket and puts it in the mailbox on her way to lunch. The written rule (mail in the outbasket by 11:30 AM) and the unwritten rule (get mail to office manager before noon) differ, but either way the mail goes out that day.

ROMANCE AND MARRIAGE BETWEEN CO-WORKERS

For better or worse, romances are very common in today's workplace. Some of these romances develop into long-term relationships and may culminate in marriage. Rules governing relationships between co-workers other than spousal relationships are not covered by labor law and are left to the discretion of employers. When it comes to marriage of co-workers, additional complexities are possible, especially in supervisory situations in which one partner is the other partner's supervisor.

If two employees marry, their employer can benefit, such as from improved job commitment from both spouses. Some married couples work well together and somehow manage to keep any personal problems out of the workplace. But if the relationship turns volatile, it may negatively impact the productivity of involved employees and their co-workers.

Employers may face complaints of invasion of privacy for inquiring into employee's off-duty romantic affairs, and they also face potential liability for sexual harassment in the workplace for ignoring these affairs. Negative effects of such affairs may include damage to the business's reputation in the community, loss of productivity, and disclosure of confidential business information. Uninvolved employees can lose confidence in a romantically involved co-worker's ability to make judgments affecting the practice or business and others around it.

For the employee, the consequences of romantic involvements between co-workers can be serious. This is especially true when the affair is between a supervisor and a subordinate; either or both may lose their job(s).

SEXUAL HARASSMENT

The courts and EEOC guidelines define *sexual harassment* as any unwelcome sexual advances or requests for sexual favors, or any conduct of a sexual nature that renders harm through work interactions when

- Submission is made explicitly or implicitly a term or condition of initial or continued employment.
- Submission or rejection is used as a basis of working conditions, including promotion, salary adjustment, assignment of work, or termination.
- Such conduct has the purpose or effect of substantially interfering with an individual's work environment or creates an intimidating, hostile, or offensive work environment.

As employers, veterinarians are not immune to claims of sexual harassment. As an example, in a recent case, a female veterinary technician won a suit in a state court in which she claimed her veterinary employer's offensive conduct created a hostile work environment. State laws apply to all employers within the state. Federal law applies only to employers with 15 or more full- or part-time employees. However, suits are often filed in both state and federal courts.

Sexual harassment can occur in veterinary practices because the care-giving aspect of practice brings people together emotionally as well as physically. In many veterinary practices, small teams of animal health care professionals frequently work long hours, under arduous conditions, and in isolated treatment and surgical rooms in close proximity to each other. In rural practices, emergency calls, especially after hours, and time-consuming treatments and nursing procedures, require team members to maintain close quarters well into the night and early morning. In these types of close-contact conditions, employees tend to form more tight-knit groups than employees of larger, less personal businesses.

Unresolved legal issues remain concerning the amount and kinds of proof required to establish certain elements of sexually harassing conduct by someone other than a managing or supervisory employee. Problems also arise in applying the law to the factual circumstances of a specific case, testing the credibility of the parties' claims and proof, conceptualizing relief, and valuing damages.

Where the conduct in question did not directly involve the abuse of authority, the employer may be liable for the acts of its employees (supervisory and nonsupervisory) and perhaps others visiting the business premises on a regular basis (including nonemployees, such as sales representatives). Liability is incurred when the employer knows or should have known of the conduct and failed to take prompt and effective remedial action.

One of the most effective ways for a veterinary employer to avoid claims of a hostile environment is to confront the issue openly and adopt a sexual harassment policy for the practice. This policy might be stated in the employee handbook or presented in another such mechanism. Repeated use of offensive language on the job creates legal grounds for a complaint. Be aware that a co-worker can file a complaint against you, as well as against the employer, for such conduct.

If you as a supervisor or employer's representative are faced with a situation in which employees in your work group are using inappropriate language, one recourse is to diplomatically point out that this behavior offends both men and women and is not appropriate for use in a business environment. Inform them that if they continue to use offensive language, they are subject to the same type of disciplinary action as that for violating other work rules (which, depending on your employer's policies, may include or contribute to the employee's being fired). Document the counseling session in the employee's file, inform your supervisor, and make a record of the incident for your own files, in case of your later involvement.

In general, unless you know someone well, other than the traditional handshake, don't hug, don't pat, and definitely do not kiss. Do unto others as they would have you do unto them. Even then, be careful and respectful. The same applies here as with other offensive things: If it looks, feels, sounds, or seems offensive, it probably is offensive.

GROUP DYNAMICS

A group is a collection of individuals who influence one another, derive some satisfaction from maintaining membership in the group, interact for some purpose, assume specialized roles, are dependent on one another, and communicate face to face. Most of us participate in three groups: primary, social, and work. *Primary groups* include one's family and closest friends. *Social groups* include neighborhood groups, fraternities, bowling partners, and hobby clubs. *Work groups* consist of a group of employees working together to produce products or provide services.

Three factors seem very important in work groups: communication within the work group; participation in the decision-making process; and democratic leadership. In work groups, the level of productivity within a company or business is set by social norms, not by physiologic capacities. Noneconomic rewards and sanctions significantly affect the behavior of the workers and largely limit the effect of economic incentive plans. (What the group defines as a "fair day's work" or how fast they work on the job determines the outcome, even if the workers could earn more if they worked faster, scheduled more appointments, or made more calls per day). Members not performing within those norms are sanctioned by other members and pressured into conformance with group rules. Workers often do not act or react as individuals but as a member of the group and adjust their actions to accommodate the group's informal standards.

COMPANY CULTURE

Productive workplaces are those where people learn and grow as they cooperate to improve an organization's performance. This creates a sense of dignity, meaning, and community. In all work settings, values are the basis for the culture within the organization. They provide a sense of common direction for all employees, are guidelines for day-to-day behavior, and provide the means to reward employee efforts. Businesses often succeed because their employees can identify, embrace, and act on the organization's values.

People just beginning their career may think that "a job is just a job." But when they choose a practice, business, and sometimes even a work group to work in, they often choose a way of life. The culture of the company shapes their responses in a strong but subtle way. The prevalent culture can make them fast or slow workers, tough or friendly managers, team players or lone rangers, and warm and friendly or guarded and distant with clients and customers.

By the time employees have worked for several years in one company culture, they may be so well conditioned by the culture they may not even recognize it. When they change jobs or employers, they may be in for a big surprise. Culture shock may be one of the major reasons why people supposedly "fail" when they leave one organization for another. Where they fail, however, is not necessarily in doing the job, but rather in not adjusting to the new company culture in which they find themselves.

To help you understand the dynamics of your work group and your company's culture, find out which behavior is rewarded and which is discouraged. If you have been working hard but have not produced the results you need, consider, "What's being rewarded?"

In the final analysis, only you can control how you think, how you feel, and how you behave on the job. With a positive attitude, you can achieve your goals for your career, your family, and your life.

RECOMMENDED READING

Anderson CI, Hunsaker PL: Why there's romancing at the office and why it's everybody's problem, *Personnel*, pp 57-63, 1985.

Burns SE: Issues in workplace sexual harassment law and related social science research, *Journal of Social Issues*, 51:195, 207, 1995.

Deal TE, Kennedy AA: *Corporate cultures, the rites and rituals of corporate life*, Reading, Mass, 1982, Addison-Wesley.

Farnham A: Are you smart enough to keep your job?, *Fortune*, pp 34-37, Jan 15, 1996.

Graen GB: *Unwritten rules for your career*, New York, 1989, John Wiley & Sons.

Henley NM: *Body politics, power, sex and nonverbal communication*, New York, 1977, Simon & Schuster.

Holzschu MA: *Complete employee handbook*, Wakefield, RI, 1996, Moyer Bell.

Lacroix CA, Wilson JF: Avoiding sexual harassment liability in veterinary practices, *J Am Vet Med Assoc*, 208:1664-1666, 1996.

LeBoeuf M: *Getting results! The secret to motivating yourself and others*, New York, 1985, Berkley Books.

Lieber RB: How safe is your job?, *Fortune* pp 72-104, April 1, 1996.

Libbin AE, Stevens CJ: Employee personal relationships, *Personnel*, pp 56-60, October 1988.

McGee-Cooper A: *You don't have to go home from work exhausted*, Dallas, Tex, 1990, Bowen & Rogers.

Palmen R: *Principles and success strategies for everyday living*, Lynnwood, Wash, 1986, The Palmen Institute.

Pell AR: *The complete idiot's guide to managing people*, New York, 1995, Alpha Books-Simon & Schuster Macmillan.

Scholtes PR: *The team handbook—How to use teams to improve quality*, Madison, Wis, 1988, Joiner Associates.

Timm PR: *50 Powerful ideas you can use to keep your customers*, ed 2, Franklin Lakes, NJ, 1995, Career Press.

Tubbs SL: *A systems approach to small group interaction*, ed 2, Reading, Mass, 1984, Addison-Wesley.

Weisbord MR: *Productive workplaces*, San Francisco, 1989, Jossey-Bass.

CLIENT RELATIONS

D.R. DOOLEY

It is easy for the staff members to get so involved with the daily operation of a veterinary practice that they may forget why the practice exists. Most of the work in a veterinary practice has to do with animals. Although the work may be done on or to the animal, it is also done for the animal's owner.

Once animal owners bring their animal to a veterinary clinic for veterinary services, they become known as *clients*. Clients decide when their animal needs the services of a veterinary practice. They decide which veterinary practice will treat their animal.

Once clients arrange for the veterinary visit, they transport their animal to and from the chosen clinic. While at the clinic they make decisions about what and how much veterinary care they want for their animal. Finally, they pay the fees for the care rendered to their animal.

DEFINING CLIENT RELATIONS

All of this activity is based on a relationship between the client and the clinic staff. Some consider client relations as concerned only with the marketing activity that brings the client to the practice. This of course is part of client relations, but equally, if not more, important are the interactions between the client and the staff that keep the client coming back to the practice.

No practice could survive for long by spending money on marketing to attract clients, only to have clients come in once and then never return. It may take just one staff member on the telephone to recruit a new client, but it takes the entire staff to keep clients coming back year after year.

All staff members are involved in client relations, including the doctor treating the animal, the technician assisting the doctor, the receptionist answering the phone, and the kennel person cleaning up an animal for return to its owner. Anything you do between the first phone call and return of the animal to its owner involves client relations.

YOUR INVOLVEMENT IN CLIENT RELATIONS

How well you relate to clients is important to the practice. It is also important to you, for a variety of reasons. Perhaps the most obvious reason is that clients are the reason you have a job. As an employee, you constitute an expense to the practice. If you were not needed to help clients, you would not be employed by the practice.

Staff job security depends on the success of the practice. Your effectiveness in relating to clients influences the number of clients patronizing the practice. You play a large role in the practice's success or failure. The number and quality of clients the practice can attract and retain dictates its success. Your job security is the first reason you must be concerned about client relations.

When a practice prospers, so does the staff. Employees who can help attract animal owners and keep them happy when they become clients are valuable and appreciated. When veterinary practices are profitable, the owner(s) of the profitable practices are usually generous with the staff.

You also have a strong influence on your personal feelings toward the job. The time you spend at the practice can be very enjoyable or it can be excruciating. You create the environment and the atmosphere in which you work. Your working hours can be very pleasant if you consider clients as friends, or work can be an endless nightmare of trying to please people who make your life miserable. You cannot control the behavior of clients, but you can control how you relate to them.

It was said many centuries ago that, "As ye sow, so shall ye reap." This is still true, especially when applied to client relations. Give a client a smile and a friendly greeting and you will be given a smile and friendly greeting in return. There are, of course, exceptions to this. After all, even the best of clients can have a bad day. However, most clients reflect the courtesies they are shown.

Incidentally, there is a way to determine whether it is you or the client that is having a bad day. If you have difficulty getting along with one out of five or more clients, it is probably that occasional client who is "off" that day. On the other hand, if you have difficulty with four out of every five of the clients you deal with that day, you are definitely having a bad day. As you read on through this chapter, you will learn how to minimize those bad days.

Consider the example of a receptionist whose telephone conversation was animated and lively. When asked if it was a personal call, her response was, "No, it wasn't a personal call. It was a new client, a friend I haven't met yet. But I'm looking forward to meeting her." As you can imagine, the hours this receptionist spent at the practice were never drudgery for her.

If you are a technician, assistant, kennel person, or anyone else who works in the back of the clinic, understand that not only the receptionists are involved with client relations. You have much more client interaction than you may realize.

For example, any time clients see you interact with an animal, they are making judgments about the practice. Even if you speak only to the receptionist when you come to the front desk to take a client's animal to the treatment area, the client is learning about you and the practice.

From your appearance and body language the client forms perceptions about the practice. Because most clients never see more than the reception area and examination rooms, you provide their only window into the mysterious back areas of the clinic, where their animal is treated.

If you enter the reception area from the back of the clinic wearing a jacket or heavy sweater in the winter, clients will assume that the wards are unheated. If your clothes are soiled and stained, they will assume the area in which you work is dirty. Torn or disheveled clothing denotes a messy, cluttered work environment.

How you look at, touch, or speak to the client's animal forms the basis of his or her perception of how the practice treats animals. So, whether you want to be or not, you are an important part of the practice's client relations team.

Understanding why you need to be concerned about client relations is a good basis for understanding why clients come to your clinic or any other veterinary clinic. Understanding why clients patronize a particular practice will help you understand how to relate to them.

The Human-Animal Bond

Clients take their animals to veterinary clinics for one very important reason: because they have a relationship with their animals and they want to maintain it as long as possible. Knowing this and being sensitive to their needs will help you in most cases automatically do the right thing.

Without this human–companion animal bond, this person would not become a client. A person may own an animal, but if his or her relationship with the animal is perceived as not important, that person will not seek veterinary services. Merely owning an animal does not automatically make a person a consumer of veterinary services or the client of any veterinary practice. It is that person's relationship with his or her animal, not the person, that is important.

This relationship between owner and animal is based on one or more physical or emotional need(s) of the owner. Dogs can help physically impaired people. Hunting dogs and sled dogs are involved in the owners' recreational activities. The emotional need for companionship may involve just about any animal from a gerbil to a horse, including fish, birds, and reptiles. Many people gain emotional stability from their animal friends. Some companion animals provide their human caretakers with a purpose in life.

People who do not *need* animals do not keep them, even if the animals were given to them. Clients do not consider their animals a luxury. Your clients own and care for their animals because they *need* them. They do not consider the money they spend on their animal friends as wasted. They bring their animals to a veterinary clinic to maintain and extend the relationship as long as possible.

What Clients Want

Before you can relate well to clients, you must know why they are at your practice and what they want from the clinic staff. Clients want two basic things: *They want someone to be concerned about their problems, and they want care for their animals.*

Finding someone who will demonstrate concern for their problems means finding someone who will listen to them. Listening is something most people do very poorly (see After the Greeting, p. 62). This is why it is so important in a veterinary practice. Clients wander from one clinic to another, trying to find a staff member and/or a veterinarian who will actually listen to them. Clients want to be listened to on the telephone and when they are at the clinic. They may not know much about animals or medicine, but they do know when they are being listened to and when they are not.

Clients also want the staff members to demonstrate that they *care* about the client's animals. They want and expect the best medical care that veterinary medicine has to offer. Unfortunately, they generally do not have the training nor the ability to judge the quality of the medical care their animal is receiving. Visible results of care are most clients' sole criteria for judgment.

They are aware of their inability to judge the quality of the medical care provided, so they compensate by being hypercritical of those things they *can* judge. Clients may ask themselves, "How did the receptionist look at my animal when we arrived?" "How did the technician touch my animal when it was taken to the treatment area or when the temperature was taken?"

Things that may seem insignificant to the clinic staff can be quite significant to a client. As mentioned above, clients pay great attention to how the staff interacts with their animals. If a guest brought a friend to your home, you would probably offend your guest if you ignored the friend. For the same reason, do not ignore what may be your client's best friend, his or her animal. Ask about the animal and speak to it in a soothing manner.

The old cliché says, "If you can't say something nice about someone, don't say anything." The revised version for the veterinary staff is, "If you can't think of anything nice to say about the client's animal, you aren't trying hard enough."

TELEPHONE ETIQUETTE
Getting Ready

The initial contact with most new clients is by telephone. Also, most established clients call before coming to the clinic. You need to be prepared to field the variety of calls you may get.

This preparation starts before you arrive at work. On your way to work each day, make a mental note of anything that could be a problem for a client driving to your clinic. For example, clients may encounter traffic problems caused by road construction, parades, and store or mall openings.

Keeping a laminated map of your area on the front counter is a good idea for two reasons. You can put adhesive notes on it to indicate areas with traffic problems noticed by the staff members on their way to work. This information can be relayed by telephone to clients coming in for an appointment that day. It is also helpful for new receptionists who may not be familiar with the immediate area around the practice so that they can give clients accurate directions.

When directing clients or prospective clients to the clinic, remember that people navigate in many different ways. Some people understand how their city is laid out and can comprehend directions of north, south, east, and west. ("Drive south 2 miles, then turn west on Highway 210.") Other people better understand left and right. ("Go 2 miles and turn left on Highway 50.") Directing people left or right means that you have to visualize left and right from *their* vantage point. Other people know the names of area streets and avenues, still others navigate by landmarks. ("Turn left at the 7-11 on the corner.")

On your way to work, it can be useful to note the distances driven on some streets and from certain landmarks to the clinic. This will help people who navigate by driving distance. ("Go 2 miles and turn left onto Center Avenue.") With a thorough knowledge of your area's streets and landmarks, you can offer new clients clear directions.

Keep some notepads and pens near every telephone. You need to be sure all of the pens work. Keep the appointment book in the same place so that all staff members can quickly locate it.

To select accurate appointment times, you must be familiar with the doctor's schedules. Check the doctor's schedule for the day and the next 2 or 3 days. You sound more intelligent to callers if you actually know which doctors are working on certain days and when they are available. Do not assume you know the doctor's schedule because you have memorized it. There is no such thing as a consistent, permanent schedule or even a temporary one to which doctors adhere. Review the schedules of each doctor every day.

Answering Promptly

Ideally, the clinic's telephone must be answered before it rings three times. The receptionist may not always be able to pick up the telephone before the third ring. Every member of the clinic support staff should be sensitive to the sound of a ringing telephone. Someone must be designated to serve as backup for the receptionist in answering the telephone. This backup person should answer the telephone before the end of the third ring. If the backup person repeatedly has to answer the phone, the receptionist must be alerted and the problem discussed.

Greeting the Caller

How do you greet the caller? There is a simple way to clear your mind and prepare your voice as you are about to answer the call. As you reach for the telephone, get in the habit of forcing yourself to smile. A smile changes your voice and can be perceived over the telephone. Also, thinking about smiling clears your mind and helps you concentrate on the incoming call. The importance of concentrating on the incoming call is explained later in this chapter.

Callers expect four things from the person answering the call:

1. They want a greeting that is friendly and one that indicates you are awake and competent. Say "good morning" or "good afternoon" with a smile on your face.
2. They want to know that they have reached the number they have dialed. Confirm this by saying the name of your clinic.
3. They want to know if they are talking to an answering machine or a person. Some answering machines are very clear and can be mistaken for a live person's greeting. Give the caller your first name and offer to be of assistance.
4. They want you to offer to help them. After giving your name, ask how you can be of help.

Putting it all together, an appropriate greeting might sound something like this: "Good morning, ABC Animal Hospital. This is Mary. How may I help you?"

This may seem like a lot to say, but it does not take as long to say as it does to read it. Depending on the name of the practice and your accent, this four-part greeting takes about five seconds.

It is sometimes necessary to put a client on hold. Before doing this, always ask the client's permission first. "Good morning, ABC Animal Hospital. May I put you on hold?" The caller must have an opportunity to respond. The call could involve an emergency. The caller could have used his or her last quarter to call from a pay phone where the wind-chill factor is 57° below zero. Or, as is very common today, the caller may be calling on a cellular phone and paying a fairly high rate for each call.

If the client consents to be put on hold, promise to get back to him or her very quickly and then do it. Being kept on hold for more than a minute is frustrating, even when the hold music is pleasant. If the caller does not

like the music or is forced to listen to commercials, remaining on hold becomes extremely frustrating.

When the caller wishes to speak to a doctor but the doctor is not available, give the client a choice. Offer to keep the client on hold until the doctor can pick up the telephone or offer to have the doctor return the call as soon as possible. If the caller chooses to wait on hold, get back to the caller every 60 or 90 seconds to see if he or she still wants to hold. If the caller wants the doctor to return the call, be sure to get a number at which he or she can be reached at the time the doctor is expected to return the call.

When you get back to a caller left on hold, thank the caller for his or her patience, give your name, and offer to be of assistance. "Thank you for waiting. This is Mary. How may I help you?" Even if you gave your name when first answering the call, repeat it when you come back on the line.

After the Greeting

After you have greeted the client, identified yourself, and offered to be of assistance, you must learn how you can help the caller and then *do it*. The caller has a question to be answered or a problem to be solved. You were hired to answer questions and solve problems.

Your ability to answer questions and solve problems is directly related to your ability to listen. You may be able to answer most questions, but for others you may need to ask another staff member. You may be able to solve many problems, but others are more complicated. In either case your success in helping the caller depends on how well you listen to the question or described problem.

Most people listen very poorly. To do it well requires a great amount of concentration. Most people are unable to avoid being distracted, and must concentrate well to become good listeners.

Depending on the amount of activity around you, you might find it necessary to close your eyes or face a blank wall away from distractions while speaking to a caller. It is better not to do something else while you are talking to a caller. You may be unable to concentrate on the call and the caller will sense that you are not listening. Failure to listen to the caller is insulting and damages any relationship you might have with a client.

If you can, use the client's name and/or the animal's name in the conversation. This helps avoid the embarrassment of forgetting who you are talking to. Also, acknowledge the caller's questions and occasionally ask questions of your own to indicate that you are listening.

Answering Questions

When answering a caller's questions, keep your answers positive. This takes a good deal of thought, but there is a positive answer to most questions. For example, a caller asks if you can bill for services rather than collect at the time the services are rendered. Instead of saying, "We don't bill," it would be better to say, "For clients who wish to be billed we accept a variety of credit cards."

"Is there anything I can do for my animal here at home?" This may be the most common question that receptionists hear. The answer is, "Yes, I'm sure there will be something for you to do at home. The doctor will explain what you will need to do at home when she sees you. Would you like to come in today or tomorrow?"

When you are asked a question you do not know how to answer, avoid getting yourself in trouble by guessing. You have two choices. If a staff member who can answer the question is available, you can say, "Just a moment please, I'll have someone who can answer your question speak with you," or "Please give me a number where I can reach you this afternoon. I'll get the answer to your question and call you." If you use the second answer, be sure to write down the question as well as the caller's name and phone number. Having made that promise to the caller, follow through with it.

When it comes to solving problems for clients, keep in mind that the place to solve medical problems is in the clinic. The telephone is not a medical instrument. Veterinarians who try to practice medicine over the telephone can make serious mistakes. It is best if receptionists and technicians not try to do something that even veterinarians cannot do well.

Making Appointments

Because the solution to the client's problem can be found in the clinic, the client will need an appointment. Some practices still see clients on a drop-in basis, but this is becoming less common. Most clients expect to be told they will need an appointment.

When making an appointment, offer the client a choice of no more than two appointment times. For example, "Would you like to come in today or tomorrow?" "Which is better for you: 2:40 or 4:00?" "If neither of those times is good, do you want the appointment earlier than 2:40 or later than 4:00?" Limiting the choices to only two appointment times makes your work easier and reduces the decision-making stress for the caller.

When making appointments, obtain a phone number where the caller can be reached, in case you need to cancel or change the appointment.

Controlling the Conversation

Anyone who answers the telephone in a veterinary clinic is aware of what it means to lose control of a conversation. Some callers have ample time and delight in giving you the life history of their beloved pets and even their own life story. This is time consuming and the information is of no use to the clinic.

Most of these calls can be controlled by asking the appropriate questions. Try to limit questions to those

that can be answered with a "yes" or "no." "Would you like to bring Charlie in today?" or "It sounds like the doctor should see Penny as soon as possible. Could you bring her in this afternoon?"

Asking the question, "What happened?" will open the floodgates and give you more information than you want to know. "How did it happen?" is another open-ended question that allows talkative clients to talk forever.

After one of these occasional nonstop telephone calls, try to determine how you lost control of the conversation. By knowing what questions to avoid and knowing how to formulate "yes" and "no" questions, you can minimize this problem.

PREPARING FOR THE VISIT

Your clinic is listed in the telephone book. You have a sign in front of the building. You answered the phone and invited the caller to come to the clinic. Your invited guests expect you to be ready for their visit.

Clinic Exterior

Preparing for guests takes some preparation. At least once a week, someone on the staff should evaluate the clinic sign, landscaping, parking lot, and building. In some clinics the employees enter through a back door and may not really notice the front of the clinic for weeks.

The owner or manager of the practice and not the staff is ultimately responsible for the exterior of the building. However, remember that the clients who are turned off by the appearance of your clinic will stay away and jeopardize your income. Take it upon yourself to mention any problems with the clinic's exterior to your manager. Practice owners appreciate employees who take an interest in the practice. Mention what needs correcting, but do not nag. Nagging is irritating and counterproductive.

Every week a different employee can be assigned the task of inspecting the sign, landscaping, parking lot, and building. If it is a lighted sign, does the illumination come on at sundown and go off after sunrise? Are any of the bulbs burned out? Is there any graffiti on the sign? Is the lettering all intact? Does the sign need repair?

Has someone been keeping up with the landscaping? The clinic's landscaping must be well maintained to convey a good impression.

Is the parking lot in good repair and clean? Can a client walk from his or her car to the front door without ruining a pair of dress shoes? Are newspapers, other trash, leaves, and dog droppings picked up at least once every day (preferably morning and afternoon)?

Is the clinic building inviting? Does it appear well maintained? There must be no peeling paint and no missing molding from the front of the building. In the evening is there light shining inside, giving evidence of life and activity in the building? Are the walk and parking lot well lit?

Having the hours posted in large type on a sign that can be read from the parking lot is a nice touch. This reduces the frustration clients feel after getting out of the car to find the clinic closed.

Clients are invited guests that deserve all of the attention and graciousness you would bestow on any guest you would invite to your home.

The Reception Area

The first thing a client sees when entering the clinic is the reception area. If clients must wait to see the doctor, the reception area must at least be comfortable. One associate veterinarian sat for 30 minutes in the reception area of the clinic where he worked to test its comfort level. He noticed several shortcomings and decided on some changes. He threw out old magazines, organized brochures, removed some pictures and posters, put up new wall hangings, discarded dead or dying plants, and purchased new plants.

Every member of the support staff ought to occasionally spend at least part of a lunch period (not eating) in the reception area. Also, when friends or relations come to the clinic to meet an employee, ask them for their assessment of the reception area: When they walked in, did they immediately feel comfortable? Was it too cold, too hot, too bright, or too dark? The comfort of clients waiting to see the doctor is very important.

Clients' facial expressions could indicate an unpleasant odor in the waiting room. Take the hint and ask them if they smell anything unpleasant. Also, ask salespeople to let you know if they smell anything unpleasant when they come in from outside. Veterinary staff members become accustomed to odors very rapidly and sometimes fail to notice them.

A great way to create an inviting smell in a reception area on a cool day is with hot cider and cinnamon. Some clients might object to an artificial room deodorizer but few people will object to the wonderful smell of cider and cinnamon, especially if they are offered some. The smell of fresh coffee is also appealing to many people. Be careful with flowers in the reception area. Some clients may have allergies to flowers. Also, employees can avoid wearing heavy perfumes and too much cologne in consideration of clients with allergies.

Clients waiting to see the doctor need some form of distraction. Though some clients are content to simply watch the receptionist and other activities in the office, others prefer to have more to do. What are the other options? Adults can read and children can read or play.

The clinic's brochure, newsletter, or product brochures can be placed in the reception area. If you want clients to read the brochures, do not make available other reading material.

Magazines are appropriate reading material in reception areas if they are carefully selected. Clients probably will not have time to read long articles. Offer magazines with lots of pictures and/or short articles.

For children there is *Ranger Rick,* the National Geographic children's magazine, and others like it. Again, the need is for many pictures and short stories.

Picture books are great for adults and children. One of the best picture books you can have is a photo album of the clinic. It is a good idea to have a professional photographer take the photos. However, many clinics have at least one staff member who is an amateur photographer who would welcome the opportunity to show off his or her ability.

Instead of or in addition to a photo album, a bulletin board can display photos of staff members. A little biographical information with each staff member's photo is a nice touch. Knowing where staff members grew up, what their interests and hobbies are, and how long they have been with the practice is interesting to clients. Photos of clients and their pets also can be very entertaining.

THE VISIT
Maintaining a Professional Demeanor

Some clients waiting in the reception area would rather observe the front desk staff than look at photographs of the staff. These clients listen as you answer the telephone and speak with other clients. They are more interested in your tone of voice and body language than in what you are saying. They picture themselves on the other end of the telephone line and are interested in your reaction to the caller. Depending on what they see and hear, either they will feel comfortable the next time they call or they may never call again.

You may feel better after making faces at the telephone and making disparaging remarks about the caller after you hang up the telephone, but such actions make nearby clients very uncomfortable. If you say anything, make only positive comments about the caller.

When speaking within earshot of clients, be very careful of the conversation between you and other staff members. You may have very good reason to be critical of your boss, one of the veterinarians, or a co-worker, but it is wrong to voice criticism where clients can hear. Save any negative comments you may have about clients or co-workers for a time when clients are not present. Negative comments can undermine the client's confidence in the practice. Also, whispering in the presence of another person is very rude.

It is important to always be pleasant while assisting clients. Tasteful humor is a part of being pleasant and also is an important part of maintaining a good attitude in the workplace. However, be sure your humor is appropriate for the audience. Much of the humor in veterinary practices is inappropriate for clients.

In addition to watching the receptionists and technicians, clients tend to observe other clients and animals as they leave the clinic. They observe the animal's appearance and the manner in which the animal is returned to its owner. Make sure every departing animal is clean and smells good.

If you are the person bringing the animal to its owner for discharge, always have something nice to say to the owner about the animal. It shows that you really cared about the animal while it was in your care. It may be difficult to think of something nice to say about a dog that tried to bite you at every opportunity or about a particularly ugly cat or dog; however, this gives you an opportunity to be creative. Try something like, "Baxter is really happy to see you!" It is worth the effort, because it is important to the animal's owner and to clients in the reception area watching your interaction with the departing client.

Informing the Client

Keep clients informed about how long they can expect to wait until they see the doctor. Offer refreshments if the wait is likely to be long. Also ask if they need any help with their animal. Do they need a carrier for their cat or a leash for their dog? Minutes seem like hours when waiting, so do everything possible to make the wait more comfortable. Be observant and aware of the client's needs, such as pointing out the location of restrooms. Have tissues handy and offer them when needed.

Ensuring Punctuality

It is inconsiderate when a doctor is not on time for appointments. A client's time is worth just as much as the doctor's, and a doctor has no right to waste the client's time. The doctor's tardiness for appointments makes the support staff's job more difficult and uncomfortable.

Of course, emergencies and unexpected developments with other patients can cause the doctor to be late. Clients are usually very understanding of such a situation. The more common reasons for delays are telephone conversations with other clients, extended conversations in the examination room, poor scheduling throughout the day, or just not being aware of the time. Another big problem is scheduling appointments every 15 minutes but spending an average of 25 minutes on each appointment.

The following are some things you can try, to keep the doctor on schedule:

- Review this part of the chapter with the doctor or doctors at a staff meeting.
- Point out to the doctors that one of the reasons clients are not on time for their appointments is

because they do not expect the doctor to be on time.

- Remind the doctors that they would have fewer irritable clients and staff members to deal with if they would be on time.
- Have new clients arrive 15 minutes before their scheduled appointment so that they can be processed and in the exam room on time. Getting a new client into the exam room 15 minutes late can upset a whole morning or afternoon schedule.
- Time the doctors when they are unaware that they are being timed to determine the average time they spend with an appointment. Some doctors need 20 minutes, whereas others may need 30 minutes.
- Be aware of time requirements. Do not schedule two appointments for complicated cases or sick animals one right after the other. Alternate short appointments for suture removals, rechecks, or vaccinations with appointments that are likely to take more time.
- When making 20-minute appointments, schedule appointments every 30 minutes until the day is full, then go back and insert another one in each hour as needed.
- Group appointments in clusters. If you only have three or four appointments for the morning, schedule them one after another. If you allow too much time between appointments, doctors are likely to become otherwise occupied and may be unavailable when the next client arrives.
- Schedule a time during the late morning and late afternoon for doctors to return phone calls. Ask callers where they can be reached at the scheduled time. Then give the information to the doctor to return the call. Organize the call backs on the doctor's desk.
- Study the reasons why the doctor tends to be late for appointments and discuss it with him or her. Work together in solving the problem. Staying on schedule is important to the doctor, to you, and of course to the client.

Preparing the Examination Room

Make sure the examination room is empty and clean. It may not be your job to clean the exam rooms, but if you are the one putting clients in the room, it is your job to make sure it is clean. There is no excuse for putting a client in a dirty exam room.

Consider the client as a guest and yourself the gracious host. A client with a 70-lb dog, 2-year-old child, and an infant in her arms needs help; provide whatever assistance is needed. An elderly client may also need your assistance.

If the client is early, and the doctor is treating an emergency case or the doctor is likely to be a few minutes late, provide the client with reading material.

Each exam room should have framed copies of the license, diplomas, and any award certificates belonging to any staff doctor that might be using the room. Most clients like to know as much as possible about the doctor who will care for their animal.

Another good idea is to have a reasonably current family picture of the doctor and his or her family, including pets. Pictures showing a doctor's outside interests are also sometimes appropriate.

Keep the waiting client informed of any unavoidable delays. Remember, minutes seem like hours to a waiting client, so do not ignore the client, even though the wait may be only 5 minutes. Some people have claustrophobia, so consider leaving the door to the reception area open. If the client appears to be distressed for any reason, ask what you can do to make him or her more comfortable. Be aware of your guest's comfort level.

Hospitalizing a Patient

The end result of some appointments is that the animal must be admitted for treatment or diagnostic procedures. At that time there are two very important things you can do: provide a written estimate and give postoperative instructions.

Written Estimates. Before the client leaves after an animal is admitted, give the client a written estimate of the charges. A written estimate eliminates most of the questions about charges that clients often ask when the animal is discharged. It may not be the receptionist's or technician's responsibility to give the estimate, but someone must be sure the client has a written estimate.

A written estimate can list two estimated dollar amounts. The first amount is the doctor's estimate. The second estimate, added by the receptionist, is 20% higher than the doctor's estimate. It is a good idea to circle both numbers with a felt tip pen and draw a line connecting them.

Tell the client that the first figure is what the doctor anticipates the charges will be. Explain that the fee could be as much as 20% higher if complications develop. Also tell the client that the charges will not exceed the second figure unless he or she is contacted and agrees to a higher figure.

Written estimates must be provided with the doctor's permission and cooperation. It is also important that the receptionists take some responsibility in seeing that this is done.

Postoperative Instructions. If the animal is being left for surgery, this is the time to give the client a sheet of postoperative instructions. Ask the client to read the sheet and offer to answer any questions when the client returns to pick up the animal. Clients often ignore instructions given verbally or sheets given to them when they return for the animal.

Status Report. Clients typically are very concerned about the status of their animal hospitalized for surgery or other treatment. Clients can be told a specific time to call for an update on their animals, or they must be asked where they can be reached by a staff member's telephone call. Ask the doctors to tell clients, "Let the receptionist know where you can be reached between 10:00 AM and noon tomorrow and we will call you to let you know how your animal is doing."

Before you or the doctor calls the client the next day, the status report must be reviewed. This status report contains the following information regarding hospitalized animals:

- The owner's name and phone numbers
- The animal's name and gender
- A one-word description of why the animal was hospitalized (e.g., ovariohysterectomy or fracture)
- Columns for functional status, such as body temperature, pulse rate, respiratory rate, and did the animal eat, drink, urinate, and have a bowel movement
- Remarks (often coded), such as doctor must talk to owner; animal can go home in the afternoon or when the owner wants to pick it up; the animal is doing better but still has fever; or we will call owner again this afternoon

With this information, the doctor or other staff member can make the phone calls as necessary and as time permits. These calls can also be made on telephone lines that do not tie up the incoming phone lines. This reduces the number of busy signals that callers get and minimizes the time they are kept on hold.

Calling clients to discuss their animals' status is preferred to asking the client to call. When clients call, they have to wait while someone is found to discuss their animal's condition. This conveys an image of chaos and inefficiency.

Discharge of Hospitalized Animals. When you tell a client his or her hospitalized animal is ready to go home, be prepared to state the total fees due. If the animal is ready for discharge, all treatment has been completed, and any medication has been packaged for dispensing, the total fee due can be calculated before the owner is called. If the client elects to pay by credit card, you can obtain the credit card number and have all of the paperwork completed before the client arrives to claim the animal.

To avoid the 4:00 to 6:00 PM rush of clients picking up animals, ask the owners if they would like to pick up their animals in the morning or early afternoon. Many can do so and appreciate the opportunity to avoid the afternoon traffic.

If all of the charges have not been calculated when you speak with the client over the telephone, at least have the final fee calculated when the client arrives. It is important to take care of all of the financial arrangements before the client and animal are reunited.

The Bill. What you say when presenting the bill to a client and how you say it are very important. Your tone of voice and body language are equally as important as what you say. If what you say, your tone of voice, or your body language is defensive or gives any hint of apology, you can expect to be challenged regarding the charges.

Remember that the client has agreed to pay the fee mentioned in the estimate; the amount is no surprise and there is no need to apologize. If the charges are more than the estimate and the client has not been informed of the increase, present this news with a positive twist. "This is your lucky day. We did $300 worth of work, but you only owe us the $250 mentioned in the estimate." (Be sure to get the practice owner's permission before you do this.) When the practice owner and the doctors become aware that they did $300 worth of work but were only paid $250, the doctors soon learn to give more accurate estimates. It is not advisable to charge a client more than the original estimate unless he or she has agreed to pay a higher amount.

Complaints About Charges. The number of complaints about charges can help identify the cause of the complaints. If there are several complaints about charges (two or three per day or more than 10% of the client visits) the reasons are probably one of the following:

- Poor communications, such as not providing estimates when extensive work is done
- The receptionists are presenting bills in a manner than invites challenges from clients
- By advertising or reputation, the practice has attracted a clientele that will complain about charges, no matter how low the fees

Ways to combat the first two problems have already been discussed. Provide accurate estimates, understand the reason for the charges, and be careful in how you present them to clients.

If your clinic has developed a reputation for low fees, you may want to recruit clients with a higher socioeconomic status. Increasing your entire fee schedule brings in higher revenues for the practice. This problem, however, may be deeply imbedded in the practice owner's "cut rate" philosophy and therefore will not be easy to change.

The best way to deal with a large number of complaints is to find the underlying cause and eliminate it. Dealing with each complaint on an individual basis is time consuming and depressing for the whole staff. Prevention is the answer.

An occasional complaint (two or three per week or less than 5% of clients seen) usually comes from a bragging client or a client who does not understand the basis of the charges.

These complaints, when merely occasional, must be dealt with on an individual basis. Complaints from bragging clients are easy to identify, once you become aware of them. Such complaints are almost always made in front of an audience of fellow clients. It sounds like this: "Oh my goodness, $1,500 for just a dog. That's more than it costs to take a child to the doctor." The translation is, "Look at me. I can afford to spend $1,500 on my dog. How about that! Don't you wish you were rich like me?"

Your response to such a complaint could be, "Barney sure is lucky to have you for an owner. Many dogs have owners that don't love them as much as you obviously love Barney." The usual response to this acknowledgment of the client's wealth and love for the animal is, "Thank you." The client acted and you applauded. This is one of the few acceptable ways in which people can brag about their wealth; do not deprive them of the opportunity.

The more serious type of complaint is made in the form of a question: "Why am I being charged for this?" "Why are these charges so high?" "What do these charges mean?"

The answer to all three questions is the same: "What is it that you don't understand about the charges? I'll try to explain it for you." Ask this calmly, with no defensiveness in your tone of voice, facial expression, or body language.

When clients tell you they do not understand the reason for the charges, provide an explanation of each fee but do not try to bluff if you do not know the answer. Tell the clients you will have a doctor answer their questions. Ask them to step into an empty exam room and ask a doctor to speak with them.

Hospital Policy. It is not acceptable to answer a client's question with, "It's hospital policy." To simply tell a client that something is or is not hospital policy actually means that you do not know the reason for the directive or there is no plausible reason. For example, if a certain client wants to visit his hospitalized animal and it is against hospital policy, tell the client why he cannot visit his animal. Clients usually are not allowed to visit their hospitalized animals, because it would be disturbing to other patients.

There is a reason for every hospital policy. Know the reason and use it to answer client inquiries. If you do not know, have someone who does know the reason speak with the client. Then learn the reasons behind the policies you do not understand.

Completing the Transaction

After the fees have been paid and the client has his or her animal (if it was an outpatient visit) or is about to be reunited with the animal after discharge, a few more things must be done.

Ask the client if he or she has any questions concerning the animal. Common concerns of clients include the following:

- "Did I cause the problem?"
- "How can I keep it from happening again?"
- "If it happens again, how can I recognize it before it progresses?"
- Can I expect this condition to get worse? Will it keep recurring?"
- Have I done the right thing for my animal?"

Do not forget to make an appointment for recheck, suture removal, or any other kind of follow-up examination that may be necessary.

Make sure that every client has several of the clinic's business cards when he or she leaves. If you have refrigerator magnets, make sure each client gets one. It is important that they have the clinic's telephone number handy to call for an appointment without having to use a telephone directory. If they open the telephone directory to the listing for veterinarians, some clients may be tempted to call another clinic if they get a busy signal or are put on hold when calling your clinic.

Let clients know that even though the clinic may seem busy, you would welcome any friends they may refer to the practice.

Finally, always *thank the client for coming to your clinic.* Remember every client brings in part of your paycheck. When you say thank you, say it like you mean it.

Client Departure

If it is raining as clients leave the clinic, hold an umbrella over them as you walk to their car. If it is not raining, ask if you can help carry any pet food, flea products, or their animal to the car. At least hold the clinic door open for clients if their hands are full.

FOLLOW-UP

It is important to maintain contact with the owners of animals that have been presented for medical treatment or that had surgery. This is done with follow-up telephone calls to inquire about the animal's condition.

The client's name can be flagged on the clinic's computer for addition to the follow-up call list. Some practices use 3×5-inch index cards, stored in a small file box, to maintain a list of clients to be called. On the index card or in the computer file, record the client's name, phone number, the animal's name, and any pertinent information you will need when you contact that client.

Follow-up calls are made for medical reasons. There may be a problem that clients are reluctant to call about. Be sensitive to any hesitancy in clients' responses when you ask how their animals are doing. Encourage them to bring the animal back to the clinic if you suspect a problem. Sometimes the client does not know what to expect after surgery or treatment and may wait too long to seek follow-up care for an animal

that is not recovering as expected. Occasionally, such a call can save an animal's life.

The other reason for making these calls is to enhance client relations. Most clients are very impressed by the clinic's concern. Few other service or retail businesses care enough to follow up and see if their client or customer is satisfied. Many clients talk to their friends about the call they received from your clinic.

Some clinics call clients again in 6 months to let them know the clinic is there if needed. Even if clients think you are making the call to bring in more business, they will be pleased. These 6-month calls are usually made only during slow times of the year or on slow days. They are good for client relations and there is also a good chance that after 6 months the animal may need veterinary attention.

File Purging

The ideal way to purge files is to start at one end and work to the other end and then start over. Call any client who has not come to the clinic for the past 15 to 18 months. These clients have ignored their vaccination reminder notices.

When you call, say you are reviewing the files and notice they have not brought their animal in for the recommended vaccinations. Ask if they still have their animal and confirm their current address. If they still have the animal and might be back in sometime in the future, note the date of the call and maintain that client's file in your active files.

If you are told that the phone number is no longer in service or another person now has the number, you can assume that client has moved. Send a first-class letter to the address listed in your files. If it is returned, with or without the new address, you will know the client has moved. If the client has moved, pull the file and store it with your inactive files.

The Importance of Persistence

Always remember that clients can obtain veterinary service for their animals from other clinics. Some of these clinics may be closer to a client's home than your clinic. If you want clients to continue patronizing your business, ensuring your paycheck and job security, you must do something to impress them by doing things for them that are unexpected. Keep your mind active and continually search for new ways to impress clients. Ask your co-workers to join you in an unending search for ways to add more perceived value to your clinic's already superior service.

Take care of your clients and they will take care of you.

RECOMMENDED READING

AAHA: *Commonly asked questions reference guide,* Denver, 1993, American Animal Hospital Association.

McCurnin DM: *Veterinary practice management,* Philadelphia, 1988, JB Lippincott.

Messonnier SP: *Marketing your veterinary practice,* St Louis, 1994, Mosby.

Messonnier SP: *Marketing your veterinary practice,* vol 2, St Louis, 1997, Mosby.

Riegger MH: *Management for results,* Cleveland, 1994, Advanstar Communications.

Riegger MH: *Management for results II,* Cleveland, 1995, Advanstar Communications.

GRIEF COUNSELING

C. BARTON ROSS
J. BARON-SORENSEN

As stated earlier, veterinary technicians play an important role in maintaining good client relations. Clients anticipating or experiencing loss of a companion animal are emotionally vulnerable. The hospital is vulnerable, also. What you do or say to a client while he or she is experiencing the loss of a companion animal can encourage or discourage his or her future relationship with the practice. At such a time, you have the opportunity to provide the best service your hospital has to offer.

The bonds people form with their pets may be as deep or deeper than those formed with friends or family members. Pets make us feel better when we are ill, comfort us when we are lonely, accept us when we have made a mistake, and love us unconditionally. This human–companion animal bond can be broken in many ways. The pet may die of natural causes, run away, or be stolen, killed accidentally, or euthanized. Clients with a deep emotional attachment to their pets can expect to grieve when they lose them.

It is important to respect the feelings of clients experiencing such loss. To do this, you must first understand the stages of grief and determine the significance of the loss to the client. Elizabeth Kubler-Ross, MD, was the first to outline predictable stages of the process of grieving in her book, *On Death and Dying,*[2] Although she wrote about human loss, the stages can be applied to the loss of pets as well.

Loss of a pet elicits a wide range of emotions in clients; these can be associated with certain stages of the grieving process. You can assist the client's smooth transition from one stage to another. The grieving process is not a steady, linear ascent from depression to joy; rather, it can be likened to a roller coaster ride, with ups and downs at every turn. At the end of the ride is a state of resolution and acceptance, in which the client is at peace with what went before.

By familiarizing yourself with the characteristics of each stage, you will recognize at what point your client is in this process and be able to shape your responses appropriately. These responses can facilitate the smooth transition from one stage to the next in the process of grieving.

STAGES OF GRIEF

The stages of grief include denial, bargaining, anger, guilt, sorrow, and resolution.[2] These stages frequently occur in this order, but they can occur in other sequences. Some stages may be repeated.

Denial

Denial, the first stage of grief, may be played out during the first 24 hours if the animal's death is sudden, or for several days if a terminal illness has been diagnosed. Denial is a coping mechanism that cushions the mind against the shock it has received.

Bargaining

Clients may bargain with God or another higher entity for the life of a pet, or bargain with the pet itself, trying to make it live. They may offer the pet vitamins, tempt it with its favorite foods, and promise never to scold or neglect it again. Bargaining is a way of keeping hope alive and buying time to fully accept the outcome of the situation. When bargaining does not yield the desired results, anger is a natural response.

Anger

When faced with the loss of a treasured pet, clients may become angry with the veterinarian, technician, office staff, family, friends, and themselves. The veterinarian who has failed to "save" the pet, or who has made the diagnosis, may be the initial recipient of the wrath. More often, it is the reception staff members who bear the brunt of the anger, either directly or indirectly. Clients may be fearful of alienating the practitioner on whom they have come to rely. If clients are angry with themselves for overlooking clinical signs or waiting too long to seek care, this self-directed anger, once dissipated, gives way to guilt.

Guilt

Guilt is an unproductive, debilitating emotion that often inhibits progress toward resolution of the loss. It is the enemy of healing and closure and, if excessive, may require the attention of a mental health professional. When guilt subsides, it opens the door for sorrow.

Sorrow

Sorrow, or deep sadness, is the core of the grieving process. Though it can be kept at bay during the early stages through the intensity of denial, anger, and guilt, sorrow eventually settles in and permeates all aspects of life.

Sorrow is, in fact, a healing emotion. This is the time when tears flow freely. Clients feel relief and release from the pent-up emotions of previous days or weeks. Tears may come at work, in the supermarket, or while driving down the freeway. Clients may report sleep and appetite disturbances at this time. The practitioner might want to remind them, soon after a terminal illness is diagnosed, that adequate rest and nutrition are important. With time, sorrow dissipates, and everyday tasks begin to dominate awareness. Tears no longer break through into daily activities but can surface at more convenient times, such as in the evening after work. Clients then feel more in control and are able to see an end to the intense pain that is true sorrow.

Resolution

In the resolution phase of grieving, clients realize that the pet is gone, that no amount of wishing will make it different, and that they will survive the loss that previously seemed engulfing. Now they can look at photographs of the pet and smile rather than cry; they can remember walks in the park in the summer, instead of anxious trips to the veterinarian; anniversaries and holidays can be recalled with tenderness rather than despair. During this stage of grief, clients may consider sharing life with another pet for the sheer pleasure of having something warm and furry to hug again.

Loneliness

Regardless of how the loss occurs and how well prepared the client is, all clients feel their lives touched by loneliness. This can occur in the presence of family and friends, as well as in the company of remaining pets at home. The client shared a relationship with the departed pet that was special and separate from other relationships. Although other pets, family members, and friends can provide company and comfort, they cannot fill the space left by the departed pet. Loneliness arises from this space, and the space fills slowly as the grief process unfolds. Clients may express anger at losing this particular pet while others to whom they are less attached are healthy and well.

An appropriate response from the staff or veterinarian might be, "Even though you have other pets at home, you may still be lonely for Taffy. While you are healing from this loss, your other pets will still be there to love you."

A Case Study

The following case study depicts the various stages of grief a client may experience. This example gives you an idea of how the stages of grief are manifested and how you may deal with them.

Mrs. Malay brings in Magic, her cat, for a yearly examination. While the cat is being examined, Mrs. Malay remarks on its distended abdomen. The veteri-

narian palpates the area and suggests an ultrasound examination. The examination reveals an abdominal tumor involving several organs.

When Mrs. Malay telephones the office the next day, the veterinarian delicately shares this sad news with her. In the course of the conversation, she says that she is having a difficult time believing the test results because Magic appears to be in good health. She asks if it is possible that the results of the ultrasound examination could be wrong. Mrs. Malay is *denying* the results of the test.

The veterinarian continues by telling her what course of action he would like to take in treating Magic. He explains the options, which range from referring her to an internist for possible treatment, to electing no treatment.

Mrs. Malay is feeling *guilty*. She is having a difficult time concentrating on what the doctor is saying to her and is instead looking to blame herself for Magic's illness. She can only focus on what she might have done to prevent it.

The veterinarian tells her that he will call her tomorrow and asks her to think if she would like a referral to an internist. When he telephones her the next day, she is very tearful. She says that she is wondering if giving Magic extra vitamins would help her to fight the disease. Mrs. Malay is *bargaining*. She begins to cry, and then falls silent.

The veterinarian suggests that she go to see Dr. McDonnell. He offers to call and arrange a consultation appointment for her and Magic. She agrees.

Shortly after this, Mrs. Malay receives her bill for the ultrasound examination and calls the front desk to express her outrage at the cost. The receptionist listens patiently but informs her that she must pay the bill. Mrs. Malay curtly responds that she will and hangs up.

Mrs. Malay is now feeling *angry*. She may be genuinely upset at the cost of the procedure, but she is also angry that she received this terrible news about her cat from your office. She probably wishes that she had never approved the ultrasound examination so that she would not have discovered the cancer.

Mrs. Malay and Magic have been seeing Dr. McDonnell for several months now. Dr. McDonnell has kept your practice abreast of the situation. The treatment bought Magic a little time, but she has now taken a final turn for the worse. Dr. McDonnell recommends euthanasia. Your office agrees to perform the euthanasia in Mrs. Malay's home.

On the day of the euthanasia, the veterinarian and technician arrive at Mrs. Malay's home. She is very calm. She takes them to the spot where Magic always suns herself. She says that this is Magic's favorite place and that she would like Magic to die peacefully here. She pets Magic lovingly. She whispers how much she loves her and what a joy Magic was in her life.

Mrs. Malay has come a long way in the process of grieving. She has now *accepted* her loss and is on the way to *resolving* her grief in learning to live without Magic.

REPLACEMENT

The decision to replace a deceased pet with a new one should be left solely to the individuals experiencing the loss. It should not be influenced by the veterinary staff in any way. Some pet owners choose to bond with new pets before their elderly pets die. Others decide that the presence of a new pet in their home would be stressful for the older pet and decide to wait. Some clients may never again adopt new pets. Everyone involved must consider the client's needs, as well as the needs of the current pet. It is important to try to not "fix" the client's loss by suggesting replacement.

If a client is trying to avoid the experience of loss by finding a replacement for the pet, bonding with the new pet usually does not occur. The new pet is not accepted as a unique being if the owner wants it to be just like the deceased pet. Often, these new pets are given away or neglected. Owners may comment that the new Max is nothing like the old Max. Occasionally, a client who had taken good care of a previous pet brings in a pet that has been neglected. This client probably has not bonded successfully with the new pet and may need support in deciding whether to keep it or find a new home for it. The client may not have resolved the loss of the previous pet and may need to see a counselor or support group that deals with pet loss issues.

ASSISTING BEREAVED PET OWNERS

Clients grieve in a variety of ways. Some demonstrate their emotions openly, whereas others may show little if any feeling in your presence. Do not assume that a stoic display means the client is not grieving.

Assess your client's feelings to determine how much support you should provide. When clients show reluctance to accept concerned overtures from you, take a minute to let them know that you care about their well-being. By acknowledging their sadness, you open the door for them to experience their emotions, giving the simple message that it is acceptable to grieve.

Veterinary staff members are in a position to encourage healthy coping skills in their clients. Clients look to the veterinary staff for support, assurance, understanding, and validation when facing a loss. If you can assist your clients in this way, you are building the foundation for natural resolution of the loss. In doing so, you continue to maintain their respect and solidify your working relationship. Recognizing the different stages of grief assists you in providing your clients with the type of support they need.

ACKNOWLEDGING THE LOSS

What a client needs and values most from the staff is their time and presence. In being present with clients during a loss, you help to legitimize the grief reaction and give them permission to verbalize their feelings. Many pet owners go to great lengths to appear stoic in the presence of others. In our society, death is often dealt with through denial, so it is vital that you validate the client's loss. The most beneficial thing a veterinary staff member can do for their clients is to let them know that grieving for the loss of a pet is perfectly normal.

Sending a card, personal note, or flowers to the client are all ways of expressing condolences. What clients will remember the most is how they were cared for during their loss. Being cared for and acknowledged is something a client will remember long after the flowers have wilted and the note or card has been discarded.

Veterinary staff members may feel uncomfortable in attending a grieving client. Some pet owners attribute unrealistic powers of control over life and death to their veterinarians. This is especially true for "last hope practitioners," veterinarians who are specialists in their fields. A client whose pet has cancer and who has been referred to an internist for treatment may have a strong need to believe that this doctor with specialized skills will be able to help the pet. This can place the veterinarian in the difficult position of conveying the limitations of treatment to the client.

Being with a client who is very tearful or angry can be an uncomfortable experience. You may worry that you will do or say the wrong thing. You may find it easier to hide behind the professional role and keep the client emotionally at a distance. This often leaves the client feeling uncared for and abandoned. A client is less likely to return to an emotionally unsupportive veterinary facility, even if the very best treatment was provided for the terminally ill pet.

Your responsibility is not to work in the capacity of a therapist or counselor. However, your relationships with your clients can be enhanced by learning and using a variety of counseling and communication skills. By communicating effectively with your clients, you help them to accept and resolve their losses sooner than pet owners whose losses have not been properly acknowledged.

Useful skills and techniques that can be used to assist your clients include attending, effective listening, reflection, and validation.

Some clients are easier to help than others, and you must make an extra effort to support the more difficult ones. Demonstrate that you are attempting to understand what the clients are expressing by responding at appropriate intervals to their comments. Avoid using clichés or telling them that you know exactly how they feel; you don't.

Try saying, "What I hear you saying is . . . ." Let the client tell you what the loss means to her. Ask the client, "How can I help you? What things have you done in the past that have supported you through a difficult time?"

A Case Study. Carley was devastated after having chosen euthanasia for her ill bird and companion of 11 years. She had centered her life around care of her bird, Poncho, and this sharply curtailed her social life.

Her associates and friends did not understand the depth of her loss. Carley talked to her veterinarian. She told him that she could not face the future without her pet.

A helpful response to such a statement would be, "You've devoted so much time and love to Poncho that you feel your life will be lonely and empty without him. It might be helpful for you to consider that while a door has closed on his life, one might be opening in yours."

This statement acknowledges the intensity of her pain while reframing the situation into one of possibilities, rather than emptiness and hopelessness.

Reflection

Summarizing what the client is expressing is called *reflection*. When you reflect clients' underlying concerns, they feel that you understand what they are saying. In addition, you can reframe the experience of loss and hopelessness into one of hope and possibility.

By establishing open communication, you will be in a position to offer the kind of help that clients need. Some clients may only need to hear that they did the right thing and want to be informed of disposing of the remains. Others need emotional support and may be referred to a group or private therapist.

Validating the Loss

When your clients tell you what the loss means to them, it is important to let them know that you understand the relationship they have shared with the pet. In validating the loss, you will discover that a pet can fulfill many needs of pet owners. Be alert for key comments, such as, "We never had any children. Kelsey was like our child," "Buttons was my whole life," or "How will I ever feel safe alone at night without Cole?" A pet may have served as a child to some, a best friend to others, or even as a bridge to the past. It may have accompanied the owner from college to career, to marriage, and on through other important life stages. It may have been a source of comfort during a stressful time: a divorce, loss of a loved one, a move, or a change in jobs.

Attending

Without realizing it, you can make it difficult for clients to express their feelings and concerns. The way in which you sit, stand, look at, or speak with them can inhibit or enhance communication.

An open posture with uncrossed arms and legs demonstrates to your clients that you are available and ready to listen. Facing them directly while maintaining comfortable eye contact sends the message that you are interested in what they have to say. Avoid standing behind the counter, desk, or exam table when clients are expressing their feelings about their pet to you.

Effective Listening

Listening effectively is much more than hearing what a client is saying. Listening effectively means giving the client your complete attention and allowing time for the client to ramble, cry, and show anger. You should learn to tolerate periods of silence from the client. You may feel a strong desire to fill in the silence with words; refrain from doing so. The client needs you to be there silently.

By recognizing the different components of grief, you can accept the client's expressions of anger and denial, and be empathetic about the guilt and deep sadness. Whether the client's initial reaction is overt despair or quiet shock, your interactions set the stage for the grieving process that follows.

The current loss can trigger remembrance of past losses. Particularly for the elderly client; this compound effect may threaten to overwhelm the client. Clients can be reminded that it is common to remember past losses while grieving a current one.

Three Case Studies. A woman who lost her baby to Sudden Infant Death Syndrome acquired a puppy to help her through the loss. The puppy was something to cuddle and make the client feel needed. Though it was by no means a replacement for the child she had lost, it helped her through the experience. When her dog died some years later, she grieved not only for the loss of the dog but also for loss of her child.

Another client who lost a dog that had been her constant companion remarked that the dog's death was more difficult for her than the recent loss of her mother, with whom she had been close.

A Vietnam veteran who had chosen euthanasia for his 17-year-old, very ill cat shared that the cat was the first living thing he was able to learn to love again after returning home from the war.

The following validating responses convey your understanding and empathy to the clients in these cases: "Losing your dog reminds you of the loss of your child. It must be a very painful time for you."

"Your dog was a significant member of your family. The unconditional love you received is a gift that people are not always able to give one another."

"It is difficult for me to imagine what Vietnam was like, but I do know that this cat was very special to you. She has given you a gift that no one else could give you."

Use your own words to convey messages of understanding and empathy toward your clients. The idea is to listen and then respond to the clients by expressing the core significance of the loss. Validating a client's loss helps to make the client feel special and cared for by the veterinarian and the hospital staff.

Achieving Closure

The perfect way to end a conversation with a grieving client is to give a directive. For example, "I would like you to go home, get some rest, and then think about the options we discussed." Or you can inform the client about a support group in your area for bereaved pet owners. For example, "There is a place you can go and meet with other pet owners who are sharing similar feelings to yours." You can give the client a brochure or offer to make an appointment for him to talk with the support group leader.

Make clients take comfort in thinking about ways in which to honor their pets. For example, clients can donate to a charity in honor of a pet, plant a rose bush near the burial site, or create a scrapbook of memories shared with the pet.

The following suggestions may be helpful in assisting your clients.

- Provide facial tissues.
- Schedule appointment times to allow for additional time to be spent with a bereaved pet owner or one whose pet is seriously ill.
- Create a brochure that includes all available support information (pet loss support groups, private therapists, hotlines, burial information, literature on pet loss, etc.). Make the brochure available to clients anticipating a loss as well as to those experiencing one.
- Send a sympathy card or flowers immediately after the loss. Late arrivals can be painful reminders for clients.
- Collect any fees owed before the euthanasia procedure is performed. A client will find it awkward to have to regain composure and pay a bill after the emotional experience of saying goodbye to a beloved pet.
- Let clients know that you and the rest of the staff are available to assist them, before and after the loss of a pet. Most pet owners have questions regarding their pets' illness and need reassurance that they did the right thing.
- If possible, maintain a private area in which clients can say goodbye to their pet, grieve, or regain composure. If such an area is not available, consider allowing extra time in the examination room before a loss or afterward.
- When attending to the patient, make certain that the owner can tell that the pet is comfortable and cared for. A simple gesture, such as placing a towel on a cold examination table, can demonstrate your compassion for the patient. If you send a final bill to the client, make sure it does not arrive on the same day as the sympathy card or flowers.

EFFECTS OF PATIENT LOSS ON STAFF

As difficult as the loss of a pet may be for a client, the loss of a patient may be difficult for the staff and veterinarian as well. Because euthanasia is an acceptable and legal means of terminating an animal's life, veterinary practitioners and their staff face a stress that is unknown to most other medical practitioners.

Each member of the staff has a personal set of beliefs and feelings regarding the issue of loss. Some may feel awkward attending a grieving client. Others may have unresolved feelings about pets they have lost themselves. Most people in the veterinary field have a love for animals and want to help them. Few consider the effect of the loss of a patient upon themselves.

When assisting bereaved pet owners, staff members may feel emotions similar to those the client experiences. Learn how to empathize and assist in a caring manner while still maintaining emotional distance. The following steps will help you in this process.

- Take a team approach to cases in which euthanasia is an option. This can alleviate some of the feelings of failure and grief regarding loss of a patient.
- Create and participate in a support group for veterinary staff. This is a forum for airing private feelings and receiving feedback from peers.
- Refer pet owners to a pet loss support group. This provides clients with a safe place to share feelings and validates the fact that loss of a patient is a real and important consideration for everyone involved.
- Encourage open communication among staff members, confrontation of personal feelings and beliefs surrounding death, and self-examination regarding the emotional reaction to loss of a patient.[1]

When a client is facing the crisis of losing a treasured pet, you can play a positive role in guiding the client through an emotionally difficult time, thereby solidifying your working relationship with the pet owner. Clients who respect the veterinarian and staff will speak highly of them to others, refer other pet owners to the practice, and return with new pets. Pet loss is an opportunity for everyone concerned to grow emotionally and to solidify working relationships.

COMPOUNDED LOSS

When faced with loss of a pet, the owner is often reminded of losses from the past, both human and animal. A compound loss can feel so overpowering that a client may respond in a way that seems out of proportion to the current facts. When this occurs, you might say, "I can see that you are troubled and concerned about Woody. Have you had other experience with loss?"

Sometimes an invitation to talk about a previous pet loss elicits information regarding past loss of family and friends, the demise of a relationship, or loss of a job. If the information is forthcoming, you can tell the client, "I know that when faced with the loss of a pet that you love, you can be reminded of other previous losses, and this can hurt more than if you were dealing with a single loss. Don't be surprised if you are suddenly recalling sad times from the past. Just know that it is very natural, at a time like this, to remember family and friends who are no longer with you. Try talking things over with a close friend, or, if you'd like, I can give you some referrals for counseling that might help you get through this difficult time."

RECOGNIZING AND RESPONDING TO SIGNALS

A client may convey feelings of deep despair either verbally or though body language. Such statements as, "Muffin is the only friend I have in the world. I don't know how I can face another day without her by my side," or "Nothing matters now that Jake is dying. It will kill me to bring him in for euthanasia. I might as well be dead, too," should alert you to the need for outside professional evaluation and treatment.

You must determine if these clients have a reliable, concerned friend or relative who can stay with them, particularly if you have doubts about their safety if left alone. Make appropriate referrals and offer to call for an appointment before they leave the office. Do this openly to encourage trust and open communication. Knowing that an appointment has been arranged can have a calming and reassuring effect. Make every effort to secure the first appointment available and, if possible, telephone the client the next day for a "welfare check" and reminder of the appointment date and time. Extract a promise from the client that he or she will contact the crisis intervention hot line if he or she experiences overwhelming loneliness and sadness. Make certain you know the telephone number and that the client leaves your office with it.

If the client refuses any referrals or assistance and you sense that the client is a danger to him- or herself, you may need to resort to police escort of this client to a local psychiatric clinic for evaluation and treatment. This may seem to be an extreme measure, but it could save a life. Let the veterinarian know about any concerns you may have regarding a client. Develop a protocol for clients experiencing emotional problems surrounding the death or illness of a pet. You might say to the client, "I know that you do not want to accept a referral for help, but I am so concerned about you that I will notify the police for assistance in getting you the help you need. I really do care about you and don't want anything bad to happen to you." Remember that extreme actions displayed by a client sometimes call for extreme reactions by the staff.

REFERRING TO MENTAL HEALTH PROFESSIONALS

Clients experiencing intense anger, despair, and guilt often benefit from professional intervention outside of your office. Maintain a list of counselors and support groups for referral of clients experiencing grief associated with pet loss. A pet loss support group can provide a client with a safe place to express his or her feelings. It offers clients the opportunity to meet with like-minded pet owners with whom to share their fears, tears, memories, and finally, smiles.

When making referrals for group or individual counseling services, you might say something like, "I know you are very sad about Mitzi's ailing health. Here is some information about a support group for people who are struggling with the loss of a pet. This may help you to sort out some of your feelings."

Your local mental health department can assist you in compiling a list of mental health professionals and support groups. The Delta Society in Renton, Washington, maintains a list of pet loss support counselors and groups throughout the country. It also can provide you with additional books and videotapes on grief counseling. Assembling a community referral file for your clients takes time and effort, but this special service conveys the hospital staff's concern for their safety and well-being.

REFERENCES

1. Hart LA, Hart BL: Grief and stress from so many animal deaths, *Companion Animal Practice* 1:20-21, 1987.
2. Kubler-Ross E: *On death and dying,* New York, 1969, Collier Books.

RECOMMENDED READING

Guntzelman J, Reiger M: Helping pet owners with the euthanasia decision, *Vet Med* 88:26-34, 1993.

Guntzelman J, Reiger M: Supporting clients who are grieving the death of a pet, *Vet Med* 88:35-41, 1993.

Kay WJ et al: *Euthanasia of the companion animal,* Philadelphia, 1988, Charles Press.

Kubler-Ross E: *On death and dying,* New York, 1969, Collier Books.

Pettit TH: *Hospital administration for veterinary staff,* St Louis, 1994, Mosby.

Ross CB: Pet loss and the human/companion animal bond. Master's thesis, Sonoma State University, 1987.

PART THREE

Basic and Clinical Sciences

CHAPTER 7

Anatomy and Physiology

T.P. Colville

Learning Objectives

After reviewing this chapter, the reader should understand the following:

Types of cells and tissues of the body
Names of tissues and structures that make up the various body systems
Ways in which organs and body systems function and interact

Differences in the digestive tract of domestic animals
Differences between exocrine and endocrine glands
Features and functions of the male and female reproductive tract

INTRODUCTION

Studying anatomy and physiology will help you better understand the wonderful machine that is the animal body. *Anatomy* describes the physical makeup of the body, including size, shape, color, and location of the various cells, tissues, organs, and systems. *Physiology*, on the other hand, describes how the body and its various components function. Although neither alone allows a complete understanding of an animal's body, examining anatomy and physiology together gives a much clearer picture of how the body is organized and how its various components function in a complex, interrelated fashion.

GENERAL TERMINOLOGY

To describe the positions and relationships of body parts, some general anatomic terms must be used. Common

words, such as *up, down, front, back, top,* and *bottom* are not useful, because their meanings depend on the orientation of both the animal and the viewer. To be useful, the meanings of directional terms used to describe anatomy must be clear and independent of the body's position or the angle from which it is viewed (Fig. 7-1).

Many directional terms come in pairs that mean opposites of each other. *Left* and *right* always refer to the animal's left and right. *Cranial* and *caudal* refer to the head (cranial) end, or tail (caudal) end of the animal. *Dorsal* means toward the backbone, whereas *ventral* means away from the backbone, toward the belly of the animal. Anything that is *superficial* is located toward the surface of the body or a part, and *deep* structures are located toward the center of the body or a part.

Some terms are used only for particular parts of the body. Although the terms *cranial* and *caudal* are useful on most of the body, when speaking of the head, *cranial* loses its meaning. The term *rostral* means toward the tip

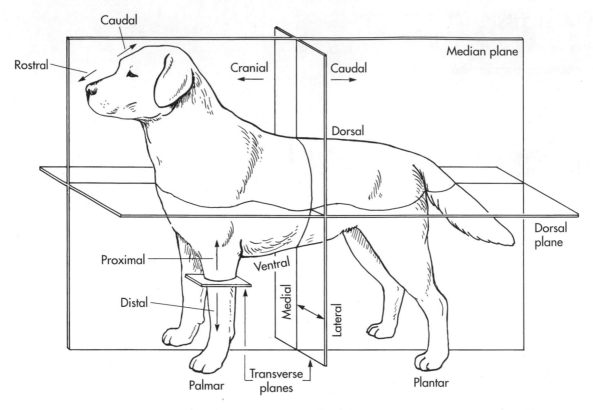

FIG. 7-1   Terms denoting position in animals. *(From McBride DF:* Learning veterinary terminology, *St Louis, 1996, Mosby.)*

of the nose and is used only when describing structures on or in the head. The terms *proximal* and *distal* are used to describe relationships on extremities. Proximal means toward the body, the attachment site of the extremity. Distal means the opposite: toward the tip of the extremity or away from the body.

Three basic planes, each at right angles to the other two, can be used to divide an animal's body and give reference points for other descriptions. A median plane divides the body into left and right parts. A *transverse* plane divides the body into cranial and caudal parts, and a *dorsal* plane divides the body into dorsal and ventral parts.

Medial and *lateral* are terms used to describe positions of structures relative to the median plane, the sagittal plane that divides the body into equal left and right halves. A medial structure is located toward the central axis and midline of the body. A lateral structure is located away from the midline, toward the side of the body.

CELLS

Cells are the basic units of life. All living things are made up of cells. An animal's body is composed of many different types of cells, each with its own place

and function. Each cell relies on the rest of the body to meet its nutritional and waste elimination needs, and the whole body relies on the contribution of all of its cells for its support. This relationship can be summarized by the following formula:

cell health ↔ tissue health ↔ organ health ↔
system health ↔ body health.

Note that the arrows point in both directions. The health of the cell depends on the health of the tissues of which it is part. In turn the tissues depend on the health of the cells that make them up, *and* the organs they are part of, and so on up the line. The degree of health at each level determines whether the body as a whole is healthy.

Unlike single-celled animals, complex (multi-celled) organisms have specialized cells that allow the whole body to operate. Groups of specialized cells make up tissues. Four basic types of tissues make up the animal body: epithelial tissue, connective tissue, muscle tissue, and nervous tissue. Functional groupings of tissues make up organs, such as the kidney, that contain elements of all four basic tissues. Systems are groups of organs that are involved in a common activity. For example, the salivary glands, esophagus, stomach, pancreas, liver, and intestines are all parts of the digestive system.

EPITHELIAL TISSUE

Epithelial tissue covers the interior and exterior surfaces of the body, lines body cavities, and forms glands. Its function includes protection from physical wear and tear as well as penetration by foreign invaders, selective absorption of substances (e.g., by the intestinal lining), and secretion of various substances.

All epithelial tissues share three common features:
- They consist entirely of cells.
- They do not contain blood vessels. Epithelial cells derive nourishment from blood vessels in the connective tissues beneath them.
- At least some epithelial cells are capable of reproducing. Epithelial tissue cells must be capable of compensating for wear and tear, as well as injuries.

The covering and lining epithelial tissue can be either simple (single cell layer thick) or stratified (more than one cell layer thick), and it can be made up of several different cell types.

The simple epithelial tissues are the following:

Epithelium	Cell shape	Example
Squamous	Flat, plate-like	Blood vessel lining
Cuboidal	Round or cuboidal	Kidney tubules
Columnar	Cylindric	Intestinal lining
Pseudostratified columnar	Irregular, nuclei not uniform in position	Upper respiratory tract lining

The stratified epithelial tissues are the following:

Epithelium	Characteristics	Example
Squamous	Deepest cells reproduce, pushing daughter cells toward the surface. They gradually die and assume a flattened shape as they move farther from their nutrient source in the underlying connective tissue.	Skin
Cuboidal, columnar	Rare in the body. Usually seen where one type of epithelium is blending into another type of epithelium.	
Transitional	Capable of considerable stretching.	Urinary bladder lining

Glandular epithelium can secrete substances directly into the bloodstream or out onto a body surface. The "ductless" glands that secrete directly into the bloodstream are the endocrine glands. They produce hormones. Exocrine glands secrete substances through ducts out onto body surfaces. They can be simple, with a single duct (e.g., sweat glands), or compound, with a branching duct system (e.g., mammary glands).

CONNECTIVE TISSUE

Connective tissue holds the body together and gives it support. If the body consisted entirely of cells, it would lie like a puddle of gelatin on the ground. Cells are, themselves, very soft in consistency. Firmer tissue, connective tissue, is necessary to support the cells and allow the body to assume an efficient shape and overall structure.

The cells of most connective tissues produce nonliving, intercellular substances that connect and give support to other cells and tissues. These intercellular substances range from various types of fibers to the firm, mineralized matrix of bone.

Six main types of connective tissues are present in the body: adipose connective tissue, loose areolar connective tissue, elastic connective tissue, dense fibrous connective tissue, cartilage, and bone. Blood is also a connective tissue; it will be discussed with the rest of the blood vascular system.

Adipose connective tissue consists of collections of lipid-storing cells, what we commonly refer to as "fat." It represents the body's storage supply of excess nutrients. When the dietary intake of nutrients exceeds the body's needs, adipose connective tissue proliferates. In leaner times, when the dietary nutrient intake is insufficient, the lipid stored in the adipose connective tissue can be mobilized to meet the body's nutritional needs.

Loose areolar connective tissue is found throughout the body wherever cushioning and flexibility are needed. It is commonly found beneath the skin and around blood vessels, nerves, and muscles. Its main components are fiber-producing cells, the fibroblasts, and two types of fibers, collagen fibers and elastic fibers. Collagen fibers are predominant and are very strong and relatively inelastic. Elastic fibers are a minor component and provide some degree of elasticity. Both sets of fibers are intertwined in a loose mesh that provides cushioning and flexibility in virtually all directions.

Elastic connective tissue is capable of stretching and returning to its original state. It consists mainly of large parallel bundles of elastic fibers, which give it a yellow color grossly. The walls of large, elastic arteries, such as the aorta, contain elastic connective tissue that helps them regulate the flow of blood from the heart.

Dense fibrous connective tissue has the same components as loose areolar connective tissue but is much more densely packed. One variety of dense fibrous connective tissue has the fibers arranged in parallel bundles. Referred to as dense fibrous connective tissue regularly arranged, it makes up tendons, which attach muscles to bones, and ligaments, which attach bones to other bones. The other type of dense fibrous connective tissue, irregularly arranged, is like a densely compacted version of loose areolar connective tissue. It is found in the capsules that surround and protect many soft internal organs.

Cartilage consists of a few cells, called *chondrocytes,* and various types and amounts of fibers embedded in a thick gelatinous intercellular substance, the matrix. Cartilage is firmer than fibrous tissue, but not as hard as bone, and contains no blood vessels. Nutrients for chondrocytes must diffuse through the matrix from the periphery of the cartilage. This limits how thick cartilage can become. Hyaline cartilage contains a few collagen fibers and is found in the tracheal rings and the articular (joint) surfaces of bones. Fibrocartilage contains large numbers of collagen fibers in its matrix, making it very durable. It makes up the majority of the intervertebral disks, which cushion the vertebrae. Elastic cartilage contains large numbers of both elastic and collagen fibers, giving it more flexibility than the other two cartilage types. It makes up parts of the larynx and most of the earflap (pinna).

Bone is second only to the enamel of teeth in its hardness. It is composed of a few cells, the osteocytes, embedded in a matrix that has become mineralized through a process called *ossification.* It is important to note that, despite its hard, dead appearance, bone is living tissue with an excellent capacity for regeneration and remodeling.

THE SKELETON

The skeleton is the framework of bones that supports and protects the soft tissues of the body. Some bones, such as the bones of the skull, which enclose and protect the delicate brain, surround sensitive tissues. Most of the bones of the skeleton, however, form the scaffolding around which the rest of the body tissues are arranged.

Common Bone Features

An articular surface is where a bone forms a joint with another bone. It is usually very smooth and is often covered with a layer of hyaline cartilage.

A condyle is a large, convex articular surface usually found on the distal ends of the long bones that make up the limbs.

A foramen is a hole in a bone through which blood vessels and nerves usually pass.

A fossa is a depression in a bone usually occupied by a muscle or tendon.

A bone head is a small, convex articular surface usually found on the proximal ends of some limb bones.

The neck of a bone is the often-narrowed area that connects a bone head with the rest of the bone.

A process, tuber, tubercle, tuberosity, or trochanter is a lump or bump on the surface of a bone. It is usually the site where the tendon of a muscle attaches to a bone. The larger the process, the more powerful the muscle that attaches at that site.

Axial Skeleton

The axial skeleton is composed of the bones located on the axis or midline of the body. It is made up of the bones of the skull, the bones of the spinal column, the ribs, and the sternum (Fig. 7-2).

The skull is made up of many irregularly shaped bones, most of which are held together by immovable joints called *sutures.* The skull bones can be divided into the bones of the cranium, which house and protect the brain; the bones of the face, which extend in a rostral direction from the cranium and house mainly digestive and respiratory structures; and the mandible, or lower jaw.

The spinal column is made up of a series of individual bones, the vertebrae, which together form a long, flexible tube dorsally that houses and protects the spinal cord. The vertebrae are divided into five groups, and each vertebra is numbered within each group from cranial to caudal (see Fig. 7-2). The *cervical vertebrae* are in the neck region. The first cervical vertebra (C1) forms a joint with the skull cranially. The *thoracic vertebrae* are dorsal to the chest region and form joints with the dorsal ends of the ribs. The *lumbar vertebrae,* which are dorsal to the abdominal region, are fairly large and heavy, because they serve as the site of attachment for the large sling muscles that support the abdomen. The sacral vertebrae, in the pelvic region, are fused together into a solid structure called the sacrum, which forms a joint with the pelvis. The caudal most vertebrae, the coccygeal vertebrae, form the tail.

The ribs support and help form the lateral walls of the thorax or chest (see Fig. 7-2). Their number varies with the species, but the number of rib pairs is usually the same as the number of thoracic vertebrae. They form joints with the thoracic vertebrae dorsally and are continued ventrally by rods of hyaline cartilage, the costal cartilages. The costal cartilages of ribs at the cranial end of the thorax are connected directly to the sternum at their ventral end. The costal cartilages of the caudal ribs do not reach the sternum; they connect to the costal cartilage cranial to them. The spaces between ribs are referred to as *intercostal spaces.*

The sternum forms the ventral portion of the thorax (see Fig. 7-2). It is composed of a series of rod-like bones called *sternebrae.* The manubrium sterni is the first (cranialmost) sternebra, and the xiphoid process is the last (caudalmost). These two bones are often used as external landmarks on the animal.

Appendicular Skeleton

The appendicular skeleton is composed of the bones of the limbs (appendages). The forelimb is referred to anatomically as the *thoracic limb* and the hind limb is termed the *pelvic limb*.

From proximal to distal, the bones of the thoracic limb are the scapula, humerus, radius and ulna, carpal bones, metacarpal bones, and phalanges (see Fig. 7-2). The scapula is the "shoulder blade." It is a flat bone with a shelf-like spine on its lateral surface. At its distal end it forms the shoulder joint with the humerus, which is the long bone of the brachium, or "upper arm."

The proximal end of the humerus is made up of the head, the smooth articular surface that forms the shoulder joint with the scapula, and the greater tubercle, where the powerful shoulder muscles attach. The distal joint surfaces of the humerus, the condyles, form the elbow joint with the radius and ulna, the bones of the antebrachium, or "forearm."

The *radius* is the main weight-bearing bone of the antebrachium, and the ulna forms much of the very snug-fitting elbow joint with the condyle of the humerus (see Fig. 7-2). At the proximal end of the ulna is the olecranon process, the point of the elbow where the powerful triceps brachii muscle attaches.

Located between the radius and ulna and the metacarpal bones is the carpus (see Fig. 7-2). It is composed of two rows of short bones and is equivalent to the human wrist. Just distal to the carpus are the metacarpal

bones, equivalent to the bones of the human hand between wrist and fingers. The phalanges are the bones of the digits, equivalent to human fingers. Each digit is composed of either two phalanges (proximal phalanx and distal phalanx), as in the human thumb, or three phalanges (proximal, middle, and distal), as in human fingers.

The bones of the pelvic limb, from proximal to distal, are the pelvis, femur, patella, tibia and fibula, tarsal bones, metatarsal bones, and phalanges (see Fig. 7-2). The pelvis is composed of three pairs of bones that are fused in the adult animal: the cranial ilium, the caudal ischium, and the medial pubis. At the junction of the three bones on each side is the acetabulum, the socket portion of the ball-and-socket hip joint.

The femur is the long bone of the thigh region (see Fig. 7-2). The head of the femur forms the ball portion of the hip joint, and the greater trochanter is the site of attachment for the powerful gluteal (rump) muscles. At its distal end are the condyles, which form the stifle joint with the tibia, and the trochlear groove, in which the patella rides.

The patella, or "kneecap," is the largest sesamoid bone in the body. Sesamoid bones are located in tendons that change direction sharply at joints. The patella helps distribute the force of the quadriceps femoris muscle, the main extensor muscle of the stifle joint.

The tibia is the main weight-bearing bone of the distal leg, and the fibula is a very small, sometimes incomplete bone that is primarily a site of muscle attachment (see Fig. 7-2).

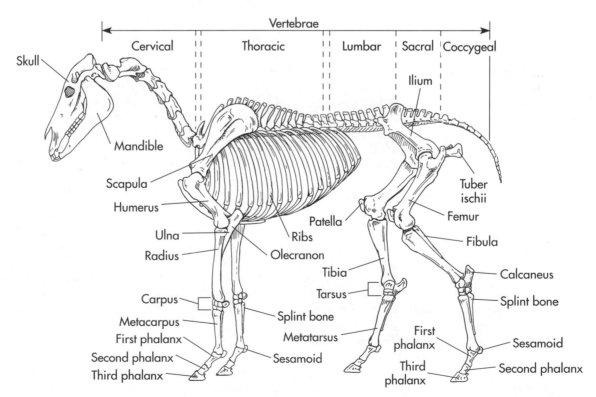

FIG. 7-2 Skeleton of a horse. *(From McBride DF:* Learning veterinary terminology, *St Louis, 1996, Mosby.)*

The tarsus is equivalent to the human ankle, and it consists of two rows of short bones. The tuberosity of the large calcaneus forms the point of the hock, equivalent to the human heel bone. The metatarsal bones and phalanges of the pelvic limb are similar to the metacarpal bones and phalanges of the thoracic limb.

Visceral Skeleton

The bones of the visceral skeleton, when present, occur in soft tissues of the body. The os penis of the dog is a well-developed bone in the penis. The os cordis forms part of the supporting structures in the heart of cattle. The os rostri helps strengthen the snout of swine.

Joints

Bones come together at joints. Our usual image of joints is that of freely movable joints, such as the elbow or hip. However, joints can be any of three main types: fibrous joints are immovable, cartilaginous joints are slightly movable, and synovial joints are freely movable.

Fibrous joints hold bones together but do not allow any movement at the joint site. The sutures that hold many of the skull bones together are immovable joints.

Cartilaginous joints allow a slight rocking movement. The cartilaginous intervertebral discs and the symphysis that unites the pubic bones of the pelvis allow a slight amount of movement.

Synovial joints are what people usually think of when they think of joints. They allow free movement between bones in several directions. Synovial joints usually have smooth articular surfaces covered by articular cartilage, and a fibrous joint capsule. Many have fibrous ligaments that hold the bones together.

Synovial joints allow some combination of six potential joint movements: flexion, extension, adduction, abduction, rotation, and circumduction. Flexion decreases the angle between two bones; extension increases the angle. Adduction moves an extremity toward the median plane, and abduction moves it away from the median plane. Rotation is a twisting movement of a part on its own axis. The shaking of the head of a wet dog is a rotation movement. Circumduction is a movement where the distal end of an extremity describes a circle.

THE INTEGUMENT

The integument is the outer covering of the body. It consists primarily of the skin, hair, claws, or hooves and horns. In nonmammals it also includes such structures as feathers and scales. In addition to its obvious protective role, the integument has several other important functions. Its multitude of sensory receptors make it one of the most important parts of an animal's sensory system. Integument also helps in regulating body temperature through its ability to adjust blood flow to the skin, adjust the position of hairs and secrete sweat. The integument also produces vitamin D and secretes and excretes a number of substances through various types of skin glands.

Skin

The skin is the largest body organ. It consists of two main layers: the superficial epithelial layer, the epidermis, and the deep connective tissue layer, the dermis.

The epidermis is composed of keratinized stratified squamous epithelium. The surface layer of the epidermis dries out and is converted to a tough, horny substance called *keratin,* which also makes up the bulk of hair, claws or hooves, and horns (antlers). Within the deepest layers of the epidermis of most animals are melanocytes, cells that produce granules of the dark pigment melanin. This pigment gives color to the skin, hair, and other integumentary structures. An albino animal has a total lack of melanin, resulting in pale, white skin and hair and unpigmented irises in the eyes.

The glands of the skin consist primarily of the sebaceous and sudoriferous glands, although the mammary and anal glands are considered skin glands also. The sebaceous glands are the oil glands of the skin. They secrete oily sebum, which helps waterproof the skin and keep it soft and pliable. Sebum is secreted directly onto the shafts of hairs in the hair follicles.

The sudoriferous glands are the sweat glands, which primarily help cool the body. Some animals, such as horses, have sudoriferous glands spread over their entire body. Others, such as dogs and cats, have only a few, clustered in the foot pad and nose areas.

Hair

Hair covers most of the body surface of most animals. Hair is composed of densely compacted keratinized cells, and produced in gland-like structures called *follicles.* Hairs are constantly shed and replaced. The visible part of each hair is referred to as the *hair shaft.* The portion within the skin is called the *hair root.* The color of hair results from granules of melanin that are incorporated into the hairs developing in the follicles. At the base of some hair roots, a tiny muscle, the arrector pili muscle, attaches. When it contracts, it pulls the hair into a more upright position. This produces "goose bumps" or "raised hackles." The purpose of erecting the hair generally is to retain heat when an animal is cold, by fluffing up the haircoat, or to make the animal look larger and more fearsome as a part of the sympathetic nervous system "fight or flight" response.

Claws and Hooves

Claws and hooves are horny structures that cover the distal ends of the digits. They are composed of parallel bundles of keratinized cells organized into an outer wall and a bottom sole.

Horns

Like claws and hooves, horns are composed of bundles of keratinized cells. They are organized around bony "horn cores," outgrowths of the frontal bones of the skull.

THE CIRCULATORY SYSTEM

The circulatory system is primarily a transport system in the body. It transports a variety of substances throughout the body, such as cells, antibodies, nutrients, oxygen, carbon dioxide, metabolic wastes, and hormones. Its two main divisions are the blood vascular system and the lymphatic vascular system.

Blood Vascular System

General Plan. The blood vascular system consists of a closed system of tubes through which a fluid connective tissue is propelled by a muscular pump. The fluid connective tissue is blood; the tubes are blood vessels; and the pump is the heart.

There are three types of blood vessels: arteries, capillaries, and veins. Arteries carry blood away from the heart to the capillaries. Arteries are quite large near the heart and gradually branch into smaller and smaller vessels as they course throughout the body. From the arteries, blood passes into the extensive networks of very tiny capillaries located throughout the body.

Capillaries are very porous and permit substances to move freely between the extracellular fluid (fluid surrounding cells) and the blood. The basic purpose of most of the blood vascular system is to deliver blood to the capillaries, where nutrients, waste products, gases, hormones, and other substances can be exchanged. Such substances as oxygen (O_2) and nutrients move out of the blood and into the cells, while metabolic wastes and carbon dioxide (CO_2) move out of the cells and into the blood. From the capillaries, the CO_2-laden, waste-filled blood passes first into small venules and then into veins for the return trip to the heart. Many veins contain tiny one-way valves along their length. These one-way valves, assisted by movement of muscles in the area, help propel the blood back toward the heart.

The Heart. The heart is the muscular pump that propels blood around the body. It comprises dense accumulations of cardiac muscle cells and connective tissue organized into two side-by-side pumps that together are composed of four chambers and four one-way valves (Fig. 7-3). The right side of the heart receives CO_2-rich blood from the systemic circulation and pumps it to the lungs for oxygenation and CO_2 elimination. The left side of the heart receives freshly oxygenated blood

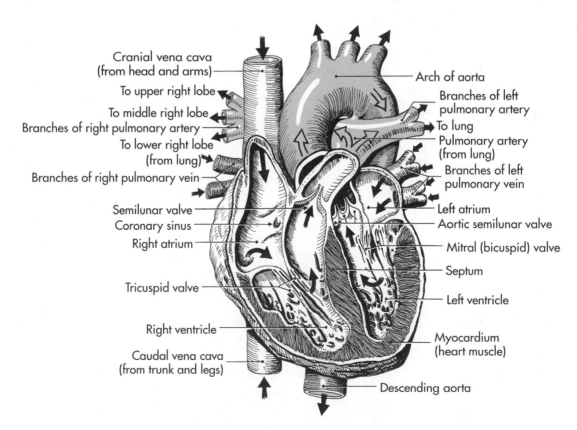

FIG. 7-3   Frontal view of the heart, with cutaway showing the heart chambers, valves, and major blood vessels. *(From McBride DF: Learning veterinary terminology, St Louis, 1996, Mosby.)*

from the lungs and pumps it to the rest of the body. Each side of the heart contains a chamber that receives blood from the large veins, a one-way atrioventricular valve that prevents backflow of blood into the receiving chamber, a pumping chamber that sends blood out through the arteries, and a one-way outlet valve that prevents blood backflow into the pumping chamber.

The receiving chamber of the right side of the heart is the right atrium. Blood flows into it from the venae cavae, the large systemic veins. When the right atrium contracts, it pumps blood through a large one-way valve, the tricuspid valve, into the right ventricle. The tricuspid valve gets its name from its three flaps, or cusps. When the right ventricle contracts, the tricuspid valve closes and blood flows out through the one-way pulmonary valve into the pulmonary artery, which carries blood to the lungs. When the right ventricular contraction is complete, the pulmonary valve closes, preventing blood from flowing back into the right ventricle.

The dynamics are similar on the left side of the heart (see Fig. 7-3). Blood flows into the left atrium from the pulmonary veins. When the left atrium contracts, it pumps blood through the mitral valve into the left ventricle. The mitral valve is named for the resemblance (in some ancient anatomist's eye) of its two cusps to the miter worn by high-ranking Catholic clergy. When the left ventricle contracts, the mitral valve closes and blood flows out through the aortic valve into the aorta, the beginning of the systemic circulation. When left ventricular contraction is complete, the aortic valve closes to prevent flow of blood back into the ventricle.

Each heartbeat is initiated and controlled by specialized areas and bundles of cardiac muscle cells. By its nature, cardiac muscle contracts without needing any external stimuli, but the activity of the many millions of individual cardiac muscle cells must be coordinated for the heart to contract in an organized, efficient manner.

Blood. Blood is a specialized connective tissue composed of fluid and cellular portions. The fluid portion is plasma, and the cellular portion is composed of red blood cells, white blood cells, and platelets.

Plasma is composed of water, some electrolytes, and some large plasma protein molecules. It serves to suspend the blood cells and dissolve the many substances that are transported in the blood. If removed from blood vessels, plasma clots. One of the proteins in plasma, fibrinogen, is converted through a complex series of steps to strands of fibrin. The fibrin strands form a meshwork that traps the rest of the cellular components and forms what is recognized as a *blood clot*. This blood-clotting process serves to temporarily obstruct leaking blood vessels and minimize blood loss caused by injury.

Red blood cells (RBCs), also called *erythrocytes*, are the most numerous of the blood cells, typically numbering in the millions per microliter of blood. In mam-

malian species, red blood cells do not normally contain a nucleus and are shaped like biconcave discs resembling tiny pillows. In birds, reptiles, and fish, they are normally nucleated and elliptic. The protein hemoglobin, which gives erythrocytes their red color, also gives them the ability to carry large amounts of O_2 to the body's cells.

White blood cells, also called *leukocytes*, typically number in the tens of thousands per microliter of blood. They are typically divided into the granulocytes (neutrophils, eosinophils, and basophils), which have stainable granules in their cytoplasm, and the agranulocytes (lymphocytes and monocytes), which lack cytoplasmic granules.

Platelets are not whole cells but rather are fragments of cytoplasm from large cells in the bone marrow. Their function is to help minimize blood loss from damaged blood vessels by adhering to the injured area and initiating the blood clotting process.

Fetal Circulation. A fetus developing in the uterus leads a parasitic existence. It derives all of its nutrition and O_2 from the mother's blood and sends its metabolic wastes and CO_2 into the mother's blood for elimination. The "life support" system of the fetus that makes this possible is the placenta, to which the fetus is connected by the umbilical cord. The placenta surrounds the fetus and attaches to the wall of the uterus so that placental and maternal blood vessels are in close proximity to each other. There is normally no direct mixing of fetal and maternal blood.

The umbilical vein carries nutrient-rich, freshly oxygenated blood from the placenta to the fetus. The fetal heart then pumps the blood throughout the developing fetus, where the blood releases its nutrients and O_2 and picks up wastes and CO_2. The umbilical arteries return this waste-filled blood to the placenta, where it exchanges its wastes for nutrients and O_2.

Because the fetal lungs are essentially nonfunctional until birth, the fetal blood vascular system has two major modifications that divert most of the blood away from the lungs. The foramen ovale is a hole in the interatrial septum of the heart, the wall between the left and right atria. This foramen allows some of the blood returning from the systemic circulation to flow from the right atrium directly into the left atrium, bypassing the lungs. The ductus arteriosus connects the pulmonary artery with the aorta. Most of the blood pumped out of the right ventricle flows through the ductus arteriosus into the aorta, and into the system circulation, again bypassing the lungs. The developing lungs need only a small amount of blood flow to meet their metabolic needs. At or soon after birth, both the foramen ovale and the ductus arteriosus normally close in response to the sudden pressure changes created by the functioning lungs.

Lymphatic Vascular System

The lymphatic vascular system basically serves to return excess tissue fluid to the blood vascular system. Along the way it filters the tissue fluid, "examines" it for foreign invaders, and manufactures defensive cells and antibodies to help keep the body healthy.

At the blood capillary level, more fluid flows out of the porous capillaries than returns to them. If not somehow removed, this excess fluid would accumulate in body tissues and cause progressive swelling. Lymph capillaries begin peripherally as blind-ended vessels that pick up this excess fluid, called *lymph,* and move it toward the thorax. The small lymph vessels merge to form larger vessels. These larger lymph channels contain small one-way valves, similar to the valves in veins. Combined with body movements, these one-way valves help propel the lymph to the thorax, where it is deposited back into the bloodstream.

Along the network of lymph vessels are small lumps of tissue called *lymph nodes.* These contain large accumulations of one type of white blood cell, lymphocytes, organized into collections called *lymph nodules.* The lymph nodes filter the lymph, removing debris and foreign invaders, and produce antibody-producing cells that are important components of the body's defense mechanisms.

Lymph nodules are also found in areas of the body other than lymph nodes. The spleen, a large, tongue-shaped organ located near the stomach, is a blood-storage organ, but it also contains large accumulations of lymph nodules. The thymus is a lymphoid organ, located in the caudal cervical/cranial thoracic region. It is of importance primarily in young animals. It helps "jump-start" their immune system and then gradually shrinks and disappears around the time of sexual maturity. Accumulations of lymph nodules are also found in the tonsils and scattered in the lining of the intestines.

THE RESPIRATORY SYSTEM

The primary function of the respiratory system is to exchange O_2 in oxygenated blood for CO_2, which is produced as a waste product by the cells. Secondary functions include vocalization (e.g., barking, mooing), body temperature regulation, and acid-base regulation.

Respiration occurs at two levels in the body. Internal respiration involves exchange of gases between the blood and the body's many cells and tissues, and it occurs at the cellular level throughout the body. Oxygen (O_2) carried in red blood cells is exchanged for carbon dioxide (CO_2) produced by tissue cells. External respiration involves exchange of gases between blood and the outside air, and it occurs in the lungs. Carbon dioxide in the blood is exchanged for O_2 from the air.

The respiratory system is made up of the upper respiratory tract, which consists of a series of tubes that connect the lungs with the external environment, and the lower respiratory tract, which consists of the structures within the lungs.

Upper Respiratory Tract

The upper respiratory tract starts at the tip of the nose. Inhaled air enters the nostrils and passes back through the nasal passages. The lining of the nasal passages contains extensive networks of blood vessels, and a ciliated epithelium that is coated with watery mucus. Blood circulating throughout the nasal lining warms the incoming air, the watery mucus humidifies it, and the cilia sweep foreign material that has become trapped in the mucus out of the nasal passages. These functions form a conditioning system that supplies the lungs with relatively pure, warm, humidified air.

From the nasal passages, inhaled air passes through the pharynx, or throat. This is a common passageway for both the digestive and respiratory systems. Through a series of intricate reflexes, the pharynx and the larynx help prevent swallowed material from entering the lower respiratory tract.

The larynx, commonly called the "voice box," is a short, irregular tube of cartilage and muscle that connects the pharynx with the trachea. In addition to its voice-producing function, it also acts as a valve to control air flow to and from the lungs. At the junction of the pharynx and the larynx is the epiglottis, a flap of cartilage that acts as a "trap door" to cover the opening of the larynx during swallowing.

Carrying air from the larynx to the lungs is the trachea, or "windpipe." Rings of hyaline cartilage prevent it from collapsing during inhalation. At its caudal end, the trachea divides into the left and right bronchi, which enter the lungs.

Lower Respiratory Tract

The bronchi enter the lungs and branch into smaller and smaller air passageways that eventually lead to tiny grapelike clusters of thin cells called *alveoli.* The alveolus is the actual site of gas exchange in the lungs. Each alveolus consists of a tiny, extremely thin-walled sac surrounded by elastic fibers and a network of capillaries.

Respiratory Mechanisms

The process of external respiration depends on physical mechanisms that allow air to move in and out of the lungs and control systems that set limits on and adjust the process.

Negative Pressure in the Thorax. Normally there is negative pressure (partial vacuum) in the thorax. Combined with the elasticity and pliable nature of the lungs, this causes the lungs to conform to the size and shape of the thoracic cavity. A small amount of pleural fluid lubricates the lung surfaces and the thoracic (pleural) lining.

Inspiration. Inspiration on inhaling is the process of drawing air into the lungs. It is accomplished by contractions of the sheet-like diaphragm and other muscles that act to increase the volume of the thoracic cavity. The lungs expand passively as the thoracic cavity enlarges, and air is drawn into them through the upper respiratory passages.

Exchange of Gases. Air that is drawn into the alveoli during inspiration contains high levels of O_2 and low levels of CO_2. Blood passing through the capillary networks around the alveoli contains low levels of O_2 and high levels of CO_2. Both gases move from areas of high concentration to areas of low concentration by a process called *diffusion*. Oxygen diffuses from the alveoli into the blood in the alveolar capillaries. Carbon dioxide diffuses the other direction, from the blood of the alveolar capillaries into the alveoli.

Expiration. Air rich with carbon dioxide from the alveoli must be eliminated from the lungs so that a fresh breath of O_2-rich air can be inspired. Expiration occurs as muscular contractions compress the thoracic cavity, expelling much of the air from the lungs.

Control of Breathing. Two systems control the process of respiration: a mechanical control system and a chemical control system. The mechanical control system sets normal limits on inspiration and expiration that allow rhythmic, resting respiration. Stretch receptors in the lungs sense when preset limits of inflation and deflation have been reached. They initiate impulses that travel to the respiratory centers in the brain, stopping inspiration or expiration and starting the opposite process. The chemical control system monitors the chemical composition of the blood. If it senses fluctuations in O_2 and CO_2 levels or pH, it initiates adjustments in respiration necessary to restore normal values.

THE DIGESTIVE SYSTEM

The digestive or alimentary system converts food eaten by an animal into nutrient compounds that body cells can use for metabolic fuel. The digestive system consists of a tube running from the mouth to the anus, with accessory digestive organs attached to it. Food moving through the tube is broken down into smaller, simpler compounds through the process of digestion. These simple compounds then pass through the wall of the digestive tract into the bloodstream through the process of absorption for distribution of nutrients to body cells.

The structure of a species' digestive system is largely dependent on its diet. Nutrients in the plant-matter diet of herbivores, such as horses and cattle, are largely incorporated within hard-to-digest cellulose. Herbivores depend on the help of microorganisms, such as protozoa and bacteria, to help break down cellulose through a process called *microbial fermentation*. At some point in their digestive tract, herbivores have a large "fermentation vat," where cellulose can be broken down into usable nutrients. In cattle this is the rumen, and in horses it is the much-enlarged large intestine. The digestive system of carnivores (meat eaters), such as dogs and cats, is much simpler. Carnivores depend on enzymes to break down their relatively easy-to-digest animal-source nutrients through the process of enzymatic digestion. Therefore, no large fermentation vat is needed. Omnivores (species eating a mixed diet), such as pigs, are somewhat intermediate. They depend primarily on enzymatic digestion, with a minor amount of microbial fermentation occurring in their large intestine.

Mouth

The mouth is where food is chewed and mixed with saliva in preparation for swallowing. Four types of teeth, arranged into upper and lower dental arcades, begin the process of digestion by cutting and crushing the food. The most rostral teeth are the incisors. Ruminants, such as cattle and sheep, do not have any upper incisors. They have a firm, fibrous "dental pad" instead. The four canine teeth, if present, are located at the rostral lateral corners of the mouth, adjacent to the incisors. The premolars are the rostral cheek teeth and the molars are the caudal cheek teeth.

Each tooth is made up of three different kinds of very firm connective tissues. The exposed portion, the crown, is covered by enamel, the hardest substance in the body. The root, which helps anchor the tooth in its bony socket, is covered by cementum. The bulk of the tooth is made up of a dense material called *dentin*.

Once the food has been chopped and ground by the teeth and moistened with saliva, it is swallowed. Muscular movements of the tongue and pharynx move the bolus of food back through the pharynx to the opening of the esophagus, where it begins its journey to the stomach and through the remainder of the digestive tract.

Esophagus

The esophagus is a muscular tube that connects the pharynx with the stomach. Food passes through it quickly on its way to the stomach; no significant digestion or absorption occurs in the esophagus. The size of the opening of the esophagus into the stomach is regulated by the cardiac sphincter. This muscular ring functions as a valve to seal the esophagus off from the stomach. In the normal digestive process, the cardiac sphincter opens only to allow swallowed food to pass into the stomach. It also relaxes to allow food to pass back up the esophagus in species that can vomit or ruminate.

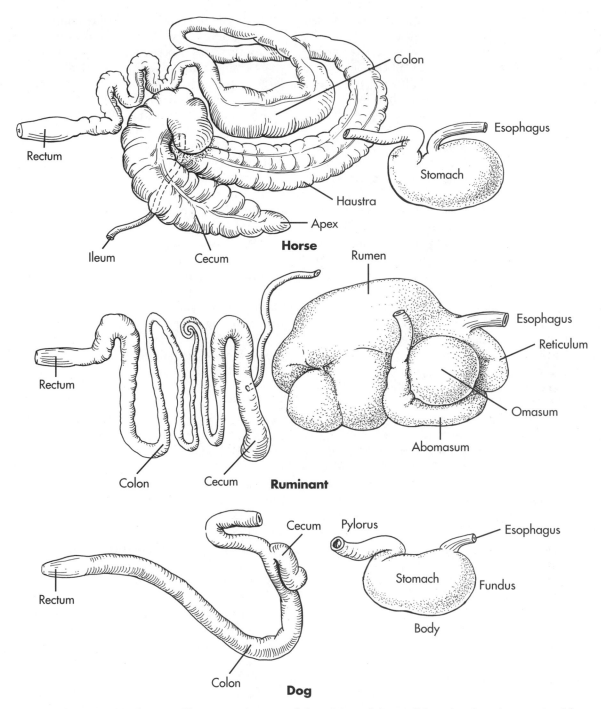

FIG. 7-4 Gastrointestinal tracts of horses, ruminants, and dogs. Most of the small intestines have been omitted for the sake of clarity. *(From McBride DF: Learning veterinary terminology, St Louis, 1996, Mosby.)*

Stomach

The stomach is an enlarged chamber where swallowed food is mixed with hydrochloric acid and digestive enzymes. In simple-stomached animals, such as horses and dogs, significant digestion of food begins in the stomach (Fig. 7-4). In animals with ruminant forestomachs, such as cattle and sheep, microbial fermentation begins before the material reaches the true stomach (abomasum).

Simple Stomach. The simple stomach of monogastric animals is a single chamber lined with large folds, the rugae, and dense accumulations of gastric glands. The gastric glands secrete hydrochloric acid and various digestive enzymes, which begin the digestion process, and mucus, which coats the stomach lining and keeps it from being digested along with the food. Very little absorption of nutrients occurs in the stomach. The stomach serves mainly to mix the food with the acid and enzymes to begin digestion. By the time the food leaves the stomach through the pyloric sphincter, it has been converted into a semi-liquid, homogeneous material called chyme.

Ruminant Forestomachs. Food swallowed by ruminant animals passes through three chambers before it gets to the true stomach. These chambers are called the forestomachs (see Fig. 7-4).

The esophagus opens into the largest forestomach, the rumen. This compartment makes up about 80% of the total stomach volume of ruminants and almost completely fills the left side of the abdominal cavity. Its main function is microbial fermentation. It is the main chamber where microorganisms break down the swallowed foods into simpler substances for absorption. Some breakdown products are absorbed into the bloodstream directly through the wall of the rumen, but the majority of the nutrient absorption takes place in the intestines.

The reticulum is the smallest, most cranial forestomach (see Fig. 7-4). It makes up about 5% of the total stomach volume of ruminants and lies against the diaphragm. Its opening is positioned directly ventral to the esophageal opening. Any heavy foreign material that is swallowed by the animal, such as wire, nails, or screws, usually drops directly into the reticulum. The honeycomb-like folds that line it serve to trap foreign material that enter the reticulum. This can irritate the reticular lining, and lead to traumatic reticulitis, commonly called "hardware disease." Normally the reticulum acts as a small fermentation vat also. Its food contents can move freely to and from the rumen.

The omasum is a dehydrating, grinding vat that makes up about 7% of the total stomach volume of ruminants. Positioned between the reticulum and the abomasum on the animal's right side, the omasum is lined by large muscular folds. Material entering the omasum from the reticulum has a very fluid consistency. Much of this fluid is absorbed from the omasum, and the muscular folds serve to further grind the food particles.

From the omasum, food enters the true stomach of the ruminant, the *abomasum*. Making up about 8% of the total stomach volume, the abomasum lies ventral to the omasum on the animal's right side. It corresponds to the simple stomach of a monogastric animal and has the same functions.

The stomach of ruminants functions somewhat differently than the stomach of monogastric animals. When ruminants graze, they swallow food that has received only a cursory chewing. In the rumen, this coarse material floats on top of the finer material. Once grazing is completed, the coarse material is periodically regurgitated back up into the mouth, mixed with saliva, chewed thoroughly, and reswallowed. This process, called *rumination*, occurs in about 1-minute cycles and is commonly referred to as "chewing the cud." The

reswallowed material is now much more finely ground and sinks into the ventral portions of the rumen, where microorganisms proceed with fermentation. In addition to releasing nutrients, the microbial action produces large quantities of gases, such as methane. These gases must be eliminated by the animal through a process called *eructation* (belching). If this gas is not regularly eructed, the rumen becomes distended with gas, resulting in a dangerous condition called *rumenal tympany,* or bloat.

Newborn ruminants, such as calves and lambs, essentially function as monogastric animals while they are nursing. Fermentation of the swallowed milk in the rumen and reticulum would likely result in digestive upsets. Closure of a structure called the *esophageal groove* enables the swallowed milk to bypass the rumen and reticulum, and pass directly into the omasum and abomasum. Closure of the groove is stimulated by the act of nursing, and by the presence of milk itself. When the maturing animal begins eating solid foods, the groove does not close, and the swallowed food enters the rumen and reticulum for microbial fermentation, as in adult animals.

Intestine

After leaving the stomach, chyme enters the tube-like intestine. Moved along by muscular contractions, the chyme is further digested by being mixed with secretions from the pancreas, liver, and glands in the intestinal wall. Most absorption of nutrients takes place in the intestines. Nutrient absorption is aided by the large surface area of the intestinal lining, which is covered by countless, tiny, finger-like processes called *villi*. Each villus contains tiny blood and lymph vessels at its center, into which nutrients are absorbed through the simple columnar epithelial covering.

The first portion of the intestine is the small intestine, so named because of its relatively small diameter. It is made up of three segments: the duodenum, jejunum, and ileum. (Note the similarity in name to, but difference in spelling from, one of the pelvic bones, the ilium.)

The duodenum is the first, relatively short segment of the small intestine. It receives the chyme through the stomach's pyloric valve. Ducts carrying bile from the liver and digestive enzymes from the pancreas enter the small intestine lumen (interior). The next segment, the jejunum, is the longest segment of the small intestine. This is where the majority of nutrient absorption takes place. The ileum is the last, relatively short segment of small intestine. It leads to the large intestine.

The large-diameter large intestine receives undigested and unabsorbed food material from the ileum. It absorbs water from the chyme and absorbs any nutrients not previously absorbed by the small intestine. The first segment of the large intestine is the *cecum* (Fig. 7-4). This blind-ended sac is small in carnivores, such as dogs, and very large in monogastric herbivores, such as horses. Next is the longest segment of the large intestine, the *colon* (see Fig. 7-4). The final intestinal segment is the rectum, which carries its contents, now called *feces*, to the anus for discharge from the body of defecation.

The anus is the caudal opening of the digestive system to the outside world. It is surrounded by ring-like sphincter muscles that allow the animal to consciously control defecation.

Accessory Digestive Organs

Several sets of salivary glands produce saliva, a watery fluid that is carried from the salivary glands to the mouth by ducts. Although saliva contains small amounts of digestive enzymes, its primary function is to moisten and lubricate food as it is chewed, making it easier to swallow. The drier the diet of the animal, the more saliva produced.

The pancreas is located near the duodenum and has both endocrine and exocrine functions. Its endocrine functions involve production of two hormones, insulin and glucagon, which help control glucose metabolism in the body. These hormones are discussed later with the endocrine system. The exocrine secretion of the pancreas, called *pancreatic juice,* is involved with digestion. Pancreatic juice is carried to the duodenum through the pancreatic duct(s). The main components of pancreatic juice are sodium bicarbonate, which helps neutralize the very acidic chyme entering the duodenum from the stomach, and a variety of digestive enzymes.

Located just caudal to the diaphragm, the liver is the largest gland in the body. Among its other important functions, it is an important "factory" that assembles simple nutrient molecules into larger compounds that can be used by the body's cells. The portal vein, which carries nutrient-rich blood from the intestines directly to the liver, supplies the raw materials for the factory. The liver also secretes bile, a greenish fluid that carries waste products of hemoglobin metabolism out of the body, and aids in breakdown and absorption of fats and fat-soluble vitamins from the intestine.

THE NERVOUS SYSTEM

The nervous system is a complex communications system in the animal body. It detects and processes internal and external information and formulates appropriate responses to the changes, threats, and opportunities that the animal continually faces. Nearly all conscious and unconscious functions of the body are controlled or influenced by the nervous system.

The basic functional unit of the nervous system is the nerve cell, the neuron. Neurons are specialized cells that respond to stimuli and conduct impulses from one part of the cell to another. Two types of fiber-like processes extend from the cell bodies of neurons: dendrites and axons. Dendrites are often multiple, and they conduct impulses received from other neurons toward the nerve cell body. Axons are usually single, and they conduct impulses away from the cell body, to other neurons or the effector organs, such as muscle cells. The junction of an axon with another nerve cell is called a *synapse.*

The branched end of an axon is called the *telodendron.* When a nerve impulse reaches the telodendron, it causes release of tiny sacs of chemicals, called *neurotransmitters,* into the narrow synaptic space. When the neurotransmitter molecules diffuse across the synapse to contact the cell membrane of the adjacent nerve cell, they induce some sort of change in the other nerve cell. Enzymes in the synaptic space then quickly inactivate the neurotransmitter molecules.

Neurons have three unique physical characteristics: they do not reproduce, their processes are capable of limited regeneration if damaged, and they have an extremely high oxygen requirement. Their lack of reproductive ability means that any loss of neurons, as from disease or injury, is permanent. Their dendritic and axonic processes sometimes regenerate if the nerve cell body is intact; this may restore function of reattached digits or limbs under some circumstances.

The high oxygen requirement of neurons makes them among the most delicate cells in the body. They begin to suffer permanent damage if deprived of blood supply for more than a few minutes. This is why cardiopulmonary resuscitation must begin within just a few minutes after cardiac arrest if there is to be any chance of complete recovery.

The main divisions of the nervous system are the central nervous system, the peripheral nervous system, and the autonomic nervous system.

Central Nervous System

The central nervous system consists of accumulations of nerve cell bodies, nerve fibers (axons), and supporting cells in the brain and spinal cord. The brain, consisting of the cerebrum, cerebellum, and brainstem, is housed in the skull (Fig. 7-5). The spinal cord is housed in the spinal canal formed by the vertebrae. Together they form the main control systems for the rest of the body.

Cross sections of the brain and spinal cord reveal two distinctly different-colored areas: the gray matter and the white matter. Areas containing accumulations of nerve cell bodies appear grayish grossly, and comprise the gray matter. Areas containing large accumulations of nerve fibers appear pale grossly, and make up the white matter.

The cerebrum is the largest, most rostral part of the brain (see Fig. 7-5). It consists of two large lateral cerebral hemispheres separated by a deep cleft. Its surface area is increased by systems of folds, the *gyri*, and grooves, the *sulci*. The cerebral cortex, or outer layer of the cerebrum is composed of gray matter. The medulla, or inner portion of the cerebrum, consists of white matter. The functions of the cerebrum are very complex and poorly understood. It is the center of higher learning and intelligence, and it functions in perception, maintenance of consciousness, thinking and reasoning, and initiating responses to sensory stimuli.

The cerebellum is located just caudal to the cerebrum (see Fig. 7-5). Its surface folds are small and packed closely together, giving it a "wrinkled" appearance. As in the cerebrum, the cerebellar cortex is made up of gray matter and its inner mudulla is made up of white matter. The cerebellum does not initiate movements but serves to coordinate, adjust, and generally fine-tune movements directed by the cerebrum.

The brainstem is the most primitive part of the brain (see Fig. 7-5). It forms the "stem" to which the cerebrum, cerebellum, and spinal cord are attached. Color distinctions between gray and white matter are difficult to observe in the brainstem. Functionally, the brainstem maintains the vital functions of the body. Centers in the brainstem control respiration, body temperature, heart rate, gastrointestinal tract function, blood pressure, appetite, thirst, and sleep/wake cycles. Severe damage to vital centers in the brainstem usually results in immediate death.

The spinal cord is the caudal continuation of the brainstem. On cross section, the gray matter forms a butterfly-shaped area in the central area of the spinal cord (Fig. 7-6). The white matter forms the outer cortex. Spinal nerves exit and enter the spinal cord between each set of adjacent vertebrae. They carry information to and from the peripheral portion of the nervous system.

Peripheral Nervous System

The peripheral nervous system consists of cord-like nerves that run throughout the body. The nerves are actually bundles of axons that carry impulses between the central nervous system and the rest of the body. Nerves that carry only information toward the central nervous system are called *sensory nerves*. Those that carry only instructions from the central nervous system out to the body are called *motor nerves*. Most nerves are *mixed nerves,* a combination of both sensory and motor nerves.

Autonomic Nervous System

The autonomic nervous system is the "self-governing" portion of the nervous system. It operates independent of conscious thought to maintain *homeostasis,* a constant internal environment in the body. Primarily a

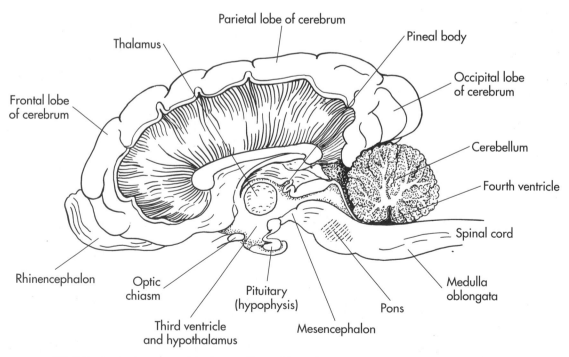

FIG. 7-5 Sagittal section of the brain. *(From McBride DF:* Learning veterinary terminology, *St Louis, 1996, Mosby.)*

motor system, the autonomic nervous system consists of two parts, the sympathetic system and the parasympathetic system, which have opposite effects and are in constant balance with each other.

The sympathetic system produces the "fight or flight" reaction in response to real or perceived threats. In a time of crisis or physical threat, the heart rate and blood pressure increase, the air passageways in the lungs and the pupils of the eyes dilate, digestive tract activity decreases, and the hairs stand on end, producing "raised hackles." The net effect is to prepare the body for intense physical exertion and to make the animal look larger and more threatening.

The parasympathetic system has the opposite effect. It is the "rest and restore" system. It predominates during relaxed, routine, business-as-usual states. The heart rate and blood pressure decrease, the air passageways in the lung and the pupils of the eyes constrict, and digestive tract activity increases. The net effect is to allow the body to relax and rejuvenate itself.

THE MUSCULAR SYSTEM

The general function of muscle is to move the body, both internally and externally. The nervous system gives the orders and the muscular system is among the most important systems that carry them out. There are three distinctly different kinds of muscle in the body: skeletal muscle, cardiac muscle, and smooth muscle.

Skeletal Muscle

Skeletal muscle derives its name from the fact that it moves the skeleton. It is also known as voluntary striated muscle because it is under conscious control, and its cells, at the microscopic level, have a striped or striated appearance.

Skeletal muscle cells (myocytes) are shaped like long cylinders or fibers. These very large cells usually have multiple nuclei. Most of their mass is made up of smaller myofibrils that are, themselves, made up of smaller protein filaments. The net effect is an intricate arrangement of filaments that can slide over each other, shortening the muscle cell when it contracts.

Skeletal muscle fibers respond to impulses delivered by nerves. The "connection" of a nerve fiber with a skeletal muscle fiber is called the *neuromuscular junction*. Each nerve fiber supplies more than one muscle fiber. A motor unit is made up of a nerve fiber and all of the muscle fibers it supplies. If there is a small number of muscle fibers per nerve fiber, fine, delicate movements are possible. The muscles that move the eyeball fall into this category. On

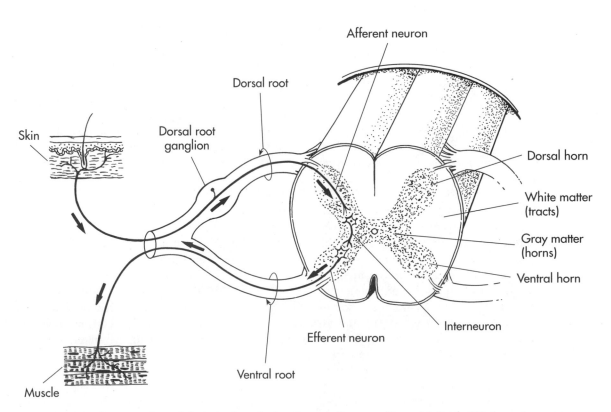

FIG. 7-6 Cross section of the spinal cord, showing a reflex arc. *(From McBride DF: Learning veterinary terminology, St Louis, 1996, Mosby.)*

the other hand, muscles that must make very large, powerful movements, such as the leg muscles, have large numbers of muscle fibers supplied by each nerve fiber.

Skeletal muscles are usually attached to bones at both ends by tendons. The more stable of the muscle's attachments is called its *origin*. The more movable of the attachments is called the *insertion*.

Cardiac Muscle

Cardiac muscle is found only in the heart. It is also known as involuntary striated muscle because it is not under conscious control and its cells are striped, or striated.

Cardiac muscle cells have no characteristic shape. Rather, they form an intricate branching network in the heart. They are firmly attached to each other, which allows considerable force to be generated as they contract.

Cardiac muscle cells each have an innate contractile rhythm that does not require an external nerve supply. The rhythmic contractions of the heart chambers are coordinated by a system of specialized cardiac muscle cells. The heart does have an autonomic nerve supply, but it does not initiate contractions of the muscle cells: it serves to modify them. Sympathetic stimulation increases the rate and force of cardiac muscle contractions. This is part of the "fight or flight" response. Parasympathetic stimulation has the opposite effect; it decreases the rate and force of contraction. Through this autonomic stimulation, the rate and force of cardiac contractions can be adjusted according to the body's needs.

Smooth Muscle

Smooth muscle is found mainly in internal organs. It is called "smooth" because its cells do not show any stripes or striations under magnification. It is sometimes called involuntary muscle because it is not under conscious control.

Cells of smooth muscle are spindle shaped, being wide in the middle and tapered at the ends. Depending on their location, they may be short and thick or long and fiber-like. Two different types of smooth muscle are found in the body: visceral smooth muscle, found in hollow abdominal organs, and multi-unit smooth muscle, found where fine contractions are needed.

Visceral smooth muscle occurs in large sheets in the walls of the gastrointestinal tract, uterus, and urinary bladder. These muscle cells are linked, so entire areas of cells act as a large unit. Nerve supply is autonomic and serves mainly to modify contractions. Sympathetic stimulation (fight or flight) decreases activity, whereas parasympathetic stimulation (rest, rejuvenation) increases it.

Multi-unit smooth muscle consists of individual muscle units that each require specific nerve stimulation to contract. Unlike visceral smooth muscle cells, these muscle cells are not linked, so their contractions are localized and discrete. Multi-unit smooth muscle is found where

fine, though involuntary, movements are needed, such as in the iris and ciliary body of the eye, the walls of blood vessels, and the walls of tiny air passageways in the lungs.

THE SENSES

The senses are the means by which the body monitors its internal and external environment. Sensory receptors are specialized nerve endings that convert mechanical, thermal, electromagnetic, and chemical stimuli from the environment into nervous impulses. When sensory impulses reach the central nervous system, they are perceived as such sensations as smell, taste, or sight.

Various sensations are received and interpreted by the central nervous system. The five senses we usually think of, hearing, smell, taste, touch, and sight, are not the only sensations perceived by the central nervous system. For our purposes, nine sets of sensations will be discussed. They are the following:

General Senses
- Tactile sense
- Temperature sense
- Kinesthetic sense
- Pain sense

Special Senses
- Gustatory sense
- Olfactory sense
- Auditory sense
- Vestibular sense
- Visual sense

General Senses

The *general senses* are so named because they are distributed generally throughout the body or over the entire skin surface. Their receptors are fairly simple, modified nerve endings. The tactile sense, or the sense of touch, perceives mechanical contact with the surface of the body. The temperature sense is a thermal sense that perceives hot and cold. The position of the limbs is monitored by the kinesthetic sense, a mechanical sense that provides information on the position of joints and the relative force exerted by muscles and tendons. The sense of pain can be set off by overloads of mechanical, thermal, or chemical stimuli.

Special Senses

The *special senses* are so named because their sensory receptors are concentrated in certain areas, rather than being generally distributed. All of the receptors for the special senses are located in the head. Also, in several cases, the sensory receptor cells are aided by some very sophisticated accessory structures.

Gustatory Sense. The gustatory sense is the sense of taste, a chemical sense. It detects chemical substances that are taken into the mouth and dissolved in saliva. The receptors are located in tiny taste buds found mainly on the tongue. Each taste bud has an opening on its surface, the taste pore, into which hair-like microvilli from the receptor cells project. When dissolved chemical substances enter the taste pore, their molecules interact with the microvilli, generating impulses that travel to the brain and are interpreted as various tastes.

Olfactory Sense. The olfactory sense, the sense of smell, is also a chemical sense. It detects chemical substances in the inhaled air. The receptor cells are located in the epithelium of the nasal passages. Hair-like microvilli from the olfactory cells project up into the mucous layer that overlies the nasal epithelium. When chemical substances dissolve in the mucus, the microvilli are stimulated and information about odors is transmitted to the brain.

Auditory Sense. The auditory sense is the sense of hearing. Through a complex set of auditory passageways and ear structures, mechanical vibrations of air molecules are converted into impulses that the brain decodes as sounds. Sound waves from the environment are collected by the external ear structures, amplified and transmitted through the middle ear structures, and converted to impulses in the inner ear. Most of the ear structures are located in the temporal bones of the skull (Fig. 7-7).

The external ear is made up of the pinna (ear flap), external auditory canal, and tympanic membrane (eardrum). The pinna is a cartilaginous funnel that collects sound waves and directs them medially into the external auditory canal, which leads to the tympanic membrane. The tympanic membrane is a thin, connective tissue membrane that is tightly stretched across the opening into the middle ear. Sound waves cause the membrane to vibrate.

Medial to the tympanic membrane is the air-filled middle ear cavity, which transmits vibrations of the tympanic membrane to the inner ear via three tiny bones, the ossicles. The first bone, the malleus, is attached to the medial surface of the tympanic membrane. It forms a tiny joint with the second bone, the incus, which forms a joint with the third bone, the stapes, which is in contact with the cochlea of the inner ear. Vibrations of the tympanic membrane are transmitted by the ossicles to the inner ear. Air pressure within the middle ear must equilibrate with the atmospheric pressure of the external air to prevent undue bulging of

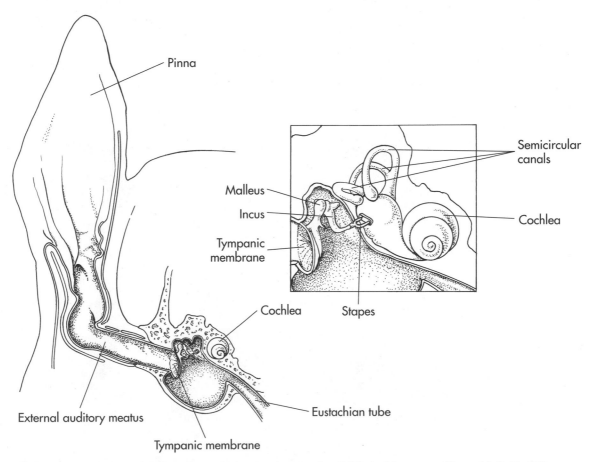

FIG. 7-7 Cross section of the canine ear, with inset showing the middle and inner ear. *(From McBride DF: Learning veterinary terminology, St Louis, 1996, Mosby.)*

the tympanic membrane. The eustachian tube, which links the middle ear with the pharynx, accomplishes this pressure equilibration as the animal swallows.

The inner ear contains the cochlea, which houses the receptor apparatus for hearing, as well as the vestibular sensory system. The cochlea is a fluid-filled space shaped like a hollow spiral snail shell. Running along its length, like a ribbon, is the organ of Corti, which contains the receptor cells for hearing. When sound wave vibrations are transmitted to the cochlear fluid, the fluid movements distort the microvilli on the receptor cells. This generates impulses that carry information on sounds to the brain.

Vestibular Sense. The vestibular sense, also a mechanical sense, monitors balance and head position. Its receptors are contained in two structures of the inner ear: the vestibule and the semicircular canals. Together with the cochlea, these structures make up the inner ear.

The vestibule consists of two fluid-filled spaces in each inner ear that contain patches of sensory epithelium on their floor. The sensory cells have hair-like microvilli that project into an overlying coat of gelatinous material. This gelatinous layer contains tiny crystals of calcium carbonate, the otoliths. Any tilting or linear motion of the head causes movement of the otoliths, which distorts the microvilli, generating ner-

vous impulses. These vestibular impulses carry information to the brain about changes in the position and linear motion of the head.

The semicircular canals are three fluid-filled canals of semicircular shape on each side of the head (Fig. 7-7). Parts of the semicircular canals are oriented in different planes, at right angles to each other, much like two walls and a ceiling join at a corner. At one end of each canal are the receptors, which contain sensory cells that are very similar to those of the vestibule. Hair-like microvilli of the sensory cells project into an overlying layer of gelatinous material. Rotation of the head in any plane moves the fluid in a semicircular canal and stimulates its sensory cells. The resulting impulses carry information to the brain about rotary motion of the head.

Visual Sense. The *visual sense* (sight) is the only well-developed electromagnetic sense of mammals. Its receptor organ, the eye, has a complex organization of component parts that function together to gather and focus light rays on photoreceptor cells (Fig. 7-8). When stimulated by light, the sensory cells of the inner eye generate impulses that the brain interprets as light.

The outer covering of the eyeball or globe is a dense, fibrous connective tissue layer that supports it and gives it shape. The clear "window" on the rostral portion of

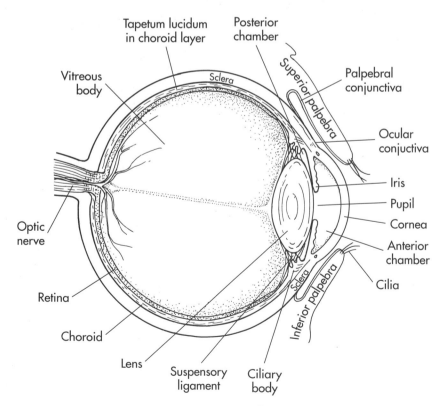

FIG. 7-8   Cross section of the eye. *(From McBride DF:* Learning veterinary terminology, *St Louis, 1996, Mosby.)*

the eye is the cornea (see Fig. 7-8). Light rays enter the eye through the cornea and are focused on the photoreceptors at the caudal portion of the eye. Although the cornea is composed of fibrous connective tissue, it normally contains just enough water to render it transparent. The sclera comprises the rest of the fibrous outer layer of the globe. Because of its white color, the sclera is commonly referred to as the "white" of the eye.

Caudal to the cornea is the fluid-filled space called the *anterior chamber,* and the colored iris (see Fig. 7-8). The watery fluid that fills the anterior chamber is called *aqueous humor* and is produced by cells caudal to the iris. The iris is a muscular diaphragm that controls the size of the aperture at its center, the pupil. In bright light, the iris contracts, reducing the size of the pupil to protect the sensitive photoreceptor cells. In dim light, the iris relaxes, enlarging the pupil to allow more light to enter.

Caudal to the iris is a transparent, biconvex, elastic, crystalline structure, the *lens* (see Fig. 7-8). The lens is responsible for the process of accommodation, focusing the light rays on the photoreceptor cells in the caudal portion of the eye to allow for near and far vision. Around its periphery the lens is connected to the ciliary body by tiny suspensory ligaments. The ciliary body contains the muscles responsible for changing the shape of the lens as required to focus the light rays. The muscles in the ciliary body are oriented such that when the animal is looking at something very close, they contract and allow the lens to assume its more natural rounded shape, focusing the close-up image on the photoreceptors. For distant objects, the ciliary muscle relaxes, allowing the globe's natural elasticity to pull the lens into a more flattened shape more appropriate for distant vision.

The area caudal to the lens is filled with a transparent, gelatinous substance called the *vitreous humor* (see Fig. 7-8). The light rays pass through this substance on their way to the photoreceptor-containing layer that lines the caudal portion of the inner eye, the retina.

The retina is where visual images are formed. It is a complex, multi-layered structure that lines most of the interior of the eye caudal to the lens. It is composed of the photoreceptor cells, called *rods* and *cones,* and several layers of nerve cell bodies and synapses that integrate and relay information from the receptor cells to the brain. The rods and cones have different shapes and different functions. The rods are long and narrow, and are more sensitive to light than the cones. They do not, however, detect colors or detail well. They are the receptors for dim light vision. The cones are somewhat "flask" shaped, and detect detail and colors well. The area of the retina where nerve fibers converge to form the optic nerve is called the *optic disc.* No rods or cones are present there; it is the "blind spot" of the eye.

The eye is a very sensitive organ that is protected by accessory structures. These include the conjunctiva, the eyelids, and the lacrimal apparatus.

The conjunctiva is a thin membrane that lines the underside of the eyelids and covers the outer aspect of the eyeball. Its transparency allows the sclera of the globe and the blood vessels of the eyelids to show through. Abnormalities, such as anemia or jaundice, can easily be seen by examining the conjunctiva.

The eyelids are dorsal (upper) and ventral (lower) folds of skin lined by conjunctiva that cover and protect the eye when the animal blinks or sleeps. The medial and lateral junctions of the eyelids are the medial canthus and lateral canthus of the eye, respectively. The third eyelid, or membrana nictitans, is a plate of cartilage covered by conjunctiva located medially between the eyelids and the eyeball.

The lacrimal apparatus is concerned with production and drainage of tears from the surface of the eye. The lacrimal glands, which produce tears, are located dorsal to the lateral canthus of the eye. Tears flow down over the surface of the eye, aided by blinking movements of the eyelids. At the medial canthus of the eye are the lacrimal puncta, two small openings, one in the upper lid margin and one in the lower lid margin, that drain tears from the eye. From the lacrimal puncta the tears drain into the lacrimal sac and then the nasolacrimal duct, which carries the tears into the nasal passages.

THE ENDOCRINE SYSTEM

The endocrine system consists of glands in various parts of the body that secrete minute amounts of chemical substances called *hormones* directly into the bloodstream, rather than through ducts. These hormones circulate throughout the body and bind to their respective target cells, causing changes in the activity of those cells.

The endocrine system and the nervous system are partners in regulating and controlling functions in an animal's body. The nervous system operates on a short time scale; it can respond rapidly to changes but is not well suited to sustained, long-term activity. The endocrine system does not respond as rapidly as the nervous system, but it can maintain secretion of hormones for very long periods.

Recent studies about the functioning of animal bodies shows that they are even more complex than we earlier thought. Nowhere is this more true than in the endocrine system. Hormones, of one sort or another, are produced throughout the body. Some work locally, whereas others circulate to distant parts of the body. For purposes of clarity and brevity, this chapter deals only with the major endocrine glands.

Hypothalamus

The hypothalamus is a part of the brainstem. Together with the pituitary gland, it controls many of the other major endocrine glands. It is extensively connected by nerve fibers to various parts of the brain dorsally, and by nerve fibers and blood vessels to the pituitary gland ventrally. It is a vital link between the nervous system and the endocrine system.

The hypothalamus influences the pituitary gland by two different mechanisms. It produces hormones, called *releasing* and *inhibiting factors,* that travel down to the anterior part of the pituitary gland through short blood vessels. Here they cause release or inhibition of the anterior pituitary's various hormones. The hypothalamus also produces two hormones that are carried down nerve fibers to the posterior portion of the pituitary gland for storage and release.

Pituitary Gland

The pituitary gland is often called the "master endocrine gland," because many of the hormones it produces direct the activity of other major endocrine glands. The pituitary is a pea-sized gland connected by a stalk to the hypothalamus. In reality it is two separate glands, the anterior and posterior pituitary glands, that are physically joined into one structure.

Anterior Pituitary Gland. The anterior pituitary gland produces and releases six hormones: growth hormone (GH), prolactin, thyroid-stimulating hormone (TSH), follicle-stimulating hormone (FSH), luteinizing hormone (LH), and adrenocorticotropic hormone (ACTH).

Growth hormone (GH), as its name implies, stimulates growth in young animals. It also plays an important role in the general metabolism of body cells in animals of any age.

Prolactin has a known effect only in females. It helps initiate and maintain milk secretion in the mammary glands.

Thyroid-stimulating hormone (TSH), as its name implies, stimulates thyroid hormone production and release.

Follicle-stimulating hormone (FSH) derives its name from its effect in females, in which it stimulates production of follicles in the ovary. In males it stimulates production of spermatozoa in the testes.

Luteinizing hormone (LH) also derives its name from its effect in females, in which it promotes ovulation of a mature ovarian follicle and the follicle's conversion into a corpus luteum. In males it stimulates the testes to produce testosterone.

Adrenocorticotropic hormone (ACTH) stimulates the cortex of the adrenal gland to produce and release its hormones.

Posterior Pituitary Gland. The posterior pituitary gland does not produce any hormones itself, but it stores and releases two hormones produced in the hypothalamus.

Antidiuretic hormone (ADH), also called vasopressin, causes the kidneys to conserve water, producing more concentrated urine. It is released when the body becomes dehydrated.

The primary effects of oxytocin, the second hormone stored in the posterior pituitary, are to promote uterine contractions at parturition and milk letdown from a lactating mammary gland.

Thyroid Gland

The thyroid gland consists of two lobes that may or may not be connected. One lobe is located on either side of the larynx in the neck region. The thyroid gland produces two hormones: thyroxine and calcitonin. Thyroxine produces an effect similar to that of growth hormone; it is necessary for normal growth and it helps regulate metabolism in the cells of animals of any age. The other thyroid hormone, calcitonin, regulates the blood calcium level and is secreted when blood calcium levels are abnormally high.

Parathyroid Glands

The parathyroid glands are several small nodules located in, on or near the thyroid gland. The effects of the hormone they produce, parathormone, oppose those of calcitonin. Parathormone acts to regulate the blood calcium level and is secreted when blood calcium levels become too low.

Adrenal Glands

The adrenal glands are located near the kidneys. They actually consist of two completely different glands, one inside the other. The adrenal cortex, the more superficial gland, produces three groups of hormones: glucocorticoids, mineralocorticoids, and sex hormones. The adrenal medulla, the inner gland, produces two hormones that are very similar to each other: epinephrine and norepinephrine.

Adrenal Cortical Hormones. Glucocorticoid hormones are the basis for cortisone-type drugs. Their primary effects are to increase the blood glucose level through a number of mechanisms, decrease inflammation, and affect metabolism of fats (mobilization), proteins (catabolism), and carbohydrates (glucose production).

Mineralocorticoid hormones, primarily aldosterone, work mainly in the kidney to promote the retention of water and sodium, which the body needs in large amounts. It does this by promoting elimination of potassium, which the body cannot tolerate in large amounts.

Sex hormones, both estrogens and androgens, are produced in the adrenal cortices of both sexes. The amounts produced are relatively minor.

Adrenal Medullary Hormones. The hormones of the adrenal medulla, epinephrine and norepinephrine, are released under control of the sympathetic nervous system as part of the body's "fight or flight" response.

Pancreas

The pancreas is mainly an accessory digestive organ whose secretions are primarily digestive enzymes. Embedded among the enzyme-secreting units, however, are small nodules of endocrine cells, the islets of Langerhans. Two hormones are produced within the islets: insulin and glucagon. Insulin is necessary for the body's cells to use glucose for fuel. It prevents abnormally high blood glucose levels and allows glucose to enter the cells for use. A defect in insulin secretion or action leads to diabetes mellitus, characterized by abnormally high blood glucose levels and many metabolic difficulties. The other pancreatic hormone, glucagon, has the opposite effect, and tends to increase the blood glucose level.

Gonads

The gonads are the sex-cell–producing organs. The male gonads are the *testes* and the female gonads are the *ovaries*. In addition to their sex cell production, the gonads are also endocrine organs.

The main hormone produced in the testes is the male sex hormone, testosterone. It is produced at a fairly constant level throughout the year. Very small amounts of the female sex hormone, estrogen, are also produced in the testes.

Levels of the hormones produced by the ovaries fluctuate in a cyclic fashion, linked to the development of follicles and corpora lutea. Under stimulation of FSH from the pituitary, follicles develop in the ovaries. The developing follicles produce *estrogen,* which is responsible for the signs of "heat," or estrus. After LH from the pituitary has caused the follicle to rupture and release its ovum, it then stimulates the empty follicle to develop into a solid corpus luteum, which produces progesterone. Progesterone is necessary for maintenance of pregnancy. If the animal is pregnant, the corpus luteum is retained. If the animal is not pregnant, the corpus luteum lasts for only a short time and then regresses.

THE URINARY SYSTEM

The many metabolic reactions that take place in the body's cells generate a variety of chemical byproducts. Some of these substances are still useful to the body and are recycled, but others would be harmful if allowed to accumulate in the body. These harmful waste products must be eliminated. The urinary system is the primary means by which waste products are removed from the blood.

The urinary system consists of two kidneys, two ureters, the urinary bladder, and the urethra.

Kidneys

The left and right kidneys are located in the dorsal part of the abdominal cavity, just ventral to the most cranial lumbar vertebrae. Most animals have smooth, bean-shaped kidneys, although bovine kidneys have a lobulated appearance. Blood and lymph vessels, nerves, and the ureter enter and leave the kidney through the indented area, the hilus.

A rough-appearing outer cortex is wrapped around a smooth-appearing inner medulla. The area deep to the hilus region is the renal pelvis, the funnel-like beginning of the ureter.

The work of the kidneys is done at the microscopic level, in tiny waste-disposal units called the *nephrons.* Depending on the animal's size, each kidney may contain from several hundred thousand to several million nephrons.

Each nephron consists of a blood filter, called the *renal corpuscle,* connected to a system of tubules surrounded by a capillary network (Fig. 7-9). Renal corpuscles are located in the renal cortex. When blood enters the renal corpuscle, a portion of the plasma, along with its wastes, is filtered out into the first portion of the tubule, the proximal convoluted tubule. The balance of the blood that was not filtered out passes into the capillary network surrounding the rest of the nephron. The filtered fluid passes slowly through the rest of the nephron and is modified as it moves along. From the proximal convoluted tubule the contents pass to the loop of Henle, which dips deep into the renal medulla. Passing superficially out of the medulla, the loop of Henle continues as the distal convoluted tubule, and finally dumps its fluid contents into the collecting tubules, which carry the solution, now called urine, to the renal pelvis.

As the fluid that was filtered out in the renal corpuscle passes through the tubules of the nephron, it is chemically altered. Useful substances, like most of the water, are resorbed back into the blood of the capillary network. Waste products that were resorbed initially are secreted from the capillaries back into the tubules. By the time the fluid in the nephron reaches the collecting tubules, it has become urine.

Ureters

From each renal pelvis, urine is transported to the urinary bladder by the ureters, muscular tubes that conduct the urine by smooth muscle contractions. The ureters enter the bladder at oblique angles, forming valvelike openings that prevent backflow of urine into the ureters as the bladder fills.

Urinary Bladder

The urinary bladder is a muscular sac that stores urine and releases it periodically to the outside in the process called urination. Urine is constantly produced by the kidneys. As it accumulates in the urinary bladder, the bladder enlarges and stretch receptors in the bladder wall are activated when the volume reaches a certain point. A spinal reflex then initiates contraction

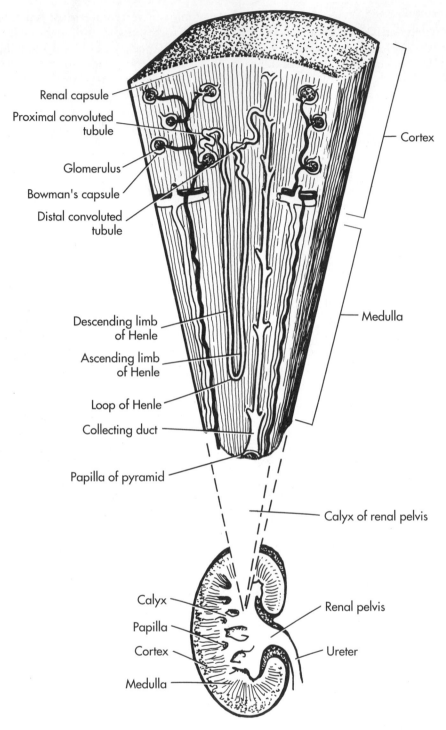

Renal capsule

Proximal convoluted tubule

Glomerulus

Bowman's capsule

Distal convoluted tubule

Cortex

Descending limb of Henle

Ascending limb of Henle

Loop of Henle

Collecting duct

Papilla of pyramid

Medulla

Calyx of renal pelvis

Calyx

Papilla

Cortex

Medulla

Renal pelvis

Ureter

FIG. 7-9 Cross section of the kidney, with wedge magnified to show renal corpuscles and collecting ducts. *(From McBride DF: Learning veterinary terminology, St Louis, 1996, Mosby.)*

of the smooth muscle in the bladder wall. A voluntarily controlled sphincter muscle around the neck of the urinary bladder enables conscious control of urination.

Urethra

The urethra is the tube that carries urine from the urinary bladder to the outside of the body. In females it is relatively short, straight and wide, and has a strictly urinary function. In males it is relatively long, curved and narrow, and serves both urinary and reproductive functions.

THE REPRODUCTIVE SYSTEM

The reproductive system is very different from other body systems. Whereas most other systems of the body contribute to the survival of the individual animal, the main function of the reproductive system is to help maintain the species. It influences other organ systems, but most parts of the reproductive system are not essential to life. Also, successful functioning of the mammalian reproductive system requires two animals, a male and a female.

Male Reproductive System

The male reproductive system is organized to produce male reproductive cells and transmit them to the female. Its main components are the testes, the vas deferens, the accessory sex glands, and the penis.

The testes are the male gonads. Their functions include production of the male reproductive cells (spermatozoa) and male sex hormones. Before birth the testes develop in the abdominal cavity. At or soon after birth they descend through slits in the abdominal muscles called the *inguinal rings,* into a sac of skin called the *scrotum* (Fig. 7-10).

The scrotum houses the testes and helps regulate their temperature. To produce viable spermatozoa, the testes must be maintained at a temperature slightly lower than body temperature. A muscle in the scrotum acts to raise or lower the testes to adjust their temperature.

Within the testes, spermatogenesis occurs in the seminiferous tubules. Each U-shaped tubule is connected at both ends to efferent ducts. When development of spermatozoa is complete in the seminiferous tubules, the spermatozoa move through the efferent ducts into the epididymis, a long convoluted tube lying along the surface of the testis. Spermatozoa are stored here until ejaculation. If spermatozoa are not expelled from the epididymis, they die there and are absorbed.

Leading from the epididymis proximally up to the pelvic portion of the urethra is the vas deferens. This muscular tube carries both spermatozoa and the fluid they are suspended in to the urethra for emission as a component of semen.

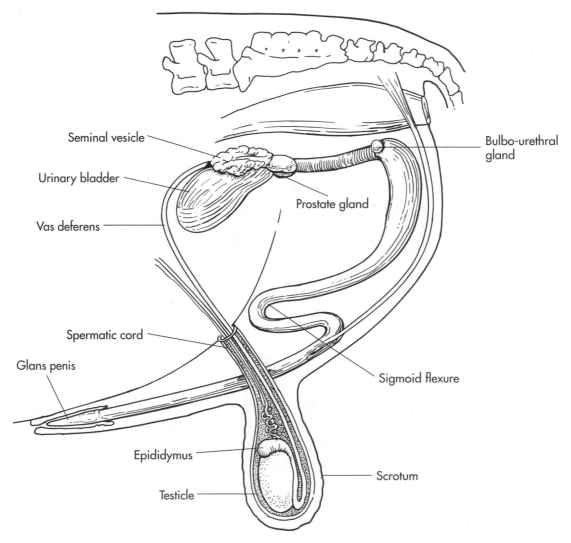

FIG. 7-10 Reproductive system of a bull. *(From McBride DF:* Learning veterinary terminology, *St Louis, 1996, Mosby.)*

Also entering the pelvic portion of the urethra are several types of accessory sex glands. The accessory sex gland found in all common mammals is the prostate gland. Other glands, such as the seminal vesicles and bulbourethral glands, are present only in certain species (see Fig. 7-10). Each is responsible for adding components of semen to the spermatozoa that are delivered by the vas deferens during ejaculation.

The *penis* is the male organ of copulation. It consists of roots, which attach it to the brim of the pelvis; a body, which consists primarily of erectile tissue; and the glans, which is the distal free end of the penis that is richly supplied with sensory nerve endings. The erectile tissue is made up of spongy networks of vascular sinuses surrounded by connective tissue.

With appropriate and adequate sensory stimulation, the penis becomes erect and ready for copulation. Through several mechanisms, more blood enters the erectile tissue than leaves it. The result is engorgement and stiffening of the penis, called *erection*.

Continued stimulation of the penis can produce ejaculation, the reflex expulsion of semen from the urethra. Ejaculation occurs in two rapidly successive stages. First, spermatozoa and seminal fluids are moved into the urethra. Second, semen is expelled from the urethra by rhythmic contractions of the muscles surrounding the urethra.

Female Reproductive System

The female reproductive system is organized to produce female reproductive cells, accept the male reproductive cells (spermatozoa), and allow one sperm cell to unite with each female reproductive cell, and then shelter and nourish the resulting developing fetuses until birth.

The ovaries are the female gonads (Fig. 7-11). Ovaries produce the female reproductive cells (ova) and hormones. Unlike spermatozoa, ova are not continually produced. At or soon after birth, the ovary contains all of the ova it will ever contain. They remain in an immature state until activated by cyclic hormonal cycles.

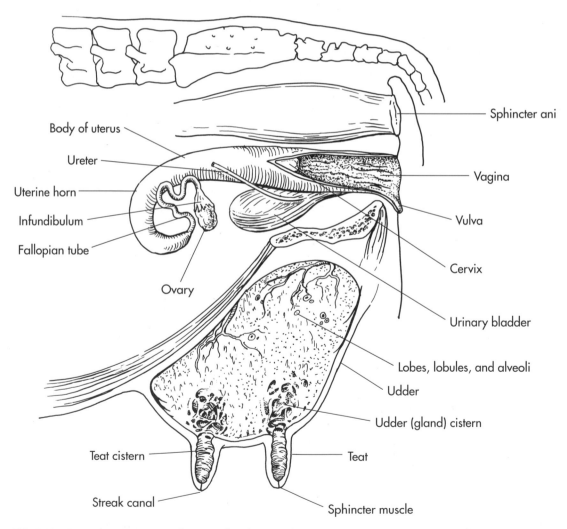

FIG. 7-11   Reproductive system of a cow, also showing the mammary gland. *(From McBride DF: Learning veterinary terminology, St Louis, 1996, Mosby.)*

Under the influence of FSH and LH from the pituitary gland, a few ova at a time develop in the *follicles* of the ovary (see Fig. 7-11). Immature ova are surrounded by a single layer of flattened follicular cells. When a particular follicle becomes activated, the follicular cells become more cuboidal and multiply to form many layers around the ovum. Spaces gradually form between follicular cells through secretion of fluid. By the time the follicle is mature, the ovum sits on a tiny hill of follicular cells and is surrounded by the fluid-filled antrum of the follicle. The mature follicle is a large, blister-like structure that protrudes from the surface of the ovary. As it develops, the follicle secretes increasing amounts of estrogen, which causes the physical and behavioral signs of heat or estrus.

Release of the ovum, called *ovulation,* usually occurs as a result of falling FSH levels and peaking LH levels. Ovulation is characterized by physical rupture of the follicle surface. As the fluid of the antrum rushes out, it carries the ovum with it. Once ovulation is complete, high LH levels cause the empty follicle to develop into the solid corpus luteum, an endocrine structure that produces progesterone, which is necessary for maintenance of pregnancy.

Partially surrounding each ovary, but not physically connected to it, are the oviducts, which are convoluted, tubular extensions of the uterus. At its ovarian end, each oviduct is flared to form the funnel-like infundibulum, which "catches" ova as they are released from the follicles.

The uterus is a hollow, muscular organ that is continuous with the oviducts cranially, and opens, via the cervix, into the vagina caudally. In most common domestic mammals, it consists of two cranial uterine horns that unite in a caudal uterine body.

The cervix is a powerful smooth muscle sphincter that functions to close off the lumen of the uterus from the lumen of the vagina most of the time. The only times the cervix is usually relaxed and partially dilated are at breeding and at parturition.

The vagina is the canal from the cervix to the vulva. It receives the erect penis during copulation and is the birth canal for the newborn at parturition.

The vulva is the external portion of the female genitalia. It consists of the vestibule, the short space between the vagina and the labia where the urethra opens; the clitoris, a small, sensitive erectile body homologous to the penis of the male; and the labia, which form the outer boundary of the vulva.

Fertilization and Pregnancy

At copulation, semen is usually deposited in the proximal vagina. Spermatozoa rapidly move through the cervix, into the uterus and up the oviducts through a combination of their own swimming actions and con-

tractions of the female reproductive tract. Normally the spermatozoa arrive at the oviduct before the ovum has entered it. They must spend some time maturing there to improve their capacity to fertilize the ovum. This final maturation process is called *capacitation.*

When the ovum arrives in the oviduct, spermatozoa swarm around it, but only one sperm cell is allowed to penetrate the ovum and fertilize it. Once a single spermatozoon has penetrated the ovum, entry of all others is blocked. Very soon after fertilization, the nucleus of the ovum and the nucleus of the spermatozoon fuse or combine. The fertilized ovum now has the full complement of chromosomes and is called a *zygote.*

The zygote immediately begins the process of cell division, called *cleavage,* as it is slowly moved distally toward the uterus by cells lining the oviduct. The single cell divides into two cells, the two cells to four, and so on. Cleavage proceeds so rapidly that the cells do not have time to grow larger between divisions. The overall size of the dividing zygote does not increase appreciably during this initial period. When it reaches the uterus, the zygote has formed into a hollow ball of cells, the *blastocyst,* which is ready to implant itself into the wall of the uterus.

Following implantation, the life-support system of the developing fetus, the *placenta,* develops. The placenta is a multi-layered, fluid-filled sac in which the embryo develops. It attaches to the uterine wall so that its blood vessels and the uterine blood vessels are intertwined. Nutrients and gases are exchanged between these maternal and fetal blood vessels. There is normally no direct mixing of fetal and maternal blood. The developing fetus is linked with the placenta via the umbilical cord, through which blood in the umbilical arteries and vein flows to and from the fetus.

The three-stage birth process, called *parturition,* occurs at the end of the gestation period (pregnancy). The first stage consists of uterine contractions that force the membrane-covered fetus distally against the cervix, causing the cervix to dilate. The second stage consists of the delivery of the newborn, accomplished by a combination of uterine and abdominal muscle contractions. The third stage is the delivery of the placenta, or afterbirth.

Milk Production. The mammary glands are specialized skin glands that produce secretions that are essential for nourishment of the newborn (see Fig. 7-11). Mammary glands are found in both males and females, but the hormone environment necessary for their full development and milk secretion only occurs near the end of pregnancy in females.

The process of milk production, called *lactation,* begins toward the end of pregnancy. Several hormones are involved, chiefly prolactin. The initial mammary secretion after parturition is called *colostrum* and differs from normal milk in composition and appearance. Colostrum has a laxative effect on the newborn and is important in transferring antibodies from the mother to the offspring. The intestine of the newborn can absorb only the large antibody molecules in the colostrum for a few hours after birth, so it is important that a newborn suckle colostrum as soon as possible after birth.

Continued production of milk is stimulated by suckling or milking. Sensory stimulation of the teat or nipple, either by the offspring's suckling or by milking, causes continued production of the hormones necessary to support lactation. Stimulation of the teat or nipple causes immediate release of oxytocin from the posterior pituitary gland. Oxytocin has the effect of squeezing milk out of the alveoli and small ducts of the mammary gland, into the large ducts and sinuses, where the newborn can extract it by suckling. The immediate effect of suckling or milking is called *milk letdown*. Cessation of suckling or milking results in the cessation of milk production; the mammary gland "dries up."

RECOMMENDED READING

Dyce KM: *Textbook of veterinary anatomy,* ed 2, Philadelphia, 1996, WB Saunders.

Frandson RD, Spurgeon TL: *Anatomy and physiology of farm animals,* ed 5, Malvern, Penn, 1992, Lea & Febiger.

McBride DF: *Learning veterinary terminology,* St Louis, 1996, Mosby.

Ruckebusch Y et al: *Physiology of small and large animals,* St Louis, 1991, Mosby.

CHAPTER 8

Pathology and Response to Disease

M.R. White

Learning Objectives

After reviewing this chapter, the reader should understand the following:

Ways in which tissues respond to injury
Phases of inflammation and the cells involved

Way in which injured tissues heal
Ways in which pathogens affect tissues
Types of immune response
Physiologic basis for vaccination
Hypersensitivity reactions

Pathology, simply stated, is the study of disease. Disease is any alteration from the normal state of health. Disease may range from a very superficial skin laceration to widely disseminated metastatic neoplasia (malignant tumors spread to many different organs). A pathologist is one who studies disease and often is responsible for accurate diagnosis of diseases, as well as determining the cause, or etiology, of those diseases. Pathologists are trained in different areas of expertise, including either anatomic pathology or clinical pathology. A veterinary pathologist is a specialist who, after receiving an advanced degree in veterinary pathology, is employed by veterinary schools, state diagnostic laboratories, or pharmaceutical companies.

The primary responsibility of a veterinary anatomic pathologist is the prosection (dissection) of cadavers (carcasses) presented for necropsy, which is analogous to an *autopsy* in humans. During necropsy the pathologist collects tissue sections from lesions, which are grossly observable diseased tissues, and examines them with a microscope. Evaluating tissues with a microscope is called *histopathology*. Histopathology may allow the

pathologist an insight into the etiology and prognosis of the disease. The prognosis is the expected outcome of the patient affected by the disease, and is usually stated as good, guarded, or poor. Veterinary anatomic pathologists also evaluate tissues that have been surgically removed by the veterinarian. Thus, these tissues are often referred to as *surgical biopsies*.

Veterinary clinical pathologists evaluate components of the blood as well as bodily fluids such as transudates and exudates. These provide valuable information regarding the causes and prognoses of diseases.

TERMINOLOGY

Pathologists use specific terms to describe the lesions observed at necropsy and with the microscope. Gross lesions are described by stating the location, color, size, texture, and appearance of the altered tissue. The diagnosis may be a morphologic (anatomic) diagnosis or an etiologic (cause) diagnosis. The morphologic diagnosis is usually limited to describing the lesion within that organ system. An example of a morphologic diagnosis is "acute necrotizing enteritis," which states that the intestine is inflamed and necrotic and that this occurred very suddenly. The corresponding etiologic diagnosis may be "enteric salmonellosis," which means that the animal had the intestinal form of infection by *Salmonella* bacteria. However, other bacterial and viral agents could also cause the lesions described in the morphologic diagnosis, so "acute necrotizing enteritis" does not always indicate a specific diagnosis of "enteric salmonellosis."

INFLAMMATION AND RESPONSE TO INJURY

Inflammation is a protective response of the animal's body to fight infection resulting from pathogens (disease-causing agents). Pathogens include viruses, bacteria, parasites, fungi, and molds. Pathogens are described in more detail later in this chapter.

Signs of Inflammation

The five cardinal signs of inflammation are *heat, redness, swelling, pain,* and *loss of function.* These signs result from complex interactions between the cells and fluids in the involved area. Initial vasodilatation (dilation of blood vessels) increases the flow of blood to the site of inflammation, resulting in an increase in temperature and redness. The swelling is caused by decreased flow of blood away from the site of inflammation, as well as possible edema, or increased fluid in the tissues. The pain and loss of function (if the inflammation is severe) are the result of pressure on the peripheral nerves at the site of inflammation. Additionally, the immune system and hemostatic (blood clotting) factors may be involved in the inflammatory process, making this a very integrated and complex series of biochemical events.

Cells of the Inflammatory Process

The cells involved in the inflammatory process are the leukocytes (white blood cells). Leukocytes include neutrophils, eosinophils, lymphocytes, and monocytes. Other cells throughout the body (but not within the bloodstream), such as mast cells and macrophages or histiocytes, also play a key role in the inflammatory process.

Neutrophils are the first leukocytes participating in the chain of events comprising an inflammatory reaction. The cells exit the blood vessels at the site by "squeezing" through the microscopic space between the endothelial cells lining the blood vessels. The primary function of neutrophils in the inflammatory process is phagocytosis, or ingestion of pathogens, as well as release of lysosomal enzymes, which destroy the pathogens. These enzymes are very toxic to certain

pathogens and include *myeloperoxidase, cathepsins,* and *proteinases.* Neutrophils are very short lived, surviving for only 24 to 48 hours once they leave the blood vessels and enter the host tissues.

Eosinophils, so named because they have eosinophilic (pink to reddish-orange) granules, also participate in inflammatory reactions. However, they are more specific than neutrophils and usually are only prominent in inflammation associated with parasitic infestations and allergic reactions. Like neutrophils, eosinophils have two major roles: (1) phagocytosis and (2) lysosomal enzyme release. Lysosomal enzymes from eosinophils include major basic protein, an enzyme that is effective against parasites, and arylsulfatase B and histaminase, which are regulators of the allergic response.

A lymphocyte is another type of important leukocyte in the inflammatory process. Like neutrophils, lymphocytes migrate to the tissue site of inflammation, but they have a very different role in the inflammatory process. They are responsible for humoral antibody production and cellular immunity. Lymphocytes can be divided into B-lymphocytes and T-lymphocytes; however, these two groups cannot be distinguished microscopically. B-lymphocytes can be transformed into plasma cells, which procure humoral entities. T-lymphocytes produce their effects by directly killing cells or by secreting lymphokines, chemical substances that allow macrophages to easily phagocytize pathogens.

Monocytes are inactivated macrophages. Once these cells leave the bloodstream and enter the tissue at the site of the inflammatory process, they become activated macrophages. Macrophages are the work horses of the inflammatory process; they contain a large number of lysosomal enzymes that kill pathogens. They are also capable of phagocytosis and may fuse together to form epithelioid cells or multinucleated giant cells. Both of these cell types may be observed in chronic inflammatory reactions. They attempt to surround and destroy the pathogens.

Inflammatory Exudates

An exudate is the visible product of the inflammatory process. It is usually composed of cellular debris, fluids, and cells that are deposited in tissues as well as on tissue surfaces, such as the serosal, mucosal, and skin surfaces. Exudates may be classified based on their primary constituent, such as serous, fibrinous, purulent (or suppurative), or others.

A serous exudate consists primarily of fluid with a low protein content. Cutaneous blisters are examples of lesions that contain a serous exudate. A fibrinous exudate is composed chiefly of fibrin, which is derived from a plasma protein, fibrinogen. Fibrinous exudate is observed in traumatic reticulopericarditis ("hardware disease"). This disease can occur when a cow ingests a metallic foreign body (nail or wire) that penetrates the forestomach (reticulum) and subsequently penetrates the diaphragm and pericardium, the membranous sac surrounding the heart. As a result, a large amount of fibrin collects in the pericardial sac. The proper morphologic diagnosis for this lesion is fibrinous pericarditis (Fig. 8-1).

Purulent or suppurative exudates are composed primarily of large numbers of neutrophils and cellular debris. Abscesses contain a purulent or suppurative exudate (Fig. 8-2).

A hemorrhagic exudate consists primarily of erythrocytes that have collected in a tissue after disruption of the vascular system. Other less common types of exudate include mucopurulent (or catarrhal), eosinophilic, and nonsuppurative. Mucopurulent exudates consist of a mixture of purulent and mucous exudates. They are commonly found in tissues that secrete mucus (i.e., have a mucous membrane), such as the intestinal tract and the respiratory tract. Eosinophilic exudates are composed primarily of eosinophils and are associated with such diseases as salt poisoning of pigs and eosinophilic myositis of dogs. Nonsuppurative exudates are composed primarily of monocytes, such as histiocytes and lymphocytes. The term *nonsuppurative* is usually restricted to exudates in only two anatomic sites: (1) the central nervous system and (2) the integumentary system (skin). Finally, exudates may consist of the combination of the above-mentioned types, such as *fibrinopurulent* or *necrohemorrhagic exudates*.

Vascular Changes Associated with Inflammation

The cellular response associated with inflammation is only a part of the inflammatory process; the blood vessels or vascular system are also involved. Blood vessels are highly dynamic structures that respond rapidly during inflammation. The first response of the blood vessel to vascular injury is dilatation, which means the diameter of the blood vessel increases, allowing more blood to flow into the affected area. This is caused by local release of histamine from mast cells. Next there is increased vascular permeability, which means the blood vessels become slightly "leaky." This is the result of contraction of endothelial cells lining the inside of blood vessels. Increased vascular permeability allows a wide array of proteins to pass through the vessel walls to the site of inflammation. Immediately after vascular permeability increases, the process of exudation allows an influx of leukocytes and red blood cells to the inflammatory site. Congestion of the blood vessels occurs in the next step, which means stasis or "sludging" of blood flow in the vessels from fluid loss through exudation.

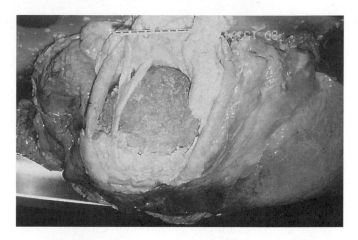

FIG. 8-1 Fibrinous pericarditis in a cow with traumatic reticulopericarditis.

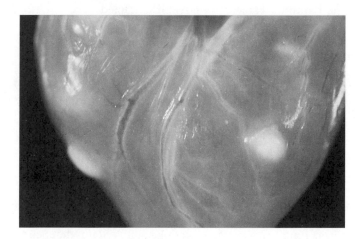

FIG. 8-2 A heart with multiple abscesses.

All of these events work in concert with the cells associated with inflammation such that the host is able to repair the injured site and defend itself against infection. The entire process occurs rapidly, beginning with vascular dilatation, which occurs within minutes of the initial insult, and ending with initiation of congestion within 8 hours of the initial vascular dilatation.

Healing and Repair of Damaged Tissues

The repair process really starts as soon as injury occurs, but healing is the last event to be completed in the inflammatory process. In almost every organ system the end result of tissue repair is fibrosis or scarring. The exception to this is in the central nervous system, which includes the brain and the spinal cord. Fibrosis does not occur in the central nervous system because it would be detrimental to the functioning of these vital tissues. Repair can take place by first-intention or by second-intention healing.

With first-intention healing of the skin, the edges of the wound surfaces close together with no discernible scarring. Proliferation of fibroblasts and endothelial cells rapidly forms a collagenous matrix. This matrix forms a bridge that brings the edges of the wound together. The last step in this process is reepithelialization, whereby the wound surface is re-covered with epithelium (cells lining the outer surface of the skin).

Wounds involving much greater tissue damage are repaired by second-intention healing. Fibroblasts and endothelial cells proliferate. Unlike first-intention healing, second-intention healing produces granulation tissue. Granulation tissue is a highly vascularized connective tissue that is only produced after extensive tissue damage. Reepithelialization eventually occurs unless excessive granulation tissue forms, a condition commonly referred to by lay people as "proud flesh." This excessive granulation tissue must be removed before the wound surface can be reepithelialized.

Fibrosis or scar tissue primarily comprises dense fibrous connective tissue and collagen and contracts when mature. In parenchymatous organ systems, such as the lungs, kidneys, liver, and spleen, scar tissue is usually characterized as a small, irregular focus that has shrunken beneath the capsule of the organ (Fig. 8-3).

PATHOGENS

Pathogens are infectious organisms that can cause disease in a host. Pathogenic agents include parasites, bacteria, fungi, rickettsiae, mycoplasmas, chlamydiae, and viruses. Many of these organisms are very specific in their ability to cause disease in only certain animal species. In most cases, they affect very specific organs or organ systems of the body.

Parasites

Parasites are organisms that have adapted to live within a host, deriving all of their nutrients from that host, ideally without killing the host. Chapter 11 contains an extensive discussion of internal and external parasites.

Bacteria

Bacteria make up another group of pathogens that cause disease in animals. Within the infected host, bacteria may be found in the interstitium (between cell layers), within inflammatory cells, or on epithelial surfaces. Bacteria are classified as either gram positive or gram negative, depending on their staining characteristics with Gram stain. As a general rule gram-negative bacteria contain endotoxins (substances that cause disease), while gram-positive bacteria contain preformed exotoxins. Some bacteria are pyogenic and cause the

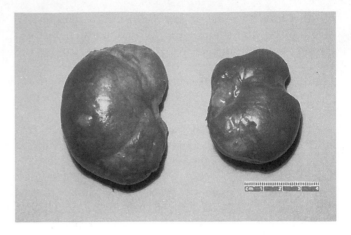

FIG. 8-3 Multiple bands of scar tissue on the outer surface of kidneys from a dog.

host to produce a purulent (suppurative) exudate (pus). See Chapter 11 for more information.

Examples of gram-negative bacteria include *Escherichia coli*, *Salmonella*, and *Klebsiella*. All three of these bacteria contain endotoxins, which are toxins that are a component of their cell walls. *E. coli*, which can be a normal inhabitant of the gastrointestinal tract, can also act as a pathogen. It can attach to the mucosal surface of the intestine and secrete toxins that are absorbed by the intestinal mucosal cells, or enterocytes. The enterocytes are metabolically altered to such an extent that they secrete fluid into the intestinal lumen, causing secretory diarrhea. The histopathologic lesions of this disease are minimal. Because there is minimal inflammatory response, diagnosis of this disease depends on culture of the particular serotype of *E. coli* responsible for the diarrhea, as well as confirmation of the bacteria attached to the intestinal surface.

Animals with bacterial infections are often febrile, lethargic, and anorexic. This is due in part to the associated endotoxins, which stimulate release of an endogenous pyrogen from neutrophils. Endogenous pyrogen is a protein that causes fever and associated lethargy and inappetence. However, this protein aids the animal by increasing the body temperature and allowing neutrophils to be more effective in killing bacteria.

Bacterial virulence factors determine the pathogenicity of bacteria. The surface of bacteria comprises such structures as pili, capsules, and the cell wall. These virulence factors allow the bacteria to more easily attach to and colonize tissues and minimize the host immune response. Additionally, bacteria may possess a wide variety of enzymes or proteins, also known as soluble factors, that inhibit host functions and provide the bacteria a "foothold" within the host.

Viruses

Viruses are extremely small organisms, ranging from 30 to 450 nm in diameter, that can cause disease in a wide variety of animals. For viruses to cause disease they must enter the animal's body, bind to the surface of a cell, enter the cell, and destroy it.

Certain viruses are specific for the type of cells they attack. For example, epitheliotropic viruses attack epithelial cells, such as respiratory, intestinal or urinary epithelium. The clinical signs of viral diseases are associated with death of the infected cells. For example, canine distemper virus, a morbillivirus, attaches to and destroys the epithelium of the dog's lungs. Dogs with distemper may develop coughing and respiratory distress because of the effect of viral infection of the lung. The result is interstitial pneumonia caused by the inflammatory infiltrates within the interstitium of the lung. Transmissible gastroenteritis (TGE) of pigs, caused by coronavirus, destroys the gastric and intestinal epithelium of preweanling pigs. Clinical signs include vomiting, diarrhea, dehydration, and death. A lesion of TGE is villous atrophy; affected intestinal villi become shortened and blunted and have an atrophic appearance (Fig. 8-4).

Viruses classified as neurotropic invade and destroy cells of the central nervous system (CNS). Examples of disease caused by these viruses include rabies and equine encephalitis. Rabies is caused by a rhabdovirus and has a worldwide distribution. Most cases of rabies are spread by animal bites; the virus is present in the saliva of infected animals. After the virus enters the body, it

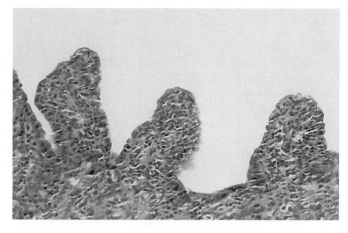

FIG. 8-4 Villous atrophy in a pig due to transmissible gastroenteritis virus (TGE). Note the blunt, short villi.

travels to the CNS by way of peripheral nerves. Once it enters the CNS it infects and destroys neurons. Animals infected with this virus develop behavioral changes and sometimes become aggressive, which may result in biting other animals or humans. The lesions of rabies are those of nonsuppurative encephalitis. Diagnosis is dependent on demonstration of the characteristic Negri bodies within affected neurons. Negri bodies are eosinophilic inclusion bodies within affected neurons.

As is the case of parasites and bacteria, a large number of viruses can infect animals. A list of some common viruses that cause disease in animals is presented in Table 8-1.

TABLE 8-1 Some viruses that cause disease in animals

Virus classification	Disease	Host	Lesions
Morbillivirus	Canine distemper	Canidae, mink, raccoon, ferret	Pneumonia, encephalitis
Herpes virus	Pseudorabies	Pig	Abortion, encephalitis
Herpes virus	Infectious laryngotracheitis	Avian	Laryngotracheitis
Adenovirus	Infectious canine hepatitis	Canidae	Acute necrotizing hepatitis
Papillomavirus	Sarcoid	Horse	Sarcoids (neoplasm)
Rhabdovirus	Rabies	Mammals	Fatal encephalomyelitis
Coronavirus	Transmissible gastroenteritis (TGE)	Pig	Enteritis, villous atrophy
Coronavirus	Feline infectious peritonitis (FIP)	Cat	Peritonitis, pleuritis
Alphavirus (*Arbovirus*)	Eastern, western Venezuelan equine encephalitis	Horse	Encephalitis

NONPATHOGENS

Disease can also be produced in animals by non-pathogens. Nonpathogenic causes of disease include trauma associated with mechanical, sonic, thermal, and electrical injuries, temperature extremes, and irradiation.

The primary effect of trauma, regardless of the initiating cause, is tissue necrosis and hemorrhage. Trauma is a physical wound or injury. A wound is an injury caused by physical means, with disruption of normal structures. An abrasion is an injury whereby the epithelium is removed from the tissue surface. A contusion is a bruise or injury with no break in the surface of the tissue. A laceration is a tear or jagged wound. A concussion is a violent shock or jarring of the tissue, a common injury to the brain after blunt trauma to the head. In all of these instances the inflammatory process occurs as described previously in this chapter, with the exception of destruction and removal of the pathogen.

THE IMMUNE RESPONSE

The immune system is another inherent protective mechanism of the body. This highly complex and complicated system has many components that, along with the inflammatory process, prevent pathogens from causing disease.

Responses of the immune system can be divided into humoral immune responses and cell-mediated immune responses. The primary components of the humoral response are antibodies, produced by plasma cells or plasmacytes, which are transformed B-lymphocytes. The other major subsets of lymphocytes, referred to as T-lymphocytes, play a major role in the cell-mediated response. B-lymphocytes are distributed throughout the body within the lymph nodes, spleen, Peyer's patches, and other organs. B-lymphocytes are so named because they were first discovered in the bursa of Fabricius, which is a lymphoid organ of birds (not mammals). T-lymphocytes are so designated because they arise from the thymus, a lymphoid organ of birds and mammals. All mammals, as well as birds, possess both B- and T-lymphocytes. These lymphocytes cannot be distinguished by their morphology because they look identical under the microscope; however, they can be differentiated by their function. They may also be differentiated by their cell surface markers, which are molecules attached to their surface, necessary for binding with antigens, antibodies, etc.

Response to Vaccination

Animals can be immunized (vaccinated) against a wide variety of diseases, ranging from blackleg in cattle to distemper in dogs. These vaccines are commonly administered by injection. The vaccine often consists of a portion of the pathogen, such as the cell wall of the causative bacterium or a small unit of the virus. After injection the vaccine does not cause disease but stimulates the cells of the immune system to develop antibodies against that particular pathogen. Upon the next exposure to that pathogen a vaccinated animal will not become infected because it has been immunized.

Humoral Immunity

Humoral immunity implies that antibodies are produced against a particular pathogen. When that pathogen enters the host's body it becomes coated with antibody, allowing it to be more easily destroyed by cells involved in the inflammatory process. Antibodies are protein molecules that can attach to the surface of cells and coat pathogens.

Antibodies can be detected in the serum of animals; the study and application of this science is known as serology. The level of antibodies present in the serum (blood) is reported as an antibody titer. Antibody titers represent the reciprocal of the highest dilution of the serum containing antibody that still gives a positive reaction to the serologic test being performed. Although a very high antibody titer to certain pathogens may indicate protection against or immunity to a specific pathogen, it may be very difficult to differentiate between vaccine-induced immunity or natural immunity. Natural immunity implies that the animal has been exposed to the pathogen by natural means rather than through vaccination. With natural immunity the animal may have previously become ill from infection with a specific pathogen and may have produced antibodies against this pathogen during the disease.

Antibodies, or immunoglobulins, can be classified by their molecular weight into immunoglobulin isotopes, including IgG, IgM, IgA, and IgE. The IgG immunoglobulin is the most common antibody and is found in the highest concentration in the blood. It helps defend tissues by opsonizing or coating the outer surface of pathogens, which allows them to be more easily phagocytized by macrophages.

The IgM immunoglobulin is the second most common antibody in the blood. It is the major immunoglobulin isotype produced in a primary immune response. It is more efficient than IgG in opsonization and neutralization of viruses. The antibody isotype IgA is of primary importance for mucosal immunity. This antibody is secreted onto the mucosal surface of such organs as the lungs and gastrointestinal tract. It binds to pathogens to prevent them from adhering to mucosal surfaces, preventing them from gaining a foothold in the body. The antibody isotype IgE is the primary immunoglobulin associated with Type-1 hypersensitivity reactions, which are discussed later in this chapter. It also plays a role in helminth infestations, along with certain cells from the inflammatory process, including eosinophils.

Cell-Mediated Immunity

The cell-mediated immune response primarily involves T-lymphocytes and macrophages. Much less is known about this type of immunity as compared with humoral immunity. Cell-mediated immunity begins when a T-lymphocyte binds the pathogen to its cell surface. The T-lymphocyte may then present the pathogen to a macrophage, which phagocytizes and kills it, or it may produce specific cytokines, also called lymphokines, such as *interleukin-1* or *interleukin-2*. These lymphokines stimulate macrophages to become more efficient in phagocytosis and pathogen destruction, and recruit more T-lymphocytes to the area.

Hypersensitivity Reactions

Abnormally severe inflammatory responses mediated by the immune system are called hypersensitivity reactions. These allergic reactions have been classified into four types: Type I (immediate); Type II (cytotoxic); Type III (immune complex); and Type IV (delayed).

Type-I hypersensitivity reactions occur within minutes after exposure to an antigen. An antigen is any foreign substance causing an abnormal immune response upon exposure to that substance. Animals may be exposed to antigens by direct contact, inhalation, ingestion, insect bites or stings, or injection. Examples of antigens include pollen, proteins (e.g., in food, milk, or bacterial cell walls), and plant resins (e.g., in poison ivy or poison oak). Antigens are often referred to as allergens when they evoke an allergic reaction.

Type-I reactions are mediated by IgE on the surface of mast cells located on mucosal surfaces (airways, intestines) and in connective tissues. Upon exposure the antigen is bound by IgE, causing the mast cells to release granules containing various factors, such as histamine, serotonin, and leukotrienes. These factors cause vasodilation, increased vascular permeability, smooth muscle contraction, and other inflammatory changes.

The severity and manifestation of a Type-I hypersensitivity reaction depend on the location and number of mast cells stimulated as well as the route of exposure and amount of antigen involved. Reactions may be relatively mild, such as *urticaria* (hives) after a bee sting or diarrhea after eating a particular food ingredient. However, Type-I reactions can also be very severe, such as acute anaphylaxis, which is characterized by profound hypotension (low blood pressure), pulmonary edema, and collapse, caused by massive exposure to an antigen.

Type-II hypersensitivity reactions involve destruction of certain cells by neutrophils and macrophages or by activation of complement. Complement is a group of enzymes that act in sequential fashion, leading to disruption of tissue or bacterial cell membranes, which results in that cell's destruction. An adverse reaction to blood transfusion is an example of a Type-II reaction.

Red blood cells contain on their cell surface antigens called *blood group antigens*. Animals of the same species tend to develop antibodies against blood groups other than their own. The red cells function normally and no immune response results if blood from one animal is transfused to a recipient with the same blood group. However, if blood is transfused into a recipient with a different blood group, the donor's red cells are destroyed by hemolysis (rupture) or phagocytosis, or become agglutinated (clumped). The first of such incompatible transfusions may be well tolerated, but it stimulates production of antibodies and red cells in a second transfusion are immediately destroyed by these antibodies.

In Type-III hypersensitivity reactions, antigens and antibodies interact to form immune complexes in various tissues, such as the skin, joints, eyes, lungs, or blood vessel walls. Macrophages gather in these areas to destroy the immune complexes, resulting in inflammation. Examples of Type-III reactions include rheumatoid arthritis and equine viral arteritis.

Type-IV hypersensitivity reactions occur hours after sensitized animals are again exposed to a particular antigen. These delayed hypersensitivity reactions reach their peak at about 24 hours after exposure and are mediated by sensitized T-cells. The tuberculin test used in cattle is a classic example of Type-IV hypersensitivity. A small volume of extract of *Mycobacterium tuberculosis* is injected into the skin of the animal. Normal cattle show no significant response to the injection. Cattle previously exposed to *Mycobacterium tuberculosis,* however, develop a large, warm swelling at the injection site within 12 to 24 hours.

RECOMMENDED READING

Carlton WW, McGavin MD: *Thomson's special veterinary pathology,* ed 2, St Louis, 1995, Mosby.

Cheville NF: *Introduction to veterinary pathology,* Ames, Iowa, 1988, Iowa State University Press.

Cottran RS et al: *Robbins' pathologic basis of diseases,* ed 5, Philadelphia, 1994, WB Saunders.

Gershwin LJ et al: *Immunology and immunopathology of domestic animals,* ed 2, St Louis, 1995, Mosby.

Jubb KVF et al: *Pathology of domestic animals,* ed 4, San Diego, 1993, Academic Press.

Tizard IR: *Veterinary immunology: an introduction,* ed 5, Philadelphia, 1996, WB Saunders.

CHAPTER 9

Preventive Medicine

R.E. Banks

Learning Objectives

After reviewing this chapter, the reader should understand the following:

General principles underlying disease prevention
Features of appropriate housing and nutrition for animals

Ways in which animals can be identified
Types and schedules of vaccinations for domestic animal species
Principles of sanitation used in disease prevention
Factors that predispose to disease

Veterinary preventive medicine is the science of preventing disease in animals. The three major components of a preventive medicine program include husbandry, vaccination or prevention through medication, and sanitation. Husbandry involves the housing, diet, and environment of animals. Vaccination involves use of vaccines or bacterins to prevent such diseases as rabies or equine encephalomyelitis; medication can be given regularly to prevent heartworms. Sanitation focuses on cleanliness and use of disinfectants to prevent infection or disease transmission.

All three of these components are interrelated; disease is prevented only by attention to all three components. For example, poor husbandry practices cannot be accommodated by over-vaccination and rigorous sanitation. Failure to properly vaccinate an animal may well result in disease, even if the husbandry is top notch, and the sanitation is impeccable. Poor sanitation frequently results in animal and human disease.

The goal of any preventive medicine program is the lowest possible incidence of disease in animals under the care of the veterinary practice. In general, the number of client visits to the hospital or the number of farm visits reflects the efficacy of the preventive medicine program. The mutual goal of veterinary professionals and animal owners should be to preserve animal health using preventive practices. Such efforts save money that otherwise would be spent for treatment of disease. Preventive medicine also prolongs the life span, improves the well-being of animals, and fosters a good client-veterinarian relationship.

Unfortunately, some clients cannot see the benefit of spending a few dollars for preventive care, such as for vaccination. These same clients then complain about the large sums of money they must spend to correct problems that could have been avoided through preventive methods. The challenge for veterinary technicians is to empathize and work with these clients for the benefit of the patient. By educating animal owners on the benefits of proper preventive medicine, you will be given the opportunity to provide the best veterinary care possible.

Tables 9-1 through 9-6 later in this chapter present preventive medicine programs recommended for various species.

HUSBANDRY
Temperature, Light, and Ventilation

For small animals, such as dogs, cats, birds, and small mammals, the ambient (room) temperature should ideally be 65° to 84° F (18° to 29° C). Birds, very young pets, old pets, and those with a sparse haircoat should be maintained at the higher end of this temperature range. Those that are well furred or overweight should be kept at the lower end of this range. Livestock can survive extremes in outdoor temperatures if sheltered from precipitation and wind; in a barn or stable, good ventilation is more important than ambient temperature. Smaller animals of any species generally require warmer temperatures, whereas larger animals, with their greater body mass, generally require cooler temperatures.

Light sufficient for humans is adequate for most animals. Excessive light can cause eye problems in albino rats. Too little light makes sanitation difficult. Rodents do well in low-light environments. Breeding stock may require adjustment of the photoperiod (periods of daylight and darkness) to maximize breeding potential. Most rodents are best housed with 14 hours of light and 10 hours of darkness. Stallions have improved breeding behavior with long light cycles. All species do better when there is a definite difference between day and night. Animals should never be kept in direct sunlight without access to shade, as they may become sunburned and overheated. Such environmental stress can also predispose to disease.

Ventilation is extremely important in maintaining good health. Inadequate air exchange in an enclosure increases urine odors, ammonia levels, and numbers of airborne bacteria and viruses. Such conditions irritate the respiratory tract and predispose to respiratory disease. Drafty conditions or excessive ventilation can be dangerous. Excessive cool air flow can cause chilling. In a low-humidity environment, as with air conditioning, high air flow can dehydrate an animal. Small pets caged indoors must be kept away from air conditioning drafts or heater vents. It is usually best to place the cage along an interior wall away from ventilation or heating ducts.

Housing

An important aspect of husbandry is housing, such as in cages, pens, or stalls. Housing should prevent contamination of the animal with feces or urine; provide for the psychosocial comfort of companion animals; be appropriate for the species; be structurally sound; be free of dangerous surfaces; be constructed so that the animal cannot escape and vermin are not allowed access; and be easy for the owner to clean. Housed animals should be dry, clean, and protected from environmental extremes.

Walls and roofing should be sufficient to protect animals from the sun, wind, rain, and snow. Rabbits held in outdoor hutches can become sunburned. Horses can develop conjunctivitis from wind-driven dust. Dogs chilled by a sudden rainstorm can develop tracheobronchitis or more severe respiratory disease. Pens and corrals must be free of exposed nails, sharp metal edges, or other dangerous features. Attention should be paid to escape-proofing cages. Rodents can squeeze through 1-inch openings; many other small pets learn to flip the latch on their cage door.

Accommodation must also be made for species-specific behavior. For example, pigs should have access to dirt lots for rooting and mud wallowing. Rodents need sufficient bedding for burrowing. Cats need scratching posts. Chinchillas require dust baths.

A major failure of many animal enclosures is that they do not allow sufficient room for normal movement or even postural changes. Cages, pens, and stalls that are too small increase the risk of disease and may predispose to abnormal behavior, such as pacing or excessive barking. Pets may be kept in close confinement for short periods, such as a dog kept for a few hours in a portable kennel or carrier; however, such enclosures should have sufficient room for normal postural movements and stretching. A useful rule of thumb for holding enclosures is a minimum of 10 times the body size of the animal. This recommendation assumes the animal will be given opportunity to exercise routinely outside of the primary enclosure. Also, housing too many animals in a single primary enclosure of insufficient size can create problems. A high concentration of animals in a primary enclosure, whether hamsters or ponies, dramatically increases the risk of stress, aggression, and disease transmission.

Animals of different species should be housed separately, or, in some cases, at least in separate rooms. Do not house natural predators and prey animals in the same room, such as cats with mice or birds, as this leads to stress and possible attack. Also there are medical reasons for housing different species separately. A disease considered inconsequential in one species may be deadly in another species. For example, healthy rabbits carry *Bordetella* and *Pasteurella* bacteria, but these agents can quickly kill guinea pigs.

Enclosures should be cleaned and sanitized frequently, from once a day to once a week. Few pet owners clean the cages or pens of their pets too often. For large animals, stalls or stanchion areas should be "mucked" daily and new straw or other bedding spread. Barn gutters and pens should be shoveled or cleared of manure with a tractor as needed and periodically hosed down. Small cages can be sanitized by hand or even in a dishwasher. Generally speaking, any good dishwashing detergent will effectively clean holding areas. Additional sanitation can be obtained with a dilute solution of laundry bleach (e.g., Clorox), using 1 part bleach to 20 parts of water. All surfaces should be rinsed thoroughly after cleaning and disinfecting. Wet items should be left to dry completely before returning the animal to the cage.

Nutrition

Animals must have free access to fresh potable water. Water in containers should be changed sufficiently to prevent accumulation of slime, algae, or dirt. Bowls should be kept clean and sanitized in a dishwasher (180° F) at least once a month. Water troughs for livestock should be periodically emptied and sanitized. Automatic watering devices must be kept clean and free of ice. Water containers should be sufficient for the number of animals in an enclosure.

Animals should be fed a wholesome, palatable diet on a regular schedule and in sufficient quantity. Feeding devices must be designed to prevent contamination by wastes. Usually this is accomplished with an appropriately sized feeder, positioned off of the floor, in close proximity to the water source. As with water containers, feeding devices should be sanitized routinely—at least monthly or more often as needed.

Clients should be encouraged to purchase good-quality feedstuffs and refrain from feeding outdated or off-brand diets. In general, commercial diets more than 3 months old should not be fed as a sole food source, because certain nutrients deteriorate with long storage. Clients should be cautioned not to buy feeds that show large amounts of oil uptake by the bag or box. Such products have likely been held for considerable time in a warehouse that was warm enough to cause oil to bleed out of the feed.

The diet fed should be formulated for that species. Cats should not be fed food formulated for dogs. Rat rations are of little value for rabbits, dogs, or cats. Guinea pigs require vitamin C in their diet. Rat or mouse diets can produce disease in guinea pigs. Pig rations, with their high carbohydrate component, can cause bloat in horses. Rabbit rations can cause metabolic disease in sheep. Feeding an improperly formulated diet produces nutritional deficiencies, excesses, or imbalances that can predispose to bacterial infections or metabolic disease. Chapter 14 contains detailed information on nutrition.

Animal Identification

An often overlooked aspect of preventive medicine is animal identification. The method of identification depends upon the species. For pets allowed outdoors, an implanted microchip or a tattoo is preferred to a collar with name tag. Collars may be removed or fall off and tags may be lost. Permanent identification ensures that a lost pet can be identified for return to its owner.

VACCINATION AND USE OF PREVENTIVE MEDICATION

Certain diseases are readily prevented by vaccination. Domestic animals should be routinely vaccinated against prevalent diseases. Such serious diseases as parvovirus infection and distemper in dogs, panleukopenia and feline leukemia virus infection in cats, and equine encephalomyelitis and tetanus in horses can be prevented by vaccination. In some cases, vaccination is beneficial to humans as well as animals. For example, animals at risk of developing rabies from the bite of rabid animals should receive regular rabies prophylaxis.

Most small mammals kept as pets (rodents and rabbits) are not routinely vaccinated because of the relatively small risk of contracting certain diseases for which vaccines are available for those species. Mice can contract rabies, but pet mice housed in a cage in a home are unlikely to encounter a rabid animal. Vaccination recommendations for some species are changing. In years past, rabies vaccination was not considered necessary for pet ferrets; with the improved rabies vaccines now available, ferret vaccination is considered appropriate.

The decision whether or not to vaccinate an animal is influenced by the risk of contracting the disease, the effects of the disease, and the benefits and cost of vaccination. Vaccination may not be warranted if the disease is unlikely to develop or causes only mild illness. For example, veterinarians do not routinely vaccinate dogs or cats against tetanus because they are unlikely to contract the disease; however, horses are vaccinated against tetanus because they are more likely to develop it. Vaccination against a very rare disease may not be necessary; however, vaccination is worthwhile if contraction of the disease poses a substantial threat to human and animal health, such as with rabies. Vaccination also benefits the offspring of vaccinated females, through transfer of maternal immunity in the dam's colostrum (first milk).

The attitude toward vaccination also varies with circumstances. Kennel and cattery owners, breeding farm managers, and ranchers are very concerned with diseases that could sweep through the animal population, with devastating economic effects. Although tracheobronchitis ("kennel cough") is a fairly mild upper respiratory infection of dogs, it could cause great harm in the form of bad public relations if it infected dogs in a boarding facility. An individual owner of a dog, however, would not be overly concerned with kennel cough in his or her pet.

Animal vaccines are available in many combinations. For example, Duramune PC (Fort Dodge) is a canine vaccine against parvovirus and coronavirus. Duramune DA2P+Pv protects against five viruses, including parvovirus, but not coronavirus. Duramune DA2PP+ CvK/LCI and Vanguard 5/CV-L (SmithKline Beecham) both protect against six viruses and two kinds of bacteria. Currently, 8 Duramune and 13 Vanguard products are available in the United States for vaccination of dogs. A similarly wide variety of vaccine products is also available for cats, horses, cattle, pigs, and other species.

Vaccination of Dogs

Dogs should generally be vaccinated against the following:

- Rabies
- Distemper
- Parvovirus infection
- Coronavirus infection
- Canine adenovirus infection (CAV-1 or CAV-2)

- *Bordetella bronchiseptica* infection
- Parainfluenza

Certain dogs, such as hunting dogs or working dogs, may also need protection against leptospirosis and borreliosis (Lyme disease). Puppies are usually immunized with one to three doses in the first few months of life and then annually as adults (Table 9-1).

Vaccination of Cats

All cats should generally be vaccinated against the following:

- Rabies
- Panleukopenia (feline distemper)
- Chlamydial pneumonitis
- Feline leukemia virus infection
- Rhinotracheitis
- Calicivirus infection

Certain cats may also receive vaccinations against ringworm and feline infectious peritonitis. Most cats begin receiving vaccines as kittens, usually around 4 to 6 weeks of age. Kittens require booster vaccinations after an original series of vaccinations. Adult cats require annual boosters against each of these diseases (Table 9-2).

TABLE 9-1   Preventive medicine programs generally recommended for dogs

6 to 8 Weeks	10 to 12 Weeks	16 Weeks or older	Annual visits
General physical examination	General physical examination	General physical examination	General physical examination
Fecal examination	Fecal examination; treat if required	Fecal examination; treat if required	Fecal examination; treat if required
Vaccinate for distemper, parainfluenza, adenovirus infection, leptospirosis, parvovirus infection, coronavirus infection	Vaccinate for distemper, parainfluenza, adenovirus infection, leptospirosis, parvovirus infection, coronavirus infection	Vaccinate for distemper, parainfluenza, adenovirus infection, leptospirosis, parvovirus infection, coronavirus infection, rabies, possibly borreliosis and tracheobronchitis	Vaccinate for distemper, parainfluenza, adenovirus infection, leptospirosis, parvovirus infection, coronavirus infection, rabies, possibly borreliosis and tracheobronchitis
Begin client education: Cage/pen care Exercise/sleep Nutrition Grooming Heartworms Viral diseases Parasites Behavior	Continue client education: Ask about cage/pen care Check on nutrition Discuss grooming practices Begin heartworm preventive therapy Recheck for parasites; treat as needed Confirm that training is working Suggest neutering if not breeding	Continue client education: Confirm cage/pen care Check on nutrition Discuss grooming practices Adjust heartworm therapy Confirm that training is working Schedule neutering	Continue client education: Confirm cage/pen care Check on nutrition Discuss grooming practices Adjust heartworm therapy Confirm that training is working Schedule neutering

TABLE 9-2 Preventive medicine programs generally recommended for cats

8 to 10 Weeks	12 to 14 Weeks	Annual visits
General physical examination	General physical examination	General physical examination
Fecal examination; treat if required	Fecal examination; treat if required	Fecal examination; treat if required
Vaccinate for feline leukemia virus infection, panleukopenia, rhinotracheitis, calicivirus infection, chlamydial pneumonitis	Vaccinate for feline leukemia virus infection, panleukopenia, rhinotracheitis, calicivirus infection, chlamydial pneumonitis, rabies	Vaccinate for feline leukemia virus infection, panleukopenia, rhinotracheitis, calicivirus infection, chlamydial pneumonitis
Begin client education: 　Exercise/sleep 　Nutrition 　Grooming 　Play 　Viral diseases 　Parasites 　Behavior	Continue client education: 　Exercise/sleep 　Nutrition 　Grooming 　Schedule for neutering 　Viral diseases 　Parasites 　Behavior	Continue client education: 　Exercise/sleep 　Nutrition 　Grooming 　Viral diseases 　Parasites 　Behavior

TABLE 9-3 Preventive medicine programs generally recommended for horses

Foals and weanlings	Yearlings and adults
Physical examination at time of vaccination	Physical examination at time of vaccination
Deworm every 2 months (rotate products)	Deworm at least every 2 months (rotate products)
Trim feet as needed	Check teeth and float as needed
Vaccinate for tetanus, EEE, WEE, VEE, equine influenza, rhinopneumonitis	Trim feet as needed
Discuss feeding regimen	Vaccinate for tetanus, EEE, WEE, VEE, equine influenza, rhinopneumonitis
Discuss exercise program	Review stall cleaning schedule
Monitor body condition	Discuss feeding regimen
	Discuss exercise program
	Monitor body condition

Vaccination of Horses

All horses should generally be vaccinated against the following:
- Rabies
- Tetanus
- Equine encephalomyelitis (eastern, western, Venezuelan)
- Equine influenza
- Rhinopneumonitis

Certain classes of horses may also require vaccination against strangles, botulism, anthrax, and Potomac horse fever. Most horses begin receiving vaccines as foals.

Horses of unknown vaccination status should receive an initial series of vaccines, which are repeated in 4 weeks for maximal antibody production. Adult horses generally require annual boosters against each of these diseases (Table 9-3).

Vaccination of Cattle

All cattle should generally be vaccinated against the following:
- Clostridial diseases
- Infectious bovine rhinotracheitis

- Parainfluenza-3 infection
- Bovine virus diarrhea
- Leptospirosis
- Vibriosis

Certain types of cattle may also require vaccination against anaplasmosis, footrot, rotavirus-coronavirus infection, brucellosis, and rabies. Most cattle begin receiving vaccines as calves, with booster doses after 6 months of age. Cattle of unknown vaccination status should receive an initial series of vaccines, which are repeated in 4 weeks for maximal antibody production. Adult cattle generally require annual boosters against each of these diseases (Table 9-4).

Vaccination of Pigs

All swine should generally be vaccinated against the following:

- Leptospirosis
- Erysipelas
- Colibacillosis
- Transmissible gastroenteritis
- Atrophic rhinitis

Certain swine herds may also require vaccination against porcine parvovirus infection, rabies, *Haemophilus* infection, and swine dysentery. Most swine begin receiving vaccines as piglets. Pigs of unknown vaccination status should receive an initial series of vaccines, which are repeated in 4 weeks for maximal antibody production. Adult pigs generally require annual boosters against each of these diseases (Table 9-5).

Vaccination of Goats

Goats should generally be vaccinated against the following:

- Clostridial diseases
- Tetanus

- Contagious ecthyma

Some goat herds are also vaccinated against anthrax, leptospirosis, caseous lymphadenitis, colibacillosis, and rabies. Most goats begin receiving vaccines as kids, usually around 4 to 6 weeks of age. Kids require booster vaccinations after an original series of vaccinations. Adult goats require annual boosters against each of these diseases (Table 9-6).

Vaccination of Sheep

Sheep should generally be vaccinated against the following:

- Clostridial diseases
- Tetanus
- Vibriosis (ewes)
- Footrot
- Bluetongue

Some sheep herds are also vaccinated against contagious ecthyma, brucellosis, caseous lymphadenitis, and colibacillosis. Most lambs are first vaccinated at 4 to 6 weeks of age. Lambs require booster vaccinations after an original series of vaccinations. Adult sheep need annual boosters against each of these diseases (see Table 9-6).

Vaccination of Llamas

Llamas should generally be vaccinated against the following:

- *Clostridium perfringens* infection
- Rabies
- Anthrax

Some llamas may also require vaccination against rabies and brucellosis. Most crias (immature llamas) are first vaccinated before 4 weeks of age. Crias require booster vaccinations after an original series of vaccinations. Adult llamas require annual boosters against each of these diseases (see Table 9-6).

TABLE 9-4   Preventive medicine programs generally recommended for cattle

Neonatal period	1 to 3 Months	5 to 6 Months	Annually
Physical examination	Physical examination	Physical examination	Physical examination
Vaccinate for bovine rotavirus and coronavirus infection (if necessary)	Deworm (rotate products)	Deworm (rotate products)	Deworm (rotate products)
Review stall cleaning schedule	Vaccinate for clostridial diseases	Vaccination for clostridial diseases, infectious bovine rhinotracheitis, parainfluenza-3, bovine virus diarrhea	Vaccinate for infectious bovine rhinotracheitis, parainfluenza-3, bovine virus diarrhea
Monitor body condition	Review stall cleaning schedule	Review stall cleaning schedule	Review stall cleaning schedule
	Discuss feeding regimen	Discuss feeding regimen	Discuss feeding regimen
	Monitor body condition	Monitor body condition	Monitor body condition

TABLE 9-5 Preventive medicine programs generally recommended for pigs

Neonatal period	1 to 3 Weeks	4 to 5 Weeks	8 to 10 Weeks	Annually
Physical examination	Physical examination	Physical examination	Physical Examination	Deworm (rotate products)
Dock tails	Vaccinate for transmissible gastroenteritis, atrophic rhinitis, porcine parvovirus infection	Vaccinate for atrophic rhinitis, erysipelas, *Haemophilus* infection, swine dysentery	Treat for ectoparasites	Check for ectoparasites
Castrate (if neccesary)			Deworm	Physical examination
Clip needle teeth			Discuss feeding regimen	Vaccinate as necessary
Iron dextran injection		Review pen cleaning schedule	Monitory body condition	Review pen cleaning schedule
Identify with ear notching	Monitor body condition	Monitor body condition		Discuss feeding regimen
	Review pen cleaning schedule			Monitor body condition

TABLE 9-6 Preventive medicine programs generally recommended for goats, sheep, and llamas

Neonatal period	1 to 3 Months	5 to 6 Months	Annually
Physical examination	Physical examination	Deworm (rotate products)	Physical examination
Vaccinate for clostridial diseases, tetanus	Deworm (rotate products)	Physical examination	Deworm (rotate products)
Review pen cleaning schedule	Vaccinate for clostridial diseases	Review stall cleaning schedule	Vaccinate as needed
Monitor body condition	Review stall cleaning schedule	Discuss feeding regimen	Review pen cleaning schedule
	Discuss feeding regimen	Monitor body condition	Discuss feeding regimen
	Monitor body condition		Monitor body condition

Use of Preventive Medication

Certain diseases can be prevented by regular administration of preventive medication. This is best exemplified by use of ivermectin, milbemycin, or diethylcarbamazine to prevent heartworm infection in dogs, or use of ivermectin, lufenuron, or pyrantel to control internal and external parasites in dogs.

SANITATION

The third aspect of the preventive medicine triad is sanitation. A good preventive medicine program involves the judicious use of selected sanitizing and disinfecting agents. Gross accumulations of dirt and organic matter must be removed by cleaning before application of disinfectants. The ideal sanitizing agent has the following characteristics: broad spectrum of antimicrobial activity; no odor; rapid microbicidal effect; no tissue toxicity; no corrosive action; no inactivation by urine or other organic matter; can be used at normal environmental temperatures; reasonably priced; readily obtainable; and easily applied. Because no single disinfectant meets all of these criteria, selection is based on the specific needs of the client's preventive medicine program.

Hypochlorites, such as in laundry bleach (e.g., Clorox), are inexpensive, widely available, and effective, and have a wide spectrum of antimicrobial activity. They are most effective in acidic solutions but less effective in the presence of organic matter or detergent residues. These agents can also damage fabrics and may be corrosive to metal. A solution of 30 ml of standard laundry bleach in 1 L of water (1 oz per quart) is an effective sanitizing agent, but it degrades quickly and a fresh batch should be made daily.

Quaternary ammonium compounds have very low toxicity to most animals, are convenient to use, and have no apparent taste or offensive odor. They are most effective against gram-positive bacteria but less effective against gram-negative bacteria. They have limited efficacy in the presence of organic matter or detergent residues and in an acidic environment. These agents are useful for sanitation of feed and water containers. All equipment and surfaces disinfected with quaternary ammonium products should be well rinsed because the residues can cause toxicity.

Phenols are good disinfecting products and effectively kill vegetative forms of both gram-negative and gram-positive bacteria. The exception is *Pseudomonas,* which can be a major contaminant in certain animal environments. (Acidification of the drinking water can prevent *Pseudomonas* contamination of water for rodents, the animals most commonly affected.) Phenols are recognized by their pine or cedar smell. Phenols are toxic to some species (e.g., cats) and so should not be used to clean feed or water containers. These agents are good for sanitizing the surfaces of pens and cages. Their strong odor, however, can mask the odor of accumulated urine or feces.

Alcohol, such as ethyl alcohol, is a poor disinfectant. To serve as an effective disinfectant, alcohol must remain in contact with the site for 15 to 20 minutes. Because it evaporates long before this, alcohol is not a good choice for most applications. Alcohol is a good solvent and helps to physically remove microorganisms when accumulated materials are wiped away.

Other agents are also used to disinfect the environment of animals (e.g., lye, formaldehyde gas, 10% ammonia), but these usually require specialized application not readily available to most animal owners. Chapter 13 contains detailed information on disinfectants and antiseptics.

A practical way to assess sanitation is to avoid use of highly scented products, such as cedar shavings, pine-scented cleaners, or perfumes, on animals or in their surroundings. Although deodorants make the animal or its enclosure smell good, they also mask odors that can be associated with poor sanitation.

FACTORS PREDISPOSING TO DISEASE

Some factors that predispose to disease can be controlled, but others cannot. Although some factors are beyond our control, we can often establish conditions so that even uncontrollable factors have only minimal impact on our animals. Animals are predisposed to disease by genetic, dietary, environmental, and metabolic factors.

Genetic Factors

Genetic factors are largely beyond our control, although they can be reduced to some extent by selective breeding. These include such things as predispositions by gender,

inherited mutations, immunodeficiencies, and the effect of inbreeding. Most male tricolored cats are sterile, whereas tricolored female cats are usually fertile. Inherited malocclusions can interfere with chewing. Immunodeficiencies may be noted by an increased incidence of infections. Inbreeding can lead to physical abnormalities or diminished mental (intellectual) capacities.

Dietary Factors

Dietary factors are generally controllable. Animal owners determine most aspects of an animal's diet, such as feed type, quality, amount, and regimen. A high-quality balanced ration is of little value if the feeder is inaccessible. This is occasionally seen with young bunnies, which are too short to reach the feeder. Limited feeding can prevent obesity but can lead to malnutrition if not applied properly. A diet formulated for one type or age of animals may not be healthful for another group of the same species. For example, hard pellets may not be chewable by aged animals. The diet must change as the needs of the animal change.

Environmental Factors

Environmental factors also require consideration in the preventive health plan. Climatic extremes or sudden climatic changes can clearly cause distress or even death. Although we cannot change the weather, we can adjust the animal's housing to reduce environmental stress. Additional bedding improves the insulation around animals housed in extremely cold conditions. Overhead cover is needed to prevent sunburn and heat prostration and shield animals from precipitation.

Inadequate ventilation increases the incidence of respiratory diseases through increased ammonia levels and large numbers of microorganisms in the air. Inadequate ventilation also impairs cooling in animals that use respiration to regulate body temperature (e.g., dogs) and prevents radiation of body heat (e.g., heat loss from the ears of rabbits). Inadequate ventilation inhibits the drying of bedding, favoring proliferation of bacteria or parasites. At the other end of the spectrum, excessive ventilation is also stressful. Drafts or excessive ventilation can cause chilling, dehydration, or inflamed ocular tissues.

The level of ventilation should be appropriate for the animal, rather than for the animal owner. We must take the time to experience the same conditions that the animal is experiencing. We must evaluate air flow not at the 5-foot level, but at the 5-inch level. A draft along the floor could lead to respiratory disease in a small mammal but may not be evident to the animal owner. A 2-hour period of sunshine directly on a hamster each day could dehydrate the pet, while the owner remained unaware of it. Inadvertent spraying of perfume or other aerosols near a fish tank could kill the fish. If the air in a poorly ventilated barn or stable causes discomfort in farm personnel, such as burning eyes or a sore throat, it is also causing discomfort in the animals.

Metabolic Factors

Metabolic factors also must be considered in preventive health programs. Factors beyond our control include the age of the animal and reproductive status; concurrent disease; and nonspecific stressors. Young, old, pregnant, and lactating animals have different physiologic needs than other animals. These needs may require alteration of the animal's diet and housing.

A common metabolic problem that influences the health of many companion animals, and that can be effectively managed by the animal owner, is obesity from overfeeding and lack of exercise. We often focus on the animal's age group and manage health problems as they relate to age; however, a much more effective preventive approach is to address factors under the client's control. Veterinary professionals should discuss proper nutrition and exercise programs with clients so that their animals can benefit from that knowledge.

RECOMMENDED READING

Birchard SJ, Sherding RG: *Saunders manual of small animal practice,* Philadelphia, 1994, WB Saunders.

Bonagura JD: *Kirk's current veterinary therapy XII, small animal practice,* Philadelphia, 1995, WB Saunders.

Harkness JE, Wagner JE: *The biology and medicine of rabbits and rodents,* ed 4, Baltimore, 1995, Williams & Wilkins.

Smith B: *Large animal internal medicine,* ed 2, St Louis, 1996, Mosby.

Veterinary pharmaceuticals and biologicals, ed 10, Lenexa, Kan, 1997, Veterinary Medicine Publishing.

CHAPTER 10

Animal Disease and People

M.E. Torrence

Learning Objectives

After reviewing this chapter, the reader should understand the following:

Ways in which animal disease can affect people
General principles of epidemiology and their application to public health

General principles of food hygiene and their application to public health
Common zoonotic diseases that pose a threat to people
Ways to control spread of zoonotic diseases

Public health is a community's effort to prevent disease and promote life and health. The effort usually includes sanitation of the environment, control of communicable infections, education of individuals in personal hygiene, and organization of medical and nursing services to ensure proper health care. Veterinary public health plays an important role in protecting and improving human well-being by using veterinary knowledge and skills to preserve the healthy relationship between humans and animals. The veterinary profession's major roles in preventing disease in people are in epidemiology, food hygiene, and zoonotic disease.

EPIDEMIOLOGY

Epidemiology is the study of the occurrences of disease and the risk factors that cause disease in a population. Some texts refer to the study of disease in an animal population as *epizootiology*, but the term *epidemiology* is appropriate for both human and animal populations and is a more widely recognized term. Descriptive epidemiology studies the frequency of disease in a population and describes the type of animals affected and how and when they are affected. In other words, it describes the disease in terms of the animal or people affected and the time and geographic region in which they are affected. This information gives epidemiologists clues about the cause of disease, allows epidemiologists to form hypotheses about the cause, and helps epidemiologists determine the risk that animals or people will become ill. Epidemiologists can then design more elaborate analytic epidemiologic studies to test these hypotheses. Once the cause of the disease and the risk factors that influence the disease are identified, programs for control or prevention of the disease can be implemented. Epidemiologists are essential professionals in veterinary and human public health efforts to study the cause and to initiate the control of disease.

FOOD HYGIENE

The field of food hygiene involves making sure that food is safe and wholesome for human consumption. Proper food hygiene is important in preventing foodborne diseases. An estimated 10 million people in the United States become ill with foodborne diseases. Primarily, veterinarians are involved in the food hygiene process through inspection and processing of animals for food. Proper inspection and processing are essential in prevention of foodborne diseases that originate from contamination with bacteria at the slaughterhouse. These organisms are the cause of significant disease in people. Some of the most common organisms involved are *Salmonella* spp., *Campylobacter* spp., and *E. coli* 0157:H7. An *E. coli* outbreak occurred recently in a number of people, particularly children, who ate undercooked hamburgers at a restaurant. *E. coli* 0157:H7 infection causes hemolytic uremia and may result in death. The most common source of *Salmonella* in the United States is poultry or poultry products, such as eggs. In fact, *Salmonella enteritidis* infection has become a highly reported foodborne disease in the United States and has generated new recommendations for the public in handling raw egg products. Proper cooking and handling of meat can help prevent serious disease. Other foodborne diseases can be caused by contamination of food and improper handling, such as *Staphylococcus* infection, *Clostridium* infection (botulism), and hepatitis.

An important step in food hygiene before an animal reaches the slaughterhouse is prevention of adulterating residues. *Residues* are hormonal compounds, antibacterials, antimycotics, anthelmintics, antiprotozoals, or pesticides in meat or milk that have accumulated to levels that are above the established safe tolerance levels. The United States Department of Agriculture (USDA) monitors foodstuffs for the presence of residues and is responsible for inspection of food. The Environmental Protection Agency (EPA) sets the residue limits for pesticides. The Food and Drug Administration (FDA) sets the limits for drug residues.

How do drugs become residues? Most drug residues are caused by misuse of drugs. Misuse of drugs includes not following label directions, using drugs in unapproved species, and not adhering to withdrawal times. Residues can occur in meat or milk through misuse of drugs in mastitis treatments or with injectable antibiotics. In addition, feed or drinking water can be contaminated with drugs or pesticides.

Residues are important to public health because they can cause toxic or allergic reactions in people. For example, penicillin residues in milk can cause a severe, life-threatening reaction in a person who is allergic to penicillin. Veterinarians and veterinary technicians are responsible for using drugs in food animals according to standard veterinary practice.

ZOONOTIC DISEASES

Zoonoses are the major area of involvement for veterinarians in public health. Zoonoses are diseases that are transmitted between animals and people. Other infectious diseases are common to but not transmitted between animals and people; these can be caused by similar exposures to the same infectious organism. Over 150 zoonoses have been reported. Zoonoses are a significant cause of human disability, hospitalization, death, and high economic cost in the United States and in underdeveloped countries. Table 10-1 lists the causative organism, hosts, and mode of transmission for some common zoonoses.

Primarily, veterinarians are concerned with monitoring and surveillance of zoonoses, evaluating risks to people, and planning and coordinating prevention and control programs with appropriate agencies and individuals. Part of that surveillance is looking for an outbreak or an epidemic of the disease. An *epidemic* is an increase over the normal expected number of disease cases in a geographic area or over a certain period. An *endemic disease* is one that has maintained a certain level of disease over time in a given geographic area. For example, rabies is endemic or always present at a certain level in raccoons in the eastern United States. However, in the late 1970s and early 1980s, when rabies began appearing in the mid-Atlantic area, it was considered epidemic. Surveillance of zoonoses or any other diseases is dependent on knowledge about the cause of the disease, transmission of the disease, and how the disease is maintained in the population.

Disease Transmission

For an infectious disease to survive in a population, the agent causing the disease must be transmitted. The mode of transmission is an important epidemiologic clue in understanding the disease. It is important for the veterinary profession to be aware of how specific diseases are transmitted so that preventive measures can be taken and the public educated. Reservoirs and hosts of a specific disease are important to identify because these are essential in transmission of a disease and its maintenance in the population. Control programs for a disease are often aimed at the reservoirs or hosts of the disease. For example, spraying programs aimed at controlling mosquito populations are initiated when there is an outbreak of encephalitis.

Reservoirs can be inanimate (e.g., soil) or animate (e.g., animals, people, birds). Reservoirs are essential and necessary for the survival and reproduction of the organism. *Hosts* are living beings that offer an environment for maintenance of the organism, but they are not necessary for the organism's survival. Depending on the disease, the infectious organism may be transmitted

TABLE 10-1   The causative organisms, animal hosts, and modes of transmission for selected common zoonoses

	Causative organisms	Small animal host	Livestock host	Wildlife host	Mode of transmission
Viral diseases					
Rabies	Rhabdovirus	Most	Most	Most	Animal bite
Encephalitis (EEE, WEE)	Togavirus		Horses, poultry	Birds, rodents	Mosquito bite
Lymphocytic choriomeningitis	Arenavirus	Mice			Varied
Contagious ecthyma (orf)	Pox virus	Sometimes dogs	Sheep, goats		Contact
Simian herpes (B virus)	Herpesvirus simiae			Primates	Animal bite, direct contact
Newcastle disease	Paramyxovirus	Domestic birds	Poultry	Wild fowl	Contact, inhalation
Yellow fever	Togavirus			Primates	Mosquito bite
Hantavirus infection	Hantavirus			Rodents	Contact
Rickettsial diseases					
Q fever	*Coxiella burnetii*		Cattle, sheep, goats	Birds, rabbits rodents	Inhalation, milk ingestion, contact
Rocky Mountain spotted fever	*Rickettsia rickettsii*	Dogs		Rodents, rabbits	Tick bite
Psittacosis	*Chlamydia psittaci*	Psittacine birds	Turkeys, ducks	Birds	Inhalation
Mycoses					
Ringworm	*Tricophyton* spp., *Micro-sporum* spp.	Cats, dogs	Cattle, horses, swine, sheep	Rodents	Contact
Parasitic diseases					
Trichinosis	*Trichinella spiralis*		Pigs	Rats, bears, carnivores	Ingestion
Scabies	*Sarcoptes scabiei*	Dogs, rodents, cats	Horses	Primates	Contact
Taeniasis, Cysticercosis	*Taenia* spp., *Cysticercus*		Pigs, cattle	Boars	Ingestion
Hydatid disease	*Echinococcus* spp.	Dogs	Herbivores	Wolves	Ingestion
Schistosomiasis	*Schistosoma* spp.	Dogs, cats	Pigs, cattle, horses	Rodents	Contact
Larva migrans	*Toxocara, Ancylostoma, Strongyloides*	Dogs, cats	Pigs, cattle	Raccoons	Ingestion
Bacterial diseases					
Anthrax	*Bacillus anthracis*	Dogs	Most	Most except primates	Contact
Brucellosis	*Brucella* spp.	Dogs	Cattle, pigs, sheep, goats	All except primates	Contact, inhalation, ingestion

Continued.

TABLE 10-1 The causative organisms, animal hosts, and mode of transmission for selected common zoonoses—cont'd

	Causative organisms	Small animal host	Livestock host	Wildlife host	Mode of transmission
Bacterial diseases—cont'd					
Plague	*Yersinia pestis*	Cats		Rodents, rabbits	Flea bite
Campylobacteriosis	*Campylobacter fetus* ss *fetus*	Dogs, cats	Cattle, poultry, sheep, pigs	Rodents, birds	Ingestion, contact
Cat-scratch disease	*Bartonella henselae*	Cats		Cats	Cat bite, scratch
Leptospirosis	*Leptospira* spp.	All, especially dogs	All, cattle, pigs	Rats, raccoons	Contact with urine
Salmonellosis	*Salmonella* spp.	All, especially dogs, cats	All, pigs, poultry, cattle	Rodents, reptiles	Ingestion
Tuberculosis	*Mycobacteria* spp.	Dogs, cats	Cattle, pigs goats, sheep, poultry	All except rodents, monkeys	Ingestion, inhalation
Tularemia	*Francisella tularensis*	All	All except horses	Rodents, rabbits	Tick bites, contact with tissue
Erysipelas	*Erysipelothrix rhusiopathiae*		Pigs, sheep, cattle, horses, poultry	Rodents	Contact
Tetanus	*Clostridium tetani*		Horses	Reptiles	Wound
Lyme disease	*Borrelia burgdorferi*	Dogs, cats	Cattle, horses	Deer, birds, rodents	Tick bite
Protozoal diseases					
Cryptosporidiosis	*Cryptosporidium* spp.	Most	Calves, sheep	Birds	Ingestion
Toxoplasmosis	*Toxoplasma gondii*	Cats, rabbits, guinea pigs	Pigs, sheep, cattle, horses	Cats	Ingestion
Balantidiasis	*Balantidium coli*		Pigs	Rats, primates	Ingestion
Sarcocystosis	*Sarcocystis* spp.	Dogs, cats	Pigs, cattle		Ingestion
Giardiasis	*Giardia lamblia*	Dogs, cats	Pigs, cattle	Beavers, zoo monkeys	Ingestion

through several hosts of different species. This is particularly true of helminth and protozoal diseases. Several hosts or reservoirs are required for the egg to develop to the larva and then to an adult. An infectious disease can be transmitted from the reservoir to a host or from one host to another host.

Direct transmission of disease requires close association or contact between a reservoir of the disease and a susceptible host. Contact with infected skin, mucous membranes, or droplets from an infected human or animal can cause disease. Examples of disease that are transmitted directly are rabies transmitted by a bite, leptospirosis by contact with contaminated urine, and brucellosis by contact with infected tissues. Another example of direct transmission is through contact with the wool, hair, or hide of an infected animal. Anthrax, although not very common in the United States, is transmitted to people through skin contact with contaminated bone meal from infected cattle or direct contact with infected wool or hair.

Animal bites can be a source of infections, trauma, and even zoonotic disease. *Pasteurella* is responsible for 50% of dog bite infections and 90% of cat bite infections. Cat bites are 10 times more likely to become infected than dog bites. Mixed infections include *Staphylococcus aureus, Staphylococcus epidermidis, Streptococcus* spp., *Bacteroides* spp., *Fusobacterium* spp., and other gram-negative bacteria that can cause fever, septicemia, meningitis, endocarditis, and septic arthritis.

Soil or vegetation contaminated with parasites, bacteria, or spores may be another source of direct transmission. Visceral larva migrans is transmitted when children eat soil or vegetables that have been contaminated with feces that contain *Toxocara* (roundworm) eggs. The eggs hatch in the individual's gastrointestinal system and the larvae migrate through the organs. The disease is usually mild and chronic, with eosinophilia, fever, hepatomegaly, and pulmonary signs. If the larvae migrate to the eye, there may be loss of vision or the eye. A similar disease occurs with *Ancylostoma* (hookworm). The signs of cutaneous larva migrans are those of dermatitis, which is caused by the hookworm larvae migrating in the skin.

Droplet spread is differentiated from airborne transmission by the fact that the droplets travel only a short distance (i.e., a few feet) and involve larger particles that often are removed by mechanisms in the upper respiratory passages. Psittacosis is an occupational risk at poultry processing plants. People are infected by inhalation of *Chlamydia psittaci* from the droppings or secretions of infected birds. People can also be infected by cage and aviary birds, especially infected large birds that are shipped into pet stores from foreign countries and not properly treated with antibiotics.

Indirect transmission of disease is more complicated and involves intermediaries that carry the agent of disease from one source to another. The intermediary may be airborne, an arthropod (vectorborne), or an inanimate object (vehicleborne through water, food, or blood). A *vector* is a living organism that transports the infectious agent. A *vehicle* is simply the mode of transmission of an infectious agent from the reservoir to the host. Indirect airborne transmission involves spread of the agent through tiny dust or droplet particles over long distances. Particles smaller than 5 microns in diameter can be inhaled into the alveoli deep within the lungs. Q fever is most commonly transmitted by airborne transmission. It is transmitted by inhalation of the rickettsia, *Coxiella burnetii*, in dust from areas that are contaminated by tissue or excreta from infected animals. Airborne particles with the infective organism can travel a long distance, which makes it difficult to locate the source of the infection. Q fever can also be transmitted by direct contact with contaminated wool, other materials, and milk. Infected individuals may have an inapparent infection or they may have chills, headache, weakness, and sweats.

Various types of arthropods may serve as vectors. These may include mosquitoes, ticks, and fleas. Each type of arthropod has its own life cycle that is often reflected by seasonal and geographic patterns in transmission of disease. For example, ticks may have two or three host maturation cycles and may take 2 years to complete a life cycle. The arthropods can merely carry the agent mechanically to a susceptible host or may be involved biologically in multiplication of the organism or in a stage of development.

Plague is the best-known vectorborne disease involving the flea as a vector. Plague still occurs in the western United States. The natural reservoir for plague is wild rodents, such as ground squirrels. Infected fleas that spend time on rabbits and especially on domestic cats are a source of infection for people. The most common source of transmission is through the bite of an infected flea. In addition, people can be infected by handling infected tissues during the hunting of small ground animals or even by airborne transmission. The *mortality* (death rate) from untreated plague can be 50%.

Several diseases are transmitted by ticks. Lyme disease (borreliosis) is the most commonly reported tickborne disease, but Rocky Mountain spotted fever (RMSF) is the deadlier disease. Other newly discovered diseases in which the role of animals is less clear are ehrlichiosis and babesiosis. RMSF causes high fever, headache, chills, severe muscle pain, and malaise. In about 50% of patients a rash occurs on the palms and soles and then spreads to the rest of the body. Mortality is about 15% to 20% if the disease is not treated. RMSF is maintained in nature by ticks, either the dog tick *Dermacentor* or the Lone Star tick *Ambylomma*. People are infected by the tick bite during outdoor activities in tick-infested areas or from contact with ticks on pets. Animal infections are usually inapparent. Tick-transmitted diseases are prevented by wearing tick repellents in areas infested with ticks and keeping pet dogs free of ticks.

Food and water are also vehicles of indirect transmission of disease. Both are sources of bacterial, viral, and parasitic diseases. Foodborne diseases are acquired by consumption of contaminated food or water. Foodborne intoxications are caused by toxins produced by certain bacteria that may contaminate food, such as *Staphylococcus aureus, Clostridium* spp., and *Vibrio* spp. The toxins may be present in the food or may be formed in the intestinal tract after the contaminated food is eaten. Foodborne infections are caused by bacterial or viral organisms that cause infection. These include *Salmonella* spp., *Campylobacter* spp., hepatitis virus, and *Vibrio* spp. The type of organism involved determines the incubation period and how quickly the clinical signs appear. Each organism also causes certain clinical signs, such as diarrhea, vomiting, or nausea. These specific incubation periods and particular clinical signs help epidemiologists determine the organism's identity and source.

Parasitic diseases are also transmitted through food and water. Nematode and trematode infections are most often transmitted either through ingestion of eggs or through ingestion of undercooked meat that contains cysts. *Giardia* is a protozoan that causes gastrointestinal disease in people; giardiasis can be quite serious in immunosuppressed individuals. Although *Giardia* is most often transmitted from person to person, it is also a source of waterborne outbreaks when people use mountain streams as community water sources without proper filtration techniques or drink the water during outdoor activities. Beavers and other domestic animals are reservoirs. Cryptosporidiosis is another disease that can be transmitted by contaminated water and is a serious disease in immunosuppressed individuals. Cattle and other domestic animals are reservoirs. Proper water filtration and treatment are essential in preventing waterborne diseases.

Pasteurization of milk is important to prevent diseases that can be transmitted through milk. Milk can transmit disease directly from animal to animal or from animals to people through ingestion of contaminated milk. Diseases directly transmitted through milk include brucellosis, Q fever, tuberculosis, toxoplasmosis, and listeriosis. Milk can be contaminated with bacteria, such as *Campylobacter* spp., *Salmonella* spp., and *E. coli,* either from the animal or from the environment. These bacteria can cause disease in people.

Maintenance of Disease

Included in the transmission cycle of disease is maintenance of disease in the human or animal population. There are several ways in which zoonotic diseases are maintained in a population. A *direct zoonosis* is transmitted by a single vertebrate species. For example, the organism that causes cat-scratch fever is maintained in the feline population. In the eastern United States, rabies virus is maintained in the raccoon population.

A *cyclozoonosis* requires several cycles of disease, usually a parasitic disease, to occur in several different vertebrate species. An example of this is hydatid disease caused by the tapeworm *Echinococcus.* The signs of echinococcosis in infected people depend on the number, size, and location of the cysts of *Echinococcus.* The primary reservoir of the adult tapeworm is the dog; eggs are produced and are shed in dog feces. The intermediate hosts are cattle, sheep, pigs, and goats. These species eat grasses and plants that are contaminated with feces. The eggs hatch and become larvae in the intermediate hosts, and cysts are formed in their organs. Dogs are reinfected by eating the organs and tissues of dead cattle, sheep, and other infected livestock, and the cycle begins again. People are infected by ingesting tapeworm eggs while handling contaminated materials or soil or infected dogs.

A *metazoonosis* is maintained by both invertebrate (tick or mosquito) and vertebrate species. An example is encephalitis. This viral disease is maintained in the vertebrate population of wild or domestic birds and horses through transmission by a mosquito. People are often infected accidentally. A *saprozoonosis* is dependent on an inanimate reservoir to maintain the cycle of infection. Visceral larva migrans, caused by *Toxocara* spp., is considered a saprozoonosis, although the disease also involves vertebrate reservoirs. Soil is essential for transmission of the disease to people and for reinfection of dogs and cats. Infected dogs and cats shed *Toxocara* eggs in their feces. Humid soil is most favorable for survival of the eggs.

Control of Zoonotic Diseases

Because of their regular contact with animals, animal tissues, animal environments, and pet owners, veterinarians and veterinary technicians are often the first to notice a zoonotic disease or the potential for one. In fact, animals can act as sentinels for a potential epidemic or outbreak of infection in people. A good example are the arboviral diseases, such as eastern equine encephalitis (EEE), western equine encephalitis (WEE), California and St. Louis encephalitis, and Japanese encephalitis (JE). Mild forms of these diseases are characterized by fever and headache; the most serious forms can cause death in people. Mortality depends on the specific type of virus involved. The diseases are transmitted by the bite of an infected mosquito. Mosquitoes acquire the infection from birds, horses, and even pigs (JE). EEE is transmitted among birds; horses and people are uncommon hosts. Both EEE and WEE viruses can cause encephalitis in horses. Venezuelan equine encephalomyelitis (VEE) rarely causes encephalitis in people but typically causes a flu-like viral infection in people. Horses are the reservoir for infection in people. Cases of encephalitis in birds or horses can signal a potential problem for humans; consequently, preventive programs can be implemented before a large outbreak of disease occurs in the human population.

Knowledge of how zoonotic diseases are transmitted and maintained in a population is important for preventing spread of diseases and preventing infection in veterinarians and veterinary technicians. Because of their close working contact with animals, veterinary professionals are at risk of contracting zoonotic diseases. It is important to determine what diseases are most common in certain animal species so that the risk of contracting a particular disease can be estimated. Certain groups of people are more susceptible and suffer more serious effects to zoonotic diseases than others. Children and the elderly are more susceptible because their immune systems function at a lower level than those of normal healthy adults. AIDS, lupus, and chemotherapeutic medications suppress function of the immune system, making an individual more susceptible to disease. Children are also likely to put contaminated soil or materials in their mouth. Pregnant women are also highly susceptible. Some diseases, such as toxoplasmosis, represent a serious disease threat to newborn infants.

Control of zoonotic diseases is aimed at the reservoir of disease or the intermediaries that transmit the disease. Control measures include spraying for mosquitoes, use of tick repellent, pasteurization of milk, adequate water filtration, and proper cooking and handling of food. Control programs also include treatment of infected animals in the reservoir population and decrease of contact with infected animals in the reservoir to prevent further transmission. Prevention programs require a thorough knowledge of the disease and how it is maintained and transmitted in order to break the cycle of disease in the population or prevent disease transmission. Prevention programs include vaccination of animals in the reservoir population, potential hosts, and people, if vaccines against that disease are available. Prevention of human infection is possible by treatment of infected animals that may transmit the disease to people. For example, treating puppies and kittens for roundworms and hookworms can prevent contamination of soil by feces containing infective eggs. Veterinarians and veterinary technicians can also test animals for infection, such as for tuberculosis and brucellosis.

The content of this chapter does not necessarily reflect the views or policies of the Department of Health and Human Services or the Food and Drug Administration, nor does the mention of trade names, commercial products, or organizations imply endorsement by the United States Government.

RECOMMENDED READING

August JR: Dog and cat bites, *J Am Vet Med Assoc* 193:1394-1398, 1988.

AVMA: *Zoonoses update,* ed 2, American Veterinary Medical Association, 1996.

Benenson AS, editor: *Control of communicable diseases in man,* ed 16, Washington, D.C., 1996, American Public Health Association.

Breitschwerdt EB: Tick-borne zoonoses, *Vet Tech* 11(5):249-251, 1990.

McCapes RH, Osburn BI, Riemann H: Safety of foods of animal origin: responsibilities of veterinary medicine, *J Am Vet Med Assoc,* 199:870-874, 1991.

National Association of State Public Health Veterinarians, Inc: Compendium of animal rabies control, *J Am Vet Med Assoc,* 208:214-218, 1996.

Laboratory Procedures

B. Hopman
E.M. Johnson
A.E. Thiessen
M. Ikram
D.J. Fisher
J. Colville

Learning Objectives

After reviewing this chapter, the reader should understand the following:

Methods used to collect samples of body tissues and fluids for laboratory examination

Ways in which diagnostic samples are prepared for laboratory examination

Hematologic examinations commonly performed on blood

Common internal and external parasites of domestic animals, and procedures used to diagnose parasitism

Chemistry assays commonly performed on blood

Assays commonly performed to assess organ function

Microbiologic tests commonly performed to identify bacterial, fungal, and viral pathogens

Procedures used in cytologic examination of body tissues and fluids

Tests commonly performed in analyzing urine specimens

Immunologic and serologic tests commonly used in veterinary practice

Methods used to maintain accuracy of laboratory test results

HEMATOLOGY

B. HOPMAN

Hematologic examination, or the analysis of blood, is a very powerful diagnostic tool. Veterinary technicians provide a valuable service by acquiring the skills necessary to perform this analysis. Only through practice and attention to detail can the veterinary technician develop the confidence and proficiency to perform these procedures.

Hematologic procedures include collecting and handling blood samples, performing a complete blood count, assisting with bone marrow examination, and helping with routine blood coagulation tests.

COLLECTING AND HANDLING BLOOD SPECIMENS

Improper handling of blood may render a blood sample unusable for analysis or result in inaccurate results. The methods and sites of blood collection depend on the species, the amount of blood needed, and personal preference.

Venous blood is frequently used in hematologic tests and is easily accessible in most species. The cephalic vein is the preferred site in dogs and cats. The saphenous vein (lateral in the dog, medial in the cat) is a reasonable substitute, especially in fractious cats. Jugular venipuncture is an efficient way to collect a large volume of blood. It is the preferred site in large domestic animals.

The wing vein is the preferred site in birds. If only a small amount of blood is needed, you may clip a nail and draw blood into a microhematocrit tube by capillary action. Vasoconstriction related to the stress of restraint may restrict blood flow after nail clipping. If this happens, it is best to let the bird calm down and try to collect again later, rather than keep clipping more nails.

The ear vein in rabbits works well for blood collection. The tail vein, infraorbital sinus, and cardiac puncture can be used in laboratory animals if the animals are anesthetized.

Ideally, clip collection site to remove the hair. The site is then cleaned with alcohol or other suitable antiseptic.

Take care not to stress the animal during blood collection. Use only the amount of restraint necessary to immobilize the animal. Excitement and stress can cause splenic contraction, which can alter the results of tests performed on red blood cells (RBCs). Results of several white blood cell (WBC) tests are also affected.

Blood may be collected in a syringe or specialized vacuum device, such as the Vacutainer system (Becton-Dickinson, Rutherford, NJ).

The amount of blood needed usually determines the size of syringe chosen. Needle size is determined by the size of the animal. For most small animals, 20- to 25-gauge needles work well. In large animals, 16- to 20-gauge needles are routinely used. Using a large syringe with a small-bore needle can result in hemolysis (rupture of red blood cells) when the syringe plunger is pulled back with great speed and force. Remove the needle before expelling the blood into the collection tube. Erythrocytes (red blood cells, or RBCs) can hemolyze (rupture) if forced back through the needle.

Vacutainers are very useful for multiple samples and when blood can be collected from a larger vessel, such as the cephalic or jugular veins. The Vacutainer system consists of a special needle, a needle holder, and vacuum-filled tubes that may be empty (clot tubes) or may contain a premeasured amount of anticoagulant. Draw a fixed amount of blood into the tube, based on tube size and amount of vacuum in the tube. Collapse of veins, especially in smaller animals, may occur because of excessive negative pressure exerted by the vacuum. Using small vacuum tubes may remedy this problem.

Fill collection tubes with the proper amount of blood, regardless of the method used to collect the sample. Unless otherwise directed, fill the tube about 2/3 to 3/4 full. This ensures a proper blood to anticoagulant ratio. Mix the blood adequately by inverting the tube *gently* for 10 to 20 seconds after transferring the blood. It is important always to try for a precise venipuncture to prevent formation of blood clots in the sample because of contamination with tissue fluids aspirated after multiple attempts at venipuncture.

The choice of blood collection tube depends on the intended use of the sample. Red-top (clot) tubes that contain no anticoagulant are used to collect blood that can then be centrifuged to yield serum. Tubes containing anticoagulant are used to preserve a whole blood sample or the anticoagulated sample can be centrifuged to yield plasma.

Several types of anticoagulant tubes are available and each has a preferred use.

Ethylenediaminetetraacetic acid (EDTA) is the most commonly used anticoagulant. EDTA binds to calcium and prevents clot formation. It is preferred for routine hematologic studies because it preserves cell morphology better than other anticoagulants. Even if collected in an EDTA tube, blood should be analyzed as quickly as possible, preferably within 2 hours after collection. Blood preserved in EDTA stays fresh for several hours or even overnight if stored in a refrigerator at 4° C; however, morphologic changes in the cells, such as cytoplasmic vacuolation, irregular cell membranes, and crenation, may occur in stored samples. This can make interpretation of observations difficult and result in inaccuracies.

It is for this reason that blood smears are best made immediately with fresh blood or within an hour after collection in an EDTA tube. If there is any delay in examining the blood, it is important to gently remix the blood by inverting it several times before making a blood smear. Crenation (shrinkage of RBCs) may occur if the tubes are not sufficiently filled, causing a relative excess of EDTA in the sample. Tubes that contain EDTA have a lavender or purple rubber stopper.

Tubes containing heparin (green-top tubes) may be used if blood smears are made immediately and tests run on whole blood are done promptly, because heparin may cause cells to clump and stain poorly. Heparin tubes may be a good choice for storing small blood samples from birds, because you can use the whole blood for hematologic tests and then collect plasma after spinning the sample.

Sodium citrate (blue-top tubes) anticoagulant is used for coagulation tests. However, it is generally not suitable for routine hematologic studies because it can cause distortion in cell morphology.

All specimen containers must be labeled with the name or number of the animal, owner's name, and the date the sample was taken. Accurate recordkeeping is paramount in preventing mistakes in sample evaluation and treatment of a patient.

The Complete Blood Count

The complete blood count, also known as the *CBC*, is a cost-effective way to obtain valuable hematologic information on a patient. CBCs may be performed by manual methods or automatically with the aid of a variety of machines. With practice and attention to detail, you can perform a CBC quickly, easily, and accurately in any veterinary hospital.

A CBC may consist of the following:
- Packed cell volume
- Total plasma protein
- Plasma fibrinogen
- Total WBC count
- Evaluation of peripheral blood smear with WBC differential count, platelet estimation, and RBC and WBC morphology
- Reticulocyte count in anemic patients

If automatic instrumentation is available or blood is processed at a commercial laboratory, other tests may be performed. These include the following:
- Total RBC count
- Hemoglobin concentration
- Erythrocytic indices, including the mean corpuscular volume (MCV), mean corpuscular hemoglobin concentration (MCHC) and mean corpuscular hemoglobin (MCH).

Packed Cell Volume. The packed cell volume (PCV), also known as the hematocrit (Hct), is an expression of the percentage of whole blood occupied by RBCs. This value is determined by centrifugation of anticoagulated whole blood placed in a capillary tube. The PCV may also be determined mathematically from the total RBC count and the mean corpuscular volume. This derivation must be performed by automated methods. The most common procedure for determining the PCV is called the *microhematocrit method.*

The microhematocrit method requires only a few drops of whole blood (Box 11-1). A blood-filled capillary tube is centrifuged for 2 to 5 minutes, depending on the type of centrifuge. The blood separates into a plasma layer, a white buffy coat composed of WBCs and platelets, and a layer of packed red cells (Fig. 11-1). Measuring the RBC layer in the capillary tube determines the PCV. The precision of a PCV is about ± 1%, making it a very accurate test.

A low PCV may indicate anemia, which is a decreased number of circulating RBCs. There are many causes of anemia, including blood loss, neoplasia, parasitism, and chronic infection. An increased PCV, known as polycythemia, has several causes, including dehydration and splenic contraction in an excited animal.

PCV values may be erroneously high because of clots in the sample, failure to adequately mix the EDTA and blood, and insufficient centrifugation time.

PCV values may be erroneously low if the microhematocrit tube contains excessive plasma because of inadequate mixing of the sample. Sample dilution because of low blood to anticoagulant ratio may also cause a spurious decrease in PCV.

Box 11-1 Microhematocrit procedure

1. Fill two microhematocrit tubes about 3/4 full with whole blood. Wipe the excess blood from the outside of the tube. Use plain (anticoagulant-free) microhematocrit tubes with anticoagulated blood. Use heparinized tubes when collecting blood from a venipuncture site.
2. Push sealing clay into one end of each microhematocrit tube. Rotate each tube as it is pressed into the clay to ensure a tight seal.
3. Put the tubes in a microhematocrit centrifuge, with the clay seal to the *outside.* Centrifuge for 2 to 5 minutes, depending on the model of the centrifuge used.
4. Determine the PCV for each tube by measuring the length of the column of RBCs using a microhematocrit tube reader. Average the two readings.

A popular tube reader is a plastic sheet known as a Critocap chart (Sherwood Medical, St. Louis, MO). Place the centrifuged tube perpendicular to the chart lines with the clay/RBC interface on the zero line. Slide the tube along the chart until the 100% line intersects the plasma/air interface in the center of the meniscus. Read the PCV (percentage) directly from the chart at the RBC/buffy coat interface (Fig. 11-2).

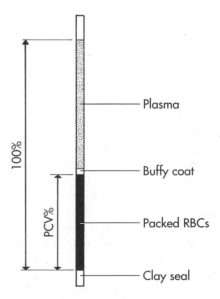

FIG. 11-1 Separated layers in a centrifuged hematocrit tube.

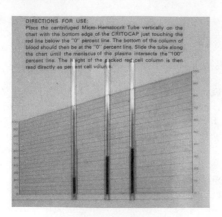

Box 11-2 Visual assessment of plasma turbidity and color

Normal: Clear and colorless to light straw yellow
Icterus: Clear and yellow
Hemolysis: Clear and red
Lipemia: Turbid and white

FIG. 11-2 Use of a Critocap chart to measure the PCV from a microhematocrit tube. The tube on the left has a PCV of 18%. *(Courtesy of Phillip Cochran, DVM.)*

After determining the PCV, evaluate the plasma for turbidity and color (Box 11-2).

An icteric, or yellow, plasma layer may occur with liver disease or hemolytic anemia. Normal adult ruminants and horses may have yellow plasma resulting from carotenes in the blood. A hemolytic, or red, sample can occur from improper sample collection and handling or with hemolytic anemia. Sometimes the buffy coat is red tinged, especially in very sick animals or if there is an increased number of immature RBCs in the circulation. Lipemic plasma appears cloudy (turbid) and white, indicating excessive lipids in the blood. This can occur if blood was collected from an animal that was not fasted, or it may be pathologic.

Icterus, hemolysis, and lipemia may be quantified as slight, moderate, or marked.

The width of the buffy coat should be assessed. With experience, you may be able to generally assess the WBC count from buffy coat width, if the total WBC count is very high or low. This is not an accurate method but can signal the technician to be on the lookout for an abnormal WBC count.

Microfilariae in heartworm-positive dogs are also observable at the buffy coat/plasma interface. The interface should be examined with a microscope at low power (100× magnification). Microfilariae can be seen wiggling, displacing plasma and buffy coat.

In certain situations, it may be valuable to microscopically examine the buffy coat for infectious agents and cell types, including cancer cells. This may be done using a process called the *macrohematocrit,* or *Wintrobe, method.* This requires a larger hematocrit tube and 1 ml of blood. The main purpose of this method is to locate cells present in very low numbers in the buffy coat. After centrifugation, make a smear of the buffy coat. Then air dry the smear and send it to a commercial laboratory for analysis. The slide may also be stained and examined for neoplastic cells or infectious agents.

Total Plasma Protein Determination. The serum or plasma total protein level can be rapidly and reliably measured using a hand-held refractometer (Box 11-3). Several types of refractometers are available. Those encountered in practice have built-in scales that you can view by looking through a viewfinder at one end of the refractometer. Most refractometers have a scale to measure both protein and specific gravity. The protein value is read directly from the scale in g/dl. This may be labeled *S.P.* on some refractometers. Urine specific gravity is discussed later in this chapter.

Sometimes refractometers must be calibrated. This involves taking a reading on distilled water at an ambient temperature of 21° to 29° C (70° to 85° F). The reading should be at 1.000 on the urine specific gravity scale. If it is not, adjust the reading by turning the zero set screw on the instrument. Refer to the manufacturer's manual for details.

Accurate plasma protein determination is difficult in lipemic samples, because the turbidity produces an indistinct line of demarcation on the scale. Hemoglobinemia caused by hemolysis can falsely increase plasma protein values because of the presence of the heme portion of hemoglobin. The yellow color of an icteric sample does not interfere with refractometry.

Normal plasma protein values vary from 6 to 8 g/dl. Common causes of increased plasma protein levels include dehydration and increased production of globulins associated with inflammation. Plasma protein values decrease with overhydration, renal disease, gastrointestinal losses, and reduced protein production by a diseased liver.

Plasma Fibrinogen Determination. Fibrinogen is a protein produced by the liver and is involved in blood coagulation. Fibrinogen synthesis increases when inflammation is present. This is especially apparent in large animals, making fibrinogen a useful indicator of inflammation in large animals. This test is based on the idea that fibrinogen becomes denatured and precipitates out of plasma heated to 56° to 58° C. This test is rapid and provides a reasonable approximation of plasma fibrinogen levels. Because only a small amount of

---

Box 11-3 Plasma protein determination

1. After centrifuging a filled microhematocrit tube, carefully break the tube just above the buffy coat/plasma interface.
2. Transfer plasma to the refractometer by allowing the sample to fill the space between the cover plate and glass surface by capillary action. You need only a very small amount of the sample. Use a syringe and needle to force the plasma onto the surface of an open refractometer. Do not tap the sample out of the tube, because this can scratch the surface of the refractometer.
3. Hold the refractometer horizontally, allowing the overhead light to reach the top of the instrument.
4. Look through the viewfinder and focus the scale by turning the eyepiece.
5. Read the protein value in g/dl at the interface of the light and shaded area (Fig. 11-3). Record the *v* value. Readings may vary slightly when different people read values on a refractometer. This results from a slight variation in an individual's perception of where the shaded line is read.
6. Clean the instrument with water and a soft, lint-free cloth or lens paper.

Box 11-4 Plasma fibrinogen procedure

1. Measure the plasma protein concentration on one of two centrifuged microhematocrit tubes.
2. Insert the remaining tube into a warm-water bath or an incubated sand-filled heat block at 56° to 58° C. Make sure the entire plasma column is immersed in the water or sand.
3. Heat the tube for at least 3 minutes. Remove the tube and examine the plasma layer for turbidity.
4. Recentrifuge to concentrate the fibrinogen in the top portion of the buffy coat.
5. Carefully break the tube at the plasma/fibrinogen interface and measure the plasma protein concentration. Subtract the second value from the first. The difference is the fibrinogen concentration. This value is measured as g/dl but may also be reported as mg/dl. (To convert from g/dl to mg/dl, move the decimal point three places to the right.)

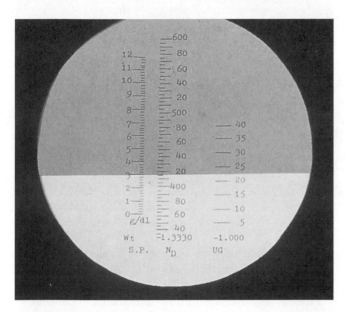

FIG. 11-3 View through a refractometer indicating 3.0 g/dl on the serum protein (S.P.) scale. *(Courtesy of Phillip Cochran, DVM.)*

fibrinogen is normally present in serum, it is much more reliable to detect increased levels than decreased levels in plasma (Box 11-4).

Normal plasma fibrinogen concentrations are 100 to 700 mg/dl, depending on the species. Severe inflamma-

tion cause increases above this value. Remember, this test is usually reserved for large animals because increases are a consistent finding in these species.

Total Blood Cell Counts. The total white blood cell (leukocyte, WBC) count is one of the most useful values determined in a CBC. Total red blood cell (erythrocyte, RBC) and platelet (thrombocyte) counts, although more difficult and less accurate, may also be performed manually with a hemacytometer or through automated methods.

Hemacytometers are counting chambers used to determine the number of cells per microliter (μl, mm³) of blood. Several models are available, but the most common type used has two identical sets of fine grids of parallel and perpendicular etched lines called *Neubauer rulings* (Fig. 11-4). Each grid is divided into nine large squares. The four corner squares are divided into 16 smaller squares and the center square is divided into 400 tiny squares (25 groups of 16 each). The area of each grid (Neubauer ruling) is designed to hold a precise amount of sample (0.9 μl). Knowing the number of cells in set parts of the grid and the amount of sample in that area is the basis for calculating the number of cells per microliter of blood. Mechanical counters are available to manually keep track of the number of each cell type observed.

Dilute the blood sample and lyse red blood cells before counting WBCs or platelets. Accomplishing this requires use of the Unopette dilution and pipette system (Becton-Dickinson, Rutherford, NJ). This system includes a pipette that holds a predetermined amount of blood and a reservoir that contains a diluting and lysing agent (Box 11-5).

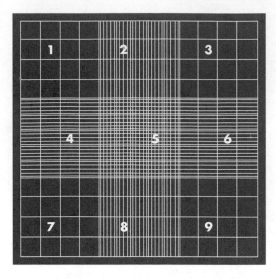

FIG. 11-4 Neubauer ruling and hemacytometer. Each *W* indicates a zone counted for the total WBC count. Each *R* indicates a square counted for the total RBC count.

The most commonly used WBC counting Unopette uses a 20-μl pipette and 3% acetic acid as the diluent (Box 11-6). The RBC counting system (Box 11-7) uses a 10-μl sample pipette and 0.85% saline as a diluent (the RBCs are not lysed in this count).

You may also estimate the total RBC count by dividing the packed cell volume by 6. For example, if the PCV is 36,

36 ÷ 6 = estimated RBC count of 6 million RBCs/μl.

The Unopette system also provides a method for manually counting platelets. The procedure is similar to counting WBCs. A 20-μl pipette is used with 1% ammonium oxalate as a diluent. The ammonium oxalate hemolyzes the RBCs but preserves the WBCs and platelets. The WBCs and platelets can be counted at the same time by this method. The platelets are counted at 400× magnification in the 25 small squares in the large center square of the grid. The number of platelets counted is then multiplied by 1,000 to calculate the number of platelets per μl of blood. Counting platelets is especially difficult because of their small size and tendency to clump together. Platelets are counted after the WBCs, because it takes about 10 minutes for the platelets to settle within the hemacytometer counting chamber.

Manual RBC and platelet counts are usually not part of routine practice, because they are less precise than the total WBC count. These counts are, however, conveniently performed at commercial laboratories and in practices with automated cell-counting machines.

Box 11-5 Blood counts with the Unopette system and hemacytometer

1. After thoroughly mixing anticoagulated blood, fill the Unopette pipette with blood by capillary action. Carefully wipe excess sample from the outside of the pipette.
2. Transfer the blood into the reservoir containing the diluting agent. Be careful not to lose any of the sample during this step. See the Unopette package insert for more detailed instructions. Thoroughly mix the sample and the diluting agent.
3. After letting the sample stand for an appropriate time (to lyse RBCs if needed), mix the sample to resuspend the cells so that a consistent sample can be delivered to the hemacytometer. Make sure the hemacytometer and its special coverslip are clean and free of dirt and fingerprints. Clean them with lens cleaner and paper.
4. After squeezing 3 to 4 drops of sample and discarding, immediately charge (fill) each side of the hemacytometer at the etched groove. Do not overfill or underfill the counting chamber. This can cause uneven distribution of cells throughout the Neubauer ruling and contributes to an inaccurate count.
5. Place the hemacytometer on the microscope stage. Lower the condenser of the microscope to increase contrast so that the cells are easier to see.
6. Count all of the cells in the appropriate squares. Cells that touch the lines between two squares are considered as within that square if they touch the top or the left-center lines (Fig. 11-5). Cells that touch the bottom or right lines are not counted with that square. Squares from each side (grid) of the hemacytometer are counted and these counts are averaged. This value is then used to calculate the count for each cell type being evaluated.

Platelet counts can be roughly estimated while viewing a blood smear with a microscope (see Evaluation of Platelets later in this chapter).

Hemoglobin Determination. Hemoglobin concentration is difficult to determine accurately without automatic instrumentation. Knowing the hemoglobin concentration offers no clinical advantage over the packed cell volume (PCV) except that the hemoglobin value is used to calculate certain erythrocytic indices. These indices are useful in describing different types of anemias and are discussed later in this chapter. The hemoglobin concentration should be about one third of the PCV if the RBCs are of normal size.

Box 11-6 Procedure for a total WBC count

1. Fill the appropriate 20-μl Unopette pipette with blood and wipe off the excess.
2. Transfer the blood to 3% acetic acid diluent (lysing agent). Make sure all the blood is transferred into the diluent by squeezing the plastic reservoir a few times. Mix the vial by inversion. The diluted sample is stable for 3 hours.
3. Let the sample stand for at least 10 minutes to allow RBCs to hemolyze.
4. Mix the sample by inversion, discard the first 3 to 4 drops and charge (fill) the hemacytometer. Let the cells settle for about a minute.
5. Under 100× magnification, count the WBCs in the nine large squares of the Neubauer grid (Fig. 11-6). Count each side separately and average these counts. The counts for the two sides should be within 10% of each other. If not, clean the hemacytometer and do the count again. With practice you can do this consistently. White blood cells appear as dark dots of varying shapes. These are the nuclei of WBCs. Be careful not to count dust particles or other contaminant debris.
6. Once you have this average count, add 10% and multiply by 100 (or multiply by 110%). This gives you the number of WBCs/μl of blood. For example, if the average count of both sides of the hemacytometer is 80, add 10% of 80 (8) to that.

$$88 \times 100 = 8,800 \text{ WBCs}/\mu\text{l of blood.}$$

Report this value to the clinician.

Box 11-7 Procedure for a total RBC count

1. Fill the appropriate 10-μl Unopette pipette with blood and wipe off the excess.
2. Transfer the blood from the pipette to the reservoir containing 0.85% saline and mix by inversion. The diluted sample is stable for 6 hours.
3. Discard the first 3 to 4 drops of sample and immediately charge (fill) each side of the hemacytometer as in the procedure for total WBC count.
4. Under 400× magnification, count the RBCs in the four corner squares and the one center square within the large center square of the grid (see Fig. 11-4). Count each side and average these counts. Erythrocytes tend to be packed tightly and are harder to count than leukocytes. It is difficult to achieve agreement within 10% of the counts for the two sides. Therefore, it is usually considered adequate if agreement is within 20%.
5. Add four zeros to the value counted in the five smaller squares on the grid. For example, if the average RBC count is 550, adding four zeros to that value would yield an RBC count of 5,500,000 RBCs/μl of blood. Another way of reporting this is $5.5 \times 10^6/\mu$l.

Preparing the Blood Smear. Examining the blood smear is one of the most valuable parts of a CBC. It can also be the most difficult to master. Patience and practice are required to develop the skills necessary to make and interpret blood films. Only one drop of blood is needed to make a smear. It is best to use blood from the tip of the needle immediately after the blood is collected. This prevents development of artifacts related to the presence of anticoagulant. If you cannot make a smear immediately, make the smear as soon as possible after collection.

The two methods of preparing blood smears are the wedge (glass slide) method and the coverslip method. Always use precleaned, glass microscope slides and coverslips. It is important to hold slides by their edges to avoid smudging with grease or fingerprints.

The wedge method is the most common type of smear used for routine hematology (Fig. 11-6). The coverslip

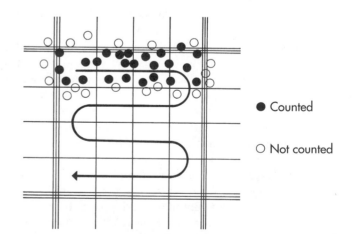

FIG. 11-5 Each area of the hemacytometer is scanned in a systematic pattern after counting blood cells. In this diagram, the solid spheres represent cells already counted, whereas the open spheres represent cells not yet counted. Count the cells that touch the top and left center lines of an individual square. Do not count cells touching the bottom and right lines of a square.

● Counted

○ Not counted

method is often preferred for avian blood smears because it renders a thinner film, which facilitates cell identification. It is also less traumatic on the fragile avian blood cells.

Coverslip smears are made by putting one drop of blood in the center of a clean, square coverslip (see Fig. 11-6). Place a second coverslip diagonally on top of the first, causing the blood to spread evenly between the two surfaces. Then pull the coverslips apart in a single smooth motion before the blood has completely spread. Wave the smears in the air to promote drying and stain them in a similar manner as described in Box 11-8 for making wedge smears.

Improper technique and inappropriate staining can result in inferior or useless blood smears. Jerky movements and dirty slides may cause streaks on the film. Using too little or too much blood results in improper smear length. Clots in the blood can cause small holes in the smear and an uneven feathered edge. If the blood is anemic (decreased PCV), increase the spreader slide angle to about 45 degrees. Conversely, the angle should be decreased to about 20 degrees if the blood is concentrated (increased PCV). Increasing the spreader slide angle makes a thicker smear, whereas decreasing it makes a thinner smear.

Table 11-1 lists problems related to staining. Cells appear dark if overstained, whereas extensive rinsing may cause them to look faded. Changing stains regularly is necessary for consistent results and preventing stain precipitation on the film. Refractile artifacts on RBCs are another common problem. These are usually caused by moisture in the fixative solution. Take care not to confuse these artifacts with cellular abnormalities.

Examining the Blood Smear

Place the slide on the microscope stage and examine the blood smear in a systematic manner. It is important to examine slides the same way each time to help avoid mistakes in counting cells and perhaps miss important observations (Fig. 11-8). Scan the smear at low power (100× magnification) to assess overall cell numbers and distribution. With practice, you can quickly estimate the total WBC count as either too high or low. Platelet clumps (aggregates) and blood parasites (microfilariae) are sometimes found at the feathered edge; note these.

A monolayer (single layer of blood cells) is located adjacent to the feathered edge. The cells should have even distribution and minimal overlapping. It is here, using the oil-immersion objective (1000× magnification), that the differential WBC count takes place. One hundred WBCs are counted, identified, and recorded during this count. Various counting devices are available to aid the differential WBC count.

A scanning pattern commonly used in performing the differential WBC count is shown in Fig. 11-8. The mor-

---

Box 11-8 Making a wedge smear

1. Place a small drop of blood at the end of a clean glass slide using a microhematocrit tube or the end of a wooden applicator stick. Place this slide on a flat surface or suspend in mid-air between the thumb and forefinger.
2. Hold a second slide (the spreader slide) at a 30° angle and pull back into contact with the drop of blood, spreading blood along the edge of the spreader slide. Push the spreader slide forward in a rapid, steady, even motion to produce a blood film that is thick at one end and tapers to a thin, feathered edge at the other (Fig. 11-7). The blood film should cover about three-quarters of the length of the slide.
3. Air-dry the smear by waving the slide in the air. This fixes the cells to the slide so that they are not dislodged during staining.
4. Label the slide at the thick end of the smear. If the slide has a frosted edge, this may be written on.
5. After drying, stain the smear with Wright's stain or a Romanowsky-type stain, available in commercial kits (e.g., Wright's Dip Stat3; Medi-Chem, Santa Monica, CA). These kits contain an alcohol fixative, a methylene blue mixture to stain cell nuclei and certain organelles bluish-purple, and eosin to stain hemoglobin and some WBC granules reddish-orange. Follow the directions packaged with the staining kit. Smears typically must be immersed in each solution for 5 to 10 seconds (5 to 10 dips).
6. After staining, rinse the slide with distilled water. Allow the slide to dry upright with the feathered edge pointed upward. This allows the water to drip off the slide away from the smear.

---

phology of RBCs and WBCs is assessed and platelet numbers are estimated. Most microscopes have a 10× ocular lens, but if a 15× ocular lens is available, you may perform the differential WBC count and evaluation of cells using the high-dry objective (600× magnification). Many objective lenses are designed for use with a coverslip in place. Resolution and sharpness are increased when coverslips are used with these types of lenses. The microscope operator's manual should be consulted for information regarding lenses.

TABLE 11-1 Some possible solutions to problems seen with common Romanowsky-type stains

Problem	Solution
Excessive blue staining	
Prolonged stain contact	Decrease staining time
Inadequate wash	Wash longer
Specimen too thick	Make thinner smears if possible
Stain or wash water too alkaline	Check with pH paper and correct pH
Exposure to formalin vapors	Store and ship cytologic preps separate from formalin containers
Wet fixation in ethanol	Air dry smears before fixation
Delayed fixation	Fix smears sooner if possible
Surface of the slide was alkaline	Use new slides
Excessive pink staining	
Insufficient staining time	Increase staining time
Prolonged washing	Decrease duration of wash
Stain or diluent too acidic	Check with pH paper and correct pH; fresh methanol may be needed
Excessive time in red stain solution	Decrease time in red stain solution
Inadequate time in blue stain solution	Increase time in blue stain solution
Mounting coverslip before preparation is dry	Allow preparation to dry completely before mounting coverslip
Weak staining	
Insufficient contact with one or more of the stain solutions	Increase staining time
Fatigued (old) stains	Change stains
Another slide covered specimen during staining	Keep slides separate
Uneven staining	
Variation of pH in different areas of slide surface (may be due to slide surface being touched or slide being poorly cleaned)	Use new slides and avoid touching their surface before and after preparation
Water allowed to stand on some areas of the slide after staining and washing	Tilt slides close to vertical to drain water from the surface or dry with a fan
Precipitate on preparation	
Inadequate stain filtration	Filter or change the stain(s)
Inadequate washing of slide after staining	Rinse slides well after staining
Dirty slides used	Use clean new slides
Stain solution dries during staining	Use sufficient stain and do not leave it on slide too long
Miscellaneous	
Overstained preparation	Destain with 95% methanol and restain
Refractile artifact on RBC (usually due to moisture in fixative)	Change the fixative

From Cowell RL and Tyler RD: *Diagnostic cytology of the dog and cat,* St Louis, 1989, Mosby.

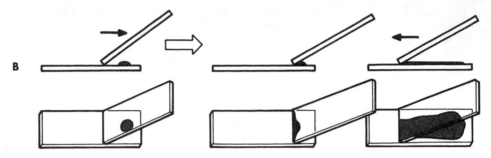

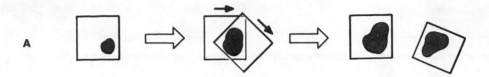

FIG. 11-6 Methods commonly used for making blood smears. **A,** Coverslip technique, **B,** Wedge-type smear. *(From Powers LW:* Diagnostic hematology, *St Louis, 1989, Mosby.)*

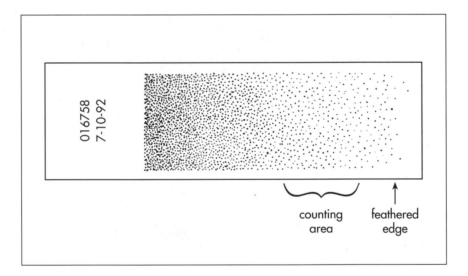

016758
7-10-92

counting area   feathered edge

FIG. 11-7 Blood smear showing the label area, monolayer counting area, and feathered edge.

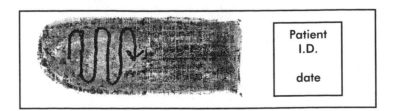

Patient I.D.

date

FIG. 11-8 Scanning pattern used for performing a differential WBC count. *(From Sirois M:* Veterinary clinical laboratory procedures, *St Louis, 1995, Mosby.)*

EVALUATION OF RED BLOOD CELLS

Red blood cells carry oxygen (bound to hemoglobin) to tissues. A decreased PCV, RBC count, or hemoglobin value is called *anemia*. Anemia has many causes and occurs in several forms, classified in a variety of ways. Anemia is the result of either decreased production or increased destruction of RBCs. Anemias are commonly classified as either *regenerative* (responsive) anemia, in which the bone marrow is responding by increasing RBC production, or as *nonregenerative* (nonresponsive) anemia, in which the bone marrow does not respond to the need for increased RBC production. These two types of anemia are distinguished from each other by the number of immature RBCs, known as *reticulocytes* or *polychromatic cells,* observed in the peripheral blood.

Anemia can also be classified with use of erythrocytic indices. These indices include mean corpuscular volume (MCV), mean corpuscular hemoglobin concentration (MCHC), and mean corpuscular hemoglobin (MCH). The erythrocytic indices are calculated using the PCV, hemoglobin concentration, and a total RBC count. The erythrocytic indices are usually not reported when performing a CBC manually.

The *mean corpuscular volume (MCV)* refers to the average size of an RBC, reported in femtoliters (fl). It is calculated by multiplying the PCV by 10 and dividing by the total RBC count. Anemia characterized by an increased MCV is called *macrocytic* (large RBC size). Regenerative anemias are typically macrocytic because immature RBCs are larger than mature RBCs. Anemias with a normal MCV are called *normocytic* (normal RBC size) and can have many causes. Most anemias are of this type. Anemia characterized by a decreased MCV are called *microcytic* (small RBC size) and are almost always the result of iron deficiency. Iron deficiency can occur from chronic blood loss or from insufficient intake of dietary iron, as is seen in young animals, especially baby pigs.

The mean corpuscular hemoglobin concentration (MCHC) is the ratio of the weight of hemoglobin in each RBC, reported in grams per deciliter (g/dl). Calculate this by multiplying the hemoglobin concentration by 100 and dividing by the PCV. The MCHC is the most accurate erythrocytic index because it does not require the less precise RBC count. Anemia characterized by a decreased MCHC is called *hypochromic* (decreased color). Hypochromic anemia may occur as a result of iron deficiency or in regenerative anemia, because the many immature RBCs do not develop their full concentration of hemoglobin. Anemia characterized by a normal MCHC is described as *normochromic* (normal color). Normochromic anemia is commonly associated with normocytic erythrocytes. An increased MCHC (hyperchromic anemia, increased color) does not occur and if detected is most likely erroneous and caused by hemolysis.

The mean corpuscular hemoglobin (MCH) is the average weight of hemoglobin found in RBCs, measured in picograms (pg). It is calculated by multiplying the hemoglobin concentration by 10 and dividing this total by the total RBC count. Many do not report MCH, because it offers no more information than the MCHC. It is also the least accurate erythrocytic index because it requires the hemoglobin concentration and total RBC count, which are not as precise as the PCV.

Anemias are often described by cell size and color. Normocytic, normochromic anemias are the most common (normal RBC size and color). Causes include chronic inflammation, infections, renal disease, neoplasia, and bone marrow destruction by toxins. Macrocytic, normochromic anemias (large RBCs of normal color) may be the result of dietary vitamin and mineral deficiencies and feline leukemia virus infection. Microcytic, hypochromic anemias (small, pale RBCs) occur after loss of much blood.

Causes of anemia include chronic bleeding disorders, parasitism, and destruction of RBCs by immune-mediated disease. Microcytic, hypochromic anemia (small, pale RBCs) may be the result of iron deficiency resulting from chronic blood loss or lack of dietary iron. Dietary copper and vitamin B_6 deficiency may also cause this type of anemia.

Reticulocyte Counts

Reticulocytes are immature RBCs that contain ribonucleic acid (RNA) that is lost as the cell matures (Plate 1 in color insert). Reticulocyte numbers increase when the bone marrow is responding to an anemic state. When reticulocytes are stained with a vital stain, such as new methylene blue, their RNA is visible as blue granules or aggregates. These cells correspond to the larger, blue-gray polychromatic RBCs seen in Wright's-stained smears.

Cats have two types of reticulocytes. The aggregate type is similar to those found in other species and is the type that is counted in all species. The punctate type has a few small, blue-stained granules (not aggregates). This type of reticulocyte may compose up to 10% of RBCs in healthy animals. Their numbers are increased in regenerative anemia but only the aggregate type is counted.

Reticulocytes do not occur in horses, even with regenerative anemia. They are not found in healthy ruminants but do increase in responding anemias. Reticulocytes are common in healthy suckling pigs. Less than 1% of the RBCs in adult pigs are reticulocytes; reticulocyte numbers increase in regenerative anemias of pigs.

To make a blood smear to examine for reticulocytes, mix a few drops of blood with an equal amount of new methylene blue stain in a test tube and allow this to stand for at least 10 minutes. Make a wedge-type smear with the mixture and allow it to air dry. Many clinicians like to counterstain this slide with Wright's or Romanowsky-type stain because the RBCs stain reddish and the aggregate granules stain a prominent blue, making the reticulocytes easier to count. Counting the reticulocytes allows the clinician to evaluate the degree of bone marrow response in anemia.

Count the reticulocytes using the oil-immersion objective (1000× magnification). Count the number of aggregate reticulocytes among an estimated 1,000 RBCs. The observed percentage can easily be calculated by dividing the number of reticulocytes counted per 1,000 RBCs by 10. Correct this percentage for the degree of anemia present by multiplying it by the patient's PCV and dividing by the normal mean PCV (45% in the dog, 37% in the cat). A corrected reticulocyte percentage above 1% in dogs and above 0.4% in cats indicates a regenerative response to anemia. For example, a dog has a PCV of 21%, with 20% reticulocytes.

$$\frac{\text{observed }\%}{\text{reticulocytes}} \times \frac{\text{patient's PCV}}{\text{normal mean PCV}} = \frac{\text{corrected }\%}{\text{reticulocytes}}$$

$$20\% \times \frac{21\%}{45\%} = 9\%$$

If a total RBC count has been performed, you can calculate an absolute reticulocyte count by multiplying the corrected reticulocyte percentage by the RBC count. This gives the number of reticulocytes per microliter (μl) of blood. In most animals (except horses), an absolute reticulocyte count above 60,000/μl indicates a regenerative response to anemia.

Red Blood Cell Morphology

Normal erythrocyte morphology varies greatly among different species (Table 11-2). Unlike the RBCs of mammals, avian RBCs are nucleated. Technicians should be able to identify normal as well as abnormal RBC morphology. Morphology is evaluated using the oil-immersion objective (1000× magnification) in the monolayer portion of the smear.

Normal canine RBCs (Plate 2 in color insert) have an obvious area of central pallor (lighter center) that represents a thin area of the cell.

Rouleaux formation (Plate 3 in color insert) is a grouping of RBCs in coin-like stacks. Increased rouleaux formation is often associated with increased levels of fibrinogen or globulin resulting from inflammation. Marked rouleaux formation is common in healthy horses.

Agglutination is a grape-bunch–like aggregation of erythrocytes that can appear similar to rouleaux (Plates 3, 4, and 5 in color insert). It occurs in some immune-mediated disorders and may be seen on the sides of blood sample tubes as hanging blood clots. Agglutination fails to dissipate in dilution with saline as rouleaux does.

Both rouleaux and agglutination may be quantified as slight, moderate, or marked.

Anisocytosis is variation in RBC size. It is normal in young animals and adult ruminants. Anisocytosis is often associated with regenerative anemias because immature RBCs (polychromatophils) are larger than mature RBCs.

Macrocytes are large cells and are usually immature polychromatic RBCs (reticulocytes if stained with new methylene blue). The MCV is increased if they occur in significant numbers.

TABLE 11-2 Characteristics of normal red blood cells in animals

Species	Diameter	Rouleaux	Central pallor	Anisocytosis	Poikilocytes	Basophilic stippling in regenerative response	Reticulocytes (normal PCV)
Dogs	7.0μ	+	++++	—	—	—	±1.0%
Pigs	6.0μ	++	±	+	++++	—	±1.0%
Cats	5.8μ	++	+	±	—	±	±0.5%
Horses	5.7μ	++++	±	±	—	—	0% (will not increase in response to anemia)
Cattle	5.5μ	—	+	++	—	+++	0% (will increase in response to anemia)
Sheep	4.5μ	±	+	+	—	+++	0% (will increase)
Goats	3.2μ	—	—	±	++ (in young)	++	0% (will increase)

Microcytes are small RBCs with a decreased MCV. They may be associated with iron deficiency from chronic blood loss. Normal Akita dogs typically have small RBCs.

Spherocytes (Plate 6 in color insert) are small, slightly darker-staining RBCs lacking central pallor. They are difficult to find in species other than the dog because canine RBCs normally have central pallor. They are observed in dogs with immune-mediated hemolytic anemia and after blood transfusions. Hemolytic, in this case, refers to accelerated destruction of RBCs.

Polychromatic cells are immature RBCs that are larger and exhibit a blue-gray tint from the persistence of residual RNA in the cytoplasm (Plate 7 in color insert). Polychromasia (many polychromatic RBCs) represents reticulocytes when smears are stained with new methylene blue. A few polychromatic cells are considered normal in the dog and cat. Increased numbers of these cells indicate a regenerative response to anemia in the same way as increased numbers of reticulocytes.

Hypochromasia (Plate 8 in color insert) is decreased staining intensity and increased central pallor of an RBC. When central pallor takes up more than 50% of the RBC's area, the cell is hypochromic and should be noted. Iron deficiency, immune-mediated hemolytic anemia, and other severe anemias may cause hypochromasia.

Basophilic stippling describes very small, dark-blue aggregates of RNA found in RBCs. It is sometimes found in ruminants and cats and represents a regenerative response similar to polychromasia. It may be detected in cases of lead poisoning when associated with nucleated RBCs without anemia.

Nucleated red blood cells (NRBCs) are immature RBCs released prematurely from the bone marrow (Plate 9 in color insert). The nucleus is usually dark and round. The cytoplasm should be the same color as in mature RBCs. Nucleated RBCs are usually metarubricytes but may be earlier stages of RBCs (rubricytes). They are considered appropriate if they are associated with a regenerative response to anemia (polychromasia and reticulocytes) but inappropriate if seen in the peripheral blood without marked evidence of response to anemia. Lead poisoning, hyperadrenocorticism, splenic disorders, fractures (bone marrow disruption), and feline leukemia virus (FeLV) infection are all causes of inappropriate NRBC response. Giant (megaloblastic) metarubricytes are sometimes observed in cats with FeLV infection.

Howell-Jolly bodies (Plate 10 in color insert) are basophilic nuclear remnants that appear very dark and round in an RBC. They are often seen in responding anemias because cells with Howell-Jolly bodies are generally young RBCs. Animals with splenic disease or that have been splenectomized have increased numbers of Howell-Jolly bodies because the spleen normally removes these remnants. A few are common in healthy animals.

Heinz bodies (Plate 11 in color insert) are round structures that represent denatured hemoglobin caused by chemical- or drug-induced oxidative injury. Acetaminophen toxicity, onion poisoning, and diabetes mellitus are some conditions that cause Heinz body formation. RBCs with Heinz bodies are more susceptible to destruction (hemolysis), leading to anemia. With Wright's or Romanowsky-type stain they appear as pale, round areas attached to the RBC membrane. Heinz bodies may vary in size and stain bluish with new methylene blue stain. Large Heinz bodies represent more severe oxidative change than small Heinz bodies and should be noted along with any increase in amount. Heinz bodies can be present in up to 5% of RBCs in normal cats. A variation of this is the eccentrocyte, which is an RBC with a large, pale area on one side of the RBC. This area also represents oxidative injury to the cell.

Poikilocytes are abnormally shaped RBCs. There are many types that are almost always associated with anemia and/or chronic disease. Only the most common are discussed here.

Crenation is shrinkage of RBCs characterized by many irregular blunt projections on the surface of an RBC. It is usually an artifact associated with slow drying of the blood film or an old sample. Cat and swine blood are especially susceptible to crenation.

Echinocytes (burr cells) are spiculated RBCs with many evenly spaced projections (Plate 12 in color insert). They often are seen in animals with kidney disease and can appear similar to crenated RBCs. In fact, crenation may be thought of as echinocytes produced as an artifact.

Schistocytes (schizocytes) are irregularly shaped RBC fragments (Plate 13 in color insert). These fragments can take on a wide variety of odd shapes. They are associated with severe anemia, immune-mediated disease, neoplasia, and disseminated intravascular coagulation.

Acanthocytes (spur or thorn cells) are spiculated RBCs with 2 to 10 blunt or rounded projections. They are associated with liver disease and hemangiosarcoma (see Plate 7 in color insert).

Stomatocytes are RBCs with oval areas of central pallor. They are seen in liver disease and severe anemia. They are also seen in hereditary stomatocytosis of Alaskan malamutes and schnauzers.

Leptocytes (target cells and folded cells) are thin RBCs with increased surface area. The membranes of these cells can fold or become deformed. Target cells are RBCs that resemble a target, having a central round area of hemoglobin surrounded by a clear area, surrounded again with a ring of hemoglobin (see Plate 7 in color insert). Folded cells have a thick, dense area of hemoglobin across the center of the cell. Both of these leptocytes can occur in a variety of conditions, including liver disease and many anemias.

It is important to be able to quantify abnormal morphology as well as identify it. Table 11-3 illustrates one method to quantify RBC morphology using the oil-immersion objective (1000× magnification). This table takes into account that RBC size varies among species; the number of RBCs per monolayer field varies accordingly. Dogs have approximately 250 to 300 RBCs per field at 1000× magnification; cats, horses, swine and ruminants have 400 to 500.

Blood Parasites

Hemobartonella felis (Plate 14 in color insert) is a common parasite of feline RBCs. Any anemic cat should be tested for this parasite. The organisms are very small, round or rod-shaped structures that stain darkly with Wright's or Romanowsky-type stain. They are often found as single organisms or pairs on the periphery of an RBC. They may also appear as chains or rings on an RBC. Because these parasites appear in the peripheral blood in cycles, the blood may need to be examined several times over 3 to 5 days before the infection can be ruled out. Be careful; do not confuse this parasite with stain precipitate or Howell-Jolly bodies. Some clinicians prefer to stain with new methylene blue, make a routine smear, and counterstain with a Romanowsky-type stain as for a reticulocyte preparation. This technique may aid in diagnosing other small blood parasites. This disease is commonly known as *feline infectious anemia (FIA)* or *hemobartonellosis*.

Hemobartonella canis is a rare blood parasite of dogs. It is observed in immunosuppressed or splenectomized dogs. This parasite resembles its feline counterpart.

Eperythrozoon occurs in cattle, sheep, and swine and appears similar to *Hemobartonella*. Coccal, rod, and ring forms are found on the RBC surface. The ring form is the most common.

Cytauxzoon felis is a very rare parasite of cats. An irregular ring form occurs within RBCs. Macrophages in the bone marrow may also contain the organism.

Anaplasma marginale (Plate 15 in color insert) is a blood parasite of cattle and wild ruminants. It can appear as a small, dark-staining spherical body at the margin of RBCs. This organism must not be confused with Howell-Jolly bodies. Early in the disease the parasite affects a large number of RBCs. Later, severe anemia develops and a smaller number of RBCs are affected. Howell-Jolly bodies usually are not observed in a large number of cells.

Babesia (Plate 16 in color insert) is a blood parasite of many species. The parasites appear as large, round, oval, or teardrop-shape bodies. They can occur singly, in pairs or in multiples of two. Infected RBCs are often seen at the feathered edge of a blood film.

Ehrlichia (Plate 17 in color insert) is an intracellular parasite of lymphocytes, monocytes, and neutrophils. The organism appears as small clusters in the cytoplasm.

TABLE 11-3 Semiquantitative evaluation of erythrocyte morphology based on average number of abnormal cells per oil-immersion (1000×) field

	1+	2+	3+	4+
Anisocytosis				
Dog	7-15	16-20	21-29	>29
Cat	5-8	9-15	16-20	>20
Cow	10-20	21-30	31-40	>40
Horse	1-3	4-6	7-10	>10
Polychromasia				
Dog	2-7	8-14	15-29	>29
Cat	1-2	3-8	9-15	>15
Cow	2-5	6-10	11-20	>20
Horse	Rarely observed			
Hypochromasia				
All species	1-10	11-50	51-200	>200
Poikilocytosis				
All species	3-10	11-50	51-200	>200
Leptocytes (target and folded cells)				
All species	3-5	6-15	16-30	>30
Spherocytes				
Dogs only	5-10	11-50	51-150	>150
Echinocytes, Heinz bodies (and eccentrocytes)				
All species	5-10	11-100	101-250	>250
Acanthocytes, schistocytes, and stomatocytes				
All species	1-2	3-8	9-20	>20

Modified from Weiss DJ: Uniform evaluation and semiquantitative reporting of hematologic data in veterinary laboratories, *Vet Clin Pathol* 13(2):27, 1984.

Infected animals are usually anemic, neutropenic, and thrombocytopenic. Examination of buffy coat smears may aid diagnosis.

Microfilariae of *Dirofilaria immitis*, the heartworm of dogs, can sometimes be found near the feathered edge of a smear. A microfilaria is about the width of an RBC.

EVALUATION OF WHITE BLOOD CELLS

White blood cells (leukocytes, WBCs) include mature and immature neutrophils, lymphocytes, monocytes, eosinophils, and basophils. Neutrophils, eosinophils, and basophils contain granules and are called *granulocytes*. Identifying and quantifying abnormal morphology of leukocytes is a vital part of a CBC, because each cell type has an important role in fighting disease and respective numbers of leukocytes reflect a patient's health status. Identifying different leukocytes is the basis for the differential WBC count.

The differential count is performed in the smear monolayer using oil-immersion (1000×) magnification. One hundred WBCs are counted and classified by type. Because 100 WBCs are counted, the number of each WBC type observed is recorded as a percentage. This is called the *relative WBC count*. Express differential counts in absolute numbers, such as cells per microliter, because percentages alone are not always diagnostically useful. Multiply the total WBC count by the percent of the individual cell type. For example,

$$\text{Total WBC count} = 6000/\mu l,$$
$$\text{with 80\% neutrophils observed}$$

$$6000 \times 80\% = 4800 \text{ neutrophils}/\mu l \text{ of blood}$$

Nucleated RBCs (NRBCs) (see Plate 9 in color insert) are also counted during the differential. They are tallied separately. If 5 or more are found per 100 WBCs, a corrected total WBC count should be calculated. The corrected total WBC count is necessary because total WBC counts performed on hemacytometers and some automatic cell counters include all nucleated cells, including RBCs. The equation used to calculate a corrected total WBC count is as follows:

$$\text{Corrected total WBC Count} = \frac{\text{Total WBCs} \times 100}{100 + \text{NRBCs}/100 \text{ WBCs}}$$

For example, the total WBC count = 9000/μl and 6 NRBCs are observed per 100 WBCs. The corrected WBC count is 9000/μl × 100/100 + 6 = 5660/μl. Note that the corrected total WBC count is always *lower* than the original WBC count. The corrected total WBC count is then used to calculate the absolute count for each type of WBC.

Segmented neutrophils, also known as "segs" or *polymorphonuclear (PMN) cells* (Plate 18 in color insert) are mature WBCs that function mainly as phagocytes and are involved in inflammation. They have an irregular, lobulated nucleus that is dark and dense. Their cytoplasm is usually colorless to pale pink in most species. Bovine neutrophils have pink to orange cytoplasm. The cytoplasm may contain very fine, diffuse, dark granules. They are the most common type of WBC found in most species.

Band neutrophils (Plates 18 and 19 in color insert) are immature neutrophils with a horseshoe- or S-shaped nucleus. The nucleus may have indentations up to 50% of its width, and that neutrophil may still be classified as

a band cell. The nucleus of band cells is smooth and is often lighter in color than that of segmented neutrophils.

Metamyelocytes (Plate 20 in color insert) and myelocytes (Plate 21 in color insert) are even earlier stages of neutrophils and are found in the bone marrow. They are not usually found in peripheral blood unless severe inflammation or infection is present. If there is any doubt about the identification of a neutrophil stage, always classify it as the more mature cell.

Toxic changes in neutrophils may indicate severe infection or inflammation. Toxic changes represent a progression of severity; more than one toxic change may be evident at the same time. Toxic cells often appear swollen and larger than normal. They may be described by number (few, moderate, many) and severity (slight, moderate, marked), as indicated in Table 11-4. Describe overall toxicity based on the most severe change observed. The toxic changes described below apply to neutrophils only. Some of these changes may occur in other WBCs, but they are usually not noted.

Döhle bodies (Plate 22 in color insert) are irregular, gray to blue cytoplasmic inclusions. They often are seen in pairs near the periphery of the cell. When alone, they represent a mild toxic change. Feline neutrophils appear to easily form Döhle bodies.

Cytoplasmic basophilia is characterized by a blue-gray cast to the cytoplasm. It may represent mild to severe toxic change, depending on intensity of color. Overstaining the slide in the blue solution or inadequate washing may cause the cytoplasm to appear basophilic. If the RBCs stain bluish, suspect this error.

TABLE 11-4 Semiquantitative evaluation of toxic changes in neutrophils by amount

Number of cells with toxic change	Percentage (%)*
Few	5-10
Moderate	11-30
Many	>30

	Severity of toxic change
Döhle bodies	Slight
Cytoplasmic basophilia	Slight to marked, depending on intensity
Cytoplasmic vacuolization (Foamy cytoplasm)	Moderate to marked, depending on amount
Indistinct nuclear membrane	Marked
Severe cell degeneration	

*If toxic changes occur in less than 5% of neutrophils, they are not reported.

Vacuolization of the cytoplasm (Plate 23 in color insert), ranging from a few vacuoles to many, causing a foamy appearance, is another toxic change in neutrophils. Vacuolization is recorded as moderate to severe, depending on the number and size of vacuoles observed. Prolonged contact with EDTA induces cytoplasmic vacuolization in neutrophils, so it is important to make blood smears soon after blood sample collection.

Toxic granulation is a moderate to severe toxic change and is particularly evident in equine blood. The granules are purplish-blue and stain quite prominently.

Nuclear degeneration and a general inability to differentiate neutrophils from other leukocytes are considered severe toxic changes.

Nuclear hypersegmentation (Plate 24 in color insert) describes the division of a neutrophil's nucleus into five or more distinct lobes. These are old neutrophils with a prolonged lifespan because of corticosteroid administration, hyperadrenocorticism, or chronic inflammation. Increased numbers of these old neutrophils is called a *right shift*. Hypersegmented neutrophils may also be an artifact caused by extended storage of anticoagulated blood.

An increase in WBC numbers is called *leukocytosis*. An increase in neutrophil numbers is called *neutrophilia*. A *left shift* describes increased numbers of immature neutrophils, as seen with inflammation and infection. A severe form of leukocytosis (more than 50,000 WBC/μl), called the *leukemoid response*, may accompany severe inflammation. Stress, excitement, and adminis-

tration of corticosteroids can cause mild neutrophilia, especially in cats, dogs, and horses. *Neutropenia* is a decreased number of circulating neutrophils. It may occur with an overwhelming infection.

Heterophils (Plate 25 in color insert) are the functional equivalent of neutrophils in rabbits, rodents, birds, reptiles, and amphibians. They have a segmented nucleus and variably sized red-brown granules. In most birds the granules are oval to needle-shaped. Heterophils may exhibit cytoplasmic basophilia and vacuolization as toxic changes.

Blood cells from exotic species can be difficult to classify and identify as abnormal. A technique for estimating the total WBC count in birds involves counting all the WBCs in at least 10 high-dry (400× magnification) fields and averaging them. This average is then multiplied by 2000 to get the number of WBCs per microliter of blood.

Lymphocytes have a round to slightly indented nucleus that almost completely fills the cell. The cytoplasm is light blue and may contain a few purple granules, especially in ruminants. Lymphocytes vary in size. Small lymphocytes (mature) (Plate 26 in color insert) have a thin rim of cytoplasm. Large lymphocytes (less mature) have larger nuclei and abundant cytoplasm. Lymphocytes are the predominant WBC type in ruminants (Plate 27 in color insert). Some bovine lymphocytes may be quite large, with nuclei that contain nucleolar rings, causing the lymphocytes to resemble neoplastic lymphoblasts (atypical lymphocytes).

TABLE 11-5 Normal hematologic values for domestic animals

	Dogs Range (mean)	Cats Range (mean)	Horses Range (mean)
PCV (%)	37-55 (45)	24-45 (37)	32-52 (42)
Hemoglobin (g/dl)	12-18 (15)	8-15 (12)	11-19 (15)
RBC ($\times 10^6$)/μl	5.5-8.5 (6.8)	5-10 (7.5)	6.5-12.5 (9.5)
Total protein (g/dl)	6.0-7.5	6.0-7.5	6.0-8.0
WBC ($\times 10^3$)/μl	6.0-17.0 (11.5)	5.5-19.5 (12.5)	5.5-12.5 (9.0)
Differential, absolute			
Segs	60-77%;3000-11,500 (7000)	35-75%; 2500-12,500 (7500)	30-65%; 2700-6700 (4700)
Bands	0-3%; 0-300 (70)	0-3%; 0-300 (100)	0-2%; 0-100 (2.0)
Lymphs	12-30%; 1000-4800 (2800)	20-55%; 1500-7000 (4000)	27-70; 1500-5500 (3500)
Monos	3-10%; 150-1350 (750)	1-4%; 0-850 (350)	0.5-7%; 0-800 (400)
Eosinos	2-10%; 100-1250 (550)	2-12%; 0-1500 (650)	0-11%; 0-925 (375)
Basos	Rare	Rare	0-3%; 0-170 (50)
Platelets ($\times 10^5$)	2.0-9.0	3-7 (4.5)	1-6 (3.3)
MCV (fl)	60-77 (70)	39-55 (45)	34-58 (46)
MCH (pg)	19-23	13-17	15.2-18.6
MCHC (g/dl)	32.0-36.0 (34.0)	30-36 (33.2)	31-37 (35)

From Pratt PW: *Laboratory procedures for veterinary technicians*, Goleta, Calif, 1992, American Veterinary Publications, Inc.

Atypical lymphocytes exhibit a wide variety of morphologic differences from large to classic small lymphocytes. These variances include divided nuclei and nucleoli. A nucleolus is a round, light-blue structure within the nucleus. A few of these lymphocytes with nucleoli may be seen in sick animals. Another atypical lymphocyte is the lymphoblast. Lymphoblasts (Plate 28 in color insert) are large, immature lymphocytes that contain a nucleolus. Large numbers of circulating lymphoblasts suggest a neoplastic disease of lymphocytes (lymphoproliferative disorders). Extreme lymphocytosis (more than 20,000/μl) may be present in these cases.

Reactive lymphocytes (immunocytes) are lymphocytes with a very dense, eccentric, irregular nucleus. Their cytoplasm typically stains intensely royal blue and may have a pale Golgi zone (Plate 29 in color insert). Reactive lymphocytes may be observed during periods of antigenic stimulation. They are occasionally present in normal animals; report them as a morphologic change only if more than 5% of lymphocytes are of this type.

Reactive and atypical lymphocytes are counted along with the other lymphocytes in the differential count. They may be quantified as *few*—5% to 10% of lymphocytes, *moderate*—11% to 30%, and *many*—more than 30%.

Increased lymphocyte numbers (lymphocytosis) occur in healthy, excited animals (especially cats) because of epinephrine release. Decreased lymphocyte numbers (lymphopenia) is a common finding in sick and very stressed animals.

Monocytes (Plate 30 in color insert) are very large WBCs with diffuse, less dense nuclear chromatin. The nucleus may vary in shape, including oval, kidney bean, bilobed, trilobed, and horseshoe shapes. The cytoplasm of monocytes is blue-gray and abundant. Vacuoles and/or fine granules may be present. Monocytes may be difficult to distinguish from toxic band neutrophils or earlier stages. Identifying an obvious band and noting its color is helpful. The cytoplasm of monocytes is usually darker than that of bands. The cell in question is most likely a monocyte if a left shift is not present.

Monocytosis (increased monocyte numbers) is common in diseases that cause chronic inflammation. Monocytopenia (decreased monocyte numbers) is not significant.

Eosinophils (Plate 31 in color insert) have a lobulated nucleus and red-orange (eosinophilic) granules in their cytoplasm. Canine eosinophils contain round granules that vary greatly in size. They usually stain the same color as RBCs. The eosinophils of sighthounds (e.g., Greyhounds) may be difficult to identify because the granules are often replaced by a colorless area. Feline eosinophils contain numerous, small, rod-shaped granules. Eosinophilic granules in horses are very large and round, and stain bright orange. The granules in swine and ruminants are uniformly small and round, and they stain pinkish-red. Increased eosinophil numbers (eosinophilia) may occur with parasitic disease or allergies.

Basophils (Plate 32 in color insert) have a lobulated nucleus and numerous dark purple (basophilic) granules

Cattle Range (mean)	Sheep Range (mean)	Pigs Range (mean)
24-46 (35)	24-50 (38)	32-50 (42)
8-15 (12)	8-16 (12)	10-16 (13)
5-10 (7)	8-16 (12)	5-8 (6.5)
6.0-8.0	6-7.5	6-7
4.0-12.0 (8.0)	4-12 (8)	11-22 (16)
15-45%; 600-4000 (7000)	10-50%; 700-6000 (2400)	28-47%; 3000-10,500
0-2%; 0-120 (20)	Rare	0-2%
45-75%; 2500-7500 (4500)	40-75%; 2000-9000 (5000)	39-62%; 4300-13,700
2-7%; 25-840 (400)	0.6%; 0-750 (200)	2-30%; 220-2200
2-20%; 0-2400 (700)	0.1%; 0-1000 (400)	0.5-11%; 0-2500
0-2%; 0-200 (50)	0-3%; 0-300 (50)	0-2%; 0-400
1-8 (5)	2.5-7.5 (4.0)	3.25-7.15 (5.2)
40-60 (52)	23-48 (52)	23-48 (33)　　50-68 (63)
14.4-18.6	9-13	16.6-22
30-36 (32.7)	31-38 (33.5)	30-34 (32)

in the cytoplasm. Canine basophils have few basophilic granules. Feline basophils have many round granules that stain mauve (grayish-purple). Equine and ruminant basophils are usually packed with granules and stain dark blue. Basophil numbers are often increased in allergies and some metabolic disorders.

Smudge (basket) cells are the nuclei of ruptured degenerative WBCs. They appear as pale-staining, amorphous bodies of stain. They are often caused by excessive pressure applied to the cells during blood smear preparations. A few smudge cells may be expected, but large numbers may indicate excessive cell fragility, which is common in very sick animals. Smudge cells are also frequently seen when old anticoagulated blood samples are used for study.

EVALUATION OF PLATELETS

Platelets (thrombocytes) play a vital role in blood clotting, or *hemostasis*. Platelets are actually fragments of megakaryocytes, which are large cells found in bone marrow. Platelets are *anuclear* (have no nucleus), and they vary in size. They are generally round or oval and may have pointed projections (see Plate 2 in color insert). Their cytoplasm stains blue and contains fine, purple granules. Platelets appear similar in most species and in cats may be larger than an erythrocyte.

Three methods for calculating platelet numbers exist: estimating on the peripheral blood smear, counting manually with a hemacytometer, or counting with an automatic cell counter. Their small size, coupled with their tendency to adhere together, can make platelet counts somewhat difficult. Feline platelets are especially prone to clumping in EDTA-preserved blood samples.

Platelet numbers are evaluated in the cell monolayer on the blood film. Platelets in 10 oil-immersion (1000× magnification) fields normally average between 10 and 30. Because each platelet in an oil-immersion field represents 15,000 to 20,000 platelets/μl of blood, the total number of platelets can then be estimated. For example, if the average number of platelets in 10 oil-immersion fields is 16, then

$$16 \times 15,000 \text{ platelets}/\mu\text{l} = 240,000 \text{ platelets}/\mu\text{l}$$

The number of platelets is normally between 100,000 and 900,000/μl, depending on the species.

If the platelet numbers appear to be decreased (less than 4 to 6/field) under oil immersion, scan the feathered edge for clumps or aggregates of platelets. If you see them, report platelets as adequate. If you find no aggregates, a platelet count (rather than an estimate) may be performed.

Increased platelet numbers (thrombocytosis) is uncommon but may occur with hemorrhage, inflamma-tion, and (rarely) neoplasia. Decreased platelet numbers (thrombocytopenia) can be caused by immune-mediated disease, disseminated intravascular coagulation (causing increased consumption of platelets), toxins, and infections. These conditions can be especially serious, because platelet counts below 50,000/μl can cause bleeding. Bone marrow evaluation may be required to diagnose the specific type of platelet disorder.

Table 11-5 lists normal hematologic reference values for domestic animals. Fig. 11-9 shows an example of a form used to report hematology values.

ASSESSMENT OF COAGULATION AND HEMOSTASIS

Coagulation tests may be appropriate if a bleeding disorder is suspected or as part of a presurgical screening protocol. These tests assess hemostasis, which is a complex interaction between blood vessel walls, platelets, and coagulation factors. The result of this interaction is formation of a blood clot (hemostatic plug) made up of platelets and fibrin. Fibrin is the end product of a complex series of chemical steps known as the *coagulation cascade*. Activation of either the intrinsic or the extrinsic coagulation pathway may trigger this cascade. The intrinsic pathway is essential for clot formation and occurs in the blood vessels. Tissue damage, such as needle puncture of a vessel wall, initiates the extrinsic pathway, which enhances coagulation. These separate pathways lead to a common pathway where the final reaction involves fibrinogen conversion to fibrin. The hemostatic plug (clot) eventually degrades as tissue heals. Many tests are available to evaluate the hemostatic process.

Platelet examination is one of the most important steps in evaluation of coagulation. As stated previously, estimations of platelet numbers are easy on a blood smear. Unopette or machine methods are also effective. The total platelet count should be between 100,000 and 900,000/μl, depending on the species. Remember to check the feathered edge for aggregates if platelets cannot be found in the monolayer area of the blood smear. Alert a clinician if you find large platelets that appear bizarre or fragmented, because they may indicate a platelet defect or neoplastic condition.

Collection of blood used for coagulation studies must involve with minimal tissue damage and sufficient blood flow to avoid clot formation and hemolysis. Sodium citrate is the preferred anticoagulant for tests of coagulation. Samples require special handling because many of the coagulation factors deteriorate rapidly.

Collect blood into a syringe by clean venipuncture. The ratio of blood to sodium citrate anticoagulant should be 9 to 1 (1.8 ml blood to 0.2 ml citrate). Blue-top Vacutainer tubes contain 0.2 ml sodium citrate and

HEMATOLOGY REPORT SHEET

Name _____   Date _____

Species, Name and History _____

Plasma Color _____   Evaluation   Normal   Abnormal

Plasma Turbidity   Clear   Hazy   Cloudy   Slight   Moderate   Marked
                                             Hemolysis   Icterus   Lipemia

		Normal	H/L
PCV % _____		_____	_____
TP g/dl _____		_____	_____
Hgb g/dl _____		_____	_____
FIB mg/dl _____		_____	_____
MCV fl _____		_____	_____
MCH pg _____		_____	_____
MCHC g/dl _____		_____	_____
TWBC/µl _____ corrected total WBC/µl _____ (thousands/cu.mm.)		_____	_____
RBC/µl _____ (millions/cu.mm.)		_____	_____

Differential	%	Absolute value	Normal	H/L
Segs (PMNs)	_____	_____	_____	_____
Bands	_____	_____	_____	_____
Lymphocytes	_____	_____	_____	_____
Monocytes	_____	_____	_____	_____
Eosinophils	_____	_____	_____	_____
Basophils	_____	_____	_____	_____
Metamyelocytes	_____	_____	_____	_____
Myelocytes	_____	_____	_____	_____
Other	_____	_____	_____	_____
TOTAL	100 cells			

Number of nucleated RBCs _____   If 5 or more are found, do a corrected TWBC count.

RBC Morphology   Normal   Crenation   Sl.   Mod.   Mrkd.
                 Abnormal   Rouleaux Agglutination   Sl.   Mod.   Mrkd.

Polychromasia	1+	2+	3+	4+	Howell-Jolly Bodies	1+	2+	3+	4+
Spherocytes	1+	2+	3+	4+	Schistocytes	1+	2+	3+	4+
Anisocytosis	1+	2+	3+	4+	Leptocytes	1+	2+	3+	4+
Poikilocytosis	1+	2+	3+	4+	Hypochromasia	1+	2+	3+	4+
Heinz Bodies	1+	2+	3+	4+	Acanthocytes	1+	2+	3+	4+
Stomatocytes	1+	2+	3+	4+	Echinocytes	1+	2+	3+	4+

Comments _____

WBC Morphology   Normal   Lymphocytes   Reac.   Atyp.   Few   Moderate   Many
                 Abnormal

Comments _____

Toxic Degeneration   Few   Moderate   Many   Severity   Sl.   Mod.   Mrkd.
Platelet Estimate _____   Adequate   Clumped

FIG. 11-9   Sample hematology report form.

are well suited for this procedure. Inspect the sample in the tube for clots and discard any that are present. If a second sample is necessary, use a new needle, syringe, and venipuncture site. Once a usable sample is ready, thoroughly mix and centrifuge it. Then, transfer the separated plasma to an empty plastic tube and freeze it. Ship the sample with frozen cold packs to a commercial laboratory unless it can be analyzed immediately. Plasma may be kept frozen and analyzed within 2 weeks of collection.

Commercial laboratories usually perform tests of the coagulation system. These tests include specific coagulation factor assays, von Willebrand's antigen assay (von Willebrand's disease is a genetic defect of platelet adhesion to blood vessels), one-stage prothrombin time (good screening test for vitamin K deficiency or rodenticide poisoning), and activated partial thromboplastin time (screening test for some hereditary and acquired bleeding disorders). Coagulation tests that may easily be performed in a veterinary hospital include whole blood clotting time, activated clotting time, and bleeding time.

The whole blood clotting time is a test of the overall function of the coagulation mechanism and especially the intrinsic system. A simplified procedure involves cleanly drawing blood into a syringe and transferring it to an empty red-top (clot) serum tube. Tilt the tube back and forth until the blood clots. Clotting should occur within 15 minutes. Although this test is insensitive, a prolonged clotting time may indicate that further testing of the coagulation system is necessary.

The activated clotting time (ACT) is a test of the intrinsic and common coagulation pathways and is easily performed in veterinary practice. ACT tubes contain diatomaceous earth, which shortens the clotting time and increases the sensitivity over the whole blood clotting time. Prewarm tubes in a 37° C water bath. Then, cleanly draw 2 ml of blood into a plastic syringe and inject it into an ACT tube. Start a stopwatch when blood first appears in the tube. Then, invert the tube a few times and place it in the water bath for 45 to 60 seconds. Remove it from the bath and tilt it (so that the blood spreads along the length of the tube) at 5-second intervals until the first sign of obvious clotting. Time of clotting is recorded; normal values are between 60 and 90 seconds. Severe thrombocytopenia and intrinsic and common pathway coagulation factor deficiencies prolong the ACT.

Bleeding time measures the ability of platelets to plug a small wound. Quickly make a small, deep puncture with a lancet, #11 Bard Parker scalpel blade, or Simplate device (Animal Blood Bank) in an area without hair, such as the nose or buccal area. Start a stopwatch when blood first appears. Without touching the area, use a filter paper or paper towel to remove the blood at 30-second intervals. When blood no longer stains the filter, record the time. Normal bleeding time is 5 minutes or less in domestic animals. Thrombocytopenia, platelet defects, increased fragility of capillaries, and von Willebrand's disease cause a prolonged bleeding time. This test is often performed when there is evidence of a bleeding disorder (e.g., hematuria, epistaxis), but platelet numbers are within the normal range.

BONE MARROW EXAMINATION

Veterinary technicians may assist the veterinarian in examination of bone marrow. This procedure is indicated when there is evidence that the bone marrow is not responding appropriately or when certain types of neoplasia are suspected. Specific indications include unexplained nonregenerative anemia, leukopenia, thrombocytopenia, and pancytopenia (decreased numbers of all cell lines). Bone marrow evaluation is also used to confirm certain infections (e.g., ehrlichiosis) and diagnose hematopoietic neoplasms (e.g., lymphoproliferative disorders).

In small animals, bone marrow is aspirated under general anesthesia or using local anesthesia. (A local anesthetic is preferred for large animals.) Follow aseptic technique throughout the procedure. The proximal end of the femur, the craniolateral portion of the humerus, and the iliac crest are common sites of bone marrow aspiration in dogs and cats. The sternum, ribs, and iliac crest are often used in large animals. Special bone marrow needles are preferred, although an 18-gauge needle may be used in cats with thin bones. Bone marrow needles have a stylet to prevent occlusion of the needle with bone and surrounding tissue as it is inserted into the marrow cavity. A syringe is used to aspirate a few drops of bone marrow, filling the needle and perhaps the distal part of the syringe. The needle is removed from the bone and the contents immediately used to make slides. Alternatively, the marrow may be placed into an EDTA tube with most of the anticoagulant shaken out so that smears may be made a short time later.

Marrow smears are prepared in a similar manner to peripheral blood. Bone marrow is thicker than blood and should contain particles or spicules. Blood contamination can be minimized by vertically positioning the slide to drain off excess blood before making the smear. The smear is air-dried and stained as described previously. You may then examine smears or send them to a commercial laboratory for analysis.

If you examine the stained smears, do so at low-power (100× magnification) for overall cellularity and megakaryocyte (immature thrombocyte) number. Cellularity is normal if the particles are composed of about 50% nucleated cells and 50% fat (Fig. 11-10). Describe the marrow as *hypercellular* or *hypocellular*, based on the proportion of cells present. There should be 2 to 3 megakaryocytes per low-power field.

At higher magnification, examine erythroid (red) and myeloid (white) cells. Ninety percent of nucleated erythroid cells should comprise rubricytes and metarubricytes. Metamyelocytes, bands, and segmenters should make up 90% of the myeloid cells. Determine the ratio of myeloid to erythroid cells (M:E ratio) by counting 500 nucleated cells and classifying them as erythroid or myeloid. Normal M:E ratios should be between 0.75:1.0 and 2.0:1.0. Notify a clinician if numbers of any cell type seem out of normal proportion.

Neoplasia is a possibility if all the cells look alike. Bone marrow status should never be evaluated without the results of a concurrent peripheral hemogram. If histologic examination of marrow is required, a special biopsy needle is used to obtain a larger core sample to be sent to a commercial laboratory for analysis.

A

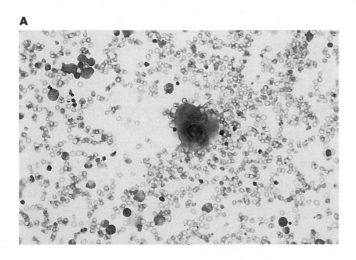

B

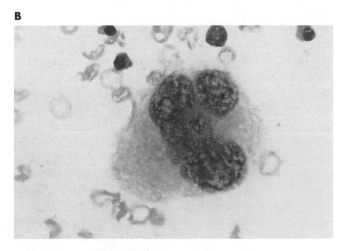

FIG. 11-10 **A,** Bone marrow smear from a normal dog, with megakaryocyte at center. **B,** High-power view of a megakaryocyte. *(Courtesy of Dr. Mary Anna Thrall.)*

HEMATOPOIETIC DISORDERS

Hematopoietic tumors (neoplasia of blood-forming tissues) are common in domestic animals. There are many types and they are broadly classified by the type of cell or cells from which the tumor originates. They are generally divided into two main groups: lymphoproliferative and myeloproliferative disorders. Lymphoproliferative disorders originate from lymphocytes or plasma cells (a tissue cell of lymphoid origin). Myeloproliferative disorders arise from nonlymphoid cells that originate in the bone marrow. Neoplasms of red blood cell and megakaryocyte origin are also included in this group. These tumors are called *leukemias* if the neoplastic cells originate in the bone marrow.

Hematopoietic disorders are often diagnosed by finding specific early stages (blast forms) of cell types in peripheral blood and/or bone marrow. Lymphoblastic leukemia may be diagnosed by finding lymphoblasts in the blood and/or some marrow. If neoplastic cells are found in the peripheral blood, the term *leukemic blood profile* is often used. Detailed descriptions of hematopoietic disorders are located in many clinical pathology or hematology textbooks.

AUTOMATED HEMATOLOGY

Automated analysis of hematologic samples has become more common in recent years. Several veterinary analyzers are currently available. CBCs performed in this manner may be cost effective if several CBCs are done each day. Advantages of automation include speed, accuracy, and consistent results. Disadvantages of certain analyzers include the need for regular maintenance and quality control. Automated hematologic examination only partially replaces a manual CBC. The veterinary technician still must perform several aspects of the CBC, usually the differential count and total protein concentration. Each instrument has a specific protocol for use; therefore, the technician should study the operator's manual or contact the manufacturer before using the equipment. Following is a brief description of two types of automation used in veterinary practice.

Electronic Cell Counters

Electronic cell counters can rapidly and efficiently count RBCs, WBCs, and platelets. They are based on the idea of counting particles (cells) as they flow past a detection device. Cells are detected by changes in electrical resistance or disruption of a laser beam. Many instruments can determine cell size as well as count blood cells. Some units also determine hemoglobin concentration and the red cell indices. These modern counters have computer-based settings for species and type of cells being counted. Because the RBCs and WBCs of animal species vary greatly in size, calibrate the instrument and set it for the proper species. Platelet clumps, especially seen in cats, can be erroneously counted as leukocytes by cell counters. Examine a blood smear if you suspect this. Proper sample collection and handling usually alleviates this problem. Two common electronic counters include those made by Coulter Electronics and CDC Technologies.

Qualitative Buffy Coat System

Qualitative buffy coat (QBC) analysis is based on measurement of a centrifuged, stained, and expanded buffy coat by a computerized automatic microhematocrit reader. The QBC Vet Autoread (Idexx Laboratories) is designed for veterinary use. A specialized microhematocrit tube, coated with stain, is filled with EDTA anticoagulated blood and then centrifuged. The centrifuged blood separates into layers based on density of the cells. RBCs are found at the bottom of the tube, as in the manual microhematocrit method. The buffy coat is expanded into several layers and the plasma is found on top. The buffy coat is divided into a granulocyte (neutrophil, eosinophil, basophil) layer, a combined lymphocyte/monocyte layer, and a platelet layer. If many reticulocytes or NRBCs are present, these may form a layer at the top of the RBC column (below the buffy coat). The tube is then placed in an optical scanning device, which measures the degree of stain fluorescence in each cell layer. The analyzer prints out a report with 12 different hematologic values and a graph illustrating cell numbers and fluorescence for each cell layer. These values include hematocrit, hemoglobin, MCHC, total WBC count, granulocyte count (percentage and absolute count), eosinophil count (absolute count, dogs only), lymphocyte/monocyte count (percentage and absolute count), platelet count, and reticulocyte/NRBC count (if present). The ability to perform separate lymphocyte and monocyte counts may be available in future upgrades.

The QBC Vet Autoread performs only a partial CBC and cannot replace blood smear evaluation. It is especially important to examine the blood smear if findings are abnormal. Total protein concentration can be measured on plasma separated in the specialized tube. An easy way to obtain plasma from the large tube is to insert a standard microhematocrit tube into the plasma layer and allow it to fill by capillary action. Refractometry is performed in the usual manner. The QBC Vet Autoread analyzer gives consistent, reliable results and is virtually maintenance free.

Acknowledgment.
I am grateful to Dr. E. Lassen, Dr. C. Andreason, Dr. M. Litner, and P. Birka, LVT, for their suggestions, and to Drs. M.A. Thrall and E. Lassen for supplying many illustrations.

RECOMMENDED READING

Benjamin MM: *Outline of veterinary clinical pathology,* ed 3, Ames, Iowa, 1981, Iowa State University.
Coles EH: *Veterinary clinical pathology,* ed 4, Philadelphia, 1986, Lea & Febiger.
Colville J: *The veterinary practice laboratory.* In Pratt P et al: *Laboratory procedures for veterinary technicians,* ed 2, Goleta, Calif, 1992, American Veterinary Publications.
Dial SM: *Clinical pathology.* In McCurnin D et al: *Clinical textbook for veterinary technicians,* ed 3, Philadelphia, 1994, WB Saunders.
Duncan JR, Prasse KW, Mahaffey EA: *Veterinary laboratory medicine, clinical pathology,* ed 3, Ames, Iowa, 1994, Iowa State University Press.
Jain NC: *Essentials of veterinary hematology,* Philadelphia, 1993, Lea & Febiger.
Jain NC: *Schalm's veterinary hematology,* ed 4, Philadelphia, 1986, Lea and Febiger.
Parry BW: *Miscellaneous laboratory techniques.* In Pratt et al: *Laboratory procedures for veterinary technicians,* ed 2, Goleta, Calif, 1992, American Veterinary Publications.
Rebar A, Metzger F: *Clinical pathology for small-animal practitioners: interpreting the hemogram,* Lenexa, Kan, 1995, Veterinary Medicine Publishing Group.
Rebar AH: *Small animal laboratory evaluation,* Trenton, NJ, 1990, Veterinary Learning Systems Co., Inc.
Sirois M: *Veterinary clinical laboratory procedures,* St Louis, 1995, Mosby.
Thrall MA, Weiser MG: *Hematology.* In Pratt et al: *Laboratory procedures for veterinary technicians,* ed 2, Goleta, Calif, 1992, American Veterinary Publications.
Tvedten H: *The complete blood count and bone marrow examination.* In Willard MW et al: *Small animal clinical diagnosis by laboratory methods,* ed 2, Philadelphia, 1994, WB Saunders.
Weiss DJ: Uniform evaluation and semiquantitative reporting of hematologic data in veterinary laboratories, *Vet Clin Pathol* 13(2):27-31, 1984.

DIAGNOSTIC PARASITOLOGY

E.M. JOHNSON

INTRODUCTION

Parasitology is the study of organisms that live in (internal parasites, endoparasites) or on (external parasites, ectoparasites) another organism, the host, from which they derive their nourishment. In a broad sense, many forms of parasitic relationships can be beneficial (commensalism, mutualism, symbiosis) or harmful (parasitism). The relationship of the parasite with its host has evolved over time and is mutually adaptive. It requires tolerance and resistance by both organisms and is influenced by ecologic factors in the environment. This discussion addresses only parasitic relationships considered harmful to the host: common parasites of domestic animals and techniques for recovery and identification of diagnostic stages.

The organism that the parasite lives in or on is called its *host.* The host may be a definitive host, sheltering the sexual, adult stages of the parasite, or an intermediate host, harboring asexual (immature) or larval stages of the parasite. There are also paratenic hosts or transport hosts for some parasites, in which the parasite survives without multiplying or developing. Some parasites can enter a state of hypobiosis (developmental arrest) within the definitive host for a time and resume development when environmental conditions for transmission and survival are optimal.

The term *life cycle* refers to maturation of a parasite through various developmental stages in one or more hosts. For a parasite to survive, it must have a dependable means of transfer from one host to another (diagnostic stage) and the ability to develop and reproduce in the host, ideally without producing serious harm to the host. This requires a mode of entry into a host (infective stage), availability of a susceptible host (definitive host), an accommodating location and environment in the host for maturation and reproduction (gastrointestinal system, respiratory system, circulatory system, urinary system, reproductive system), and a mode of exit from the host (feces, sputum, blood, urine, smegma), with dispersal into an ecologically suitable environment for development and survival.

There are six major categories of parasites of domestic animals: protozoa, nematodes, trematodes, cestodes, acanthocephalans, and arthropods. Each category contains a variety of different groups of organisms and each group may demonstrate a diversity of life-cycle patterns. It is beyond the scope of this chapter to discuss each group of parasite and individual species in detail. More information can be found in the recommended reading listed at the end of this section.

CLASSIFICATIONS OF PARASITES
Protozoa

Protozoa are single-celled organisms with one or more membrane-bound nuclei containing DNA and specialized cytoplasmic organelles. The bodies of protozoans are covered by a triple-layered unit membrane (surface membrane or cell wall). Membranous organelles, which function in energy production, nutrition, excretion, and reproduction, consist of mitochondria, Golgi apparatus, endoplasmic reticulum, and vesicles. The cytoplasm is composed of an inner, fluid endoplasm and an outer rigid ectoplasm. Organelles for locomotion consist of flagella (long whiplike structures), cilia (short flagella usually arranged in rows or tufts), pseudopodia (temporary extensions and retractions of the body wall), and undulatory ridges (small snakelike waves that form in the cell membrane and move posteriorly). Locomotor organelles and modifications of them are frequently used to help identify the type of protozoa recovered

from animals. Protozoan parasites, important as agents of disease in domestic animals, are usually recovered from the gastrointestinal tract in feces, from the circulatory system in blood or lymph, and from the reproductive system in smegma, semen, or vaginal mucus.

The life cycles of protozoa can be simple or complex. Reproduction may be asexual (binary fission, schizogony, budding) or sexual (syngamy, conjugation). With certain groups of protozoa, reproductive stages are useful in identification. Many protozoa can go into a resting, resistant stage called a *cyst* by production of a heavy wall around the whole organism. Cyst formation is common in protozoa that will be subjected to harsh, environmental conditions, such as desiccation (drying). The cyst stage also serves as a site for reorganization and nuclear division, followed by multiplication upon entry and excystment in a new suitable host. The cyst is the infective stage for many parasitic protozoa. *Oocyst* is the name given to the cyst stage of a group of intestinal protozoa known as coccidia (see Fig. 11-15). The normal feeding, motile form of a protozoan is called a *trophozoite* (Fig. 11-11). The trophozoite is often too fragile to survive transfer to a new host and generally is not infective. However, some protozoa do not produce a cyst stage and have adapted to direct transfer by trophozoites to a new host (*Tritrichomonas foetus*).

Four main groups of protozoa commonly produce disease in domestic animals: flagellates, such as *Tritrichomonas foetus*, *Giardia duodenalis* (see Fig. 11-11), *Trypanosoma* spp., and *Leishmania* spp.; amoebae, such as *Entamoeba histolytica*; ciliates, such as *Balantidium coli*; and apicomplexa, such as *Eimeria* spp. (Fig. 11-12), *Isospora* spp. (Fig. 11-13), *Cryptosporidium* spp. (Fig. 11-14), *Sarcocystis* spp., *Toxoplasma gondii* (Fig. 11-15), *Neospora caninum*, *Plasmodium* spp., *Haemoproteus* spp., *Leucocytozoon* spp., *Babesia* spp. (Fig. 11-16), and *Theileria* spp.

Nematodes
Nematodes are multicellular, cylindric organisms commonly referred to as *roundworms*. The body wall of nematodes consists of an external, acellular, protective layer called the *cuticle*; a cellular layer beneath the cuticle called the *hypodermis*; and a layer of longitudinal, somatic muscles that function in locomotion. The digestive tract and reproductive organs of roundworms are tubular and are suspended in the body cavity (pseudocoelom). The digestive tract is a straight tube that runs the length of the body from the mouth to the caudal end (anus). The sexes for most nematodes are separate. The reproductive organs are also tubular but typically are longer than the body and coil around the intestinal tract of the worm. Nematodes have a nervous system and an excretory system, but no respiratory system.

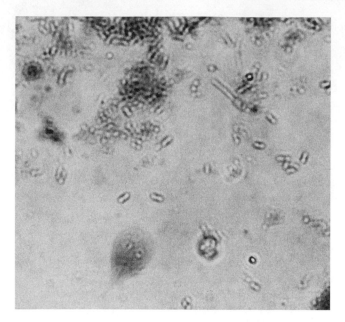

FIG. 11-11 *Giardia duodenalis* trophozoite (Romanowsky-stained impressions smear of duodenum).

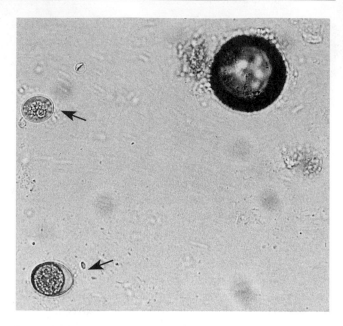

FIG. 11-13 *Isospora* sp. oocysts (fecal flotation).

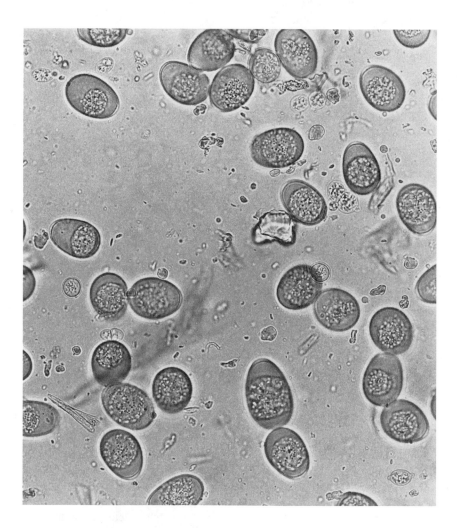

FIG. 11-12 *Eimeria* spp. oocysts (fecal flotation).

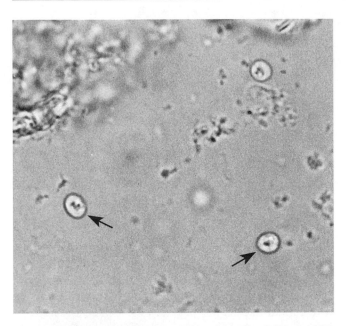

FIG. 11-14 *Cryptosporidium parvum* oocysts (fecal flotation).

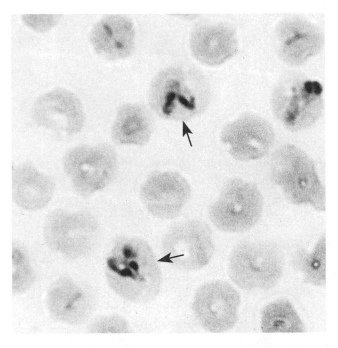

FIG. 11-16 *Babesia gibsoni* (Romanowsky-stained blood smear).

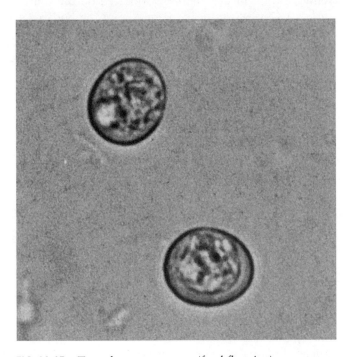

FIG. 11-15 *Toxoplasma* sp. oocysts (fecal flotation).

The life cycle of nematodes follows a standard pattern consisting of several developmental stages: the egg, four larval stages that are also wormlike in appearance, and sexually mature adults. The infective stage may be an egg containing a larva, a free-living larva, or a larva within an intermediate host or transport host. A life cycle is considered *direct* if no intermediate host is necessary for development to the infective stage. If an intermediate host is required for development to the infective

stage, the life cycle is considered *indirect*. Transmission to a new definitive host (host harboring sexually mature adults) can occur through ingestion, skin penetration of infective larvae, ingestion of an intermediate host, or deposition of infective larvae into or on the skin by an intermediate host.

Once a nematode gains entry into a new host, development to the adult stages may occur in the area of their final location or may occur after extensive migration through the body of the definitive host. The diagnostic stages of parasitic nematodes are typically found in feces, blood, sputum, or urine. Most parasitic nematodes are found in the intestinal tracts of their respective definitive hosts, but some are found in the lungs, kidney, urinary bladder, or heart.

There are 11 major superfamilies (taxonomic groupings) of nematodes important in veterinary medicine: Ascaroidea (*Toxocara* spp., *Toxascaris* spp., *Ascaris* spp., *Parascaris equorum, Toxocara vitulorum*), Strongyloidea (*Strongylus* spp., *Ancylostoma* spp., *Bunostomum* spp., *Uncinaria* sp., *Syngamus* spp., *Chabertia ovina, Oesophagostomum* spp.), Trichostrongyloidea (*Haemonchus* spp., *Ostertagia* spp., *Trichostrongylus* spp., *Cooperia* spp., *Nematodirus* spp., *Ollulanus tricuspis, Dictyocaulus* spp.), Metastrongyloidea (*Metastrongylus* spp., *Protostrongylus* spp., *Muellerius capillaris, Filaroides* spp., *Aelurostrongylus abstrusus, Crenosoma* spp.), Oxyuroidea (*Oxyuris equi, Skrjabinema ovis*), Trichuroidea (*Trichuris* spp., *Capillaria* spp., *Trichinella spiralis*), Filaroidea (*Dirofilaria immitis, Dipetalonema reconditum, Onchocerca* spp., *Setaria* spp., *Elaeophora schneideri, Stephanofilaria stilesi*), Rhabditoidea (*Strongyloides* spp.), Spiruroidea (*Habronema* spp., *Thelazia* spp., *Spirocerca lupi, Ascarops strongylina, Physocephalus sexalatus, Physalopetera* spp.), Dracunculoidea (*Dracunculus* spp.), and Dioctophymoidea *(Dioctophyma renale)*.

Cestodes

Cestodes (tapeworms) are multicellular organisms that lack a body cavity. Their organs are embedded in loose cellular tissue (parenchyma). The body of tapeworms is long and dorsoventrally flattened, and consists of three regions. The head (scolex) is modified into an attachment organ and bears two to four muscular suckers, or bothria. The suckers may be armed with hooks. There may also be a snout (rostellum) on the head, which can be fixed or retractable. The rostellum can also be armed with hooks. Caudal to the head is a short neck of undifferentiated tissue, followed by the body (strobila). The body is composed of segments (proglottids) in different stages of maturity. Those near the neck are immature, followed by sexually mature proglottids, and terminating with gravid segments containing eggs. Gravid proglottids break off and pass out of the body of the definitive host in the feces. New proglottids are continually formed from the undifferentiated tissue of the neck. Cestodes lack a digestive tract and nutrients are absorbed directly through the body wall. The most prominent organs in cestodes are the organs of the reproductive system. Both male and female reproductive organs occur in an individual tapeworm. Cestodes also have a nervous system and an excretory system.

The cestode egg contains a fully developed embryo, which has six hooks in three pairs (hexacanth embryo or oncosphere), or a zygote that develops into a ciliated embryo (coracidium). The life cycle of tapeworms is always indirect and involves one or two intermediate hosts. The intermediate hosts may be arthropods, fish, or mammals. Domestic animals can be definitive hosts and/or intermediate hosts for tapeworms. The larval stages of some tapeworms found in domestic animals are called "bladder worms" because they resemble fluid-filled sacks with one or multiple scoleces. When ingested by a definitive host, the "bladder worms" are released from the tissue of the intermediate host and develop into adult tapeworms within the digestive tract of the definitive host. Some cestodes have larval forms that are solid bodies *(procercoid, plerocercoid, tetrathyridium)*. Domestic animals become infected with the larval stages of tapeworms by ingestion of the cestode egg or procercoid.

Two major groups of tapeworms are important in veterinary medicine: cyclophyllidean tapeworms, which typically have one intermediate host (such as *Dipylidium caninum, Taenia* spp., *Echinococcus* spp., *Moniezia* spp., *Anoplocephala* spp., *Thysanosoma actinoides)* (see Figs. 11-24 and 11-31); and pseudophyllidean tapeworms, which have two intermediate hosts (such as *Diphyllobothrium latum* and *Spirometra mansonoides*). Typically the larval stages of cestodes in domestic animals are more harmful (pathogenic) than the adult stages in the intestinal tract. However, the adult stages are the source of eggs, especially for cestodes, which can use people as an intermediate host and pose a risk to human health (zoonotic).

Trematodes

The trematodes (flukes) are flatworms that, like cestodes, lack a body cavity. They are unsegmented and leaflike. The organs are embedded in loose tissue (parenchyma), and they also possess two muscular attachment organs or suckers. One sucker, the anterior sucker, is located at the mouth. The other sucker, the ventral sucker or *acetabulum,* is located on the ventral surface of the worm near the middle of the body or at the caudal end. There are three main groups of trematodes: monogenetic trematodes, aspidogastrid trematodes, and digenetic trematodes. Only digenetic trematodes are parasites of domestic animals.

Digenetic trematodes have an outer body wall or cuticle. They have a simple digestive tract consisting of a mouth, pharynx, esophagus, and an intestine that divides into two blind sacs (ceca). The main organs visible in trematodes are the reproductive organs. Most trematodes have both male and female reproductive organs in the same individual, but a few have separate sexes (schistosomes). A nervous system and an excretory system are also present.

The life cycle of digenetic trematodes is very complicated. They pass through several different larval stages (miracidium, sporocyst, redia, cercaria, metacercaria) and typically require one or more intermediate hosts, one of which is nearly always a mollusk (snail, slug). Multiplication takes place in both the definitive (sexual) and intermediate (asexual) hosts. The eggs of digenetic trematodes are capped (operculated) and they contain a ciliated embryo called a *miracidium*. The miracidium gains access to a suitable snail, through penetration or ingestion, and develops through several stages that eventually give rise to a motile, tailed stage referred to as a *cercaria*. Cercariae are released from the snail and swim actively. Sometimes, depending upon the species of fluke, the cercariae encyst on vegetation. This encysted stage, the metacercaria, is infective for the definitive host. In other species, the cercaria may penetrate the skin of the definitive host or encyst in another intermediate host. Examples of digenetic trematodes of domestic animals are *Fasciola hepatica* (see Fig. 11-31), *Heterobilharzia americana, Paramphistomum cervi, Nanophyetus salmincola* (see Fig. 11-26), and *Paragonimus kellicotti.*

Acanthocephalans

Acanthocephalans are commonly referred to as "thorny-headed worms." This group of intestinal parasites is rarely encountered, but occasionally they can be found in pigs and dogs. They are worm-like in appearance after fixation, and have a spiny, protrusible snout *(proboscis)*. They have a body cavity and lack a digestive tract; the sexes are separate.

The life cycle of acanthocephalans is complex and involves an intermediate host, usually a crustacean or an insect. Mature adults produce eggs that are shed through the feces of the definitive host. The eggs contain an embryo, the *acanthor,* which is surrounded by three to four envelopes. This gives the eggs a layered appearance, which is useful for identification. When an aquatic crustacean or insect ingests the eggs, continuous development through two stages occurs to produce the infective stage *(cystacanth)*. Infection of the definitive host occurs by ingestion of the intermediate host. The main acanthocephalan of concern is *Macracanthorhynchus hirudinaceus* (see Fig. 11-33) which is found in the small intestines of pigs. *Oncicola canis* is an acanthocephalan found in dogs. Other hosts for acanthocephalans are aquatic birds, fish, amphibians, and monkeys.

Arthropods

Arthropods are a large group of animals characterized by the presence of jointed legs. They have a chitinous exoskeleton composed of segments. In the more advanced groups, some segments have fused together to form body parts, such as a head, thorax, and abdomen. Arthropods have a true body cavity *(coelom),* a circulatory system, a digestive system, a respiratory system, an excretory system, a nervous system, and a reproductive system. The sexes are separate and reproduction is by means of eggs. Only certain groups of arthropods are parasitic. Members of other groups may act as intermediate host for the other parasites previously discussed. When a parasite resides on the surface of its host, it is called an *ectoparasite*. Most ectoparasites are either insects (fleas, lice, flies) or arachnids (ticks, mites).

The two major classes of arthropods of veterinary importance can be differentiated by the following general characteristics: Insects have three pairs of legs, three distinct body regions (head, thorax, abdomen), and a single pair of antennae; Arachnids (adults) have 4 pairs of legs, a body divided into two regions (cephalothorax, abdomen), and no antennae. Pentastomids (tongue worms) are another group of parasitic arthropods rarely encountered in the respiratory passages of vertebrates. They resemble worms rather than arthropods in the adult stage. Adults have two pairs of curved, retractile hooklets near the mouth. Immature stages are mitelike, with two or three pairs of legs.

The mouthparts of insects vary in structure, depending on feeding habits, with adaptations for chewing-biting, sponging, or piercing-sucking. The thorax may have one or two pairs of functional wings, in addition to the three pairs of jointed legs. The sexes are separate and reproduction results in production of eggs or larvae. Development often involves three or more larval stages called *instars,* followed by formation of a pupa and a change in form or transformation *(complete metamorphosis)* to the adult stage. In other insects development occurs from the egg through several immature stages *(nymphs),* which resemble the adult in form but are smaller *(incomplete metamorphosis)*. Fleas and flies demonstrate complete metamorphosis and lice demonstrate incomplete metamorphosis. Insects may produce harm to their definitive host as adults and/or larvae.

The arachnids include ticks, mites, spiders, and scorpions. Ticks and mites are the more important groups of arachnids in veterinary medicine, although some spiders and scorpions can harm domestic animals by way of toxic venoms. Arachnids are generally small, often microscopic. Their mouth parts are borne on a structure called the *basis capituli* and consists of a pair of mobile digits adapted for cutting *(chelicerae)* and a pair of sensory structures (palps). There is a structure (hypostome) with recurved teeth for maintaining attachment to the host and bears a groove that permits the flow of arthropod saliva and host blood or lymph. Life cycle stages consist of egg, larva, nymph, and adult. There can be more than one nymphal instar. Nymphs resemble the adult in form but are smaller. There is usually only one larval stage, which differs from the nymphs and adults in size and has only three pairs of legs.

DIAGNOSTIC TECHNIQUES IN PARASITOLOGY

Parasites may be located in the oral cavity, esophagus, stomach, small and large intestines, internal organs, and skin of animals. Diagnostic stages can be found in sputum, feces, blood, urine, secretions of the reproductive organs, and epidermal layers of the skin. Samples collected for examination should be as fresh as possible and examined as soon as possible, preferably within the first 24 hours after collection. The clients can collect samples and store them in any clean, sealable container, or collection can occur at the clinic. Refrigeration or fixation may be necessary if prompt examination is not possible. A sample of 5 to 50 grams (g) (the size of a pecan or walnut) may be needed, depending on which procedures are necessary. Pooled samples from a herd or kennel can be used, but generally it is better to examine several samples from individual animals.

Take proper precautions when working with samples to prevent contamination of the work environment and to ensure personal health when handling agents transmissible to people. Wear gloves and/or wash your hands frequently with warm water and soap. Clean and disinfect work areas after examinations. Also, clean equipment frequently.

Maintenance of good records is important. Label samples with the owner's name, date of collection, species of host, and identification of the animal. Records should include identification information, procedures performed, and the results. An adequate history, including clinical signs, duration of signs, medications given, environment, vaccinations, stocking density, and number of animals affected, should accompany the sample.

Parasitologic examination begins with gross examination of the sample, noting consistency, color, presence of blood, mucus, odor, adult parasites or foreign bodies, such as string. Normal feces should be formed yet soft. Diarrhea or constipation can occur with parasitic infections. Most secretions are clear and moderately cellular. A yellowish discoloration with excessive mucus could signal infection. Blood in a sample can be fresh and bright red or partially digested (hemolyzed), appearing dark reddish brown to black and tarry. Excessive mucus in a sample generally indicates irritation to a mucosal membrane, with proliferation of mucus-producing cells. This is common in parasitic infections of the respiratory system and lower digestive tract. Adult parasites, such as roundworms and tapeworm proglottids, can be found in vomitus or feces, and can be identified.

Microscopic examination of samples is the most reliable method for detection of parasitic infections. A binocular microscope with 10×, 40×, and 100× objectives is needed. A stereo microscope is also helpful for identifying gross parasites. A calibrated ocular micrometer is necessary to determine sizes and specific differentiation of some parasitic stages, such as microfilariae. Samples are generally mounted on a glass slide in a fluid medium with a coverslip on top. The sample should be thoroughly and systematically viewed, beginning at one corner of the coverslip and ending at the opposite end using the 10× objective. Parasite stages usually are in the same plane of focus as air bubbles or the edge of the coverslip. Any materials or objects observed can be viewed and verified with more powerful objectives. A good working knowledge of the parts of the binocular microscope and adjustments to produce Kohler illumination is essential for parasitologic examinations.

Parasitologic Procedures

Feces, sputum, urine, smegma, and blood can be observed with the technique described in Box 11-9. It requires a minimum amount of equipment and materials and is a rapid scan for parasite stages. It is especially useful for finding motile trophozoite stages of protozoa, which lyse in concentration procedures using saturated salt solutions. Unfortunately, a direct smear by itself is not an adequate examination for parasites, because only a small quantity of sample is examined and parasitic infections can be missed. However, it should be incorporated as a routine part of any parasitologic examination.

Flotation methods are based on differences in the specific gravity of life cycle stages of parasites found in feces and fecal debris. Simple fecal flotation is an example of a flotation method (Box 11-10). Specific gravity (sp. gr.) refers to the weight of an object as compared with the weight of an equal volume of water. Most parasite eggs have a specific gravity between 1.10 and 1.20

Box 11-9 Direct smear of feces

Materials:

75 × 25-mm glass microscope slides

22-mm^2 #1 glass coverslips

wooden applicator sticks

water or saline

Procedure:

1. Dip the applicator stick into the feces (only a small amount should adhere to the stick).
2. Place a drop of saline on a slide.
3. Mix the feces with the saline to produce a homogeneous emulsion that is clear enough to read newsprint through it. A common mistake is to make the smear too thick.
4. Place the coverslip over the emulsion.
5. Examine the slide at 100× and 400× magnification for eggs, cysts, trophozoites, and larvae.

Optional: A drop of Lugol's iodine (10 g potassium iodide/100 ml distilled water; then add 5 g iodine crystals = 5% Lugol's stock solution, which must be stored in an amber bottle away from light; dilute 1 part 5% Lugol's stock solution to 5 parts distilled water to make a staining solution) can be added to demonstrate diagnostic features of protozoa.

<table>
<tr><td></td></tr>
</table>

Box 11-10 Simple fecal flotation

Materials:

75 × 25-mm glass microscope slides

22-mm^2 #1 glass coverslips

wooden tongue depressors

waxed paper cups (90-150 ml)

cheesecloth or gauze squares (10 × 10 mm) or metal screen tea strainer

shell vial (1.25-2.0 cm × 5.0-7.5 cm) or 15-ml conical centrifuge tube

saturated salt or sugar flotation solution

Procedures:

1. Place approximately 2-5 g of feces in the paper cup.
2. Add 30 ml of flotation solution.
3. Using the tongue depressor, mix the feces to produce an evenly suspended emulsion.
4. If using cheesecloth, bend the sides of the cup to form a spout and cover the top with the cheesecloth squares while pouring the suspension into the shell vial. If using a metal strainer, pour the suspension through the metal strainer into another cup and fill the shell vial with the filtered solution.
5. Fill the shell vial to form a convex dome (meniscus) at the rim. Do not overfill the vial! Fresh solution can be used to form this dome.
6. Place a coverslip on top of the filled shell vial.
7. Allow the coverslip to remain undisturbed for 10 to 20 minutes.
8. Pick the coverslip straight up and place it on a glass slide, fluid side down.
9. Systematically examine the surface under the coverslip at 100× magnification.

---

ered using this technique. Nematode larvae can be recovered but frequently are distorted from crenation, making identification difficult. If the specific gravity of the flotation solution is too high, a plug of fecal debris floats and traps parasite stages in it, obscuring them from view.

Commonly used flotation solutions are sugar, sodium chloride, sodium nitrate, magnesium sulfate, and zinc sulfate. Each solution has advantages and disadvantages, including cost, availability, efficiency, shelf life, crystallization, corrosion of equipment, and ease of use. Selection is often determined by the type of practice and common parasites encountered in the area. Some companies (Synbiotics Corporation, San Diego, CA) have packaged flotation kits (Ovassay Plus) using prepared solutions of sodium nitrate or zinc sulfate, disposable plastic vials, and strainers. They are convenient but more expensive. Supplies to conduct simple flotations can be acquired through suppliers of scientific equipment and chemicals (e.g., Scientific Products, McGaw Park, IL). Formulas for making flotation solutions are as follows.

Sugar Solution (sp.gr. 1.275)
454 g granulated sugar
355 ml water
1 g crystalline phenol/100 ml solution

Heat the water and add the sugar. Continue heating until all the sugar is dissolved. Add the phenol as a preservative. Sugar is thick and viscous, and eggs take longer to float. It is also sticky and attracts ants and flies. However, it is readily available, inexpensive, and efficient. Slides can also be stored for a longer time in sugar. Some protozoan cysts collapse rapidly in sugar. It is a recommended flotation solution for recovery of *Cryptosporidium* oocysts.

Sodium Chloride Solution (sp.gr. 1.20)
360 g sodium chloride (better to use crude salt than refined salt)
1000 ml water

Heat the water and add the salt. An excess of crystals in the container ensures a saturated solution. Brine solution is inexpensive and clean to use. It crystallizes rapidly, collapses some protozoan cysts and nematode larvae, and fails to float some heavier nematode eggs. It is also corrosive.

Sodium Nitrate Solution (sp.gr. 1.39)
850 g sodium nitrate
1000 ml water

Add the sodium nitrate to the water and allow the solution to sit overnight at room temperature, stirring often. The water may also be heated before adding the salt. This solution is very efficient at floating eggs, even heavier eggs, such as ascarid eggs, trichurid eggs, and some fluke eggs. It tends to form air bubbles and floats more fecal debris. It also crystallizes rapidly and is more expensive.

---

g/ml. A liquid with a specific gravity greater than that of the eggs is required for the eggs to rise and float on the surface of the solution. Saturated solutions of sugar and various salts are used as flotation solutions and have specific gravities ranging between 1.18 and 1.40.

Fecal debris and eggs with a specific gravity greater than that of the flotation solution do not float. Fluke eggs are generally heavier than the specific gravity of most routinely used flotation solutions, with a few exceptions *(Paragonimus, Nanophyetus)*, and are not usually recov-

Magnesium Sulfate Solution (sp.gr. 1.285)

920 g magnesium sulfate

1000 ml water

Add the magnesium sulfate to the water and allow the solution to sit overnight at room temperature, stirring often. Magnesium sulfate is economical, accessible, and more efficient than sodium chloride at floating some of the heavier eggs. It also crystallizes fairly rapidly.

Zinc Sulfate Solution (sp.gr. 1.18)

336 g zinc sulfate

1000 ml water

Add the zinc sulfate to the water and allow to sit overnight at room temperature, stirring frequently. Zinc sulfate solution floats protozoan cysts and nematode larvae without distorting them. It is the recommended solution for recovery of *Giardia* cysts and *Filaroides* larvae.

Sodium Dichromate Solution (sp.gr. 1.40)

700 g sodium dichromate

1000 ml water

Add the sodium dichromate crystals to the water and shake well. Allow the solution to sit at room temperature overnight. Sodium dichromate is expensive, toxic, and not readily available. However, it is an excellent flotation solution for recovery of *Cryptosporidium* oocysts and floats some fluke eggs. Because of the higher specific gravity of this solution, more debris floats as well.

The specific gravity of flotation solutions can be checked using a hydrometer and adjusted by adding more salts or more water to the solution. Leaving extra crystals of salt on the bottom of the solution ensures that the solution is saturated.

The centrifugal flotation is more sensitive than a simple flotation, recovering more eggs and cysts in a sample in less time (Box 11-11). However, it requires access to a tabletop centrifuge with a head for rotation buckets. Fixed-angle heads do not work for this procedure as described. They can be adapted for this procedure by not filling the tubes and using a bacteriologic wire loop to collect the eggs from the surface of the solution. The centrifugal force holds the coverslips in place during spinning, provided the tubes are balanced.

Sedimentation concentrates parasite stages as well as fecal debris (Box 11-12). Because of the debris, parasite stages may be obscured from view; this technique is also more laborious. Sedimentations are used primarily when fluke infections are suspected. Most fluke eggs do not float or they are distorted by flotation solutions having higher specific gravities, making it difficult to recognize them. A few drops of liquid detergent can be added to the water as a surfactant to help remove excess fats and debris from the sample.

The modified McMaster technique provides an estimate of the number of eggs or oocysts per gram of feces, primarily with livestock species and horses (Box 11-13). Originally it was adapted from a technique used in peo-

---

Box 11-11 Centrifugal flotation

Materials:

75×25-mm glass slides

22-mm^2 #1 glass coverslips

waxed paper cups

cheesecloth or a metal tea strainer

funnel

15-ml conical centrifuge tubes

test tube rack

flotation solution

centrifuge with rotating buckets

wooden tongue depressors

balance scale

Procedure:

1. Prepare a fecal emulsion using 2-5 g of feces and 30 ml of flotation solution.
2. Strain the emulsion through the cheesecloth or tea strainer into the centrifuge tube. Suspending a funnel over the tube facilitates filling the tube.
3. Fill the tube to create a positive meniscus with flotation solution.
4. Place a coverslip on top of the tube.
5. Create a balance tube of equal weight, containing another sample or water.
6. Place the tubes in the centrifuge buckets and weigh them on a balance. Water may be added to the buckets to make them equal weights.
7. Centrifuge the tubes for 5 minutes at 400-650 gravities (approximately 1500 rpm).
8. Remove the coverslips from the tubes by lifting straight up and place them on a slide.
9. Systematically examine the slides at $100\times$ magnification.

---

ple infected with hookworms to estimate the worm population in the host. However, it is impossible to calculate the actual worm population in a host, especially in livestock and horses, because many factors influence egg production, and the number of eggs produced varies with the species and number of worms present.

Typically, livestock and horses are infected with several species of worms at one time, and some species are more prolific and pathogenic than others. Also, lesions often result from damage produced by immature stages

Box 11-12 Fecal sedimentation

Materials:

waxed paper cups (90-150 ml)

wooden tongue depressors

cheesecloth or gauze pads (10 × 10 cm) or a metal tea strainer

funnel

50-ml conical centrifuge tubes

disposable 2-ml pipettes

75 × 25-mm glass microscope slides

22-mm² #1 glass coverslips

Procedure:

1. Mix 2-5 g of feces in a cup with 30 ml of water.
2. Strain the fecal suspension through the cheesecloth or tea strainer into a 50-ml conical centrifuge tube. Suspending a funnel over the tube facilitates filling the tube.
3. Wash the sample with water until the tube is filled.
4. Allow the tube to sit undisturbed for 15 to 30 minutes.
5. Decant the supernatant off and resuspend the sediment in water.
6. Repeat steps 4 and 5 two more times.
7. Decant the supernatant without disturbing the sediment.
8. Using a pipette, mix the sediment and transfer an aliquot to a slide.
9. Place a coverslip over the sediment and systematically examine the slide with 100× magnification.
10. Repeat steps 8 and 9 until all of the sediment has been examined.

Box 11-13 Modified McMaster quantitative egg counting technique

Materials:

McMaster slides (Olympic Equine Products, 5003 228th Avenue South, Issaquah, WA 98027)

waxed paper cups (90 to 150 ml) or beakers

graduated cylinder

balance scale

saturated sodium chloride solution

wooden tongue depressors

disposable pipettes

rotary stirrer (optional)

Procedure:

1. Using the scale, weigh 5 g of feces into a cup.
2. Add a small amount of the flotation solution to the cup.
3. Mix the feces and flotation solution together thoroughly with a tongue depressor to make an even suspension.
4. Add sufficient flotation solution to bring the total volume to 75 ml.
5. Turn the rotary stirrer on and place the cup containing the fecal suspension in it. If a rotary stirrer is not available, the fecal suspension can be mixed with a tongue depressor.
6. Using a pipette, withdraw a portion of the mixing suspension and fill the chambers of the McMaster slide.
7. Allow the slide to sit undisturbed for 10 minutes.
8. Using the 10× objective, focus on the grid etched in the McMaster slide. Count all of the eggs or occysts seen in the six columns of the etched square, keeping a separate count for each different species of parasite seen.
9. Multiply the numbers counted by the appropriate dilution factor (dependent upon the number of squares counted) and record the results as eggs per gram (epg) of feces. The volume under the etched area is 0.15 ml. If 5 g per 75 ml total volume equals 1 g per 15 ml total volume, then 0.01 g is contained in 0.15 ml. Therefore, if one chamber is counted, multiply by 100. If two chambers are counted, multiply by 50 to arrive at the total number of eggs per gram of feces.

of the parasites. In ruminants, the parasites of interest are coccidia and trichostrongyles. In horses, the parasites of interest are large and small strongyles. Both trichostrongyles and strongyles infect ruminants and horses. The eggs of trichostrongyles and strongyles cannot be readily distinguished from one another and are referred to as *strongyle eggs* (see Fig. 11-30). Nevertheless, counts in excess of 1000 are considered indicative of heavy infections, whereas those greater than 500 indicate moderate infections. A low egg count can indicate a low level of infection, or severe infections in which the parasites are just becoming mature. Egg counts must always be interpreted in view of the clinical signs observed, age, sex and nutritional level of the animals, and stocking density of a herd or flock.

More recently, egg counts have been used in epidemiologic investigations and herd health management programs as predictors of peak pasture contamination and transmission potential for different geographic regions and individual farms. This information is applied toward prevention programs involving strategic use of broad-spectrum anthelmintics and pasture rotation schemes aimed at reducing the infective levels of pastures and exposure rates. When herd studies are conducted, individual samples are taken from at least 10% of the herd. Egg counts are also used to monitor development of resistance to anthelminthics. Egg counts are done before treatment and again 3 weeks after treatment to determine the effectiveness of the anthelminthic used and development of resistance in a given worm population.

The Baermann technique is used to recover nematode larvae from feces, fecal culture, soil, herbage, and animal tissues (Box 11-14). The warm water stimulates larvae to migrate out of the sample and relax. They then sink to the bottom of the apparatus, where they can be collected relatively free of debris. Free-living larvae must be distinguished from parasitic ones, especially if the sample is collected off the ground, from soil, or from herbage. This may require the expertise of an experienced helminthologist. Preserve samples by adding 5% to 10% formalin to the pellet for submission to an expert. Kill free-living larvae by adding 1% hydrochloric acid to the pellet and examine the preparation without heat fixation. Unfortunately, identification of motile larvae is more difficult.

The Baermann technique is routinely performed on feces of domestic animals when lungworm infections (*Dicytocaulus, Aelurostrongylus, Filaroides, Crenosoma, Muellerius, Protostrongylus*) are suspected. Ideally, samples should be fresh and collected rectally. In dogs and cats, a Baermann technique should be conducted when *Strongyloides* spp. infections are suspected. If the sample is not fresh, a fecal culture may be needed to distinguish first-stage hookworm larvae from first-stage larvae of *Strongyloides*. The third-stage filariform larva of *Strongyloides* is diagnostic and characterized by an esophagus that is half the length of the larva and a forked (bipartite) tail. Care should be taken when handling *Strongyloides* fecal cultures because of the zoonotic potential.

Fecal culture is used to differentiate parasites whose eggs or larvae are not easily distinguished by examination of a fresh fecal sample (Box 11-15). Trichostrongyle eggs in ruminant feces are indistinguishable from strongyle eggs. Small strongyle eggs in a horse sample cannot be distinguished from large strongyle eggs. First-stage hookworm larvae in a dog or cat sample and some free-living nematode larvae in soil or on grass cannot be easily distinguished from first-stage *Strongyloides* larvae. After fecal culture, the third-stage larvae of many of these parasites can be identified to

---

Box 11-14 Baermann technique

Materials:

Baermann apparatus (ring stand, ring, funnel, rubber tubing, clamp, wire screen)

cheesecloth or Kimwipes

disposable pipettes

15-ml centrifuge tubes or Petri dishes

pinch clamps

Procedure:

1. Construct a Baermann apparatus by fastening the ring to the ring stand. Attach 3 to 4 inches of rubber tubing to the narrow portion of the funnel. Make sure there is a good seal (tubing can be glued on). Place the funnel in the ring. Place the wire screen in the top portion of the funnel to support the feces. Put several layers of cheesecloth or Kimwipes over the wire screen. Place the pinch clamps at the end of the rubber tubing and check, using water, to ensure a tight seal. Put 30 to 50 g of feces on top of the Kimwipes and fill the funnel with warm water (not hot) to a level above the fecal sample. (An alternative method, which is more practical in a practice setting, is to use long-stem, plastic champagne glasses with hollow stems. The feces are wrapped in several layers of Kimwipes, similar to a tea bag. The fecal pouch is then set in the glass. Fill the glass with warm water to a level above the fecal sample.)
2. Allow the apparatus to remain undisturbed for a minimum of 1 hour up to 24 hours.
3. Collect the fluid in the rubber tubing (stem of the glass) and transfer to a Petri dish or centrifuge tube.
4. Examine the Petri dish for larvae using a stereo microscope or centrifuge the solution to pellet the larvae. Remove the supernatant from the centrifuge tube and place the pellet on a microscope slide.
5. Examine the slide for larvae and identify them. The slide can be passed over the flame of a Bunsen burner several times to kill the larvae in an extended position before identification.

Box 11-15 Fecal culture

Materials:

glass jar with tight-fitting lid

charcoal or vermiculite

wooden tongue depressors

Procedure:

1. Moisten 50 g of charcoal or vermiculite with water. The charcoal or vermiculite should be damp but not wet.
2. Using the tongue depressor, mix an equal amount of feces with the moistened substrate.
3. Place the fecal mixture in a glass jar and seal with the jar lid.
4. Place the jar in indirect light at room temperature for up to 7 days.
5. Check the jar periodically to make sure the contents remain moist. A spray bottle of water can be used to moisten the fecal mixture if it becomes too dry. Make sure not to saturate the material.
6. Do a Baermann technique on the fecal culture at 48-hour intervals to recover developing stages. Some larvae migrate up the wall of the jar and congregate in condensation droplets. These can be collected by flushing the sides of the jar with water and collecting the excess fluid in a centrifuge tube or Petri dish.
7. Identify the larvae recovered.

Box 11-16 Sporulation of coccidian oocysts

Materials:

beaker or waxed paper cups

Petri plates

2.5% potassium dichromate solution

wooden tongue depressors

15-ml centrifuge tubes

75×25-mm glass slides

22-mm^2 #1 glass coverslips

Procedure:

1. Mix 20 to 30 g of fresh feces with 60 ml of 2.5% potassium dichromate solution in a beaker or waxed paper cup.
2. Homogenize the feces with the tongue depressor.
3. Pour the fecal suspension into Petri dishes and cover. Allow the plates to incubate at room temperature for 3 to 7 days. Label the plates with the date and identification informaiton.
4. Open the plates daily and gently swirl the contents to aerate the sample.
5. After 3 to 7 days of incubation, pour the contents of the plates into centrifuge tubes and centrifuge for 5 minutes at 1500 rpm.
6. The sediment can be examined microscopically or resuspended in a flotation solution for centrifugal flotation.

---

genus level. Because the life cycles, pathogenicity, and epidemiology of some species may differ, identification may be necessary for proper treatment and control. Usually identification requires the help of an experienced helminthologist.

Most coccidian oocysts in fresh feces are unsporulated (single-celled zygote) and appear similar to one another. *Sporulation* is a process of development the oocyst undergoes to become infective (Box 11-16). Sporulated oocysts of *Eimeria* spp. (see Fig. 11-28) and *Isospora* spp. can be distinguished from one another, as well as those of other genera. *Eimeria* oocysts contain four sporocysts each having two sporozoites, while *Isospora* oocysts contain two sporocysts each having four sporozoites. *Cryptosporidium* oocysts (see Fig. 11-14) are sporulated when freshly passed and contain four sporozoites. Sporulated *Sarcocystis* oocysts or sporocysts can be recovered from fresh fecal samples. Oocysts have two sporocysts each containing four sporozoites.

Cellophane tape preparations are used to detect pinworm infections (Box 11-17). Pinworms can be found in primates, horses, and ruminants. The adult female worms migrate out of the anus and deposit their eggs on the skin around the anus (perianal region). The activity of the female worms is irritating and produces itching. Pinworm eggs are not consistently found on fecal flotations and are suspected when animals rub their tails on objects, resulting in loss of hair. *Oxyuris equi*, the pinworm of horses, can be a problem. Pinworm species of domestic animals are not transmissible to people. People can be infected with *Enterobius vermicularis* through direct contact with another infected person or premises contaminated with *Enterobius* eggs. Frequently, infected people are misinformed and believe that their infections came directly from their animals.

Blood Smears

Thin or thick blood smears are prepared in the same way that smears for a WBC differential count are prepared. (Preparation of smears for a white blood cell differential count is described earlier in this chapter.) Most parasites are carried with the laminar flow to the feathered edge of the slide. Parasites may be located between cells, on the surface of cells, or in the cytoplasm of cells. Thin blood films are most effectively used to study the morphology of protozoan and rickettsial parasites. If the parasitemia is low, infections can be missed, and a thick blood film or a buffy count smear is more effective because it concentrates a larger volume of cells (Box 11-18).

The buffy coat smear is a concentration technique for detection of protozoa and rickettsiae in white blood cells. Microfilariae and some protozoa in the plasma are also trapped in the buffy coat. A large number of cells can be examined rapidly. Some cells become smudged. The technique is quick and can be done in conjunction with a packed cell volume.

Impression smears can be used for diagnosis of intracellular parasites (Box 11-19). They can be useful for diagnosis of parasitic, neoplastic, and fungal diseases antemortem and postmortem. Frequently, protozoal organisms produce systemic disease and are located in the reticuloendothelial cells of lymph nodes, liver, lung, bone marrow, spleen, brain, kidneys, or muscles. Also, the liver, lung, lymph nodes, bone marrow, and spleen filter out damaged and abnormal cells of the blood, collecting parasitized cells. Toxoplasmosis, leishmaniasis, ehrlichiosis, and babesiosis are examples of parasitic diseases that can be diagnosed using this technique.

The modified Knott's technique is a rapid method for detection of microfilariae (heartworm larvae) in the blood (Box 11-20). It is used primarily for differentiating *Dirofilaria immitis* and *Dipetalonema reconditum* infections in dogs. The technique concentrates microfilariae while fixing them and lyses red blood cells. When preparing the 2% formalin solution, it is important to remember that 37% formaldehyde is equivalent to 100% formalin. It is also important to use water, not physiologic saline, to prepare this solution because physiologic saline does not lyse red blood cells. For accurate differentiation of the microfilariae, the micro-

---

Box 11-17 Cellophane tape preparation

Materials:

transparent adhesive tape

wooden tongue depressors

75 × 25-mm glass microscope slides

Procedure:

1. Place the adhesive tape in a loop around one end of the tongue depressor, with the adhesive side facing out.
2. Press the tape firmly against the skin around the anus.
3. Place a drop of water on the slide. Undo the loop of tape and stick the tape to the slide, allowing the water to spread out under the tape.
4. Examine the taped area of the slide microscopically for the presence of pinworm eggs.

Box 11-18 Buffy coat smear

Materials:

hematocrit tubes

sealant

hematocrit centrifuge

75 × 25-mm glass microscope slides

22-mm² #1 glass coverslips

file

Permount

Procedure

1. Fill the hematocrit tube with the blood sample and plug one end with sealant.
2. Centrifuge for 5 minutes.
3. The buffy coat is located in the middle of the centrifuged sample, between the red blood cells and the plasma.
4. Use the file to etch the glass below the buffy coat. Snap the tube by applying pressure opposite the etched spot.
5. Take the end of the tube containing the buffy coat and plasma and tap the buffy coat onto a glass slide with a small amount of plasma. If too much plasma is released, use a clean Kimwipe to wick away excess.
6. Apply a clean slide over the buffy coat and rapidly pull the two slides across one another in opposite directions.
7. Allow the slides to air dry and stain with Romanowsky stain.
8. After staining, apply mounting medium and a coverslip.
9. Examine the slides microscopically at 400× and 1000× magnification.

scope must have a calibrated ocular micrometer. Table 11-6 lists the characteristics used to distinguish microfilariae. Figs. 11-19 and 11-20 show these microfilariae.

The most accurate characteristics are body width, body length, and shape of the cranial end. The other characteristics are not consistent. The modified Knott's technique cannot detect occult heartworm infections. *Occult infections* occur if the infection is not yet *patent*, if the population of adult heartworms consists of only one sex, and if immune reactions of the host to microfilariae eliminate this stage from the bloodstream. Occult infections can also occur if animals infected with adult

heartworms are given heartworm preventative medications of the avermectin group. These interfere with oogenesis and sterilize the worms.

The filter technique is another method for concentration of microfilariae in blood (Box 11-21). The principles

---

Box 11-19 Impression smear

Materials:

paper towels

75×25-mm^2 glass microscope slides

22-mm^2 #1 glass coverslips

Romanowsky stain

scalpel blade or single-edged razor blade

forceps

Procedure

1. With tissues from necropsy or a lesion on an animal, either make a fresh cut of the tissue or remove any crust or scabs over the lesion.
2. Lightly blot the tissue or lesion with a clean paper towel.
3. Press the fresh edge of the tissue or lesion to a glass slide.
4. Stain the slide and examine it microscopically for parasites at 400× and 1000× magnification.

Box 11-20 Modified Knott's technique

Materials:

blood collection materials

15-ml conical centrifuge tubes

2% formalin (2 ml 37% formaldehyde and 98 ml water)

2.5% methylene blue (2.5 g methylene blue/100 ml water)

tabletop centrifuge

75×25-mm glass microscope slides

22-mm^2 #1 glass coverslips

pipettes

Procedure:

1. Mix 1 ml of blood with 9 ml of 2% formalin in a centrifuge tube. Agitate the tube and mix well.
2. Centrifuge the tube at 1500 rpm for 5 minutes.
3. Pour off the supernatant and add 1 to 2 drops of the methylene blue stain to the pellet at the bottom of the tube.
4. Using a pipette, mix the stain and sediment, and transfer the mixture to a glass slide.
5. Apply a coverslip and examine the sediment microscopically for microfilariae at 100× and 400× magnification.

TABLE 11-6 Differential characteristics of *Dirofilaria immitis* and *Dipetalonema reconditum* microfilariae

Characteristic	*Dirofilaria immitis*	*Dipetalonema reconditum*
Body shape	Usually straight	Usually curved
Body width	5-7.5μ	4.5-5.5μ
Body length	295-325μ	250-288μ
Cranial end	Tapered	Blunt
Caudal end	Straight	Curved or hooked
Numbers	Numerous	Sparse
Movement	Undulating	Progressive

Box 11-21 Millipore filtration procedure

Materials:

5-μ millipore filters

millipore filter holders

2.5% methylene blue stain

2% formalin

75 × 25-mm glass microscope slides

22-mm^2 #1 glass coverslips

12-ml disposable syringes

Procedure:

1. Assemble the filter holder with a millipore filter.
2. Place 1 ml of blood in the syringe.
3. Add 9 ml of 2% formalin to the blood in the syringe and insert the plunger.
4. Connect the syringe to the filter apparatus and slowly apply pressure to the syringe plunger.
5. Remove the syringe and fill it with tap water. Allow a few milliliters of air to remain in the syringe. Flush the water through the filter apparatus.
6. Remove the filter from the filter holder and place top side up on a glass slide.
7. Place a drop of the methylene blue stain on the filter and add a coverslip.
8. Examine the slide microscopically at 100× magnification for microfilariae.

Box 11-22 Heartworm antigen ELISA

Materials:

Commercial kits provided by Pitman-Moore, Mundelein, IL; IDEXX, Portland, ME; and Synbiotics Corporation, San Diego, CA

Procedure:

Follow the instructions provided by the manufacturer.

---

applied are similar to those of the modified Knott's test, except that the blood is passed through a millipore filter (5-μ pores), which collects the microfilariae. Supplies can be purchased from Scientific Products. Commercial kits use a detergent lysing solution and a different stain. This procedure is quicker and easier than the modified Knott's test, but the differential characteristics of the microfilariae are not as obvious. Identification using the characteristics listed in Table 11-6 is not possible with the commercial kits, because the characteristics of the microfilariae are based on fixation with 2% formalin.

Approximately 25% of heartworm-infected dogs have occult infections. For diagnosis of occult infections, enzyme-linked immunosorbent assays (ELISAs) have been developed. In ELISA, monoclonal antibodies are used to detect antigens of adult heartworms in the serum or plasma of dogs. These procedures are rapid and easy to perform (Box 11-22). They are also more sensitive and specific than the microfilariae detection methods. Only 1% of infected dogs have microfilaremia without circulating adult antigens. The American Heartworm Society currently recommends using antigen-detection methods for routine screening. Antigen-detection methods are preferred to microfilariae concentration methods in cats because such aberrant hosts circulate microfilariae only for a very short time. However, antigen levels in the blood of infected cats may also be too low to detect. Other methods, such as radiography, may be employed to make a diagnosis in cats.

Skin scrapings are used as a diagnostic tool for dermatologic conditions, especially mange in domestic animals (Box 11-23). Because some mange mites dwell in burrows and hair follicles deep in the epidermis, superficial scrapings are not productive. Other mites live in the more superficial layers of the skin and produce crusty or scaly lesions; deep scrapings are not required to diagnose these infestations. Sometimes the thick crusts interfere with seeing the mites.

Soaking the crust in a 10% potassium hydroxide solution helps to dissolve the keratinized skin and releases the mites. Mite infestations (*mange*) usually localize in specific locations (ear margin, tail head) initially, depending on the species of mite involved. Later they may become generalized and more difficult to diagnose. *Sarcoptes* (see Fig. 11-49) and *Cheyletiella* mites can be transmitted to people and produce pruritic reactions requiring attention. Specific identification of mites can be accomplished with the aid of taxonomic keys.

Cheyletiella infestation can be diagnosed by combing the coat of infested animals over a piece of black paper and observing the paper for "moving dandruff" (see Fig. 11-49). *Otodectes cynotis* (ear mite, see Fig. 11-48) infestations of the external ear canal can be diagnosed

Box 11-23 Skin scrapings

Materials:

75 × 25-mm glass slides

22-mm² #1 glass coverslips

#10 scalpel blades

10% potassium hydroxide solution (10 g potassium hydroxide/100 ml water)

Procedure:

1. With one hand, pinch the skin at the periphery of the lesion.
2. Apply a small amount of mineral oil to the area of skin to be scraped and a drop of oil to the center of a glass slide.
3. With the scalpel blade held between the thumb and index finger, scrape the skin until serum and a small amount of blood ooze from the area. Hold the blade perpendicular to the skin so as not to cut the skin.
4. Transfer the hair and epithelial debris from the blade to the oil on the slide.
5. Place a coverslip over the slide and examine microscopically at 100× and 400× magnification.

Box 11-24 Tritrichomonas foetus culture

Materials:

lactated Ringer's solution or phosphate buffered saline

pipettes

disposable gloves

diamond's culture medium or In Pouch TF (Biomed Diagnostics, San Jose, CA)

Procedure:

1. Wear gloves to prevent contamination of the sample to be collected.
2. Perform a preputial wash of the bull or collection of vaginal, cervical, or uterine secretions of the cow, using the Ringer's or saline solution.
3. Transfer the sample immediately to a clean tube and allow the sample to settle.
4. Inoculate the Diamond's medium or In Pouch with 1 to 2 ml of the sediment.
5. Incubate the medium at 37° C.
6. Examine the medium within the first 48 hours microscopically for growth of trichomonads. Allow the medium to incubate for 5 days and reexamine periodically for organisms.
7. If trichomonads are cultured, transfer 3 to 5 drops of the lower (deeper) portion of the medium containing the organisms to a new tube or pouch of culture medium and repeat the process of incubation and observation for growth.
8. Withdraw a small amount of a positive culture with a pipette and transfer to a slide to observe motility and morphology microscopically (0.5% formalin can be used to kill the flagellates for viewing with a phase microscope).

by otoscopic examination or by taking a swab of the dark waxy debris found in the ear and microscopically examining it in mineral oil.

Tritrichomonas foetus is a flagellated protozoan parasite of the reproductive tract of cattle that causes early-term abortions and repeat breeding (Box 11-24). Bulls remain permanently infected and must be identified and slaughtered to prevent spread of this organism. The organism can be found in fluid from the abomasum of aborted fetuses, uterine discharges, and vaginal and preputial washes. However, the numbers present are usually low and culture of these materials facilitates diagnosis. Occasionally, intestinal flagellates can contaminate a sample. These must be differentiated from *Tritrichomonas foetus*. *T. foetus* has three cranial flagella and one caudal flagellum attached to an undulating membrane. Isolates of *T. foetus* can be propagated through several passages of culture medium, whereas intestinal flagellates usually cannot. Materials may also be collected and shipped to diagnostic facilities for culture and identification. In Pouch TF (Biomed Diagnostics, San Jose, CA) is an excellent transport medium.

Total worm burden estimates provide the most accurate information regarding whether pathogenic levels of parasites are present in an animal or herd (Box 11-25). This technique is used most frequently in grazing animals, but can be used in small animal practices as well. It is frequently employed in scientific studies investigating the epidemiology of parasitic helminths and in drug efficacy studies.

Specific identification of gross parasites recovered from domestic animals is beyond the scope of this book and often requires the expertise of experienced helminthologists, protozoologists, and entomologists. Government, academic, and private diagnostic labora-

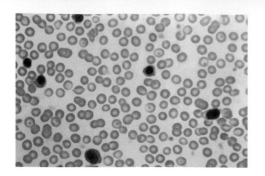

PLATE 9 Nucleated red blood cells in a smear from a dog with lead poisoning. *(Courtesy of Dr. E. Lassen.)*

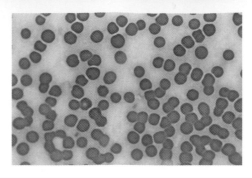

PLATE 10 Howell-Jolly bodies and basophilic stippling in feline red blood cells. *(Courtesy of Dr. E. Lassen.)*

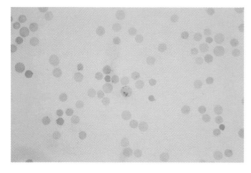

PLATE 11 Heinz bodies and aggregate reticulocytes in a smear from a cow with onion poisoning. *(Courtesy of Dr. E. Lassen.)*

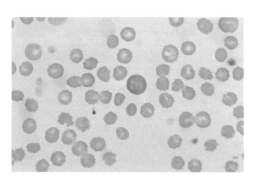

PLATE 12 Echinocytes in a canine blood smear. Note the polychromatophil in the center. *(Courtesy of Dr. Mary Anna Thrall.)*

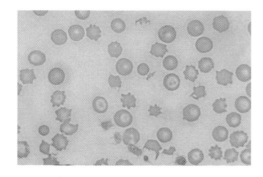

PLATE 13 Schistocytes in a smear from a dog with iron deficiency. Target cells and red cells with other membrane abnormalities (keratocytes) are also present. *(Courtesy of Dr. Mary Anna Thrall.)*

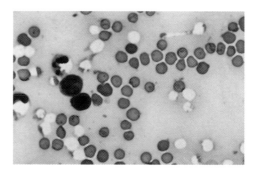

PLATE 14 *Hemobartonella felis* in feline red blood cells (new methylene blue, counterstained with Wright's stain). *(Courtesy of Dr. E. Lassen.)*

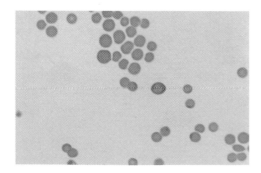

PLATE 15 *Anaplasma marginale* in bovine red blood cells. *(Courtesy of Dr. Mary Anna Thrall.)*

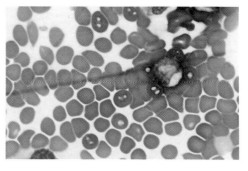

PLATE 16 *Babesia canis* in a canine blood smear. *(Courtesy of Dr. Mary Anna Thrall.)*

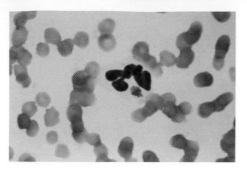

PLATE 17 Morula of *Ehrlichia equi* at the five o'clock position in a neutrophil *(center)* in an equine blood smear. *(Courtesy of Dr. Mary Anna Thrall.)*

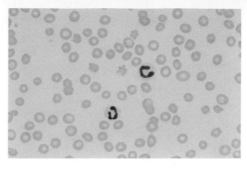

PLATE 18 Canine blood smear showing a band neutrophil *(top)* and a segmented neutrophil *(bottom)*. *(Courtesy of Dr. E. Lassen.)*

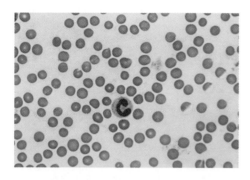

PLATE 19 Band neutrophil in a feline blood smear. *(Courtesy of Dr. E. Lassen.)*

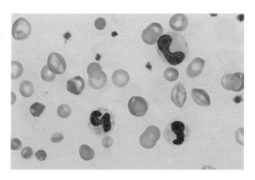

PLATE 20 Metamyelocyte *(upper right)* in a canine blood smear. The two segmented neutrophils at bottom center are toxic and contain Döhle bodies. *(Courtesy of Dr. Mary Anna Thrall.)*

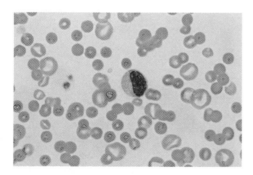

PLATE 21 Myelocyte *(center)* in a canine blood smear. *(Courtesy of Dr. Mary Anna Thrall.)*

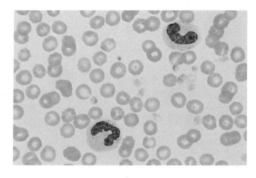

PLATE 22 Toxic neutrophils containing Döhle bodies in a canine blood smear. *(Courtesy of Dr. Mary Anna Thrall.)*

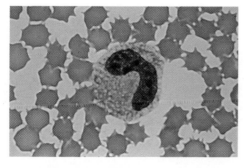

PLATE 23 Cytoplasmic vacuolization in a toxic neutrophil in a feline blood smear. *(Courtesy of Dr. Mary Anna Thrall.)*

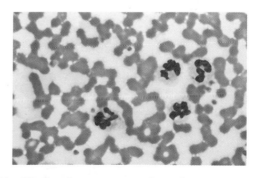

PLATE 24 Nuclear hypersegmentation of canine neutrophils. *(Courtesy of Dr. E. Lassen.)*

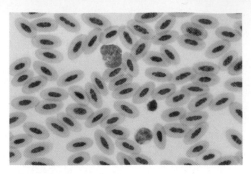

PLATE 25 Heterophil *(top center)* in an avian blood smear. Also present are a thrombocyte *(center)* and a lymphocyte *(bottom center)*. *(Courtesy of Dr. Mary Anna Thrall.)*

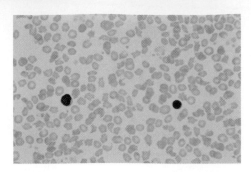

PLATE 26 Lymphocytes in a feline blood smear. *(Courtesy of Dr. E. Lassen.)*

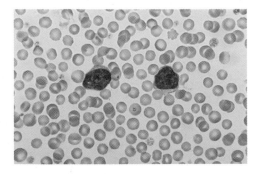

PLATE 27 Large lymphocytes *(center)* with nucleolar rings in a bovine blood smear. *(Courtesy of Dr. Mary Anna Thrall.)*

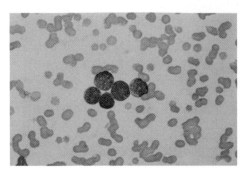

PLATE 28 Atypical lymphocytes (lymphoblasts) in a feline blood smear. *(Courtesy of Dr. E. Lassen.)*

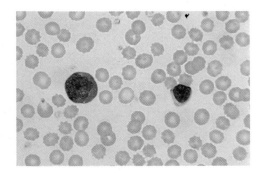

PLATE 29 Reactive lymphocyte *(left)* and normal lymphocyte *(right)* in a canine blood smear. *(Courtesy of Dr. Mary Anna Thrall.)*

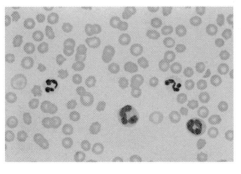

PLATE 30 In this canine blood smear, the two larger cells are monocytes; the smaller cells are segmented neutrophils. *(Courtesy of Dr. E. Lassen.)*

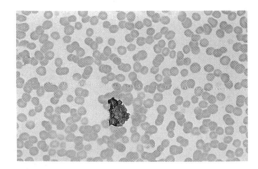

PLATE 31 Eosinophil in an equine blood smear. *(Courtesy of Dr. E. Lassen.)*

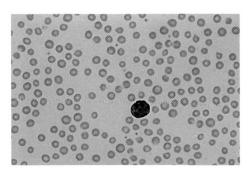

PLATE 32 Basophil in a bovine blood smear. *(Courtesy of Dr. E. Lassen.)*

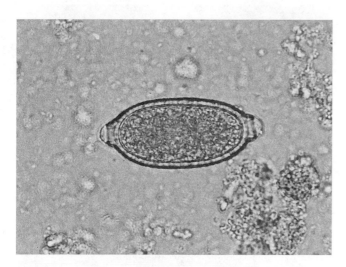

FIG. 11-23 *Capillaria aerophilus* egg (fecal flotation).

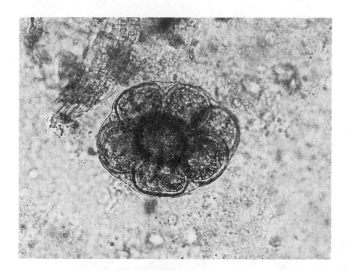

FIG. 11-24 *Dipylidium caninum* egg packet (recovered from gravid proglottid).

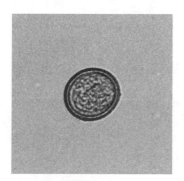

FIG. 11-25 *Taenia* sp. egg (recovered from gravid proglottid).

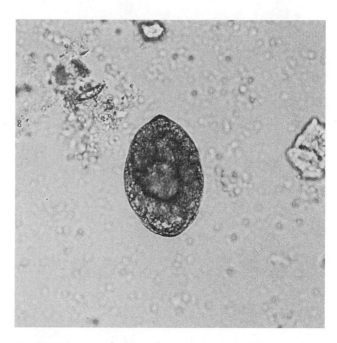

FIG. 11-26 *Nanophyetus salmincola* eggs (sedimentation).

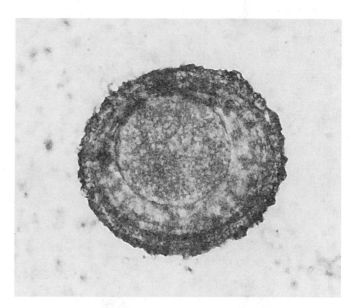

FIG. 11-27 *Parascaris equorum* egg (fecal flotation).

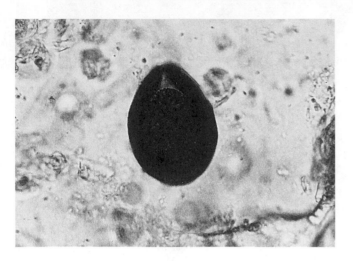

FIG. 11-28 *Eimeria leuckarti* oocyst (fecal flotation).

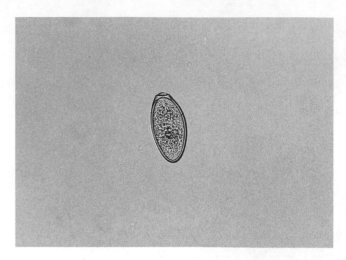

FIG. 11-29 *Oxyuris equi* egg (fecal flotation).

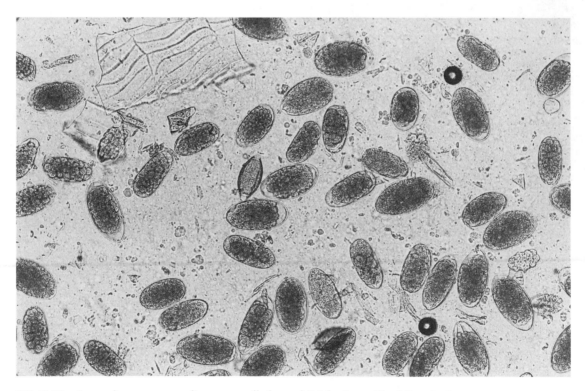

FIG. 11-30 Strongyle eggs surrounding a centrally located *Trichuris* egg (fecal flotation).

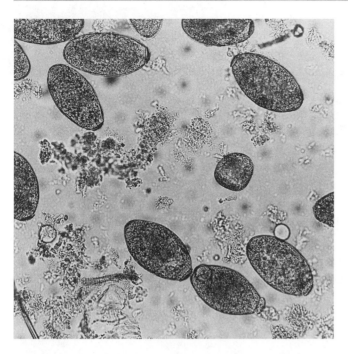

FIG. 11-31 *Fasciola hepatica* eggs surrounding a centrally located *Moniezia* egg (sedimentation).

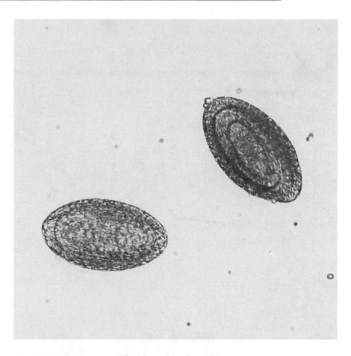

FIG. 11-33 *Macracanthorhynchus hirudinaceus* eggs (fecal flotation).

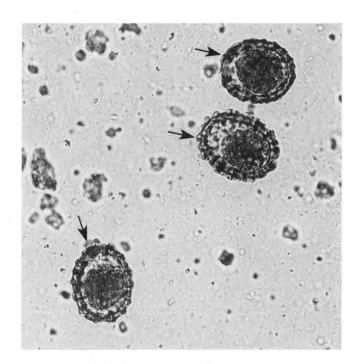

FIG. 11-32 *Ascaris suum* eggs (fecal flotation).

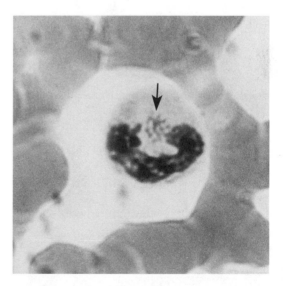

FIG. 11-34 *Ehrlichia* morula in a white blood cell (Romanowsky-stained blood smear).

TABLE 11-7 Diagnostic characteristics of internal parasites of domestic animals

Parasite	Location	Prepatent period	Diagnostic stage	Test
Dogs				
Toxocara canis (see Fig. 11-17)	Small intestines	3-5 weeks	Dark brown, thick-walled egg, with a pitted egg shell; zygote single-celled 90-75μ	Fecal flotation
Ancylostoma caninum (see Fig. 11-18)	Small intestines	2-3 weeks	Clear, smooth, thin-walled hook-worm egg; zygote 8 to 16-cell morula; 55-65 × 27-43μ	Fecal flotation
Uncinaria stenocephala	Small intestines	2 weeks	Hookworm egg; 63-93 × 32-55μ	Fecal flotation
Trichuris vulpis	Large intestines	3 months	Smooth, amber, thick-walled, barrel-shaped egg with bipolar plugs; zygote single-celled; 72-90 × 32-40μ	Fecal flotation
Eucoleus bohmi	Nasal sinuses	Unknown	Smooth, yellow-brown, thick-walled egg with a striated shell and asymmetric bipolar plugs; zygote single celled	Fecal flotation
Filaroides spp.	Lungs	5-10 weeks	L1 with S-shaped tail lacking a dorsal spine; esophagus 1/3 length of body; 230-266μ long	Fecal flotation, Baermann
Crenosoma spp.	Lungs	19-21 days	L1 with a straight, pointed tail; esophagus 1/3 length of body; 265-330μ long	Baermann
Spirocerca lupi	Esophagus	5-6 months	Clear, smooth, thick-walled, paper clip-shaped, larvated egg; 30-37 × 11-15μ	Flotation
Dirofilaria immitis (see Fig. 11-19)	Heart	6-8 months	Microfilaria (L1) lacks an esophagus	Modified Knott's millipore filtration, ELISA, antigen test
Dipetalonema reconditum (see Fig. 11-20)	Subcutaneous tissue	9 weeks	Microfilaria	Modified Knott's millipore filtration
Dioctophyma renale	Kidney	5 months	Dark brown, thick-walled, barrel-shaped egg with a pitted shell and an operculum at each pole; zygote single celled; 71-84 × 46-52μ	Sedimentation of urine
Dracunculus insignis	Subcutaneous tissue	309-410 days	Comma-shaped larva with an eso-phagus and a straight tail; 500-750μ long	Direct smear of fluid in blister
Cats				
Toxocara cati (see Fig. 11-21)	Small intestines	8 weeks	Dark brown, thick-walled, pitted egg; zygote single celled; 65-75μ	Fecal flotation
Ancylostoma	Small intestines	3 weeks	Hookworm egg; 55-76 × 34-45μ	Fecal flotation
Aelurostrongylus abstrusus (see Fig. 11-21)	Bronchioles alveoli	4-6 weeks	L1 with S-shaped tail and a dorsal spine; 360μ long; esophagus 1/4 length of body	Baermann

TABLE 11-7 Diagnostic characteristics of internal parasites of domestic animals—cont'd

Parasite	Location	Prepatent period	Diagnostic stage	Test
Cats–cont'd				
Platynosomum fastosum	Liver	8-12 weeks	Dark amber, oval, operculated egg containing a miracidium; 34-50 × 20-35μ	Sedimentation of feces
Toxoplasma gondii (see Fig. 11-15)	Small intestines	1-3 weeks	Clear, smooth, thin-walled spherical oocyst; zygote single celled; 8-10μ	Fecal flotation
Dogs and Cats				
Toxascaris leonina (see Fig. 11-22)	Small intestines	11 weeks	Clear, smooth, thick-walled egg shell with wavy internal membrane; zygote single celled and does not completely fill the egg shell; 75 × 85μ	Fecal flotation
Ancylostoma braziliense	Small intestines	3 weeks	Hookworm egg; 75-95 × 41-45μ	Fecal flotation
Uncinaria stenocephala	Small intestines	15 days	Hookworm egg; 63-93 × 32-55μ	Fecal flotation
Capillaria aerophilus (see Fig. 11-23)	Trachea Bronchi	6 weeks	Rough, granular, thick-walled, barrel-shaped, straw-colored egg with asymmetric bipolar plugs; zygote single celled; 58-79 × 29-40μ	Fecal flotation
Capillaria plica	Urinary bladder	60 days	Rough, striated, thick-walled, barrel-shaped, amber-colored egg with asymmetric bipolar plugs; zygote single celled; 60-68 × 24-30μ	Sedimentation of urine
Strongyloides stercoralis	Small intestines	8-14 days	L1 with a rhabditiform esophagus and a straight pointed tail;	Baermann
			L3 with a filariform esophagus and a bipartite tail	Fecal culture
Physaloptera spp.	Stomach	56-83 days	Smooth, clear, thick-walled, larvated egg; 45-53 × 29-42μ	Fecal flotation
Dipylidium caninum (see Fig. 11-24)	Small intestines	3 weeks	Proglottid with bilateral genital pores; eggs containing six-hooked hexacanth embryos in packets; 35-60μ	ID proglottids fecal flotation
Taenia spp. (see Fig. 11-25)	Small intestines	2 months	Dark brown, thick, radially striated egg shell; six-hooked hexacanth embryo; 32-37μ; rectangular proglottids with unilateral genital pore	ID proglottid
Echinococcus spp.	Small intestines	47 days	Similar to *Taenia* eggs	Fecal flotation
Mesocestoides spp.	Small intestines	16-20 days	Smooth, thin egg capsule containing six-hooked hexacanth embryo; 20-25μ; globular proglottid with parauterine body	Fecal flotation ID proglottid
Spirometra mansonoides	Small intestines	10-30 days	Unembryonated, thin-walled, smooth, amber-colored egg; operculated; 70 × 45μ	Fecal flotation
Paragonimus kellicotti	Lung	1 month	Smooth, golden brown, urn-shaped, operculated egg; 75-118 × 42-67μ	Sedimentation of urine

Continued

TABLE 11-7 Diagnostic characteristics of internal parasites of domestic animals—cont'd

Parasite	Location	Prepatent period	Diagnostic stage	Test
Dogs and Cats–cont'd				
Nanophyetus salmincola (see Fig. 11-26)	Small intestines	1 week	Rough, brown, operculated egg; 52-82 × 32-56μ	Sedimentation of feces
Isospora spp. (see Fig. 11-13)	Small intestines	4-12 days	Clear, spherical to ellipsoid thin-walled oocyst, size varies with species	Fecal flotation
Sarcocystis spp.	Small intestines	7-33 days	Thin-walled oocyst with 2 sporocyst containing 4 sporozoites each or sporocyst; size varies with species	Fecal flotation
Horse				
Parascaris equorum (see Fig. 11-27)	Small intestines	10 weeks	Rough, brown, thick-walled, spherical egg; zygote single celled; 90-100μ	Fecal flotation
Eimeria leukarti (see Fig. 11-28)	Small intestines	15-33 days	Dark brown, piriform, thick-walled oocyst; 70-90 × 49-69	Fecal flotation
Cyathostomes (small strongyles)	Large intestines	2-3 months	Smooth, thin-walled, clear strongyle egg; zygote 8 to 16-cell morula; size varies with species	Fecal flotation
Strongylus spp. (large strongyles)	Large intestines	6-12 months	Strongyle egg	Fecal flotation
Oxyuris equi (see Fig. 11-29)	Large intestines	5 months	Clear, smooth, thin-walled egg with one side flattened; operculated; 90 × 42μ	Cellophane tape preparation
Anoplocephala spp.	Small and large intestines	1-2 months	Clear, thick-walled, square eggs with a pear-shaped (piriform) apparatus containing a hexacanth embryo	Fecal flotation
Trichostrongylus axei	Stomach	25 days	Strongyle egg	Fecal flotation
Dictyocaulus arnfieldi	Lung	2-4 months	L1 with dark, granular intestines; esophagus ⅓ length of larva; tapered tail	Fecal flotation Baermann
Habronema and *Draschia* spp.	Stomach	2 months	Thin-walled, larvated egg (rarely seen)	ID adults at necropsy
Strongyloides westeri	Small intestines	8-14 days	Smooth, thin-walled, larvated egg; 40-50 × 32-40μ	Fecal flotation
Onchocerca spp.	Ligaments of legs and neck	1 year	Unsheathed microfilaria in the skin of ventral midline; 200-370μ long	Skin biopsy
Setaria equina	Peritoneal cavity		Sheathed microfilaria in the blood; 190-256μ long	Blood smear ID adults at necropsy
Gasterophilus spp. (see Fig. 11-40)	Stomach		2.5 cm, robust grub with rows of spines and straight spiracular slits (breathing tubes)	ID 3rd instar at necropsy

TABLE 11-7 Diagnostic characteristics of internal parasites of domestic animals—cont'd

Parasite	Location	Prepatent period	Diagnostic stage	Test
Cattle, Sheep, Goats				
Trichostrongyles *Haemonchus, Ostertagia, Cooperia, Trichostrongylus* (see Fig. 11-30)	Abomasum, small intestines	15-28 days	Strongyle egg	Fecal flotation
Dictyocaulus spp.	Lungs	3-4 weeks	L1 with dark granular intestines; esophagus ⅓ length of larva; straight pointed tail; 550-580μ long	Baermann
Strongyloides spp.	Small intestines	3-4 weeks	Thin-walled egg with parallel sides; 40-60 × 20-25μ	Fecal flotation
Oesophagostomum spp.	Large intestines	45 days	Strongyle egg	Fecal flotation
Skrjabinema spp.	Large intestines	25 days	Clear, smooth, thin-walled egg with one side flattened, zygote single celled	Fecal flotation
Eimeria spp. (see Fig 11-12)	Small and large intestines	10-30 days	Smooth or rough, thin-walled, clear to yellowish brown oocysts; zygote single celled; size varies with species	Fecal flotation
Moniezia spp. (see Fig. 11-31)	Small intestines	6 weeks	Thick-walled, clear, triangular to square egg with a piriform apparatus containing a hexacanth embryo	Fecal flotation
Thysanosoma actinoides	Bile ducts		Thin-walled egg with hexacanth embryos in packegs; 21-45μ	Fecal flotation
Fasciola hepatica (see Fig. 11-31)	Liver	10-12 weeks	Dark amber, oval, operculated egg; 130-150 × 63-90μ	Sedimentation of feces
Dicrocoelium dendriticum	Liver	10-12 weeks	Dark brown, operculated egg; 36-45 × 22-30μ	Sedimentation of feces
Paramphistomum spp.	Rumen	7-10 weeks	Light greenish, oval, operculated egg; 114-176 × 73-100μ	Sedimentation of feces
Bunostomum spp.	Small intestines	2-3 weeks	Strongyle egg	Fecal flotation
Chabertia ovina	Large intestines	47-63 days	Strongyle egg	Fecal flotation
Toxocara vitulorum	Small intestines	3 weeks	Thick-walled, pitted egg shell; single-celled zygote; 90-100μ	Fecal flotation
Setaria labiatopapillosa	Peritoneal cavity		Sheathed microfilaria in the blood; 240-260μ	Blood smears; adults at necropsy
Trichuris spp. (see Fig. 11-30)	Large intestines	2-3 months	Dark, brownish, thick-walled, smooth egg with symmetric bipolar plugs; single-celled zygote; size varies with species	Fecal flotation
Capillaria spp.	Small intestines		Brownish, thick-walled striated egg with asymmetric bipolar plugs; single-celled zygote; 45-52 × 21-30μ	Fecal flotation

Continued

TABLE 11-7 Diagnostic characteristics of internal parasites of domestic animals—cont'd

Parasite	Location	Prepatent period	Diagnostic stage	Test
Cattle				
Onchocerca spp.	Ligamentum nuchae	1 year	Unsheathed microfilaria in the skin of ventral midline; 170-265μ	Skin biopsy
Stephanofilaria stilesi	Skin along ventral midline		Microfilaria in the skin along ventral midline; 45-60μ	Skin biopsy
Cryptosporidium muris	Abomasum	4-10 days	Clear, smooth, thin-walled oocyst containing 4 sporozoites; 5 × 7μ	Fecal flotation
Sheep				
Elaeophora schneideri	Arteries	4-5 months	Microfilaria in skin of the poll; 207 × 13μ	Skin biopsy
Protostrongylus rufescens	Lungs	30-37 days	L1 with a straight, pointed tail 48 × 56μ long without a dorsal spine; 340-400 × 19-20μ	Baermann
Mullerius spp.	Lungs	6 weeks	L1 are 300-320 × 14-15μ with S-shaped tail bearing a dorsal spine	Baermann
Pigs				
Eimeria spp.	Small intestines	4-10 days	Smooth or rough, thin-walled oocyst; zygote single celled; size varies with species	Fecal flotation
Isospora suis	Small intestines	5 days	Smooth, clear, thin-walled oocyst; zygote single celled; 17-25 × 16-21μ	Fecal flotation
Balantidium coli	Large intestines		Thin-walled, greenish cyst with hyaline cytoplasm; 40-60μ	Fecal flotation
			30-150 × 25-120μ trophozoite with rows of cilia	Direct smear
Ascaris suum (see Fig. 11-32)	Small intestines	7-9 weeks	Brownish yellow, thick-walled, mammilated egg; single-celled zygote; 50-80 × 40-60μ	Fecal flotation
Strongyloides ransomi	Small intestines	3-7 days	Smooth, thin-walled, larvated egg with parallel sides; 45-55 × 26-35μ	Fecal flotation
Oesophagostomum spp.	Large intestines	32-42 days	Strongyle egg	Fecal flotation
Stephanurus dentatus	Kidney	3-4 months	Strongyle egg	Sedimentation of urine
Hyostrongylus rubidus	Stomach	15-21 days	Strongyle egg	Fecal flotation
Metastrongylus spp.	Lungs	24 days	Rough, clear, thick-walled, larvated egg with a corrugated surface; 45-57 × 38-41μ	Fecal flotation
Ascarops strongylina	Stomach	6 weeks	Oblong, clear, smooth, thick-walled, larvated egg; 34-40 × 18-22μ	Fecal flotation
Physocephalus sexalatus	Stomach	6 weeks	Clear, smooth, thick-walled, larvated egg; 31-45 × 12-26μ	Fecal flotation
Trichuris suis	Large intestines	2-3 months	Brownish yellow, smooth, thick-walled egg with symmetric bi-polar plugs; single celled zygote 50-56 × 21-25μ	Fecal flotation

TABLE 11-7 Diagnostic characteristics of internal parasites of domestic animals—cont'd

Parasite	Location	Prepatent period	Diagnostic stage	Test
Pigs–cont'd				
Trichinella spiralis	Small intestines	2-6 days	L3 encysted in striated muscles; espophagus composed of sticho-cytes (single cells stacked on top of one another); cysts are 400-600 $\times 250\mu$	Squash prepara-tion of muscle
Macracanthorhynchus hirudinaceus (see Fig. 11-33)	Small intestines	2-3 months	Dark brown, thick-walled egg with 3 membranes; zygote an acanthor with anterior hooks; 67-110 $\times$ 40-65μ	Fecal flotation
Dogs, Cats, Cattle, Horses, Sheep, Goats, Pigs				
Thelazia californiensis	Eye	3-6 weeks	Adult worm in conjunctival sac and tear duct	ID adult
Giardia duodenalis (see Fig. 11-11)	Small intestines	7-10 days	Smooth, clear, thin-walled cyst with 2-4 nuclei; 4-10 $\times$ 8-16μ	Fecal flotation
			Piriform, bilaterally symmetric greenish trophozoite with 2 nuclei and 4 pair of flagella; 9-20 $\times$ 5-15μ	Direct smear
Trichomonads	Digestive tract		Spindle-shaped to piriform tropho-zoite with 3-5 anterior flagella, an undulating membrane and one posterior flagellum	Direct smear
Cryptosporidium spp. (see Fig. 11-14)	Small and large intestines	4-10 days	Clear, thin-walled, spherical oocyst containing 4 sporozoites; 5 $\times$ 5μ	Fecal flotation

TABLE 11-8 Diagnostic characteristics of blood parasites of domestic animals

Parasite	Definitive host	Location	Prepatient period	Diagnostic stage	Diagnostic test
Babesia spp. (see Fig. 11-16)	People, dogs, cattle, horses	Blood (erythrocytes)	10-21 days	Paired piriform (tear-shaped) merozoites in erythrocytes	Romanowsky-stained blood film, indirect fluorescent antibody test
Trypanosoma spp.	People, dogs, cats, cattle, sheep, horses	Blood and lymph, heart, striated muscle, reticuloendothelial muscle	Acute and chronic disease	Trypanosome form, spindle-shaped flagellate with undulating membrane, central nucleus and kinetoplast, found in blood Amastigote form, intracellular spherical bodies with single nucleus and rod-shaped kinetoplast, found in myocardium, striated muscle cells, and macrophages	Blood smears; xenodiagnosis (clean vector allowed to feed on suspect patient and organism isolated from the vector), biopsy, animal inoculation, serology
Leishmania donovani	People, dogs	Intracellular in cytoplasm of macrophages of reticuloendothelial system	Several months up to a year	Amastigote form, oval, single nucleus, with a rod-shaped kinetoplast, in clusters within the cytoplasm of macrophages	Impression smears and biopsy of skin, lymph nodes, and bone marrow

TABLE 11-9 Zoonotic internal parasites

Parasite	Host	Reservoir	Infective stage	Condition
Toxocara spp.	Dogs, cats	Dogs, cats	Egg with L2	Visceral larva migrans
Ancylostoma spp.	Dogs, cats	Dogs, cats	L3	Cutaneous larva migrans
Uncinaria stenocephala	Dogs, cats	Dogs, cats	L3	Cutaneous larva migrans
Toxoplasma gondii	Cats	Cats, raw meat	Sporulated oocyst, bradyzoite, tachyzoite	Toxoplasmosis Toxoplasmosis
Strongyloides stercoralis	Dogs, cats, people	People, dogs, cats	L3	Strongyloidiasis
Dipylidium caninum	Dogs, cats, people	Flea	Cysticercoid	Cestodiasis
Taenia saginata	People	Bovine muscle	Cysticercus	Cestodiasis
Taenia solium	People	Porcine muscle	Cysticercus	Cestodiasis
	People	People	Egg	Cysticercosis
Echinococcus granulosus	Dogs	Dogs	Egg	Hydatidosis
Echinococcus multilocularis	Dogs, cats	Dogs, cats	Egg	Hydatidosis
Spirometra mansonoides	Dogs, cats	Unknown	Procercoid in arthropod	Sparganosis
Sarcocystis spp.	People	Cattle, pigs	Sarcocyst in muscle	Sarcocystiasis
	Dogs, cats	Dogs, cats	Oocyst	Sarcosporidiosis
Cryptosporidium parvum	Mammals	Mammals	Oocyst	Cryptosporidiosis
Balantidium coli	People, pigs	People, pigs	Cyst, trophozoite	Balantidiasis
Ascaris suum	Pigs	Pigs	Egg with L2	Visceral larva migrans
Trichinella spiralis	Mammals	Porcine and bear muscle	Encysted L3	Trichinellosis
Thelazia spp.	Mammals	Fly	L3	Verminous conjunctivitis
Giardia duodenalis	Mammals	Mammals	Cyst	Giardiasis
Babesia microti	Rodents, people	Hard tick	Sporozoite	Babesiosis
Trypanosoma	Mammals	Reduviids	Trypanosomal form in kissing bug	Chagas' disease
Leishmania donovani	Mammals	Phlebotomine fly	Leptomonad form in sandfly	Leishmaniasis

COMMON ECTOPARASITES OF DOMESTIC ANIMALS

Fleas

Fleas are blood-sucking parasites of dogs, cats, rodents, birds, and people. They are vectors of several diseases, such as bubonic plague and tularemia. Cat and dog fleas, *Ctenocephalides felis* (Fig. 11-35) and *C. canis*, respectively, can act as intermediate hosts for the common tapeworm, *Dipylidium caninum*. Heavy infestations with fleas, especially in young animals, produce anemia. Flea saliva is antigenic and irritating, causing intense pruritus (itching) and hypersensitivity, known as *flea-bite dermatitis* or *miliary dermatitis*.

Fleas are laterally compressed, wingless insects with legs adapted for jumping. They move rapidly on the host and from host to host. Flea infestations are encountered most frequently on dogs and cats. They can be detected around the tailhead, on the ventral abdomen, and under the chin.

Fleas demonstrate complete metamorphosis. Eggs deposited on the host fall off and develop to larvae in the environment. The larvae (Fig. 11-36) can occasionally be found in the animal's bedding, on furniture, or in cracks and crevices of the animal's environment. The larvae are maggot-like, with a head capsule and bristles. Flea larvae feed on organic debris, including the excrement of adult fleas. Flea droppings are reddish brown, comma-shaped casts of dehydrated blood. Flea droppings in the animal's haircoat indicate flea infestation.

Specific identification of fleas requires the expertise of an entomologist. Other fleas of veterinary importance are *Pulex irritans*, *Xenopsylla cheopis*, *Tunga penetrans*,

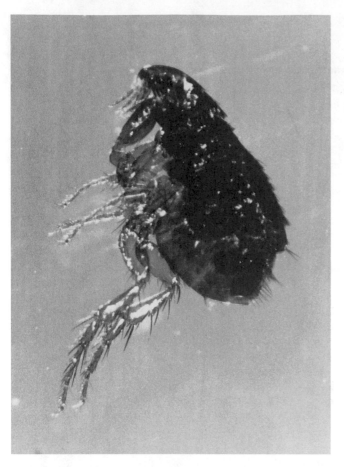

FIG. 11-35   *Ctenocephalides felis* adult.

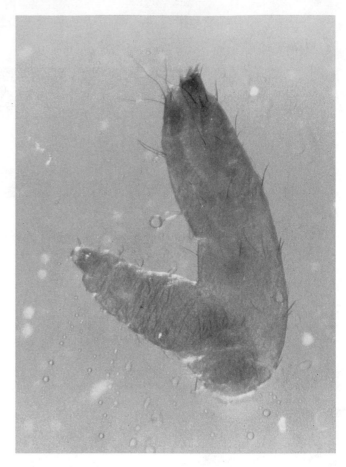

FIG. 11-36   Flea larva.

Ceratophyllus gallinae, and *Echidnophaga gallinacea.* Fleas have preferred hosts, but they attack any source of blood if the preferred host is not available. Adult fleas can also survive for extended periods off the host and can heavily infest premises.

Lice

Lice are dorsoventrally flattened, wingless insects with clawed appendages for clasping to the host's hairs. Lice are separated into two Orders, based on whether their mouth parts are modified for chewing (Mallophaga, Fig. 11-37) or sucking (Anoplura, Fig. 11-38). Sucking lice feed on blood and move slowly on the host. They have a long, narrow head. Biting lice feed on epithelial debris and can move rapidly over the host. They have a broad, rounded head. Lice are very host specific, remain in close association with the host, and have preferred locations on the host. Lice glue their eggs or *nits* (Fig. 11-39) to the hairs or feathers of the host. Transmission is usually by direct contact but can occur through equipment contaminated with eggs, nymphs, or adults.

Louse infestations *(pediculosis)* tend to be more severe in young, old, or poorly nourished animals, especially in overcrowded conditions and during the colder months. Sucking lice produce anemia, whereas biting lice are irritating and disturbing to the animal. Common biting lice of domestic animals include *Trichodectes canis* (dog), *Damalinia equi* (horse), *D. bovis* (cow), *D. ovis* (sheep), *D. caprae* (goat), and *Felicola subrostratus* (cat). Common sucking lice of domestic animals include *Linognathus setosus* (dog), *Haematopinus asini* (horse), *Haematopinus vituli, Haematopinus eurysternus, Solenopotes capillatus, Haematopinus quadripertusus* (cow), *Linognathus ovillus, Linognathus pedalis* (sheep), and *Haematopinus suis* (pig). Identification of lice beyond their Order is difficult, but not usually necessary.

Flies

Flies are a diverse group of insects that undergo complete metamorphosis. They have one pair of wings, which may be scaled or membranous, and a pair of balancing structures called *halters.* The mouth parts may

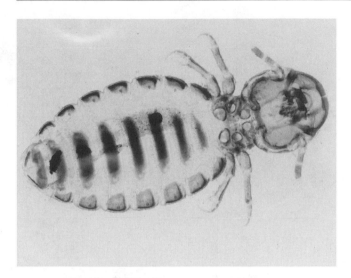

FIG. 11-37   Chewing louse, *Damalinia equi.*

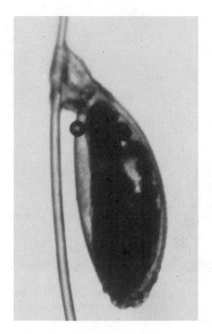

FIG. 11-39   Louse egg (nit).

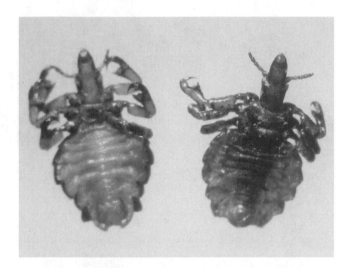

FIG. 11-38   Sucking louse, *Haematopinus* sp.

be adapted for sponging or piercing-sucking. Flies produce harm by inflicting painful bites, blood sucking, producing hypersensitive reactions, depositing eggs in sores, migration of larval stages through the tissues of the host with escape through holes in the skin (warbles), causing annoyance, and acting as vectors and intermediate hosts to other pathogenic agents.

Biting midges (no-see-ums), *Culicoides* spp., are small flies. The females are blood suckers that inflict a painful bite. Some species cause allergic dermatitis and others transmit helminths, protozoa, and viruses. Blackflies (buffalo gnats) are small flies with a characteristic humped back. They produce similar harm as no-see-ums and in great numbers can exsanguinate (bleed out) a host. Sandflies (phlebotomine flies) are moth-like flies,

known primarily for their role in the transmission of leishmaniasis and viral diseases. The females suck blood. *Mosquitoes* are a large and important group of flies known for the annoying bites of the females, which suck blood, and also for their role in transmission of numerous protozoal, viral, and nematode diseases to animals and people. Horse flies and deerflies are large flies with serrated mouthparts that inflict a painful bite. Only females suck blood. They are serious pests of livestock, can transmit filarial nematodes, and act as mechanical vectors of bacterial, viral, and rickettsial disease agents.

Muscid flies include the house fly, face fly, horn fly, and stable fly. The house fly and face fly do not suck blood, but are annoyances because they are attracted to excrement and secretions. Both act as intermediate hosts for spirurid parasites (*Habronema* spp., *Thelazia* spp.) and can mechanically transmit bacteria. The horn fly and the stable fly inflict painful bites and suck blood. *Horn flies* spend most of their life on the host, cattle. *Stable flies* feed intermittently and rest on fences and in barns. The stable fly can spread bacterial and viral diseases to cattle and horses and is an intermediate host for the stomach worm of horses *(Habronema).*

Blowflies, flesh flies, and screwworm flies are larger flies with bright coloration. The adults do not suck blood but deposit their eggs in decaying organic matter, septic wounds, or living flesh. The larvae of *Callitroga hominovorax* (Fig. 11-40) and *Wohlfahrtia opaca* are the only primary invaders of living tissue in North

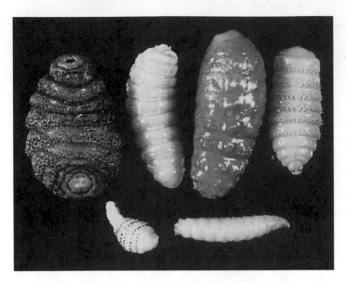

FIG. 11-40   Fly larvae (*left* to *right, top row: Cuterebra* sp., *Oestrus ovis, Hypoderma* sp., *Gastrophilus* sp.; *left* to *right, bottom row: Dermatobia hominis, Callitroga* sp.).

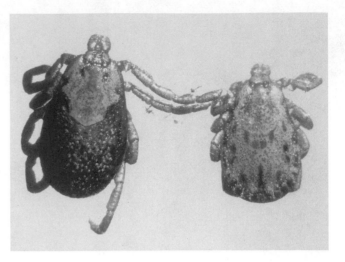

FIG. 11-41   Hard tick, *Dermacentor occidentalis.*

America. Other members are attracted to septic wounds and are known as secondary invaders. *Botflies (Gastrophilus* spp., *Hypoderma* spp., *Cuterebra* spp., *Oestrus ovis)* are bee-like flies, the adults of which do not feed. The adult flies glue their eggs to the hairs of the host or deposit them at the entrance of animal burrows. The larvae (see Fig. 11-40) hatch and penetrate the skin of the host. Some migrate extensively through the host's body and others develop locally. They produce large pockets in the subcutaneous tissues of the host with air holes in the skin, and are known as *warbles.* Hippoboscids or sheep keds *(Melophagus ovinus)* are dorsoventrally flattened, wingless flies that resemble ticks. They suck blood and spend their entire life on the host, sheep. They cause pruritus and damage the wool.

Ticks

Ticks are blood-sucking arachnids. They are dorsoventrally flattened in the unengorged state. There are two types of ticks: hard ticks (Ixodidae, Fig. 11-41) and soft ticks (Argasidae, Fig. 11-42).

Hard ticks are important vectors of protozoal, bacterial, viral, and rickettsial diseases. The saliva of female ticks of some species is toxic and produces flaccid, ascending paralysis in animals and people *(tick paralysis).* The adults, larvae, and nymphs attach to the host and feed on blood. Eggs are deposited in the environment. Hard ticks are dorsoventrally flattened, with well-defined lateral margins in the unengorged state. They have a hard, chitinous covering *(scutum)* on the dorsal surface of the body. Hard ticks may have grooves, margins, and notches *(festoons),* which are

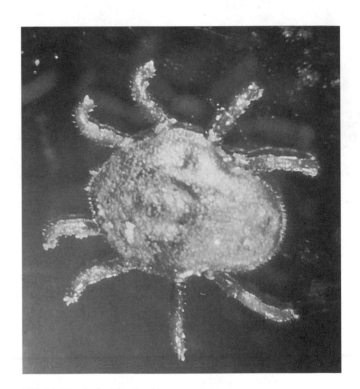

FIG. 11-42   Soft tick, *Otobius megnini.*

useful for identification purposes. They may attach to and feed on one to three different hosts during a life cycle and are referred to as *one-host, two-host,* or *three-host ticks.*

Important hard ticks in North America include *Rhipicephalus sanguineus, Dermacentor variabilis, Dermacentor andersoni, Dermacentor occidentalis, Dermacentor albipictus, Ixodes scapularis, Ixodes cookei, Ixodes pacificus, Amblyomma americanum, Amblyomma maculatum, Haemaphysalis leporispalustris, Ano-*

centor nitens, and *Boophilus annulatus. R. sanguineus* is unusual in that it can become established in indoor dwellings and kennels.

Soft ticks lack a scutum and the mouth parts are not visible from the dorsal surface. The lateral edges of the body are rounded. The females feed often and eggs are laid off the host. Soft ticks are more resistant to desiccation than hard ticks, and they can live for several years in arid conditions. There are three genera of veterinary importance: *Argas* spp., *Otobius megnini,* and *Ornithodoros* spp.

Argas spp. are ectoparasites of birds. The larvae, nymphs, and adults live in cracks and crevices of poultry houses and feed at night about once a month. They cause restlessness, loss of productivity, and severe anemia. They also serve as a vector for bacterial and rickettsial diseases of birds. *O. megnini,* the spinose ear tick, occurs on housed stock, dogs, and even people. Only the larval and nymphal stages are parasitic. They live in the external ear canal and suck blood, causing inflammation and production of a waxy exudate. *Ornithodoros* spp. live in sandy soils, in primitive housing, or in shady areas around trees. This genus is probably more important on people and rodents than on domestic animals, but *Ornithodoros coriaceus* is known to transmit the agent of foothill abortion in California.

Mites

Mites are arachnids that occur as parasitic and free-living forms, some of which act as intermediate hosts for cestodes. Most parasitic mites are obligate parasites, which spend their entire life cycle on the host and produce the dermatologic condition referred to as *mange.* A few species found on birds and rodents live off the host and visit the host only to obtain a blood meal *(Dermanyssus gallinae, Ornithonyssus bacoti).* Most mite infestations are transmitted through direct contact with an infested animal. Burrowing mite infestations are diagnosed with deep skin scrapings at the periphery of lesions.

Mites can be divided into two main groups: burrowing mites and nonburrowing mites. Another group of mites is parasitic only as larvae, the trombiculid mites or "chiggers." The burrowing mites include: *Sarcoptes scabiei* (Fig. 11-43), *Notoedres cati* (Fig. 11-44), and *Knemidokoptes* spp. These mites tunnel into the superficial layers of the epidermis and feed on tissue fluids. Infestations begin as localized areas of inflammation and hair loss, but they spread rapidly to become generalized. Females deposit their eggs in the tunnels. Mating occurs on the surface of the skin. Sarcoptic mange caused by *S. scabiei* can affect most animal species, including people, but it is most commonly seen on dogs and pigs. It is characterized by loss of hair and intense pruritus. Each animal species has its own variety of *S. scabiei,* and cross transmission does not occur. However, temporary infes-

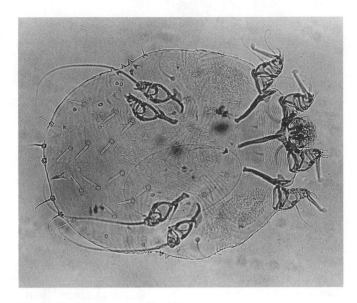

FIG. 11-43 *Sarcoptes scabiei* (skin scraping).

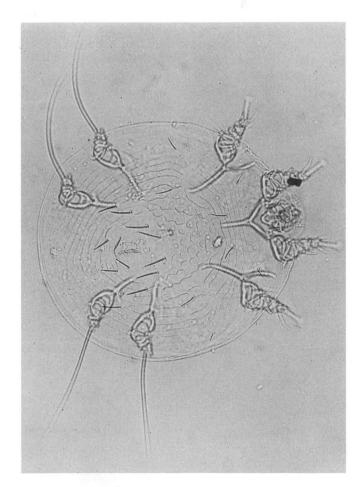

FIG. 11-44 *Notoedres cati* (skin scraping).

tation may take place without colonization of the skin. Notodectic mange (caused by *Notoedres*) is more restricted in host range and occurs in cats and occasionally rabbits. *Knemidokoptic mange* (caused by *Knemidokoptes)* affects birds.

Demodex spp. (Fig. 11-45) are also burrowing mites that live in the hair follicles and sebaceous glands of the skin. They are considered part of the normal skin fauna of most mammals. *Demodectic mange* is most common in dogs and can be localized or generalized. Immunodeficiency, both genetic and induced by the mites, is necessary for an infestation to become clinically apparent. The disease is characterized by loss of hair, thickening of the skin, and pustule formation. Pruritus is not a manifestation of this type of mange. Deep skin scrapings are used to recover the cigar-shaped mites for diagnosis.

Nonburrowing mites live on the surface of the skin and feed on keratinized scale, hair, and tissue fluids. *Psoroptes* spp. (Fig. 11-46), *Chorioptes* spp. (Fig. 11-47), *Otodectes cynotis* (Fig 11-48), *Psorergates ovis,* and *Cheyletiella* spp. (Fig. 11-49) are examples of nonburrowing mites. *Psoroptic mange* is important in sheep. The mites are active in the superficial keratinized layer of the skin but also pierce the skin with their mouth parts. Vesicles develop, with crusting and intense pruritus. *Chorioptic mange* is less severe and tends to remain localized. *Chorioptes bovis* is the more important species and a common parasite of cattle.

Cheyletiella and *Otodectes* are parasites of dogs and cats. *Cheyletiella* produces a mild condition referred to as "walking dandruff." *Otodectes cynotis* lives in the external ear canal of dogs and cats. A brownish, waxy exudate accumulates, with crust formation, ulceration, and secondary bacterial infections. Infested animals scratch frequently at the ears and shake their head. Head-shaking can result in rupture of blood vessels and hematomas of the pinna. The mites can be found in the waxy exudate and crust within the ear canal.

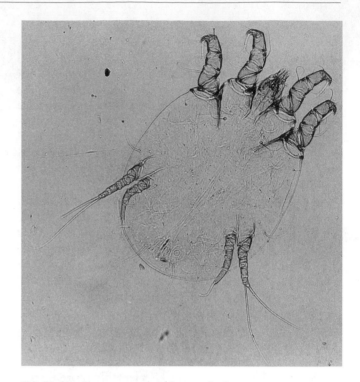

FIG. 11-46 *Psoroptes ovis* (skin scraping).

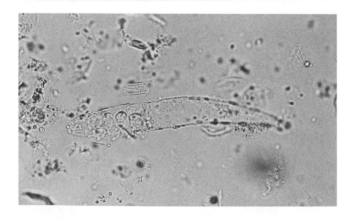

FIG. 11-45 *Demodex canis* (skin scraping).

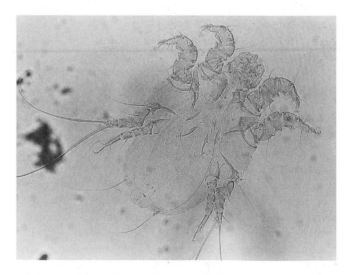

FIG. 11-47 *Chorioptes* sp. (skin scraping).

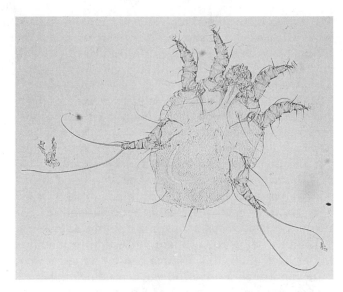

FIG. 11-48 *Otodectes cynotis* (swab of external ear canal).

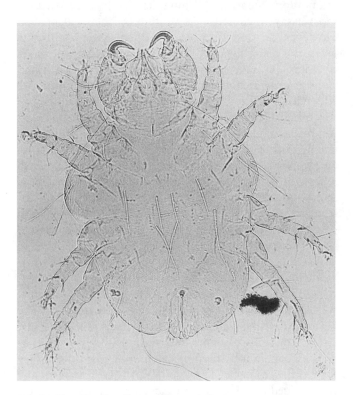

FIG. 11-49 *Cheyletiella* sp. (skin scraping).

RECOMMENDED READING

Bowman DD: *Georgi's parasitology for veterinarians,* ed 6, Philadelphia, 1995, WB Saunders.

Colville J: *Diagnostic parasitology for veterinary technicians,* St. Louis, 1991, Mosby.

Harwood RF, James MT: *Entomology in human and animal health,* ed 7, New York, 1979, Macmillan Publishing.

Levine ND: *Veterinary protozoology,* Ames, Iowa, 1985, Iowa State University Press.

Pratt PW: *Laboratory procedures for veterinary technicians,* ed 3, St Louis, 1997, Mosby.

Sloss MW, Kemp RL, Zajac AM: *Veterinary clinical parasitology,* ed 6, Ames, Iowa, 1994, Iowa State University Press.

Soulsby EJL: *Helminths, arthropods and protozoa of domestic animals,* ed 7, Philadelphia, 1982, Lea & Febiger.

BLOOD CHEMISTRY

A.E. THIESSEN

Laboratory analysis of blood biochemical constituents is performed for a variety of reasons. A blood sample might be collected from a patient as part of a general, nonspecific screening process, to confirm or rule out a specific disease, as part of management of a particular clinical case to evaluate the status of a previously diagnosed condition, or as part of emergency medical therapy.

Biochemistry profiles, or groups of tests, are routinely performed using serum as the preferred sample type, although heparinized plasma may also be used. If questions arise such as which is the proper sample for the desired test(s), or what are proper sample handling procedures, it is always best to check with the laboratory that will be performing the test(s) or to check the protocol of the specific test(s).

SAMPLE COLLECTION

Unless the purpose of the test is to monitor therapy, always collect the blood sample before any treatment is given. It is important to remember that treatments, such as fluid therapy, may affect results, such as total serum protein concentration, albumin concentration, and blood urea nitrogen (BUN) concentration. Fasted samples, or samples from an animal that has not eaten for some time, are ideal. Postprandial samples, or samples collected after the animal has eaten, may produce many erroneous results. For example, after meals, the blood glucose concentration frequently increases. Also, an increased BUN concentration may be present if the meal was high in protein. Increased amounts of lipid *(lipemia)* may also be present in postprandial blood samples.

Depending on which tests are to be performed, the type of sample desired determines which tube is used to collect the blood. If any uncertainty exists concerning the proper sample, always review the test protocol or ask personnel at the laboratory performing the test.

Serious errors may result if a sample is not labeled immediately after it has been collected. Label the tube with the date and time of collection, the owner's name, the patient's name, and the patient's clinic identification number. If submitted to a laboratory, include with the sample a request form that includes all necessary sample identification and a clear indication of which tests are requested.

Collection Site

Make venipuncture with the least tissue injury possible to minimize contamination with tissue fluid, which acts as a procoagulant, and to minimize hemolysis. Use of a vacuum tube (Vacutainer, Becton-Dickinson, Rutherford, NJ) or syringe is determined by the size of the animal (and vein) and the quantity of sample desired. All blood samples collected in a tube containing anticoagulant should be gently inverted several times immediately after collection to distribute the anticoagulant. If a Vacutainer is used, fill the tube to capacity to ensure the proper blood to anticoagulant ratio. If a syringe and needle are used, remove the needle from the syringe before transferring the blood to the vial, as forcing blood through the needle may result in hemolysis.

Small Animals. In adult dogs and cats, the jugular vein is the preferred site for collection of blood samples. It is relatively easy to locate, and the size of the vein allows adequate quantities of blood to be collected. Alternate sites include the cephalic and saphenous veins in dogs, and the cephalic and femoral veins in cats. Vacutainers may be used with large dogs, but in very small animals the vacuum in the tube can collapse the vein. Blood samples from small animals are routinely collected with a calibrated syringe and a needle of appropriate size. If the needle bore is too small or too large, it may cause disruption of erythrocytes (hemolysis). Needles of 20 to 25 gauge work well for collection of samples from dogs and cats.

Large Animals. The jugular vein is a suitable site for collection of blood samples in most large animals. In adult cattle, the subcutaneous abdominal (milk) vein and coccygeal (tail) vein are alternate sites. Alternate sites for sample collection from horses include the cephalic, lateral thoracic, and saphenous veins. Vacutainers work well, but needles and calibrated syringes can also be used. Needle gauges range from 16 to 20, with lengths of 1.5 to 2 inches; 20-gauge needles of 1.5 to 4 inches are used to obtain samples from the cranial vena cava of pigs. Because the blood of goats is easily hemolysed if collected with a Vacutainer, a syringe and a 20-gauge needle are recommended for collection of caprine blood samples.

Sample Type

Whole Blood. Whole blood is composed of cellular elements (erythrocytes, leukocytes, platelets) and a fluid called *plasma*. A whole blood sample is collected by placing the appropriate amount of blood into a container with the proper anticoagulant (discussed later) and gently mixing the sample by inverting the tube mul-

tiple times. Whole blood may be refrigerated if analysis is to be delayed, but it should never be frozen unless the plasma has been separated from the cellular elements. If the blood has been refrigerated, warm the sample to room temperature and mix gently before analysis.

Plasma. To obtain a plasma sample, collect the appropriate amount of blood in a container with the proper anticoagulant and gently mix well. Centrifuge the closed container for 10 minutes at 2000 to 3000 rpm to separate the fluid from the cells. After the sample is centrifuged, remove the plasma from the cells, being careful not to contaminate the plasma with any of the pelleted cells, and transfer the plasma into another appropriately labeled container. Separate plasma from the cellular elements as soon as possible after collection to minimize any artifactual changes. Plasma can be refrigerated or frozen until analysis is performed, depending on the specific requirements of the desired test(s).

Plasma collected in tubes containing heparin as the anticoagulant (sodium heparin, potassium heparin, ammonium heparin, or lithium heparin) can be used for most assays included on a routine biochemical profile. However, do not use potassium heparin if electrolyte levels are being measured, because artifactual increases of potassium concentrations can occur. Heparin functions as an anticoagulant by activation of antithrombin III, which prevents conversion of prothrombin to thrombin. Heparin is not a permanent anticoagulant; it inhibits coagulation for only 8 to 12 hours. When biochemical analysis must be performed quickly, as in an emergency situation, collection of a blood sample with a heparin anticoagulant is indicated. The plasma can be harvested immediately after collection and centrifugation, rather than the time delay (necessary for the blood to clot and the clot to retract) required to harvest a serum sample.

Plasma collected in tubes containing ethylenediaminetetraacetic acid (EDTA) as the anticoagulant, which is routinely used for complete blood counts, should not be used for serum biochemical analysis, because spurious values for electroyltes, trace elements, and many serum enzymes will result. EDTA functions as an anticoagulant by binding calcium, which is necessary for clotting to occur. Because EDTA binds calcium, any test procedure that requires calcium cannot be performed on samples collected in EDTA. All other anticoagulants, such as potassium oxalate and sodium citrate, also function by binding calcium, and therefore should not be used to collect plasma for biochemical analysis.

Serum. Serum is plasma that has had the coagulation proteins, such as fibrinogen, removed during the clotting process. A serum sample is obtained by placing blood in a container with no additives and allowing it to clot at room temperature. Once sufficient time has passed for the clot to retract (approximately 30 to 120 minutes), the closed container is then centrifuged at 2000 to 3000 rpm for 10 minutes, and the serum is harvested. Centrifugation for longer periods can result in hemolysis.

If the serum is not separated from the clot, numerous artifactual changes can result in erroneous laboratory values. An artifactual decrease in glucose concentration can occur due to glucose metabolism by blood cells. Release of inorganic phosphorus from high-energy phosphate bonds results in artifactual increases in serum phosphorus concentrations. Leakage of potassium from RBCs occurs in large animal species and in some small animal species, resulting in erroneously high potassium concentrations. Artifactual increases of some serum enzymes may also occur. such as aspartate aminotransferase (AST) and alanine aminotransferase (ALT).

Once harvested, the serum may be refrigerated or frozen. Freezing may affect some test results, so check the test protocol prior to freezing the sample.

Blood can also be collected in serum tubes containing a gel substance that, during centrifugation, moves into a position between the clot and the serum. Using this type of serum tube, called a *serum separator tube,* does not necessarily prevent artifactual changes. The benefit of a serum separator tube is that the gel substance facilitates removal of serum without accidental aspiration of clot elements, which would contaminate the serum sample.

All of the above-mentioned artifactual changes can occur without the problems of hemolysis or lipemia being present. Hemolysis can result from difficult blood collection, mixing too vigorously after sample collection, forcing the sample through a needle when transferring it to a tube, or freezing a whole blood sample. The syringe must be completely dry before it is used, because water in the syringe can cause hemolysis. Also, it is beneficial to remove the needle from the syringe before transferring the blood into a tube. Cells can be ruptured when blood is forced through the needle. To reduce the chance of hemolysis occurring when transferring blood to a tube, expel the blood slowly from the syringe without causing bubbles to form. Hemolysis may cause errors in testing resulting from direct interference, dilution, and/or release of substances found in high concentrations within erythrocytes.

Hemolysis may not be apparent until after the blood sample has been centrifuged. Visibly hemolytic serum (slight pink discoloration) can be detected by the trained observer at hemoglobin concentrations as low as 20 mg/dl. Mild to moderate hemolysis has minimal effect on most routine serum chemistry assays, but bilirubin and ALT levels are often increased. Also, lipase activity is inhibited by hemolysis, resulting in falsely decreased values. If marked hemolysis is present, the results of most assays, especially total bilirubin, direct bilirubin, indirect bilirubin, creatinine, total protein, inorganic phosphorus, calcium, potassium, gamma-glutamyl-

transferase (GGT), ALT, lactate dehydrogenase (LDH), and AST, are likely to be affected, resulting in falsely elevated values.

Lipemia also affects the results of serum biochemical assays, resulting in erroneous values. *Lipemia* describes the milky appereance of serum or plasma resulting from increased concentrations of triglyceride-containing lipoproteins. Transient lipemia is common approximately 4 to 6 hours after a meal. Ideally, collect blood samples from an animal that has been fasted for at least 12 hours. This should eliminate any lipemia resulting from ingestion of food. Water need not be withheld. Lipemia can cause erroneous results for all routine clinical chemistries. Light scattering is the most common source of error in testing of lipemic samples. Light scattering may result in falsely increased or decreased values, depending upon whether lipemia in the sample results in an increase or decrease in light absorbance measured by the spectrophotometer.

Endpoint enzymatic assays are generally more severely affected by lipemia than are kinetic enzymatic assays. However, results are invalid in markedly lipemic samples and should be interpreted with caution even in mildly lipemic samples. Lipemia can result in falsely decreased values of electrolytes if a flame photometer is used to measure the electrolytes. If an ion-specific electrode is used to determine electrolyte concentrations, lipemia does not affect results (see Electrolytes later in this chapter).

Laboratory Selection

There are several choices of where to obtain clinical chemistry results. Veterinary reference laboratories, human hospitals, or in-clinic chemistry machines are the most common choices. There are advantages and disadvantages to each of these choices. Price, service, and quality are the main variables to consider.

The main benefit to choosing a veterinary reference laboratory is that the staff members should be familiar with and should have established reference ranges ("normal values") for domestic species. Some laboratories may have reference ranges for certain exotic animal species, as well. In addition to providing chemistry profiles, these laboratories may also offer endocrine testing, microbiology, cytology, and histopathology services. Using a single laboratory for all services can be very convenient. Also, many of these laboratories offer consultations with specialists, such as internists, clinical pathologists, or anatomic pathologists. These laboratories are generally only available in larger cities. Some reference laboratories may have arrangements with an overnight mailing service so that results are available the next day. Most of these laboratories provide results via telephone or fax, in addition to mailing a printed copy of the results. One disadvantage is that quality assurance standards have not been established for veterinary laboratories, in contrast to the standards that have been established for human laboratories.

Laboratories in human hospitals provide an alternative for obtaining clinical chemistry results. Unlike veterinary reference laboratories, these laboratories must adhere to rigorous quality-control standards, and the testing methods are of high quality. Human hospital laboratories are not likely to have established reference ranges for animal species. The cost of having animal samples analyzed at a human hospital may be quite reasonable because of the high volume of human samples assayed. Most of the assays included in routine chemistry profiles performed at human hospital laboratories are valid for animal species.

It is important not to assume, however, that every assay is valid. Certain reagents that human hospitals use in their testing methods may not provide accurate or reliable results for animal species. If the validity of any assay is in question, check to confirm the proper testing protocol for that assay and possibly for the animal species. Keep in mind that the technicians at human hospitals may or may not be aware of which procedures are invalid for animals species.

Chemistry machines designed for in-clinic use are increasing in quality and becoming more affordable and easier to use. One of these machines may or may not be practical for a particular veterinary clinic. A great advantage of in-clinic chemistry analyzers is that the results can be obtained very quickly. Also, performing these tests in-clinic can be a source of profit. Factors to consider are the initial cost of the machine, cost of the reagents, anticipated use of the machine, and amount of maintenance the machine requires. Quality-control procedures are essential for any test that is performed on an in-clinic basis. The machine must be kept calibrated and regular control samples that contain known quantities of a substance or substances must be assayed. If these are not done, the potential for erroneous results is great.

Certain tests can be performed using commercially available dry chemistry strips. Some examples include blood urea nitrogen (Azostix, Bayer, Elkhart, IN) and blood glucose (Chemstrip bG, Boehringer Mannheim, Indianapolis, IN).

LIVER ASSAYS

The liver is a large organ with many functions, including metabolism of amino acids, carbohydrates, and lipids, synthesis of albumin, plasma proteins, clotting factors, and cholesterol, secretion of bilirubin (bile), detoxification of toxins, and metabolism of many drugs.

Tests for Hepatocellular Damage

Enzymes are normally present in the cytoplasm of hepatocytes and appear in the serum after the cell has experienced some injury that altered the permeability of its membrane. Therefore, detection of elevated levels of these enzymes in the serum indicates that hepatocellular injury is occurring. The magnitude of elevation is dependent on the number of liver cells affected, not on the severity of the injury to the cells. It is very important to remember that reversibility of the lesion cannot be predicted by the magnitude of enzyme elevations. A routine serum biochemistry file usually includes the following enzymes.

Alanine Aminotransferase. Alanine aminotransferase (ALT) was formerly known as serum glutamate-pyruvate transaminase (SGPT).

Reason for test. This enzyme is considered a liver-specific enzyme and a good indicator of hepatocellular damage in dogs, cats, and primates because the primary/major source of serum ALT is the hepatocyte. It is not useful in large animal species, such as horses, cattle, sheep, and pigs, because the hepatocytes of these species contain insignificant amounts of ALT.

Sample type. Serum or plasma may be used. EDTA and citrated plasma give similar results. Heparinized plasma should not be used if this buffer is used in the assay because the results may be as much as 70% lower.

Handling specifications. Avoid hemolysis and lipemia, because these can result in false elevations of enzyme activities.

Stability. If the serum or plasma is separated from the red blood cells, this enzyme is stable in serum or plasma for several days at 0° to 4° C.

Aspartate Aminotransferase. Asparate aminotransferase (AST) was formerly known as serum glutamate oxaloacetate transaminase (SGOT).

Reason for test. Hepatocytes are one source of serum AST, but there are other sources. Both skeletal and cardiac muscle contain significant amounts of AST. Other sources include erythrocytes, kidneys, and pancreas. Increased levels of AST indicate liver or muscle damage. It is important to remember that AST is not considered a liver-specific enzyme.

Sample type. Serum, plasma, or any anticoagulant may be used.

Handling specifications. Hemolysis and lipemia can result in elevated concentrations and should be avoided.

Stability. If the serum or plasma is removed from the red blood cells, samples for AST analysis can be stored for 2 days at 20° C, for 2 weeks at 0° to 4° C, and for several months at -20° C. Storage of whole blood results in elevated concentrations.

Lactate Dehydrogenase

Reason for test. Lactate dehydrogenase (LDH) values are frequently included in biochemistry profiles. This enzyme is not considered organ specific, because it has many sources and the concentrations in each tissue are not high enough to result in significant elevations. LDH is found in the liver, skeletal muscle, cardiac muscle, kidney, leukocytes, erythrocytes, and skin.

Sample type. Serum or plasma may be used. Anticoagulants containing EDTA or oxalates should not be used, because these compounds inhibit LDH activity.

Handling specifications. Hemolysis and storing the sample in contact with blood cells result in falsely elevated values. Storing the sample below 10° C falsely decreases LDH values.

Stability. This enzyme appears to be most stable at room temperature or refrigerator temperature. Freezing deactivates LDH.

Sorbitol Dehydrogenase

Reason for test. Sorbitol dehydrogenase (SDH) is found in high concentrations in hepatocytes of all species, including large animals, and is considered a liver-specific enzyme.

Sample type. Serum is preferred. If plasma is used, heparin should be used as the anticoagulant.

Handling specifications. Hemolysis does not appear to affect results.

Stability. SDH is unstable and serum activity decreases rapidly. Samples should be analyzed within 12 hours of collection.

Other Enzymes. Other enzymes can leak from damaged or dead liver cells, but no standard methodology has been developed for laboratory testing and enzymes are not routinely measured. Following are enzymes that are occasionally assayed.

Arginase. Arginase is present in significant concentrations in the liver of mammals. Studies evaluating arginase levels in dogs, cats, horses, sheep, and pigs have been published. It is considered a liver-specific enzyme and increased serum values indicate hepatic necrosis.

Glutamate dehydrogenase. Glutamate dehydrogenase (GD) is highly concentrated in the liver of cattle and sheep, as well as in the liver of other species. Increased serum values of GD indicate hepatic necrosis. GD is considered a liver-specific enzyme.

Ornithine carbamoyltransferase. Similar to GD, ornithine carbamoyltransferase (OCT) is a liver-specific enzyme that indicates liver necrosis. Studies have been conducted on cattle, swine, and dogs.

Tests for Cholestasis

Cholestasis is cessation of the flow of bile from the liver and gallbladder through the bile ducts, and into the intestine.

Certain enzymes are present within liver cells but are bound to membranes and do not leak out of the cells when membrane damage occurs. Several levels of these enzymes may be increased because of an increased rate of synthesis by the liver cells, with escape of enzymes from the cell into systemic circulation. Biliary obstruc-

tion can also cause increased enzyme levels. The following enzymes are usually included in routine biochemistry profiles.

Alkaline Phosphatase

Reason for test. Alkaline phosphatase (ALP) comprises a group of isoenzymes that are present in many tissues. High concentrations are found within the liver, bone (osteoblasts), intestinal mucosa, kidney, and placenta. The half-lives of the intestinal and renal isoenzymes are extremely short (minutes), as compared with the half-lives of hepatic enzymes (hours to days). Because of this, the intestinal and renal isoenzymes of ALP are not usually found in serum (or plasma) in high concentrations. Special analytic methods in commercial or research laboratories can be used to determine which isoenzyme is increased.

ALP is most often used to detect cholestasis in dogs and cats. Production of ALP is induced by increased pressure within the biliary system during any form of cholestasis. The cholestasis may be *intrahepatic* because of tumors, swelling, inflammation, or anything blocking bile flow, or it may be *extrahepatic* because of bile duct obstruction. ALP is a sensitive indicator of cholestasis in dogs and cats, but it is not useful in large animals because of the wide variation of ALP concentrations found in normal large animal species.

In dogs, certain drugs induce ALP synthesis. The magnitude of increase may be great. The most commonly used drugs that induce ALP synthesis are glucocorticoids, such as prednisone or cortisone. Exogenously administered or endogenous (due to hyperadrenocorticism) glucocorticoids stimulate this effect. It occurs through induction of a unique isoenzyme of ALP. Anticonvulsants, such as phenobarbital, primidone, and diphenylhydantoin, also induce synthesis of ALP (hepatic isoenzyme). These increases in ALP are due to drug induction and do not necessarily indicate liver disease.

ALP levels can be increased in young growing animals because of bone remodeling and increases in the bone isoenzyme. Other causes of increased osteoblastic activity, such as primary hyperparathyroidism, fracture healing, and neoplasia, can also result in increased serum ALP activity.

Placental ALP is present in mares and queens during pregnancy.

Sample type. Serum or heparinized plasma may be used. Anticoagulants containing oxalates or EDTA inhibit ALP activity, resulting in falsely decreased values.

Handling specifications. Hemolysis or storage at room temperature for up to 24 hours has little effect on results. If the serum sample is kept at room temperature for more than 24 hours, ALP values may be increased.

Stability. Samples can be stored for 8 days at 20° C (a slight rise may be evident after 2 to 3 days), 8 days at 0° to 4° C, and 8 days at -20° C.

Gamma Glutamyltransferase

Reason for test. Gamma-glutamyltransferase (GGT) is similar to ALP in that it is bound to microsomal membranes within the cell. Serum levels of GGT are increased when the cell is stimulated to increase synthesis. GGT is present in most cells but is found in high concentration in liver, pancreatic, and renal tubular cells. GGT from renal tubular cells is released into the urine during renal tubular damage, not into the blood. Pancreatic GGT is apparently secreted into the intestines and also does not cause elevated serum concentrations. Therefore, serum GGT is considered a liver-specific enzyme. As with ALP, the major inducer of hepatic GGT is cholestasis. This occurs in all species. GGT is an excellent indicator of cholestasis in horses, ruminants, and swine. GGT can also be used in dogs and cats, although it offers no advantage over ALP for these species.

Sample type. Serum or plasma may be used. Any anticoagulant is acceptable.

Handling specifications. Hemolysis does not affect results, but prolonged contact with erythrocytes may affect results.

Stability. Samples can be stored for 2 days at 20° C, for 1 week at 0° to 4° C, and 1 month at -20° C.

Tests of Hepatic Function

Bilirubin

Reason for test. Bilirubin is a breakdown product of the *heme* molecule. The majority of heme originates from hemoglobin, although small amounts come from other sources. Bilirubin exists in two forms in serum: unconjugated and conjugated. Heme is first converted to biliverdin and then to bilirubin. This initial form of bilirubin is termed *unconjugated (indirect) bilirubin* and is lipid soluble. Unconjugated bilirubin is bound to serum proteins (mainly albumin) and carried to the liver. Unconjugated bilirubin is taken up by the liver and conjugated, primarily to glucuronic acid, to make it water soluble and more easily cleared from the body. This *conjugated (direct) bilirubin* is secreted by hepatocytes into the bile, where it eventually is delivered to the intestines. A small portion of this conjugated bilirubin (direct) is "regurgitated" back into the hepatic sinusoids (and therefore into the systemic circulation) from the biliary system before being passed through the bile ducts into the intestine. Because conjugated bilirubin is water soluble and not bound to serum proteins, it can pass through the glomerulus into the urine.

In the intestines, bilirubin is converted by the intestinal flora to urobilinogen and eventually oxidized to stercobilins. Some urobilinogen is resorbed by the intestine and enters the portal circulation. Most of this is cleared during the first pass through the liver, but a small amount enters the systemic circulation and is cleared by the kidneys (and can be quantified in the urine).

Both unconjugated and conjugated bilirubin are found in plasma (and serum). Assays can directly measure total bilirubin (conjugated plus unconjugated) and conjugated bilirubin. Conjugated bilirubin is also referred to as *direct bilirubin,* because test methods directly measure the amount of conjugated bilirubin in the sample. Unconjugated bilirubin is also referred to as *indirect bilirubin,* because it reacts with test substrates only after addition of alcohol (indirect reacting). Measuring the color produced before addition of alcohol gives the concentration of conjugated bilirubin (direct reacting); measuring the color after addition of alcohol gives the concentration of total bilirubin. The concentration of unconjugated (indirect) bilirubin is determined by subtracting the conjugated (direct) bilirubin concentration from the total bilirubin concentration.

Bilirubin is assayed to determine the cause of jaundice (icterus), to evaluate liver function, and to check the patency of bile ducts. Blood levels of conjugated bilirubin are elevated with hepatocellular damage or bile duct injury and/or obstruction. Excessive erythrocyte destruction often results in production of more unconjugated bilirubin than the liver can clear. Initially the elevated bilirubin levels in the blood are primarily composed of unconjugated bilirubin; however, with time, more and more conjugated bilirubin appears.

Serum appears grossly icteric (yellow-tinged) when the bilirubin level rises to approximately 1.5 to 2.0 mg/dl or greater. Icterus can be grossly detected in the patient (sclera of the eye) when the bilirubin level is 3 to 4 mg/dl or greater.

Sample type. Serum or plasma may be used. Any anticoagulant is acceptable.

Handling specifications. Hemolysis produces artificially low values if the diazo assay method is used (check the test protocol). Avoid using lipemic blood samples. Store samples in the dark, because bilirubin is very sensitive to light. Direct exposure to sunlight or artificial light can result in decreases in concentration of up to 50% an hour. Unconjugated bilirubin is more light sensitive than conjugated bilirubin.

Stability. Samples for bilirubin concentrations are not stable when stored at 20° C. Samples protected from light can be stored for 2 weeks at 0° to 4° C and for up to 3 months at -20° C.

Bile Acids

Reason for test. Bile acids are synthesized in the liver from cholesterol. They are secreted in the bile and stored in the gallbladder (in species that have a gallbladder). Following a meal, gallbladder contraction results in flow of bile acids into the intestine, where they function in the digestion of fat. Most of the bile acids are resorbed in the small intestine and enter the portal circulation. Most of the bile acids are then extracted by the liver on the first pass. This recirculation functions to conserve bile acids and is so efficient that the entire pool of bile acids is generally recirculated three to five times after every meal, with only small amounts being lost in the feces or bypassing the liver into the systemic circulation. Because of this, blood levels of bile acids in normal animals are very low, especially in fasted animals. Serum bile acid (SBA) concentrations are increased when there is decreased hepatic function and bile acids are not cleared from the blood effectively. This occurs with decreased functional hepatic mass (cirrhosis), abnormalities of portal circulation (portosystemic shunting of blood), and cholestatic disease (bile acids in the blocked bile ducts are regurgitated into the systemic circulation).

Collect serum samples for SBA assay after a 12-hour fast (preprandial sample) and then two hours after a meal (postprandial sample). The purpose of the second sample is to increase the sensitivity of the test. Animals with portal shunts or reduced functional hepatic mass may clear the bile acids to normal levels after a prolonged fast, and therefore have a normal SBA level in the preprandial sample. A patient with a normal fasting SBA concentration may have markedly elevated SBA concentrations 2 hours after eating. This would still indicate reduced hepatic mass or altered portal blood flow. In horses, only a fasting sample is collected because horses have no gallbladder to contract following a meal.

Bile acid assays are useful in animals with suspected defects in hepatic function in whom all other hepatic indicators (bilirubin, serum enzymes) are normal or only slightly elevated. If an animal is icteric and has an increased serum bilirubin level (and hemolysis can be ruled out as the cause), then measuring SBA levels does not provide any additional information, because compromised liver function has already been documented.

Sample type. Serum is the sample of choice.

Handling specifications and stability. Samples for serum bile acid determination are stable once the serum has been removed from the red blood cells. Freezing does not affect results to a significant degree.

Ammonia

Reason for test. Ammonia is produced in the intestine (primarily in the colon) from the action of bacteria on dietary proteins. Ammonia is absorbed in the intestine and carried in the portal vein to the liver, where it is effectively cleared from the circulation. The hepatocytes convert ammonia to urea via the urea cycle. Much like bile acids, blood ammonia levels are increased with reduced hepatic mass and abnormalities in portal circulation. Ammonia levels have been measured in cases of suspected hepatic encephalopathy.

Sample type. Heparinized plasma, using ammonia-free heparin, is required.

Handling specifications and stability. Samples for ammonia determination are not stable and must be stored on ice immediately after collection, centrifuged in a refrigerated centrifuge, separated from the red blood cells, and assayed as soon as possible (preferably within 15 minutes). Sample collection must be as smooth as possible, because occlusion of a vein for prolonged periods results in ammonia accumulation.

Sulfobromophthalein Excretion Test. The sulfobromophthalein (BSP) excretion test was used primarily before the bile acid assays became available. It is now very rarely performed. BSP dye is not widely available because the test is no longer used in human medicine because of severe adverse reactions (fatal anaphylactic reactions).

KIDNEY ASSAYS

The kidneys are a pair of complex organs that perform a multitude of vital functions. These include conservation of or increased elimination of water and electrolytes relative to the body's needs; excretion or conservation of hydrogen ions to maintain blood pH within normal limits; elimination of metabolic waste products, such as urea, creatinine, and allantoin; conservation of nutrients, such as glucose and proteins, that are vital to normal body functions; production of renin, an enzyme that aids in controlling blood pressure; production of erythropoietin, a hormone that is involved with erythrocyte production; production of prostaglandins, which are involved in smooth muscle contractility, regulation of blood pressure, inflammation, and other processes; and activation of vitamin D.

Blood Urea Nitrogen. Blood urea nitrogen (BUN) is also referred to as serum urea nitrogen (SUN) or urea nitrogen (UN), because this test is not always performed on whole blood.

Reason for test. Urea is produced by hepatic conversion of ammonia (from protein catabolism) via the urea cycle. The urea formed is primarily cleared by the kidneys. It is freely filtered through the glomerulus, but a significant amount is resorbed as urine flows through the tubules. The amount resorbed is dependent on the rate of urine flow through the tubules. At maximal flow, 40% is resorbed; at lower rates, considerably more is resorbed. Levels of urea in the blood are increased (called *azotemia*) if the glomerular filtration rate (GFR) is reduced; therefore, BUN is used a test of renal clearance. If BUN levels are increased because of decreased renal function *(renal azotemia)*, this indicates that approximately 75% of the nephrons are nonfunctional.

BUN levels can be increased from nonrenal causes *(prerenal azotemia* and *postrenal azotemia)*. Causes of prerenal azotemia include anything that reduces renal perfusion and therefore results in a decreased GFR. This most commonly occurs because of reduced blood volume from moderate to severe dehydration. It may also occur with reduced effective circulating volume, such as poor perfusion because of cardiac insufficiency. Postrenal azotemia results from an abnormality in the urinary system distal to the kidneys; urea cannot be eliminated from the body. Urinary obstruction (e.g., urethral obstruction in a male cat) and rupture of the urinary tract (e.g., rupture of the urinary bladder in newborn foals) are common causes of postrenal azotemia.

Sample type. Use serum or plasma. Any anticoagulant except ammonium oxalate and sodium fluoride is acceptable. The nitrogen component of ammonium oxalate results in falsely elevated BUN values. Plasma preserved with sodium fluoride cannot be used, because fluoride interferes with the enzyme urease, which is used in the test procedure.

Handling specifications. Hemolysis has little effect on results. Lipemia may result in a turbid final solution if a "wet" chemistry assay system is used.

Stability. Samples can be stored for up to 3 days at 20° C, for 10 days at 0° to 4° C, and for several months at -20° C.

Creatinine

Reason for test. Serum creatinine is produced from metabolic breakdown of phosphocreatine in muscle tissue. The day-to-day rate of creatinine production is relatively constant in any animal and is dependent on muscle mass. Creatinine is also primarily cleared by the kidney. Glomerular filtration is the primary mode of elimination. Creatinine is minimally resorbed by the tubules and so it is not influenced by the rate of urine flow, as is BUN.

Creatinine is used to evaluate renal function based on the ability of the glomeruli to filter creatinine from the blood and eliminate it in urine. Like BUN, if serum creatinine values are increased because of decreased renal function, this indicates that approximately 75% of the nephrons are nonfunctional.

Sample type. Serum or plasma may be used. Heparinized and EDTA plasma samples produce similar results.

Handling specifications. Hemolysis has little effect on results.

Stability. Samples can be stored for 2 to 3 days at 20° C, for 1 week at 0° to 4° C, and almost indefinitely at -20° C.

PANCREAS ASSAYS

The pancreas is composed of two organs, one with endocrine function and one with exocrine function, contained within one stroma. The endocrine portion functions in carbohydrate metabolism through secretion of insulin (which lowers blood glucose levels) and glucagon (which elevates blood glucose levels). The exocrine portion functions to aid digestion through secretion of digestive enzymes into the small intestine. Two conditions that can occur as a result of abnormal exocrine pancreas function are acute pancreatitis and exocrine pancreatic insufficiency (insufficiency of digestive enzymes).

The enzymes amylase and lipase are used to detect pancreatitis. Both of these enzymes are produced by the pancreas in their inactive proenzyme form and are normally secreted into the intestines. During acute pancreatitis, these enzymes may be present in the blood in increased concentrations. Neither enzyme is truly specific for the pancreas, and therefore other causes of increased amylase and lipase must be considered. It is best to measure both enzymes if pancreatitis is suspected, because often one is elevated while the other is normal. Amylase is more easily assayed and is usually included in a routine chemistry profile. Lipase assays are more time consuming and usually must be requested separately.

Amylase

Reason for test. The sources of amylase activity are the pancreas, small intestine, and liver. Amylase functions in the breakdown of starches and glycogen in sugars to form such sugars as maltose and residual glucose. Increased levels of amylase can occur with acute pancreatitis, flareups of chronic pancreatitis, and obstruction of the pancreatic ducts.

Nonpancreatic disease may also increase serum amylase levels. Most commonly, amylase levels are elevated with renal disease. Renal disease can cause amylase levels that are approximately 2.5 times the upper limit of normal. Increased amylase levels have also been reported with certain liver and intestinal diseases (intestinal obstructions).

Amylase levels can be determined by two methods: amyloclastic or saccharogenic. Amyloclastic methods measure the rate of disappearance of starch and should be used for canine serum. Saccharogenic methods, which measure the rate of appearance of reducing sugars and are valid for humans, give falsely elevated results in canine samples because of other enzymes found in canine serum.

Sample type. Serum or heparinized plasma may be used.

Handling specifications. Do not use calcium-binding anticoagulants, such as EDTA, because amylase requires calcium for activity. Hemolysis may result in falsely elevated amylase levels. Lipemia may reduce amylase activity. Because normal canine and feline amylase values can be up to 10 times higher than those in people, samples may have to be diluted if tests designed for human samples are used. The saccharogenic method should not be used for canine samples.

Stability. Samples can be stored for up to 7 days at 20° C and for up to 1 month at 0° to 4° C.

Lipase

Reason for test. The pancreas is the primary source of serum lipase. Lipase functions to break down the long-chain fatty acids of lipids. In experimental pancreatitis, lipase levels rise rapidly and are elevated for more than a week. Clinical cases are not as consistent and not all animals with pancreatitis have elevated lipase levels. Some studies suggest that lipase is more valuable than amylase because it is more consistently elevated.

Lipase activity may also be elevated by nonpancreatic factors, such as chronic renal failure, exploratory surgery, and corticosteroid use.

Test methods for determining lipase activity are usually based on hydrolysis of an olive oil emulsion into its constituent fatty acids. The quantity of NaOH required to neutralize the fatty acids provides a measure of lipase activity.

Sample type. Serum or heparinized plasma may be used.

Handling specifications. Do not use calcium-binding anticoagulants, such as EDTA. Hemolysis and lipemia should be avoided; however, hemolysis does not affect results of turbidimetric methods (check the test protocol).

Stability. Samples for lipase assay can be stored for 1 week at 20° C and for 3 weeks at 0° to 4° C.

Glucose

Reason for test. The blood glucose level is used as an indicator of carbohydrate metabolism in the body. It also can be used as a measure of endocrine function of the pancreas. The blood glucose level reflects the net balance between glucose production (dietary intake, conversion from other carbohydrates) and glucose utilization (energy expended, conversion to other products). It also reflects the balance between blood insulin and glucagon levels.

Glucose utilization depends on the amount of insulin and glucagon being produced by the pancreas. As the blood insulin level increases, so does the rate of glucose utilization, resulting in decreased blood glucose levels. Glucagon acts as a stabilizer to prevent blood glucose levels from becoming too low. As the insulin level decreases (as in diabetes mellitus), so does glucose utilization, resulting in increased blood glucose concentration.

Sample type. Serum is preferred over plasma. Any anticoagulant is acceptable when obtaining a plasma sample. If a plasma sample is used, it should be separated from the erythrocytes immediately after sample collection.

Handling specifications. Separate serum and plasma from the erythrocytes immediately after blood collection. If the sample is left in contact with the erythrocytes, the blood glucose levels can drop up to 10% an hour at room temperature. Erythrocytes use glucose for energy and in a blood sample may decrease the glucose level enough to give false normal results if the original sample had an elevated glucose level. If the sample originally had a normal glucose level, a falsely low level may result. If the blood sample cannot be centrifuged and the serum or plasma is not separated from the erythrocytes, collect the sample in a sodium fluoride tube. This anticoagulant tube contains potassium oxalate. The sodium fluoride inhibits utilization of glucose by erythrocytes and therefore stabilizes glucose levels in the sample. Glucose levels remain stable for 12 hours at room temperature and for 48 hours if the sample is refrigerated. Fill this tube at least half full of blood; otherwise the fluoride concentration may be high enough to interfere with glucose analysis.

Refrigeration slows glucose utilization by erythrocytes. Hemolysis does not affect results. Because eating raises the blood glucose level and fasting decreases it, a 12-hour fast is recommended when possible for all animals, except for mature ruminants, before the blood sample is collected.

Stability. Samples of serum or plasma that have been separated from the erythrocytes can be stored for 8 hours at 20° C and for 72 hours at 0° to 4° C. The stability of frozen samples has not been determined. Do not thaw and refreeze a sample more than once.

MUSCLE ASSAYS

Creatine Kinase

Reason for test. Creatine kinase (CK, CPK), also referred to as *creatine phosphokinase*, is a cytoplasmic enzyme that appears in the serum in increased concentrations after cellular injury. This enzyme consists of three isoenzymes: CK_1, CK_2, and CK_3. CK_1 is found in neurologic tissue, cerebrospinal fluid, and viscera. This isoenzyme is not present in serum and/or plasma. CK_2 is found mainly in cardiac muscle. CK_3 is found in skeletal and cardiac muscle. The last two isoenzymes are present in serum and/or plasma. Therefore, changes in CK concentrations are specific for muscle (skeletal and cardiac) injury or necrosis.

CK is a very sensitive enzyme and serum levels can be dramatically increased after relatively minor insults to muscle. Intramuscular injections are enough to raise CK levels several times above the normal range. Other causes of muscle damage include inflammatory myopathies from infectious causes (e.g., *Clostridium*) or noninfectious causes (e.g., immune-mediated, eosinophilic), traumatic myopathies (e.g., accidental, postoperative, downer animals, CNS diseases, seizures), degenerative myopathies (e.g., muscular dystrophy, myotonia, hyperadrenocorticism, hypothyroidism, equine rhabdomyolysis, transport myopathy, malignant hyperthermia, capture myopathy), nutritional myopathies (e.g., vitamin E/selenium deficiency), or ischemic myopathies (e.g., bacteria endocarditis, heartworm disease, thrombosis).

Sample type. Serum or heparinized plasma may be used. Do not use EDTA as an anticoagulant, because it may cause falsely elevated results.

Handling specifications. Hemolysis, icterus, or contamination of serum with fluid from muscle during difficult venipuncture can cause falsely elevated results.

Stability. CK is an unstable enzyme when stored at 20° C, 0° to 4° C, or -20° C. Analyze the sample as soon as possible.

Aspartate Aminotransferase

Reason for test. AST is a cytoplasmic enzyme found in most tissues, but is in highest concentrations in the liver and muscle. Increased serum AST levels are due to hepatic injury (as previously discussed), muscle cell injury, or hemolysis. Elevations of AST along with elevations of CK suggest muscle damage. Elevations in AST with normal CK levels suggest hepatocellular injury or prior muscle injury in which the CK level has returned to normal.

Sample type. Serum or plasma may be used. Any anticoagulant is acceptable.

Handling specifications. Hemolysis and lipemia result in elevated blood AST levels.

Stability. Samples for AST determination can be stored for 2 days at 20° C, for 2 weeks at 0° to 4° C, and for several months at -20° C.

Lactate Dehydrogenase

Reason for test. Like CK, LDH is a serum enzyme with many isoenzymes. Different amounts of isoenzymes are present in different tissues. Almost all tissues have LDH, although liver, muscle, and erythrocytes are the major sources of increased blood LDH levels. As compared with CK, the magnitude of LDH rise is less dramatic following muscle injury.

Sample type. Serum or plasma may be used. Do not use anticoagulants containing EDTA or oxalates, because these substances inhibit LDH activity.

Handling specifications. Hemolysis and storing the serum in contact with the clot or the plasma in contact with blood cells can falsely elevate LDH levels.

Stability. LDH appears to be most stable at room temperature or refrigerator temperature. Freezing the sample deactivates LDH activity.

ELECTROLYTE ASSAYS

Electrolytes are minerals that exist as positively charged or negatively charged particles in an aqueous solution. Positively charged particles are called *cations* and negatively charged particles are called *anions*. These particles play essential roles in processes that are vital to normal physiologic function and life. Some of the functions

of electrolytes include maintenance of water balance and fluid osmotic pressure, normal conduction of nervous impulses, normal contraction of muscles, and maintenance and regulation of body fluid pH. Electrolytes also function as vital cofactors in many enzymatically mediated metabolic reactions.

The electrolytes that are most commonly measured are sodium, potassium, chloride, calcium, inorganic phosphorus, and magnesium. Electrolytes can be measured using serum or heparinized plasma. It is important to remember that different salts of heparin are available: sodium heparin, potassium heparin, ammonium heparin, and lithium heparin. When selecting an anticoagulant, do not choose a form of heparin that contains the substance that is being measured.

Sodium

Reason for test. Sodium (Na) is the major cation of plasma and interstitial fluid. Plasma and interstitial fluid make up what is known as *extracellular fluid.* Sodium plays an important role in maintaining extracellular fluid and vascular volume, because it is the most important contributor to effective osmolality. *Effective osmolality* is a term used to describe the number of particles that cannot easily cross cellular membranes (impermeant particles) in a solution. Effective osmolality is the major factor in determining fluid shifts between intracellular fluid and extracellular fluid. *Hyponatremia* (decreased sodium) causes hypoosmolality and movement of fluid from the vascular space to the intracellular space. This causes vascular hypovolemia and may result in cellular swelling. *Hypernatremia* (increased sodium) results in hyperosmolality and movement of intracellular water into the extracellular space, leading to cellular dehydration.

There are two commonly used methods of measuring sodium: flame photometry and ion-specific electrodes. Flame photometry has been the standard for many years and is still used in some laboratories. This method measures concentrations of electrolytes relative to the entire plasma volume. Ion-specific electrodes, which more recently have achieved wider use, measure the concentration of electrolytes relative to the amount of plasma water. Plasma is approximately 93% water, with the remaining percentage composed of lipids and proteins; electrolytes are distributed only in the water phase. In samples that are hyperlipemic or hyperproteinemic, plasma sodium concentrations measured by flame photometry may be artifactually low because of displacement of plasma water by lipids or proteins, a phenomenon that decreases total water content of plasma.

Sample type. Serum is the sample of choice. If plasma is used, lithium heparin or ammonium heparin are the best anticoagulants.

Handling specifications. Use of the sodium salt of heparin as an anticoagulant may falsely elevate the results. Hemolysis does not significantly alter results, but it may dilute the sample with erythrocytic fluid, causing falsely decreased values.

Stability. Serum or plasma may be stored at 4° C or -20° C for delayed analysis.

Potassium

Reason for test. Potassium (K) is the major intracellular cation. Because potassium is found predominantly intracellularly, measures of plasma potassium concentration are not necessarily a good indicator of total body potassium. Potassium distribution across the cell membrane is important in normal function of cardiac and neuromuscular tissues. *Hypokalemia* (decreased potassium) decreases cell excitability, causing weakness and paralysis. *Hyperkalemia* (increased potassium) increases cell excitability; the most serious manifestation is abnormal cardiac rhythm.

Sample type. Serum or heparinized plasma (lithium heparin or ammonium heparin) may be used.

Handling specifications. If heparin is used as the anticoagulant to obtain a plasma sample, either lithium heparin or ammonium heparin will work. Using potassium heparin as the anticoagulant may result in falsely elevated values. Hemolysis may falsely elevate the results in large animal species (cattle, horses, pigs, some species of sheep) because intraerythrocytic potassium concentrations are higher than potassium concentrations in plasma (or serum). This is not true for cats and most species of dogs. Mild hemolysis in cats and dogs does not affect plasma or serum potassium concentration. One notable exception is the Akita. This breed of dog has high intraerythrocytic potassium concentrations. Platelets and leukocytes have enough intracellular potassium to affect plasma potassium levels only if they are present in markedly increased numbers and the plasma is not separated from the clot quickly.

Stability. Information concerning stability of samples for potassium determination is not available.

Chloride

Reason for test. Chloride (Cl) is the predominant extracellular anion and is an important component of serum osmolality. It also helps to maintain electroneutrality (equal number of positive and negative charges) for all of the sodium present.

Increases in chloride are termed *hyperchloremia;* decreases are termed *hypochloremia.*

Sample type. Serum is the sample of choice. Heparinized plasma is preferred over EDTA plasma.

Handling specifications. Hemolysis may affect results by diluting the sample with erythrocytic fluid. Prolonged storage without first separating the serum or plasma from the blood cells can cause slightly low results.

Stability. Samples for chloride determination are stable at room, refrigerator, and freezer temperatures if the serum or plasma is separated from the blood cells.

Calcium

Reason for test. Approximately 99% of calcium (Ca) in the body is found in bones. Only a small percentage of calcium is present in extracellular fluid (including blood), but its presence is essential. Calcium ions are required for preservation of skeletal structure, muscle contraction, blood coagulation, activation of several enzymes, transmission of nerve impulses, and decreasing cell membrane and capillary permeability. Calcium in whole blood is found primarily in plasma (or serum), as erythrocytes contain very little calcium.

Hypercalcemia is an elevated blood calcium concentration; *hypocalcemia* is a decreased concentration.

Sample type. Serum or heparinized plasma may be used.

Handling specifications. Do not use EDTA or oxalate anticoagulants, because they bind calcium and therefore make it unavailable for assay. Hemolysis may result in a slight decrease because of dilution with erythrocytic fluid.

Stability. Samples for calcium determinations can be stored for 10 days at 20° C, 0° to 4° C, or -20° C.

Inorganic Phosphorus

Reason for test. More than 80% of the phosphorus (P) in the body is found in bones, with less than 20% in extracellular fluids. These extracellular phosphorus ions play an important role in carbohydrate metabolism as metabolic intermediates and high-energy phosphate bonds. Phosphorus is also a component of nucleic acids, phospholipids, nucleotides, and body fluid buffers.

Most of the phosphorus in whole blood is found within erythrocytes as organic phosphorus (phosphoric esters). The phosphorus in plasma and serum is inorganic phosphorus and is what is usually measured in the laboratory.

Hyperphosphatemia is an increased serum or plasma phosphorus concentration; *hypophosphatemia* is a decreased serum or plasma phosphorus concentration.

Sample type. Serum or heparinized plasma may be used.

Handling specifications. Hemolysis may artifactually increase results because of release and hydrolysis phosphoric esters to inorganic phosphorus. Prolonged contact of serum or plasma with blood cells may also result in artifactually elevated values. Therefore, separate the serum or plasma from the blood cells as soon as possible after blood collection and before the sample is stored.

Stability. Samples for phosphorus determinations can be stored for 3 to 4 days at 20° C, 1 week at 0° to 4° C, and 3 weeks at -20° C.

Magnesium

Reason for test. Magnesium (Mg) is the fourth most common cation in the body and the second most common intracellular cation. Magnesium is found in all body tissues, although approximately 60% is found in bones. It is an activator (catalyst) for many biological enzymes, and the actions of magnesium extend to all major anabolic and catabolic processes. Magnesium balance is primarily affected by absorption from the gastrointestinal tract and excretion by the kidney. Clinical disorders related to magnesium deficiency are primarily seen in cattle and sheep, although disorders of magnesium metabolism have been reported in cats, horses, and goats.

Hypermagnesemia refers to an elevated blood magnesium level; *hypomagnesemia* is a decreased blood magnesium level.

Sample type. Serum or heparinized plasma may be used.

Handling specifications. Anticoagulants other than heparin may artificially decrease the results. Hemolysis may elevate the results through release of intraerythrocytic magnesium.

Stability. Samples for magnesium determination are stable when stored at 20° C, 0° to 4° C, and -20° C.

PROTEIN ASSAYS

The liver and the immune system (primarily plasma cells) are the source of plasma proteins. These proteins have a wide range of functions, including maintenance of osmotic pressure; acid-base regulation; basic structure of cells, organs, and tissues; catalysts (enzymes) in biochemical reactions; nutritive functions; regulators (hormones); blood coagulation; body defense as antibodies; and transport of plasma constituents.

Total Protein

Reason for test. Total plasma protein measurements include fibrinogen values. Total serum protein concentrations include all plasma proteins except fibrinogen and certain other coagulation proteins, which have been removed during the coagulation process. Total protein concentrations are affected by changes in hydration status (dehydration and overhydration), changes in hepatic synthesis, changes in protein distribution, and changes in protein breakdown or excretion.

Determination of total protein concentration can be useful when evaluating a patient's hydration status. Dehydrated animals usually have elevated total protein values; overhydrated animals usually have decreased total protein values. Other conditions in which total protein concentrations may be helpful include coagulation (clotting) abnormalities, hepatic disease, renal disease, weight loss, diarrhea, edema, and ascites.

The refractometric method measures the refractive index of serum or plasma using a refractometer. This is a good screening test because it is quick, inexpensive, and accurate. This is done often during hematologic examination to measure the total plasma protein to include in complete blood counts.

The biuret method measures the peptide bonds of the proteins in serum and plasma. This colorimetric method is commonly used by analytic instruments in laboratories. The biuret method is very accurate in the ranges usually found in serum (1 to 10 g/dl) but is not precise at low levels (less than 1 g/dl).

Precipitation (trichloroacetic acid) and dye-binding (Coomassie blue) methods have been used to measure the low levels of protein found in such fluids as cerebrospinal fluid and urine.

Sample type. Serum is used if the total serum protein concentration is to be measured; plasma is used if the total plasma protein concentration is to be measured. The total plasma protein concentration includes the fibrinogen concentration, whereas the total serum protein concentration does not.

Handling specifications. Marked hemolysis falsely increases total protein values. Do not use lipemic samples, especially if the refractometric method is used. Moderate icterus has no effect on the refractometric method. Heat, ultraviolet light, surfactant detergents, and chemicals can break down proteins, leading to artifically low results.

Stability. Information concerning stability of samples for total protein determination is not available.

Albumin

Reason for test. Albumin is one of the most important proteins in plasma or serum. It makes up approximately 35% to 50% of the total serum protein concentration. Albumin is synthesized by the liver; severe hepatic insufficiency is a cause of decreased albumin levels. Albumin levels are also influenced by dietary intake, renal disease, and intestinal protein absorption. Albumin is a major transport and binding protein of the blood and is responsible for maintaining osmotic pressure of plasma.

Sample type. Serum or plasma may be used. Heparin and EDTA are the anticoagulants of choice.

Handling specifications and special considerations. Hemolysis may increase the apparent albumin level if the bromcresol green method (commonly used in veterinary laboratories) is used. Methods of measurement used in some human laboratories (those that use bromcresol purple) can be unreliable. Check the test protocol for the method used. Keep the sample covered to prevent dehydration, which can falsely elevate protein levels.

Stability. Samples for albumin determination can be stored for 1 week (2 days on the clot has no effect) at 20° C, for 1 month at 0° to 4° C, and indefinitely at -20° C.

Globulins

Reason for test. Globulins are a complex group of proteins that include all of the proteins (plasma or serum) other than albumin. The globulins are separated into three major classes by electrophoresis: alpha, beta, and gamma globulins. Most alpha and beta globulins are synthesized by the liver. The proteins in these groups include complement, transferrin, ferritin, and other acute-phase proteins of inflammation, and lipoproteins. The gamma globulins (immunoglobulins) are synthesized by plasma cells and are responsible for the body's immunity provided by antibodies. Immunoglobulins identified in animals include IgG, IgD, IgE, IgA, and IgM.

Serum protein assays can be performed with serum protein electrophoresis. Electrophoretic separation of serum protein is based on differential migration of protein molecules within an electrical field. Direction and rate of migration of the different proteins are determined by the type of charge (positive or negative) of the protein, strength of the charge, size of the protein, intensity of the electrical field, and support medium through which the proteins are induced to migrate. To compare results of serum protein electrophoresis, the support medium, pH, buffer, and electric current should be known. Electrophoretic techniques are not normally employed in a practice laboratory.

Because direct assay methods for globulins are often beyond the capabilities of a practice laboratory and not performed on a routine basis in most laboratories, indirect measurements are often used. The total serum globulin concentation is determined by subtracting the serum albumin concentration from the total serum protein concentration.

Albumin-to-Globulin Ratio. The albumin:globulin (A:G) ratio may be reported on chemistry profiles. The normal A:G ratio is approximately 0.5 to 1.5 across species. An increased A:G ratio may occur with any condition that increases albumin (e.g., dehydration) and/or decreases globulin. A decreased A:G ratio may occur with any condition that decreases albumin and/or increases globulin (e.g., inflammation). Although A:G ratios are frequently reported, they are of little significance without knowledge of the absolute total protein, albumin, and globulin values.

Fibrinogen

Reason for test. Fibrinogen is synthesized by hepatocytes. It is one of the factors necessary for clot formation and is the precursor of fibrin, which is the insoluble protein of blood clots. Clot formation is impaired when fibrinogen concentrations are decreased. Because fibrinogen is removed from plasma when a blood clot forms, no fibrinogen is present in serum. Acute inflammation or tissue damage can elevate fibrinogen levels.

Fibrinogen concentration is usually determined by a heat precipitation method. When plasma is heated to 56° C, fibrinogen precipitates out. Fill two pairs of microhematocrit tubes with anticoagulated blood. Spin one pair of microhematocrit tubes in a microhematocrit centrifuge and read the total plasma protein level with a refractometer. Heat the second pair of tubes in a 56° C incubator or water bath for 3 minutes to precipitate the

fibrinogen. After incubation, spin the heated pair of microhematocrit tubes and read the total plasma protein level with a refractometer. Calculate the fibrinogen value by subtracting the total plasma protein value of the heated tubes (this value should be the lower value as fibrinogen has been removed from the plasma) from that of the unheated tubes. This method is too insensitive to detect decreased levels of fibrinogen.

Sample type. Plasma is required; serum does not contain fibrinogen. EDTA plasma is preferred. Heparinized plasma may yield falsely low results.

Stability. Samples for fibrinogen determination can be stored for several days at 20° C and for several weeks at 0° to 4° C.

MISCELLANEOUS CHEMISTRY ASSAYS

Cholesterol

Reason for test. Cholesterol is produced in almost every cell in the body and is especially abundant in hepatocytes, adrenal cortex, ovaries, testes, and intestinal epithelium. The liver is the primary site of synthesis in most animals.

Cholesterol levels are frequently elevated in animals with hypothyroidism, although other conditions may also result in increased cholesterol levels. These include hyperadrenocorticism, diabetes mellitus, and nephrotic syndrome. Dietary causes of hypercholesterolemia are rare but may include very-high-fat diets or postprandial lipemia. (*Note:* Cholesterol alone does not cause the grossly lipemic plasma seen after eating. This lipemia is due to the presence of triglycerides.)

Sample type. Serum or heparinized plasma may be used. All anticoagulants decrease cholesterol levels to some degree, but heparin produces the least effect.

Handling specifications. Hemolysis may affect colorimetric test results. Fluoride and oxalate anticoagulants may elevate enzymatic method results.

Stability. Blood samples for cholesterol determination can be stored for 48 hours at 20° C without separating serum or plasma from the cells. Samples are very stable at 20° C if serum or plasma is removed for the cells, and they are stable for weeks at -20° C.

RECOMMENDED READING

Coles EH: *Veterinary clinical pathology,* ed 4, Philadelphia, 1986, WB Saunders.

Duncan JR, Prasse KW, Mahaffey EA: *Veterinary laboratory medicine,* ed 3, Ames, Iowa, 1994, Iowa State University.

Kaneko JJ: *Clinical biochemistry of domestic animals,* ed 4, San Diego, 1989, Academic Press.

Pratt P: *Laboratory procedures for veterinary technicians,* ed 3, St Louis, 1997, Mosby.

MICROBIOLOGY

M. IKRAM

SPECIMEN COLLECTION AND HANDLING

The use of laboratory tests enhance the veterinarian's ability to diagnose, evaluate, and manage microbial diseases. The accuracy and value of these tests depend on the quality of clinical specimens. No matter how good the methods used in the laboratory, it is impossible to obtain satisfactory results with samples that are collected improperly.

The specimen selected must contain the organism causing the problem. Normal flora and contaminants can complicate sample collection and subsequent interpretation of results. The following guidelines should be kept in mind for proper specimen collection and handling:

1. *Submit a complete history and sufficient clinical date to help select procedures most appropriate to isolate organisms that may be present.* Required data include animal's name or number, species, age, and sex; source, date and time of collection; number of animals affected and duration of problem; major signs observed and degree of severity; summary of clinical and necropsy findings; tentative diagnosis and organism suspected; treatment given, particularly antibiotics because such drugs may temporarily reduce the number of bacteria; and type of laboratory investigation required, especially if unusual microorganisms are suspected.

2. *Collect the specimen aseptically.* Specimen contamination is the most common cause of diagnostic failure. The importance of aseptic collection of microbiologic specimens cannot be overemphasized. Collect samples as soon as possible following the onset of clinical signs.

3. *Collect tissue samples that are at least 5 to 15 cm²* (block or wedge-shaped) so that the microbiologist can sear the outside surface of tissue with a hot spatula, section with a sterile scalpel, and obtain a sample by inserting a swab into the tissue through the incision.

4. *Keep multiple specimens separate from each other to avoid cross contamination.* This is essential for intestinal specimens because of the normal flora found there. Sections of intestines should be tied off at both ends.

5. *Label the specimen container, especially if a zoonotic condition is suspected,* such as anthrax, rabies, leptospirosis, brucellosis, or equine encephalitis.

Tissues from animals with suspected zoonoses should be submitted in a sealed, leakproof, unbreakable container.

6. *Keep the specimen cool during transport.* Any sample that can be frozen should be frozen (especially in summer). Swabs must be sent in transport medium. Bacteriologic, virologic, and *Mycoplasma* tests require separate swabs for each. Tissues for anaerobic culture must be submitted cool or frozen.

7. *If shipping involves dry ice, seal the container or swab to prevent entry of CO_2 into container.* Carbon dioxide released by dry ice may kill bacteria and viruses.

8. *Swabs placed in viral transport medium cannot be used for bacterial culture.* Use duplicate bacterial transport medium.

9. *Do not freeze samples for which you may require histopathologic examinations.*

10. *Contact the reference laboratory for advice on specimen collection.* If there is uncertainty about the most appropriate selection of specimen or a submission procedure, contact the laboratory for their suggestions.

11. *Avoid hurrying to obtain results quickly at the expense of accuracy.*

12. *Send the specimen to the diagnostic laboratory by the fastest possible means.* If the sample will be arriving during a weekend, inform the laboratory ahead of time so that arrangements can be made for pickup.

13. *Discuss the results with the veterinarian promptly,* in a clear, concise manner. Failure to do so reflects adversely on both the veterinarian and the laboratory.

Fig. 11-50 shows the typical sequence of procedures used in processing microbiologic specimens.

Materials for Submitting Samples to a Diagnostic Laboratory

The following materials should be kept on hand for submitting microbiologic samples to a diagnostic laboratory.

- sterile cotton-tip swabs
- culturette swabs in transport medium
- plastic specimen bags
- sterile screw-cap containers (100-200 ml)
- sterile screw-cap tubes or bottles (10 ml)
- scissors, forceps, scalpel with blades (stored in 70% alcohol and flamed to sterilize)
- "discard jar" containing disinfectant for contaminated instruments
- small hacksaw to cut bone specimens
- wooden tongue depressors for handling fecal specimens

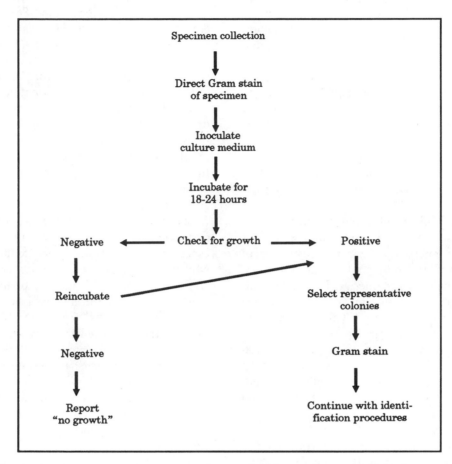

FIG. 11-50 Sequence of procedures used in microbiologic examination. *(From Pratt PW: Laboratory procedures for veterinary technicians, ed 3, St Louis, 1997, Mosby.)*

- Bunsen burner (natural gas or propane gas)
- racks to hold tubes and bottles
- refrigerator
- "cold packs" and polystyrene shipping containers
- polystyrene box, slide mailers, unbreakable containers, waterproof marker pens

Collecting Specimens

Abortion Specimens. A good range of specimens is particularly important in cases of abortion. Specimens should include a small piece of placenta with one or two cotyledons, fetal stomach contents, amniotic fluid, and a piece each of fetal liver, lungs, and spleen. For large animal fetuses aborted before 7 months of gestation, send the entire fetus. Pack the specimens in a leakproof container with several cold packs. If no placenta is

available, submit 5 ml of uterine discharge. For histopathologic examination, submit cotyledons, fetal lesions, liver, and lungs in 10% buffered formalin. If infectious bovine rhinotracheitis is suspected, submit pieces of lung and liver, and a nasal wash.

Sometimes seroconversion coincident with abortion, as in bovine virus diarrhea or brucellosis, may provide more conclusive evidence of the cause than isolation of pathogens. Thus, paired serum samples, one collected at the time of abortion and the other 10 to 14 days later, are required. If leptospirosis is suspected, a midstream urine sample and clotted blood sample should be submitted with placenta and fetal urine.

Leptospirosis Specimens. In diagnosing leptospirosis in cattle, a midstream urine sample is preferred to one collected by catheter. To induce cows to urinate, massage the vulva. Another method is to ask the farmer to hold the cows in a nearby corral until you arrive. When the cows are run into the shed, a few will urinate spontaneously. It is easiest to collect a midstream urine sample in a plastic 200-ml container and then decant 20 ml of this into a screw-capped bottle containing 1.5 ml of 10% formalin. This should be done within 10 minutes of collection or the *Leptospira* organisms may die and disintegrate. Formalin kills the leptospires but preserves their morphology.

When attempting to diagnose leptospirosis, urine and kidney are the samples of choice. In all cases, paired serum samples (acute and convalescent sera) should be submitted to demonstrate positive results despite negative culture results. Where *Leptospira* or *Camplylobacter* is suspected, rapid transport of samples is essential. *Handle suspected brucellosis and leptospirosis samples with caution.*

Milk Specimens. Milk is cultured to identify the organisms that cause mastitis. If milk samples are not collected aseptically, microorganisms from the skin of the udder and from the air may contaminate the specimen, and culture results are erroneous. If possible, collect milk samples from the cow after mastitis is noticed and before treatment is commenced. Culturing samples within 3 days of the last treatment usually results in a negative culture and meaningless findings. Do not wash the udder before obtaining samples unless it is very dirty. If the udder must be washed, use warm water and disinfectant at the recommended strength. Dry the udder and teats thoroughly with single-service paper towels.

Using 70% ethyl alcohol or 70% to 90% isopropyl alcohol, wipe the two teats farther from you first and then the two nearer teats. Carefully swab the teat sphincters. Use sterile bottles or tubes with screw caps for collection. Fisher-brand sterile vials (Fisher Scientific, Springfield, NJ) are useful, because they can be conveniently snapped shut. Containers such as Zipper Seal Sample Bags (Fisher Scientific) are not satisfactory.

Hold the collection tube as near to horizontal as possible. Discard the first few squirts of milk from each teat and then direct a little milk from each quarter into a separate tube that has been labeled. Sample the two teats nearer to you first and then those farther from you so that your arm does not accidentally brush against the disinfected teats before sampling. Collect the samples as quickly as possible, taking care not to contaminate the cap of the container. Hold your forefinger against the palm of the hand taking the sample, while using the thumb to collect the milk. Screening of samples with the California mastitis test before culturing is recommended.

Refrigerate the milk samples as soon after collection as possible until they can be cultured. Do not freeze the samples. If mastitis from *Mycoplasma* is suspected, ampicillin can be added at 1 to 10 mg/ml of milk sample to control contaminant bacteria. Keep these milk samples at room temperature so that the *Mycoplasma* organisms can multiply in the sample. Another milk sample should also be taken without adding antibiotics so as to check for the more common mastitis-causing organisms, such as *Streptococcus agalactiae, Staphylococcus aureus, Streptococcus uberis, Escherichia coli,* and *Nocardia.*

Urine Specimens. Normal voided urine may contain small numbers of bacteria. It is important to differentiate these small numbers from significant bacteriuria. Urinalysis thus must be quantitative to yield meaningful results. Be careful to avoid contamination with preputial or vulvar flora. Ideally the vulva or prepuce should be thoroughly cleaned with detergent, after which at least 5 ml of a midstream sample are collected in a sterile tube. Infection is determined from the number of organisms present. A bacterial count of $\geq 10,000/\mu l$ suggests an active infection. For diagnostic purposes, however, 1 to 2 ml of urine must be collected aseptically by catheter or cystocentesis. Cystocentesis is the method of choice, especially for samples from female dogs and cats. Midstream samples or samples collected by manual compression of the bladder are unacceptable.

Additional specimens should be submitted 72 to 96 hours after the start of antimicrobial therapy so as to monitor the response to treatment. Common pathogens isolated from urine samples include *E. coli, S. aureus, Streptococcus, Proteus,* and *Pseudomonas.*

Fecal Specimens. Collect feces in a fecal cup when freshly voided or directly from the rectum using aseptic precautions. In large animals, a disposable rubber glove or sleeve is useful. Once inverted and tied off, the entire sleeve can be submitted containing the specimen. At least 1 to 2 g of fresh feces is the preferred specimen for fecal culture. Submit three consecutive specimens. Fecal swabs are less effective for fecal culture because of the small volume of samples. However, in small animals, a sterile cotton swab can be used to collect samples from the rectum while avoiding contamination of the swab with anal skin microflora, but usually swabs do not provide enough volume. Where delay is unavoidable, the specimen should be put into a standard transport medium. It is important to remember that a single negative fecal culture does not rule out involvement of infectious agents (e.g., intermittent excretion of *Salmonella*); at least three fecal samples should be cultured to rule out most enteric pathogens. The most common organisms associated with intestinal infection are members of the family Enterobacteriaceae.

Specimens from Abscesses and Wounds. If the abscess has not ruptured, shave the area, swab liberally with alcohol and allow it to dry. If possible, collect 3 ml of pus with a sterile syringe and wide-bore needle. When possible, obtain scrapings from the wall of the abscess, as causative organisms are more likely to be viable there. Collect several milliliters of material for culture rather than relying on a swab sample.

To culture samples from wounds, the surrounding area should be disinfected and superficial debris lifted away. The surface of open wounds frequently contains contaminating bacteria. Gross observation of pus for color, odor, and presence of "sulfur granules" can be helpful, as is a direct smear for Gram staining. The swab must be taken near the edge of a wound, as the center frequently contains only necrotic debris. For draining abscesses, aspirate as deeply as possible, avoiding the surface of the wound. The most common pathogens involved with abscesses and wounds are *Staphylococcus, Streptococcus, E. coli, Proteus, Pseudomonas, Nocardia, Actinomyces, Fusobacterium,* and *Clostridium.*

Specimens from the Eye. Organisms from the eye are often fastidious, such as *Moraxella, Streptococcus,* and *Mycoplasma.* It is best to culture corneal scrapings, a swab rolled into the conjunctival sac, or lacrimal secretions collected with a sterile swab by applying the specimen directly onto a blood agar plate or transporting the swab immediately to the laboratory. If this is not possible, deposit the end of the swab into about 2 ml of sterile saline and culture within 2 hours of collection. Use of topical anesthetics is discouraged, because they may inhibit bacterial growth. Pathogens isolated from the eye include *Staphylococcus, Pasteurella, Pseudomonas, Chlamydia,* and *E. coli.*

Genital Specimens

Cervicovaginal mucus aspirate. The normal vagina contains numerous resident flora. Use a vaginal speculum to avoid vaginal microorganism contamination. Cervical mucus may be collected in a sterile artificial insemination pipette introduced through the speculum. A syringe attached to the pipette by a short length of rubber tubing is used to aspirate the mucus. About 3 ml should be collected and expressed into vials containing Cary-Blair medium, a transport broth used for culture of *Campylobacter fetus* and other genital organisms. If *Taylorella (Hemophilus) equigenitalis* is suspected, use Amies transport medium containing charcoal.

Vulvar swab. The culture swab should be applied to the vulvar mucosa, particularly around the clitoral fossa. The swab is then cultured for *Ureaplasma diversum* and *Mycoplasma* spp. Swabs that cannot be sent to the laboratory on the same day of collection should be stored at 4° C and shipped at 4° C with an ice pack. If the sample is to be held more than 2 days, it should be stored and shipped frozen at -70° C. *Mycoplasma* is very sensitive to drying; therefore, *do not submit dry swabs.* If mycoplasmal infection is suspected, tissue specimens are the preferred specimen. If swabs are submitted, they should only be submitted in Stewart agar medium.

Specimens from the Ear. Ear swabs are most often collected from dogs. Usually both ears should be individually swabbed, as comparison of the cultured organisms helps differentiate normal from abnormal flora. Organisms commonly involved in ear infections are *S. aureus, P. aeruginosa, Proteus, Streptococcus,* and *Malassezia pachydermatis (Pityrosporon canis).*

Blood Samples. Before blood is obtained for culture, the skin over the site of venipuncture must be shaved, cleaned, and disinfected first with antiseptic solution applied in widening circles from the site, followed by chlorhexidine solution. Do not touch the site with ungloved fingers after it has been prepared. Usually 5 to 10 ml of blood are collected for culture. The blood should be collected into a sterile Vacutainer with sodium polyanethole sulfonate (yellow top). Blood collected in tubes containing EDTA or heparin (blue or lavender tops) is not suitable for culture.

Skin Scrapings. The skin typically maintains a normal resident bacterial flora that rarely contributes to skin lesions. To minimize contamination of bacteriologic specimens with normal skin flora, observe strict asepsis. Harvest the contents of intact postules or vesicles by sterile fine-needle aspiration after disinfecting the skin with 70% alcohol.

Joint Samples. Joint infections in dogs and cats are caused by bite wounds, whereas in large animals joint infections are due to injuries. Aseptically aspirate synovial fluid for culture and transport into a syringe or tube. Do not submit synovial fluid samples on swabs, because they do not provide enough volume for culture. The pathogens most commonly involved in joint infections include *Staphylococcus, Streptococcus, Actinomyces, Mycoplasma, Hemophilus,* and *E. coli.*

Cerebrospinal Fluid Samples. Observing aseptic precautions, collect cerebrospinal fluid into a sterile tube. A minimum of 0.5 ml is required. The sample should be transported immediately to the laboratory, where it will be centrifuged and plated.

Tracheal Washes. For pulmonary infection, collect tracheal and bronchial aspirates directly into a syringe for culture. If secretions cannot be obtained initially, flush with lactated Ringer's solution and aspirate.

Culture of Anaerobes

Because most anaerobes can survive exposure to air for less than 20 minutes, collection of samples for anaerobic culture on swabs is completely useless. Acceptable anaerobic specimens include blocks of tissue (2-inch cube minimum) in a closed sterile container; material placed in Becton Dickinson's Anaerobic Specimen Collector; and pus and exudate collected in a sterile syringe, with the air expelled and the needle plugged with a rubber stopper or bent backward on itself.

Specimens should be cultured as soon as possible after collection. The specimen is inoculated onto a blood agar plate and into thioglycollate broth, which is a liquid medium used to grow anaerobes. The blood agar plates are put into an anaerobe jar, which provides an anaerobic environment during incubation. A self-contained system, such as Gas Pack (Oxoid), can be used. A commercial anaerobe culture system, such as API Anaerobic system, is also available. In cases where demonstration of specific toxin is required, at least 20 ml of ileal contents or a loop of ileum with contents should be submitted.

Conditions in which isolation of anaerobes might be significant include soft-tissue abscesses, postoperative wounds, peritonitis, septicemia, endocarditis, endometritis, gangrene, pulmonary infection, and footrot in cattle, sheep, and swine. The isolated anaerobe may be the sole etiologic agent or a partner in a synergistic relationship with another bacterium. For example, liver abscesses seen at slaughter in otherwise healthy feedlot cattle commonly yield the anaerobe *Fusobacterium necrophorum* and the aerobe *Actinomyces (Corynebacterium) pyogenes.*

For conditions involving *Clostridium chauvoei, Cl. septicum, Cl. novyi,* and *Cl. sordellii,* most laboratories use the fluorescent antibody technique in diagnosis. Specimens include affected muscle and a rib containing bone marrow, because bone marrow appears to be one of the last tissues to be invaded by contaminating microorganisms.

Table 11-10 summarizes bacterial pathogens of veterinary importance, species affected, resultant diseases or lesions, and specimens required for diagnosis.

Collecting Specimens for Mycologic Examination

Superficial Mycoses. Clean the affected area with 70% alcohol, pluck any hair attempting to retain the roots, and scrape deeply with a blunt scalpel (drawing blood) on the edge of a lesion. A Wood's (ultraviolet) lamp may help detect hairs that are fluorescent, although not all ringworm organisms cause fluorescence.

Specimens from pigs, particularly, are often contaminated with saprophytic fungi. Lesions can be swabbed with 70% isopropyl alcohol and allowed to dry before specimens are taken.

Collect hairs and skin scrapings in paper envelopes. The specimens tend to stay drier and less contaminated in envelopes than when placed in a closed container.

Organisms commonly involved in superficial mycoses are called *dermatophytes.*

Deep Mycoses. Send a frozen tissue specimen, including the wall and center of the lesion. Tissues should be marked "caution," because deep-seated mycoses are potential zoonotic agents.

Fluids. Submit at least 0.5 ml of an aspirate, blood, cerebrospinal fluid or other fluid sample in a sterile screw-capped tube or container.

Swabs. Generally, swabs are an inappropriate submission for mycotic examination and should only be submitted from nasal sources or when yeast infection is suspected. Table 11-11 contains a list of pathogenic fungi of veterinary importance, species affected, resultant diseases/lesions, and specimens required for diagnosis.

Collecting Specimens for Virologic Examination

Viruses are often present in the nasal or pharyngeal secretions early in the acute stage of respiratory diseases. Take mucosal scrapings rather than just swabs of the secretions. Sterile wooden tongue depressors are useful for mucosal scrapings. Attempted isolation from blood samples might be considered in generalized catarrhal diseases that tend to have a viremic stage. Poxviruses can often be demonstrated by electron microscopy in fluid from early vesicular lesions, and sometimes in scabs from early lesions.

Do not neglect also to select specimens for indirect studies, such as serologic, hematologic, histologic, and bacteriologic examinations. Viral diseases are often complicated by pathogenic bacteria acting as secondary invaders. These often turn a mild viral infection into a serious disease.

Viral specimens should be refrigerated at 4° C when possible, because viral titers decrease rapidly as temperature increases. In necropsy and biopsy specimens, temperature higher than 4° C facilitates autolysis, destroying viral infectivity and/or antigenic properties. If specimens cannot be delivered to the virology laboratory within 24 hours, snap-freeze at -70° C and ship on dry ice, except for parainfluenza and influenza viruses, in which case -20° C is best, because the integrity of these viruses is preserved best at this temperature. Specimens must be shipped in an air-tight container to prevent entry of CO_2 into the containers. CO_2 gas from the dry ice can lower the pH of fluid, killing any pH-sensitive viruses. Also, repeated freezing and thawing should be avoided.

Containers. The most typical containers and materials used for collection of virologic samples include sterile swabs, vials containing virus transport medium, bottles for feces or other samples that do not require transport medium, blood collection equipment for both serum and plasma samples, and bottles containing fixative for histologic examination.

Timing. Collect the specimen for virologic analysis as soon as possible after the onset of clinical signs. For serologic tests, collect two blood samples, one during the acute phase, usually when the animal is examined and clinical signs are obvious, and the second during the convalescent phase, usually 2 weeks after the first specimen is taken. An increased antibody titer may be observed in the second sample.

TABLE 11-10 Summary of some veterinary bacterial pathogens, species affected, resultant disease or lesions, and specimens for diagnosis

Organism	Species affected	Disease or lesion	Specimens
Actinomyces	Cattle, pigs, dogs	Mandibular osteomyelitis, chronic granulomatous and suppurative mastitis in sows, periodontal disease	Fresh tissue, pus
Actinobacillus	Cattle, sheep, foals, pigs, chickens	Granulomatous lesions containing pus; most commonly affects tongue (wooden tongue); found in rumen and on tongues of normal animals, "sleepy foal" disease; abortion, navel infections	Fresh tissue and pus
Bacillus	Cattle, sheep, pigs, people	Anthrax, fatal septicemia in sheep, cattle, pigs; acute pharyngitis with hemorrhagic swelling of throat region	Fresh blood smear from ear vein; collect tissues with great caution
Bacteroides	Sheep	Foot rot in conjunction with *Fusobacterium necrophorum*	Fresh smear from lesion
Bordetella	Pigs, dogs, lab animals	Atrophic rhinitis in pigs; respiratory infection in dogs, associated with distemper virus; snuffles in rabbits and guinea pigs	Fresh nasal swabs or lungs
Brucella	Cattle, pigs, sheep, goats, horses, dogs	Abortion, orchitis	Fresh fetal stomach contents, placenta, blood serum, milk, testes
Campylobacter	Cattle, sheep, pigs	Abortion, infertility, venereal infection	Fresh vaginal mucus
Clostridium	Many species	Botulism, malignant edema, septicemia, tetanus	Fresh serum obtained before death. At necropsy: heart blood and intestinal contents; suspect feed; presence of toxin must be demonstrated.
Chlamydia	Sheep, cats, birds, cattle	Enzootic abortion, feline pneumonitis (conjunctivitis, fever, ocular discharge), psittacosis/ornithosis	Fresh conjunctival scrapings, liver, spleen, kidney, lungs
Corynebacterium	Pigs, cattle, sheep, goats	Suppurative pneumonia, wound and surgical infections, arthritis, mastitis, navel infections	Fresh pus (scrape abscess wall); affected tissue, milk
Dermatophilus	Cattle, horses, goats, sheep	Dermatitis with scab formation	Swab exudate, fresh plucked hair, scab
Erysipelothrix	Pigs, sheep, cattle	Diamond skin disease (septicemia, endocarditis, arthritis)	Fresh liver, spleen, heart, synovial fluid
Escherichia	Young of many species	Calf scours; mastitis; piglet diarrhea; edema disease; hemorrhagic enteritis	Fresh feces, milk, urine, affected tissue
Fusobacterium	Cattle, sheep, goats, pigs, horses	Principal agent of foot rot; necrobacillosis of liver in feedlot cattle (associated with *Actinomyces pyogenes*); calf diphtheria	Fresh pus or affected tissue; fixed affected tissue
Taylorella (H) equigenitalis	Horses	Contagious equine metritis; possible abortion	Fresh cervical or uterine swabs; sheath swabs; place in Amies transport medium

TABLE 11-10 Summary of some veterinary bacterial pathogens, species affected, resultant disease or lesions, and specimens for diagnosis—cont'd

Organism	Species affected	Disease or lesion	Specimens
Hemophilus	Cattle, pigs	Infectious thromboembolic meningoencephalitis; pneumonia and polyserositis, contagious and pleuropneumonia, Glasser's disease	Fresh and fixed affected tissue
Klebsiella	Pigs, cattle, horses, dogs	Mastitis, cervicitis and metritis, setpicemia in foals, pneumonia	Fresh milk, fresh liver, spleen, bone marrow, fresh lung
Leptospira	Cattle, sheep, pigs, horses	Hemoglobinuria and jaundice, abortion, infertility and agalactia	Fresh kidney taken within 4 hours of death, urine
Listeria	Cattle, sheep	Abortion, encephalitis	Fresh abortion specimens, brain or liver
Moraxella	Cattle	Infectious keratoconjunctivitis (pink eye)	Fresh swab of eye discharges
Mycobacterium	Cattle, pigs, sheep	Tuberculosis, paratuberculosis, granulomas with caseation	Fresh and fixed lesions and affected tissue
Mycoplasma	Cattle, pigs, sheep, goats	Contagious bovine pleuropneumonia, pneumonia, mastitis, arthritis	Fresh swabs containing exudates from eye, nostril, trachea, and genitalia
Pseudomonas	Many species	Wound infections, bovine mastitis, otitis in dogs and cats	Fresh swabs or affected tissue
Pasteurella	Many species	Frequently a secondary invader or opportunist, associated with shipping fever complex in cattle, snuffles in rabbits, enzootic pneumonia in pigs	Fresh and fixed lung and spleen or other tissue with lesions
Rickettsia	Dogs, horses, sheep	Recurrent tick-borne fever, Potomac horse fever	Blood smear
Staphylococcus	Many species	Suppurative wound infections, abscesses, mastitis	Fresh milk, wound, skin or abscess swabs
Salmonella	All animal species	Acute septicemia, gastroenteritis, abortion	Fresh feces, mesenteric lymph nodes, liver, rib with bone marrow, intestines, pus, abortion specimen
Streptococcus	Cattle, horses, pigs	Mastitis, strangles, endocarditis	Fresh milk, pus, lymph nodes, affected tissue, uterine or cervical swabs
Serpula (Treponema)	Pigs	Swine dysentery	Rectal swabs, spiral colon

Modified from Ikram M: *Diagnostic microbiology.* In Pratt PW, ed: *Laboratory procedures for veterinary technicians,* ed 2, St Louis, Mosby, 1992.

Collection Site. The collection site depends upon the clinical signs and knowledge of the suspected virus, such as nasal swabs for respiratory diseases, feces for gastroenteritis, or vaginal mucus for abortion.

Blood Samples. Collect approximately 5 ml of blood in heparin or EDTA Vacutainers (lavender or blue top). Submit samples maintained at 4° C to prevent hemolysis. Do not freeze blood samples, because freezing causes hemolysis and may render serum samples useless for serologic examinations.

Smears. Use a clean slide. Air-dry the smear thoroughly. *Do not fix the smear.*

Swabs. Swabs should be collected using sterile swabs and placed in virus transport medium immediately with conjunctival swabs; remove any exudate before swabbing the everted conjunctiva.

Vesicle Fluid. Collect fluid from vesicles using a small-bore needle and syringe. Leave the fluid in the syringe and transport the specimen to the laboratory at 4° C.

Urine. Send approximately 5 ml of aseptically collected urine in a sterile container. *Do not use virus transport medium.* Maintain the sample at 4° C if the specimen is to arrive at laboratory within 24 hours of collection; otherwise, snap freeze at -70° C and ship on dry ice.

TABLE 11-11 Summary of pathogenic fungi, species affected, resultant disease or lesions, and specimens for diagnosis

Organism	Species affected	Disease or lesion	Specimens
Microsporum	Dogs, cats, horses, pigs	Ringworm	Fresh plucked hair and skin scrapings from edges of lesions; send to laboratory in paper envelopes
Trichophyton	Most animal species	Ringworm	Fresh plucked hair and skin scrapings from edges of lesions; send to laboratory in paper envelopes
Candida albicans	Chickens, turkeys, other birds	Infection of mouth, crop, esophagus	Fresh affected tissue or scrapings from affected tissue
Malassezia pachydermatis (Pityrosporon canis)	Dogs	Chronic otitis externa	Fresh ear swabs
Cryptococcus neoformans	People, dogs, cats	Frequently affects nervous system	Fresh nasal discharges, milk
Cryptococcus neoformans (worldwide distribution)	Cattle	Sporadic cases of mastitis	Fixed affected tissue, brain, lung
Coccidioides immitis SW USA and South America; occurs in soil	People horses, cattle, sheep, dogs, cats, captive feral animals	Disease characterized by granulomas, often in bronchial and mediastinal lymph nodes and lungs; can cause lesions in brain, liver, spleen, kidneys	Fresh and fixed lesions and affected tissue
Histoplasma capsulatum NE, central, and S central USA; occurs in soil	People, dogs, cats, sheep, pigs, horses	Disease that generally affects reticuloendothelial system; dogs, cats: ulcerations of intestinal canal; enlargement of liver, spleen, lymph nodes; can get TB-like lesions	Fresh and fixed lesions or affected tissue
Histoplasma farciminosum Mediterranean, Asia, Africa, and parts of Russia	Horses, mules, donkeys	Epizootic lymphangitis, African farcy or Japanese glanders	Fresh pus and discharges from lesions
Blastomyces dermatitidis USA, Canada, and Africa; occurs in soil	People, dogs, cats, sea lions	Granulomatous lesions in lungs and/or skin and subcutis	Fresh and fixed lesions and affected tissue
Sporothrix schenckii	People, horses, dogs, pigs, cattle, fowl, rodents	Subcutaneous nodules or granulomas that eventually discharge pus; can get involvement of bones and visceral organs	Fresh and fixed pus, granulomas
Rhinosporidium seeberi (not yet cultured in vitro)	Horses, dogs, cattle, people	Characterized by polyps on the nasal and ocular mucous membranes	Fresh nasal discharge and polyps; fixed polyps
Aspergillus	Many animal species and birds	Air sac infection, mycotic abortion and mastitis, guttural pouch mycosis	Fresh deep scrapings or affected tissue
Petriellidium boydii (Allescheria boydii)	Cattle, horses	Abortion, mastitis, metritis, infertility	Fresh milk, uterine discharges, affected tissue Fixed affected tissue

From Ikram M: *Diagnostic microbiology.* In Pratt PW, ed: *Laboratory procedures for veterinary technicians,* ed 2, St Louis, 1992, Mosby.

TABLE 11-12 Common viral infections of domestic animals

Virus	Disease or lesion	Specimens
Cattle		
Bovine herpesvirus 1	Infectious bovine rhinotracheitis and infectious pustular vaginitis	Mucosal scrapings; whole aborted fetus or fresh and fixed fetal kidney and liver; paired serum samples
Bovine herpesvirus 2	Bovine mammillitis; dermatitis, often hemorrhagic, of udder and teats, muzzle esions in sucking calves	Vesicular fluid from early lesions or deep scrapings from older lesions; fixed biopsy; scabs of no value
Alcelaphine herpesvirus 1	Malignant catarrhal fever	Fixed liver, brain, kidney, lymph nodes, adrenals, and lesions from alimentary tract
Flavivirus	Bovine virus diarrhea-musocal disease	Fresh spleen, lymph nodes and blood clot; serum; fixed portions of lesions
Retrovirus	Bovine leukosis	Lesions, fresh and fixed; EDTA blood
Picornaviruses	Neonatal disease, upper respiratory tract infection, foot and mouth disease	Feces and serum. Nasal mucosal scrapings, serum, vesicle fluid
Parvovirus	Diarrhea in young calves	Feces
Reoviruses	Respiratory and enteric conditions in young calves	Nasal mucosal scrapings; feces; serum. Feces
Adenoviruses	May cause upper respiratory tract infections	Nasal scrapings
Paramyxovirus	Upper respiratory tract infections, diarrhea	Nasal scrapings, whole blood, lung, serum
Papovavirus	Papillomas (warts)	Fixed and fresh excised tumors
Poxviruses	Pseudocowpox (paravacinia, milker's nodules), dermatitis on udder and teats with "horseshoe" scab formation	Deep scrapings of early lesions
	Papular stomatitis	Deep scrapings of several oral ulcers; fixed tissue from lesion
Horses		
Herpesvirus	Rhinopneumonitis; abortion, coital exanthema	Nasal scrapings; fresh, whole aborted fetus or fresh and fixed fetal liver; kidney and lung
Papovavirus	Papillomas (warts)	Fresh and fixed excised tumors
Orthomyxovirus	Upper respiratory tract infection	Nasal scrapings; lung; whole blood
Paramyxovirus	Upper respiratory tract infection	Nasal scrapings from very early cases; serum
Picornavirus	Upper respiratory tract infection, mainly in young horses	Nasal scrapings and exudates
Togaviruses	Arteritis, edema of the limbs and eyes, abortion, encephalomyelitis	Nasal or conjunctival exudates, fresh and fixed brain
Sheep		
Herpesvirus	Chronic progressive lung disease in sheep >4 yr; no metastases	Fixed lung lesion
Paramyxovirus	Signs referable to respiratory tract, with pneumonia in young animals	Nasal scrapings very early in diease; isolation often difficult from pneumonic lesions; serum
Picornavirus	Foot and mouth disease	Vesicle fluid, serum
Togavirus (closely related to BVD virus of cattle)	Border disease of lambs or "hairy shaker" disease (hairy coat, nervous signs, poor growth)	Serum

TABLE 11-12 Common viral infections of domestic animals—cont'd

Virus	Disease or lesion	Specimens
Sheep–cont'd		
Rotavirus	Diarrhea in lambs	Feces and serum
Pigs		
Herpesvirus	Inclusion-body rhinitis, pseudorabies (Aujeszky's disease)	Whole, recently dead pig carcass or sick live pig; head of older pigs or fixed nasal mucosa
Picornavirus	Talfan or Teschen's disease, encephalomyocarditis, stillbirths, mummification, embryonic deaths, infertility	Fresh and fixed whole brain; serum, recently dead pigs or fresh heart, spleen, aborted fetuses; serum
Parvovirus	Reproductive failure	Freshly aborted fetuses, especially mummified fetuses; serum
Rotavirus	Acute gastroenteritis in piglets	Feces
Orthomyxovirus	Bronchopneumonia and lung edema	Respiratory exudates or lung; serum
Coronavirus	Transmissible gastroenteritis	Live affected piglets or fresh and fixed small intestine; serum; feces are valueless
Cats		
Herpesvirus 1	Rhinotracheitis, occasionally abortion in queens and some fatalities in neonates	Nasal scrapings early in disease
Parvovirus	Panleukopenia or feline infectious enteritis	Fresh spleen, fixed portions of intestine, lymph nodes, thymus, bone marrow, EDTA blood
Dogs		
Herpesvirus	Deaths in neonatal pups, rhinitis and pharyngitis in pups >6 wk old, vaginitis, and abortion	Whole puppy carcass or fresh and fixed kidney, spleen, lungs, liver, and nasopharynx; serum
Rhabdovirus	Rabies	Consult with state veterinarian
Papovavirus	Oral papillomas (warts)	Fixed and fresh excised tumors
Paramyxovirus	Distemper	Fresh whole lung; fixed lung, brain, bladder, kidney, liver, gallbladder
	Parainfluenza: upper respiratory tract infection	Respiratory exudates
Adenovirus	Infectious canine hepatitis	Whole puppy carcass or fresh nasopharyngeal scraping, and fresh and fixed lung, kidney, spleen, liver, brain; feces and urine from live pups; serum
Parvovirus	Enteritis, myocarditis, leukopenia	Fresh feces; serum; mesenteric lymph nodes; ileum; spleen
Coronavirus	Vomiting, diarrhea	Feces
Reovirus	Mild upper respiratory infection	Nasal exudate; feces
Rotavirus	Gastroenteritis in young pups	Feces

Modified from Ikram M: *Diagnostic microbiology.* In Pratt PW, ed: *Laboratory procedures for veterinary technicians,* ed 2, St Louis, 1992, Mosby.

Necropsy and Biopsy Tissues. Collect tissue samples while avoiding bacterial contamination, particularly from the gastrointestinal tract. *Place the specimen immediately into the virus transport medium.* Maintain at 4° C and submit to the laboratory as soon as possible. Cubes of tissue of approximately 1 cm² are recommended, as small pieces of tissue can be snap-frozen uniformly, eliminating the problem of autolysis at the sample's center. When lesions are visible to the unaided eye, collect samples for virus isolation from the edge of the lesion, rather than from the center.

Special Precautions. If exotic or zoonotic viruses are suspected, special packaging and appropriate permits are necessary for interstate and international transport. This information is available from the postal service, shipping companies, and government veterinary and public health authorities.

Table 11-12 indicates the type of specimens usually collected for diagnosis of common viral diseases of domestic animals.

Collecting Specimens for Histologic Examination

All tissues taken for routine histopathologic examination should be fixed in 10% buffered formalin. This is prepared as follows:

10% Buffered Formalin

Formalin (37-40% formaldehyde gas)	1000 ml
Sodium phosphate dibasic	65 g
Sodium phosphate monobasic	40 g
Distilled water	9000 ml

pH should be between 6.8 and 7.0

Soft tissue for fixation should be cut into small slices approximately 6 mm in maximum thickness. When possible, use wide-mouth jars, as large pieces of fresh tissue forced through the narrow mouth of a jar cannot be easily removed after fixation is complete. One part tissue to 10 times volume of 10% buffered formalin is ideal. For tissues that float, such as aerated lung, a piece of crumpled paper toweling should be placed in the formalin to keep these tissues submerged to ensure complete fixation. Never freeze sections for histologic examination, because this causes tissue artifacts that may be difficult to differentiate from a pathogenic process.

RECOMMENDED READING

Ikram M, Hill E: *Microbiology for veterinary technicians,* St Louis, 1991, Mosby.

Ikram M: *Microbiology* In Pratt P: *Laboratory procedures for veterinary technicians,* ed 3, St Louis, 1997, Mosby.

Quinn PJ et al: *Clinical veterinary microbiology,* St Louis, 1994, Mosby.

CYTOLOGIC EXAMINATION

D.J. FISHER

Cytologic examination is used for microscopic assessment of cells that have exfoliated from tissues, either freely or by mechanical methods. Cytologic examination has become a common diagnostic tool in many veterinary practices. The advantages of cytologic examination include relatively low risk during sample acquisition (sedation is rarely necessary and there is minimal risk of life-threatening hemorrhage), low cost, and quick turnaround of results as compared with histopathologic examination. In addition, most veterinary practices already have on hand all of the materials and equipment necessary to perform cytologic examinations (Box 11-27). One disadvantage is that,

---

Box 11-27 Basic equipment used for cytologic examination

- Binocular microscope (Nikon, Olympus, American Optical, Swift)
- Immersion oil
- 20- or 22-gauge, 1.5-inch needles (some prefer 25 gauge for some types of specimens)
- 6- and 12-ml syringes
- Glass slides (frosted end is helpful in labeling) and coverslips
- Stains: Diff-Quik (Scientific Products), Hema-Quik (Curtis Matheson Scientific), Quik Stain II (Scientific Products) new methylene blue, Gram stain
- Coplin staining jars
- Specimen tubes: red-top tubes contain no anticoagulant; lavender-top tubes contain EDTA as anticoagulant
- Forceps, scalpel blades
- Refractometer
- Hemacytometer

---

unlike histologic evaluation, cytologic examination does not allow assessment of tissue architecture.

The goal of cytologic examination is, at the minimum, to classify a pathologic process as inflammatory, infectious, reactive, hyperplastic, or neoplastic. In some cases, cytologic examination is not very revealing or may even be nondiagnostic. At its most definitive, however, it can reveal an etiologic agent (e.g., *Blastomyces dermatitidis*) or a specific diagnosis (e.g., mast-cell tumor).

Specimens can be obtained by fine-needle aspiration of masses, lymph node, spleen, liver, and other internal organs. Other specimens suitable for cytologic examination include tracheal washes, bronchoalveolar lavages, cerebrospinal fluid, abdominal or thoracic fluid, synovial fluid, bone marrow aspirates, and various other tissue swabs and/or scrapings. Cytologic evaluation of these specimens can provide relatively accurate and reliable diagnostic information in experienced hands. To gain the most information from a cytologic specimen and minimize nondiagnostic samples, however, requires collecting an adequate sample and processing the material in an appropriate manner for cytologic evaluation. In addition, staining quality of the slides can greatly enhance or diminish the diagnostic information gained from a sample. The final step is cytologic diagnosis or interpretation of the slide. Although the experienced practitioner or technician can interpret many cytologic slides, evaluation by a veterinary cytopathologist occasionally may be necessary.

EQUIPMENT FOR CYTOLOGIC EXAMINATION

Microscope

A good microscope and its proper care are essential for the best cytologic results. A binocular microscope with a substage condenser and an internal light source is preferred. Usually, there is room for four or five objective lenses. Most veterinary practices use 4×, 10×, 40×, and 100× (oil) objective lenses. These lenses are adequate for most cytologic examinations. If examination of cytologic and hematologic slides is the primary use of the microscope, a 50× (oil-immersion) objective instead of the 40× lens should be considered. The advantage of the 50× oil lens is that it typically has increased resolution. In addition, it allows for going back and forth between high and low power without worrying about getting oil on a high-dry lens (40×). On the other hand, an oil-immersion lens is difficult to use with coverslipped wet preparations, such as fecal flotations. If this is how the practice microscope is most commonly used, a 40× lens would be a more appropriate choice. In addition to these lenses, the 100× oil-immersion lens is helpful when examining for bacteria or cellular inclusions. The low-power 4× and 10× lenses are used for quick scans of the slides and detecting large organisms or cell clusters.

Two important concepts relating to microscopes are magnification and resolution. The magnification of a specimen is determined by the ocular lenses (typically 10×) multiplied by the objective lens (e.g., 10× ocular × 40× objective = 400× magnification). *Resolution,* or resolving power, refers to the ability of a lens to distinguish two closely placed particles as separate. The resolving power or resolution is related to the numeric aperture (N.A.) of the lenses (usually printed on the side of the lens). A higher N.A. indicates a greater resolving power. Oil-immersion lenses generally have a higher N.A.; therefore, they typically have better resolution than another lens with comparable magnification. For example, a 50× oil-immersion lens with an N.A. of 0.85 would be better able to distinguish two closely placed bacterial cocci than a 40× lens with an N.A. of 0.66.

When using oil-immersion lenses, a coverslip is not required; however, most high-dry lenses (40×) are designed to be used with a coverslipped slide to obtain the top resolving power of the lens. If the objective lens has 0.17 engraved on its side, this lens requires a 0.17-mm–thick coverslip for top resolution. Lenses also vary in quality, in particular, relative to how well they correct for chromatic and spherical aberration. An achromatic lens is satisfactory for most cytologic specimens.

Clean the microscope and lenses after every use with commercial lens cleaning solution and lens paper.

Leaving oil on the lenses eventually ruins them. Cover the microscope when not in use. Keep replacement bulbs and fuses in stock.

On occasion, you may have trouble getting the microscope to focus properly. If you have difficulty focusing on the slide, check the following:
- The eyepieces are in focus.
- The condenser is all the way up next to the slide stage, except if viewing slides with very low contrast (fecal flotation smears, other wet preparation slides).
- The condenser is centered.
- Diaphragms are typically located at the light source and on the condenser. In general, they should be open.
- The appropriate (specimen) side of the slide is on top (especially if you can focus on low power but cannot focus on high power).

Stains

Many different types of cytologic stains are available. The most commonly used are Romanowsky-type stains, including quick stains, Wright's stain, and Giemsa stain. Quick stains (e.g., Diff-Quik) are most commonly used in veterinary practice because of their relatively low cost and fast staining time (approximately 30 to 60 seconds). Routine Wright's or Giemsa staining takes longer, generally 15 to 20 minutes, but typically gives better and more consistent staining quality. All of these stains are *polychromatic,* meaning they stain specimens pink to purple to blue. They are meant to be used on air-dried smears. Cytologic smears do not require fixation before staining unless more than 72 hours will elapse between the time of slide preparation and staining. All of these stains provide excellent cytologic quality when used properly.

Although quick stains are advantageous in terms of convenience and time, they have some drawbacks. They tend to give a bluer color than routine staining, they may not stain metachromatic granules (mast-cell or basophil granules), and they are somewhat inconsistent in staining quality from slide to slide. Also, some quick stains use a single solution for dipping; others use three. Although one-solution quick stains are the most convenient, they are the least flexible in trying to correct a staining problem.

The typical problems associated with Romanowsky-type stains include excessive pink or blue staining, uneven staining on the slide, and precipitate on the slide. Excessive blue staining is caused by overstaining, inadequate washing, overly thick smears, excessively alkaline pH of the stain, or exposure to formalin fumes. Excessive pink staining is caused by understaining, prolonged washing, or an acidic stain. Uneven staining of the slide is typically due to variable thickness of the smear, variation of slide surface pH (e.g., dirty slides) and inadequate mixing of the stain and buffer. Finally, precipitate on slides is typically caused by inadequate stain filtration and/or washing of slides. Most stains typically are supplied with good instructions on how the stain should be used, including preparing slides, dipping slides, and filtering and changing stains. These instructions should be followed closely to avoid the problems noted previously.

Other types of stains that may be useful in a veterinary practice include new methylene blue (NMB) and Gram stain. NMB is most commonly used to stain reticulocytes. However, it may also be used on air-dried smears as a wet preparation to quickly assess slides for cellularity, to examine for fungal elements, or to assess nuclear morphology, particularly when thick cell clusters are present. The slides are stained by putting a drop or two of NMB on an air-dried smear and covering the area with a coverslip for immediate examination. The drawback to this technique is that cytoplasmic staining is minimal and the staining is not permanent.

Gram stain is used to identify bacteria and classify them as gram negative (stain pink) or gram positive (stain blue). Most bacteria can also be found with Wright's or quick stains, but they always stain blue and cannot be classified as gram positive or gram negative. This is not a big problem in that all bacterial cocci of veterinary importance are gram positive, whereas most, but not all, bacterial bacilli are gram negative. Gram stain is not useful for evaluating the morphology of cells.

Papanicolaou (Pap) stains and Sano trichrome stains are used on wet-fixed specimens, that is, the slides are *fixed* before drying. These stains require immediate fixation with 95% ethanol before the sample dries on the slide. Although used routinely in human medicine, they are used infrequently in veterinary medicine.

CYTOLOGIC PROCEDURES

Fine-needle aspiration is used to collect material from lymph nodes, cutaneous or subcutaneous masses, and thoracic or abdominal viscera or masses (Box 11-28). Various methods for collecting fine-needle aspirates exist, but they all basically require inserting a needle into a mass, lymph node, or organ and aspirating a small amount of material. Needles of various sizes may be used; the smaller needles (22 or 25 gauge) are less likely to cause hemorrhage but also are less likely to collect large numbers of cells. Larger needles (18 to 20 gauge) typically collect larger numbers of cells but are more likely to cause hemorrhage. In addition, a large-bore needle may collect only tissue cores that are unsuitable for cytologic evaluation. The type of tissue being aspirated (likely to exfoliate cells or likely to bleed) should dictate what size of needle is used. If the sample is to be cultured, surgically prepare the site before aspi-

ration. Otherwise, do the same type of site preparation as is done for venipuncture or vaccination.

Attach the needle to a syringe (6 to 12 ml) so that negative pressure is applied when aspirating or the needle may be redirected through the tissue by hand. In tissues likely to exfoliate large numbers of cells (lymph nodes, round-cell tumors, some epithelial tumors), simply redirecting a needle through the tissue by hand may collect enough cells for evaluation (Fig. 11-51). In other cases, it is helpful to apply negative pressure (suction) with the syringe plunger while collecting material to increase the yield of cells (Fig. 11-52). If you use a syringe, it is important to apply negative pressure (by pulling back on the plunger) only while the needle is embedded in the tissue. Take care not to remove or push the needle out of the mass before release of negative pressure. This avoids contaminating the sample with the surrounding tissue or sucking the aspirated material into the barrel of the syringe, where it cannot be recovered.

Preparing Slides

After you collect cells in the needle, they must be applied to a slide in a layer thin enough to evaluate but still intact. If the sample is bloody or contains more than a few drops of proteinaceous fluid, prepare the slide quickly, before the sample clots. Various techniques have been described for making cytologic smears.

For most samples, *squash preparation* is adequate (Box 11-29) (Fig. 11-53). Attach the needle containing the aspirated material to a 6- or 12-ml syringe with the

---

Box 11-28 Fine-needle aspiration

Materials:

20-, 22-, 25-gauge needles

1- to 1.5-inch needles

6- to 12-ml syringes

glass slides

Procedure:

1. Clean the site.
2. Immobilize the mass or lymph node with one hand.
3. Insert the needle into the mass and redirect through the mass while aspirating to collect cells.
4. Release pressure from the syringe plunger before removing the needle from the mass.
5. Prepare squash or push smears immediately.

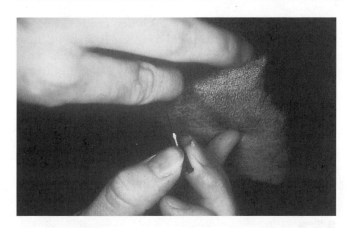

FIG. 11-51 Fine-needle apsiration using only a needle. The cutaneous and/or subcutaneous mass is usually immobilized using one hand. In this case, the mass is so large both hands are needed. The hair has been clipped to better visualize the area. After redirecting the needle through the mass, the needle is removed from the mass, then attached to a syringe with the plunger withdrawn in preparation for making a squash smear. *(Photo courtesy of Dr. Anthony Carr, University of Wisconsin, Madison).*

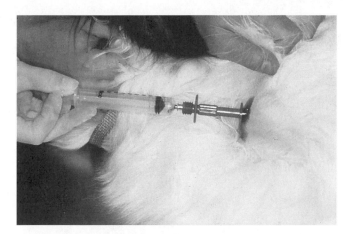

FIG. 11-52 Bone marrow aspiration. A syringe is used to apply negative pressure (suction) while the needle is embedded in the marrow cavity. The same type of negative pressure is used when using a syringe for fine-needle aspiration of masses. Negative pressure must be released before the needle is removed from the mass (marrow in this case). *(Photo courtesy of Dr. Anthony Carr, University of Wisconsin, Madison).*

plunger pulled back. If the needle was already on the syringe from sample collection, remove the needle from the syringe before drawing back on the plunger. Then reattach the needle to the syringe. Gently expel the material in the needle onto one end of a glass slide. Place a second slide over this material, either at a right angle or in a parallel but offset fashion. Minimal pressure is applied to this second slide; it should gently compress the aspirated material into a monolayer of cells. If the slides are too forcefully pushed together, many of the cells will be ruptured. The second slide is then quickly pulled across the first slide to spread the sample. The goal is to make an oval smear with a feathered edge that occupies the middle two-thirds of the slide. This technique works for most samples except those that are very bloody or contain a lot of fluid. In those cases, it is typically better to make a *push smear* (see following page).

After the smears are made, allow the slides to air dry. In general, even if the slides are to be reviewed by a cytopathologist, it is a good idea to stain at least one slide to assess for adequate cellularity and good smearing technique. A properly prepared slide contains few ruptured cells and an area on the smear that is thin enough so that cytomorphologic features can be evalu-

---

Box 11-29 Preparing squash smears

Materials:

glass slides

Procedure:

1. Place one drop of aspirated material on one end of a slide.
2. Place a second slide gently on top of and parallel or at a right angle to the first.
3. Pull the second slide across the surface of the first slide.
4. Allow the slides to air dry.

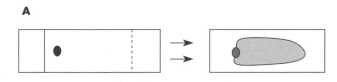

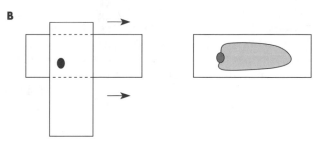

FIG. 11-53 Squash smear. The second slide may be placed in a parallel, **A,** or perpendicular, **B,** orientation. Care should be taken not to push forcefully on the two slides, because most of the cells would be ruptured.

ated. Frequently, this area is located toward the feathered edge of the smear, but all areas of the slide should be evaluated.

As opposed to solid-tissue aspirates, fluid samples must be prepared as *push smears* in the same way as blood smears are made (Box 11-30) (Fig. 11-54). Although making good-quality push smears seems difficult at first, with practice it is relatively easy to master. The key is to practice the technique before you need to make good smears for a clinical case.

Place a drop of fluid at one end of a slide. Place a second slide's short edge at an angle, approximately 45 degrees, onto the surface of the first slide and back into the drop. The fluid spreads along the edge of the slide. Advance the second slide across the first slide. Advance the slide in a smooth manner, the speed of which is determined by the viscosity of the fluid. With thin, low-protein fluids, advance the slide rapidly; thicker, high-protein fluids require a slower speed. As with the squash preparation, the goal of a push smear is to have an oval smear filling two-thirds of the slide, with the far edge feathered. If the smear continues all the way to the edge of the first slide, cells may be lost for evaluation. In this situation, either too much fluid was used or the smear was not made quickly enough. Remake the smear with a smaller drop of fluid or quicker motion of the spreader slide. Alternatively, the angle of the spreader slide may be changed. Increasing the angle shortens the smear, whereas decreasing the angle lengthens it.

Impression smears may be made directly from an oozing lesion or from biopsied tissue specimens (Box 11-31). The value of impression smears is they allow immediate evaluation of the type of pathologic process occurring in a lesion or quick identification of infectious agents. When you make impression smears from biopsied tissue samples, follow the ensuing procedure. Hold the tissue with forceps and lightly blot it against a gauze sponge or paper towel to remove excess fluid or blood. Repeat this as often as necessary until the specimen does not leave a bloody mark. Then lightly touch the specimen to the surface of a clean glass slide, with repeated multiple impressions made along the length of the slide. If the sample is particularly bloody, alternate blotting with the impression smears. Resist the temptation to forcefully smash the tissue onto the slide or smear it, because this results in smudged and ruptured cells. Some types of tissue samples, such as biopsies from mesenchymal tumors, are less likely to exfoliate cells in this manner. In these cases, it may be useful to scrape the tissue with the edge of a scalpel blade and then use the material collected on the blade to make a squash preparation on a glass slide.

Fluid analysis involves assessing the physical properties of the fluid (color, transparency, odor), counting cells, measuring protein content, and performing a cyto-

logic examination (Box 11-32). When fluid is collected from a cavity, save some of the sample in a sterile, non-anticoagulated (red-top) tube in case culture is later deemed necessary. In addition, it may be helpful to put some fluid in a tube containing anticoagulant (lavender top). You may perform cytologic evaluation on the sample in either tube, but reserving an anticoagulated sample is helpful if the sample contains a lot of blood or fibrin. Even if a cytopathologist will examine this fluid, prepare slides immediately so that cell morphology is preserved until examination.

Box 11-30 Preparing push smears

Materials:

glass slides

Procedure:

1. Place one drop of aspirated fluid on one end of a slide.
2. Put a second slide at 45-degree angle on the first slide in front of the material.
3. Draw the second slide back into the drop and allow it to spread along the edge of the second slide.
4. Push the second slide across the surface of the first.
5. Allow the slides to air dry.

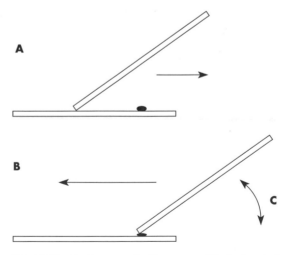

FIG. 11-54 Push smear. **A,** The upper slide is slowly drawn back into the drop of fluid. The fluid is allowed to spread along the edge of this slide until it nearly reaches the edges. **B,** This slide is then pushed along the surface of the first slide to make the smear. **C,** The length of the smear can be varied by altering the pushing speed, changing the amount of fluid on the slide, or changing the angle of the top slide.

Box 11-31 Preparing impression smears

Materials:

scalpel

forceps

paper towels and/or gauze sponges

glass slides

Procedure:

1. Hold the tissue fragment with forceps.
2. Blot excess fluid on a paper towel or gauze sponge.
3. Gently touch the tissue to the surface of a slide repeatedly down the length of the slide.
4. Allow the slide to air dry.
5. Place the tissue fragment in formalin for histologic evaluation.

Box 11-32 Fluid analysis

Materials:

hemacytometer

WBC Unopette (Becton Dickinson)

refractometer

glass slides

Procedure:

1. Collect a fluid sample in an aseptic manner.
2. Count the cells using a hematocytometer. If the fluid is turbid, a WBC Unopette may be helpful.
3. Make air-dried push smears.
4. If the fluid is turbid, spin it in a centrifuge and separate off the supernatant.
5. Measure the specific gravity and/or protein concentration of the fluid or supernatant using a refractometer.
6. If the cell count is low, make air-dried sediment smears.

If the fluid is not very cellular, prepare sediment smears for cytologic evaluation. If the fluid is not turbid, it is likely that cell counts are low enough for a sediment smear to be prepared. In this case, spin the fluid down in a centrifuge at 150 to 300 G for 2 to 5 minutes (as with urine sediment). In most urine centrifuges, a speed of 500 to 1500 RPM is satisfactory for making sediment smears. Then decant the supernatant off and gently resuspend the sediment at the bottom in the remaining few drops of fluid. Use this material to make a push smear. Occasionally, in fluids with very low protein concentrations, it is helpful to add a drop of bovine serum albumin or a drop of serum from any animal to the resuspended cells. This added protein helps protect the cells from rupturing when making the smear.

In addition to making smears for cytologic evaluation, cell counts, specific gravity, and protein concentration are assessed in complete fluid analyses. Manual cell counts are possible using a Unopette (Becton Dickinson) WBC diluter and a hemacytometer. These items are used in the identical manner in which manual cell counts are made on a complete blood count (CBC). If a very low cell count is expected (less than 500 cells/μl), as with cerebrospinal fluid, make direct counts of the fluid using the hemacytometer. If a hemacytometer is not available, an alternative is to make rough estimates by counting the cells observed in each 40$\times$ or 50$\times$ field for approximately 10 fields. Although every microscope must be standardized for these kinds of estimates, a rough guide is to estimate approximately 1000 to 1500 cells/μl for every cell counted using the 40$\times$ or 50$\times$ lens. For example, an average of 7 cells/40$\times$ field is roughly equivalent to 7000 to 10,500 cells/μl.

A refractometer assesses the protein concentration of the fluid. Refractometry is based on both the size and number of particles in solution. For this reason, if the fluid is turbid or cloudy, perform the refractometer reading on the supernatant fluid after centrifugation to avoid artificially high protein readings because of cells or other suspended particulate matter. A chylous effusion invariably gives a high protein measurement from the interference caused by lipids in the fluid.

Fluid analysis is important for any fluid in which cell counts and refractometer readings, in addition to cytologic analysis, would be helpful in determining the pathologic process causing the fluid accumulation. In particular, this can be helpful for abdominal and thoracic effusions. Other fluids in which complete fluid analysis is helpful include synovial and cerebrospinal fluids. For fluid collection from a subcutaneous mass, such as a seroma or hematoma, fluid analysis (cell counts and refractometer readings) is typically not helpful, although cytologic evaluation of a smear may be.

Fluid accumulation in the thoracic or abdominal cavity is abnormal. When excessive fluid is present in these cavities, fluid is collected from them for both diagnostic and therapeutic purposes (Box 11-33). Analysis of the fluid may help to determine whether the accumulation is due to heart failure, liver disease, neoplasia, inflammatory disease, sepsis, or hemorrhage. To best make this determination, do a complete fluid analysis. If an

Box 11-33 Abdominocentesis and thoracentesis

Materials:

surgical prep materials

local anesthetic

18- or 20-gauge, over-the-needle catheter or needles (cats, dogs)

2- or 3-inch teat cannula, bitch catheter, 18-gauge, 1½-inch needle (cattle, horses)

6- to 12-ml syringe

red-top, lavender-top tubes

3-way stopcock (thoracentesis)

sterile IV extension tubing (horses)

Procedure:

1. Anesthetize or tranquilize the animal as necessary.
2. Surgically prepare the site (thorax: cranial rib ventral to the fluid line; abdomen: ventral midline). Local anesthetic may be used to infiltrate site the site of catheter, needle, or cannula insertion.
3. Insert the needle or catheter in the appropriate location. If using a needle, use care to avoid lacerating internal organs. Attach the needle or catheter to a three-way stopcock or syringe when entering the thoracic cavity to avoid causing pneumothorax.
4. Use a three-way stopcock between the catheter and syringe if you are collecting multiple syringefuls from thoracic cavity. IV extension tubing is also helpful, particularly when draining large volumes of thoracic fluid from a horse. Collect samples in a red-top and lavender-top tube if the sample is very bloody.
5. Catch the fluid as it falls from the needle into a red-top and lavender-top tube for abdominocentesis. Withdraw fluid with a syringe for thoracentesis.
6. Prepare push smears from the fluid samples. If sediment smears are required, also prepare these. Allow the slides to air dry.
7. Perform a cell count. Assess specific gravity (protein content) using a refractometer on the supernatant after centrifugation.

inflammatory or septic process is a consideration, save some fluid in a sterile, non-anticoagulated (clot) tube (red-top).

Cerebrospinal fluid (CSF) is collected to assess the functional status on the central nervous system (Box 11-34). Changes in cell numbers, nucleated cell differential counts, and protein content are used to differentiate among neoplastic, degenerative, or inflammatory diseases. Cell numbers and protein content in CSF are generally quite low, even with significant disease. For this reason, although the same general type of approach is done regarding fluid analysis, special instrumentation is helpful in assessing CSF. If possible, use a cytocentrifuge to make concentrated smears. The cytocentrifuge sediments cells from an aliquot of fluid directly onto a slide, minimizing ruptured cells and also concentrating the cells to a greater degree than can be achieved with regular sediment smears. Protein content of CSF must be measured by a chemical method because a refractometer generally cannot measure the small amounts of protein found in CSF.

As previously mentioned, it is usually necessary to make very concentrated smears for cytologic analysis of CSF. In a referral laboratory, this is usually accomplished by using a cytocentrifuge. Most practices do not have this piece of equipment, but this type of technique can be approached by making a sedimentation chamber out of a 16-mm-diameter test tube with the ends cut off. One end of this barrel is seated onto a glass slide with petroleum jelly. Add fluid to the barrel (approximately 0.5 ml) and allow cells to sediment onto the surface of the slide by gravitation for at least 30 minutes. Remove the supernatant by aspiration, remove the tube, and quickly wick away residual fluid with filter paper. Allow the slide to air dry and clean off the petroleum jelly before staining. If slides are not prepared within 30 to 60 minutes, it may be helpful to preserve cells for cytologic evaluation by adding 8 to 10 drops of CSF to 1 ml of 40% ethanol. If the sample is to be submitted to a laboratory, contact the laboratory before sample collection to determine how the CSF should be handled.

Synovial fluid analysis is most useful in distinguishing inflammatory from noninflammatory causes of joint disease. On rare occasions, the analysis may identify etiologic agents, such as bacteria. Synovial fluid is handled in a similar way as other fluids, although the sample obtained may be of low volume, depending on the species and joint sampled. As with analysis of other fluids, joint fluid analysis entails a three-part examination: assessment of physical properties, cell counts, and cytologic examination (Box 11-35). Assessment of physical properties include color, transparency, specific gravity and/or total protein content, viscosity, and a mucin clot test.

Cell counts should include both red and white blood cell counts; these may be done with a hemacytometer.

Box 11-34 Cerebrospinal fluid smears

Materials:

surgical prep material

20- or 22-gauge, 1½- to 3-inch spinal needle with stylet (dogs, cats)

18-gauge, 7- or 8-inch spinal needle (horses)

18-gauge, 3½-inch spinal needle (most ruminants)

red-top tube, lavender-top tube

Procedure:

1. Induce general anesthesia, lateral recumbency (dogs, cats); standing and sedated (horses, cattle).
2. Surgically prepare the dorsal cervical area (small animals) or lumbosacral area (large animals).
3. Advance the needle into the subarachnoid space at the cisterna magna or lumbar cistern.
4. Remove the stylet and collect fluid in a red-top tube and a lavender-top tube (if bloody).
5. Collect approximately 1 to 3 ml in dogs, 0.5 to 1 ml in cats, 3 ml in large animals.
6. Prepare a cytospin or sedimentation smear or submit the fluid directly to a laboratory.

Box 11-35 Synovial fluid smears

Materials:

WBC Unopette (Becton Dickinson)

3- to 6-ml syringe

20-gauge, 1-inch needles

red-top tube, lavender-top tube

Procedure:

1. Tranquilize or sedate the animal as necessary.
2. Prepare the site using aseptic technique.
3. Attach the needle to the syringe and insert the needle into the joint.
4. Aspirate fluid.
5. If the sample is bloody, put some of the fluid in a lavender-top tube; otherwise use a red-top tube.
6. Prepare two push smears immediately and air dry.
7. Handle the fluid aseptically if culture may be indicated.

If only a small amount of fluid is available, prepare smears for cytologic examination before cell counts, because you may then estimate cell numbers off of the slide. Smears are made in the same manner as other fluids. Read total protein content or specific gravity from a refractometer. If the fluid is turbid, do this reading on the supernatant fluid after centrifuging. Assess viscosity in a subjective manner by evaluating how the fluid strings out between the thumb and index finger. Synovial fluid of good viscosity should string out to a length greater than 2 cm before breaking. The mucin clot test assesses the amount of mucin in the fluid. Add a few drops of synovial fluid to 2 ml of 2.5% acetic acid. Normal synovial fluid forms a thick, ropy precipitate, whereas abnormal synovial fluid forms little or no precipitate. If the volume of synovial fluid collected is limited, making smears and saving some for culture should have the highest priority.

Tracheal washes and bronchoalveolar lavages procedures are performed to assess the upper and lower respiratory tract for disease, as well as to identify infectious agents or neoplastic disease. Tracheal washes are collected via endotracheal tube or through a catheter inserted through the skin into the trachea (transtracheal) (Box 11-36). The transtracheal procedure is done in a sterile manner and the recovered fluid should be suitable for culture because it is not contaminated by the oral flora. A good tracheal wash produces a small volume of cloudy fluid containing flocculent material. The fluid should be put in a sterile container (test tube, red-top tube, other sterile collection devices) and can be used both for cytologic and microbiologic examination. If there are no suspended flecks and the fluid looks clear, it is likely that cytologic analysis will not be very revealing.

Multiple types of smears can be made with this fluid. As with fluid analysis, even if the cytologic analysis is to be done elsewhere, smears should be prepared immediately to preserve cytologic detail. Remember to save some of the fluid and flecks for microbiologic examination. Pick out a small fleck of material with a pipette and make a squash preparation in the same manner as described for fine-needle aspirates. If no flecks are apparent, a sediment or cytocentrifuge smear can be made of the fluid. Direct smears of clear fluid, as mentioned previously, are usually not revealing.

Bronchoalveolar lavage is used to assess a localized area of the lower respiratory tract (bronchi, alveoli). Fluid recovered from this procedure may also be cultured, but the results may not be dependable. The procedure is not sterile because the oropharynx must be traversed by a catheter or endoscope to collect a sample.

Box 11-36 Tracheal wash and bronchoalveolar lavage

Materials:

surgical prep materials

local anesthetic

18-gauge jugular catheter

sterile polyethylene tubing and trocar (horses)

sterile scalpel blade

20- to 30-ml syringe

sterile buffered saline

endotracheal tube

Procedure:

1. A standing animal is preferred; sedation may be necessary. If an endotracheal tube is used, general anesthesia is necessary.
2. The transtracheal approach requires surgical preparation over the cricothyroid area.
3. Infiltrate a local anesthetic agent over the cricothyroid membrane and skin (dogs, cats) or over the tracheal rings (horses, cattle).
4. Make a stab incision with the scalpel blade in the anesthetized area.
5. Insert the catheter (or trocar) into the trachea and direct toward the tracheal bifurcation.
6. Attach a saline-filled syringe (approximately 10 ml for small dogs and cats, 20 ml for large dogs, 30 ml for large animals) and flush into the trachea. An unanesthetized animal typically coughs.
7. Bronchoalveolar lavages are done with an endoscope or through an endotracheal tube. Move the catheter or endoscope as far down the trachea as possible (until wedged in a bronchus) before infusing the fluid and aspirating.
8. Aspirate fluid into the syringe by pulling back on the plunger while gently pulling the catheter back and forth within the trachea. Only a portion of the fluid will be recovered.
9. Make two squash smears as soon as possible.

Bronchoalveolar fluids are typically less cellular than tracheal washes and sometimes do not have mucus flecks associated with them. Very commonly, only cytocentrifuge smears are prepared from these samples. Some reports have indicated that cell counts on bronchoalveolar lavage fluid are useful, as well as differential cell counts. To add more significance to the cell counts, note the amount of fluid infused into the lung and the amount recovered.

Bone marrow aspiration is generally done to assess nonregenerative anemia or other persistent cytopenias, leukemia, lymphoma, metastatic tumor cells, or infectious agents (Box 11-37). For the most complete evaluation, both marrow aspiration and core biopsy should be done at the same time, although many veterinarians biopsy only if aspiration does not yield any marrow. Because the marrow cavity is quite vascular, it is not unusual to obtain a moderate to large amount of blood contamination when aspirating. For this reason, it is essential to immediately make smears. In addition, some marrow may be saved in diluted EDTA.

Marrow smears are made in a similar manner as other aspirate smears. Expel the marrow aspirate onto a glass slide or Petri dish. Hold the slide or dish at an angle to allow excess blood to drain off and expose the coarse, grain-like marrow spicules. These can be transferred to another slide with a pipette or broken wooden swab. Place a second slide on top of the particle and allow it to gently squash the material. Then gently and smoothly slide this second slide across the surface of the first slide. Multiple slides should be made in this manner and allowed to air dry. Interpretation is generally done by a cytopathologist, but stain at least one slide to examine for cellularity and the presence of spicules.

Vaginal smears are used most commonly in dogs to detect estrus but can also be used to detect some pathologic processes (Box 11-38). In general, the smears are evaluated for increasing numbers of superficial squamous epithelial cells as estrus progresses. When the superficial cells make up more than 90% of all the epithelial cells on the smear, the bitch is in late estrus, is about to ovulate, and should be bred.

Submitting Slides to a Laboratory

Because cytologic evaluation typically involves examining relatively few cells, the yield of diagnostic information can be low, depending on the sample type. To maximize the chances of receiving a specific or etiologic diagnosis when submitting slides to a cytopathologist, pay particular attention to sample handling. Follow these recommendations when submitting samples for cytologic examination:

- Make multiple air-dried smears if possible. Slides do not have to be fixed before submission. Stain at least one slide to make sure the smears contain something to evaluate.
- Do not refrigerate slides after they have been prepared. Refrigeration allows moisture to condense on the smears, resulting in disruption of cells.
- Label all samples and/or slides with the number of the animal or owner's name and site of sample collection if multiple samples are submitted.
- If smears were prepared in a special manner, such as sediment smears prepared from fluid, be sure to note this on the submission form or on the slide.

Box 11-37 Bone marrow aspiration

Materials:

16- to 18-gauge, 1-inch bone marrow needles

sterile scalpel blade

Petri dish

glass slides

12- to 20-ml syringe

surgical prep materials

local anesthetic

Procedure:

1. Heavy sedation or anesthesia may be necessary but is not required.
2. Surgical preparation: different sites are used for marrow aspiration, including the iliac crest, trochanteric fossa of the proximal femur, proximal humerus, and sternebrae (horses).
3. Infiltrate a local anesthetic into the skin and periosteum.
4. Make a stab incision through the skin.
5. Advance the marrow aspiration needle into the bone in a twisting fashion until the tip is in the marrow cavity.
6. Remove the stylet and attach the syringe.
7. Apply negative pressure; stop when blood appears in the needle hub.
8. Make squash smears immediately. Save some marrow in diluted EDTA.
9. Stain at least one slide (the quickest way is with wet preparation NMB) to assess for cellularity. If the slide contains only blood but no marrow flecks, then reaspirate, perhaps at a different site.

- Do not package slides together with samples preserved in formalin. Formalin fumes can partially fix cells, altering their staining characteristics.
- Describe the animal (age, breed, sex, species), sample type, and clinical data on the submission form. This information is used by the pathologist to help interpret the sample. Omitting this information reduces the chances of accurate cytologic interpretation. If you have specific questions about the smears, write them on the submission form.
- Package the slides in a slide mailer to prevent breakage.

Box 11-38 Vaginal smears

Materials:

sterile saline

gauze sponges

cotton-tipped wooden swabs, 5-7 inches in length

glass slides

Procedure:

1. Gently clean the vulva and surrounding area.
2. Spread the labia and insert a cotton-tipped swab craniodorsally into the vaginal vault.
3. Redirect the swab more cranially and advance it.
4. Rotate the swab to collect cells, then remove.
5. Immediately roll the cotton tip the length of a glass slide at least twice.
6. Air dry the smear. Stain and evaluate.

RECOMMENDED READING

Ramsey DT: Cytologic examination of the eye, *Vet Technician* 15:131-139, 1994.

Tyler RD, Cowell RL: *Diagnostic cytology of the dog and cat*, ed 2, St Louis, 1997, Mosby.

URINALYSIS

A.E. THIESSEN

Complete examination of urine is a relatively simple, rapid, and inexpensive diagnostic procedure that can provide crucial information to the veterinarian. A complete urinalysis includes estimation of its solute concentration, evaluation of the physical properties (e.g., color, turbidity), and evaluation of the chemical constituents (e.g., protein, pH, glucose). Abnormalities in the urinalysis may reflect diseases in a variety of body systems, not only the renal and lower urinary tract.

URINE COLLECTION

Collect urine samples in clean glass or plastic containers. Sterile containers are not necessary unless you are performing a urine culture.

Voided Sample. A voided, free catch sample can be easy to obtain and is satisfactory for routine analysis but is the least desirable method for obtaining urine for culture. Before collection, wash the prepuce or vulva to decrease sample contamination. Urine voided during mid-stream flow is the optimum voided sample.

Manual Compression of the Urinary Bladder. Urine collected in this manner is also unsatisfactory for urine culture. After outlining the bladder by abdominal palpation, using one or both hands, exert moderate, gentle, steady pressure over as large an area of the bladder as possible to express the urine.

Catheterization. Catheterization of the urinary bladder is one of the two preferred methods of urine collection, especially if the urine is required for culture (cystocentesis is the other preferred method). Sterile rubber or flexible plastic catheters may be used. Catheterization must be done as aseptically and atraumatically as possible to avoid introduction of bacteria and other contaminants to the urinary tract and to avoid increased numbers of epithelial cells and erythrocytes in the sample.

Cystocentesis. This is the optimal method of urine collection if a culture is to be done because contact with the lower urogenital tract is completely avoided. Cystocentesis involves collection of a sterile urine sample by inserting a needle, attached to a syringe, directly into the urinary bladder through the ventral abdominal body wall.

SPECIMEN PRESERVATION

Once the urine sample has been obtained, perform the analysis as soon as possible to ensure accurate results. If the urine cannot be analyzed within 30 minutes of collection, refrigerate the sample in an air-tight container to slow the rate of artifactual changes. If the sample is refrigerated, allow it to come to room temperature before performing the urinalysis.

Color

Normal urine is pale yellow to amber and transparent. Normal equine urine is cloudy and darkens if allowed to stand. Red or reddish-brown urine indicates the presence of RBCs *(hematuria)*, hemoglobin *(hemoglobinuria)*, or possibly myoglobin *(myoglobinuria)*.

Odor

An ammonia odor in a freshly voided sample may occur with cystitis caused by urease-producing bacteria that have broken urea down to ammonia. A sweet, fruity odor suggests the presence of ketones and most often occurs with diabetes mellitus, acetonemia (ketosis) in cows, and pregnancy disease in ewes.

Specific Gravity

Urine specific gravity is defined as the weight of a quantity of urine relative to the weight of an equal amount

of distilled water. Colorless, pale yellow urine generally has a lower specific gravity than dark yellow urine. Specific gravity is most often determined using a refractometer or total solids meter.

The following tests can be performed using commercially available dry chemistry strips (e.g., Multistix, Bayer, Elkhart, IN).

Protein

Protein is normally present in very low quantities in the urine (at or below the limit of sensitivity of the urine reagent strips). Physiologic (nonpathologic) proteinuria can occur with fever or strenuous exercise that results in increased permeability of the glomeruli to plasma proteins. Postrenal proteinuria is the result of serum proteins being added from hemorrhage or inflammation in the lower urinary tract (bladder) or genital tract. Renal proteinuria is fairly common and may be due to glomerular damage.

Glucose

Glucose is normally not present in the urine in quantities detectable on dipsticks. The presence of glucose in the urine is called *glucosuria* or *glycosuria*. Glucosuria occurs with any condition that causes the blood glucose level to exceed the renal threshold for resorption. Diabetes mellitus is a common cause of glucosuria resulting from excessive blood glucose concentrations.

Ketones

Ketonuria can occur with diabetes mellitus in small animals, during lactation in cows, and during pregnancy in cows and ewes. It also occurs with high-fat diets, starvation, fasting, anorexia, and impaired liver function.

pH

The pH is an indication of the hydrogen ion (H+) concentration, and it is a measure of the degree of acidity or alkalinity of urine. A pH greater than 7.0 is alkaline; a pH below 7.0 is acidic. High-protein diets produce a lower urine pH, whereas vegetable diets result in high urine pH. Carnivores typically have acidic urine, whereas herbivores have alkaline urine. Nursing herbivores have acidic urine from consumption of milk.

Bilirubin

Normal dogs occasionally have small amounts of bilirubin in their urine. Any bilirubinuria is abnormal in other species. Bilirubinuria can be seen with a number of diseases, including hemolytic diseases, hepatic insufficiency, and diseases that cause obstruction of bile flow.

Occult Blood

The occult blood reagent detects both myoglobin and hemoglobin in urine. The hemoglobin may be free hemoglobin *(hemoglobinuria)* or within intact erythrocytes *(hematuria)*. Hematuria is detected by a positive occult blood test, along with observation of intact red blood cells on urine sediment examination. Moderate to large amounts of blood impart a cloudy red, brown, or wine color to urine. Similar colors, but with a transparent appearance, that remain after centrifugation indicate hemoglobinuria. Hemoglobinuria is usually due to intravascular hemolysis. Myoglobin is a protein found in muscle. Myoglobinuria is usually seen in horses with rhabdomyolysis. A positive occult blood reading is most commonly associated with hematuria, rather than with hemoglobinuria.

URINARY SEDIMENT

Microscopic examination of urinary sediment is an important component of a complete urinalysis and should be included with every urinalysis. If the sediment cannot be examined within 30 minutes after collection, refrigerate the urine in an air-tight container. Centrifuge the sample at approximately 100 G (1000-2000 RPM) for 3 to 5 minutes. Carefully remove the supernatant from the test tube, leaving approximately 0.3 ml, by decanting or with a pipette and saved for chemical analysis. Allow the remaining urine to run back to the bottom of the centrifuge tube, and resuspend the sediment by gently flicking the bottom of the tube. The sediment may be microscopically examined either stained or unstained.

Erythrocytes (RBCs)

Up to five RBCs per high-power field (Fig. 11-55) is considered normal. RBCs are smaller than WBCs or epithelial cells, so they are round and slightly refractile and lack internal structure.

In concentrated urine, the RBCs crenate (shrivel); in dilute urine they swell and lyse, and appear as colorless rings (ghost cells) that vary in size and shape.

Leukocytes (WBCs)

Up to five WBCs per high-power field can be found in the urine sediment of normal animals (see Fig. 11-55). These cells are round and granular, larger than RBCs, and smaller than epithelial cells. They degenerate in old urine and may lyse in hypotonic or alkaline urine.

Epithelial Cells

Epithelial cells are usually found in small numbers in the urine (see Fig. 11-55). Transitional epithelial cells originate from the bladder, ureters, renal pelvis, and proximal urethra. These cells are variably sized; oval, spindle, or caudate in shape; and granular. Squamous epithelial cells originate from the distal urethra, vagina, vulva, and pre-

puce, and are present normally in voided samples. They are large cells with irregular, angular margins, and a small nucleus. Renal epithelial cells originate from renal tubules and are the smallest epithelial cells seen in urine. They are small, round, and slightly larger than WBCs. These cells usually degenerate and are difficult to identify and are different than leukocytes.

Casts

Urinary casts are molds of proteins that form in the loop of Henle and distal tubules of the kidney (Fig. 11-56). Cast types include cellular casts, hyaline casts, granular casts, and waxy casts, depending on the material trapped in the protein matrix at the time of formation and the age of the casts. Casts dissolve in alkaline urine, so identification and quantitation are best done with fresh urine samples. Casts may also be disrupted with high-speed centrifugation and rough urine handling. A small number of hyaline casts or granular casts (1 or 2/lower-power field) may be seen in normal urine, but larger numbers of casts (called *cylindruria*) localize a disease process to the kidneys.

Crystals

The presence of crystals in the urine is called *crystalluria* (Fig. 11-57). Formation of crystals is dependent on the amount of the substance in the urine, the solubility of the particular crystal type, urine pH, and urine temperature. Triple phosphate crystals are commonly found in the slightly acidic urine of dogs and cats. They may be found in the urine of normal animals or in the urine of animals with urinary stones *(urolithiasis)*. Amorphous phosphate crystals are common in alkaline urine. These crystals appear as a granular precipitate. Calcium carbonate crystals are commonly found in the urine of normal horses and cattle. These crystals resemble colorless "dumbbells" and can be seen in neutral or alkaline urine.

Amorphous urate crystals, seen in acidic urine, resemble amorphous phosphates (a granular precipitate), but amorphous phosphates are seen in alkaline urine. Ammonium biurate crystals are round and brownish, with long spicules (thorn apple–shaped) and are not present in the urine of normal animals; they are seen in the urine of animals with liver disease or portosystemic shunts.

Calcium oxalate dihydrate crystals can be found in the urine of normal animals. They are seen in acidic, neutral, or alkaline urine, and appear as small squares or "envelopes" containing an X. These crystals can be associated with oxalate ingestion in large animals and ethylene glycol (antifreeze) poisoning in small animals. Calcium oxalate monohydrate crystals are most commonly associated with ethylene glycol (antifreeze) poisoning but can also be seen in the animals with cal-

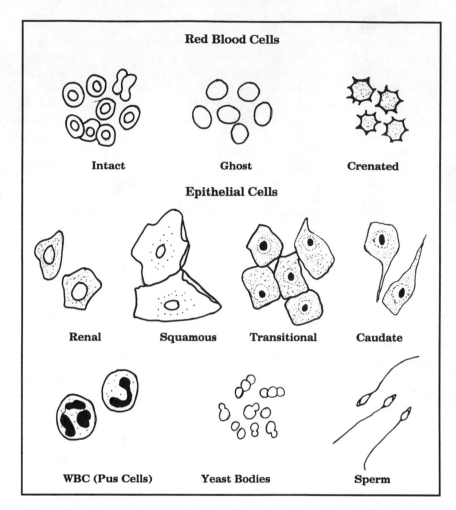

FIG. 11-55 Cell types that may be observed in urine. *(From Pratt PW: Laboratory procedures for veterinary technicians, ed 2, St Louis, 1992, Mosby.)*

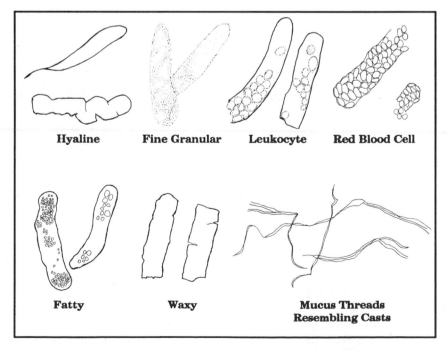

FIG. 11-56 Types of casts that may be observed in urine. *(From Pratt PW: Laboratory procedures for veterinary technicians, ed 2, St Louis, 1992, Mosby.)*

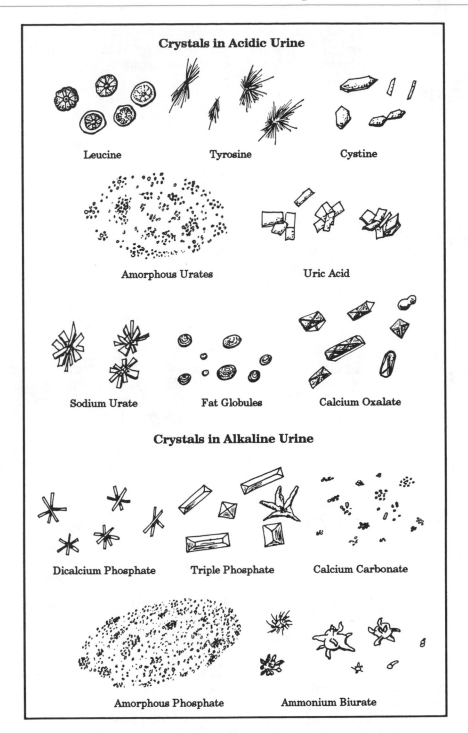

FIG. 11-57 Types of crystals that may be observed in urine. *(From Pratt PW: Laboratory procedures for veterinary technicians, ed 2, St Louis, 1992, Mosby.)*

cium oxalate urolithiasis. Uric acid crystals can be seen in alkaline urine and are associated with a metabolic defect (most common in Dalmatians) and formation of uroliths. Cystine crystals are seen in acidic urine and appear as flat, hexagonal (six-sided) plates. These crystals are associated with a metabolic defect in cysteine metabolism and may be associated with uroliths.

Bacteria

Bacteria may be present as the result of infection or contamination. Normal urine is free of bacteria but may be contaminated by bacteria from the distal urethra and genital tract. Urine obtained by cystocentesis is the preferred sample for evaluation of bacteria because contamination is avoided. Bacteria numbers are reported as few, moderate, or many. Because bacteria often proliferate in urine that has been left standing for some time, it is important to examine a fresh sample.

RECOMMENDED READING

Duncan JR, Prasse KW, Mahaffey EA: *Veterinary laboratory medicine*, ed 3, Ames, Iowa, 1994, Iowa State University Press.
Ling GV: *Lower urinary tract diseases of dogs and cats,* St Louis, 1995, Mosby.
Pratt PW: *Laboratory procedures for veterinary technicians,* ed 3, St Louis, 1997, Mosby.
Pringle J: *Pathophysiology and diagnosis of urinary diseases.* In Kobluk CN, Ames TR, Geor RJ, eds: *The horse: diseases and clinical management,* Philadelphia, 1995, WB Saunders.

IMMUNOLOGY AND SEROLOGY

D.J. FISHER

The immune system is important in protecting an animal from developing diseases, as well as in combating diseases once they have been contracted. Immunity can generally be divided into two types: passive and active. Passive immunity includes maternal antibodies from colostrum and physicochemical barriers, such as the skin and mucous membranes. Active immunity is developed or acquired and is classified as humoral or cell-mediated immunity.

Humoral immunity is mediated by production of unique proteins *(antibodies),* which are responsible for specific recognition and elimination of antigens. *Antigens* are foreign substances, usually proteins, that can be bacterial, viral, fungal, or altered host cells. When an antibody encounters an antigen it recognizes, it binds to the antigen and forms a complex, facilitating its removal from the host. Cell-mediated immunity is dependent upon cells, in particular lymphocytes. Like antibodies, these lymphocytes recognize specific antigens, such as those of fungi, para-

sites, intracellular bacteria, or tumor cells, and help remove them from the animal by lysing the infected/cancerous cell or organism.

IMMUNOLOGIC TESTS

Dysfunction of the immune system can lead to an overactive immune system that produces immune-mediated disease, or an underactive immune system that produces immunodeficiency disorders. These disorders can involve any component of the immune system (passive, humoral, or cell-mediated). In addition, the cellular components of the immune system can undergo neoplastic transformation, resulting in lymphoma or plasma-cell tumor. Some routine tests in veterinary medicine to detect these disorders include the Coombs' test, antinuclear antibody test, serum protein electrophoresis, and immunoglobulin quantitation.

Coombs' Test

The Coombs' test detects immunoglobulin (IgG or IgM) or complement (C3) bound to the surface of erythrocytes. It is used to confirm the diagnosis of immune-mediated hemolytic anemia. In this test, RBCs from the patient are incubated with a species-specific antiglobulin reagent. The sample is then evaluated for agglutination (irregular clumps of 3 to 5 or more RBCs). Agglutination occurs if the erythrocytes have enough antibody or complement on their surface to allow cross linking between the cells. Although the Coombs' test is fairly simple to perform, the expense of stocking the species-specific Coombs' reagent for only occasional tests makes this test somewhat impractical to run in-house. An EDTA blood sample is required for a Coombs' test.

Antinuclear Antibody Test

The antinuclear antibody (ANA) test is an example of an indirect fluorescent antibody (IFA) test. This test is used to rule out the diagnosis of systemic lupus erythrematosus, a systemic autoimmune disorder. The patient's serum is serially diluted and the dilutions are added to slides coated with cells, such as mouse liver or tissue-culture cell lines. If the patient's serum contains antinuclear antibodies, these bind to the cells on the slides. The slides are washed to remove unbound antibody and are then further treated with species-specific antiglobulin, which is fluorescein-labeled. The fluorescein-labeled antibodies bind to antibody from the patient's serum that is now bound to the cells. The slides are then evaluated using a fluorescence microscope. A positive result is determined to the highest dilution, which is reported as a *titer.* Results from different laboratories should not be compared, as there may be variation in reagents used and the interpretation of fluorescence by different technicians.

The ANA test takes some expertise to run and requires specific reagents and special instrumentation and is thus not practical to run in-house. The ANA test requires a serum sample that may be kept refrigerated if the test is to be done soon or frozen if there will be a delay in testing.

Serum Protein Electrophoresis

Serum protein electrophoresis is occasionally done to help assess the cause of severe hyperproteinemia, in particular, hypergammaglobulinemia. The test requires approximately 0.5 ml of serum, which may be refrigerated or frozen. The serum is placed on a gel preparation and subjected to an electrical current. The size and charge of the various proteins (albumin, globulins) determine how far they migrate across the gel. These bands are then visualized by applying a protein-binding dye and the density of these bands (assessed by a densitometer) corresponds to the amount of protein present. A very sharp, dense band in the beta- or gamma-globulin region is called a *monoclonal spike,* typically associated with a lymphoid or plasma-cell tumor. On the other hand, a wide band in this region is associated with a polyclonal gammopathy, typically caused by chronic antigenic stimulation, such as feline infectious peritonitis or some types of chronic liver disease.

Immunoglobulin Measurement

Many tests are available for measurement of serum immunoglobulin levels. Some of the tests used to assess immunoglobulin levels are available in kit form for use in the clinic or in the field (Table 11-13). These tests are most useful for detection of failure of passive transfer of maternal antibodies (failure of a newborn to ingest adequate colostrum). They are most often used in large animal species. Two types of tests are generally available: field tests (refractometry, zinc sulfate precipitation, glutaraldehyde precipitation) and clinic or laboratory tests (radial immunodiffusion). Refractometry and precipitation tests provide semiquantitative estimates of immunoglobulin concentration within a few minutes. Radial immunodiffusion takes longer (24 to 48 hours) but measures levels of specific immunoglobulins. These tests generally require a small serum sample.

SEROLOGIC TESTS

Serologic testing is based on the ability to detect antibody-antigen interactions. Some ways in which antibody-antigen interactions are measured are listed in Table 11-14. Some of these methods apply to the tests mentioned previously. For example, the Coombs' test is an agglutination reaction and the ANA test is an immunofluorescence test. Serologic testing is used most frequently to detect an antibody response to a particular infectious agent. In some cases, the organism itself or, more specifically, an antigen from the organism may be detected. Serologic tests formerly required a reference laboratory; however, many kits are now available for in-house testing for a variety of infectious agents (see Table 11-13). Many of the kits are based on enzyme-linked immunosorbent assay (ELISA) technology and may detect either antigens (organism) or antibodies (humoral immune response), depending on the kit.

Enzyme-Linked Immunosorbent Assay

Enzyme-linked immunosorbent assay (ELISA) is based on the ability to produce monoclonal or polyclonal antibodies to a specific antigen or isolation and production of a specific antigen. In kits to detect antigens, antibody specific for the antigen is bound to the wall of a test well, wand, or membrane. The patient's sample (serum, plasma, or whole blood) is added. Any antigen present binds to the antibody. Thorough washing removes any unbound antibody. A second enzyme-labeled antibody is added and this also binds to the antigen of interest. A second thorough washing removes any unbound second antibody. Finally, a substrate (chromogen) is added to develop a specific color if the antigen is present. The ELISA to detect antibodies is similar, but a specific antigen is bound to the well, wand or membrane, rather than a specific antibody.

A drawback to these tests, when first introduced, was the numerous steps necessary and the precise timing involved to obtain accurate results. Most kits now have fewer steps, reducing the chance of human error (Fig. 11-58). Nevertheless, following the directions for each kit carefully is crucial to obtaining accurate results. Many of these test kits also include positive and negative controls to further improve the accuracy of the test. ELISA kits have great sensitivity and specificity, but only if the test procedures are followed completely. This includes storing the kit as described, rewarming reagents if necessary, using only the samples as specified, avoiding interfering agents (such as hemolysis) as specified, and disposing of expired kits and outdated instruction.

Latex Agglutination

Latex agglutination is commonly used to diagnose brucellosis in dogs. Latex particles are coated with *Brucella* antigen. Serum from the patient is added to these particles. If the animal's serum contains antibodies to *Brucella,* they form complexes with the latex particles, causing agglutination. The serum can further be manipulated to detect separate classes (IgG versus IgM) of antibody. Other kits using this methodology include tests for organisms that cause mastitis and for canine rheumatoid factor.

TABLE 11-13 Commercially available immunologic and serologic test kits

Product name	Detects/measures	Test type*	Specimen type	Manufacturer†
Bovine				
CITE *Brucella abortus* Antibody Test Kit	*B. abortus* antibodies	ELISA	Serum Plasma	IDEXX
D-tec *Brucella A*	*B. abortus* antibodies	Microwell ELISA	Serum Plasma	Synbiotics
Gamma-Check-B	Semiquantitative immunoglobulin	Glutaraldehyde precipitation	Whole blood serum	V.D.I.
Leukassay B	Antibody to bovine leukemia virus	AGID	Serum	Synbiotics
Rapid Johne's Test	Antibody to *Mycobacterum pseudotuberculosis*	AGID	Serum	ImmuCell
RMT (Rapid Mastitis Test)	*Strep aglactiae, Staph aureus*	Latex agglutination	Milk	ImmuCell
Canine				
Assure/CH	Adult heartworm antigen	Wand ELISA	Serum Plasma	Synbiotics
Canine *Borrelia burgdorferi* Antibody Test	Antibody to *B. burgdoferi* (Lyme disease)	ELISA	Serum Plasma	Remel
CITE *Borrelia burgdorferi* Antibody Test Kit	Antibody to *B. burgdoferi* (Lyme disease)	ELISA	Whole blood Serum Plasma	IDEXX
CITE Canine Parvovirus Test Kit	Parvovirus antigen	ELISA	Feces	IDEXX
CITE Probe Canine Parvovirus Antigen Test Kit	Parvovirus antigen	ELISA	Feces	IDEXX
CRF	Canine rheumatoid factor	Latex agglutination	Serum	Synbiotics
D-Tec CB	Antibody to *Brucella canis*	Slide agglutination	Serum	Synbiotics
DiroCHEK	Adult heartworm antigen	Microwell ELISA	Canine or feline serum plasma	Synbiotics
Gamma-Check-C	Semiquantitative immunoglobulins	Glutaraldehyde precipitation	Whole blood Serum	V.D.I.
ICT Gold HW	Adult heartworm antigen	ELISA	Whole blood Serum Plasma	Synbiotics
LymeCHEK	Antibodies to *B. burgdorferi*	Microwell ELISA	Whole blood Serum Plasma	Synbiotics
PetChek Canine Heartworm Antigen Test Kit	Adult heartworm antigen	ELISA	Canine or feline serum plasma	IDEXX
Snap Heartworm Antigen Test Kit	Adult heartworm antigen	ELISA	Serum Plasma	IDEXX
Uni-Tec CHW	Adult heartworm antigen	Membrane ELISA	Canine or feline serum plasma	Synbiotics
VetRED Canine Heartworm Antigen Test Kit	Adult heartworm antigen	RBC agglutination	Whole blood	Rhone Merieux

TABLE 11-13. Commercially available immunologic and serologic test kits—cont'd

Product name	Detects/measures	Test type*	Specimen type	Manufacturer†
Equine				
CITE Foal IgG Test Kit	Semiquantitative IgG concentration	ELISA	Whole blood Serum Plasma	IDEXX
D-Tec EIA	Antibody to equine infectious anemia virus	AGID	Serum	Synbiotics
Equine RID Test	Quantify IgG concentration	RID	Serum Plasma	V.D.I.
Gamma-Check-E	Semiquantitative immunoglobulin concentration	Glutaraldehyde precipitation	Whole blood Serum	V.D.I.
Feline				
Assure/FeLV	FeLV antigen	Wand ELISA	Whole blood Serum Plasma	Synbiotics
CITE Anti-FIV	FIV antibody	ELISA	Whole blood Serum Plasma	IDEXX
CITE Feline Leukemia Virus Test Kit	FeLV antigen	ELISA	Whole blood Serum Plasma	IDEXX
CITE Probe Combo FeLV AG/FIV Ab	FeLV antigen and FIV antibody	ELISA	Whole blood Serum Plasma	IDEXX
CITE Probe Feline Leukemia Virus Test Kit	FeLV antigen	ELISA	Whole blood Serum Plasma	IDEXX
DiaSystems FeLV Flex II Test Kit	FeLV antigen	ELISA	Saliva, tears Whole blood Serum Plasma	IDEXX
DiaSystems FIP Antibody Test Kit	Antibody to feline coronavirus	ELISA	Fluids including serum	IDEXX
PetChek FeLV	FeLV antigen	ELISA, 12-well setup	Serum Plasma	IDEXX
Uni-Tec FeLV	FeLV antigen	Membrane ELISA	Whole blood Serum Plasma	Synbiotics
ViraCHEK/FeLV	FeLV antigen	Microwell ELISA	Whole blood Serum Plasma	Synbiotics

*Abbreviations: ELISA = enzyme-linked immunosorbent assay; AGID = agar gel immunodiffusion; RID = radical immunodiffusion.
†Manufacturers' addresses:
  IDEXX Laboratories, Inc., One Idexx Drive, Westbrook, ME 04092; (207) 856-0300
  ImmuCell Corporation, 56 Evergreen Street, Portland, ME 04103; (207) 878-2770
  Remel L.P., 3351 Wrightsboro Road, Suite 502, Augusta, GA 30909
  Rhone Merieux Inc., 115 Transtech Drive, Athens, GA, 30601; (706) 548-9292
  Synbiotics Corp., 11011 Via Frontera, San Diego, CA 92127; (800) 228-4305
  V.D.I., 2671 Carpenter Canyon Road, San Luis Obispo, CA 93401; (805) 549-8066

TABLE 11-14 Methods used to detect antibody-antigen interactions

Test method	Principle	Use	Comments
Precipitation	Occurs between large soluble proteins and antibodies	Identify/quantify immuno-globulins; also identify bacterial, fungal, viral antigens	Cannot measure very low antigen or antibody concentration
Agglutination	Occurs between antibody and particles (RBCs, bacteria, beads)	Detects antibody on cells (specifically Coombs' test), identify bacteria or antibody to infectious agents	Antibody excess may cause false-negative results (prozone reaction)
Complement fixation	Complement plus antibody-antigen complexes lyse red cells	Detects complement-fixing antibody in serum; used in serodiagnosis of many viral, bacterial and mycotic diseases	Does not require purified antigen; most efficient at detecting IgM antibody (early phase)
Immunofluorescence	Antibody tagged with fluoro-chrome binds to immuno-globulin or infectious agent antigen	Used to diagnose immune-mediated disease directed at various tissues; detects infectious agents or specific antibodies in serum	Direct IFA detects antibody or antigen in tissue samples from patient; indirect IFA detects antibody or antigen in the serum
Enzyme-linked immunosorbent assay (ELISA)	Specific antibody or antigen bound to a surface binds to corresponding antigen or antibody; complex is detected by enzymatic reaction	Used to diagnose a wide variety of infectious diseases	Very sensitive technique

Immunodiffusion

Immunodiffusion is a type of precipitation test that detects antibody-antigen complexes (precipitates) that form as antigen and immunoglobulin diffuse through an agar gel plate. Wells are cut in this plate and the patient's serum is placed in one well and antigen is placed in the other. The two components diffuse toward one another and form a line of precipitation if specific antibody is present in the patient's serum. Antibodies to equine infectious anemia virus are detected and immunoglobulin levels measured with immunodiffusion tests.

Antibody Titers

Results of some antibody tests may be reported as positive or negative. In other words, the test indicates the presence or absence of antibody to the particular infectious agent in the animal's serum. Results of other antibody tests may be reported as antibody *titers*, or levels. The animal's serum is serially diluted to different concentrations, such as 1:10, 1:40 and 1:160, meaning one part of serum in nine parts of saline, one part of serum in 39 parts of saline, and one part of serum in 159 parts of saline. A test to detect antibodies (e.g., hemagglutination test, complement-fixation test, or IFA test) is done on each of these dilutions and the greatest dilution that

tests positive is reported. For example, if 1:10 and 1:40 are positive and 1:160 is negative, the titer is reported as 1:40. If none of the dilutions is positive, the titer may be reported as negative or the test may be repeated at lesser dilutions, such as 1:2, 1:4, or 1:8. A higher titer (positive at greater dilutions) indicates that more antibody is present. More antibody is present in a sample with a titer of 1:160 than in a sample with a titer of 1:40.

Note that antibody titers are conventionally expressed in terms of dilution. It is important to also note that when measuring titers of antibodies to infectious agents, typically titers are measured in two samples collected over a 2- to 4-week period to assess for a fourfold increase in antibody titer. An antibody titer in a single sample may indicate only that the animal has been previously exposed to an infectious agent; the animal may not currently have an active infection. A rising titer in two or more samples indicates an active infection. Usually it is best to run both titers at the same time to minimize the error in measuring antibody at two different times. This requires that the first sample be drawn, separated, frozen, and stored in such a way that it can be easily retrieved when the second sample is collected.

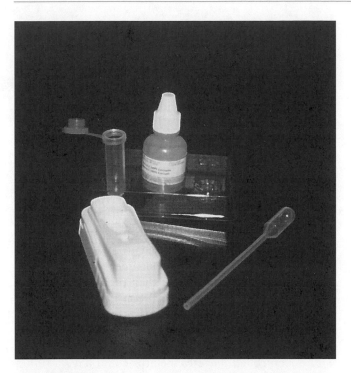

FIG. 11-58 Feline leukemia virus test kit (IDEXX). The kit provides all the materials necessary for detection of feline leukemia virus antigen in blood, serum, or plasma. The patient's sample is mixed with the conjugate in the provided tube. The contents are then placed in the white device. This device is activated by snapping it closed. The positive and negative controls and the patient sample on the device membrane are monitored for color development.

RECOMMENDED READING

Gershwin IJ, et al: Assays for humoral immunity including serology. In Gershwin L, Olsen RG, Krakowka S: *Immunology and immunopathology of domestic animals,* St Louis, 1995, Mosby.

Gorman NT, Halliwell REW: The immunoglobulins: structure, genetics, and function. In: *Veterinary Clinical Immunology,* Philadelphia, 1989, WB Saunders.

Hill E: Immunology and serology. In Pratt PW, ed: *Laboratory procedures for veterinary technicians,* ed 3, St Louis, 1997, Mosby.

Tizard I: Serology: the detection and measurement of antibodies. In Tizard I: *Veterinary immunology: an introduction,* ed 4, Philadelphia, 1992, WB Saunders.

QUALITY CONTROL

J. COLVILLE

Veterinarians expect veterinary technicians to present them with dependable analytic results. Through a well-planned and carefully controlled quality-control program, veterinary technicians can provide veterinarians with accurate laboratory results. *Quality control* (also called *quality insurance*) is a series of steps and procedures to ensure that the analytic results from a laboratory are representative of the state of the animal from which a sample was taken. If these *in vitro* results are to be of any value to a veterinarian, they must match as closely as possible the *in vivo* values of the animal at the time the sample was obtained.

IMPORTANCE OF QUALITY CONTROL

Inaccurate test results can lead a veterinarian to make an incorrect diagnosis. Based on inaccurate test results, the veterinarian might prescribe medications that are contraindicated or might withhold medications that are essential for recovery.

ACCURACY, PRECISION, AND RELIABILITY

Accuracy, precision, and reliability are terms frequently used to describe quality control. They form the basis of a quality-control program in a clinical laboratory setting. *Accuracy* refers to how closely the results a veterinary technician reports match the true quantitative value. Are the results correct? *Precision* is the extent of random errors and the reproducibility of measurements. In other words, if the technician repeated the analysis, would the results be the same? *Reliability* refers to the consistency of a method in producing accurate results. Also, are the analytic methods used in the laboratory appropriate for the type of testing being done? If they are, the results obtained by the veterinary technician will accurately reflect the state of health of the patient.

Instrument Maintenance

Proper instrument maintenance is essential to sustain peak instrument performance. All analytic instruments come with an operator's manual that outlines maintenance procedures to prolong the life of the instrument and prevent expensive down time when the instrument cannot be used. If a maintenance manual is not available for each instrument in the laboratory, contact the manufacturer for a replacement. The manual lists the instrument components that must be inspected and serviced regularly. These components can include the light source, rubber gaskets, plastic tubing, O rings, or thermocuvettes. Some of these components may need replacing, whereas others may need only cleaning. Whatever the case, timely maintenance in accordance with the manufacturer's recommendations is crucial. Any component of the instrument that is not functioning at 100% capacity can affect the results produced by the instrument.

The most efficient method of making sure maintenance is regularly performed is to set up a maintenance notebook containing a schedule of maintenance, listing each instrument in the laboratory on a separate page. Each page should include the instrument name, serial number and model number, components to be checked, frequency of checks, and a space for the date and initials of the technician performing the maintenance. The purchase date and price of the instrument can be included if that information is available (Fig. 11-59).

Samples

Commercially available solutions can be used in a quality-control program. Chemistry analyzers and electronic cell counters use control solutions as a means of instrument calibration and technician assessment. Control serum consists of pooled serum samples from numerous patients. Assayed control serum has been analyzed repeatedly by the manufacturer for each of the constituents present in the serum (e.g., glucose, blood urea nitrogen, calcium, enzymes). The results are statistically analyzed and a range of acceptable values for each constituent is established. The manufacturer then creates a chart that lists the range (lowest acceptable value to highest acceptable value obtained during the assays) and mean (average value) for each constituent. The pooled serum is then freeze-dried and packaged for sale to human and veterinary clinical laboratories for use in their quality-control programs.

Lyophilized (freeze-dried) control serum must be carefully rehydrated according to the manufacturer's directions if it is to produce accurate calibration. Once the powder is rehydrated, small aliquots of the control serum can be placed in small tubes, covered tightly, and frozen. The frozen aliquots can be thawed and used one at a time as needed. Control serum is analyzed in the veterinary clinical laboratory at the same time a patient sample is analyzed. It is handled exactly like patient serum. After the assay is completed, the control value is checked against the manufacturer's acceptable range. If the control value falls within the accepted range, the chances of the test results being accurate and precise are increased. If the control value does not fall within the acceptable range, the assay for both the control serum and the patient serum should be repeated.

The frequency with which control serum is analyzed is determined by each clinical laboratory. Ideally, control serum should be analyzed with every batch of tests. This sometimes becomes impractical, so the control serum is analyzed less frequently. Some clinical laboratories run control samples once a day; some only once a week. To ensure reliability, controls *must* be tested when a new assay is set up, a new technician runs the test, a new lot number of reagents is used, or an instrument is known to perform erratically.

In the same manner as control serum, control samples of whole blood are used to evaluate electronic cell counters. These controls are treated like patient samples when they are analyzed by the electronic cell counter. Again, the manufacturer analyzes pooled samples numerous times to determine the normal range and mean value of the control. To ensure reliability, the control sample must be tested when a new assay is set up, a new technician runs the test, a new lot number of reagents is used, or the cell counter is known to perform erratically.

Samples with normal and abnormal concentrations of constituents are available commercially. This is because an assay method may not perform the same at all concentrations tested by a particular analytic method. Abnormal control serum has constituent concentrations that are either higher or lower than the normal concentrations. If there is an abnormal constituent concentration in a patient sample, the results are more reliable if the abnormal control serum concentration produced results within the acceptable range. For example, a dog with uncontrolled diabetes mellitus could have a serum glucose level of 450 mg/dl. By using an abnormal control serum that contains glucose at an abnormally high concentration, one can feel more confident that the elevated glucose level in the patient's sample is accurate if the control serum assays were within the acceptable range.

Record Keeping

The results of assays of control samples should be recorded, graphed, and kept in a permanent file (Fig. 11-60). If the results of a control assay do not fall within the acceptable range, the sample should be reassayed. If the results are not within the acceptable range for the second assay, the instrument and the technician's technique must be evaluated. Factors that should be evaluated include instrument maintenance, housekeeping procedures, errors in labeling and transcription, pipetting technique, pipette performance, storage and handling of the patient sample, storage and handling of reagents and supplies, and instrument calibration. When the control sample values continually fall outside the acceptable range, there has been a shift of the mean itself and a systematic error is involved.

Graphing the control results enables the laboratory personnel to detect changes or trends in assay results. Fig. 11-60 shows an example of a control serum graph used in a clinical laboratory that assays control serum once a day.

Some manufacturers provide a quality-control service in which test samples are sent to many clinical laboratories for assay each month. The results from all the laboratories are collected and compared. From these results the manufacturer can identify laboratories with accuracy problems.

DUPONT ANALYST ROUTINE MAINTENANCE SCHEDULE
SERIAL #A61651.2.020 NDSU #140616

Month/Year

Day of the Month	1	2	3	4	5	6	7	8	9	10	11	12	13	14	15	16	17	18	19	20	21	22	23	24	25	26	27	28	29	30	31
Daily																															
Analyst																															
ensure surfaces are clean																															
Pipettor/Dilutor																															
prime with water when not in use																															
ensure fluid is present in lines																															
check unit for leaks/check air gap size																															
keep rotor prep station and unit clean																															
check aspirate tubing tip on handprobe																															
check purified water diluent level																															
Weekly																															
Pipettor/Dilutor																															
prime with recommended detergent																															
flush 10 times with purified water diluent																															
Monthly																															
calibrate with each method																															
analyst fan screen/filter maintenance																															

FIG. 11-59 Example of an instrument maintenance log sheet for use in a veterinary clinical laboratory.

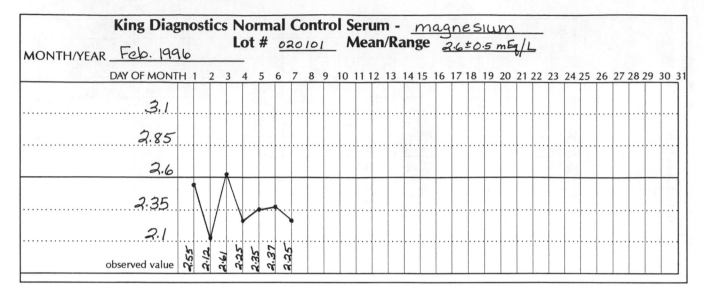

FIG. 11-60   Example of a graph used to chart normal control values.

Blanks and Standards

Some analytic instruments require the use of a blank to prepare them for assays. A blank is a solution made at the time of assay. It contains all the reagents used in the assay *except the patient serum*. The instrument is adjusted to read 100% light transmission (or zero absorbance) using the blank. In effect the blank tells the instrument to ignore chemicals or colors contained in the reagents that might interfere with the assay. This is called "blanking the instrument." A standard solution is a solution that contains an exact, known amount of a consitutent. A standard solution is used to calibrate some instruments.

Many newer instruments no longer require a blank or a standard. However, control samples are absolutely necessary for any successful quality-control program in a veterinary clinical laboratory.

ERRORS

Three types of errors can affect a quality-control program: clerical, systematic, and random.

Clerical errors include incorrect labeling, delays in transporting of samples, inappropriate handling of samples, incorrect calculations, transcription errors, and sampling the wrong patient. These errors are avoidable. A well-educated and conscientious veterinary technician produces few clerical errors. Some of the most common problems related to sample handling are mislabeling samples and incorrectly filling out requisition forms. All tubes, slides, and sample containers should be labeled with the patient's name (and the owner's last name), species, identification or clinic number, and the date.

Systematic errors cause shifts or trends in results obtained with a specific assay method. They often result in gradual changes, causing the mean value of assay results to increase or decrease. These types of errors can be detected by using commercially available controls. Some factors causing systematic errors are using improper standards or controls, reagent instability, and using an assay method that is unsuitable for the constituent being assayed.

Random errors, such as variations in the thickness of glassware and pipettes, electronic and optical variations of instruments, and temperature and timing control variations, can occur in all facets of a testing system. These random errors increase the variability of results. Many random errors can be prevented with routine maintenance of the instruments.

RECOMMENDED READING

Operator's manual for the DuPont analyst, Wilmington, Del, 1993, DuPont Company.

Operator's manual for the Kodak Ektachem DT60 analyzer, Rochester, NY, 1986, Eastman Kodak Company.

Pratt PW: *Laboratory procedures for veterinary technicians,* ed 3, St Louis, 1997, Mosby.

CHAPTER 12

Euthanasia Methods, Specimen Collection, and Necropsy Techniques

L.J. Brown

Learning Objectives

After reviewing this chapter, the reader should understand the following:

Importance of and reasons for necropsy
Methods used to euthanize animals before necropsy
Methods to collect and preserve body tissues for laboratory examination

Appropriate packaging and transport of body tissues for laboratory examination
Necropsy procedures for domestic animals
Appropriate ways to dispose of animal carcasses

EUTHANASIA METHODS

The term *euthanasia* is derived from the Greek *eu-*, meaning good, and *thanatos-*, meaning death. The goal is to provide the animal with a quick and painless death, while minimizing stress and anxiety. Considerations that help determine the method of euthanasia include safety of the individual performing the task and of the animal, ability of the agent to produce rapid loss of consciousness and death without pain, distress, or anxiety, reliability and availability of the agent, and age and species limitations, Depending on the technique used, death is produced by hypoxia, depression of neurons vital for life's function, or disruption of brain activity.

Animals can be euthanized by inhalation, injection, or physical methods. An enclosed chamber or induction mask is used to deliver inhalant anesthetics (halothane, ether, isoflurane) or another gas (carbon dioxide). Often the animal is placed in an enclosed chamber containing cotton or gauze soaked with the anesthetic agent. The vapors from the anesthetic are inhaled until respiration

ceases and death ensues from hypoxia. Inhalant anesthetics can also be used to render an animal unconscious while a second method is used to cause death.

Intravenous injection of an anesthetic (barbiturates) is the most rapid, the most reliable, and a very desirable method for performing euthanasia. An animal that is wild and aggressive, or that poses a threat to the handler should be sedated before intravenous administration of any euthanasia agent. In small animals (less than 7 kg), intraperitoneal injection is acceptable, provided the euthanasia agent is nonirritating. Intracardiac injection is acceptable in an animal that is heavily sedated, anesthetized, or comatose.

Physical methods of euthanasia include captive bolt, gunshot, cervical dislocation, electrocution, exsanguination, and stunning or pithing. The last two methods should not be used as a sole method of euthanasia but should be used in conjunction with another technique or agent. Although some individuals may find these methods displeasing, they may be more rapid, practical, and painless than other methods. Physical methods of euthanasia are appropriate for easily handled small animals. They may also be appropriate for large farm, wild, or zoo animals, and animals in research when other forms of euthanasia may interfere with laboratory results or cause tissue changes.

When it becomes necessary to euthanize any animal, death should be induced as quickly and painlessly as possible. It should be carried out by individuals trained and qualified to do so. When a necropsy is to be performed immediately after euthanasia, the method of euthanasia should be one that causes the least amount of artifactual changes in the tissues and leaves the animal as intact as possible.

SPECIMEN COLLECTION AND PRESERVATION

Proper specimen collection at the time of necropsy can affect the diagnostic results. A complete case history should accompany all specimens. Each individual specimen must be properly identified as to the body site from which it was collected and the date collected. In addition, each specimen must be placed in a separate container.

Specimens collected for microbiology should be collected soon after death and sent to the diagnostic laboratory as soon as possible. Many pathogenic bacteria die in decaying tissues, whereas contaminating environmental microbes thrive under these conditions. Tissues collected for bacterial testing should be collected with sterile instruments and placed in sterile Petri dishes or other sterile containers. Before any handling of tissues during necropsy, these specimens should be collected.

Many toxicologic tests require large quantities of tissue or specimen. In addition, many toxins are organ specific, making the appropriate choice of specimens very important. If the exact toxin is not known, samples of liver, kidney, heart, urine, brain (one half), serum or blood (collect heart clot if necessary), eyes, feed, stomach contents, skin, and body fat should be collected and frozen. When testing for a certain toxin, always consult with the testing lab before shipping the tissues. Unless specifically requested, do not add any type of preservative to the tissues.

Fecal samples should be collected from the colon and rectum when looking for parasite ova. Once collected, these specimens should be kept cold. When an animal is presented alive for necropsy, blood should always be collected, whether or not testing will be immediately performed. If possible, collect three 10-ml samples of blood in EDTA, heparin, and clot tubes before euthanasia.

Histopathology is the examination of the structure, composition, and function of diseased and nondiseased tissues using a light microscope. Many lesions not evident to the unaided eye can be observed with a microscope. As a general rule, tissue samples should be collected from all organs, whether or not a lesion or abnormality is obvious. A checklist should be established so that the same tissues are collected at every necropsy. Collected tissues may be cut into thin sections and quickly placed in 10% neutral buffered formalin or formaldehyde to prevent postmortem change. Fixation retards the autolysis (self-digestion) that begins immediately after death. Tissue sections should be no thicker than 5 mm. The amount of fixative used is also very important. At the minimum the ratio of the fixative volume to tissue should be 10:1. Before shipping formalin-fixed tissues, fix the tissues for 24 to 48 hours.

PACKAGING AND SHIPPING SPECIMENS

Individual tissues should be packaged separately and placed in a sealed, leak-proof bag or container and kept sterile if necessary for microbiologic testing. Each container or bag should be labeled as to its contents and the date collected. Any container with fluids, whether formalin fixative or tubes of blood, should be double bagged and sealed tightly. Other than formalin-fixed tissues, specimens for microbiology should be kept cold (not frozen), and then placed in an insulated container. Because time is important, specimens should be shipped by the quickest service possible and should not be in transit for more than 24 hours.

NECROPSY PROCEDURE

Necropsy (postmortem examination) is an excellent diagnostic tool that should be used as often as possible. The course of a disease can be better understood if a necropsy is performed. In addition, the knowledge gained from a necropsy can be applied to future circumstances involving similar conditions or disease processes. When an unexpected death occurs in a cattery, kennel, or herd situation, it is especially important to perform a necropsy. If there is a possibility of litigation, or an animal dies while under veterinary care, a necropsy should be performed by a qualified laboratory or institution. A written consent form signed by the owner authorizes a postmortem examination.

Before beginning a necropsy, obtain a complete clinical history. This information should include the owner's name and address, and complete identification of the animal, including species, breed, age, sex, weight, and name or number. The cause of death, if known, dictates which tissues to collect for testing. Develop a checklist and follow it (Box 12-1). In addition to the tissues listed on the checklist, any abnormal tissue must be collected with attached adjacent normal tissue.

Necropsy Equipment

Most of the instruments required to perform a necropsy are readily available in veterinary clinics (Fig. 12-1). These include a scalpel handle with replaceable blades, sharp scissors, rat-tooth thumb forceps, a broad-blade knife with a curved edge (similar to a butcher's knife), sharpening stones, a chisel and mallet and/or an electric oscillating (Stryker) saw, a medium pair of pruning shears, and a cutting board. In addition, you should have on hand a ruler, No. 2 pencil, a permanent marking pen, sterile instruments, sterile Petri dishes, measuring cup for measuring large amounts of body fluids and syringes for measuring small quantities, blood tubes, a method for taking notes during the postmortem examination (notebook or tape recorder), 10% neutral buffered formalin, and a camera.

Just as important as the instruments is personal protective clothing to protect against exposure to infectious agents. Protective clothing should include washable or disposable coveralls or something comparable, rubber gloves, rubber or plastic boots, safety glasses and, at the discretion of the prosector, a surgical mask. Because most of the work is done with the hands, the gloves should be of highest quality and should fit comfortably so that small tissues may be easily manipulated. Overly large or small gloves may lead to accidents, such as cutting oneself. Always have an extra pair of rubber gloves available during the necropsy.

A well-lit, well-ventilated area with a water source is ideal for necropsies. A sturdy, slatted rack placed over a tub or large sink works well. A water source should be available and kept running at all times beneath the slatted rack during the necropsy procedure. A drain trap should be used to prevent large pieces of tissues from clogging the drain.

Before the Necropsy

Before beginning the postmortem examination, make sure that all instruments and required materials are readily available. Review the clinical history carefully and make a list of tissues that must be collected for diagnostic testing and be familiar with methods for collection. Label the appropriate vials and bags with the tissue type, date collected, and animal identification.

Beginning the Necropsy

Using a dog as an example, the following is one method of postmortem examination. The necropsy should begin with a thorough external physical examination. If broken bones or gunshot are suspected, radiographs should be

---

Box 12-1 Sample checklist for tissue collection at necropsy

Primary incision
- ☐ Peripheral lymph node
- ☐ Muscle

Thoracic cavity
- ☐ Thyroid glands with parathyroid gland
- ☐ Esophagus (can remain attached to trachea)
- ☐ Upper trachea
- ☐ Thymus
- ☐ Bronchial lymph node (collect with section of trachea)
- ☐ Lung
- ☐ Right atrium
- ☐ Right ventricle
- ☐ Left ventricle

Other
- ☐ Brain with hypophysis
- ☐ Femoral bone marrow

Abdominal cavity
- ☐ Liver with section of gallbladder
- ☐ Kidney (cut left kidney longitudinally and right kidney transversely)

Adrenal glands
- ☐ Spleen
- ☐ Stomach
- ☐ Duodenum with attached pancreas
- ☐ Jejunum with attached mesenteric lymph node
- ☐ Ileum with cecum
- ☐ Colon
- ☐ Urinary bladder
- ☐ Ovary
- ☐ Uterus
- ☐ Testis

Optional
- ☐ Eyes
- ☐ Tonsils
- ☐ Prostate
- ☐ Spinal cord

---

obtained to identify these sites. Note the overall body condition, skin and haircoat condition, mucous membrane color, and normal anatomic associations. With the animal in left lateral recumbency, use a knife to make a ventral midline incision, cutting through the skin from the mandibular symphysis, around any external genital organs, to the area of the pubis. It is helpful to insert the tip of the knife just under the skin and make the cut from beneath while directing the knife outward.

Next, cut the pectoral muscles of the accessible (right) front leg. Continue to cut through these muscles until the leg can be reflected dorsally and is resting without support. This cut exposes the axillary lymph nodes (Fig. 12-2). Repeat this technique with the accessible (right) rear leg while disarticulating or separating and exposing the coxofemoral joint at the round ligament. Note any joint fluid and its color. Also note the smoothness of the joint surface.

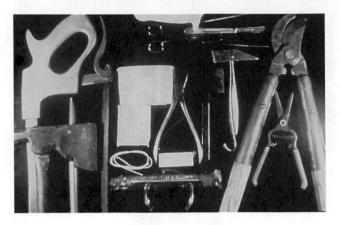

FIG. 12-1   Some instruments used to perform a necropsy.

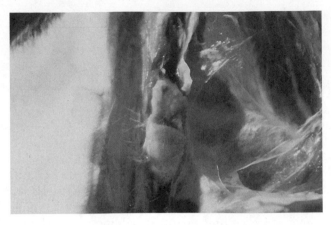

FIG. 12-2   The axillary lymph nodes are exposed when the accessible front leg is reflected laterally.

From the ventral midline incision, reflect the skin dorsally from the right side of the animal. Note any changes or abnormalities in the underlying subcutaneous tissue, such as hemorrhage, jaundice, or edema. Next, reflect dorsally the skin from the neck and face. Be careful not to cut the jugular vein in this area. This exposes the prescapular and mandibular lymph nodes; note their size and color. At this point, the body should be completely skinned over its right lateral side, with both accessible (right) front and rear limbs reflected dorsally, exposing the axilla and coxofemoral joint. The next step is to open the abdominal cavity.

Abdominal Cavity. Make a vertical cut (dorsal to ventral) through the abdominal muscles, parallel to the last rib. Next make a midline incision from the point of the xiphoid cartilage to the pubis. When making this cut, remember to stay shallow so as not to puncture the intestine or stomach. Continue this cut dorsally along the pelvis. Next, reflect this muscle wall dorsally, exposing the abdominal viscera. Note the placement and condition of all abdominal organs. Note any fluid within the abdominal cavity and its color. Before further examination of the abdominal cavity, open the thoracic cavity.

Thoracic Cavity. Before opening the thoracic cavity, puncture the diaphragm with the tip of a knife. Under normal circumstances, this causes the lungs to collapse. As this occurs, the negative pressure within the thoracic cavity is neutralized, causing the diaphragm to outpouch.

Using pruning shears, remove the right side of the rib cage. With the shears, cut from the point of the xiphoid cartilage to the thoracic inlet (cranially). Using the shears, begin cutting at the point of the last rib just a few centimeters from the vertebrae, toward the thoracic inlet. During this procedure, use a knife to cut away any soft tissue that may interfere with the cutting action of the pruning shears. To free the rib cage from the thorax, cut away the diaphragm.

Note the placement, color, and condition of all thoracic organs, including the lungs, pericardium, and mediastinum. The mediastinum is the mass of tissue that separates the two halves of the thoracic cavity in the area of the thoracic inlet. Note the color and volume of any fluid. With both the thoracic and abdominal cavities open and before any tissue is handled, all specimens for microbiologic testing should be collected at this time. Next, examine the costochondral junctions (area on each rib where bone and cartilage meet).

Often the thoracic organs are removed intact as a group to maintain normal anatomic orientation. This method is often preferred over removing one organ at a time. Begin by inserting a knife at the mandibular symphysis. Incise on either side of the tongue. Free the tongue of all its attachments. Next, grasp the tongue and pull in the direction of the thoracic inlet (caudally) while cutting all dorsal attachments. As this is done, gradually strip the larynx, esophagus, and trachea away from the neck. As these are being stripped, you will encounter the hyoid bone at the base of the tongue, which supports the larynx. Use a knife to cut the hyoid bone at this cartilaginous joint on both sides of the larynx. Continue to strip out the larynx caudally. Note the condition of the tonsils within the dorsal wall of the pharynx (Fig. 12-3). While pulling caudally on the tongue, continue dissecting caudally down the neck. As the dissection continues, salivary glands, deeper lymph nodes, and the thymus can be seen.

Continue pulling the tongue caudally while cutting away any dorsal attachments. This frees the lungs, pericardium, heart, aorta, and vena cava. This large mass of tissues can be completely free from the cavity once it is cut away from the diaphragm. This mass or group of tissues is often referred to as the "thoracic pluck" and

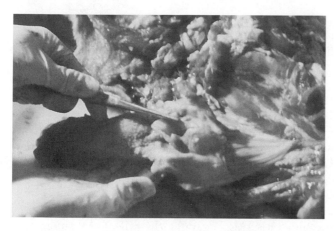

FIG. 12-3 The condition of the tonsils is noted while removing the thoracic pluck.

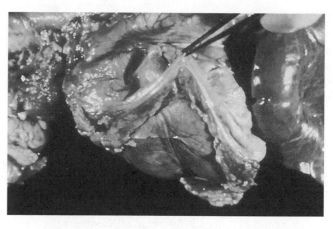

FIG. 12-4 Before examining the heart, remove the pericardial

includes the tongue, esophagus, trachea, thyroid glands, lungs, heart, great vessels, and thymus.

In examining the thoracic viscera, follow a consistent routine, beginning with the tongue. Examine the surface or mucosa of the tongue for ulcers and areas of necrosis or dead tissue. Next, incise the tongue transversely, noting any color changes within the muscle. Then examine and remove the thyroids, parathyroids, and thymus. In most animals, the thyroid and parathyroid glands lie adjacent to the trachea, just caudal to the larynx, at the point of the fifth or sixth tracheal ring. The thyroid gland appears ovoid and is reddish brown. The parathyroid gland lies so closely to the thyroid that it is often difficult to differentiate; it is somewhat paler than the thyroid and much smaller. The thymus is a lymphoid organ located in the mediastinum. The thymus should be examined for its size in relation to the age of the animal. The thymus is relatively large in young animals but is usually very difficult to identify in older animals.

Use scissors to open the entire length of the esophagus. Examine its mucosal surface for parasites, ulcers, and marked changes in color. Next, incise the dorsal wall of the larynx with a knife. Use scissors to extend this incision into the trachea caudally as far as the two main bronchi of the lung. Examine the contents of the trachea. Often, if death was agonal (not sudden), large amounts of foam are noted along the entire length of the trachea.

Next, make a visual inspection of the lungs, noting their color. Carefully palpate all lobes of the lungs for firmness, crepitation, foreign bodies or abnormal masses, and weight. Going back to the main bronchus, use scissors to extend the incision into the bronchioles as far as possible. Incise into as many bronchioles as possible, looking for such abnormalities as excessive fluid and any lung parasites that may favor these terminal airways.

After the lungs have been completely examined, examine the heart. Carefully assess the transparency of the pericardium and its fluid content. Under normal circumstances, a small amount of clear fluid is present within this sac. Pericardial fluid of abnormal color and/or consistency or present in large volume is a significant finding. Next, incise into the pericardial sac and remove this covering from the heart (Fig. 12-4). Examine the heart, along with its vessels, for size, symmetry, color, and hemorrhage. Palpate the heart for firmness. The right and left sides of the heart can be differentiated by the thickness of the ventricular walls. The right side is much thinner and more flaccid than the left.

The heart is most often examined by tracing the flow of blood. Begin on the right side and cut into the right auricle using a pair of scissors. This exposes the right atrium. Cutting parallel to the ventricular septum, continue this cut into the right ventricle, cutting toward the apex. Rotate the heart so that this cut can be directed parallel to the coronary groove. Continue to cut in this direction and cut through the tricuspid valve. Continue cutting past the tricuspid valve and into the pulmonary artery. Remove any clotted blood that may be present. Rotate the heart back to its original position and carefully examine the endocardium, valve leaflets, and major vessels. Trace the pulmonary artery, looking for heartworms.

Examine the left side of the heart by first cutting into the left auricle, exposing the left atrium. Next, make a single cut through the center of the left ventricular wall in the direction of the apex. With the apex oriented toward yourself, identify the septal leaflet of the atrioventricular valve. Cut through this leaflet and proceed through the bicuspid valves and into the aorta. Once again, carefully examine the endocardium, valves, and great vessels. After examining the heart, make several incisions into the myocardium, looking for any changes in color or texture.

Once the thoracic cavity has been completely examined and all necessary tissues collected, examine the abdominal cavity. Examine the liver first. Examine for size, color, and firmness. In addition, note the borders of the liver lobes. These borders should have sharp edges, as opposed to rounded edges. Next, gently squeeze the gallbladder. As you squeeze the gallbladder, bile should flow freely through the bile duct and into the duodenum. If this does not occur, there may be some type of biliary obstruction. Note any resistance to the outflow of bile. Next, remove the liver from the abdomen. Examine the hepatic parenchyma by making multiple parallel incisions (like slicing bread) into each lobe. There should be a lobular pattern throughout the liver.

Next, remove the spleen by cutting it away from the stomach. Examine the spleen for size, shape, color, and texture. Keep in mind that if the animal was euthanized with a barbiturate, the spleen will be somewhat enlarged. As with the liver, make multiple parallel incisions throughout the length of the spleen.

Before continuing with the kidneys, it is best to remove the entire alimentary tract from the abdominal cavity. The intestines should be set aside and examined later in the necropsy procedure. Now locate each kidney. The ovoid adrenal glands are often buried in fat and can be located by palpating dorsal and medial to the cranial poles of each kidney. The left adrenal gland is situated somewhat lateral to the aorta, while the right adrenal gland is situated near the dorsolateral aspect of the caudal vena cava. Carefully dissect through the fat and remove both adrenal glands. Make a transverse incision through each gland and examine for color, size, and shape. In addition, note the proportion of the tan adrenal cortex to the reddish-brown adrenal medulla.

Examine the kidneys next, noting their size, shape, and color. Before removing the kidneys, use blunt dissection to locate the ureters. Follow the ureters and examine distally to the point where they enter the bladder. Examine for stones, hydroureter, constrictions, and hemorrhage. Remove the left kidney and make a longitudinal incision through the entire organ with a knife. Examine the renal cortex, medulla, and pelvis. From the cut surface of the kidney, peel away its closely adhered transparent capsule. This capsule must be removed from the kidney to allow for fixation. This cut surface will demonstrate pinpoint indentations or tears, which represent normal vasculature. Examine the subcapsular surface. Repeat the same procedure for the right kidney.

Inspect the urinary bladder and its contents. The contents of the bladder may be withdrawn using a needle and syringe or expressed into a beaker. Incise the thick-walled bladder and examine its mucosal surface. Make impression smears of the bladder if you suspect canine distemper. These smears can be examined for inclusion bodies.

Examine the reproductive system next. In the female, locate the oviduct and follow each uterine horn. Note the size of the ovaries and presence of follicles, corpora lutea, and cysts. Next, use the pruning shears and make a cut through the pubis. Separate these bones to expose the underlying vagina and rectum. Cut between the vulva and anus to free the caudal end of the vagina. Gently pull the vagina ventrally while severing the connective tissue that lies between it and the rectum. Continue to carefully dissect the area of the cervix while cutting away at its dorsal attachments.

In the male, incise the scrotum and examine both testes for comparable size and tumors. Note any cryptorchid testis. Also examine the tail of the epididymis and the prostate gland (Fig. 12-5). As in the female, use the pruning shears to cut through the pubic bones and expose the urethra and rectum. Open the urethra, beginning at the penile orifice, and trace it proximally to the prostate and into the bladder. Examine all serosal and mucosal surfaces.

Intestinal Tract. To better visualize the segments of intestine, cut the entire mesentery at the point of the mesenteric lymph nodes, close to their attachment to the intestines. Note the size of these lymph nodes. This procedure frees the loops of the intestine from each other, allowing them to be laid out as one, long, tubular structure. Examine the serosal surface of the entire length of the intestines. Then, beginning at the esophageal opening, use a pair of scissors and cut along the greater curvature of the stomach. Examine the stomach contents as well as the mucosal surface of the stomach. Depressions on the mucosal surface may be erosions or ulcers. Also examine for parasites and foreign bodies. Next, remove the pancreas from the duodenum and note its color and size. Examine the pancreas for tumors or hemorrhage.

If sections of intestine are to be cultured, tie them off and remove these unopened segments before any further examination. As the remainder of the small and large intestines is opened, carefully examine their mucosal surfaces. Using scissors, continue cutting from the greater curvature of the stomach into the duodenum, followed by the jejunum, which makes up most of the small intestine. Continue this cut into the ileum and its attached cecum. This comma-shaped, blind sac marks the beginning of the large intestine. Continue cutting into the colon and proceed into the rectum. Collect any fecal samples at this terminal end.

Central Nervous System. Every necropsy should include examination of the central nervous system. The clinical history dictates whether both the brain and spinal cord should be examined or the brain alone. Remove the head by using a knife to make a transverse cut through the muscle immediately caudal to the occipital protuberance and deep enough to expose the atlanto-occipital joint. Place the tip of the knife between

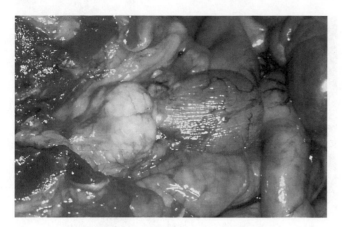

FIG. 12-5 In males, always examine the prostate gland as well as the urinary bladder.

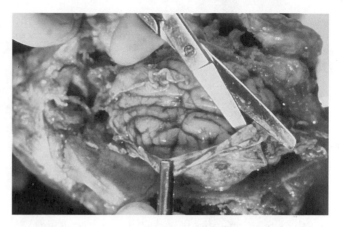

FIG. 12-6 Remove the dura mater to expose the brain for examination.

the atlas and axis and sever the spinal cord. Place the head over the edge of the working surface and hyperextend the neck. This disarticulates the atlanto-occipital joint. Detach the head from the body by cutting the loose muscle and skin that keep the head attached.

Once the head is separated from the body, cut and reflect all remaining skin toward the eyes, completely exposing the skull. Cut and remove the temporal muscles on either side of the skull. To remove the calvaria, up to three cuts are needed. Using a hammer and chisel, make a single transverse cut just caudal to the eyes, extending to both lateral margins of the orbits. At the lateral termination of this cut, make a second cut that extends caudally to the foramen magnum. Repeat this cut at the other lateral termination of the first cut. This third cut frees the calvaria from attachment so it can be easily removed. The exposed dura mater on the surface of the brain is visible as a semitransparent film. Carefully examine for opacity and hemorrhage. Use scissors to remove the dura mater covering both cerebral hemispheres and the cerebellum (Fig. 12-6). Next, examine the surface of the exposed brain for hemorrhage and tumors.

Use extreme care when removing the fragile brain. Begin by making a transverse cut across the olfactory lobes. Next, tip the skull so that the nose is pointed toward the ceiling and the head is resting on its occipital condyles. Allow gravity to pull the brain out of its cavity. Beginning at the olfactory lobes, use the handle of the scalpel to scoop out the brain. Once the optic nerves are visible, use the scalpel blade to cut them. With careful scooping, allow the brain to continue to fall out of its cavity. Remove the hypophysis, or pituitary gland, as intact as possible and attached to the brain. It can be removed from the fossa in which it sits

with careful dissection using the scalpel blade. This takes some practice to achieve. As the brain continues to fall away, cut any nerves and attachments that prevent complete removal. At the point of the cerebellum, support the brain with one hand to prevent it from falling to the floor. Examine the freed brain for size and shape. Unless indicated otherwise, fix the brain whole in formalin and do not section it.

If the spinal cord is to be examined, it can be removed by performing a dorsal laminectomy. Once the vertebrae are removed, the nerves must be cut to free the spinal cord. Before fixing the spinal cord in formalin, open the dura mater to expose the cord.

ANATOMIC VARIATIONS
Pigs

The two thyroid glands are somewhat fused, giving the appearance of one large gland. The deep purple thyroid glands of pigs are located in the area of the thoracic inlet. The tonsils of pigs are diffuse and located in the area of the epiglottis. This tissue is important for testing if pseudorabies is suspected. Always examine the nasal turbinates for evidence of atrophic rhinitis.

Cattle

The kidneys of cattle are lobulated and embedded in large amounts of fat, termed capsula. The four stomach compartments of cattle and other ruminants are the rumen, reticulum, omasum, and abomasum. The rumen occupies most of the left half of the abdominal cavity. It is the first stomach compartment, where food is temporarily stored while undergoing fermentation before regurgitation and remastication. The rumen wall has folds that divide it into two sacs. The reticulum is the second of the four stomach compartments. It is the most cranial and the smallest. It has the appearance of a honeycomb. The omasum is the third compartment. From the greater curvature of the omasum extend hundreds of longitudinal folds. The abomasum is the fourth or "true" stomach of ruminants. The heart of cattle contains a bony structure called the ossa cordis. These bones develop in the aortic fibrous rings.

Horses

The guttural pouch is a ventral diverticulum of the eustachian tube, which drains the middle ear. This is often the site of mycotic or bacterial infections (Fig. 12-7). Horses do not have a gallbladder. The large intestine of horses is divided into several anatomic areas. The cecum, about 120 cm in length, is curved somewhat like a comma, and is located to the right of the median plane. Four longitudinal bands along the cecum form four rows of sacculations. The great or large colon begins at the cecocolic orifice (located at the lesser curvature of the cecum) and terminates at the small colon. *In situ* (in the normal position), the great colon is folded and divided into four portions, all of which are identified according to their position. The first portion is the right ventral colon, which begins at the lesser curvature of the base of the cecum, forming an initial curve passing dorsally and caudally. Then it passes ventrally and cranially, along the floor of the abdomen. It then bends sharply to the left and caudally, forming the sternal flexure. The second part, the left ventral colon, passes caudally on the abdominal floor, to the left of the first part of the cecum. Once it reaches the pelvic inlet, it turns sharply dorsally and cranially, forming the pelvic flexure. The left dorsal colon passes cranially, dorsal or lateral to the left ventral colon. Once it reaches the diaphragm and left lobe of the liver, it turns to the right and caudally, forming the diaphragmatic flexure. The fourth portion is the right dorsal colon. It passes caudally, dorsal to the first part. Once it reaches the medial surface of the base of the cecum, it turns left and dorsally, caudal to the stomach, where it becomes constricted and joins the small colon below the left kidney. The cranial mesenteric artery should be examined for possible strongyle migration.

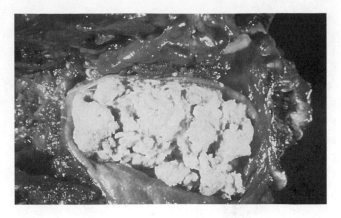

FIG. 12-7   The guttural pouch of horses is often the site of mycotic and bacterial infections.

RECOMMENDED READING

Alden CL: *Color atlas for small animal necropsy,* Lenexa, Kan, 1981, Veterinary Medicine Publishing.

Jones TC, Gleiser CA: *Veterinary necropsy procedures for the dog and cat,* Philadelphia, 1954, Lippincott.

Report of the AVMA panel on euthanasia, *J Am Vet Med Assoc* 202:231-246, 1993.

Strafuss AC: *Necropsy: procedures and basic diagnostic methods for practicing veterinarians,* Springfield, Ill, 1988, Charles C Thomas.

CHAPTER 13

Pharmacology and Pharmacy Practices

R.L. Bill

Learning Objectives

After reviewing this chapter, the reader should understand the following:

Various categories of drugs and their clinical uses
Dosage forms in which drugs are available
Ways in which drug dosages are calculated

Routes by which various types of drugs are administered
Ways in which drugs exert their effect and affect body tissue
Procedures used to safely store and handle drugs
Primary drugs affecting various body systems

DRUG NAMES

Drugs are generally referred by three different names. Their *chemical name,* such as D-alpha-amino-p-hydroxy-benzyl-penicillin trihydrate, describes the drug's chemical composition. The *nonproprietary name* (sometimes called the *generic name*) is a more concise name given to the specific chemical compound. Examples of nonproprietary names are aspirin, acetaminophen, and amoxicillin. The *proprietary* or *trade name* is a unique drug name given by a manufacturer to its particular brand of drug. Examples of proprietary or trade names include Excedrin™, Tylenol™, and Amoxitabs™. Because the trade name is a proper noun, it is capitalized and the superscript © or TM is added to signify that the trade name is a registered trademark and cannot be legally used by other manufacturers. Because many drug manufacturers produce similar products, a single generic drug can be sold under multiple trade names. For example, the antibiotic amoxicillin is manufactured by several different companies, each of which has its own trade name for amoxicillin (e.g., Amoxi-Tabs, Robamox-V, Amoxil).

When a drug company develops and patents a new drug (not just a new trade name for an old drug, but a new chemical), and obtains FDA approval to sell the new drug, the company has the exclusive rights to manufacture this drug for a number of years. During that time, no other drug manufacturer can produce this same drug. This allows the drug company to recover, at the expense of the consumer, the costs of the research, development, and testing the company has invested to bring this drug to market. After these patent rights expire, other companies can legally produce the drug. These "copy cat" drugs are called *generic equivalents,* because they have properties equivalent to those of the original compound. Generic equivalents are usually sold at a much lower price than the original manufacturer's product, because the generic manufacturer has not had to underwrite development of the original drug.

DOSAGE FORMS

Drugs are also described by their *dosage form*. Solid dosage forms include tablets, which are powdered drugs compressed into pills, disks, or capsules, which are powdered drugs enclosed within gelatin capsules. Enteric-coated tablets have a special covering that protects the drug from the harsh acidic environment of the stomach and prevents dissolving of the tablet until it enters the intestine. Suppositories are inserted into the rectum, where they dissolve and release the drug to be absorbed across the membranes of the intestinal wall. Sustained-release forms of oral drugs release small amounts of the drug into the intestinal lumen over an extended time.

A *solution* is a drug dissolved in a liquid vehicle that does not settle out if left standing. In contrast, a *suspension* contains drug particles that are suspended, but not dissolved, in the liquid vehicle. These drug particles usually settle to the bottom of the container when the container is left standing, so one must shake it back into suspension before administration so as to ensure consistent dosing. *Syrups,* such as cough syrups, are solutions of drugs with water and sugar (e.g., 85% sucrose). *Elixirs* are solutions of drugs dissolved in sweetened alcohol. Elixirs are used for drugs that do not readily dissolve in water. It is therefore important that you do not dilute an elixir with water, because the water will stratify into a layer separate from the elixir solution.

Tinctures are alcohol solutions meant for *topical application* (applied onto the skin). Topical products are available as liniments, which contain a drug in an oil base that are rubbed into the skin, or lotions, which are drug suspensions or solutions that are dabbed, brushed, or dripped onto the skin without rubbing (e.g., poison ivy medications). *Ointments, creams,* and *pastes* are semi-solid dosage forms that are applied onto the skin (ointments, creams) or given orally (pastes). Ointments and creams are designed to liquefy at body temperatures, whereas pastes tend to keep their semi-solid form at body temperature.

Injectables are administered via a needle and syringe. Repository forms of injectable drugs are formulated to prolong absorption of the drug from the site of administration and thus provide a more sustained effective drug concentration in the body. *Implants* are solid dosage forms that are injected or inserted under the skin and dissolve or release a drug over an extended period.

PRESCRIPTIONS AND DISPENSING MEDICATION
Writing Prescriptions

A *prescription* is an order from a licensed veterinarian directing a pharmacist to prepare a drug for use in a client's animal. When writing prescriptions, veterinarians must adhere to the following guidelines:
- Veterinary prescription drugs must be used only by or on the order of a licensed veterinarian.
- A valid veterinarian/client/patient relationship must exist.
- Veterinary prescription drugs must meet proper requirements for labeling.
- Appropriate records of all prescriptions issued must be maintained.
- Veterinary prescription drugs must be appropriately handled and stored for safety and security.

Components of a Prescription

A hypothetical prescription is shown in Fig. 13-1. Fig. 13-2 shows common abbreviations used in prescriptions and their meanings. Valid prescriptions must contain the following items:
- Name, address, and telephone number of the person who wrote the prescription.
- Date on which the prescription was written.
- Owner's name and address and species of animal (animal's name is optional).
- Rx symbol (abbreviation of *recipe*, Latin for "take thou").
- Drug name, concentration, and number of units to be dispensed.
- *Sig* (abbreviation of *signa*, Latin for "write" or "label"), indicating directions for the client in treating the aminal.
- Signature of the prescriber.
- DEA registration number if the drug is a controlled substance.

Containers for Dispensing Medication

Many veterinary practices dispense tablets and capsules in plastic containers with a childproof lid. If medication is dispensed in a paper envelope and a child becomes poisoned, the veterinarian could be found negligent in dispensing the medication in a manner that placed the child "at risk."

HOMETOWN VETERINARY ASSOCIATES

2000 West Chelsea Ave., Momack, PA
(324) 555-4313

Date: November 22, 1995

Patient: Cricket   Species: Canine

Owner: Lee Ann Wozniak   Phone: 555-0127

Address: 929 Christopher Robin Lane, Brookside, PA 13235

℞   Amoxicillin tablets 100 mg #30 tabs
      Sig: 1 tab q8h PO PRN until gone

                                    _____ Robert L. Bill **D.V.M.**

FIG. 13-1 A typical prescription for a veterinary drug.

BID	twice a day	**po**	by mouth
cc	cubic centimeter	**prn**	as needed
disp	dispense	**q**	every
g	gram	**q8h**	every 8 hours
gm	gram	**qd**	every day
gr	grain	**QID**	four times daily
h	hour	**QOD**	every other day
lb	pound	**SID**	once a day
mg	milligram	**stat**	immediately
ml	milliliter	**TID**	three times daily
od	right eye	**tsp**	teaspoon
os	left eye		

Note: SID is rarely used or recognized by pharmacists
outside of the veterinary profession.

FIG. 13-2 Abbreviations commonly used in prescriptions. *(From Bill RL: Pharmacology for veterinary technicians, St Louis, 1993, Mosby.)*

CALCULATING DRUG DOSES

Calculating the dose of drug to be administered involves the following steps:

1. Weigh the animal and convert the weight in pounds to kilograms (if necessary).
2. If the veterinarian has not specified the dose to administer, consult the drug package insert or a drug reference to determine the correct dosage (e.g., mg/kg body weight). Then use the animal's weight to calculate the correct dose (i.e., in mg, ml, units, g, etc.).
3. Based upon the concentration of the drug (e.g., mg of drug/ml of solution or mg of drug/tablet), determine what volume or number of tablets to administer. Simple algebra helps calculate the amount (dose) of drug to be given (e.g., mg or ml), along with the animal's weight and the recommended drug dosage (e.g., mg/kg). You can also calculate the number of units to give (e.g., tablets or ml) if you know the amount of drug in each unit (e.g., mg/ml or mg/tablet) and the duration of treatment (days). Common metric conversion factors used in calculating drug doses are listed in Fig. 13-3.

Step 1. Set up an equation so that the units (kg, lb, etc.) are the same on the top (numerator) and bottom (denominator) on both sides of the equation. Then solve for X (e.g., kg of body weight), as shown in Step 1 of Fig. 13-4.

Step 2. Once the animal's weight has been converted to the appropriate units (in this case, kg), determine the amount of drug (dose) to be given. On the left of the equation is the drug dosage (e.g., milligrams of drug/kilogram body weight) and the X you are solving for is the total drug dose (in milligrams of drug). This is shown in Step 2 of Fig. 13-4.

Step 3. After the total dose is determined (in mg or some other measure), calculate the volume (e.g., ml) or number of solid units (tablets, capsules) to be administered using the concentration of drug in the solution (mg of drug/ml of solution) or in each solid unit (mg of drug/tablet), solving for ml of liquid or number of tablets. This step is shown in Step 3 of Fig. 13-4.

When dispensing solid units (tablets, capsules), round to the nearest unit (or half or quarter tablet if the tablet is designed to be broken and greater accuracy is essential). The steps for calculating the total number of solid units required during a course of treatment are detailed in Fig. 13-5.

---

1 kg = 1000 g = 100,000 milligrams (mg)

1 kg = 2.2 lb

1 gram = 1 gm = 1000 mg = 0.001 kg

1 gram = 1 g = 15.43 grains (gr)

1 grain = 64.8 milligrams (usually rounded to 60 or 65 mg)

1 lb = 0.454 kg = 16 ounces (oz)

1 mg = 0.001 g = 1000 micrograms (μg or mcg)

1 liter (L) = 1000 ml = 10 deciliters (dl)

1 ml = 1 cc = 1000 microliters (μl or mcl)

1 tablespoon (tbsp) = 3 teaspoons (tsp)

1 tsp = 5 ml

1 gallon (gal) = 3.786 L

1 gal = 4 quarts (qt) = 8 pints (pt) = 128 fluid ounces (fl oz)

1 pt = 2 cups (c) = 16 fl oz = 473 ml

FIG. 13-3 Metric conversion factors. *(From Bill RL: Pharmacology for veterinary technicians, St Louis, 1993, Mosby.)*

What volume of a drug solution should we give to a 44-lb dog if the recommended dosage is 5 mg/kg and the concentration of the solution is 50 mg/ml?

Step 1: Convert pounds to kilograms.

$$X \text{ kg} = 44 \text{ lb} \times \frac{1 \text{ kg}}{2.2 \text{ lb}} = \frac{44}{2.2} = 20 \text{ kg}$$

Step 2: Calculate the total drug dose.

$$X \text{ mg} = \frac{5 \text{ mg}}{\text{kg}} \times 20 \text{ kg} = 5 \times 20 = 100 \text{ mg}$$

Step 3: Calculate the volume of solution needed.

$$\frac{50 \text{ mg}}{\text{ml}} = \frac{100 \text{ mg}}{X \text{ ml}} = \frac{100 \text{ mg}}{50 \text{ mg/ml}} = 2 \text{ ml}$$

FIG. 13-4 Simple algebraic calculation used to calculate a drug dose.

How many 25-mg tablets should we dispense for a 10-lb cat if the recommended dosage is 5 mg/lb twice daily for 7 days?

Step 1: Calculate the number of tablets needed per dose.

$$10 \text{ lb} \times \frac{5 \text{ mg}}{\text{lb}} = 50 \text{ mg per dose}$$

$$50 \text{ mg} \times \frac{1 \text{ tablet}}{25 \text{ mg}} = 2 \text{ tablets per dose}$$

Step 2: Calculate the number of tablets needed daily.

2 tablets per dose × twice daily = 4 tablets daily

Step 3: Calculate the number of tablets needed for 7 days.

4 tablets daily × 7 days = 28 tablets

FIG. 13-5 Calculating the number of tablets to dispense.

STORING AND HANDLING DRUGS IN THE PHARMACY

Drugs that are improperly stored (e.g., exposed to extreme temperature or light) can degenerate or become inactivated, providing little or no benefit to the animal in which they are used. Drugs still on the pharmacy shelf after the listed expiration date on the container may be less effective. In some cases, such as with tetracycline, these expired drugs can become hazardous to the animal. Store drugs at their optimum temperature to prevent damage. Temperatures used for drug storage, according to label specifications, are as follows:

Cold: not exceeding 8°C (46°F)
Cool: 8° to 15°C (46° to 59°F)
Room temperature: 15° to 30°C (59° to 86°F)
Warm: 30° to 40°C (86° to 104°F)
Excessive heat: greater than 40°C (104°F)

Drugs that are sensitive to light are usually kept in a dark amber container. Tablets and powders tend to be sensitive to moisture, and their containers usually contain silica packets to absorb moisture. Some drugs are destroyed by physical stress, such as vibrations. Some forms of insulin can be inactivated by violent shaking of the vial.

Storing and Prescribing Controlled Substances

A *controlled substance* is defined by law as a substance with potential for physical addiction, psychological addiction, and/or abuse. Controlled substances must be stored securely under lock and key to prevent access by unauthorized personnel. By law, a written record must be kept describing when, for what purpose, and how much of the controlled drug was used. These records must include receipts for purchase or sale of controlled substances and must be maintained for 2 years. Although ketamine is not listed as a controlled drug, its hallucinogenic characteristics increase the potential for abuse; ketamine should therefore be handled as a controlled substance.

Drug manufacturers and distributors are required to identify a controlled substance on its label with a capital C, followed by a Roman numeral, which denotes the drug's theoretical potential for abuse.

C-I   Extreme potential for abuse; no approved medicinal purpose in the United States; includes such drugs as heroin, LSD, and marijuana.

C-II   High potential for abuse; use may lead to severe physical or psychological dependence; includes such drugs as opium, pentobarbital, and morphine.

C-III Some potential for abuse, but less than for C-II drugs; use may lead to low to moderate physical dependence or high psychological dependence.

C-IV Low potential for abuse; use may lead to limited physical psychological dependence; includes such drugs as phenobarbital and diazepam (Valium).

C-V   Subject to state and local regulation; low potential for abuse.

For veterinarians to legally use, prescribe, or buy a controlled substance from an approved manufacturer or distributor, they must have obtained a certification number from the Drug Enforcement Administration (DEA). This DEA certification number must be included on all prescriptions or any order forms for Schedule (controlled) drugs. Even with a valid DEA number, veterinarians cannot prescribe Schedule I (C-I) drugs. Prescriptions for Schedule II (C-II) drugs, which have the most potential for abuse, must be in written form (many states have special forms for C-II drug prescriptions) and cannot be telephoned to a pharmacist. In the event of an emergency, when the prescription must be ordered by telephone, the verbal prescription must be followed by a written order within 72 hours. Schedule II drug prescriptions may not be refilled; a new prescription must be written for each treatment period.

Handling Toxic Drugs

Veterinary professionals may be exposed to toxic drugs in various ways, including the following:

- Absorption through the skin via spillage from a syringe or vial, or other contact.
- Inhalation of aerosolized drug as the needle is withdrawn from a vial pressurized by injection of air to facilitate removal of the drug.
- Ingestion of food contaminated with drug via aerosolization or direct contact.
- Inhalation resulting from crushing or breaking of tablets and subsequent aerosolization of drug powder.
- Absorption or inhalation during opening of glass ampules containing antineoplastic agents.

The best way to avoid exposure is to educate all involved personnel in safe handling or storage of these drugs. The training may be in-house or through formal training available in many communities. Such safety training should be periodically repeated to emphasize the importance of handling precautions and as a refresher for staff members.

THE THERAPEUTIC RANGE

The concentration of a drug in the body must be such that the detrimental effects are minimized and benefits are maximized. This ideal range of drug concentration is referred to as the *therapeutic range*. If an excessive dose results in accumulation of too much drug in the body, drug concentrations are said to be *toxic,* and signs of toxicity develop. If a small drug dose does not produce drug concentrations within the therapeutic range, drug concentrations are said to be at *subtherapeutic levels,* and the drug's beneficial effect is not achieved.

DOSAGE REGIMEN

There are three components of therapeutic administration of drugs: the dose, the dosage interval, and the route of administration. Altering any of these three components can result in drug concentrations that are too high or too low.

A drug's *dose* is the amount of drug administered at one time. For accuracy and clarity in communicating with pharmacists or other veterinary professionals, always state the dose in units of mass (e.g., mg, g, gr), as opposed to number of product units (e.g., tablets or capsules) or volume (ml, L), because manufacturers may produce the same drug in solid dosage forms of various sizes or solutions with various concentrations. For example, writing in an animal's record that the animal received "1 tablet of amoxicillin" is of no value because amoxicillin is available in tablet sizes ranging from 50 mg up to 400 mg. The same is true if you state, "Give 3 ml of xylazine," because 3 ml of a xylazine

solution with a concentration of 20 mg/ml contains much less xylazine than 3 ml of a solution with a concentration of 100 mg/ml.

The time between administration of separate drug doses is referred to as the *dosage interval.* Dosage intervals are often expressed with the Latin abbreviations shown in Fig. 13-2.

The dose and the dosage interval together are often referred to as the *dosage regimen.* The total amount of drug delivered to the animal in 24 hours is the *total daily dose* and is determined by multiplying the dose by the frequency of administration (e.g., 100 mg given 4 times daily results in a total daily dose of 400 mg).

ROUTES OF ADMINISTRATION

The amount of a drug that reaches the target tissues in the body can be significantly altered if the proper route of administration is not used. The route of administration is how the drug enters the body. Drugs given by injection are said to be *parenterally administered.* Drugs given by mouth, or *per os (PO),* are said to be *orally administered.* If a drug is applied to the surface of the skin, as with lotions and liniments, it is said to be *topically administered.*

Parenteral administration of drugs is further broken down into specific routes. Intravenous (IV) administration involves injecting the drug directly into a vein. Intravenous injections can be given as a single volume at one time, called a *bolus,* or they can be slowly injected or dripped into a vein over several seconds, minutes, or even hours as an intravenous infusion. The differences in drug concentrations achieved by these variations of intravenous administration are shown in Fig. 13-6.

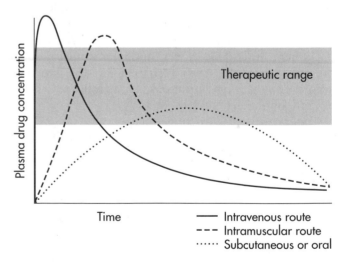

FIG. 13-6 Plasma drug concentrations attained after intravenous, intramuscular, subcutaneous, and oral administration.

Note that *intravenous* injection is not the same as *intraarterial* injection. Drugs given by intraarterial injection are injected into an artery (not a vein), quickly producing high concentrations of drug in tissues supplied by that artery. After intravenous injection, blood containing the drug passes to the heart and is mixed and diluted with the remaining blood in circulation before it is delivered to body tissues. Inadvertent injection of drugs intraarterially (e.g., injection into the carotid artery instead of the jugular vein) delivers a bolus of a drug directly to tissues. These accidental intraarterial injections can produce severe effects, such as seizures or respiratory arrest. Injection of a drug outside of the blood vessel (not within the vessel lumen) is an extravascular or perivascular injection. Some drugs cause extreme local inflammation and tissue death if accidentally injected extravascularly.

Intramuscular (IM) administration involves injecting the drug into a muscle mass. *Subcutaneous (SC or SQ) injections* are administered deep to (beneath) the skin, into the subcutis. *Intradermal (ID) injections* are administered within (not beneath) the skin with very small needles. The intradermal route is usually reserved for skin testing procedures, such as testing for tuberculosis or reaction to allergenic substances. *Intraperitoneal (IP) injections* are administered into the abdominal body cavity and are frequently used when IV or IM injections are not practical (as in some laboratory animals) or large volumes of solution must be administered for rapid absorption.

MOVEMENT OF DRUG MOLECULES IN THE BODY

Pharmacokinetics describes how drugs move into, through, and out of the body. Knowledge of a drug's pharmacokinetics facilitates understanding of why the drug must be given by different routes or dosage regimens to achieve therapeutic success under different clinical circumstances. Pharmacokinetics involves absorption, distribution, metabolism, and elimination.

Movement of drug molecules from the site of administration into the systemic circulation is called *absorption*. After a drug has been ingested, injected, inhaled, or applied to the skin, it must be absorbed into the blood and travel to the body areas where it will have its intended effect (target tissues). IV injections almost instantaneously achieve their peak concentration (highest level) in the blood (Fig. 13-6). Drugs given by IM administration take some time to diffuse from the injection site in the muscle, into the systemic circulation. Drugs given by PO administration and SC injection take longer to be absorbed because they must diffuse farther to reach the systemic circulation (SC injection) or they

must pass through several barriers to be absorbed (PO administration). Drugs given IM, SC, or PO attain therapeutic concentrations more slowly than drugs given IV.

Distribution describes movement of a drug from the systemic circulation into tissues. Drugs generally are distributed most rapidly and in greater concentrations to well-perfused (rich blood supply) tissues. Examples of well-perfused tissues include active skeletal muscle, the liver, kidney, and brain. In contrast, inactive skeletal muscle and adipose (fat) tissue are relatively poorly perfused, so it takes more time for drugs to be delivered to these tissues. Some drugs bind to proteins in the blood; these protein-bound drug molecules are unable to leave the systemic circulation and so are not distributed to tissues. Thus, a significant portion of a highly protein-bound drug remains in systemic circulation, where these protein-bound drug molecules act as a "reservoir" of additional drug.

Many drugs are altered by the body before being eliminated. This process is referred to as *biotransformation* or *drug metabolism*. The altered drug molecule is referred to as a *metabolite*. The liver is the primary organ involved in drug metabolism or biotransformation. However, other tissues, such as the lung, skin, and intestinal tract, may also biotransform drug molecules. The product of biotransformation (metabolite) is usually readily eliminated by the kidney or liver. Removal of a drug from the body is called *drug elimination* or *excretion*. The two major routes of elimination are via the kidney (into the urine) and via the liver (into the bile and subsequently into the feces). Inhalant anesthetics and other volatile agents are mostly eliminated via the lungs, although some inhalant anesthetics (methoxyflurane and halothane) have some hepatic biotransformation and renal excretion. Drug elimination is greatly affected by dehydration; kidney, liver, or heart disease; age; and a variety of other physiologic and pathologic (disease) conditions.

By law, all drugs approved for use in food animals have mandated withdrawal times. The *withdrawal time* is the period after drug administration during which the animal cannot be sent to market for slaughter, and the eggs or milk must be discarded.

HOW DRUGS EXERT THEIR EFFECT

For cells to respond to a drug molecule, usually the drug must combine with a specific protein molecule on or in the cell, called a *receptor*. A given receptor combines only with the molecule of certain drugs, based upon their shape or molecular make-up. This concept is illustrated by a key and lock, where the drug is the key and the receptor is the lock into which only the correct key will fit (produce an effect). The effect of the correct drug molecule-receptor combination is some cellular change, such as causing the cell to secrete substances, muscle cells to contract, or neuronal cells to depolarize (fire). Cells do not have receptors for all drugs; only certain cells respond to certain drugs.

Drugs Affecting the Gastrointestinal Tract

Drugs or functions related to the stomach are called *gastric,* as in gastric ulcers, gastric blood flow, or gastric emptying. Drugs or functions related to the duodenum, jejunum, or ileum are usually referred to as *enteric.* Drugs and functions related to the colon are termed *colonic.*

Emetics. *Emetics* are drugs that induce vomiting. The complex process of emesis is controlled by a group of neurons in the medulla of the brainstem, known as the *vomiting center.* Emetics are most often used to induce vomiting in animals that have ingested toxic substances. They should not be used in all cases of poisoning, however, because the risk of aspiration (inhalation) of stomach contents into the lungs may outweigh the benefit of induced vomiting. Also, vomiting should not be induced if a corrosive substance or volatile liquid was ingested.

Apomorphine quickly causes emesis in dogs when given by IV or IM injection, or when an apomorphine tablet is placed in the conjunctival sac of the eye. Apomorphine is a less effetive emetic in cats. An effective emetic for cats is the sedative xylazine (Rompun, Anased, and others), which produces emesis within minutes of injection.

Syrup of ipecac does not produce vomiting until 10 to 30 minutes after administration. This is because the ipecac must pass from the stomach into the intestine to produce the required local irritation (local effect) and also to be absorbed (central effect on the vomiting center). The 10- to 30-minute lag time between ipecac administration and the onset of vomiting can lead uninformed clients or veterinary professionals to believe the initial dose was ineffective, causing them to administer multiple doses of the drug before vomiting begins. Other local emetics include hydrogen peroxide; a warm, concentrated solution of salt and water; and a solution of powdered mustard and water. These emetics do not work consistently.

Antiemetics. Antiemetics are drugs that prevent or decrease vomiting. Antiemetics should only be used when the vomiting reflex is no longer of benefit to the animal. Phenothiazine tranquilizers, such as acepromazine (PromAce), chlorpromazine (Thorazine), and prochlorperazine (Compazine, Darbazine), are commonly used to combat vomiting caused by motion sickness. The antihistamines dimenhydrinate (Dramamine) and diphenhydramine (Benadryl) are also used occasionally for prevention of motion sickness.

Atropine, aminopentamide (Centrine), and isopropamide (combined with prochlorperazine in Darbazine) are anticholinergic drugs that prevent vomiting by blocking the impulses traveling to the CNS via the vagus nerve and the motor impulses traveling via the vagus nerve to the muscles involved with the vomiting reflex.

Metoclopramide (Reglan) is a centrally acting antiemetic that also has local antiemetic activity. Metoclopramide has been useful in otherwise healthy dogs that intermittently vomit small amounts of bile-tinged fluid, usually in the morning. Cisapride (Propulsid) has been used to reduce regurgitation in dogs with megaesophagus (dilated esophagus) and in cats with chronic constipation or cats that frequently vomit hairballs.

Antidiarrheals. Antidiarrheals are drugs used to combat various types of diarrhea. Narcotics commonly used to combat diarrhea include diphenoxylate (Lomotil), paregoric (tincture of opium), and loperamide (Imodium). A disadvantage of narcotics when used as antidiarrheals is that their analgesic effect can mask pain that otherwise could be used to monitor progression or resolution of disease. Another disadvantage is that narcotics can cause excitement in cats ("morphine mania").

The anticholinergics atropine, isopropamide (Darbazine), and aminopentamide (Centrine) are used as antispasmodics because they decrease spastic colonic contractions and combat diarrhea associated with these contractions. These drugs are not particularly effective for most small bowel diarrhea.

Bismuth subsalicylate, the active ingredient in Pepto-Bismol, breaks down in the gut to bismuth carbonate and salicylate. The bismuth tends to coat the intestinal mucosa, perhaps protecting it from enterotoxins, and seems to have some antibacterial activity. The major antisecretory effect, however, is probably from the salicylate (an aspirin-like compound), which decreases inflammation and blocks formation of prostaglandins that would normally stimulate fluid secretion.

Adsorbents and Protectants. Locally irritating substances, such as bacterial endotoxins, can produce acute diarrhea. Any drug that prevents these agents from contacting the intestinal mucosa could theoretically reduce the diarrheal response. That is the underlying principle of adsorbents and protectants. An adsorbent causes another substance to adhere to its outer surface, thus reducing contact of that substance with the intestinal tract wall.

Activated charcoal adsorbs enterotoxins to its surface, preventing them from contacting the bowel wall. The charcoal and the adsorbed enterotoxin then pass out in the feces. Kaolin and pectin (Kaopectate) are often used together for symptomatic relief of vomiting or diarrhea. The kaolin-pectin combination is thought to adsorb enterotoxins. It is questionable as to whether kaolin-pectin has any significant effect in controlling diarrhea in veterinary patients.

Laxatives, Lubricants, and Stool Softeners. Laxatives, cathartics, and purgatives facilitate evacuation of the bowels. Laxatives are considered the most gentle of this class of drugs, whereas cathartics are more marked in their evacuating effect, and purgatives are quite potent in their actions. *Irritant laxatives,* including castor oil and phenolphthalein, work by irritating the bowel, resulting in increased peristaltic motility.

Bulk laxatives are much more gentle than irritant laxatives. These drugs osmotically pull water into the bowel lumen or retain water in the feces. Hydrophilic colloids or indigestible fiber (bran, methylcellulose, Metamucil) are not digested or adsorbed to any degree and therefore create an osmotic force to produce their laxative effect. Psyllium is a hydrophilic compound that has gained popularity for its supposed health benefits. Hypertonic salts, such as magnesium (Milk of Magnesia, Epsom salts) and phosphate salts (Fleet Enema), are poorly absorbed and create a strong osmotic force to attract water into the bowel lumen.

Lubricants (mineral oil, cod liver oil, white petrolatum, glycerin) are given to make the stool more "slippery" for easy passage through the bowel. Mineral oil is most commonly used for horses with impactions and is administered by stomach tube. The greatest danger associated with use of this oil is aspiration into the lungs, with subsequent pneumonia. Glycerin is most commonly used as a suppository.

Docusate sodium succinate (Colace) is a stool softener that acts as a "wetting agent" by reducing the surface tension of feces and allowing water to penetrate the dry stool. Docusate sodium succinate and related calcium and phosphate compounds may also stimulate colonic secretions, resulting in increased fluid content of feces.

Antacids and Antiulcer Drugs. Antacids reduce acidity of the stomach or rumen. *Nonsystemic antacids,* in liquid or tablet form, are composed of calcium, magnesium, or aluminum, and they directly neutralize acid molecules in the stomach or rumen. Such over-the-counter products as Tums and Rolaids are nonsystemic antacids made primarily of calcium. Other nonsystemic antacids include magnesium products (Riopan, Carmilax), aluminum products (Amphojel), and combinations of magnesium and aluminum products (Maalox).

Systemic antacids decrease acid production in the stomach. Systemic antacids include cimetidine (Tagamet), ranitidine (Zantac), and famotidine (Pepcid). Sucralfate (Carafate) is an antiulcer drug used to treat ulcers of the stomach and upper small intestine. The drug has been called a "gastric Band-Aid" because it forms a sticky paste and adheres to the ulcer site, protecting it from the acidic environment of the stomach.

Ruminatorics and Antibloat Medications. *Ruminatorics,* such as neostimine (Stiglyn), are drugs used to stimulate an atonic ("limp") rumen. *Antibloat medications* act by reducing numbers of gas-producing rumen microorganisms or by breaking up the bubbles formed in the rumen with frothy bloat. Mineral oil or ordinary household detergents mixed with mineral oil are often used to decrease the viscosity of the rumen contents, decrease the stability of the bubbles, and remove the froth. Some commercial antibloat preparations contain poloxalene. Dioctyl sodium succinate (DSS) also reduces the viscosity of rumen contents, allowing the foam to dissipate.

Drugs Affecting the Cardiovascular System

Antiarrhythmic Drugs. An *arrhythmia* is any abnormal pattern of electrical activity in the heart. Arrhythmias are divided into two general groups: arrhythmias that result in an increased heart rate (tachycardia) and those that cause a decreased heart rate (bradycardia). Once the type of arrhythmia has been determined, an effective antiarrhythmic drug is used to reestablish a normal conduction sequence (called a *sinus rhythm).*

Lidocaine, quinidine, and procainamide reverse arrhythmias primarily by decreasing the rate of movement of sodium into heart cells. Lidocaine, which is also used as a local anesthetic under the name of Xylocaine, is only available in injectable form. Veterinary technicians must realize that lidocaine is packaged in vials with or without epinephrine. Lidocaine with epinephrine is designed for use as a local anesthetic, *not* as an antiarrhythmic drug. Accidental IV injection of lidocaine containing epinephrine in an animal with an arrhythmia could cause death. For this reason, it is important to always check the lidocaine bottle before use in treating arrhythmias to be sure it does not contain epinephrine.

Procainamide and quinidine have been used for supraventricular arrhythmias in horses, but they are not very effective against atrial fibrillation in dogs or cats. Hence, they are more commonly used for their ventricular antiarrhythmic effects. Because quinidine and procainamide are available in oral forms, they are used for long-term maintenance of patients with ventricular arrhythmias.

When stimulated by the sympathetic nervous system or by sympathomimetic drugs (drugs that mimic the effects of the sympathetic nervous system), beta-1 receptors in the heart cause the heart to beat more rapidly and with greater strength. Such beta-1 stimulation can produce arrhythmias. Drugs that block beta receptors are known as beta-blockers. Beta blockers cause the heart to contract with less force. Propranolol (Inderal) stimulation of beta-1 receptors by epinephrine, norepinephrine, and other beta-stimulating drugs. It decreases the heart rate and prevents tachycardia in response to stress, fear, or excitement.

Calcium channel blockers include verapamil, nifedipine, and diltiazem. Although calcium channel blockers are not commonly used to treat arrhythmias in veterinary patients, verapamil and diltiazem have been used successfully for treatment of supraventricular tachycardia, atrial fibrillation, and atrial flutter. A more common use of diltiazem is in cats with hypertrophic cardiomyopathy, in which the heart becomes very thickened and enlarged to the point where it cannot contract very efficiently. All of these drugs combat arrhythmias by blocking calcium channels of cardiac muscle cells, resulting in decreased conduction of depolarization waves and decreased automaticity of parts of the conduction system.

Positive Inotropic Agents. Drugs that increase the strength of contraction of a weakened heart are referred to as *positive inotropic drugs (positive inotropes).* Digoxin is the drug of choice for maintaining long-term positive inotropic effects. Digoxin exerts its positive inotropic effect primarily by making more calcium available for the contractile elements within cardiac muscle cells. Digoxin, available as tablets and an elixir, is often used to control supraventricular tachycardia caused by atrial fibrillation. Digoxin has a small *therapeutic index,* meaning that therapeutic concentrations are very close to toxic concentrations. Early signs of digoxin toxicity include anorexia, vomiting, and diarrhea. Owners of animals receiving digoxin should be instructed to watch for these early signs of toxicity and to contact the veterinarian immediately if they should occur.

Vasodilators. Vasoconstriction of peripheral blood vessels is a normal physiologic response to the drop in blood pressure caused by congestive heart failure, hemorrhage, and dehydration. *Vasodilators* open (dilate) constricted vessels, making it easier for the heart to pump blood through these vessels.

Hydralazine is a vasodilator that causes arteriolar smooth muscle to relax, which benefits animals with a poorly functioning left atrioventricular (mitral) valve (mitral insufficiency). Hydralazine allows more blood to flow into the aorta and less to flow back into the left atrium. Although the valve itself remains poorly functional, blood flow through the left heart is improved.

Nitroglycerin relaxes the blood vessels on the venous side of the circulation; it may also help dilate coronary arterioles. The drug is well absorbed through the skin and mucous membranes. In animals, nitroglycerin cream and nitroglycerin in patch form are applied to the skin to improve cardiac output and reduce pulmonary edema and ascites (abdominal fluid accumulation). Nitroglycerin cream is applied every 8 to 12 hours to the hairless inner aspect of the pinna, thorax, or groin. A nitroglycerin patch provides drug diffusion for 24 hours and can be cut into small pieces to adjust the dose for smaller patients.

Other vasodilators are enalapril (Enacard) and captopril, which block angiotensin-converting enzyme and prevent formation of angiotensin II (potent vasoconstrictor) and aldosterone. For this reason, they are sometimes referred to as *angiotensin-converting enzyme (ACE) inhibitors.* Enalapril and captopril are "balanced" vasodilators that relax the smooth muscles of both arterioles and veins, so they are useful in treating animals with cardiac disease that involves the right and the left ventricle (e.g., severe cardiac valvular disease, cardiomyopathy).

Diuretics. Diuretics are drugs that increase urine formation and promote water loss (diuresis). In animals with congestive heart failure, sodium retention from aldosterone secretion and concomitant retention of water in the blood and body tissue lead to pulmonary edema, ascites, and an increased cardiac workload. Removing water from the body with diuretics reduces these deleterious conditions. Diuretics should be used cautiously in animals with hypovolemia (low blood volume) or hypotension (low blood pressure), because they further decrease the fluid component of blood and reduce blood pressure.

Loop diuretics, such as furosemide (Lasix), produce diuresis by inhibiting sodium resorption from the loop of Henle in nephrons. Retention of sodium in the forming urine osmotically retains water in the urine and prevents its resorption. In the distal convoluted tubule, potassium is exchanged for sodium so that sodium is still resorbed and conserved by the body to some degree. Because loop diuretics cause potassium to be excreted in the urine, prolonged use of loop diuretics may result in hypokalemia (low blood potassium).

Thiazide diuretics, such as chlorothiazide, are not often used in veterinary medicine because of the safety and effectiveness of furosemide. Thiazides are less potent than loop diuretics because of their site of action in the distal convoluted tubule. Thiazide diuretics can cause loss of potassium, with resultant hypokalemia.

Spironolactone is a diuretic that is a competitive antagonist of aldosterone, the hormone that normally causes sodium resorption from the distal renal tubules and collection ducts. When aldosterone is inhibited, more sodium remains in the lumen of the renal tubules, osmotically retaining water and preventing its resorption. Because sodium is excreted and potassium is conserved in the body, drugs like spironolactone are called *potassium-sparing diuretics.*

Mannitol is a carbohydrate (sugar) used as an *osmotic diuretic.* Mannitol is poorly resorbed from the renal tubule, thus providing a solute that osmotically retains water in the renal tubular lumen. Mannitol is not used in treatment of cardiovascular disease but is used to reduce cerebral edema associated with head trauma and as a diuretic for flushing absorbed toxins from the body.

Drugs Affecting the Respiratory System

Antitussives. Antitussives are drugs that block the cough reflex, which is coordinated by the cough center in the brainstem. A *productive cough* refers to a cough that produces mucus and other inflammatory products that are coughed up into the oral cavity. A *nonproductive cough* is "dry" and "hacking," and no mucus is coughed up. Antitussives suppress the coughing that normally removes mucus, cellular debris, exudates, and other products that accumulate within the bronchi as a result of infection or inflammation. For this reason, in animals with a very productive cough (much mucus produced), antitussive drugs should be used cautiously and large doses should be avoided. In such situations, suppression of coughing with cough suppressants can result in accumulation of excessive mucus and debris.

Antitussives should be used in animals with a dry, nonproductive cough producing little or no inspissated mucus. Often these coughs keep the animal (and owner) awake, preventing the animal from getting rest it needs to recover. Anititussives are commonly used in treating uncomplicated tracheobronchitis ("kennel cough") in dogs. This "retching" type of cough is often punctuated by gagging up small amounts of mucus the owner interprets as vomitus. This type of cough is extremely irritating to the upper airway mucosa; such irritation stimulates more coughing, which further irritates the airway. This pattern can continue for weeks if the cough is not treated.

Butorphanol (Torbutrol) is a centrally acting opioid cough suppressant that, unlike most other opioid cough suppressants, is not classified as a controlled substance in most states. In antitussive doses, butorphanol causes little sedation, as compared with stronger opioid drugs.

Hydrocodone (Hycodan) is a C-III narcotic available only by prescription from a veterinarian with a Drug Enforcement Administration (DEA) clearance for writing C-III prescriptions. Sedation is often noted in treated animals, and long-term administration can result in constipation.

Codeine is a relatively weak opioid/narcotic that is a component of many cough suppressant preparations. Most products containing codeine are prescription preparations with a C-V controlled substance rating. The sedative effect of codeine is similar to that of hydrocodone, and use of the compound can become habit forming.

Dextromethorphan is a common ingredient in over-the-counter (OTC) nonprescription cough, flu, and cold preparations. Its actions are similar to those of the more potent, narcotic antitussives but it is not a controlled substance. Dextromethorphan is generally not as effective in controlling coughs in veterinary patients as butorphanol or other prescription antitussives; however, owners often initially use human cold products containing dextromethorphan to curtail coughing in their pets. Although dextromethorphan in OTC products is

fairly harmless, the other compounds in cold or flu preparations can cause significant harm to animals (e.g., acetaminophen can be very toxic in cats); therefore, it is unwise to recommend that pet owners use OTC products to control coughing in their animals.

Mucolytics, Expectorants, and Decongestants. *Mucolytic agents* are designed to break up ("lyse") mucus and reduce the viscosity of mucus so that the cilia can move it out of the respiratory tract. Acetylcysteine (Mucomyst) is a mucolytic agent that decreases the viscosity of mucus. Acetylcysteine may be administered by nebulization (inhalation of a fine mist containing the drug) or given PO (although the taste is awful and the taste must be masked with flavoring agents or it must be administered by feeding tube). Nebulized saline and other fluids are used to increase the fluid content of respiratory mucus in the lower airways.

Expectorants are compounds that also increase the fluidity of mucus in the respiratory tract by generating liquid secretions by respiratory tract cells. Guaifenesin (glycerol guaiacolate) and saline expectorants (ammonium chloride, potassium iodide, sodium citrate) are given PO. The volatile oils, such as terpin hydrate, eucalyptus oil, and pine oil, directly stimulate respiratory secretions when their vapors are inhaled.

Many OTC human cold preparations that contain expectorants also contain *decongestants*, such as phenylephrine or phenylpropanolamine, for relief of nasal congestion. Decongestants reduce congestion (vascular engorgement) of the mucous membranes.

Bronchodilators. Bronchoconstriction is caused by contraction of smooth muscles surrounding the small terminal bronchioles deep within the respiratory tree. Drugs that inhibit bronchoconstriction are called *bronchodilators*. Terbutaline and albuterol are available in an oral dosage form and as an inhaler. The methylxanthines include such bronchodilators as theophylline and aminophylline. The difference between theophylline and aminophylline is that aminophylline is approximately 80% theophylline and 20% ethylenediamine salt. Because 100 mg of aminophylline contains only 80 mg of active theophylline, the dose of theophylline must be adjusted if the animal is switched to aminophylline or vice versa based upon the amount of active ingredient (theophylline) in the compound.

Drugs Affecting the Endocrine System

Drugs Used to Treat Hypothyroidism. Drugs used to treat hypothyroidism (insufficiency of thyroid hormone) include levothyroxine (T_4) and synthetic liothyronine (T_3). Supplementing a hypothyroid animal with levothyroxine (T_4) provides the various organs and tissues with the appropriate amount of thyroid hormone, as each organ or tissue converts T_4 to T_3. With T_3 supplementation, the local tissue regulation of thyroid hormone converstion is bypassed. Another advantage of synthetic levothyroxine is its ability to trigger the natural negative-feedback mechanism, thus emulating the normal regulatory mechanism for thyroid hormone production. Levothyroxine (e.g., Synthroid, Soloxine) is usually the drug of choice for treating hypothyroidism. Also, T_3 products (e.g., Cytomel) are generally more expensive than T_4 products and must be administered three times daily, rather than once daily.

Drugs Used to Treat Hyperthyroidism. *Hyperthyroidism* is an increase in thyroid hormone production. It is most common in cats and is associated with a hormone-secreting thyroid tumor. Hyperthyroidism is best treated by surgical removal of the thyroid gland. However, some animals may be treated with drugs that decrease thyroid hormone production or destroy the thyroid tissue (antithyroid drugs).

Methimazole (Tapazole) and propylthiouracil have been used to control hyperthyroidism in cats by blocking the thyroid tumor's ability to produce T_3 and T_4. Of the two drugs, methimazole causes fewer complications and is preferred over propylthiouracil for decreasing thyroid hormone production.

If the owner is reluctant or unable to give oral medication to the hyperthyroid cat, or if the risk of side effects is unacceptable to the owner, use of radioactive iodine (I-131) is an alternative to oral treatment of hyperthyroidism. The radioactive iodine is injected IV. The iodine, a normal component of thyroid hormone, is taken up and concentrated by the active thyroid tumor cells, which are then destroyed by the radioactivity.

Endocrine Pancreatic Drugs. Insulin is responsible for movement of glucose from the blood into tissue cells. Lack of insulin results in diabetes mellitus, a condition characterized by high blood glucose levels (hyperglycemia) and passage of glucose in the urine (glucosuria). Blood glucose levels can be controlled by one or two SC insulin injections a day. The insulins of choice for maintaining diabetic dogs are NPH insulin and lente insulin, which are of intermediate duration. Diabetic cats require the longer-acting ultralente insulin, which is administered once or twice daily. Regular insulin is not commonly used to maintain diabetic cats or dogs because its short duration of activity requires multiple doses during a 24-hour period. However, because regular insulin is the only type that can be given IV, it is used initially to stabilize the glucose concentrations of animals with severe, uncontrolled diabetes or diabetic ketoacidosis.

Drugs Affecting Reproduction

Hormone drugs, either natural or synthetic, are used in food animals and horses to synchronize estrous cycles, terminate pregnancies, and induce ovulation. In dogs and cats they are used primarily to prevent pregnancy or alter the state of the uterus.

Gonadotropin-releasing hormone (GnRH) drugs (e.g., Cystorelin) stimulate release of luteinizing hormone (LH) and/or follicle-stimulating hormone (FSH) from the pituitary gland, causing the ovary to develop follicles. *Gonadotropins* is another name for FSH and LH produced by the pituitary gland. In addition to pituitary gonadotropins, some species produce chorionic gonadotropins from the placenta. These can be used as drugs and include human chorionic gonadotropin (HCG), a hormone produced by pregnant women, and equine chorionic gonadotropin (eCG), formerly known as pregnant mare serum gonadotropin (PMSG). These drugs are sometimes used in food animals to induce superovulation (release of ova from multiple follicles) and occasionally in dogs and cats to induce estrus.

Estrogens, such as estradiol cypionate, have been used to induce estrus in anestrual mares. Their most common use in small animals is to prevent pregnancy after "mismating."

Progestins are reproductive hormones that are similar to progesterone. Progestins can prevent an animal from coming into full estrus. The progestins used in veterinary medicine include altrenogest (Regu-Mate) and norgestomet.

In livestock breeding systems, the estrous cycles of females can be synchronized so that many animals can be artificially inseminated at the same time. Injecting cows with prostaglandins during diestrus lyses the CL, causing return to estrus within 2 to 5 days. Prostaglandin drugs used include *dinoprost tromethamine* (Lutalyse), *cloprostenol* (Estrumate), *fluprostenol* (Equimate), and *fenprostalene* (Bovilene).

Because equine breed registries encourage birth of foals as soon as possible after January 1, veterinarians are often asked to help mares conceive during the spring. To stimulate more predictable ovulation during this period of transitional estrus, progesterone or a progestin is given for 10 to 14 days to mimic diestrus. Drug use is then halted to mimic lysis of the CL. Such hormonal therapy is often coupled with exposing the mares to artificial lighting to artificially lengthen the photoperiod. This causes the mare to cycle as though it were summer.

Pregnancy can be prevented (contraception) by suppressing the estrous cycle or by preventing implantation of the fertilized ova in the uterine wall. Megestrol acetate (Ovaban) is an oral progestin used for contraception in female dogs and cats. Megestrol use increases the risk of cystic hyperplasia of the endometrium, endometritis, or pyometra. Prolonged use of megestrol can result in mammary hyperplasia (proliferation of mammary tissue). Mibolerone (Cheque Drops) is another contraceptive used in female dogs. Because mibolerone is a testosterone analog (similar structure), it produces effects similar to those of high levels of testosterone, including increased production of anal sac secretions, masculinization of developing female fetuses, and increased vulvar discharge.

Estradiol cypionate (ECP) is an injectable estrogen used after mismating in dogs. Estrogens prevent pregnancy by increasing the number and thickness of folds within the oviducts, preventing passage of the ova to the uterus. Because there are safer alternatives to estradiol therapy, such as ovariohysterectomy (spaying), many theriogenologists (specialists in animal reproduction) do not recommend use of estradiol in dogs.

Prostaglandin administration causes lysis of the corpus luteum, resulting in a decrease in progesterone levels and subsequent fetal death. Fluprostenol (Equimate) and dinoprost tromethamine (Lutalyse) are both approved for termination of pregnancy in mares. Prostaglandins are only effective in cows if given before the fourth month of pregnancy. Corticosteroids (e.g., dexamethasone) may induce abortion in mares or cows by mimicking the elevated levels of cortisol that occur at the beginning of normal parturition.

Oxytocin is commonly used to increase uterine contractions in animals with dystocia (difficult birth) related to a weakened or fatigued uterus. Anabolic steroids, such as testosterone and progesterone, have been used to increase the weight and conditioning of feedlot cattle. Progestins (e.g., megestrol acetate) have been used to modify behavior in cats.

Drugs Affecting the Nervous System

Anesthetics. Barbiturates are frequently used to produce short-term anesthesia, induce general anesthesia, control seizures, and euthanize animals. Thiobarbiturates contain a sulfur molecule on the barbituric acid molecule; oxybarbiturates contain an oxygen molecule. Thiamylal and thiopental are thiobarbiturates; methohexital, pentobarbital, and phenobarbital are oxybarbiturates. Thiobarbiturates have a more rapid onset but shorter duration of action than oxybarbiturates.

Propofol is usually injected as an IV bolus and provides rapid injection of anesthesia and a short period of unconsciousness. It is relatively expensive and may cause pain when injected IV.

Ketamine and tiletamine are short-acting injectable anesthetics that produce a rather unique form of anesthesia in which the animal feels dissociated (apart) from its body. This dissociative effect is characterized by retention of laryngeal, pharyngeal, and corneal reflexes, lack of muscular relaxation (often rigidity), and an increased heart rate. The lack of muscular relaxation makes ketamine unsuitable as a sole anesthetic agent for major surgery. Ketamine and tiletamine produce good somatic (peripheral tissue) analgesia

(pain relief) and are suitable for superficial surgery; however, they are much less effective in blocking visceral (internal organ) pain and should not be used alone as anesthesia for internal procedures. Tiletamine is included with zolazepam, a benzodiazepine tranquilizer, in a product marketed as Telazol. Zolazepam reduces some of the CNS excitation and side effects produced by tiletamine.

Nitrous oxide, also referred to as "laughing gas," is very safe when used properly and has much weaker analgesic qualities than other inhalant anesthetics. The major role of nitrous oxide is to decrease the amount of the more potent inhalant anesthetics needed to achieve a surgical plane of anesthesia.

Methoxyflurane (Metofane, Penthrane) is an inhalant anesthetic characterized by good muscle relaxation, a relatively slow rate of anesthetic induction (as compared with halothane and isoflurane), and a prolonged recovery period. Unlike halothane and isoflurane, methoxyflurane does not require a precision vaporizer for administration.

Like methoxyflurane, halothane (Fluothane) is a nonflammable, nonirritating inhalant anesthetic that can be used in all species. Anesthesia is induced much more rapidly with halothane than with methoxyflurane. Because of its chemical and physical properties, halothane should be administered with a precision vaporizer.

Isoflurane (Forane, AErrane) is an inhalant anesthetic that has gained popularity in veterinary practice because of its rapid, smooth injection of anesthesia and short recovery period. Other inhalant agents with similar properties of isoflurane include enflurane (Ethrane), desflurane (Suprane) and sevoflurane (Ultane). Chapter 20 contains detailed information on anesthetic agents.

Tranquilizers and Sedatives. Acepromazine maleate is a phenothiazine tranquilizer that reduces anxiety and produces a mentally relaxed state. It is often used to calm animals for physical examination or transport. Unlike xylazine or detomidine, phenothiazine tranquilizers have no analgesic effect (do not relieve pain).

Droperidol is a butyrophenone with much more potent sedative effects than most phenothiazine tranquilizers. Droperidol has been combined with fentanyl, a strong narcotic analgesic with emetic activity, and marketed as a neuroleptanalgesic product called Innovar-Vet.

Diazepam (Valium), zolazepam (contained in Telazol), midazolam (Versed), and clonazepam (Klonopin) are benzodiazepine tranquilizers often used with other agents as part of a preanesthetic protocol for their calming and muscle relaxing effect.

Xylazine (Rompun, Anased), medetomidine (Domitor), and detomidine (Dormosedan) produce a calming effect and somewhat decrease an animal's ability to respond to stimuli. These drugs also have some analgesic activity. A disadvantage of xylazine is that sedative doses produce vomiting in about 90% of cats and 50% of dogs.

Analgesics. *Analgesics* are drugs that reduce the perception of pain without loss of other sensations. Oxymorphone (Numorphan) is commonly used for preanesthesia and anesthesia. Butorphanol (Torbutrol, Torbugesic) is used for cough control in small animals and for reducing colic pain in horses. Fentanyl has an analgesic effect 250 times greater than that of morphine. Meperidine (Demerol) is a fairly weak analgesic/sedative and is often injected SC to restrain cats. Pentazocine (Talwin) is a weak analgesic used in horses with colic and dogs recovering from painful surgery. Buprenorphine (Buprenex) is commonly combined with sedatives or tranquilizers (acepromazine, xylazine, detomidine). It is also used alone in dogs and cats as an analgesic, both for its potency (30 times the analgesic potency of morphine) and its long duration of analgesia (8 to 12 hours). Etorphine (M-99) is an extremely potent narcotic (1000 times the analgesic potency of morphine) used to sedate and capture wildlife or zoo animals. Butorphanol, pentazocine, and buprenorphine are sometimes used to partially reverse some of the respiratory depression and sedation caused by stronger narcotic agents. Nalorphine is another reversal agent.

Neuroleptanalgesia refers to a state of CNS depression (sedation or tranquilization) and analgesia induced by a combination of a sedative (e.g., xylazine) or tranquilizer (e.g., acepromazine), and an analgesic (oxymorphone). Phenothiazine tranquilizers or butyrophenone tranquilizers (droperidol) calm the animal and also decrease or block the emetic (vomiting) side effect of a narcotic analgesic. Innovar-Vet is a neuroleptanalgesic product containing droperidol and fentanyl (a narcotic analgesic).

Anticonvulsants. *Seizures* are periods of altered brain function characterized by loss of consciousness, altered muscle tone or movement, altered sensations, or other neurologic changes. Drugs used to control seizures are called *anticonvulsants*. Phenobarbital is the drug of choice for long-term control of seizures in dogs and cats. This barbiturate is inexpensive and, because of its long half-life, may be given orally once or twice a day. The dose of phenobarbital is often measured in grains (1 grain = approximately 60 mg). Although primidone itself has some anticonvulsant activity, most of its efficacy is attributable to phenobarbital, produced by metabolism of primidone.

Phenytoin (Dilantin) is a human anticonvulsant that was once popular for use in treating epilepsy in animals. The major disadvantage of phenytoin is that it is difficult to maintain therapeutic plasma concentrations in dogs. Diazepam (Valium) is the drug of choice for emergency treatment of convulsing animals. Diazepam is very effective when given IV, but it is poorly effective when given PO and is absorbed irregularly if injected SC or IM. Clonazepam (Klonopin) is occasionally used with phenobarbital in animals in which plasma concentrations of barbiturate are in the therapeutic range, but the seizures are not adequately controlled.

Central Nervous System Stimulants. Central nervous system (CNS) stimulants are primarily used to stimulate respiration in anesthetized animals or to reverse CNS depression caused by anesthetic or sedative agents. The active ingredient in chocolate is theobromine. A dosage as low as 90 mg/kg (41 mg/lb) can produce toxicity in dogs. For a 10-lb dog, it would take two or three chocolate bars to produce serious toxicity. Fortunately, ingestion of that much chocolate by such a small dog would likely produce vomiting, thus decreasing the amount of theobromine absorbed.

Doxapram (Dopram) is a CNS stimulant that increases respiration in animals with apnea (cessation of breathing) or bradypnea (slow breathing). Doxapram is most often used in animals that have received large amounts of these respiratory depressant drugs. Yohimbine, tolazoline, and atipamezole increase respiration through reversal of CNS depression caused by such drugs as xylazine, detomidine, and medetomidine.

Antimicrobials

Antimicrobials are drugs that kill or inhibit the growth of microorganisms or "microbes," such as bacteria, protozoa, viruses, or fungi. The term *antibiotic* is often used interchangeably with the term *antimicrobial*. An antimicrobial can be classified by the type of microorganism against which it is effective and whether the antimicrobial kills the microorganism or prevents the microorganism from replicating and proliferating. The suffix *-cidal* generally describes drugs that kill the microorganism (e.g., bactericidal). The suffix *-static* usually describes drugs that inhibit replication but generally do not kill the microorganism outright (e.g., fungistatic). Examples include the following:

bactericidal	kills bacteria
bacteriostatic	inhibits bacterial replication
virucidal	kills viruses
protozoistatic	inhibits protozoal replication
fungicidal	kills fungi

Antimicrobials work by different mechanisms to kill or inhibit bacteria and other microorganisms. Antimicrobials generally exert their effects on the cell wall, cell membrane, ribosomes, critical enzymes or metabolites, or nucleic acids of microorganisms.

Some microorganisms have developed the ability to survive in the presence of antimicrobial drugs. This ability to survive is referred to as *resistance*. Bacteria may become resistant to certain drugs because of genetic changes inherited from previous generations of bacteria, or they may acquire resistance by spontaneous mutations of chromosomes.

A *residue* is an accumulation of a drug or chemical or its metabolites in animal tissues or food products, resulting from drug administration to an animal or contamination of food products. Use of drugs in animals intended for food (meat, egg, milk, etc.) must be stopped a specific number of days (the withdrawal period) before the animal is slaughtered or the food products are to be marketed as food for people. *Most antimicrobial residues in food are not degraded by cooking or pasteurization.*

Penicillins. Penicillins are bactericidal and can usually be recognized by their *-cillin* suffix on the drug name. The most frequently used penicillins in veterinary medicine include the following: the natural penicillins, penicillin G and penicillin V; the broad-spectrum aminopenicillins, ampicillin, amoxicillin, and hetacillin; the penicillinase-resistant penicillins, cloxacillin, dicloxacillin, and oxacillin; and the extended-spectrum penicillins, carbenicillin, ticarcillin, piperacillin, and others. Penicillins are generally effective against gram-positive bacteria and varying types of gram-negative bacteria. Penicillins are generally well absorbed from injection sites and the gastrointestinal tract. A penicillin that should not be given PO is penicillin G. Pencillin G is inactivated by gastric acid and so is used only in injectable form.

Cephalosporins. Cephalosporins are bactericidal beta-lactam antimicrobials with a *ceph-* or *cef-* prefix in the drug name. Cephalosporins are classified by generations, according to when they were first developed. *First-generation cephalosporins* are primarily effective against gram-positive bacteria *(Streptococcus, Staphylococcus).* They are less effective against gram-negative bacteria than the *second-* or *third-generation cephalosporins.* Veterinary products include cefadroxil (first generation, Cefa-Tabs), cephapirin (first generation, Cefa-Lak and Cefa-Dri intramammary infusions), and ceftiofur (third generation, Naxcel injectable). Human products used in veterinary medicine include cephalothin (first generation, Keflin), cephalexin (first generation, Keflex), cefoxitin (second generation, Mefoxin), and from cefotaxime (third generation, Claforan). First-generation cephalosporins are well absorbed from the GI tract.

Bacitracins. Bacitracins are a group of polypeptide antibiotics, of which bacitracin A is the major component. Bacitracin is a common ingredient in topical antibiotic creams or ointments. It is often combined with polymyxin B and neomycin to provide a broad spectrum of antibacterial activity.

Aminoglycosides. Aminoglycosides used in veterinary medicine include gentamicin, amikacin, neomycin, streptomycin, dihydrostreptomycin, apramycin, kanamycin, and tobramycin. With the exception of amikacin, most aminoglycosides can be recognized by the *-micin* or *-mycin* suffix in the nonproprietary name.

Aminoglycosides are bactericidal and are quite effective against many aerobic bacteria (bacteria that require oxygen to live), but are not effective against most anaerobic bacteria (those that do not require oxygen). Aminoglycosides are potentially nephrotoxic (toxic to the kidney) and ototoxic (toxic to the inner ear), even at "normal" dosages.

Fluoroquinolones. Fluoroquinolones are bactericidal antimicrobials that are gaining favor for a variety of uses in veterinary medicine. Enrofloxacin (Baytril) is approved for use in dogs and cats. It has also been used extra-label (in unapproved ways) to treat neonatal diseases in swine. Sarafloxacin (Saraflox) was the first quinolone approved for use in food animals (poultry only). Ciprofloxacin is approved only for use in people, and any use in animals is unapproved. The fluoroquinolones are effective against common gram-negative and gram-positive bacteria found in skin, respiratory, and urinary infections. Baytril (enrofloxacin) is available in injectable and oral (tablets) forms. Saraflox (sarafloxacin) is marketed as a water-soluble powder for oral administration and as an injectable product.

Tetracyclines. Tetracyclines are bacteriostatic drugs with a nonproprietary name ending in *-cycline.* Tetracycline and oxytetracycline have similar spectra of antibacterial activity and actions in the body. The newer and more lipophilic doxycyline and minocycline are human drugs that are being used more frequently in animals (unapproved use) because of their longer half-life (increased duration of activity), broader spectrum of antibacterial action, and better penetration of tissues than the older tetracyclines. After oral administration, doxycycline and minocycline are absorbed better than oxytetracycline or tetracycline. Oxytetracycline is the most commonly used injectable tetracycline because of its good absorption from IM injection sites.

Sulfonamides and Potentiated Sulfonamides. Because sulfonamides ("sulfa drugs") have been in use for many years, many strains of bacteria have become resistant to them. To increase the efficacy of sulfonamides and convert them from bacteriostatic to bactericidal drugs, they are sometimes combined with other compounds, such as trimethoprim and ormetoprim, to *potentiate* (increase) their antibacterial effects. Some of the more common sulfonamides used in veterinary medicine include sulfadimethoxine (combined with ormetoprim in Primor), sulfadiazine (combined with trimethoprim in Tribrissen), sulfamethoxazole (combined with trimethoprim in Septra), sulfachlorpyridazine (used in livestock and poultry), and sulfasalazine (used for its antiinflammatory effect in inflammatory bowel disease). Potentiated sulfas used in veterinary medicine have a fairly broad spectrum of antibacterial activity, including many gram-positive organisms (e.g., *Streptococcus, Staphylococcus, Nocardia*). Although sulfas and potentiated sulfas are not very effective against gram-negative organisms, they are the drugs of choice for treating some protozoal infections, including *Coccidia* and *Toxoplasma*.

Lincosamides. Lincosamide antibiotics, including linocomycin and clindamycin (Antirobe), can be bacteriostatic or bactericidal, depending upon the concentrations attained at the site of infection. The lincosamides are generally effective against many gram-positive aerobic cocci. Lincomycin is approved for use in a variety of species (dogs, cats, swine, poultry), but clindamycin is approved only for use in dogs.

Macrolides. The macrolide antibiotics erythromycin and tylosin (Tylan) are approved for use in a variety of companion animals and food animals, including dogs, cats, swine, sheep, cattle, and poultry. Although tylosin is approved for use in dogs and cats, its primary use is in livestock. Both drugs are bacteriostatic and share similar spectra of antibacterial activity and bacterial cross-resistance. *Tilmicosin* (Micotil) is a macrolide approved for SC administration for treatment of bovine respiratory diseases.

Metronidazole. Metronidazole (Flagyl) is a bactericidal antimicrobial that is also effective against protozoa that cause intestinal disease, such as *Giardia* (giardiasis), *Entamoeba histolytica* (amebiasis), *Trichomonas* (trichomoniasis), and *Balantidium coli* (balantidiasis).

Nitrofurans. The nitrofurans are a large group of antimicrobials, of which nitrofurantoin (Furadantin) is most commonly used in veterinary medicine. Nitrofurantoin is bacteriostatic or bactericidal, depending upon concentrations attained at the site of infection. Because about half of the drug administered is secreted into the renal tubule, it is used to treat infections of the lower urinary tract (bladder, urethra) in dogs, cats, and occasionally horses.

Chloramphenicol and Florfenicol. Chloramphenicol is an antimicrobial that is bacteriostatic at low concentrations but may become bactericidal when used at higher dosages. Chloramphenicol has produced fatal aplastic anemia in humans. For this reason, *chloramphenicol is totally banned from any use in food animals.* Fluorfenicol is a new drug similar to chloramphenicol but without the risk of aplastic anemia. It is approved for treatment of respiratory disease in cattle.

Rifampin. Rifampin is a bactericidal or bacteriostatic antimicrobial belonging to the rifamycins. It is primarily used with or without erythromycin for treatment of *Rhodococcus equi* infections in young foals, and sometimes in conjunction with antifungal agents for treatment of aspergillosis or histoplasmosis in dogs and cats.

Amphotericin B and Nystatin. Amphotericin B is an antifungal that is administered IV for treatment of deep or systemic mycotic infections. Nystatin, because of its toxicity to tissues, is used only to treat *Candida* infections (candidiasis) on the skin, mucous membranes (e.g., mouth, vagina), and lining of the intestinal tract in dogs, cats, and birds.

Ketoconazole and Itraconazole. Ketoconazole and itraconazole are imidazole antifungals with fewer side effects than amphotericin B. Of the two imidazoles, itraconazole has fewer side effects than ketoconazole and is apparently safe for use in cats.

Griseofulvin. Griseofulvin is a fungistatic drug used primarily to treat infections with *Trichophyton*, *Microsporum*, and *Epidermophyton* dermatophytes (superficial fungi) in dogs, cats, and horses. These fungi usually infect the skin, hair, nails, and claws, causing the condition known as *ringworm*. Griseofulvin is available as a veterinary product (Fulvicin) for oral use as a powder (for horses) or tablets.

Disinfectants and Antiseptics

Disinfection is the destruction of pathogenic microorganisms or their toxins. *Antiseptics* are chemical agents that kill or prevent the growth of microorganisms on living tissues. *Disinfectants* are chemical agents that kill or prevent growth of microorganisms on inanimate objects (surgical equipment, floors, tabletops). Antiseptics and disinfectants may also be described as *sanitizers* or *sterilizers*. Sanitizers are chemical agents that reduce the number of microorganisms to a "safe" level, without completely eliminating all microorganisms. Sterilizers are chemicals or other agents that completely destroy all microorganisms. As with antimicrobials, it is important to know against what organisms the antiseptic or disinfectant is effective (Table 13-1).

Phenols. Phenols are used as scrub soaps and surface disinfectants. Phenols are also the main disinfecting agents found in many household disinfectants (Lysol, pine oil, and similar cleansers). They are very effective against gram-positive bacteria but generally not effective against gram-negative bacteria, viruses, fungi, or spores. Hexachlorophene is a phenolic surgical scrub that has decreased in popularity because of its suspected neurotoxicity (damage to the nervous system) and teratogenic effects (birth defects) in pregnant nurses who performed hexachlorophene scrubs on a regular basis.

Alcohols. Alcohols, such as ethyl alcohol or isopropyl alcohol, are among the most common antiseptics applied to skin. Solutions of 70% alcohol are used to disinfect surgical sites, injection sites, and rectal thermometers. Nonenveloped viruses are not susceptible to the virucidal effects of alcohol. Alcohol is also ineffective against bacterial spores and must remain in contact with the site for several seconds to be effective against bacteria (several minutes for fungi). Therefore, a cursory swipe with an alcohol-soaked swab on an animal's skin, especially if the skin is encrusted with dirt or feces, does little to disinfect an injection site.

TABLE 13-1 Relative efficacy of disinfectants and antiseptics*

	Chlorhexidine	Quaternary ammonium compounds	Alcohol	Iodophor	Chlorine	Phenols
Bactericidal	3+†	2+	2+	3+	2+	2+
Lipid-enveloped virucidal	3+	2+	2+	2+	3+	1+
Nonenveloped virucidal	2+	1+	(–)‡	2+	3+	(–)
Sporicidal	(–)	(–)	(–)	1+	1+	(–)
Effective in presence of soap	1+	(–)	2+	2+	2+	2+
Effective in hard water	1+	1+	1+	2+	2+	1+
Effective in organic material	3+	1+	1+	(–)	(–)	(–)

*Ratings are relative indicators, and the effectiveness is dependent upon concentration of compound used.
†The higher the positive number, the greater the efficacy.
‡Hyphens (–) indicate lack of efficacy.

Quaternary Ammonium Compounds. Quaternary ammonium compounds are used to disinfect the surface of inanimate objects. One of the most commonly used quaternary ammonium compounds in veterinary medicine is benzalkonium chloride. Quaternary ammonium compounds are effective against a wide variety of gram-negative and gram-positive bacteria, but they are ineffective against bacterial spores and have poor efficacy against fungi. Although quaternary ammonium compounds can destroy enveloped viruses, they are ineffective against nonenveloped viruses, such as parvovirus. They act rapidly at a site of application and are not normally irritating to the skin or corrosive to metals.

Chlorine Compounds. Chlorine compounds, such as sodium hypochlorite (Clorox, household bleach), can kill enveloped and nonenveloped viruses and are the disinfectant of choice against parvovirus. Chlorines are also effective against fungi, algae, and vegetative forms of bacteria. Like many other disinfectants, chlorine is not effective against bacterial spores.

Iodophors. Iodophors are used as topical antiseptics before surgical procedures or for disinfection of tissue. An iodophor is a combination of iodine and a carrier molecule that releases the iodine over time, prolonging the antimicrobial activity. The most common iodophor is iodine combined with polyvinylpyrrolidone, more commonly known as *povidone-iodine*. Iodophors are bactericidal, virucidal, protozoicidal, and fungicidal.

Biguanides. Chlorhexidine, a biguanide antiseptic, is commonly used to clean cages and to treat various superficial infections in animals. Its wide variety of uses is likely related to its low tissue irritation and its virucidal, bactericidal (both gram positive and gram negative), and fungicidal activity. Because chlorhexidine binds to the outer surface of the skin, it is thought to have some residual activity for up to 24 hours if left in contact with the site.

Antiparasitics

Anthelmintic is a general term used to describe compounds that kill various types of internal parasites (helminths or "worms"). A vermicide is an anthelmintic that kills the worm, as opposed to a vermifuge, which only paralyzes the worm and often results in passage of live worms in the stool. Antinematodal compounds are used to treat infections with nematodes (roundworms). Nematodes include hookworms, ascarids, whipworms, and strongyles. Anticestodal compounds are used to treat infections with cestodes (tapeworms or segmented flatworms). Antitrematodal compounds are used to treat infection with trematodes (flukes or unsegmented flatworms), including *Paragonimus, Fasciola,* and *Dicrocoelium*. Antiprotozoal compounds are used to treat infection with protozoa (single-celled organisms), including *Coccidia, Giardia,* and *Toxoplasma*. Coccidiostats are drugs that inhibit the growth of coccidia specifically.

Internal Antiparasitics. Piperazine, a vermicide and vermifuge, is the active ingredient in most of the "once-a-month" dewormers sold in grocery stores and pet shops. Piperazine is very safe but is only effective against ascarids. The benzimidazoles include fenbendazole (Panacur), mebendazole (Telmin, Telmintic), thiabendazole (Equizole, Tresaderm Otic), oxibendazole (Anthelcide EQ, Filaribits-Plus), albendazole, oxfendazole, and cambendazole.

Organophosphates are used as internal antiparasitics (Task, Combot), as well as external antiparasitics to combat fleas, ticks, and flies. The organophosphates most commonly used internally are dichlorvos and trichlorfon. Ivermectin (Ivomec, Eqvalan, Heartgard-30) is an avermectin widely used in almost every species treated by veterinarians. Ivermectin can produce adverse reactions in Collies and Collie-cross breeds. Anticestodals used in animals include praziquantel (Droncit) and epsiprantel (Cestex).

Anthelmintics containing pyrantel (Strongid, Nemex, Banminth, Imathal) safely remove a variety of nematodes in domestic species. They are marketed as pyrantel pamoate and a more water-soluble salt, pyrantel tartrate. Morantel tartrate (Nematel) is very similar to pyrantel and has similar uses. Febantel is marketed in a palatable paste formulation for horses or in combination with the anticestodal drug praziquantel (Vercom) for dogs and cats or with the organophosphate trichlorfon (Combotel) for horses.

Thiacetarsamide sodium (Caparsolate) for years had been the only drug approved for treatment of adult heartworms; thiacetarsamide is given by IV injection. In 1996, melarsomine dihydrochloride (Immiticide) was approved as an adulticide; it is given by IM injection. After adulticide treatment, a microfilaricide can be administered to eliminate circulating heartworm microfilariae. Ivermectin (e.g., 1% Ivomec injectable, approved for use in livestock) is the microfilaricide of choice. Milbemycin oxime (Interceptor), a drug very similar to ivermectin, is also used as a microfilaricide. After microfilariae have been cleared from the blood, the animal can begin receiving heartworm preventive to prevent reinfection. Diethylcarbamazine (DEC), marketed as Caricide, Nemacide, and Filarbits, is given daily during seasons when an animal could be bitten by a mosquito and for 2 months thereafter. Because they must be given only once a month, ivermectin (Heartgard-30) and milbemycin (Interceptor) have captured a significant percentage of the heartworm preventive market. Ivermectin is also available as a heartworm preventive for cats (Heartgard-30 for Cats).

Antiprotozoals are most commonly used against coccidia, *Giardia,* and other protozoa. They include sulfonamide antimicrobials, such as sulfadimethoxine (Albon, Bactrovet), metronidazole, and amprolium (Corid).

External Antiparasitics. Chlorinated hydrocarbons constitute one of the oldest group of the synthetic insecticides. The only chlorinated hydrocarbon currently used in veterinary medicine is lindane, which is incorporated in some dog shampoos. Lindane is easily absorbed through the skin and can produce harmful side effects if absorbed in sufficient quantities.

Organophosphates and carbamates are usually grouped together because of their similar mechanism of action, effects on insects, and toxic effects. Unlike the chlorinated hydrocarbons, organophosphates and carbamates decompose readily in the environment and do not pose a significant threat to wildlife. Included in this group are chlorpyrifos, carbaryl (Sevin), and propoxur (Baygon).

Pyrethrins and pyrethroids (synthetic pyrethrins) constitute the largest group of insecticides marketed for use against external parasites and as common household insect sprays. They are generally quite safe. Pyrethrins and pyrethroids produce a quick "knockdown" effect, but the immobilized flies or fleas may recover after several minutes. Pyrethroids include resmethrin, allethrin, permethrin, tetramethrin, bioallethrin, and fenvalerate.

Amitraz is a diamide insecticide that was one of the first effective agents available for treatment of demodectic mange in dogs. Since its introduction, amitraz has been incorporated into other insecticidal products. Amitraz is toxic to cats and rabbits, so it should not be used in those species. The liquid form, available as a dip or sponge-on bath product (Mitaban), is used to treat demodectic mange in dogs. Amitraz is also available as the Preventic, a tick collar for dogs, and as Taktic, a liquid topical or a collar for use in cattle.

Imidacloprid (Advantage) is a chloronicotinyl nitroguanidine insecticide used topically to kill adult fleas on dogs and cats. Imidacloprid is applied to the back of the neck in cats or between the shoulder blades in dogs (and over the rump area of large dogs), and kills adult fleas upon contact. Fipronil (Frontline and Top Spot) is a once-a-month flea spray and topical application that resembles ivermectin in its insecticidal activity.

Rotenone (Derris Powder) is a natural insecticide derived from derris root. It may be included with other insecticides in dips, pour-ons, and powders. D-limonene, derived from citrus peels, purportedly has some slight insecticidal activity. When included in insecticidal products, it imparts a pleasant citrus smell to the haircoat. Sulfur is sometimes included in "tar and sulfur" shampoos to help reduce skin scaling and to treat sarcoptic mange. These products are usually recognized by their strong sulfur odor.

Insect growth regulators are compounds that affect immature stages of insects and prevent maturation to adults. They are insecticidal without toxic effects in mammals. Methoprene (Siphotrol, Ovitrol) and fenoxycarb (Basus, Ectogard, and others) were some of the first insect growth regulators incorporated into topical products or flea collars. These compounds are distributed over the animal's skin. Female fleas absorb the drug and it is incorporated into the flea eggs. The drug-impregnated eggs hatch and the larvae do not mature to adult fleas. Lufenuron (Program) is an insect development inhibitor given once a month as a tablet for dogs and cats and as an oral liquid for cats. Lufenuron interferes with development of the insect's chitin, which is essential for proper egg formation and development of the larval exoskeleton. If flea larvae survive within the egg despite a defective shell, they will be unable to hatch. Because lufenuron is orally ingested and distributed throughout the animal's tissue fluids, a flea must bite the animal to be exposed to the drug.

Insect repellents are used to repel insects and keep them off of animals. Butoxypolypropylene glycol (Butox PPG) has been incorporated into flea and tick spray products for use in dogs and cats. It is also used in equine fly repellents. Diethyltoluamide (DEET) is a common ingredient in repellent products formulated for use in people.

Antiinflammatories

Drugs that relieve pain or discomfort by blocking or reducing the inflammatory process are called *antiinflammatories*. There are two general classes of antiinflammatories: *steroidal antiinflammatory drugs* (glucocorticoids) and *nonsteroidal antiinflammatory drugs (NSAIDs)*. Most of these drugs relieve pain indirectly by decreasing inflammation; however, some also have direct analgesic (pain-relieving) activity.

Glucocorticoids. When veterinarians use the terms "cortisone" or "corticosteroids," they are usually referring to glucocorticoids. A glucocorticoid that exerts an antiinflammatory effect for less than 12 hours, such as hydrocortisone, is considered a *short-acting glucocorticoid*. Many of the glucocorticoids used in veterinary medicine are classified as *intermediate-acting glucocorticoids*, with activity for 12 to 36 hours. These include prednisone, prednisolone, triamcinolone (e.g., Vetalog), methylprednisolone, and isoflupredone. *Long-acting glucocorticoids*, such as dexamethasone, betamethasone, and flumethasone, exert their effects for more than 48 hours.

Glucocorticoids are generally available in three liquid forms: aqueous solutions, alcohol solutions, and suspensions. Glucocorticoids in aqueous (water) solution are usually combined with a salt to make them soluble in water. Dexamethasone sodium phosphate (Azium SP) and prednisolone sodium succinate (Solu-Delta-Cortef) are aqueous solutions of glucocorticoids. The advantage of aqueous forms is that they can be given in large doses IV with less risk than alcohol solutions and suspensions (suspensions should never be given IV). The aqueous forms are often used in emergency situations (shock, CNS trauma) because they can be delivered IV in large amounts and have a fairly rapid onset of activity. If the label of a vial of dexamethasone specifies the active ingredient as dexamethasone, without mention of sodium phosphate, it is likely an alcohol solution. Suspensions of glucocorticoids contain the drug particles suspended in the liquid vehicle. Suspensions are characterized by their opaque appearance (after shaking), the need for shaking the vial before use, and the terms *acetate, diacetate, pivalate, acetonide,* or *valerate* append-

ed to the glucocorticoid name. When injected into the body, the drug crystals dissolve over several days, releasing small amounts of glucocorticoid each day and providing prolonged action. Topical preparations of glucocorticoid suspensions using the acetate ester are used in topical ophthalmic medications.

Overuse of glucocorticoid drugs can produce Cushing's syndrome. The signs of Cushing's syndrome are related to the effects of glucocorticoids and include alopecia (hair loss), muscle wasting, pot-bellied appearance, slow healing of wounds, polyuria, polydipsia, and polyphagia. Physical changes (alopecia, muscle wasting) do not become apparent until the animal has been treated for weeks.

Nonsteroidal Antinflammatory Drugs. The advantage of nonsteroidal antiinflammatory drugs (NSAIDs) over glucocorticoids centers around the many side effects of glucocorticoids as compared with the few adverse effects associated with NSAIDs. NSAIDs decrease protective prostaglandins in the stomach and kidney. In large doses or in sensitive animals, NSAIDs can produce gastric ulcerations or decreased blood flow to the kidneys.

Phenylbutazone is given PO or IV to horses for relief of musculoskeletal inflammation. Aspirin (acetylsalicylic acid) is a fairly safe NSAID in most animal species. Like other NSAIDs, aspirin is metabolized by the liver. Aspirin is metabolized much more slowly in cats than in other species. Aspirin has a half-life of 1.5 hours in people, approximately 8 hours in dogs, and 30 hours in cats. Thus, as with many other drugs, the aspirin dosage for cats is lower than dosages used in other species and usually consists of one "baby aspirin" tablet (81 mg) every 2 or 3 days. If used prudently, however, aspirin is one of the safest and most effective NSAIDs for cats.

Ibuprofen, ketoprofen, and naproxen are available as OTC medications (ibuprofen is marketed as Advil, naproxen is marketed as Aleve, ketoprofen is marketed as Orudis). Naproxen is marketed as the veterinary product Naprosyn. A ketoprofen product, Ketofen, is approved for use in horses. Flunixin meglumine (Banamine) is also is a potent analgesic used primarily in equine medicine for treatment of colic; dogs are very sensitive to the GI side effects of flunixin. Carprofen (Rimadyl) is a new veterinary NSAID that decreases prostaglandins associated with inflammation but does not significantly reduce the protective prostaglandins of the stomach and kidneys.

Meclofenamic acid (Arquel) is commonly administered to horses as granules mixed in the feed. Dimethyl sulfoxide (DMSO) is used topically and parenterally, primarily in horses. DMSO is also a component of some otic (ear) preparations used in dogs and cats. Orgotein (superoxide dismutase) is most commonly used to treat horses with joint and vertebral disease.

Other Antiinflammatories. Although acetaminophen is not an antiinflammatory drug, it is included here because its analgesic and antipyretic (fever reducing) properties often cause it to be grouped with NSAIDs. Acetaminophen (e.g., Tylenol) does not cause the GI upset, ulcers, or interference with platelet clumping associated with NSAIDs. Unfortunately, the metabolites of acetaminophen can have other severe side effects, especially in cats. A single "extra-strength" acetaminophen tablet (500 mg) can kill an average-sized cat. In dogs, a higher dosage (above 150 mg/kg) is required before signs of hepatic necrosis, weight loss, and icterus (jaundice) become evident.

Phenacetin is a compound found in many "cold preparations." This drug is metabolized to acetaminophen and thus can produce acetaminophen toxicity in susceptible species and individual animals. Gold salts, such as aurothioglucose, have been used to treat severe immune-mediated skin problems, such as the various forms of pemphigus. The antiinflammatory activity of dipyrone is weak compared with its analgesic properties and its ability to decrease fever.

RECOMMENDED READING

Adams HR: *Veterinary pharmacology and therapeutics,* ed 7, Ames, Iowa, 1995, Iowa State Univ Press.

Allen DG: *Handbook of veterinary drugs,* Philadelphia, 1993, JB Lippincott.

Bill RL: *Pharmacology for veterinary technicians,* ed 2, St Louis, 1997, Mosby.

Duran SH, Lin HC: *Mosby's Veterinary drug reference,* St Louis, 1997, Mosby.

Gilman AG et al: *Goodman and Gilman's The pharmacological basis of therapeutics,* ed 7, New York, 1985, MacMillan.

Physicians' Desk Reference, Oradell, NJ, 1997, Medical Economics.

Physician's GenRx, St Louis, 1997, Mosby.

Plumb DC: *Veterinary drug handbook,* ed 2, Ames, Iowa, 1995, Iowa State Univ Press.

Veterinary Pharmaceuticals and Biologicals 1997/1998, ed 10 Lenexa, Kans, 1997, Veterinary Medicine Publishing.

Wanamaker BP, Pettes CL: *Applied pharmacology for the veterinary technician,* Philadelphia, 1996, WB Saunders.

CHAPTER 14

Nutrition

S.R. Grosdidier
S.A. Berryhill
R.J. Van Saun
J.A. De Jong

Learning Objectives

After reviewing this chapter, the reader should understand the following:

Basic energy-producing and non–energy-producing nutrients

Considerations for feeding young and adult dogs
Considerations for feeding young and adult cats
Nutritional peculiarities of livestock
Methods used in feeding livestock

NUTRITION OF DOGS AND CATS

S.R. GROSDIDIER
S.A. BERRYHILL

ENERGY-PRODUCING NUTRIENTS

A *nutrient* is any constituent of food that is ingested to support life. The six basic nutrients are proteins, fats, carbohydrates, water, vitamins, and minerals. *Energy-producing nutrients* (proteins, fats, carbohydrates) have a hydrocarbon structure that produces energy through digestion, metabolism, or transformation. Energy is used for all metabolism, cell rejuvenation, maintenance of homeostasis, and production of new cells. *Non–energy-producing nutrients* (water, vitamins, minerals) play an important role throughout the body system and are often called the "gatekeepers of metabolism."

Proteins

Dietary protein is used to build body tissues. Amino acids, the building blocks of protein, are categorized into essential and nonessential types. *Essential amino acids* (arginine, histidine, isoleucine, leucine, lysine, methionine, phenylalanine, threonine, tryptophan, valine, and taurine in cats) cannot be synthesized in the body and so must be supplied by the diet. *Nonessential amino acids* are synthesized in the body. The proportion of essential and nonessential amino acids largely determines the quality, or biologic value, or a particular protein source. A protein's biologic value is reflected by the amount that is retained by the body after ingestion. A protein with a 100% biologic value is entirely retained by the body after ingestion. A protein of very low biologic value, such as 5%, is almost entirely excreted by the body after ingestion.

Fats

Vegetable and animal fats, oils, and lipids are composed of fatty acids and contain more energy per unit of weight than any other nutrient. There is a direct correlation between fat content and caloric density in a diet; the more fat in a diet, the more calories it contains. Cats require three essential fatty acids in their diet (linoleic, linolenic, arachidonic), whereas only two are essential in dogs (linoleic, linolenic).

Carbohydrates

Carbohydrates are classified as *soluble* or *insoluble,* based upon their digestibility. Mammals cannot digest insoluble carbohydrates, such as fiber, although bacteria can degrade fiber in the stomach of herbivores. Fiber decreases a diet's digestibility and caloric density. Fiber is added to a diet for treatment of obesity or management of gastrointestinal disorders. Soluble carbohydrates, such as sugar and starches, can be readily digested and are metabolized for energy needs.

NON–ENERGY-PRODUCING NUTRIENTS
Water

Water provides the foundation for metabolism of all nutrients in the body. Minor alterations in the body's water content and distribution can result in dramatic alterations in nutritional requirements. Water balance in the system affects the ability to excrete waste into the urine by the kidneys. Water is also essential for absorption and metabolism of water-soluble vitamins B and C. Access to fresh, clean water is imperative for all animals. An animal's water needs may not be met if the water source freezes during inclement weather or if the water container is tipped over. It is important to educate clients on providing access to fresh, clean water in all seasons.

Vitamins

Vitamins play a very important role in maintaining normal physiologic functions. These organic molecules are required only in minute amounts to exert their function as coenzymes, enzymes, or precursors in metabolism. *Water-soluble vitamins* are passively absorbed from the small intestine and excess amounts are excreted in the urine. Water-soluble vitamins include thiamin, riboflavin, niacin, pyridoxine, pantothenic acid, folic acid, cobalamin, vitamin C, choline, and L-carnitine. *Fat-soluble vitamins* are metabolized in a manner similar to fats and stored in the liver. Because of this storage mechanism, toxicity from excessive intake of fat-soluble vitamins can occur. A deficiency of fat-soluble vitamins is not as common as with water-soluble vitamins. The fat-soluble vitamins are A, D, E, and K.

Minerals

Within the body, minerals are often distributed in ionized form as a cation or anion electrolyte. In this form they are involved with acid/base balance, clotting factors, osmolality, nerve conduction, muscle contraction, and a variety of other cellular activities.

Deficiencies or excesses in mineral intake can lead to problems through imbalances. Minerals are closely interrelated and an imbalance in one mineral can affect several others. Dietary minerals include calcium, phosphorus, potassium, sodium, chloride, magnesium, iron, zinc, copper, manganese, selenium, iodine, and boron.

FEEDING CONSIDERATIONS FOR DOGS

Contrary to popular belief, domestic dogs do not need variety in their diet. Frequent changes in diet have few positive effects, encourage finicky eating, and precipitate digestive disorders. It is best to consistently feed a diet formulated to meet the animal's needs at each stage of life. Regular assessment of weight can help determine the amount of feed. Weight loss or gain indicates a need to reevaluate the amount being fed or diet selection.

Feeding Methods

Portion Control. This is currently the most popular way to feed dogs. After determining the animal's nutritional requirements, the daily portion is offered to the animal, either in a single feeding or divided into several portions offered several times a day. The animal is then allowed to consume the food throughout the day or during 5 to 10 minutes for each divided portion.

Free Choice. In free-choice feeding, the animal is allowed access to food 24 hours a day. The food supply is replenished as needed. It may be difficult to detect subtle changes in food intake with this method. Free-choice feeding is not recommended for puppies and obese dogs, but it works well in cats.

Time Control. In time-controlled feeding, a portion of food is offered and the animal is allowed access for only 5 or 10 minutes. Any remaining food is taken away after that time. Puppies are commonly fed in this manner.

Feeding Puppies

With puppies born by cesarean section or if the bitch has no milk, the veterinary technician must intervene and provide nutritional support to neonatal puppies. Fortunately, they can be raised successfully on canine milk replacers. Cow's milk is not an acceptable substitute, because it contains inappropriate levels of protein and lactose. Initially, it may be necessary to use orogastric intubation or a feeding syringe and then gradually adopt a regular small animal feeding bottle as the puppies begin to thrive.

Daily or twice-daily weighing and physical examination of the puppies helps identify problems early enough to adjust feeding protocols or begin other therapeutic measures to avoid mortality. Puppies typically gain 2 to

4 g/kg of anticipated adult weight each day; any variance in weight demands closer investigation.[7] Some neonatal puppies fail to gain weight when nursing the bitch because they cannot compete with siblings for a nipple. Puppies in this situation tend to be restless and whimper inordinately. Normal weight can be restored by allowing such puppies to nurse the bitch without competition three to four times daily.

Weaning begins around 3 to 4 weeks of age in large-breed puppies and at 4 to 5 weeks of age in smaller breeds. To facilitate the transition to solid foods, begin by making a gruel or "slurry" of a growth type of diet. A gruel is created by mixing equal parts of food and water together to form a homogeneous consistency. The mixture should have the texture of cooked oatmeal. Puppies initially may play with or walk through the slurry, but eventually they consume it in increasing volumes. Gruel should be offered three to four times daily during the weaning process. Feed the puppy increasing amounts until the puppy can be maintained without nursing, at 5 to 7 weeks in large-breed puppies and at 6 to 7 weeks in smaller breeds. Once weaning is complete, decrease the volume of water added to the mixture until the puppy is eating the desired diet and voluntarily drinking water.

Feeding Adult Dogs

As a dog matures, monitor activity level and predisposition to obesity to preserve a neutral energy equilibrium. Reassess feeding methods, because inappropriate techniques commonly result in excessive nutrient intake and obesity. Review feeding habits with clients to preclude future problems (Box 14-1).

Most dogs are managed efficiently through time-restricted meal feeding. Some dogs nibble throughout the day when offered food free choice. Care should be taken in these situations to ensure that optimal body condition is maintained, with weight neither lost nor gained.

Feeding Active Dogs

Active dogs require energy to sustain hunting, obedience trial, or other activities. The diets for active dogs must have enhanced levels of fat, the most energy-dense nutrient, as well as increased total digestibility. Dogs that are only slightly more active than others need slightly more food, but working dogs with significant energy demands require a substantial increase in food portions. Any increase in food portions, to condition a dog for work, should be gradually instituted over a 7- to 10-day period. Hunting dogs should be fed just before a period of increased activity so as to avoid hypoglycemia.

Feeding Geriatric Dogs

Older dogs are less able to adjust to prolonged periods of poor nutrition. Any changes in an older dog's diet should be based upon careful patient assessment and not solely on the dog's age. Dietary protein should be of high

---

Box 14-1 Recommended feeding practices for dogs and cats

- Match the diet to the animal's stage of life.
- Feed for the ideal body weight.
- Measure the amount of food fed.
- Adjust the amount fed to the animal's body condition.
- Don't feed table scraps.
- Don't overfeed.
- Don't change the diet frequently.
- If the diet is to be changed, do so gradually, over 3 to 5 days.
- Don't feed multiple animals from a single bowl.
- Treats should not comprise more than 10% of the diet.
- Use dry food ("kibble"), ice chips, and vegetables as treats.
- Deduct the amount fed as a treat from the total amount fed daily.

---

biologic value to reduce the level of metabolites that must be excreted through the kidneys. Dietary fats must be sufficiently digestible to provide adequate levels of essential fatty acids without an excess that could lead to obesity. Because of its detrimental effects on the kidneys, dietary phosphorus should be limited. Increased levels of zinc, copper, and vitamins A, B-complex, and E may be required in the diet of older dogs.

Feeding Overweight Dogs

Obesity is the most common nutritional disorder of pets. Obesity places significant stress on the body system and may predispose to diabetes mellitus, cardiovascular disease, and skeletal problems. Early counseling of owners can alert them to weight gain. Educate clients on the potential adverse effects of weight gain.

FEEDING CONSIDERATIONS FOR CATS
Feeding Kittens

Kittens that are orphaned or born to queens unable to nurse must be hand fed. Weaning should not commence until 7 weeks of age. Kittens can be gradually introduced to a diet by first offering a slurry of canned food mixed with kitten milk replacer. As with puppies, the amount of liquid is gradually reduced. Later they can be offered a dry diet if preferred.

Feeding Adult Cats

Adult cats typically eat several small meals throughout a 24-hour period. Unfortunately, many clients provide food to their cats in unlimited amounts, filling the food dish each time their cat empties it. Such free-choice feeding predisposes to obesity. Overfeeding can be prevented by offering limited amounts of food throughout the day. This gives the cat the opportunity to nibble throughout the day while avoiding excessive caloric intake.

Caution owners against offering a constantly changing diet, such as various brands and types of commercial diets, because this can result in undesirable eating behavior.

Feeding Cats with Lower Urinary Tract Disease

Lower urinary tract disease, also known as *feline urologic syndrome,* is a complex disease characterized by bouts of frequent painful urination, bloody urine, and, in males, possible urethral obstruction. It tends to occur more often in obese, sedentary cats. Factors other than diet are involved in lower urinary tract disease, but careful attention to the diet of affected cats can help prevent future episodes.

Depending on the type of uroliths (small stones composed of cellular debris and mineral crystals) present in the urinary tract (struvite or calcium oxalate), prevention involves manipulation of dietary mineral, fiber, and water intake. Special commercial diets are available for dietary management of feline urologic syndrome.

Feeding Geriatric Cats

Because aging can diminish the senses of smell and taste, it is sometimes necessary to enhance the aroma and taste of foods to improve their palatability for aged cats. Successful techniques include warming canned food to body temperature in the microwave to improve the aroma, applying garlic powder to canned food before it is warmed, and addition of aromatic foodstuffs, such as clam juice or bits of canned fish.

FEEDING DEBILITATED OR ANORECTIC PATIENTS

Diseased patients that are anorectic face a state of accelerated starvation in as little as 48 hours. Aggressive, early nutritional intervention can alleviate the potentially devasting effects of accelerated starvation or hypermetabolism. The adverse effects of anorexia can also occur in sick animals that are obese.

The most effective, practical, and economical method of feeding anorectic patients is through *enteral nutrition* (administering nutrients into the gastrointestinal tract). Nutrients provided by enteral feeding are easily assimilated by the body and enteral feeding causes fewer detrimental side effects than *parenteral* (intravenous) *feeding* (see Chapter 24).

Enteral methods include encouraging voluntary eating with highly palatable food; forced oral feeding; orogastric tube feeding; nasogastric tube feeding; pharyngostomy tube feeding; esophagostomy tube feeding; gastrostomy tube feeding; and jejunostomy tube feeding. In all of the tube feeding methods, a commercial or custom-mixed diet is slowly injected into the feeding tube. The required daily amount is calculated and the total daily dose is divided into several, small feedings. A successful enteral feeding method is to begin by feeding 1/3 of the total daily requirement on the first day of enteral feeding. On day two, 2/3 of the total daily requirement is given. On day three, the total amount of diet is administered in several small, frequent enteral feedings. The total daily dose is usually divided into five to six equal feedings early in the regimen and then tapered down to three to four feedings as the patient becomes accustomed to enteral feeding.

RECOMMENDED READING

Case LP et al: *Canine and feline nutrition,* St Louis, 1995, Mosby.
Kelley NC, Wills JM: *Manual of companion animal nutrition and feeding,* Ames, Iowa, 1996, Iowa State University Press.
Morris ML et al: *Small animal clinical nutrition III,* Topeka, Kan, 1987, Mark Morris Assoc.
Schaeffer MC et al: *Nutrition of the dog and cat,* Cambridge, Mass, 1989, Cambridge University Press.

LIVESTOCK NUTRITION

R.J. VAN SAUN
J.A. DE JONG

NUTRITIONAL PECULIARITIES OF LIVESTOCK

Livestock species (cattle, horses, pigs, sheep, goats) require certain essential nutrients to meet metabolic and physiologic needs. Essential nutrients include water, energy, amino acids (proteins), fatty acids, minerals, and vitamins; these are discussed in the first part of this chapter.

There is a unique feature to protein nutrition in ruminants (e.g., cattle, sheep, goats). As a result of their pregastric fermentation system, nonprotein nitrogen (e.g., urea), in addition to rumen-degradable dietary protein, can be used by the resident microbes as a nitrogen source of synthesis of microbial proteins. Microbial protein then passes into the abomasum (true stomach) and is digested like any other dietary protein. Microbial protein can account for a significant amount of dietary protein in ruminants.

Dietary fiber is required to maintain adequate gastrointestinal function in herbivores (plant-eating animals) with active microbial fermentation chambers. These include ruminants (cattle, sheep, goats) and hind gut fermenting animals (horses). Therefore, gastrointestinal anatomy has a very critical role in the animal's ability to derive essential nutrients from the feedstuffs available. Domestic livestock extract essential nutrients from plant materials. The plant material consumed by livestock species contains cellulose, hemicellulose, pectin, and lignin compounds that are indigestible by people and carnivorous predators. These plant compounds are used by microbes within the gut and the animal uses the end-products of microbial fermentation. Animals have evolved in many different ways to take advantage of microbial fermentation in their digestive process.

The alimentary tract includes the mouth and associated structures, esophagus, stomach, small intestine, cecum, and colon (large intestine). The rumen of cattle, sheep, and goats functions as a pregastric fermentation vat (Fig. 14-1). This allows ruminants to efficiently derive nutrients from plant material. In hind gut fermenters, such as horses, a greatly enlarged colon serves as a fermentation vat. These animals can also digest plant material, but not to the same extent as ruminants. As a result of differences in their anatomy, ruminants digest prefermented feed material, whereas hind gut herbivores ferment predigested feed material. Pigs are considered omnivores, which means that they can digest materials of both plant and animal origin, although they are primarily fed less bulky plant materials. Pigs have some microbial fermentation capacity in their enlarged, sacculated colon (see Fig. 14-1), but not to the extent of hind gut fermenters or ruminants.

Feedstuffs

A *feedstuff* is any dietary component that provides some essential nutrient or serves some other function. Nonnutritive feedstuffs may provide bulk, flavor, odor, or color, or act as an antioxidant to protect other dietary components. More than 2000 different feedstuffs have been fed to domestic livestock throughout the world. The variety of feedstuffs available for use in a given geographic area depends on the crops grown locally. Potential feedstuffs must be matched with the appropriate livestock species, based on nutrient requirements and gastrointestinal tract capabilities. Feedstuffs may be divided into a number of categories, based on their source and nutrient concentration. General categories include forages (roughages), concentrates, by-products, mineral and vitamin supplements, and nonnutritive additives.

Forages are feeds made up of most or all of the plant. Forages generally have large amounts of fiber, low ener-

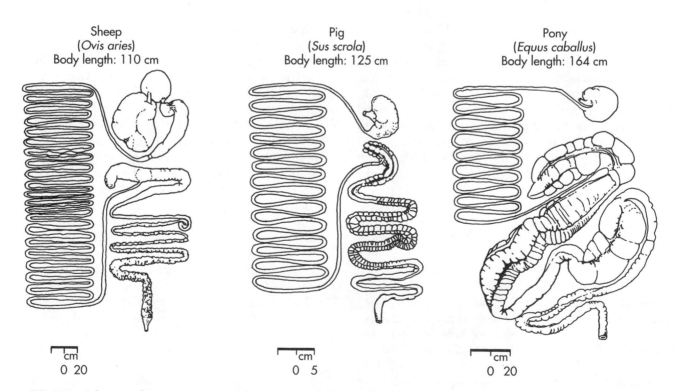

FIG. 14-1 Schematic diagrams comparing the gastrointestinal tract of ruminants (sheep), horses, and pigs. *(From Stevens CE: Comparative physiology of the vertebrate digestive system, New York, 1988, Cambridge University Press.)*

gy density, and high bulk (low weight per unit volume). This is a direct result of the amount of plant cell wall material present. Plant cell walls are composed of cellulose, hemicelluose, lignin, and other compounds. A forage's protein content depends upon the type of plant and stage at harvesting. For example, alfalfa hay has much higher protein levels than grass hays at a comparable stage of plant growth. Within plant species, protein and energy content, as well as overall digestibility, declines and fiber content increases with advancing maturity of the plant. The decline in digestibility with maturity is due to increasing lignin content of the plant. Lignin is an inert compound that increases rigidity of the plant cell wall. Straw represents the most mature and indigestible form of forages.

Forages fed to livestock belong to either the legume or grass plant families. Legumes commonly used for forage production include alfalfa, red and white clover, bird's foot trefoil, and vetch. Grasses offer much more variety for forage production and include bahia grass, bermuda grass, bluegrass, bromegrass, fescue, timothy, orchard grass, reed canary grass, ryegrass, and Sudan grass. Other grass forages that may be used for cereal grain production include corn, wheat, rye, oats, and sorghum. Of these, corn is the most important forage and cereal grain product grown for livestock.

Forage products are harvested and stored for livestock feeding purposes in a number of ways. Grasses, legumes, and other broadleaf vegetation (forbs and browse) may be grazed by livestock. Allowing livestock to harvest forage avoids costs incurred in mechanical harvesting and storage. However, forage quality and quantity can be extremely variable, depending upon plant maturity and environmental conditions. A more controlled method of grazing being adopted is intensive rotational grazing. In this method, animals are allowed to graze restricted areas of forage for limited periods and are then moved to another area; the forage in the grazed area is allowed to regrow until the animals are returned for grazing. With highly managed rotational grazing, forage quality can be maintained at a very high level.

Forage crops can also be mechanically harvested, stored, and fed using various methods. *Green chop* or *spoilage* represents forage harvested at a given stage of development and fed directly. Green chop contains a high level of water (75% to 85%) and available nutrients; however, it must be harvested daily to avoid rapid deterioration with storage. Ensiling is a harvesting process by which a forage is chopped and placed into a storage unit (e.g., silo), which excludes oxygen. The forage ferments, producing lactic acid (lowers pH) and effectively "pickling" the forage material in a partially fermented state, called *silage*. Good-quality silage can be stored indefinitely in upright silos, bunker silos, or plastic bags, the important feature being exclusion of

oxygen. Silage has an intermediate water content (55% to 75%) and has the least loss of nutrients from harvesting and storage. Grass, legume, and corn silages are the most common ensiled forages fed to livestock. *Hay* is forage that is cut and allowed to dry before being collected into bales for storage. Hay should have less than 15% water to be stable in storage. Harvesting losses are high in hay making, but storage losses are usually minimal if it is properly dried.

Concentrates are generally low in fiber and high in energy and/or protein. Cereal grains, such as barley, corn, millet, oats, rye, sorghum, and wheat, are the seeds of many of the grass species. Corn is the most common grain fed to livestock and the standard with which others are compared. Cereal grains contain large amounts of energy in the form of starch and are added to diets to increase energy density. Other feed products used as energy concentrates include molasses, root crops (e.g., turnips, beets, carrots), and potatoes. Fats and oils of plant or animal origin contain 2.25 times the energy density of carbohydrates and are also used as energy concentrates.

Concentrate feeds that contain more than 20% crude protein are subclassified as *protein supplements*. Protein supplements may be of plant or animal origin, including marine fish. Plant-based protein products are derived from oilseed crops, such as soybean, canola, cottonseed, sunflower, and peanut seed meals. Of these, soybean meal is by far the most common oilseed meal fed to livestock. Oil from the seeds is harvested for a variety of industrial and nutritional uses; the remaining seed contains more than 40% crude protein. Animal-based protein supplements are derived from rendered animal or fish tissues or from dried milk products. Animal proteins generally range from more than 50% crude protein to 90% crude protein. As compared with plant-based protein sources, animal protein sources have a better amino acid composition relative to requirements. However, there is much variability in the quality of animal-based products and the way in which they are manufactured.

Byproduct feeds are residues of the feed processing industry and span a wide array of feedstuffs. Examples of byproduct feeds include sugar beet pulp, bakery waste, blood, meat, fish, and bone meal, brewer's grains, tallow, and whey. Many byproduct feeds contain substantial amounts of fermentable fiber, energy, and protein.

Mineral and *vitamin supplements* are sources of individual or combination of minerals, with or without vitamins. Fat-soluble vitamins are supplemented primarily in the form of premixes. Fat-soluble vitamins are sensitive to oxidation, sunlight, heat, and fungal growth. Certain water-soluble vitamins may be supplemented in swine and horse diets; they are not routinely supplemented in ruminant diets. Yeast cultures are good sources of B-complex vitamins and are commonly added to livestock diets.

Nonnutritive feed additives can include buffers, hormones, binders, and medications. Feed medications may include antibiotics, antifungals, anthelmintics, antiparasitics, and ionophores (antibiotics with growth-promoting effects). Their use is regulated by the Food and Drug Administration in an effort to prevent tissue residues (see Chapter 13). Nonnutritive additives are used to stimulate animal performance, improve feed efficiency, and improve animal health or metabolic status.

Feed Analysis

Different classes of feedstuffs contribute variable amounts of the essential nutrients (Table 14-1). Even within certain feed groups, such as forages, nutrient composition can vary tremendously. *Feed analysis* is a procedure by which chemical analysis determines the proportion of specific components of a feedstuff. The *proximate analysis* includes determinations of dry matter (DM), crude protein (CP), ether extract (EE, crude fat), crude fiber (CF), and ash. The nonfiber carbohydrate portion of the feed, termed *nitrogen-free extract* (NFE), is determined using the equation NFE = 100 − CP − CF − EE − ash. More recently, crude fiber analysis has been replaced with neutral and acid detergent fiber analysis, improving our estimate of cell wall components and their availability. Feed analysis should be routinely completed in any nutritional diagnostic problem.

Feeding Management

The goal of any livestock feeding management program is to provide sufficient daily amounts of the essential nutrients for optimal (cost-effective) productivity. Because feed costs account for the greatest amount of total production costs in the livestock industry, we must minimize feed costs to ensure profitability. Byproduct feeds are so widely used when available, because they usually are of lower cost.

Dairy Cattle. Dairy cattle are segregated and housed by production stages and fed according to specific nutrient requirements. Typical feeding groups on a dairy farm include milk-fed calves, growing replacement heifers, nonlactating pregnant cows (dry cows), and lactation groups. Lactation groups are usually based on level of milk production, parity (first lactation vs. older cows), days in milk, or some combination of these factors.

Feeding systems and housing facilities vary among dairy farms, depending upon prevailing environmental conditions. Smaller family dairies with fewer than 100 cows generally have individual tie stalls, and cows are fed individually. The amount of forage and concentrates are fed according to production level and body condition score (see Table 14-3). These farms are predominantly found in the northeastern and midwestern United States as a result of the cold winters. In larger dairies, cows are generally housed in free-stall barns or in open drylots, depending upon environmental conditions. Drylots are found primarily in the southern and western United States, whereas free-stall barns are found anywhere in the United States. In larger dairy management systems, cattle are fed in groups at a common feedbunk, rather than individually. Feedbunks may be located within the free-stall facility or along one side of the drylot.

Although feeding management of dairy cattle depends upon the type of facilities available, there are some options as to how feed is delivered to the animals. Forage (hay, silage) may be fed separate from the concentrates in any of the feeding management systems

TABLE 14-1 Relative nutrient content of various feedstuffs for livestock

| | Relative Nutrient Content | | | | | | |
| | Protein | Energy | Minerals | | Vitamins | | Fiber |
Feedstuff Group			Macro	Micro	Fat-Sol.	B-Complex	
High-quality roughage	+++	++	++	++	+++	+	+++
Low-quality roughage	+	+	+	+	−	−	++++
Cereal grains	++	+++	+	+	+	+	+
Grain millfeeds	++	++	++	++	+	++	++
Fats and oils	−	++++	−	−	−	−	−
Molasses	+	+++	++	++	−	+	−
Fermentation products	+++	++	+	++	−	++++	±
Oil seed proteins	++++	+++	++	++	+	++	+
Animal proteins	++++	+++	+++	+++	++	+++	+

From Church DC: *Livestock feeds and feeding*, ed 3, Englewood Cliffs, NJ, 1991, Prentice Hall.
+ to ++++: low to very high content
± : may or may not be present in significant amounts
− : not present

described. Concentrates may be fed separately in the milking parlor or from computerized feeders. Parlor grain feeding and computerized feeding are becoming more common with current interest in pasture grazing management systems. In larger dairies, the most common method of feed delivery is by total mixed ration (TMR). In this system, all individual feed ingredients are mechanically mixed in a feed wagon and presented as a single mixture to the cows. This allows cows to consume the same blend of nutrients in each bite and minimizes selectivity. Some dairies feed what might be termed a partial TMR in that dry hay is fed separate from the rest of the diet.

Beef Cattle. Beef cattle management can be divided into cow-calf and cattle feeding (feedlot) operations. Cow-calf enterprises produce calves that enter the breeding herd or are sent to cattle feeding operations (feedlots). Forage use is the basis of cow-calf enterprises. Feed costs account for more than 60% of production costs and therefore must be minimized. Cows are allowed to graze pasture or range land, depending upon availability, and then are supplemented with energy, protein, and vitamin-mineral supplements as necessary to meet specific nutritional requirements. Depending upon geographic location and season, pasture grazing may be replaced with feeding of dry hay or silage. Supplementation programs depend upon prevailing forage quality relative to nutrient requirements of the various production units. Cow-calf operations may have feeding groups for bulls, replacement heifers, growing calves, maintenance, and pregnant or lactating cattle.

Cattle feeding enterprises involve feeding calves from weaning to slaughter and include backgrounding, stocker, and feedlot systems. In backgrounding and stocker feeding systems, weanling calves are placed on low-cost pasture and supplementation feeding programs to gain weight at a moderate rate and then are sold to feedlot operations. The goal of a feedlot enterprise is to maximize rate of gain and feed conversion efficiency for lowest cost. New arrivals at the feedlot are initially fed a high-forage, low-concentrate diet to acclimate the animal to the operation. The proportion of forage is gradually reduced and concentrate increased to facilitate the desired rate of gain. To minimize feeding costs, a wide variety of byproduct feeds and grain products is fed. To ensure animal health with high-grain feeding, ionophores, buffers, and antimicrobial agents are incorporated into the feedlot diet. Generally, the feedlot diet is fed as a TMR similar to the method for daily cattle.

Horses. Horse feeding management is primarily designed to meet the nutritional requirements of individual horses. Although horses are not ruminants, they require a substantial amount of dietary fiber, in the form of forage, to maintain a healthy digestive tract. Forages fed to horses are primarily hay and pasture. Ensiled forage (silage) is not commonly fed to horses because of their sensitivity to the molds and mycotoxins potentially found in silage. Many varieties of grasses and legumes can be suitable hay forages for horses. Energy, protein, and mineral-vitamin supplementation depends upon forage quality and nutrient requirements of the horse. Corn, barley, and oats are common grain supplements fed to horses for added energy. Recently, fat supplementation has been advocated to provide energy for growing, lactating, and working horses. Such protein sources as linseed, canola, and soybean meal are commonly used. Byproducts containing fermentable fiber, such as rice bran and beet pulp, are becoming more popular.

Many commercial horse feeds are available to horse owners. These range from complete feeds (no supplementation required) to specific vitamin-mineral supplements. Various grain supplements containing energy, protein, minerals, and vitamins are available. These commercial grain supplements may be formulated specifically for growing foals, lactating mares, or geriatric horses, or they may be more generic in purpose. Horse owners should match the concentrate to their forage relative to energy, protein, mineral, and vitamin requirements. A proper horse feeding program would provide adequate amounts of water and provide sufficient energy to achieve and maintain proper body condition. The diet must then be balanced for protein, minerals, and vitamins according to the National Research Council recommendations. Appropriate dental care and parasite management programs should accompany all horse feeding systems.

Pigs. Pig feeding management is similar to beef cattle management in that there are breeding-farrowing (reproductive) and growing enterprises. The farrowing unit produces baby pigs as reproductive replacements or to enter the growing unit for feeding to slaughter weight. The pig industry is one of the most intensively managed agricultural enterprises. Current pig production units are moving to total confinement farrow-to-finish operations containing many animals. Within these operations, feeding groups are segregated according to nutrient requirements, with diets for lactating and gestating sows and gilts, boars, nursery pigs, and growing pigs. For the most part, animals in the farrowing unit are housed and fed as individuals to better control body weight and condition. Within the feeding operation, starting with the nursery pigs, all animals are group housed and fed according to age and moved between groups as an entire unit.

As omnivores, pigs have a digestive tract that can accommodate a certain level of dietary fiber. Given the economics of rate of gain from forages versus grains, pig diets consist primarily of concentrates, along with energy, protein, mineral, and vitamin supplements. All feed ingredients are thoroughly mixed and provided as a single diet, like the TMR for cattle. Dietary ingredients depend upon the nutritional requirements of the specific group of animals being fed. The classic pig diet consists of corn grain and soybean meal, with a vitamin-mineral premix. Learning more about the specific nutrient requirements of pigs has resulted in more sophisticated diets for pigs. Crystalline amino acids, high-quality animal byproduct protein meals, fiber sources, and vitamin-mineral supplements have been incorporated into specific pig diets to improve growth efficiency.

Sheep. Sheep are managed similarly to beef cattle in that there are reproductive and lamb growing enterprises. Sheep are raised under a wide variety of conditions, ranging from large flocks on western rangelands to small flocks in confinement. The basis of any sheep production system is forage. The advantage of feeding sheep is their ability to selectively graze. This allows sheep to consume a diet of higher nutritional value than the quality of the total forage. A variety of forage types including harvested and stored forages can be used for feeding sheep. As ruminants, sheep can also use a wide variety of byproduct feeds efficiently.

For the most part, sheep diets consist of vitamin-mineral supplements added to the base forage. The composition of the vitamin-mineral supplement depends upon the forage. Grazing sheep are provided with minerals as a block ("salt lick") or loose from a feeder. Additional energy and protein supplementation may be used for late gestation, lactation, and growing diets. A wide variety of feed sources may be used, with cost being of primary concern. These supplements may be top dressed on (spread on top of) the forage or fed by themselves in a feed bunk. Commercial concentrate pellets are also available for ewes and growing lamb diets. Growing lambs may be sent to slaughter directly from grazing high-quality forage or after feeding in a feedlot. Lamb feedlots are similar in organization and feeding practices to beef feedlots. Lambs are acclimated from a high-forage to high-concentrate TMR diet to increase grain and feed efficiency.

Goats. Goats are managed similarly to dairy cattle because of their milk production. However, some breeds of goats are primarily used for mohair (wool) or meat production. Forage is the primary component of goat feeding programs. Like sheep, goats can selectively graze the more nutritious parts of plants. Goats raised for mohair and meat are managed with grazing or browsing rangeland or pasture and appropriate energy and protein supplementation when necessary. Dairy goats are managed more intensively because of their higher nutritional requirements for milk production.

Dairy goats are usually housed in smaller areas and fed stored forages, such as dry hay. Pasture grazing alone cannot support milk production, so supplements are necessary. The energy and protein feed supplements for goats are similar to those of dairy cattle. Many of the commercial concentrate products used for horses, sheep, and dairy cattle can also be fed to goats. The amount and nutrient composition of the supplement depend on the nutrient requirements of the animal being fed and on forage quality. Lactating does require substantial energy supplementation and should be fed the highest-quality forages. Supplements may be top dressed on forage in a feedbunk or provided in the milking parlor.

CLINICAL NUTRITION

A basic understanding of nutrition can be applied to medical management of livestock. The most important part of clinical nutrition is obtaining an appropriate nutritional history. This is used to determine the potential role of nutrition in a medical problem. Questions one should ask in obtaining a nutritional history are outlined in Table 14-2.

Following the history taking, assess the nutritional status of the animal through physical assessment of the animal and via blood chemistry determinations. Physical assessment of the animal involves obtaining an accurate body weight, height measurement, and body condition score. Body height at the shoulders (withers) can be used to assess frame size and growth. Body weight and height measurements can be compared with those in standardized growth charts to assess growth performance.

Body condition scoring is a method of subjectively quantifying subcutaneous body fat reserves. Animals are scored on a scale of 1 to 5 or 1 to 9, with the low and high scores representing emaciated and obese animals, respectively (Table 14-3). Changes in body condition score represent either a positive (increased) or negative (decreased) energy balance. A negative energy balance suggests that the diet contains insufficient energy to meet needs and body fat reserves are being mobilized.

Beyond this quantitative measure, physical assessment of the animal may include observations of haircoat, hoof quality, hydration status, manure consistency, and attitude. Assess these factors and record them in the animal's records daily for hospitalized patients. Indirect measures of nutritional status may be evaluated through metabolite concentrations in blood.

TABLE 14-2 Nutritional history in livestock (specific information depends on the species of livestock)

General categories of information	Specific information
Identify the people involved	Names and telephone numbers of the owner, herdsman, veterinarian, nutritionist, others
Owner's primary concern	Pertaining to the presenting problem
Historical information about the agribusiness	Ask questions relating to years of ownership, number of hired hands, new animal purchases, acreage, other farms, etc.
Herd information	Function, breeds, average weights, and age distribution of animals on the farm
Production information	Level of performance (milk production, weaning weights, litter size, etc.) in the herd over time; use production record systems if available
Housing facilities	Type of housing, stall surfaces, and bedding used for each group of animals; adequacy of ventilation
Feeding system	Feed storage facilities, feeding system used, feed and water availability, bunk space per animal, number of times fed per day, etc.
Dietary information	Feed ingredients and their nutrient analyses, specific feeds for each feeding group; obtain feed samples if feed analysis or feed tag information is unavailable
Herd disease information	Disease prevalence for pertinent disease problems, animal culling and mortality rates over the past month, 6 months, and year
Reproductive information	Measures of fertility, pregnancy losses, etc.
Preventive medicine practices	Vaccinations, treatments, and dewormings administered and when; ask if routine herd health visits are made by the veterinarian

TABLE 14-3 Body condition scoring classifications for livestock

Body condition scoring scale*		Generalized animal description†
1.0	1	*Emaciated.* All bones obviously protruding; no subcutaneous fat evident
1.5	2	*Very thin.* Bones visible and easily palpated; minimal subcutaneous fat
2.0	3	*Thin.* Thin, flat musculature; prominent ribs, pelvic bones, and spinal processes
2.5	4	*Moderately thin.* Minimal subcutaneous fat; individual ribs not obvious
3.0	5	*Moderate.* Smooth musculature; bones not visible but palpable
3.5	6	*Moderately fleshy.* Fat palpable; soft fat over ribs and covering pelvis
4.0	7	*Fleshy.* Fat visible; ribs barely visible; spinal processes buried in fat
4.5	8	*Fat.* Thick neck; ribs difficult to palpate; rounded appearance to pelvis
5.0	9	*Grossly obese.* Bulging fat all over; patchy fat pads around tailhead

*The body condition scoring scale used depends upon the species. Dairy cattle, sheep, pigs, and goats are typically scored on a scale of 1 to 5, whereas beef cattle and horses are scored on a scale of 1 to 9.
†When determining body condition score, evaluate for the presence or absence of fatty tissue over the neck, ribs, spine, and pelvis, independent of animal body weight and frame size.

RECOMMENDED READING

Cheeke PR: *Applied animal nutrition: feeds and feeding,* New York, 1991, Macmillan.

Church DC: *Livestock feeds and feeding,* ed 3, Englewood Cliffs, NJ, 1991, Prentice-Hall.

Ensminger ME, Olentine CG, Heinemann WW: *Feeds and nutrition,* ed 2, Clovis, Cal, 1990, Ensminger Publishing.

Jurgens MH: *Applied animal feeding and nutrition,* Dubuque, Iowa, 1973, Kendall/Hunt Publishing.

National Research Council: *Nutrient requirements of beef cattle,* ed 7, Washington, DC, 1996, National Academy Press.

National Research Council: *Nutrient requirements of dairy cattle,* ed 6, Washington, DC, 1988, National Academy Press.

National Research Council: *Nutrient requirements of goats: angora, dairy, and meat goats in temperate and tropical countries,* Washington, DC, 1981, National Academy Press.

National Research Council: *Nutrient requirements of horses,* ed 5, Washington, DC, 1989, National Academy Press.

National Research Council, *Nutrient requirements of sheep,* ed 6, Washington, DC, 1985, National Academy Press.

National Research Council: *Nutrient requirements of swine,* ed 9, Washington, DC, 1988, National Academy Press.

Pond WG, Church DC, Pond KR: *Basic animal nutrition and feeding,* ed 4, New York, 1995, John Wiley & Sons.

CHAPTER 15

Reproduction

S.D. Van Camp

Learning Objectives

After reviewing this chapter, the reader should understand the following:

Normal reproductive cycles of female domestic species
Patterns of hormone secretion during pregnancy

Ways in which pregnancy is diagnosed
Stages and events of parturition
Ways in which males are evaluated for breeding soundness
Techniques of artificial insemination

NORMAL REPRODUCTIVE PHYSIOLOGY
Nonpregnant Animals

Unlike women and other female primates that have *menstrual cycles*, with variable levels of sexual receptivity, the mammals commonly dealt with in veterinary medicine have an *estrous cycle*, in which the period of sexual receptivity, *estrus*, is concentrated during a short period lasting from one to several days. During the reminder of the estrous cycle, the female does not accept the male's sexual advances nor allow mating.

The estrous cycle is made up of four or five stages, depending on the species and whether the animal is *polyestrous* (cycles repeatedly) or is *monestrous* (cycles only once during the breeding season). The following are the stages of estrus:

Anestrus: The period of ovarian inactivity, with no behavioral signs of "heat" or estrus.

Proestrus: Under the influence of gonadotropin-releasing hormone (GnRH) produced in the hypothalamus, fol-

licle-stimulating hormone (FSH) is released from the pituitary to act on the ovary to cause initial follicle development. These growing follicles produce estrogen, which causes the genital and behavioral changes that attract the male and prepare the female's reproductive tract for mating. Although the proestrous female may show signs of interest in the male, she will not allow mating.

Estrus: The period of true heat, during which the female allows mating. The estrogen levels peak early in estrus and cause the pituitary to release luteinizing hormone (LH), which further matures the follicles and results in release of the egg(s) at ovulation.

Metestrus: A short stage during which the female may still attract males but no longer allows mating. During this stage, ovulated follicles metamorphose into corpora lutea, which begin to secrete progesterone. Metestrus is so short in some species that it is not even discussed as a separate stage and is included in diestrus.

Diestrus: A stage of ovarian activity without signs of heat. The corpus luteum (CL) develops fully and produces maximum levels of progesterone to ready the uterus for the conceptus and maintain pregnancy.

273

If the female does not become pregnant, prostaglandins are released from the uterus, destroying the CL and stopping progesterone production. The female then either enters anestrus (if it is a monestrous species, such as the dog) or reenters proestrus (if it is a polyestrous species, such as the cow). Some polyestrous animals cycle throughout the year (cow), whereas other animals are seasonally polyestrous (mare, ewe, and doe) in response to changing day length. Seasonally polyestrous animals enter anestrus at the end of the breeding season.

Reproductive Physiologic Patterns

Cows. The normal cow is a polyestrous animal that cycles throughout the year (Table 15-1). Heat lasts about 18 hours of the 21-day cycle (range 18 to 23 days). The signs of approaching heat in cows include nervousness, vocalization, and attempting to mount and ride other animals. A cow in "true" heat stands to be ridden by other cows. A thick, clear, tenacious string of mucus can often be seen hanging from the vulva of cows in heat. Unlike other animals, cows ovulate about 12 hours after going out of heat. Cows that are to be bred artificially should be bred 12 hours after heat is first detected, if the herd is watched 20 to 30 minutes twice daily for estrual animals (Fig. 15-1). Obviously, cows to be bred naturally must still be in standing heat. Cows often show metestrous bleeding in the mucus 1 to 2 days after they have ovulated. It is too late to breed cows that have evidence of metestrual blood in their vulvar mucus.

Mares. The mare is a seasonally polyestrous animal (see Table 15-1). Most mares stop cycling (become anestrual) during the winter; however, a few mares continue to cycle during the winter. The mare's natural breeding season is in the late spring and summer. However, breed registration rules require breeding mares in February and March. During the natural breeding season (May through August), the mare's estrous cycle is about 21 days long. They are in standing heat for about 5 days and then out of heat for 16 days.

Estrual mares (in heat) seek out the stallion. They squat and urinate frequently in the presence of the stallion, raise the tail to the side, and evert (wink) the clitoris. Estrual mares stand to be mounted by the stallion. Mares that are not in heat squeal, kick, switch the tail from side to side, pin their ears back, and may attempt to bite the stallion.

Mares enter and leave the natural breeding season with very erratic cycles. They often have prolonged or erratic heats in the early spring. These early-season erratic periods result in extra labor and ineffective breedings. Rectal examinations by a veterinarian can be used to predict the optimum time for breeding. Mares usually ovulate 24 to 36 hours before going out of heat. The best time to breed a normally cycling mare is on the second day of heat and again every other day until she goes out of heat. In the early spring, when mares have prolonged heats, breeding all mares every other day may exhaust the stallion.

The veterinarian can predict ovulation, based upon changes in the follicles, as palpated rectally, and on changes in the cervix. The follicles become large and soft before ovulation and the cervix changes from a dry, firm, tight, pale organ to a very pink, edematous, soft, amorphous mass on the floor of the vagina before ovulation. Ultrasonography helps predict ovulation. The follicular wall thickens and its shape changes from round to pointed. After ovulation the collapsed follicle fills with blood and becomes a corpus hemorrhagicum (CH), which is converted quickly to a corpus luteum (CL), which produces progesterone until it regresses if the mare is not pregnant, and becomes a nonfunctional corpus albicans (CA) just before the next heat.

Sows. Gilts (young females) reach puberty at about 6 to 7 months of age, although this varies with the breed and time of year they are born (see Table 15-1). Pigs are nonseasonally polyestrous animals; however, in hot, humid climates they may show a reduction in cyclicity during the summer. Pigs are unique in that they show an early postpartum heat but do not ovulate during this heat. They then undergo a true lactational anestrus, at which time they do not resume cyclicity until the litter is weaned. After resumption of cycling, the sow demonstrates heat for 2 to 3 days every 21 (18 to 24) days. Heat is recognized in sows by a slightly swollen, reddened vulva. They are restless, seek out the boar, and assume a characteristic braced stance when the boar mounts. The "riding test" uses this stance to detect sows and gilts in heat. A female in heat assumes the same braced stance if pressed on the back by a person.

Sows ovulate in the last half of heat. They should be bred on the first day of heat and 24 hours later for maximum conception rate and litter size.

Bitches. The bitch (female dog) is a seasonally monestrous animal with a definite anestrous period between cycles (see Table 15-1). Most bitches come into season about once every 6 to 7 months. The heats can occur at any time of the year; however, they seem to be concentrated in the spring and fall. Some female dogs may cycle only once a year, as is the case with the Basenji breed. Other individual dogs may cycle every 4 months and still be considered normal. Bitches reach puberty at 6 to 24 months of age, with an average of 10 to 12 months. Small breeds usually reach puberty earlier than large breeds. Vaginal smears can be used to determine the stage of the cycle (Fig. 15-2). Owners say a bitch has come into "heat" when they notice attraction of males and dripping of blood from the vulva. This is actually proestrus, not estrus.

TABLE 15-1 Reproductive data for various domestic species

	Cycle pattern	Cycle length	Heat length	Ovulation time	Time to Breed — Natural Heat	Time to Breed — AI	Gestation length	Puberty	Age to first breeding
Cow	Polyestrous	21 days	18 hours	12-18 hours after heat	Heat	12 hours after first see heat	280 days	6-16 months	14-22 months
Mare	Seasonally polyestrous (long day)	21 days	5 days	24-36 hours before end of heat	Day 2 and every other day of heat	Same as natural	330 days (320-360 days)	18 months	2-3 years
Sow	Polyestrous	21 days	2-3 days	36 hours after onset of heat	Daily when in heat	Same as natural	115 days	7 months	8-9 months
Bitch	Seasonally monestrous	4-7 months	7-9 days	Day 2-3 of heat	Days 1, 3, and 5 of heat	Same as natural			
Queen	Seasonally polyestrous	21 days	4-10 days	Induced	In heat	In heat	63 days	7-12 months	12-18 months
Ewe	Seasonally polyestrous (short day)	17 days	1-1.5 days	Toward end	In heat	In heat	150 days	6-16 months*	6 months
Doe	Seasonally polyestrous (short day)	21 days	1-3 days	12 hours before end of heat	In heat	In heat	150 days	6-16 months*	6 months

*Lambs and kids born early in the year may reach puberty at their first breeding season. Those born late may wait until the next year's breeding season.

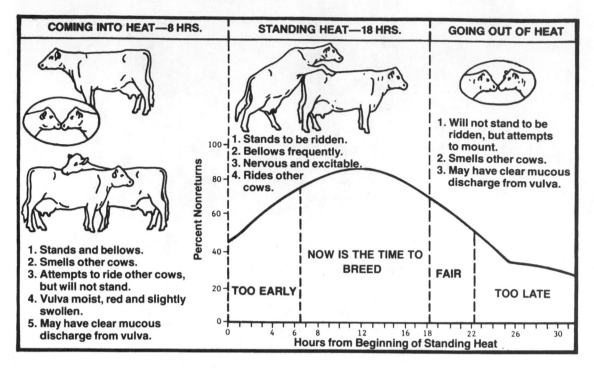

FIG. 15-1 Signs of estrus and timing of breeding in the cow. *(From Herrick JB: Estrus detection in the bovine,* Large Animal Veterinarian, *May/June 1988, courtesy of Watt Publishing Co.)*

Proestrus. This stage is characterized by increased vulvar swelling, a bloody vulvar discharge, attraction to males, and courtship play, such as spinning, crouching in front, nuzzling, and even mounting the male. However, proestrous females do not stand to be mounted by males. The vaginal smear at this stage shows a variable amount of red blood cells (RBCs) and white blood cells (WBCs), and initially contains predominantly small, round parabasal and small intermediate vaginal epithelial cells (see Fig. 15-2). Parabasal and small intermediate cells are distinguishable by their round shape and relatively large nucleus in proportion to the amount of cytoplasm.

As the bitch progresses through proestrus, the number of RBCs in the smear remains variable. The number of WBCs declines and vaginal cells increasingly tend toward large intermediate and superficial cells, both of which are thin, large, and angular cells, having small pyknotic (dense) nuclei or no nucleus at all. The vaginal cells are becoming keratinized or cornified. The vulva is still large and edematous at this stage. Proestrus lasts an average of 9 days (range 3 to 17 days). By the end of proestrus, more than 50% of the vaginal cells are anuclear (no nucleus), keratinized superficial cells (see Fig. 15-2). A short-lived LH peak causes progesterone levels to begin to rise at the end of proestrus, or early estrus before ovulation. Kits are available to detect the LH or progesterone rise and predict the time of ovulation for maximum breeding efficiency.

Estrus. The onset of estrus is marked by the bitch standing to be mounted by the male. Estrus averages 9

days in the bitch but can be as short as 3 or as long as 21 days. During estrus, the bitch lifts the tail and deflects it to the side, arches the back, and elevates the vulva.

The vulva is less turgid than in a proestrus; this facilitates copulation (mating). The estrual vulvar discharge may remain red or become straw colored. As mentioned earlier, the estrual vaginal smear consists almost entirely of superficial and large intermediate cells (see Fig. 15-2). The WBCs are no longer present in the smear; RBCs may or may not be present. The presence or absence of RBCs is not a significant finding when trying to determine the stage of the cycle.

Bitches ovulate early in estrus. The best time to breed a bitch is on the first, third, and fifth days of standing heat. Breeding bitches on the ninth and eleventh or eleventh and thirteenth days after the onset of vulvar bleeding is less than satisfactory because of the variable duration of proestrus and estrus. Breeding bitches on these predetermined days assumes the owner noticed the first day of vulvar discharge. However, this is often not the case. Breedings based upon the preovulatory rise in LH or progesterone levels are the most effective. The kit directions (mentioned earlier) should be followed for predicting the most fertile period, because the exact days on which to breed vary with the kit.

During breeding, it is important to be sure that the stud (male dog) has inserted the penis completely and that the bulbus glandis (enlarged portion of the penis) is completely inserted into the vagina, producing the

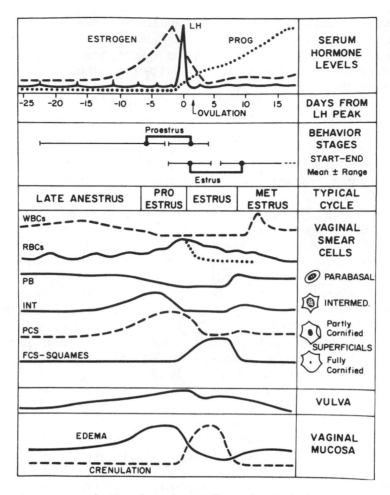

FIG. 15-2 Events during the canine estrous cycle. Note that vulvar swelling and vaginal edema are greatest in proestrus and reduced in estrus. As the vaginal edema subsides, wrinkling (crenulation) of the vaginal mucosa can be detected with vaginoscopy. *(From Kirk RW: Current veterinary therapy VIII small animal practice, Philadelphia, 1983, WB Saunders.)*

coital lock or "tie." The tie is important for stimulating contractions that help move the semen into the uterus and up the oviducts. A normal tie can last 15 to 30 minutes. The dogs should not be disturbed at this time. Efforts to physically separate the bitch and stud may injure the penis or the vagina. At the end of estrus, the bitch no longer accepts the stud dog, even though he may continue to show interest in her. The bitch then enters metestrus.

Metestrus. Metestrus is a short stage, marked by the female's refusal of the male's sexual advances and reappearance of WBCs and noncornified parabasal and small intermediate cells in vaginal smears. Vulvar swelling and discharge decrease rapidly during this stage. Metestrus rapidly progresses into diestrus. The wide range of days during which breeding can take place in the dog makes accurate prediction of whelping difficult. The whelping date can be predicted to occur 56 to 58 days after the vaginal smear reverts to predominantly noncornified small intermediate and parabasal cells typical of diestrus.

Diestrus. This is the longest stage of the canine estrous cycle; it lasts about 60 days, which is nearly the same length as a normal pregnancy. There is no vulvar discharge after the first few days of diestrus. The vaginal smear contains predominantly noncornified parabasal and small intermediate cells, with a few WBCs.

Toward the end of diestrus, about the time a pregnant bitch would be ready to whelp, the nonpregnant bitch often shows *pseudopregnancy,* or "false pregnancy," as progesterone levels decline. The abdomen may enlarge and the mammary glands may swell and fill with milk. The bitch may start building a "nest" and even undergo a false first stage of labor (see below). Pseudopregnant bitches often "adopt" socks, stuffed toys, or kittens as their surrogate puppies. They may have a behavior change at this time and become aggressive if attempts are made to remove their "puppies." Pseudopregnant bitches have been known to raise an orphaned litter of kittens. Not all bitches show clinical signs of pseudopregnancy; however, they all undergo the same hormonal changes that could make them exhibit these signs.

Anestrus. After diestrus or pregnancy, the uterus undergoes a period of regeneration or repair during anestrus. Anestrus may last 1 to 11 months, depending on the breed, with 4 to 5 months being the average. The vaginal smear at this time comprises primarily noncornified parabasal and small intermediate cells, with variable numbers of WBCs. At times, WBCs can be quite numerous, making it difficult to rule out infection. Anestrous females do not attract males, nor do they allow courtship or mating behavior by the stud. After anestrus, the bitch reenters proestrus and the cycle repeats itself.

Queens. The queen (female cat) is different from other animals previously discussed in that the others are *spontaneous ovulators.* That is, they release their eggs at the predetermined time in their cycle, after the appropriate hormonal changes. The queen, on the other hand, is an *induced ovulator,* meaning coitus (mating) is necessary to stimulate ovulation. The queen is a seasonally polyestrous animal (see Table 15-1). If not induced to ovulate, she will have several cycles of sexual behavior before either being bred and induced to ovulate, or having the follicles regress. Queens have a short anestrous period between October and January, but they then cycle regularly the rest of the year if they do not conceive. Because the cat is an induced ovulator, CLs are not produced unless coitus has occurred. The cycle lasts about 14 days and is composed of 1 to 2 days of proestrus, 3 to 6 days of estrus (heat), and about 7 days of metestrus before proestrus occurs again.

Estrus. Estrus in queens is recognized by behavioral changes. They become more affectionate, vocalize, and rub up against inanimate objects and people. When petted, they arch their back, elevate the hindquarters, and laterally displace the tail. Treading of the hind feet is often evident at this time.

Queens do not show the vulvar bleeding as do dogs, but they have similar changes in vaginal cells. Reappearance of WBCs in the smear marks the end of estrus and the beginning of metestrus. Natural breeding can successfully take place at any time during estrus, because the eggs are not ovulated until breeding. Many owners find the recurrent estrous behavior of their cat annoying. It can be stopped by inducing ovulation and pseudopregnancy after a sterile mating or false mating using a glass rod (e.g., a sanitized rectal thermometer) to gently stimulate the queen's vagina. Ovulation can also be induced by injection of the appropriate luteinizing hormone or releasing factor. Overaggressive probing for a vaginal smear for estrus detection can also stimulate ovulation. Induced ovulation should keep a queen out of heat for 40 days or longer if winter is approaching.

Ewes and Does. Ewes (female sheep) and does (female goats) are photosensitive, seasonally polyestrous animals (see Table 15-1). They begin to cycle in response to shortening of the day length and thus are fall and winter breeders. Some breeds of sheep and goats vary from this pattern and can be bred at other times of the year. Estrus in the ewe is often unapparent and a ram wearing a mount marking harness is usually necessary to detect ewes in heat. Does, on the other hand, are more demonstrative of their sexual receptivity. They bleat frequently, approach the male, wiggle their elevated tail, and may urinate in the male's presence. The odor of the buck (male goat) often stimulates cycling and estrous behavior. Does in estrous can be detected by their teasing a male or by exposing a doe to the male's odor on a rag rubbed in his scent glands near the horns.

Although these small ruminants are similar in size and seasonality, their estrous cycles are very distinct. Does have a cycle length similar to the cow's, ranging from 19 to 24 days, with an average length of 21 days. The cycle is often shorter in the early part of the breeding season. Unlike cows, does ovulate 12 hours or so before the end of heat. Heat lasts an average of 28 hours, but it may be as long as 3 days. The doe should be bred on the days she is in heat.

The ewe's estrous cycle is shorter than the doe's and cow's. Ewes cycle about every 17 days (range 14 to 19 days). Heat averages 26 hours in length (range 20 to 36 hours) and the ewe ovulates toward the end of heat. It is best to breed on the day the ewe is noted to be in heat.

Gestation lasts about 150 days for both the doe and ewe, and parturition (birth) is followed by a period of anestrus until the next breeding season.

Pregnancy Diagnosis

One of the indicators of pregnancy in large animals is failure to return to heat after breeding during their breeding season. However, this is not true for dogs because, as seasonally monestrous animals, they will not return to heat for 4 to 7 months, even if they fail to conceive after mating. Mated but nonpregnant cats will not return to heat for several months after breeding. Seasonally polyestrous animals do not return to heat at the end of their breeding season. Traditionally, animals are examined for pregnancy by palpation (manual examination) of the uterus through the abdominal wall or by rectal palpation. Various histologic, chemical, electronic, ultrasonic, and radiographic techniques can also be used to identify the pregnant animal.

PARTURITION

After the preparatory changes of late pregnancy, which ready the dam and fetus for birth, parturition begins. Parturition has several common names, depending upon the species involved. The terms *calving, lambing, kid-*

TABLE 15-2 Stages of labor in various domestic species

Stage	Cow	Mare	Sow*	Bitch*	Queen
I	1-4 hours (longer in heifers); restless; off feed; isolates self; allantois protrudes	1-4 hours; colic; sweats; isolates self; defecates; urinates; placenta ruptures	2-12 hours; 1-2° F drop in rectal temp; builds nest	6-12 hours; 1-2° F drop in rectal temp; builds nest	2-12 hours; 1-2 ° F drop in rectal temp; builds nest
II	1/2-4 hours; abdominal straining; amnion ruptures; calf delivered	5-40 minutes; forceful abdominal straining; amnion ruptures; foal delivered	1-5 hours; amnion ruptures; straining; pigs delivered	3-6 hours; amnion ruptures; pups delivered	3-6 hours; amnion ruptures; kittens delivered
III	1/2-8 hours; uterine contractions; passes placenta	1/2-3 hours; rests between uterine contractions; ± mild colic	1/3-4 hours; eats; drinks	1/2-1 hour; greenish-black fluid passed	1/2-1 hour; brownish fluid passed

*Several fetuses may be passed before a placenta is passed.

ding, and *foaling* are self-explanatory. However, parturition in the sow or gilt is called *farrowing,* and in the bitch, it is called *whelping.* In the cat, it is called *kittening* or *queening.*

Parturition is divided into three stages (Table 15-2). *Stage 1* is preliminary to expulsion of the fetus. During this stage, the uterine muscles undergo rhythmic contractions, which reposition and advance the fetus toward the cervix. In response to these contractions and the pressure of the fetus, the cervix relaxes fully and dilates. The dam in first-stage labor often is anxious and restless and shows evidence of abdominal cramps. Stage 1 ends with delivery of the fetus into the pelvic canal and rupture of the fetal membranes.

Stage 2 is the stage of expulsion of the fetus from the birth canal. Uterine contractions are stronger and accompanied by abdominal straining to help expel the fetus. The importance of abdominal straining versus uterine contractions in the birth process varies among species. Abdominal pressing is very important in foaling, but uterine contractions are relatively more important in farrowing. With successful delivery of the fetus, the dam completes stage 2 and rests during the first part of stage 3.

Stage 3 of parturition is characterized by expulsion of the placenta. Uterine contractions continue but are not as severe as those in stage 2. The uterus begins to shrink toward its nonpregnant size. In polytocous (litter-bear-

---

Box 15-1 Guidelines for intervention in dystocia in various species

Bitch, Queen

- Intense straining that does not produce a pup or kitten in 30 minutes
- Weak, intermittent straining that does not produce a pup or kitten in 2-3 hours
- An interval of over 4 hours between pups or kittens, without further labor
- Illness in the dam
- A bloody, malodorous or greenish vulvar discharge
- Prolonged pregnancy (overdue)
- Obvious difficulty in delivering the pup or kitten (e.g., a fetus halfway out)

Sow

- Prolonged pregnancy (over 115 days)
- Malodorous or bloody vulvar discharge
- Expulsion of fetal feces (meconium) without expulsion of a fetus
- Weak labor or cessation of labor before delivery of all fetuses
- Incomplete expulsion of a fetus

Cow

- First-stage labor lasting more than 6 hours, without abdominal pressing
- Second-stage labor, with abdominal pressing, lasting over 2-3 hours without progress
- Rupture of the waterbag (amnion) without expulsion of the calf within 2 hours
- Fetal malposition (backwards, legs retained, etc.)
- Fetal monstrosity (malformed fetus)

Mare

Parturition, especially stage 2, in mares is quicker and more violent than in other species. Furthermore, foals seem more susceptible to the adverse effects of dystocia than other neonates. Therefore, differentiation between a normal birth and dystocia is especially important in mares. Delivery should be assisted when any of the following occur:

- Appearance of the red unruptured placenta at or outside the vulva at the start of second-stage labor, with evident straining
- Failure of the clear amnion to appear soon after the start of second-stage labor
- Failure to locate the foal's head and legs in the pelvic inlet at the beginning of second-stage labor
- Rolling, repeated getting up and down, and reversing of the recumbent position by the mare, without progressing through stage 2 of labor and delivering a foal
- Repeated straining without delivery of a partially expelled foal
- Fetal malposition (backwards, legs retained, etc.) or other abnormality in delivery
- Fetal fecal (meconium) staining on the foal

ing) species, the cycle of stages 1 to 3 repeats itself with each fetus. Stages 1 and 2 may occur several times and result in passage of several fetuses before a placenta is passed in stage 3 in these species.

After delivery of the fetus, the dam rests and begins to care for the newborn. She licks it dry, which helps stimulate breathing. She chews off any amniotic membrane remaining on the fetus. The bitch and queen usually chew the umbilical cord to sever the placenta. The cord usually ruptures spontaneously during delivery of the calf or during the mare's or foal's efforts to rise.

Calves and foals are usually delivered front feet first, in a "diving" position. Most pigs, pups, and kittens are also delivered head first, but frequently one or both front legs are retracted alongside the body. However, in these small species, rear-end (breech) delivery is common and results in normal, live offspring. Most dams deliver while lying down, but occasionally a cow or mare may deliver while standing up. This can be dangerous to the fetus.

It is often difficult to tell when a dam has finished delivering all of its offspring. Prepartum radiographs made one week before the due date can determine the exact number of pups or kittens in the dam. Twins in mares and cows are uncommon and can be detected by manual exploration of the vagina and uterus. However, this is not as easily accomplished in sows, bitches, and queens, so other signs or tests may be necessary. The bitch's abdomen may be palpated for more pups, or a finger in a sterile glove may be introduced into the vagina to feel for another pup. Radiographs of the abdomen may be necessary. Some bitches and queens eat their neonatal pups, so care must be taken to differentiate fetuses in the stomach from those in the uterus. Sows often get up to drink and may eat some feed after a period of rest once the last pig is delivered.

One of the most difficult situations encountered in theriogenology is to decide when parturition is not proceeding normally and the dam is in *dystocia* (difficult birth) and requires assistance. Box 15-1 contains helpful guidelines.

BREEDING SOUNDNESS EXAMINATION OF MALES

Breeding soundness examination of males should include a good physical examination, evaluation of the reproductive organs, and examination of the ejaculate's quantity, percentage of motile sperm, and percentage of normally shaped sperm. Procedures used in such examinations vary with the species (Table 15-3). Semen can be collected by electroejaculation in the bull, ram, tom, and anesthetized boar. An artificial vagina can be used in the dog, bull, tom, boar, and stallion. Manual stimu-

lation of the penis is effective in producing an ejaculate in the boar and dog and some stallions. After collection of a semen sample, be careful to prevent the sperm from becoming cold or heat shocked, which decreases motility and produces large numbers of secondary abnormalities in the sperm.

Sperm motility is evaluated subjectively as soon after semen collection as possible, using prewarmed slides, preferably on a microscope stage warmed to about 37° C. The motility score is the percentage of individual sperm with rapid progressive motility when examined under high power. Ruminant semen is very concentrated and should be diluted with saline or sodium citrate to see individual motile sperm.

After evaluating motility, stain a smear of the semen and evaluate it for morphologic abnormalities. A smear for morphologic evaluation can be made by staining the sperm with any number of stains, such as eosin-nigrosin, Cassarett's or fine-grain India ink (positively

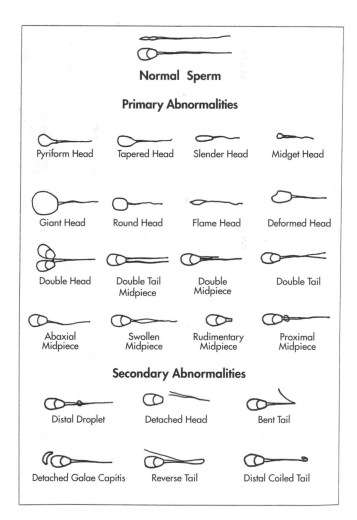

FIG. 15-3 Characteristics of normal and abnormal sperm. Primary abnormalities are of testicular origin. Secondary abnormalities occur during epididymal transport or ejaculation or subsequent to poor semen handling techniques.

TABLE 15-3 Semen evaluation in some domestic species

| | Collection Methods | | | Volume (ml) | Concentration (million/ml) | Sperm per ejaculate (billion) | Scrotal measurement | Progressively motile sperm (minimum % acceptable) | Abnormal sperm (maximum % acceptable) |
	Manual	Electro-ejaculator	Artificial vagina						
Dog	Yes	No	40-42° C	10 (1-25)	125 (20-540)	1.25	Yes‡	70%	20%
Stallion	Yes	No	41-50° C	70 (30-250)	120 (30-600)	8.4	Yes‡	70%	35%
Boar	Yes	Yes*	45-50° C	250 (125-500)	150 (25-1000)	37.5	Yes‡	85%	30%
Bull	Yes†	Yes	40-52° C	4 (1-15)	1200 (300-2500)	4.8	Yes∥	30%§	30%§

*Must be anesthetized.
†By rectal massage of prostate and seminal vesicles.
‡Scrotal width and testes dimension measured by caliper.
∥Scrotal circumference measured with tape: 30 cm at ≤ 15 mo.; 31 cm at 15-18 mo.; 32 cm at 18-21 mo.; 33 cm at 21-24 mo.; 34 cm at > 24 mo. old.
§General oscillation or better.

silhouettes sperm). Smear the stained sample onto a slide to produce a thin layer of sperm so that individual cells can be seen in their entirety for counting. Examine several hundred sperm and categorize them as normal or affected by a primary abnormality or secondary abnormality (Fig. 15-3). Record the percentage of each type of sperm. Acceptable levels of these abnormalities for each of these species are listed in Table 15-2. *Primary abnormalities* of sperm occur in the testis, whereas *secondary abnormalities* are produced in the extra-testicular ducts (epididymis) or are artifacts produced by careless semen handling techniques. Primary abnormalities are predominantly abnormalities of the head and midpiece but include some tail abnormalities (see Fig. 15-3).

After morphologic evaluation, the concentration of sperm in the sample should be evaluated in all species except the bull. In bulls, sperm production is estimated by measuring scrotal circumference. In the other species, the concentration of sperm in the sample is determined by counting the sperm with a hemacytometer, Coulter counter, Spectronic 20 calibrated for sperm, or densimeter. When using a hemacytometer, an RBC pipette can be used for concentrated samples and a WBC pipette for more dilute semen; a Unopette WBC platelet chamber can be used, but care must be taken to be sure the proper dilution factors are used when calculating the concentration.

ARTIFICIAL INSEMINATION

Successful artificial insemination (AI) depends upon accurate determination of the appropriate time to breed, use of high-quality semen, and careful attention to semen handling and insemination techniques.

Cows. Cows' behavior should be properly observed so as to determine the optimal time of breeding. It is advisable to take at least 30 minutes twice a day, early and late in the day, for observing cows for heat. Cows in heat stand to be mounted by other cows, are usually less interested in eating, act nervous, and vocalize frequently (see Fig. 15-1). A long strand of clear mucus is commonly seen draining from the vulva or smeared on the tail or perineum. Although standing heat is the time to breed naturally, AI requires use of the "AM/PM rule." That is, cows first seen in heat in the morning should be inseminated that evening and vice versa (see Fig. 15-1).

Handle frozen semen carefully to avoid killing or damaging the sperm in the insemination straw or ampule. The thawing procedure varies and should be carried out in accordance with the recommendation of the company packaging the frozen semen. In general, ampules of frozen semen are thawed in ice water for 10 minutes. The straws (0.5 cc) are thawed in warm water (32.2° to 35° C) for 45 seconds. However, follow the recommendations of the company processing the semen. Because thawing and refreezing damage the sperm, straws or ampules not being used should not be raised above the "frost line" in the neck of the tank of liquid nitrogen used to store the frozen semen.

Once semen is out of the storage tank and thawed, deposit it in the cow within 15 minutes to ensure viability. Dry the straw or ampule before loading the semen into the insemination gun or pipette, because water kills sperm. Before artificially inseminating the cow, make sure the vulva is wiped clean and dry.

Placing a plastic-sleeve–covered hand just inside the rectum, apply ventral (downward) pressure to open the labia. This helps prevent contamination of the pipette and semen during passage of the pipette into the vagina. Once the pipette is 3 to 4 inches into the vagina, extend the hand in the rectum cranially (forward) to identify and grasp the cervix, a firm cylindric structure. Encircle the cervix with the hand or hold it against the pelvis with the fingers, and extend the vagina to its full length to eliminate any folds in it, which could interfere with passage of the pipette through the cervix. Use your fingers as a guide to make sure the pipette is in the cervix and not in the fornix (along the thinner vaginal wall, beside the cervix).

The pipette must pass through three to five constrictions in the cervix. While passing the pipette through these "rings," always keep your fingers in contact with the end of the pipette to guide it, as well as to protect the uterine wall from being punctured as it enters the uterus. After the pipette enters the uterus 1/4 inch or so, depress the plunger slowly, depositing the semen. Withdraw the pipette and examine for pus or blood.

Mares. Artificial insemination of mares is not as widely practiced as in cows, because of breed regulations and the limited availability of frozen equine semen. However, AI may be used in addition to natural breeding to "reinforce" a service (breeding) in Thoroughbreds and some other breeds. In Quarterhorses, Standardbreds, and a few other breeds, AI is used when several mares must be bred at one time, and the stallion's ejaculate can be diluted and still have sufficient numbers of viable sperm. Regulations for most breeds that allow AI require that the stallion and the mare be on the same farm at the time of AI. In Hanoverians and some other breeds, freezing and shipping of semen to other locations for AI are permitted. Overnight shipping of cooled, extended (diluted) semen is allowed by some breeds, as long as strict recording and animal identification standards are met. Starting on day 2 of heat and breeding every other day until the mare goes out of heat produces satisfactory results with natural breeding or fresh extended semen that is artificially inseminated. However, use of cooled, extended, or frozen semen requires close attention to the time of insemination and should be used in conjunction with follicle checks to ensure that insemination precedes ovulation as closely as possible. Frozen semen works best if inseminated within 6 hours before ovulation.

Semen is collected with the aid of an artificial vagina. The temperature inside the vagina should be about 40.6° C at the time of collection. A mare in heat or a "dummy" that the stallion is trained to mount is required to collect semen.

Fresh semen samples should be kept as close to 35° C as possible to ensure sperm viability. The collection container is often equipped with a filter to assist in separating the gel from the remainder of the semen. Raw semen can be placed in a warm syringe and deposited into the mare's uterus through an infusion pipette, or semen extender can be added to the semen if desired.

Extending (diluting) the semen allows more mares to be inseminated and protects the sperm for a short time until deposition into the uterus. There are several acceptable commercially available semen extenders. They often contain antibiotics to help control any bacteria that have contaminated the semen during collection or that may have been introduced into the uterus during insemination. The semen can be diluted 1:1 or 1:4 with the extender, depending on the sperm concentration in the semen. It is desirable to have 100 to 500 million live normal sperm per insemination dose. Extended semen can be stored or shipped for use several days later.

Stallion semen may be frozen in 0.25-cc to 5-cc straws, in plastic pouches, or as pellets. Follow meticulously the handling precautions mentioned for bull semen and the thawing instructions provided with the semen.

Sows. Sows can be inseminated with fresh or frozen semen. AI is growing in acceptance in commercial swine production. Some reasons for reluctance of the swine industry to extensively use AI are a lack of reliable means of synchronizing heat in gilts and sows, the amount of time and work involved, and the high level of management required. Heat detection and record keeping must be very accurate.

The optimum time to artificially inseminate sows depends on the heat detection techniques used. Sows checked for heat once daily should be bred every day they stand to be mounted, for at least 3 days. If heat detection is used twice daily, sows should be inseminated 12 and 24 hours after the onset of heat.

After estrus is detected, semen is collected in an artificial vagina or directly in a prewarmed thermos by manually massaging the boar's penis. Semen can be collected while the male is mounted on an estrual female or boars can be trained to mount dummies constructed for this purpose. The semen can be extended 1:4 or 1:5. One ejaculate usually contains enough sperm to inseminate 6 to 8 females. A minimum of 2 billion live normal sperm is needed for adequate conception and large litter sizes. Frozen extended semen is available from at least one commercial source in the U.S. and one in Canada.

When AI is used, relatively large volumes (50 to 100 ml) of semen are deposited with the aid of a spiral-tipped pipette or an infusion pipette that has the last (distal) inch bent at a 30-degree angle. These pipettes are actually "screwed" into the cervical rings of the sow.

Bitches. Artificial insemination in the dog is usually carried out with fresh, undiluted semen. However, in the last few years, the American Kennel Club has approved registration of litters using shipped, cooled, extended, or frozen dog semen when collection, storage, transfer, and insemination are done under very strict rules and regulations.

Canine semen is usually collected by manual massage of the penis. Most dogs do not require an estrual bitch present when this is done; however, some timid males may need teasing by a bitch in heat before collection. Collect semen in a quiet room, with good footing for the dog and no distractions. Aerosol bitch scent containing pheromones may be helpful in stimulating the male. The male can also be allowed to smell the vaginal swab from an estrual bitch.

The dog ejaculates in three fractions. The first fraction is clear and contains no sperm; discard this. Collect the second fraction, the sperm-rich fraction. The third fraction (prostatic fluid) is clear. Collect a few drops and discard the rest. There may be a 15- to 60-second delay between passage of fractions.

The semen is protected from cold and heat shock and transferred to a prewarmed syringe and deposited in the cranial vagina through 6- to 12-inch infusion rod. The rear of the bitch should be elevated during and for a few minutes after insemination. Some veterinarians prefer to introduce the index finger, covered with a sterile, powder-free glove, into the vagina with the infusion rod. The finger is left in the vagina a few minutes and the dorsum of the vaginal vault is stroked gently to simulate the coital tie between the male and female. It is thought that this induces waves of uterine and vaginal contractions that help the sperm move into the uterus.

Canine sperm is usually not diluted because of a lack of ability to synchronize heat in females. Bitches usually are artificially inseminated because of a lack of ability or desire by the selected male to copulate. Bitches should be inseminated on the first, third, and fifth day of standing heat or as determined by vaginal cytology and progesterone determination, if available.

RECOMMENDED READING

Feldman EC, Nelson RW: *Canine and feline endocrinology and reproduction,* ed 2, Philadelphia, 1996, WB Saunders.

Hafez ESE: *Reproduction in farm animals,* ed 6, Philadelphia, 1993, Lea & Febiger.

Hayes KEN: *The complete book of foaling,* ed 1, New York, NY, 1993, Howell Book House.

McKinnon AO, Voss JL: *Equine reproduction,* ed 1, Philadelphia, 1993, Lea & Febiger.

Siegal M: *Book of dogs,* ed 1, New York, NY, 1995, Harper Collins.

Smith MC, Sherman DM: *Goat medicine,* ed 1, Philadelphia, 1994, Lea & Febiger.

CHAPTER 16

Behavior

S. Hetts

Learning Objectives

After reviewing this chapter, the reader should understand the following:

Role of veterinary professionals in managing behavior problems

Ways in which behavior problems can be prevented in companion animals

Ways in which behavior problems can be treated by the veterinary practice

Appropriate procedure for referring clients for resolution of their animals' behavior problems

PREVENTING BEHAVIOR PROBLEMS IN COMPANION ANIMALS

Most behavior problems are easier to prevent than to correct. Many pet owners are annoyed when their animals damage household belongings with destructive and housesoiling behavior. Techniques based on scientifically valid ethologic and learning principles minimize such behaviors. Unfortunately, much of the information in the popular literature to which owners have easy access does not always meet these criteria. Thus, technicians can be an important source of scientifically accurate information on preventing behavior problems.

Housetraining

Dogs and cats can be encouraged to eliminate reliably in locations that are acceptable to their human owners. Dogs can learn to eliminate outside of the "den." Cats, as well as pigs and rabbits, learn to use litterboxes. Other species of domestic companion animals are either caged or kept outside because their elimination behavior is not restricted to specific locations.

Dogs. People have probably been training dogs not to eliminate in the house for almost as long as dogs have been domesticated. You might assume that thousands of years of practice have resulted in good housetraining techniques. Surprisingly, this is not the case.

Misconceptions and oversimplifications about the process of housetraining seem to be relatively common. Perhaps the one most often encountered concerns the use of crates. A common belief is that dogs will not soil their sleeping areas. The popular theory continues that therefore a dog, when confined to a crate (its sleeping area), will not eliminate in it.[1] This assumption is then used as a basis for confining a dog to a crate as the primary tool in housetraining.

These ideas seem to be an oversimplification of the literature on behavioral development. In many species of canids, including dogs, beginning at birth, the dam stimulates her pups to eliminate by licking their anogenital area.[13] They begin to eliminate without such stimulation between 3 and 4 weeks of age. At about 6 weeks of age, *if given the opportunity,* the pups tend to move away from their nesting, sleeping, or den area to eliminate.[22] This developmental finding does not imply that confinement magically prevents a dog from eliminating. This means that, if given a choice, a puppy will move away from the nesting area to eliminate. If not given a choice (i.e., confined), the puppy will eliminate where confined. This is often seen when dogs are consistently confined in small areas, such as in cages in pet stores. Such confinement interferes with the dog's developmental tendencies. When dogs eliminate in their crates or cages because of the inability to move somewhere else, this may make later housetraining more difficult. If a dog is eliminating in its crate, this is an indication that something is wrong. Possible problems include excessively long confinement periods, disease or illness, or fear or anxiety problems.

The developmental finding that dogs tend to eliminate away from the nest area has been oversimplified to imply that confinement is the sole technique required for housetraining. Many owners, either because they are given incorrect or more probably insufficient information, limit their housetraining procedures to confining the puppy or dog in a crate and then taking it outside at intervals. Reliance on these procedures alone at best delays housetraining and at worst makes housetraining impossible.

Owners must be made aware of several important points when housetraining their dog. First, a puppy or dog's confinement to a crate must not exceed the time the animal can control its bladder and bowels. For young puppies, this can be as little as an hour, or sometimes as much as 2 or 3 hours at a time. In addition, many puppies need to eliminate at least once during the night.

Second, the dog must be actively taught, by reinforcing correct behavior, the desired location for elimination. Owners should reward elimination outside with verbal praise and petting, and possibly a special tidbit. The timing of this reward, however, is critical. Research in animal learning suggests that a delay of longer than 0.5 seconds between the behavior and the subsequent reinforcement significantly decreases the effectiveness of the reinforcement.[2,17] Thus, if the owner waits by the door to reinforce the puppy as it returns from eliminating in the yard, the behavior that has been reinforced is returning to the house. In these cases, owners often complain that all the puppy does when taken outside is to stand by the door. This should come as no surprise because it is what the puppy has inadvertently been rewarded for doing. To reinforce the elimination behavior, the owner must go outside with the puppy and provide reinforcement *immediately* following elimination at the location where it occurs.

Third, although supervision during the housetraining process is imperative to ensure the dog does not develop unacceptable location or surface preferences, a crate is not the only one, or sometimes even the best, means of supervision. Confinement in a small room, such as a laundry room or kitchen, or in an exercise pen, may work equally well. If the dog is to be left for longer than it can maintain bladder or bowel control, a place to eliminate must be provided. Alternatively, when the owner is home, supervision can also be accomplished by keeping the dog in sight at all times, by using a Hands-Away Leash Belt (Fig. 16-1) or by simply tying the leash to one's belt.

Confinement of any kind should never prevent the dog's needs for social interaction and physical exercise from being met. Inappropriate guidelines for confinement suggest the dog be confined except when being taken outside for elimination. Not only does this interfere with other needs but it also prevents the dog from becoming familiar with the rest of the house. The theoretical basis for housetraining is for the dog to view the entire house as its "den" or living area and therefore an inappropriate area for elimination.[10] Perhaps this lack of familiarity is one of the reasons why housesoiling behavior sometimes occurs in areas of the house used

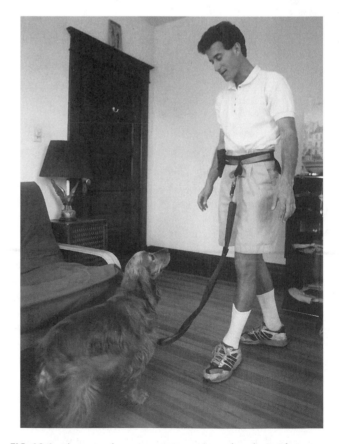

FIG. 16-1 A convenient way to supervise a dog during housetraining is to keep the dog with you at all times using a Hands-Away Leash Belt. *(Courtesy of Woof Whirled, Boulder, Co.)*

infrequently, such as formal dining rooms. An alternative explanation is that the dog is less likely to be caught eliminating there and thus avoids punishment.

Finally, use of physical punishment in housetraining is never appropriate. Interactive punishment that involves the owner (even if delivered at the time of housesoiling) may cause the dog to become reluctant to eliminate in the owner's presence at other times. This interferes with the owner's attempts to appropriately reinforce elimination outside. Remote punishment, such as a loud noise or other startling but harmless stimuli, should be sufficient to temporarily interrupt the behavior. The dog can then be taken outside in a positive, nonthreatening manner.

In an ideal housetraining program, the dog's environment and behavior should be so well managed that correct behavior is reinforced with 100% consistency, and opportunities for inappropriate behavior never occur. In reality, this ideal is seldom met, but if owners are made aware of it through your educational efforts, it may give them a much more accurate perspective on the time and effort required for housetraining. As can be seen, educating owners about housetraining dogs should be much more detailed than simply telling them to "get a crate and put the dog in it when you can't watch him."

Cats. The process of encouraging cats to consistently use litterboxes is based on different developmental events than is housetraining dogs. Like bitches, queens stimulate the kittens to elminate until 3 to 4 weeks of age. At this time, the kittens become increasingly active and begin to play and investigate any loose, particulate material that is available.[2] Shortly thereafter, they begin to use these substrates for elimination. This normal developmental phase occurs even in the absence of observational learning.[5] Kittens, therefore, do not need to observe the queen eliminating or have the owner demonstrate part of the process by raking the cat's paws in the litter. Providing a clean, easily accessible litterbox with an acceptable substrate is sufficient. However, the accessibility of the litterbox and suitability of the substrate must be examined from the kitten's or cat's perspective.

Because kittens are physically and behaviorally immature, a litterbox should be within easy access at all times. This may mean providing several litterboxes at strategic locations in the house or initially limiting the cat's access to only portions of the house. The litterbox should be easily accessible but also should afford some privacy. High-traffic areas are not a good choice, but neither is locating the box in a basement with a cold cement floor. Close proximity to appliances that make unexpected, startling noises, such as the washer, furnace, or hot water heater, should also be avoided.

One study found that cats seem to prefer the softer texture of fine-grained substrates.[3] Thus, a cat is less likely to develop an aversion to a clumping litter comprising very small particles. However, cats develop idiosyncratic preferences for substrates and locations for elimination for reasons that are not well understood. These changing preferences are often the basis of many inappropriate elimination problems in cats. Sometimes these preferences can be influenced by the condition of the litter material. Cats may avoid litter that is consistently dirty, too deep, or scented. One study found that cats with elimination problems were more likely to have scented than unscented litter as compared with cats without such problems.[12]

Owners are sometimes under the impression that the more litter they put in the box, the less often they need to clean it. General guidelines are to keep the litter depth at no more than 2 inches, remove feces and urine clumps daily, and change the litter frequently enough to prevent odors from developing and to ensure that the majority of the litter is always dry.

Another consideration influencing the cat's perception of litterbox accessibility is the presence of other cats in the household. A litterbox may be temporarily unavailable because another cat is either using it or "guarding" it. Thus advise owners to provide at least as many litterboxes as there are cats, and to keep the boxes in different locations so that a single cat cannot block the other cats' access to the litterbox area. In addition, the litterbox location should allow the cat using it to be aware of the presence of other cats in order to prevent any surprise attacks that may occur during elimination.

Preventing Destructive Scratching by Cats

Probably more owners recognize the need to provide their cats with litterboxes than to provide scratching posts. Because cats scratch for a variety of reasons, cats may want to scratch in different locations for different reasons. One of the most important motivations for cats scratching objects with their front claws is territorial marking.[10] Scratching leaves a visual as well as an olfactory mark that serves as an indication of the cat's presence. In addition to marking, scratching may also serve to stretch the muscles and tendons of the legs and remove the worn outer sheaths from the claws. It may also be used as a greeting or play behavior.

Scratching objects should be provided in locations in which the behavior is likely to be triggered. Even if the cat scratches objects when allowed outdoors, it still should have access to an acceptable object indoors. Merely providing a scratching object does not guarantee the cat will use it preferentially to carpet, drapes, or furniture. The scratching objects must match the cat's preferences for desirable locations, and with regard to height, orientation, and texture.

Height. Many scratching posts available commercially do not permit the cat to reach vertically to its full height to scratch, as many cats like to do. For larger cats using relatively short posts, this means they are scratching almost with their abdomen on the floor (Fig. 16-2). It may be a good idea to talk to owners about the desirability of taller, or even floor-to-ceiling scratching poles. If the back of the couch allows the cat to reach to its full height to scratch but the scratching post does not, it is easy to guess which surface the cat will prefer.

Orientation. Not all cats scratch vertically all of the time. Some cats may prefer to stretch their legs out in front and rake backward in a horizontal motion. If this is the case, the cat may be more likely to use a flat, horizontal object (Fig. 16-3) than a vertical post. Some cats may use both, depending on where, when, and why they scratch. One unusual cat was reported to only scratch upside down by pulling herself along on her back as she scratched the underside of the couch.

Texture. This may be the most frequently overlooked aspect of providing an acceptable scratching object. As with other aspects of the behavioral pattern of scratching, cats vary in textures they prefer. Cats that like to rake their claws in long, vertical motions may be more likely to use an object with a texture that permits this. If the cat scratches vertically and the texture is not conducive to those motions, the cat may not use the object. Other cats use more of a "picking" motion and may prefer items covered with sisal, wrapped horizontally. It has been proposed that an object that has been scratched repeatedly, with the result that the covering is somewhat shredded and holds the cat's scent, will be preferred over a new, unused object.[11] If this is true, it suggests owners should not replace scratching posts that are well worn, even if they appear unsightly to the human eye.

The scratching object should be placed in a location where the cat is likely to be motivated to scratch, or adjacent to an unacceptable item the cat is already using. To encourage the cat to use the desirable object, it can be scented with catnip, or a toy can be attached to the top to entice the cat to reach high up the post. Raking the cats feet up and down the post is not necessary and may actually have adverse effects. The most reliable way to discourage scratching of inappropriate objects is to first provide an appropriate substitute and then change the texture of the "off-limit" items. This can be done by covering them with plastic, sandpaper, or any other covering with an unpleasant (from the cat's perspective) texture.

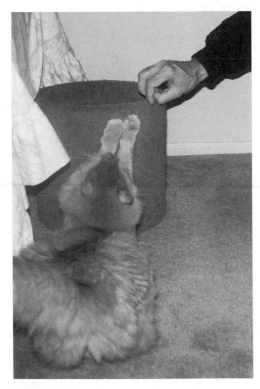

FIG. 16-2 This scratching object is not tall enough to allow this cat to stretch to its full vertical height while using it.

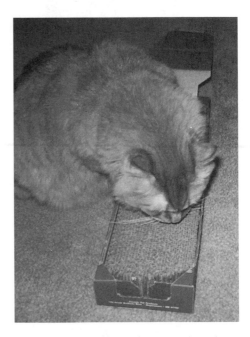

FIG. 16-3 Horizontal scratching objects, such as this cut cardboard pad scented with catnip, are preferred over vertical objects by some cats.

Preventing Destructive Behavior by Dogs

Destructive behavior is a classification of behavior based more on the owner's view of the result (destruction) than on the actual behavior that caused it. Digging, chewing, tearing, scratching, moving objects from one place to another, and removing the contents from the trash all fall within the broad, somewhat anthropomorphic category of destructive behavior.

Dogs show these behaviors for a variety of reasons. Destructive behavior that is the symptomatic manifestation of other problems, such as separation anxiety or noise phobias, may not be preventable. In these cases, the underlying problem must be resolved, rather than trying to treat the symptom. However, destructive behavior that occurs as the result of normal, developmental process, such as teething, play, and investigative behavior, can often be prevented or at least minimized.

Dogs vary in their need for physical activity and play. Some dogs are content to lead relatively inactive lives, whereas others seem to be on the move constantly. Just as with cats' scratching, the goal in minimizing problem destructive behavior due to teething, play, and investigative behavior is not to eliminate the behavior, but to direct it toward acceptable objects by making acceptable toys more attractive than household items. This can be difficult to do on a consistent basis. Thus, it may also be helpful to remind owners that, realistically, they can expect to lose one or more valuable (either monetarily or sentimentally) items to normal canid chewing behavior.

Appealing Toys. The attractiveness of acceptable toys can be maximized by first rewarding the dog every time it plays with them. The toy should also elicit the play patterns that the dog is likely to exhibit. For example, dogs that like to shake toys may be more satisfied with one made of lambskin than with a tennis ball. Toys should be available for chewing and tearing, as well as for carrying and chasing, if the dog displays both patterns of play behavior. It may be helpful to establish a toy rotation so that different toys are available each day to make them more appealing.

If the dog is caught chewing an unacceptable item, the item should be taken away and replaced with one that is acceptable. To decrease the dog's interest in household items, even when the owner is not present, attempts can be made to lessen their appeal. Commercial products, such as Bitter Apple, are available to give objects a bad taste. Motion detectors (Fig. 16-4) or Snappy Trainers (modified mousetraps that do not harm the animal) can discourage animals from bothering specific items or areas, or items can also be "booby-trapped" in other creative ways. Remind owners of the advisability of "dog-proofing" the house just as they would for a young child.

Dogs that insist on digging outside can be provided with their own area in which to do so. This area should

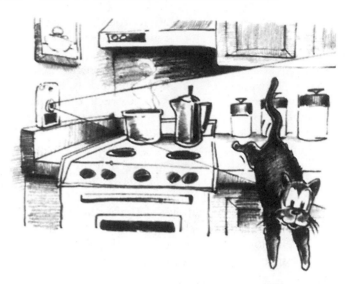

FIG. 16-4 This motion detector emits a series of short, high-pitched beeps when its heat or motion sensors are triggered by an animal's presence. This startling noise discourages animals from approaching the area. The device resets itself automatically and is triggered repeatedly if the animal returns. *(Courtesy of Amtek, San Diego, Calif.)*

consist of loose soil or sand to facilitate digging. Owners can shallowly bury enticing items in this area to attract the dog.

Preventing Aggressive Behavior Problems

Aggressive behavior is normal behavior for most species of animals, including companion animals. Aggression, defined as behavior that is intended to harm another individual, is only one aspect of agonistic behavior. Agonistic behaviors are those behaviors that animals show in situations involving social conflict.[18] Submission, avoidance, escaping, offensive and defensive threats, and offensive and defensive aggression are all part of the agonistic behavior system. Dogs, cats, birds, pigs, and other animals can display a variety of types of aggression behavior.[4] Because the factors that determine when and where an animal will display aggressive or threatening behavior are not fully understood, it is unlikely that preventing problems will be a simple process.

Puppy Tests. One way to prevent aggression problems in animals would theoretically be to select pets that are unlikely to develop such problems. The popular literature has descriptions of a variety of "puppy tests" that supposedly predict a puppy's likelihood for dominant behavior or aggression problems as an adult.[21] Several scientific studies have demonstrated that these tests are not predictive of adult behavior.[1,13,25] This may be because dominance relationships within a litter of puppies can change from day to day and probably do not reflect a rank order based on status.[6] The developmental course of territorial aggression has not been well studied and there are no selection procedures that allow owners to select puppies that would have a high threshold for this behavior.[23]

No such selection tests have ever been devised for cats and other species of companion animals. However, a study currently in progress at Cornell University is attempting to develop a "kitten personality test" based on expectations of the pet as an adult.[15]

Dominance Exercises. Several authors have suggested that puppies should be restrained in a variety of subordinate positions on a regular basis, and any struggling should be firmly reprimanded.[21] These exercises supposedly teach the puppy to be subordinate and prevent biting, especially that directed toward children. No scientific evidence exists to support these claims and, from an ethologic viewpoint, they may not be conceptually valid.

Castration. Castrating male animals clearly reduces some forms of aggressive behavior in many species of animals, including dogs, cats, and horses.[10] Postpubertal castration seems to be as effective as prepubertal. Reports on dog bite statistics show that male dogs are more often involved in serious attacks, and the majority of these dogs are not castrated.[16,24] Therefore, selection of female animals as pets may reduce problems with aggressive behavior.

Socialization Experiences. Many species of mammals and birds have sensitive periods of development of normal species-typical social behavior. This sensitive period in dogs has been well studied, and to a lesser degree in cats and horses.[9,14,22] The sensitive socialization period usually occurs fairly early in life. For example, in dogs it is from 4 to 12 weeks of age and in cats from 2 to 7 weeks.

Companion animals must have a variety of pleasant experiences with different types of people and environments during these sensitive periods so that they are able to accept humans as their social peers later in life. Poorly socialized animals are typically fearful of people or may attach strongly to one or two individuals but are unable to generalize this acceptance to unfamiliar individuals. This fear of people can sometimes develop into defensive aggression problems. Veterinary technicians can encourage dog owners to enroll puppies in puppy classes and to expose both puppies and kittens to a variety of gentle handling and play sessions with people outside the family. A procedure for developing good social relationships between people and horses has also been used.[19]

Providing Problem Prevention Services

Knowing *what* to tell clients to prevent problems is a separate issue from finding sufficient time to do so. It may not be realistic to expect the veterinary professional to do so during a 15-minute office visit when the time is allocated to addressing the presenting medical concern, or in a brief telephone call while greeting clients at the front desk or searching for a client record. Veterinarians and technicians must purposely decide how the valuable information regarding problem prevention can be disseminated. One obvious way is to make it a policy to schedule extra time for appointments involving new animal examination and to charge accordingly. These are often new puppy and kitten appointments, but not always. The fee structure for new animal appointments can include an extra 15 to 20 minutes of staff time, even if the problem prevention discussion takes place separately from the medication examination and vaccination time. Talking to clients about these issues is preferable to relying on written materials alone. However, written materials can be of value because they reinforce what was said and allow clients to read them as often as needed and at their convenience. It can also be argued that the expenses for the time required for problem prevention, even if not charged directly as a fee, may be recouped indirectly. Problem prevention sessions could improve the chances that the animal will remain in the home and thus continue being a patient. Also, the owner's perception of the clinic is enhanced, making word-of-mouth referral of new clients more likely.

Providing Problem Resolution Services

Problem resolution is almost always a more complex process than is problem prevention. It requires first arriving at a behavioral diagnosis for the type of problem. The presenting complaint, whether it be excessive barking, housesoiling, or aggression, can be thought of as behavioral signs similar to medical signs, such as vomiting, limping, or a poor haircoat. Each of these signs can potentially be related to a variety of problems. In the case of behavior problems, medical conditions that could account for the behavioral signs should first be evaluated. This is especially important with aggressive and housesoiling behavior. Once this is done, arriving at a behavioral diagnosis requires obtaining a complete behavioral history and ideally observing the animal and its environment. For some types of problems, such as feline elimination problems, seeing the animal in its home environment may make it possible to identify physical features of the environment that are contributing to the problem. Behavioral diagnosis can sometimes require several hours to interview the owner and observe the animal.

Once the type of problem has been narrowed down to one or a few possibilities, a *behavior modification plan* must be devised. The specific procedures used are dictated by the type of problem. Time is required to explain these procedures to the owner, write them down, demonstrate them if necessary, and have the owner practice them, if appropriate. Once treatment begins, the case must be followed up with either additional in-home or clinic visits or regularly scheduled telephone calls. These follow-up contacts can be relatively brief, sometimes less than 15 minutes, or they may be more lengthy in more difficult or complex cases.

The process of problem resolution cannot be collapsed into "25 words or less" solutions. This oversimplified approach to problem solving trivializes the importance of the problem and omits the scientific knowledge required to successfully modify behavior. Because technicians often have the opportunity to solve behavior problems but may not have the time or expertise to do so, it is important to be aware of the veterinary practice's policies regarding referrals and to become proficient in referring cases to behavior specialists.

Referring Cases to Behavior Specialists. Before referral of an animal to a behavior specialist, evaluate medical conditions that could contribute to the problem behavior. Behavior referrals should be based on the same model of professionalism as are medical case referrals. This includes determining the qualifications of the referral resource, learning the preferred method of referral, facilitating contact between the client and the specialist, and informing the client of what type of services to expect from the referral.

Evaluating referral resources. Many different types of professionals offer to assist pet owners with animal behavior problems. These can range from self-taught dog trainers to academically trained, degreed, and certified behavior specialists. The Behavior College of the American Veterinary Medical Association offers board certification in behavior to veterinarians who meet the established criteria. The Animal Behavior Society, which is the largest organization in North America dedicated to the study of animal behavior, offers two levels of certification to individuals holding a master's or doctoral degree in the behavioral sciences and who meet educational, experiential, and ethical criteria. Although veterinary behaviorists can be board certified, and applied behaviorists can be certified by the Animal Behavior Society, anyone, regardless of academic training, can legally use the professional title of animal behaviorist.

The National Association of Dog Obedience Instructors (NADOI) and the Association of Pet Dog Trainers (APDT) are two professional organizations that dog trainers can join. NADOI membership is open only to trainers who meet the organization's qualifications. APDT encourages and promotes use of positive reinforcement in training, but its membership is open to anyone training dogs.

Because certification does not guarantee competence and professionally trained, qualified people may not be certified, it is the referring professional's responsibility to evaluate the credentials, knowledge, competence, and

philosophies of individuals considered as potential referral resources for the clinic. This may include not only interviewing these individuals but also observing their classes and/or behavior consulting sessions. Gathering information about the individuals from others who offer behavioral assistance can be a valuable service the technician can perform for the clinic.

When choosing a referral resource for behavior cases, technicians should be aware that obedience or command training does not resolve behavior problems. Teaching a dog sit, down, and/or stay does not address separation anxiety problems, housesoiling problems, or other types of problems unrelated to obedience performance. However, obedience classes can be a useful tool in helping dog owners exert better verbal control over their dogs and establishing a more consistent relationship. You may want to identify referral resources for dog obedience classes as well as for behavior counseling for whatever species of animal the clinic provides medical care. You may need to select several different individuals. Certified behavior specialists consult only on those species with which they have experience. Thus, a behaviorist may work with cats and dogs but not birds or horses.

Making the Referral. Handle behavior referral cases as you would medical referrals. When referring a client to a veterinary medical specialist, such as a cardiologist or oncologist, a veterinary professional probably would not instruct the client to call the specialist for some "tips" or "advice." Unfortunately, all too often this is the way clients are referred to behavior specialists. Find out whether the behavior specialist prefers the initial contact to be from the client or from the veterinary medical professional. If contact from the veterinary professional is preferred, be prepared to provide a pertinent medical and behavioral history during that initial conversation.

Give the client a reasonable set of expectations about the referral. Discuss with the client information about the fee structure, where the consultation will take place, how to schedule the appointment, and the amount of time required. You can also encourage the client to seek behavioral help without giving false expectations. Although most animal behavior problems can benefit from professional assistance, not all problems can be completely and permanently resolved.

Dealing with behavior referrals in a professional manner may help clients to view the behavior consulting process as a legitimate aspect of health care and overcome some of their embarrassment about seeking "psychological help" for their pets. It may also help them to better understand why behavior specialists charge fees for professional services, just as veterinarians do. The veterinary clinic can facilitate referrals by having business cards, brochures, and other information about the behavior specialist available to give to clients at the clinic.

REFERENCES

1. Beaudet R, Chalifoux A, Dallaire A: Predictive value of activity level and behavioral evaluation on future dominance in puppies, *Appl Anim Beh Sci* 40:273-294, 1994.
2. Beaver BV: *Feline behavior: a guide for veterinarians,* Philadelphia, 1992, WB Saunders.
3. Borchelt PL: Cat elimination behavior problems, *Advances in Companion Animal Behavior: Vet Clin North Am, Small Anim Pract:* 21(2):257-264, 1991.
4. Borchelt PL, Voith VL: *Aggressive behavior in dogs and cats.* In Voith VL, Borchelt PL, editors: *Readings in companion animal behavior,* Trenton, NJ, 1996, Veterinary Learning Systems.
5. Borchelt PL, Voith VL: *Elimination behavior problems in cats.* In Voith VL, Borchelt PL, editors: *Readings in companion animal behavior,* Trenton, NJ, 1996, Veterinary Learning Systems, pp 179-190.
6. Bradshaw WS, Nott HMR: Social and communication behaviour of companion dogs. In Serpell J, editor: *The domestic dog: its evolution, behaviour and interactions with people,* New York, 1995, Cambridge University Press, pp 115-130.
7. Campbell WE: *Behavior problems in dogs,* Santa Barbara, Calif, 1975, American Veterinary Publications.
8. Colflesh L: *Making friends: training your dog positively,* New York, 1990, Howell Book House.
9. Fraser AF: *The behaviour of the horse,* Wallingford, UK, 1992, CAB International.
10. Hart BL: *The behavior of domestic animals,* New York, 1985, WH Freeman.
11. Hart B, personal communication.
12. Horwitz D: Factors affecting elimination behavior problems in cats: A retrospective study (submitted for publication), JAAHA.
13. Houpt KA: *Domestic animal behavior for veterinarians and animal scientists,* ed 2, Ames, Iowa, 1991, Iowa State University Press.
14. Karsh EB, Turner DC: The human-cat relationship. In Turner DC, Bateson P, editors: *The domestic cat: the biology of its behaviour,* New York, 1988, Cambridge University Press.
15. Kitten personality test could predict adult behavior, *J Am Vet Med Assoc* 208(5):644+, 1996.
16. Lockwood RL: Canine aggression. In Serpell J, editor: *The domestic dog: its evolution, behaviour and interactions with people,* New York, 1995, Cambridge University Press, pp 132-138.
17. Marder A, Reid PJ: *Treating canine behavior problems: behavior modification, obedience and agility training.* In Voith VL, Borchelt PL, editors: *Readings in companion animal behavior,* Trenton, NJ, 1996, Veterinary Learning Systems, pp 56-61.
18. McFarland D: *Agonistic behaviour.* In McFarland D, editor: *The Oxford companion to animal behavior,* New York, 1981, Oxford University Press, p 13.
19. Miller RM: Imprint training the newborn foal, *Large Animal Vet* 44(4):21, 1989.
20. Reid PJ, Borchelt PL: *Learning.* In Voith VL, Borchelt PL, editors: *Readings in companion animal behavior,* Trenton, NJ, 1996, Veterinary Learning Systems, pp 62-71.
21. Riegger MH, Guntzelman J: Prevention and amelioration of stress and consequences of interaction between children and dogs, *J Am Vet Med Assoc* 196(11):1781-1785, 1990.
22. Scott JP, Fuller JO: *Dog behavior: the genetic basis,* Chicago, 1965, University of Chicago Press.
23. Serpell J, Jagoe JA: Early experience and the development of behaviour. In Serpell J, editor: *The domestic dog: its evolution, behaviour and interactions with people,* New York, 1995, Cambridge University Press, pp 79-102.
24. Wright JC: Canine aggression toward people: bite scenarios and prevention. *Advances in Companion Animal Behavior: Vet Clin North Am Small Anim Pract,* 21(2):299-314, 1991.
25. Young MS: Aggressive behavior. In Ford RB, editor: *Clinical signs and diagnosis in small animal practice,* New York, 1988, Churchill Livingstone, pp 135-150.

PART FOUR

Clinical Applications

CHAPTER 17

Physical Restraint

R. Quinn

Learning Objectives

After reviewing this chapter, the reader should understand the following:

Psychological principles underlying physical restraint techniques

Safety precautions taken before and during physical restraint

Methods used to restrain dogs, cats, small mammals, birds, horses, pigs, cattle, and sheep

Typical behavior responses of animals to physical restraint

Correct use of mechanical devices for physical restraint

RESTRAINT AND HANDLING OF DOGS
Restraining Techniques

Removing Dogs from Cages or Runs. It takes practice and sensibility to remove fearful or aggressive dogs safely from cages or runs. Common sense says *never expose your face to an unfamiliar dog*, even if it is acting friendly. Make certain that all escape routes are closed, because many dogs bolt out of a cage or run if given the opportunity. To prevent this, the animal handler should block the cage door with a knee.

Nonaggressive, Nonfearful Dogs. Small dogs can usually be grasped by the collar and then lifted out of the cage with one hand, using the other hand to support the dog's body. Alternatively, a leash can be placed over the dog's head and the dog can be led out. Medium-sized to large dogs are usually led out with a leash.

Fearful Dogs or Aggressive Dogs. Ideally, dogs that are likely to bite should be sedated before they are stored in the cage or run. The dog is easily removed when it is time for the clinical procedure. If this is not possible, proceed with caution. Do not corner the dog. Calmly encourage the dog verbally with praise and place a leash over the dog's head if possible. Another alternative is to call the dog. When it begins to exit the run, squeeze it quickly with the gate and loop the leash over its head. Be careful not to injure the animal.

A small dog in a cage can be captured by placing a leash around its body and quickly swinging it onto the floor. This allows enough time to get another leash around its neck. A small dog can also be removed from a cage by carrying it in a towel or blindfolding it with a towel for removal.

Lifting a Dog. Grasp medium-sized dogs around the abdomen and around the chest. Carry the dog close to your body and place it onto the table. Large dogs should be lifted by two people.

Standing Restraint. This technique allows restriction of movement without causing defensiveness in most

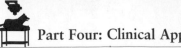

dogs. It is used for such procedures as urinary catheterization, anal sac expression, measuring the rectal temperature, and obtaining vaginal smears. The dog may be placed on an examination table or, if the dog is large, it may stay on the floor. Place one arm around the dog's chest and the other around the abdomen (Fig. 17-1).

Crowding. This technique may be used with very large dogs. Using a corner of a room, push the dog's rear into the corner so it cannot back away.

Sitting or Sternal Recumbency. This technique is usually used on the examination table, and sometimes on the floor with large dogs. This technique is useful for blood collection, intravenous injection, nail trimming, some types of radiography, and oral examination.

For restraint in sternal recumbency, allow the dog to rest on its sterum. Then cradle the dog's body between the arms. The forelegs or jugular vein can then be used for blood collection.

For restraint in the sitting position, place one arm around the dog's chest and one around the neck or muzzle (Fig. 17-2). Pull the dog close and turn the dog's face away to protect against biting. A thumb can be placed in the intermandibular space to discourage biting. You may also need to abduct one of the dog's forelegs for venipuncture.

Lateral Recumbency. This technique is usually used on the examination table but also can be used on the floor. It is useful for radiographs, suture removal, and other procedures of short duration. Place the dog on its left or right side. Hold the legs closer to the table (left legs in left recumbency, right legs in right recumbency), lifting them slightly. Put one arm across the dog's neck and the other across the flank. This prevents the dog from getting up (Fig. 17-3).

Dorsal Recumbency. This technique is used for blood collection from the jugular vein, radiography, cystocentesis, etc. It sometimes requires two persons. Place the dog on its back. If it is a very deep-chested dog, a V-trough may be necessary to keep the dog from rolling. The forepaws are stretched cranially and back paws are stretched caudally, exposing the thorax and abdomen.

Mechanical Devices for Restraint

Muzzle. A muzzle can be made simply with a length of roll gauze. Many commercially made varieties are also available. Apply a muzzle when biting is likely or certain. Remain as far from the dog as possible if it is aggressive. Using a 4-foot–long piece of gauze, make a loop and flip it around the dog's muzzle. Quickly tighten it over and then under the dog's muzzle (Fig. 17-4). Move in closer and make a pass under the dog's chin and tighten. Tie the muzzle behind the ears using a quick-release knot. Keep scissors close by in case the muzzle must be quickly cut off.

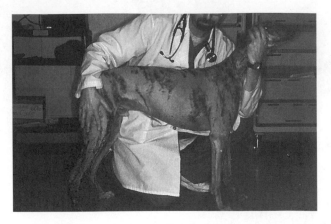

FIG. 17-1   Holding a dog in standing position. One arm is placed in front of the chest and the other supports the abdomen, which prevents sitting. *(Courtesy of Cathy Winters, LVT.)*

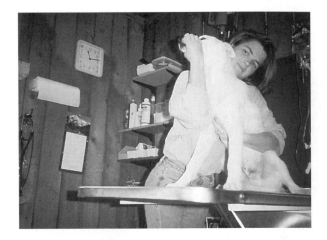

FIG. 17-2   Holding a dog in the sitting position. Both the jugular vein and the cephalic vein are exposed.

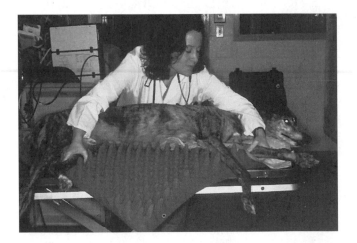

FIG. 17-3   Holding a dog in lateral recumbency. One arm is placed across the dog's neck and the other across the dog's abdomen. The feet closer to the table are held to prevent rising. *(Courtesy of Cathy Winters, LVT.)*

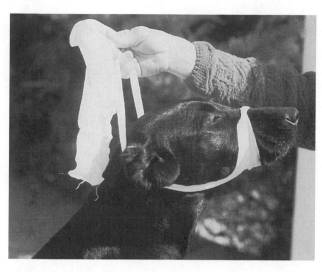

FIG. 17-4   After wrapping around the snout, the gauze muzzle is tied behind the head.

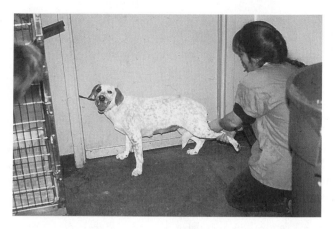

FIG. 17-6   Snubbing a dog to a door. The rope has been run through a crack in the door near the hinges and then the dog is pulled toward the door.

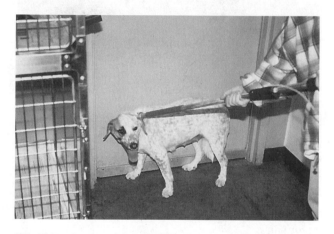

FIG. 17-5   Catch pole applied to a dog.

Catch Pole. Many types of catch poles are available commercially. A catch pole is used to move an aggressive dog to or from a run or cage. The rigid pole separates the restrainer and dog, and a quick-release handle is used to prevent strangulation (Fig. 17-5).

Snubbing. This method prevents an aggressive dog from getting too close to the restrainer. In one variation, one end of the leash is run through an eyebolt anchored in a wall. The leash is then pulled, snugly forcing the dog's lead up to the eyebolt. In another variation, one end of the leash is run through the crack of a door near the hinges. The leash is then pulled so the restrainer is on one side of the door and the dog on the other. This technique is used for vaccinating or injecting dogs that cannot be restrained by other means (Fig. 17-6).

RESTRAINT AND HANDLING OF CATS
Feline Behavior

Before restraining a cat for a procedure, it is best to become friendly with it. Relax the cat by removing fearful stimuli. If you take the time to establish a good relationship, the cat is less likely to resent restraint.

A very important concept to understand in restraint of cats is that *minimal restraint is always desirable*. If the cat begins to struggle and vigorously resist physical restraint, release it and consider use of chemical restraint after it has calmed. Rough handling, extreme physical restraint, and a hot temper are counterproductive and have no place in restraint of cats. If you are uncomfortable working with cats, consider asking another person, of appropriate temperament, to help restrain the animal.

Minimal Restraint Techniques

Nonmanipulative Physical Restraint. For a routine physical examination, quietly pet and stroke a cat from head to tail repeatedly while gently keeping it in place with your hands. This works well with most cats.

Rubber Band around the Base of the Ears. Some cats can be restrained by placing a medium-sized rubber band around the base of the ears (see Fig. 17-12). This technique is useful for clipping nails, bandaging, measuring the rectal temperature, rapid physical examination, or flushing drains.

Fetal Hold or "Scruffing." This technique is useful for giving intramuscular injections to fractious cats. As the cat sits, grasp as much of the skin on the nape of the neck as possible. When this hold is applied properly, a reflex causes the cat's tail to curl ventrally toward its abdomen and the legs tend to be relaxed.

Small cats held in this position can be lifted with one hand. If the cat is large, its body can be supported against the arm that is holding it or with the other hand placed under its hindquarters.

Intermediate Restraint Techniques

Lateral Recumbency. Cats can be restrained in lateral recumbency for many procedures, including intravenous injection, ear examination, and radiography. Place the cat on its left or right side, and place one arm across the cat's neck and gently hold the forelegs. With the other hand, gently hold the cat's hind legs.

Stretching. This method combines "scruffing" and lateral recumbency. With the cat in lateral recumbency, grasp the scruff with one hand and extend somewhat the head and neck. The other hand is free to occlude the femoral vein or hold the hind legs and tail (Fig. 17-7).

Sternal Recumbency. This technique is useful for blood collection, nail trimming, radiography, and oral examination. With the cat resting on its sternum, cradle the cat's body between your arms or grasp the scruff. The forelegs can be restrained for blood collection (Fig. 17-8).

Dorsal Recumbency. This technique is used for blood collection from the jugular vein, radiography, and cystocentesis. It sometimes requires two persons. Place the cat on its back. Stretch the forelegs cranially and the back legs caudally, exposing the thorax and abdomen.

Wrapping. Cats can be restrained by wrapping them in a large terrycloth towel or small blanket. Typically, the forelegs are extended caudally and the head is left protruding. The legs can be withdrawn as necessary (Fig. 17-9). This is a good technique for fractious cats for quick procedures, such as vaccination or venipuncture.

Cat Bag. Cats can be restrained in commercially made cat bags. These cloth or canvas bags have zippered or Velcro closures, with holes in various areas for limb exposure. They serve the same purpose as wrapping and are available in a variety of sizes.

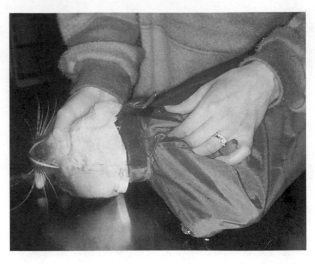

FIG. 17-8   Cat restrained in sternal recumbency for jugular venipuncture. *(Courtesy of Cathy Winters, LVT.)*

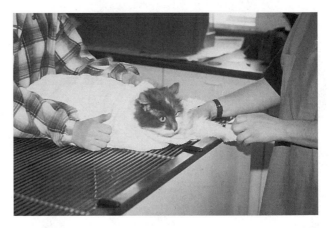

FIG. 17-9   Cat wrapped in a towel, with the head and one foreleg protruding.

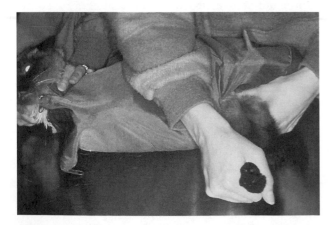

FIG. 17-7   Cat restrained in lateral recumbency for femoral venipuncture. *(Courtesy of Cathy Winters, LVT.)*

RESTRAINT AND HANDLING OF SMALL MAMMALS

If small mammals (rabbits, gerbils, guinea pigs, rats, mice) are restrained correctly, the chances of your being bitten are minimal. Many of these "pocket pets" are frequently played with by children and do not resent being handled. If, however, the restrainer is fearful and mishandles the animal, it may become fearful as well. The first impulse of a frightened small animal is to flee. If it is being held, however, it is likely to bite if it is alarmed and unable to escape.

Gerbils

Gerbils are friendly, curious rodents that are not prone to biting, although that is their best defense. They can also scurry quite quickly if loose on the floor.

Restraint. A gerbil's tail can be grasped at the base (*not* at the end) and the animal can be lifted and placed on the examination table. Be aware that gerbils' tail skin is easily pulled off of the caudal vertebrae, so this method should be used sparingly and carefully. Very tame or sick gerbils can be scooped up with two hands. Once on the examination table, the gerbil can be held in the scruffing position for examination.

Guinea Pigs

Guinea pigs are one of the easiest animals to restrain, because they rarely bite, do not move as quickly as smaller rodents, and tend to remain very still when frightened.

Restraint. Grasp the guinea pig under its forelegs or around the chest and set it on its tailless rear (Fig. 17-10). They can be hand-held near your body for examination or wrapped in a towel. Guinea pigs *cannot* be "scruffed," because they have almost no loose skin on their neck. Scruffing can be very painful for a guinea pig.

Hamsters, Mice, and Rats

Hamsters are tailless, nocturnal rodents that tend to be grumpy when handled in the daylight hours. Hamsters can be scooped up and held in the hand, and they can be "scruffed" by the nape of the neck.

Mice can be handled and restrained like gerbils. They can be carefully picked up by the tail base but may be able to twist around and bite. Other methods for picking up mice are scooping with the hands or wrapping in a soft cloth. Once on the examination table, they can be gently pressed to the table. Mice can also be held by the scruff.

Rats kept as pets can be held in the hand. Rats enjoy attention and generally do not require much more restraint than distraction and simple holding. Place your hand over the rat with your thumb under the rat's chin and forefinger encircling the rat's neck. Rats can also be grasped by the tail base for a short time, but their bodies should also be supported.

Rabbits

Rabbits can be difficult to restrain; they tend to be nervous and fragile. Rabbits have been known to struggle and kick violently, breaking their own spine. Although rabbits rarely bite, they do have long nails that can inflict painful scratches. When very frightened, rabbits emit high-pitched screams.

Picking Up a Rabbit. Do not use the ears or scruff to lift a rabbit. Using the scruff for handling damages the subcutaneous tissues; this is painful and devalues the animal. Place one hand around the rabbit's chest and

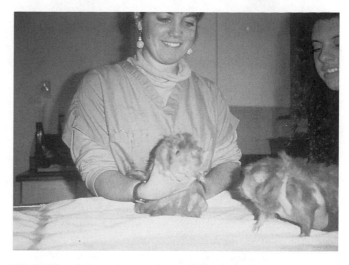

FIG. 17-10 Guinea pigs can be cradled in your hands while you support their bodies.

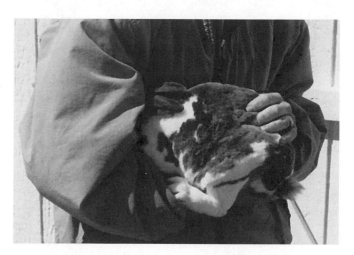

FIG. 17-11 A rabbit can be safely carried by tucking its head into the crook of your elbow while supporting its body along your forearm.

support the hindquarters with the other hand. Face the rabbit away from your body to prevent scratching.

Head Tuck. An easy way to carry a rabbit is by carrying it backward, with its head tucked under your arm (Fig. 17-11).

Sternal Recumbency. Rabbits can be restrained in sternal recumbency for most procedures. Place the rabbit on the examination table, preferably giving the rabbit good footing. Place an arm on either side of the rabbit to restrain it.

Wrapping. Like guinea pigs, rabbits can be wrapped up in towels for simple restraint. When using this method, do not allow the rabbit to overheat.

Set Up with Limb Restraint. Rabbits that do not struggle can be set on their hindquarters, with their backs supported against the restrainer. The limbs can be restrained two in each hand.

Ferrets

The only defense of the ferret is to escape or bite. Ferrets may "hiss" as a warning sign, but they usually do not bite unless distressed. When they do bite, however, they may not let go. If a ferret should bite and remain attached, put the ferret under running water. This is the best way to release a ferret's grip. Ferrets can easily become hyperthermic. Panting is an indication of over-heating; these animals must be quickly cooled.

Picking Up a Ferret. Never pick up ferrets by the tail or neck. Use two hands to pick up a ferret. One hand should firmly grasp the ferret behind the front legs. The other hand should support the animal's hindquarters. As the ferret is picked up, move slowly and turn it to face you. Always talk to the ferret to reassure it.

Distraction. This is a good restraint method for short, nonpainful procedures, such as nail trimming, simple examination, vaccination, auscultation, or mea-suring the rectal temperature. One method of distrac-tion is to place a dab of liquid treat on the ferret's stom-ach. The ferret will be engrossed in cleaning it off. You can also keep the ferret in place on the examination table with your hands, stroking and petting it.

Scruffing. Scruffing can be applied for restraint dur-ing procedures that require no movement, such as radi-ography or cystocentesis. As with cats, grasp the loose skin around the shoulders and neck. Completely sup-port the hindquarters with your other hand. The ani-mal's mouth will open and the face takes on a grimace. This method is recommended for dental examinations but not for oral drug administration, because the ferret cannot swallow when held by the scruff.

Wrapping. Towels can be used to wrap a ferret for short procedures. If the ferret struggles and begins to pant, this indicates overheating. If this occurs, quickly unwrap the animal.

RESTRAINT AND HANDLING OF BIRDS

Birds can be a challenge to restrain; the larger parrots may be the most difficult. Restraint of tiny, fragile song-birds and finches requires very careful planning and execution as well.

Restraint of Psittacines

The main defense of birds is flight and biting. The larg-er parrots can inflict injury to hands with their claws and by biting. Before applying restraint, carefully check to be sure that all potential escape routes are closed.

If possible, have the bird's owner remove it from the cage, because many birds are territorial and may be more tolerant of the owner than a stranger. Also, because many birds are possessive, do not attempt to remove a bird from an owner's arm or shoulder. Have the owner place the bird on the floor. When the bird is on the floor, it feels vulnerable and is more agreeable to being picked up. Do not use your hands to capture birds.

Dowel. If the owner does not remove the bird from its cage, gently place a wooden dowel (rod or perch) against the bird's legs. The bird typically hops onto the dowel, which can then be withdrawn from the cage.

Towel. Procedures can be performed on a large bird if it is wrapped in a towel. These procedures include examining the bird, collecting blood, trimming the nails and beak, and clipping wing feathers. With the bird on the floor, spread the towel like a curtain and drop it over the bird. Locate the head by feeling through the towel. Grasp the bird behind the head, placing one fin-ger beneath the beak. Be careful not to twist the neck or occlude breathing by compressing the trachea or tho-rax. Place the other hand around wings and tail, avoid-ing the thorax. This allows the sternum to move freely (Fig. 17-12). The towel can be totally or partially removed to perform medical procedures.

Gloves. Use of heavy gloves to restrain large psitta-cines is not recommended. Gloves cause fear, can spread disease, and are too thick to allow a sensitive touch. Birds held in gloved hands could be unintentionally crushed.

Restraining Small Songbirds

Songbirds have delicate legs and wings. Most are unac-customed to being handled and are best caught in a semi-illuminated room. A soft cloth can be used to seize the bird in the cage. If the bird escapes, a net with a long handle works best for capture. Avoid stressful stimuli, such as barking dogs, loud music, and hurried activity, if possible.

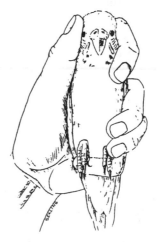

FIG. 17-12 When restraining small or medium-sized birds, posi-tion the fingers so as not to compress the thorax or trachea. (*From Sonsthagen:* Restraint of domestic animals, *St Louis, 1991, Mosby.*)

Small birds can be held in one hand for examination. The restrainer must always be careful not to compress the thorax. Some procedures, such as nail trimming and jugular venipuncture, can be done with one person holding the bird.

RESTRAINT AND HANDLING OF HORSES
Equine Behavior

Horses naturally live in groups and develop strong social relationships. If separated from its herdmates, a horse can become nervous, agitated, distracted, and uncooperative. The horse uses numerous vocal sounds and a variety of body language to communicate with offspring, to indicate social position in the herd, and to signal fear and nervousness. Horses have well-developed senses to detect possible threats.

Horses have keen binocular, stereoscopic vision. Their eyes are situated on the sides of their heads (as in most prey animals) to see in two directions at once. Although this is very advantageous for horses, it also makes them shy from objects located directly in front of them, in their "blind spot." A horse cannot see directly in front of its head nor directly behind it. The horse's depth perception is also very poor. Horses cannot distinguish between a shadow on the ground and a deep hole.

Horses have excellent hearing and can recognize each other's calls from great distances. By watching a horse's ears, you can locate the origin of sounds. Although most domestic horses are accustomed to certain amounts of noise, sudden loud sounds can startle a horse into flight.

The sense of touch is well developed in the horse. Horses are very sensitive on the body surface, especially under the belly and in the flank area.

If a horse cannot run away from a threatening situation, it will resort to jumping, then kicking, bucking, rearing, and biting. Although unprovoked aggression is rare in horses, defensive biting and kicking are relatively common.

Body Language. A horse's temperament and intentions are often signaled by its "body language."

- *Ears:* Pinned-back ears indicate aggression or threat. Forward-pointing ears indicate listening or attentiveness. One ear pointed forward and the other pointed backward indicate listening in two directions.
- *Mouth:* An open mouth with teeth exposed may signal attack. Lifting of the upper lip to expose the gums, with teeth together, is the *Flehmen response,* a type of sexual behavior in males.
- *Head:* A lowered head and pinned-back ears are threatening gestures, as in a mare protecting its foal. An elevated head with eyes widely opened signals fright.
- *Feet:* Pawing at the ground indicates impatience. Lifting of a rear foot with slight kicking indicates a possible defensive kick. Elevation of both front feet off of the ground signals the intent to rear defensively.
- *Tail:* Tucking of the tail tight against the hindquarters signals fear. Swishing of the tail back and forth signals agitation.

Initial Restraint Methods

To restrain a horse, the handler must first demonstrate dominance. Fortunately, horses are easily dominated. This is demonstrated by the fact that small children can safely ride 1000-lb horses. The horse must be convinced that it is not being threatened.

Approaching the Horse. It can be dangerous to approach a horse from the rear. When approaching a horse in a stall, it is best to persuade the horse to turn until its head is facing the handler. Although most horses are accustomed to being approached from the left (near) side, horses that are handled frequently can be approached from either side.

Catching the Horse. If the horse is standing quietly, place an arm or the lead rope over the neck. This signals capture and typically results in immediate submission. Place the halter over the bridge of the nose and buckle it on the left side. The halter should not fit too snugly. Two fingers should easily slip under the nose band.

Leading the Horse. Never wrap the lead rope around a hand. This is extremely dangerous because of the possibility of injury if the horse bolts. Even seasoned horse handlers should keep this in mind.

Lead the horse from the left side. Gather the lead rope in the left hand. Use the right hand to hold the lead rope 6 to 9 inches from the snap on the halter. If the horse tries to pull ahead, take the tail of the lead rope and twirl it in front of the horse's nose. If it touches the horse several times, it is likely to settle down. If the horse refuses to be led, turn its head toward the rear. This forces the horse to move its front feet. Keep turning the horse off of its forequarters until it submits to the lead.

Tying the Horse. Because horses tend to frighten easily, never tie them to anything that could be torn loose and dragged behind them. Always tie the lead rope with a quick-release knot. A horse should be tied with its head in a comfortable position. Depending on the horse's height, tie the head at least 3½ feet above the ground, with approximately 2½ feet of slack in the lead rope. There should not be enough slack to allow the horse to put its foot over the rope and become entangled.

Halter Tie. Tie the lead rope with a quick-release knot. The knot must release immediately when you pull on the free end of the lead rope. The proper type of lead rope is also important. Heavy braided cotton rope is best.

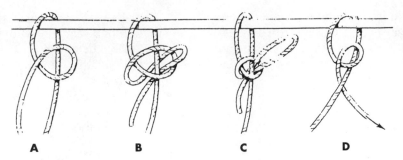

FIG. 17-13 Tying a quick-release knot. **A,** The free end of the rope is run behind the post and a loop is formed in the free end and is brought up over the long end of the rope. **B,** The free end is pushed up through the loop. **C,** The free end of the rope is pulled up through the loop. **D,** The long end of the rope is pulled to complete the knot. The knot can be released quickly by pulling on the free end of the rope. *(From Sonsthagen: Restraint of domestic animals, St Louis, 1991, Mosby.)*

Using a stout post or another appropriate hitching post, place the free end of the rope behind the post. Bring the free end around and make a loop over the long end (the part attached to the horse) (Fig. 17-13, *A*). Make another loop with the free end. From underneath, push this loop up and through the first loop (Fig. 17-13, *B* and *C*). This traps the long end of the rope and forms a slip knot. Test the knot by pulling the free end of the rope (Fig. 17-13, *D*). The knot should release easily.

Distraction Techniques. Minimal restraint can be used for short procedures to divert the horse's attention. Distraction techniques are most useful for suture removal, injections, radiography, and oral administration of paste dewormers.

A horse can be restrained somewhat by holding up one of its legs in a flexed position. Usually the restrainer stands on the same side as the person performing the procedure. The horse should not be tied. A front foot is the most convenient to use, because the restrainer is usually holding the lead rope as well. Facing the horse's rear, pick up a front foot and hold the foreleg in a flexed position. If the horse begins to resist, flex the foreleg a bit more.

Skin Twitch. The skin twitch is another method of minimal restraint. The horse's sensitivity to touch is used to distract its attention away from other procedures. The restrainer usually stands on the same side as the person performing the procedure. Grasp a handful of loose skin on the lateral aspect of the neck or shoulder. Roll the skin under and pull it taut. Some people use two hands when applying this method. After release, scratch and pet the area.

Ear Hold. A horse's ears should never be used for restraint, because it causes pain and causes the horse to become head shy.

Restraining Foals. Foals can be restrained by placing one arm in front of the foal's chest and the other behind the foal's hindquarters. The foal can also be backed into the corner of a stall and gently held in position with an arm placed in front of the chest. Foals are sometimes held by the base of the tail and around the neck, with a hand gently grasping an ear. The ear is pulled down but never twisted or abused. This is an advanced technique and must be done very carefully so as not to adversely affect future handling.

Blindfolding. Horses often become docile when blindfolded with a soft towel, jacket, or other large piece of clean cloth. Halter the horse; do not tie it. Standing on the same side as the person performing the procedure, slip the cloth underneath the halter and over the eyes, and secure it. Make sure the horse cannot see around the blindfold.

Intermediate Restraint Techniques

The following techniques are useful for procedures of longer duration or causing some pain. They are most useful for such procedures as floating teeth, eye treatments, cleaning superficial wounds, changing bandages, and nasogastric intubation.

Stocks. Horse stocks are the ideal piece of equipment for most procedures requiring the horse to stand still for some time. Stocks protect the people treating the horse and protect the horse from injury. Walk the horse into the stocks and close the head and tail gates. Adjust any parts, such as side rails, as necessary to accommodate the horse. Tie the horse's head with a halter tie quick-release knot.

Leg Hobble. A hobble strap can be applied to a front leg to provide restraint (Fig. 17-14). Use this technique in an area where the ground is soft and there is no danger of injury to the horse's knee (carpus), should it fall while struggling. Untie the horse. Pick up the front leg and flex the carpal joint. Slip the leg hobble around the flexed leg and buckle securely. Back away, because the horse may struggle for a moment.

Chain Shank Under the Chin. Horses can be restrained by running a chain shank through the halter,

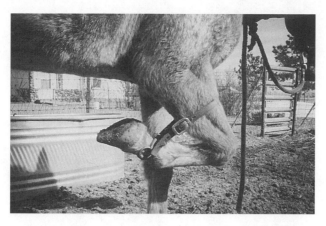

FIG. 17-14 Hobble strap applied to the front leg of a horse.

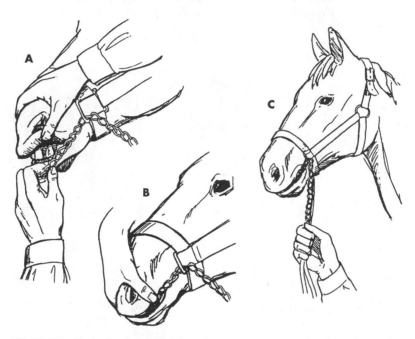

FIG. 17-15 Chain shank applied over the upper gums. **A,** The chain shank is moved between the upper lip and the upper front teeth. **B,** The slack is taken up in the shank. **C,** Both the shank and the lead are grasped in the same hand. *(From Sonsthagen: Restraint of domestic animals, St Louis, 1991, Mosby.)*

beneath the horse's chin. A halter is applied and a chain shank is run from one side ring of the halter and under the horse's chin, and connected to the other side ring. As the horse jerks or rears, the chain tightens against the mandible, causing discomfort. If the chain tightens during struggling, it should be immediately released.

Chain Shank Against the Gingivae. A more severe form of restraint involves use of a chain shank to apply pressure on the upper gums. The chain shank is run from one side ring of the halter, under the upper lip and over the upper gums, and connected to the other side ring (Fig. 17-15). As with the chain shank under the chin, struggling causes discomfort. The tightened chin shank should be quickly loosened as needed.

Lip Twitch. A lip twitch is a mechanical device attached to a horse's upper lip for restraint. When applying a lip twitch, do not stand in front of the horse; stand to one side. Grasp as much of the horse's upper lip as possible, place the clamp twitch around the bunched lip, and close the clamps on the lip (Fig. 17-16). If the twitch has been applied properly, the horse should begin to look drowsy. The procedure can be performed at this point. After the clamp twitch has been released, gently massage the lip.

Tail Tie. By tying the tail up, the horse cannot swish it or tuck it under. Procedures such as rectal palpation, Caslick's surgery, and artificial insemination can be performed on the hindquarters. Grasp the tail in one hand and lay the loose end of a heavy braided cotton rope

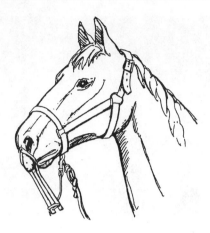

FIG. 17-16   Humane (clamp) twitch applied to a horse's upper lip. *(From Sonsthagen: Restraint of domestic animals, St Louis, 1991, Mosby.)*

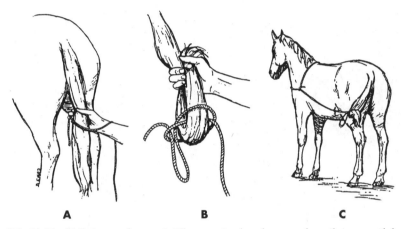

A   **B**   **C**

FIG. 17-17   Tail tie on a horse. **A,** The rope is placed across the tail, just caudal to the least coccygeal vertebra. **B,** Position of the rope in forming a tail tie. **C,** The long end of the rope can be tied around the horse's neck. *(From Sonsthagen: Restraint of domestic animals, St Louis, 1991, Mosby.)*

across the tail hairs, just distal to the last coccygeal vertebra (Fig. 17-17). Fold the rope over the horse's tail, then flip the tail hairs up and over the rope. Wrap the rope around the tail hairs twice. Finish with a quick-release half hitch (like tying a shoe with just one loop).

RESTRAINT AND HANDLING OF CATTLE
Bovine Behavior

Rough or inappropriate handling of cattle can reduce conception rates, the immune response, and rumen function. Understanding cattle behavior will help you predict how they are likely to respond to handling. In addition, understanding bovine behavior can facilitate handling, reduce stress on the animal, and improve handler safety and animal welfare.

Cattle have wide-angle vision that can be used to the handler's advantage in finding their defensive zone. Always stay caudal to the shoulder of cattle, whether standing or approaching to move an animal or herd.

Cattle also have a natural tendency to move in a circle. As prey animals, cattle are easily frightened and have sensitive hearing. Keep noise and introduction of strange objects to a minimum when working with cattle. Solid walls in alleyways and chutes are the ideal when cattle are to be moved.

Cattle should not be shouted at, whipped, or beaten, because it is cruel and this will adversely affect their response to handling in the future. Herdsmen who understand cattle behavior will not tolerate ill treatment of their animals.

Restraint

Squeeze Chute.   The ideal cattle restraint device is the squeeze chute. Nearly all medical procedures can be facilitated by use of a properly constructed chute. A

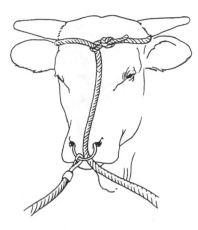

FIG. 17-18 Applying a tail jack to a cow in a stanchion. *(From Sonsthagen: Restraint of domestic animals, St Louis, 1991, Mosby.)*

chute usually has three mechanical working parts: the head catch, the tail gate, and the squeeze. An animal is run into a chute by means of an alley, preferably of solid panel construction.

Once the cow is in the chute, the proper adjustments are made with the head catch to secure the head. Close the head catch tight enough so that the animal cannot put a foot through, but not so tight as to clamp the cow's neck. Adjust the squeeze snugly, but not too tightly against the cow's sides. Cows remain more calm if they feel they are confined in this way. Closing the tail gate prevents other cattle from entering the chute.

Cattle Halter. Once the cow is in the chute, a cattle halter can be applied and the cow's head tied to the side of the chute. Such restraint allows jugular venipuncture, jugular injection, ear tag placement, oral drenching, or use of a balling gun.

Tail Jacking. Cattle can be encouraged to move forward in a chute by grasping the tail at the base and elevating it vertically (Fig. 17-18).

Nose Tongs. Nose tongs are outdated pieces of equipment that inflict unnecessary pain and can damage the nasal septum. These pincer-like instruments should not be used to lead or restrain cattle.

Electric Prod. Battery-powered prods are sometimes used to deliver a shock to the hindquarters. These instruments should be used sparingly and only by experienced people.

RESTRAINT AND HANDLING OF GOATS
Caprine Behavior

Goats are gregarious, ruminant animals. Although they are herd animals, they do not move together as easily as sheep. Also, goats become very vocal when separated

from herdmates. It is usually easier for all involved if a companion goat is kept near the patient during a procedure. Goats that are used to being handled are docile and enjoy attention and petting.

Goats cannot be treated like sheep or controlled by force. They are much more agile and resistant to restraint. Although goats can withstand more stress than sheep, rough handling is unnecessary. Goats also tolerate heat fairly well. Goats become agitated and tend to struggle against restraint after a certain point. When handling goats, it is best to keep untrained dogs away, because goats make a game of attacking a dog. Although goats do not bite or kick, they do rear and charge humans and dogs, especially rams and does defending kids. Goats are also excellent at escape by climbing and jumping.

Restraint

When you work with a herd of goats, the ideal restraint is to use a small pen, with access to a high, solid-paneled race or run. Chutes and tables are not used with goats.

Catching and Holding. Untamed goats must be cornered in a pen using 5-foot-wide wooden panels or gates. Once confined, individual goats can be caught by placing an arm around its neck or grabbing its collar. Some goats that are handled frequently can be held by placing one arm around the front of the goat's chest and one hand on the dock of the tail.

Halter. A goat halter can be used on some goats. Goats that are milked or shown can usually be led easily. A goat will stand quietly for short periods if tied securely to an object using a collar or halter and lead. These techniques can be used for such procedures as hoof trimming, vaccination, and blood collection.

Stanchion. Dairy goats that are accustomed to the stanchion can easily be restrained for most procedures in this manner. Grain can be fed as a distraction.

RESTRAINT AND HANDLING OF SHEEP
Ovine Behavior

Sheep are herd animals that prefer to move in a flock. Because sheep do not like to be separated from herdmates, it is easier to work with a flock of sheep rather than with individuals. Sheep are generally not calmed with a soothing voice, nor do they enjoy being petted. When handling sheep, it is best to keep noise to a minimum and keep untrained dogs away.

Sheep become hyperthermic (overheated) very easily because of their wool and normally high body temperature (103° F). Use caution when working with sheep in ambient temperatures above 60° F.

Sheep have a frail skeletal system and their necks can be injured easily if they are chased into fences. Their

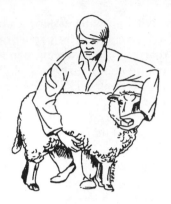

FIG. 17-19   Correct placement of the hands in preparation for setting a sheep up on its rump. *(From Sonsthagen:* Restraint of domestic animals, *St Louis, 1991, Mosby.)*

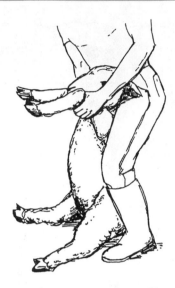

FIG. 17-20   Setting a sheep up on its rump. *(From Sonsthagen:* Restraint of domestic animals, *St Louis, 1991, Mosby.)*

back and legs can be broken by rough handling. Wool is easily pulled out and sheep's skin tears easily; this causes bruising and blemished pelts. Therefore, never grab sheep by the wool; it is painful and devalues the carcass and pelt.

Although uncommon, at times a ram or wether may charge and butt a person. Ewes protecting lambs and other adult sheep sometimes charge dogs. Usually sheep that are behaving defensively face the assumed "predator" and stamp their feet. Sheep can bound over obstacles or people when feeling threatened.

Restraint

When you work with a sheep flock, the ideal restraint is to use a race or run. The sheep are driven to a catch gate with a sheep squeeze chute.

Catching and Holding. Sheep are cornered in a pen using 4-foot-wide wooden panels or gates. Confine the sheep to a small area with the panel or gently force the sheep against a fence with your knees. Single out the sheep that is needed. Place one hand on the tail base and the other under the jaw. Sheep can also be caught by crowding them in a small pen and using a shepherd's crook to catch a sheep by the hock.

Halter. A sheep halter can be applied after a sheep is caught. Take care not to occlude the nostrils with the nose band. Some show sheep can be led by a halter, whereas others must be coaxed and pushed from behind.

Setting Up. Sheep are often set on their hindquarters for shearing and other procedures, such as hoof trimming, if a sheep restraint table is not available. The restrainer stands with his or her legs against the sheep's side and flank. The sheep's head is pulled laterally and then back to its shoulder (Fig. 17-19). After a few moments, the sheep will begin to slowly sag. At this point, the restrainer uses his or her knee as a pivot point to set the sheep on its rump (Fig. 17-20).

Sheepdogs. A well-trained sheepdog is a valuable asset in moving sheep and isolating individual sheep. All other dogs should be kept away from sheep.

RESTRAINT AND HANDLING OF PIGS
Porcine Behavior

Pigs are not herd animals but they tend to follow other pigs. When one pig becomes distressed and screams, the others may react as a group and panic. Pigs have a good memory, remembering how humans have treated them in the past.

Pigs can become hyperthermic if chased or roughly handled in hot weather. Overheated pigs must be cooled immediately or they are likely to die of heat stroke.

The main defensive weapon of pigs is their teeth. They can tear flesh easily and have very strong jaws. Young pigs that see humans frequently are easier to handle, but the tusks of boars can be very dangerous. Also, sows with young should be approached with caution. Enter all adult swine enclosures with caution and be prepared to exit quickly.

Exerting dominance over pigs may be a good idea before handling. Pigs dominate one another by biting on the dorsal aspect of the neck. Handlers can demonstrate dominance by pressing on the pig's neck with a board, cane, or pole.

Restraint

Driving and Catching. Pigs can be difficult to drive. Solid-paneled chutes work well to move pigs, because they cannot see outside distractions. Pigs stop when confronted with a barrier. Pigs can be driven or caught in a small area with panels at least as high as the pig's shoulder. Pigs can easily be moved with a solid panel, but they can thrust their nose under the panel and knock a person down.

Directing a Single Pig. When moving a single pig, place a bucket or blindfold over the pig's head. Pigs respond to this by moving backward. By continuing to hold the bucket over the pig's head, the pig can be directed backward to the chosen area. A cane or stick can also be used to direct pigs by tapping it on the flank and shoulder. A rope harness can be made for small pigs. Place a loop over the pig's head and tighten it gently. Form a half hitch, and put this over the animal's head. Let the pig walk through the loop until the loop is caudal to the shoulders and tighten the loop.

Hog Snare. A hog snare is sometimes used for restraining a large pig. The snare is usually a metal pipe with a cable loop on one end. The free end of the cable runs through the hollow pipe, so the size of the loop can be controlled. Manipulate the loop over the snout. When the cable is caudal to the tusks, carefully tighten the loop over the snout. Excessive tightening can injure the pig. A rope can be used in place of the pipe and cable snare.

Restraining Piglets. Baby pigs weighing less than 30 lb are restrained by holding them upside down by the hind legs or placing them in a V-trough for such procedures as castration and cutting teeth.

Restraining Potbellied Pigs. Potbellied pigs are usually kept as pets and have a docile temperament; however, some potbellied pigs may show aggression. Small pet pigs tend to squirm, jump, and climb on whomever is trying to restrain them. They can squeal as loud as a full-sized pig. Chemical restraint is sometimes the best choice.

RECOMMENDED READING

Fowler F: *Restraint and handling of domestic and wild animals,* ed 2, Ames, Iowa, 1995, Iowa State University Press.

Grandin T: *Livestock handling and transport,* Wallingford, UK, 1993, CAB International.

Houpt KA: *Domestic animal behavior for veterinarians and animal scientists,* ed 2, Ames, Iowa, 1991, Iowa State University Press.

O'Farrell V: *Manual of canine behavior,* ed 2, 1992, Shuadington, UK, British Small Animal Veterinary Association.

O'Farrell V: *Manual of feline behavior,* 1994, Shuadington, UK, British Small Animal Veterinary Association.

CHAPTER 18

Patient History and Physical Examination

A.M. Rivera
P.J. Gaveras

Learning Objectives

After reviewing this chapter, the reader should understand the following:

Importance of clear communication with the client
Components of the patient's history

Appropriate ways to elicit information from the client
Approaches used for physical examination
Components of a physical examination
Ways to assess patients in emergency situations

A patient's history and physical examination are the foundations upon which sound medical and nursing interventions are based. Animal patients cannot verbally communicate the ailments or discomforts caused by disease. Therefore, pay meticulous attention to the observations and concerns voiced by the animal owner, who provides information from which you may formulate the patient's history. Astute observation from both the veterinarian and the nursing staff is crucial when performing the physical examination.

The variety of patients and idiosyncrasies of species mandate that the veterinary team address the areas of both history and physical examination. Paying close attention to details allows the team to notice subtleties that otherwise might be missed. Technicians who can perform a thorough physical evaluation can use these skills to assess and monitor hospitalized patients.

In the emergency setting, the concepts of *triage* and *primary* and *secondary survey* (discussed later in this chapter) are used when addressing life-threatening conditions.

TECHNICIAN-CLIENT INTERACTION
Communicating with Clients

Communication is the key to a successful interview and productive physical examination. The interviewer must be able to ask questions that are easily understood and are geared to the medical sophistication of the animal owner. If necessary, slang words describing certain conditions may be used to facilitate communications and avoid misunderstanding.[28,40]

The interview is most successfully conducted when the technician is professional but cheerful, friendly, and genuinely concerned about the patient (Fig. 18-1). A dry, inquisitional approach, consisting of rapid-fire questions, is typically less effective in unearthing important details of the history. A key technique employed in obtaining a history is to *allow animal owners to express the information in their own words.*[40]

The ability to listen without interrupting the client requires patience, competence, and practice. Many owners disclose their animal's problems spontaneously. Often,

311

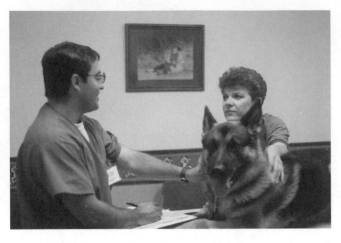

FIG. 18-1 The interview should be conducted in a professional yet friendly manner, while displaying genuine concern for the animal and client. The appearance, attire, and attitude of the veterinary staff set the tone of the visit and convey an impression of the quality of veterinary services being rendered.

an interview will fail to reveal all the clues because the interviewer did not listen closely to the owner.[21,28,40]

The best clinical interview focuses on the *patient*, not the technician's agenda. When speaking with the owner, determine not only the primary medical problem (presenting or chief complaint) but also how the animal is manifesting the illness. An important interviewing technique employs *reflective listening* methods that incorporate active listening, infrequent interruption, limited speaking, and asking for clarification when needed. Interrupting an animal owner may disrupt his or her train of thought and prevent the owner from reporting important facts.[28,40]

Allow the owners to control the interview, at least in part. Once they have reported the facts, repeat important information to them, indicating that you have heard them and understand their concern. If the history given is vague, use direct questioning. Asking "how," "where," and "when" is generally more effective than asking "why."[29,40]

The technician's appearance influences the success of the interview. Neatness counts.[40] An untidy interviewer wearing a soiled smock will be viewed as unprofessional, careless, or incompetent by the animal owner. Some owners may view a sloppy appearance as a sign of uncaring, and as such will taint their expectations and impressions of the entire veterinary team.

The *rule of five vowels* is useful in conducting an interview. This rule states that a good interview contains elements of Audition, Evaluation, Inquiry, Observation, and Understanding. *Audition* means listening carefully to the animal owner's story. *Evaluation* refers to the sorting of data to determine which is important and which is irrelevant. With *inquiry*, the interviewer probes into the

significant areas requiring more clarification. *Observation* refers to the importance of nonverbal communication, body language, and facial expressions, regardless of what is said. *Understanding* the owner's concerns and apprehensions enables the interviewer to play a more emphatic role.[40]

The physical setting of an interview can enhance or hinder it. Ideally, the interview should take place in a quiet, properly lighted room or with lighting adjusted to produce optimal illumination, although this is not always possible in field situations. Make the owner feel as comfortable as possible. If feasible, you and the owner should be seated on an even level, allowing for direct eye contact. Maintain a distance of 3 to 4 feet between yourself and the owner. Distances greater than 5 feet are impersonal, whereas distances less than 3 feet intrude on the owner's "comfort zone."[40] Sit in a relaxed position and avoid crossing your arms across your chest, because this body language projects an attitude of superiority and may interfere with communication. A key to successful history taking is to *put the owner at ease.*

Obtaining a thorough history by a medical interview depends upon the technical knowledge and communication skills of the interviewer. The interview should be flexible and spontaneous, not interrogative. The major goal of the interview is to sort through the reported signs associated with the illness to better understand the pathophysiology of the disease in question. Although the novice may have limited knowledge of the signs associated with various diseases, with experience and education, one can learn to recognize the history and signs as they relate to various injuries and illnesses.

Obtaining a History

The information gathered when obtaining the history should alert the veterinary team to potential problems and direct the technician's attention to certain of the patient's body areas during the examination.[27]

Any given disease tends to be characterized by a certain group of signs.[28,39,40] With only one isolated clinical sign, be careful not to jump to conclusions nor to allow premature assumptions or preconceptions to affect your objectivity when making additional assessments.[40]

Obtaining a thorough history from an owner includes an introductory statement, a review or clarification of preliminary data (e.g., patient characteristics, geographic origin, any prior ownership, current environmental conditions, diet, past medical history, and vaccination status), and the history and nature of the presenting complaint.

The Introductory Statement. Review the preliminary data (e.g., animal's name and sex) before introducing yourself to the owner. If the patient is a new animal to the household or farm or a geriatric patient not seen recently, or if the owner is a new client, confirm this and note it in the medical record. Greet the owner by name, make eye contact, shake hands firmly, and smile.[40] Always address the client by an honorific (e.g., Mrs., Mr.) and his or her last name.

For example you might say: "Good morning, Mrs. Schwartz. My name is Joe Smith. I'm a veterinary technician and I'll be obtaining a history and performing a preliminary examination on Buffy. Could you please tell me the reason for Buffy's visit today?" You can then validate the preliminary data if needed and go on to obtain the history for the presenting complaint.

Some technicians prefer to address the presenting complaint first, and then validate or confirm the preliminary data. Regardless of which approach you prefer, develop a consistent routine that is comfortable for you and the client and that obtains the necessary data (Box 18-1).[19,28,29,40]

Patient Characteristics. The receptionist can obtain certain preliminary data, such as patient characteristics (age, breed, sex, reproductive status). The technician should verify that the patient's age, breed, sex, and reproductive status have been correctly recorded and note any changes since the patient's last visit (i.e., has the patient been spayed or castrated).[21,28,29,39]

Pay close attention to the patient's age. Congenital and infectious diseases, parasitism, ingestion of foreign bodies, and intussusceptions are usually predominant in young animals. Degenerative diseases and neoplasia are more common in adult animals.[28,29]

Certain species or breeds are predisposed to particular problems. For example, toy breeds of dogs (e.g., Chihuahuas, Pomeranians) are predisposed to patellar luxation and hydrocephalus. Brachycephalic (short-nosed) dogs are predisposed to respiratory problems. Combined immunodeficiency affects Arabian horses. Any predispositions should be considered when formulating a list of *differential diagnoses* (diagnostic possibilities).[28,29]

The patient's sex and reproductive status are important, because certain conditions are gender specific and determine what areas should be given special attention in patient evaluation.[29] For example, in a 10-year-old intact (not spayed) female dog with a history of excessive water consumption and urination, vomiting, and lethargy, pyometra (uterine infection) would be an important differential diagnosis. In a 5-year-old spayed female with the same history, however, diabetes mellitus would be an important differential diagnosis.[28,29] The incidence of some diseases decreases markedly as a result of ovariohysterectomy (spay) or castration. Dogs spayed at an early age are less likely to develop mammary tumors, and castrated male dogs are at lower risk of developing perianal adenomas.[28]

Geographic Origin and Prior Ownership. Determine where the patient originated (e.g., home raised, breeder, pet shop, animal shelter, neighboring farm, livestock auction), where it has recently traveled, and if it was recently boarded or shown. This information may indicate if the patient has been exposed to infectious or parasitic diseases enzootic to (prevalent in) certain regions but not in the current environment.[19,21,39]

Current Environment. Obtain information about the animal's environment and activities. Is it an indoor or outdoor animal? Is the patient free-roaming or confined to the yard or house? Is it housed in a pasture or in a stable? Free-roaming or pastured animals are at higher risk of being exposed to toxins or trauma. Determine if the patient shares the environment with other animals.[21,29,36] For example, multiple-cat households and catteries have a higher prevalence of infectious respiratory diseases and feline leukemia virus infection.[39]

Diet. Information about the animal's diet can help rule out nutritional disease. When obtaining dietary information, question the owner about the patient's appetite, any gain or loss of weight, type of diet (e.g., dry, moist, table food, total mixed rations, supplements), brand name of food, method of feeding (free choice or individual meals), and amount fed daily.[21,29,36]

Box 18-1 Checklist for physical examination

Introduction to the client
Obtain a history
- ❑ Patient characteristics
- ❑ Geographic origin
- ❑ Current environment
- ❑ Diet
- ❑ Previous medical history and vaccination status
- ❑ Presenting complaint(s)
- ❑ History of chief presenting complaint
- ❑ Conclusion

Physical examination
General observation
Recording vital signs
- ❑ Level of consciousness
- ❑ Respiratory rate and effort
- ❑ Heart rate and rhythm
- ❑ Indications of perfusion

Systematic physical examination (visual inspection, palpation, percussion, auscultation)
- ❑ Examination of the head and neck
- ❑ Examination of the trunk and forelimbs
- ❑ Examination of the thorax
- ❑ Examination of the abdomen
- ❑ Examination of the skin and lymph nodes
- ❑ Examination of the hind limbs
- ❑ Examination of the external genitalia and perineum

Past Medical History. The past medical history provides information about the patient's health before the current illness. Carefully inquire about and record the dates of previous illnesses and treatment, hospitalization, and surgeries, followed by a brief description of each problem, how it was managed, and how the patient responded to treatment. Ask the client to describe any allergies (environmental, ingestible, or drug related) and how these were diagnosed. Note any medications the patient is currently receiving. It is important to determine if the owner is giving the medications as prescribed.[21,29,36]

Vaccination Status. Question the owner about the animal's vaccination status and when any vaccinations were given.[21,29] Some owners are not familiar with vaccination schedules and may simply report that their animal "has been vaccinated." You could easily presume that the patient is up to date on vaccinations, when in fact the vaccinations were given several years previously. Be aware of recommended intervals for vaccinations and diagnostic tests. For example, inquire when the cat was last assessed for exposure to feline leukemia virus and feline immunodeficiency virus. Ask if the dog has been checked for heartworm infection in the past year, and if and what type of preventive is being used.[21,29]

The Presenting Complaint. The *presenting complaint* is the reason the owner has sought veterinary care for the animal. For example, the owner might say a cow has had diarrhea for 3 days, is not eating, and is depressed. It is important to remember that *the presenting complaint is what the owner perceives the patient's problem to be.* Although the owner's fears or anxieties may influence your observations of the animal, pay attention to these owner concerns. Allow the client to communicate these observations, and then continue with the interview. This tends to relieve a client's anxieties about the animal.[28,29,36]

Another important interviewing skill is the ability to assess the source and reliability of the information obtained.[40] A history obtained from second parties presenting the animal for evaluation (friends, neighbors, children) may lack important information that only the owner can provide.

It is also important to determine if the client understands the meaning of any medical terms he or she might use in describing the problem. Ask the owner to define such terms. For example, "What do you mean when you say the cat regurgitated?" An owner might bring in a dog and say that it "just had a stroke." To an experienced veterinary professional, the patient's ataxia, incoordination, head tilt, and horizontal nystagmus might indicate vestibular disease rather than a cerebrovascular accident ("stroke"). It is important to *record the clinical signs observed and not an owner's presumptive diagnosis.* Be aware that the owner's comments, observations, and conclusions are based on his or her experience. We must interpret those comments, observations, and conclusions in light of our professional experience.[28]

Once the presenting complaint is listed, record the information gathered in chronologic order to clarify areas of possible confusion. Separate the owner's observations from his or her conclusions and amplify certain portions of the complaint that may be important.[28,40]

History of presenting complaint. The history of the current complaint helps determine when the animal was last normal, if the condition is acute or chronic, what medications and dosages were used previously, how the patient responded to previous therapy, and the duration and progression of clinical signs.[29,39,40] The history is best recorded by chronology (i.e., in the order in which events occurred). This provides a better understanding of the sequence and development of the problem. Begin with the first sign of illness observed by the owner and follow its progression to the present (see Box 18-1).[40]

It is important to determine when the owner first noticed the presenting complaint, apart from any other health problems. Some patients might have other ongoing health problems (e.g., flea-bite dermatitis, food allergies) unrelated to the current complaint.[40] Ask for specific information that described the signs observed (e.g., color, odor, consistency, and volume of vomitus or diarrhea). When the owner uses such terms as "somewhat," "a little," "sometimes," or "rarely," ask for clarification. Remember, precise communication is important.

Some owners simply cannot remember when the signs first developed. You may be able to help the owner relate the onset of signs to some event.[40] For example, ask, "Was the horse's lameness evident around the Thanksgiving or Christmas holidays?" When obtaining information on the presenting complaint, use open-ended questions that allow the client to describe the problem, rather than simple "yes" or "no" questions. The following example illustrates a series of open-ended questions that elucidate the sequences of events and the nature of the problem:

Why is Buffy being presented? This identifies the presenting complaint.

When did you first notice the problem? This determines the onset of the problem.

What was the first sign that you observed, and what did you notice after that initial sign? This helps establish progression of the problem.

Can you describe in detail the signs you observed? This helps identify clinical signs observed, rather than the owner's diagnosis.

Was there any change in routine or anything new, unusual, or different in Buffy's routine at the time of onset? This helps determine precipitating events.

Has Buffy been treated for this problem before? How did she respond? This determines the response to previous treatment.

Concluding the History. If any part of the history needs further clarification, it should be done after all of the initial information has been gathered. At this point, you may wish to summarize for the owner the most important parts of the history. Encourage the owner to correct any misinterpretations and discuss any additional concerns; allow the owner the final say. At the conclusion of the interview, thank the owner and say that you will now perform a physical examination of the animal.[40]

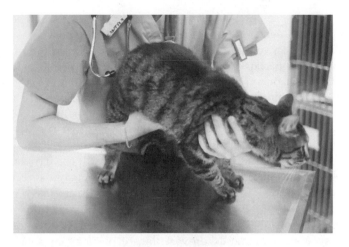

FIG. 18-2 Because of patient size and personal safety, abdominal palpation is used more commonly in small animals than in large animals. In cats and small dogs, one hand can be used to restrain the animal while the other is used for palpation.

PHYSICAL EXAMINATION

The physical examination confirms the information elucidated by the history and assesses the animal's current state of health. The validity and extent of physical examination findings depend on the technician's clinical experience. The four primary techniques employed during physical examination are *inspection, palpation, percussion,* and *auscultation.*[24,28,34,41]

Primary Techniques for Physical Examination

Inspection. Inspection begins with the technician's first contact with the patient and continues throughout the data collection. Early in the physical examination, the technician visually examines the patient's entire body for structure and function, paying close attention to deviations or abnormalities. Inspection is an active process, not a passive one. The technician must know what to look for and where. It should be done in a systematic manner so that nothing is missed.[24,28,29,34,41]

Observe closely the patient's general body condition, behavior, attitude, posture, ambulatory ability, and the respiratory effort and pattern.[21,29] You, the technician, should be able to recognize signs of inflammation, such as swelling, heat, redness, pain, and disturbance of function. Swelling is a result of edema or congestion in local tissues. Heat and redness are the result of increased circulation to the affected area. Pain is often the result of swelling that causes increased pressure on nerves.

Palpation. Palpation involves using the hands and the sense of touch to detect tenderness, altered temperature, texture, vibration, pulsation, masses or swellings, and other changes in body integrity (Fig. 18-2). The sense of touch is most acute using light, intermittent pressure; heavy, prolonged pressure causes loss of sensitivity in the hands of the examiner.[24,34]

One's fingertips are highly sensitive to tactile discrimination. The pads of the fingertips are used to assess turgor (e.g., skin), texture (e.g., hair), position, size, consistency, mobility (e.g., mass or organ), distention (e.g., urinary bladder), pulse rate and quality, tenderness, and pain. Temperature of a skin area is best assessed using the dorsum (back) of a hand or finger. The palm of the hand is more sensitive to vibrations, allowing one to feel such abnormalities as crepitus ("grinding") in a joint.[24,34]

Palpation can be classified as light or deep. *Light palpation* of structures such as the abdomen is performed primarily to detect areas of tenderness. *Deep palpation* is used to assess underlying organs (e.g., liver), while giving careful consideration to the discomfort the procedure may cause the patient.[9,29]

Terms used to describe structures palpated include *doughy* (soft, malleable), *firm* (normal texture of organs), *hard* (bone-like consistency), *fluctuant* (soft, elastic, and undulant, as with a cyst or abscess), and *emphysematous* (air or gas in tissue planes).[29]

Percussion. Percussion is tapping of the body's surface to produce vibration and sound. The sound reflects the density of underlying tissue and size and position of organs. Percussion is most commonly used on the thorax for examining the heart and lungs. It helps determine if a tissue is fluid-filled, air-filled, or solid.[24,28,34,41] Percussion elicits five types of sounds: *flatness* (extremely dull sound produced by very dense tissue, such as muscle or bone), *dullness* (a thud-like sound produced by encapsulated tissue, such as liver or spleen), *resonance* (a hollow sound, such as that produced by air-filled lungs), *hyperresonance* (a "booming" sound heard over a gas-filled area, such as an emphysematous lung; this is always abnormal), and *tympany* (a musical or drum-like sound produced by an air-filled organ, such as with gastric dilatation-volvulus).[24,28,34,41]

Thoracic percussion in the standing patient can be used to detect a fluid line, as found in hydrothorax. Percussion ventral to the fluid line produces a dull thud, whereas percussion dorsal to the fluid line produces a resonant or hyperresonant sound.[28]

Abdominal percussion can detect large volumes of air or fluid in the peritoneal cavity. Rhythmic palpation of a fluid-filled abdomen elicits a fluid wave that is transmitted to the opposite side.[24,28,34,41]

Auscultation. Listening to sounds produced by the body is termed *auscultation*. Auscultation may be direct (with the ear and no instrument) or indirect (using a stethoscope to amplify sounds). The stethoscope allows auscultation of specific areas within a body cavity for assessment of the cardiovascular, respiratory, and gastrointestinal systems (Fig. 18-3).[24,34]

Abnormal sounds can be recognized only after one has learned to identify the types of sounds normally arising from each body structure and the location in which they are most commonly heard. Proficiency at auscultation requires good hearing, a good-quality stethoscope, and knowledge of how to use a stethoscope correctly. The technician should become familiar with this instrument before attempting to use it with the patient.[24,34]

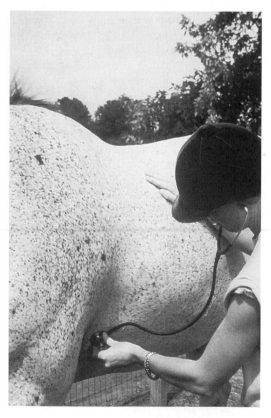

FIG. 18-3 Thoracic auscultation should be performed systematically, evaluating the lungs first and then the heart. The abdomen can also be auscultated to evaluate gastrointestinal sounds.

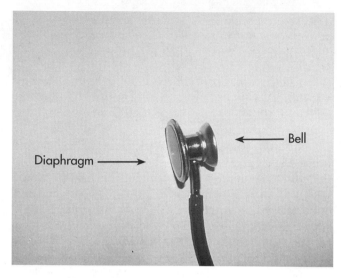

FIG. 18-4 The diaphragm of the stethoscope is used to detect high-pitched sounds, such as heart, bowel, and lung sounds. The bell is used to detect lower-frequency sounds, such as the third and fourth heart sounds.

The stethoscope's chestpiece should have a stiff, flat diaphragm and a bell (Fig. 18-4). The *diaphragm* is the flat, circular portion of the chestpiece covered by a thin, resilient membrane. It transmits high-pitched sounds, such as those produced by the bowel, lungs, and heart. The *bell* is not covered by a membrane. It facilitates auscultation of lower-frequency sounds, such as third and fourth sounds of the heart, or what is most commonly termed a "gallop rhythm."[39]

Aspects of Physical Examination

General Survey. The physical examination begins from the moment the owner and the animal enter the examination area. While obtaining the history, the technician should generally observe the patient to note certain characteristics:[21,28,29,41]

Mentation. The patient's attentiveness or reaction to its environment provides a basis to evaluate the degree of consciousness, depression, excitement, or overreaction to stimuli. The patient's ability to walk or avoid objects can be used to assess vision and balance.

General appearance. Assess the patient's facial expression, size and position of the eyeballs, general body condition (flesh and haircoat), response to commands, and temperament.

State of nutrition. Note if the patient appears in normal body condition, or is thin and frail, or obese. Most patients with chronic disease appear cachexic (wasted). Sunken eyes, temporal muscle atrophy, and excessively loose skin turgor are signs of poor nutrition in chronically ill patients. Long-standing disease, such as renal failure, hyperthyroidism, and cancer, can result in marked wasting.

Symmetry. The body is normally symmetric; note any asymmetry. Observe closely for complementary ("balanced") or noncomplementary conformation of the thorax and abdomen. Note any difference in size or shape of the extremities.

Posture and gait. Walking requires coordination and integrity of the nervous and musculoskeletal systems. Note if the patient can walk and any abnormalities in the gait. Proprioception (sense of body part position), soundness (lack of lameness), and coordination can be quickly assessed.

Vital Signs. Vital signs include the level of consciousness, respiratory rate and effort, heart rate and rhythm, and indications of perfusion. These reflect overall patient status; changes in any vital sign can warn the medical team of impending complications. Vital signs are monitored at regular intervals. The initial findings are used as the baseline and subsequent findings help establish trends indicating improvement or deterioration. To identify abnormalities, technicians must know the normal ranges for each species, age group, and, sometimes, breed (Table 18-1).

Vital signs should be evaluated in relation to the presenting complaint, history, and current health status. Technicians must know the normal ranges for each vital sign and understand which variations might be considered "normal" with regard to a particular patient's status. Remember that vital signs reflect function of various body systems. For example, when assessing the level of consciousness, pupillary light response, and eye position, to some degree we are assessing the nervous system. All body systems (e.g., neurologic, cardiovascular, and respiratory) contribute to overall function of the individual; failure of one system can lead to compromise of others. For example, in patients with heart disease, a drop in blood pressure can compromise kidney function.

Level of consciousness. A declining level of consciousness suggests progressive brain damage and a worsening prognosis. In order of declining consciousness, the levels of consciousness are alert and responsive; depressed; uncontrolled hyperexcitability; stupor; and coma. A depressed patient is conscious but slow to respond to stimuli. A semiconscious patient that can respond to noxious (painful) stimuli is considered stuporous. An unconscious patient that does not respond to any stimuli is in a coma.[7,33] Of these levels, coma warrants the worst prognosis.

A patient might be conscious yet have abnormal mentation (mental function). These mentation changes can include slow but appropriate responses to stimuli (suggesting severe depression) and inappropriate responses to stimuli (suggesting dementia). Bizarre behavior (e.g., biting at imaginary flies) may also be seen. Patients that are mentally dull exhibit slow responses and are unaware of stimuli.

TABLE 18-1 Normal ranges of heart rate, respiratory rate, and rectal temperature in adults of some domestic species[17,23,32,36]

	Heart rate (beats/min)	Respiratory rate (breaths/min)	Rectal temperature
Dogs	70-160	8-20	37.5°-39° C
Cats	150-210	8-30	38°-39° C
Hamsters	250-500	35-135	37°-38° C
Guinea pigs	230-280	42-104	37.2°-39.5° C
Rabbits	130-325	30-60	38.5°-40° C
Horses	28-50	8-16	37.5°-38.5° C
Cattle	40-80	12-36	38°-39° C
Sheep	60-120	12-72	39°-40° C
Pigs	58-100	8-18	38°-40° C

Changes in level of consciousness or mentation can be caused by metabolic problems (e.g., liver failure, portacaval shunts, hyperglycemia, hypoglycemia, hypernatremia, hyponatremia), hypoxia, hypotension, iatrogenic rapid elevation in serum osmolality (e.g., mannitol overdose, total parenteral nutrition), trauma, toxicity (e.g., ethylene glycol), brain damage (e.g., tumors, infection, inflammation), and drugs (e.g., sedatives, anesthetics).[7] Any pathologic change can lead to brain edema or hemorrhage and result in increased intracranial pressure. When this occurs, the brain is compressed and it malfunctions.

Stupor and coma result from an interruption in ascending pathways in the brainstem and midbrain, terminating in the cerebral cortex. Localizing the lesion to the cerebral cortex or midbrain-brainstem is important to formulate a prognosis and detect deterioration in clinical status. Diffuse cortical damage generally carries a better prognosis than midbrain or brainstem injuries.

Changes in behavior, the response to stimuli, or posture may be significant. Unconscious patients can be tested by toe pinching to detect their response to this painful stimulus. Any decline in the level of consciousness suggests worsening pathologic changes and warrants immediate neurologic examination and medical or surgical intervention.

In the conscious patient with altered mentation, the cerebral cortex and diencephalon are the sites of injury.

The patient can show behavioral changes, dementia, circling toward the side of the lesion, seizures, stupor, or coma. The animal may also show slight weakness in the limbs.

Neurologic evaluation of the unconscious patient can localize and determine the progression of the injury. Pupillary size and response to light are noted. Normal, responsive pupils, or equally constricted (miotic) pupils are associated with damage to the cerebral cortex or subcortical structures. Dilated or midrange fixed pupils are most commonly related to midbrain injury and are a grave sign. Eye position is noted, with ventral or lateral strabismus (crossed eyes) indicating a midbrain lesion. Nystagmus (repeated sweeping movement) is caused by a vestibular problem, either in the inner ear or within the brainstem.[44] In an unconscious patient, changes in posture, with the forelimbs and neck in extensor rigidity (decerebrate rigidity), are a grave neurologic sign, indicating a midbrain lesion.[7]

Respiratory changes in an unconscious patient imply serious central nervous system damage. A rhythmic waxing and waning of respiration (Cheyne-Stokes respiration) is due to severe, diffuse cortical injury. Apneustic breathing (holding the breath) and uncontrolled hyperventilation indicate a brainstem lesion.[7]

Respiratory rate and effort. The lungs, airways, larynx, pharynx, and nasal passages make up the respiratory tract. The rate, pattern, and effort of breathing are controlled by the brain and respiratory muscles (intercostal muscles and diaphragm).[42,44]

Respiratory rate and effort can be affected by disease of the respiratory tract, respiratory center of the brain, or respiratory muscles. Thoracic trauma (e.g., diaphragm rupture, pressure on the diaphragm, rib fractures, intercostal muscle damage) can hinder respiration from pain and by disrupting the mechanics of breathing. Metabolic changes leading to acid-base imbalances and pain can cause abnormal breathing.

When blood carbon dioxide levels increase or bicarbonate levels decrease, the brain responds by increasing pulmonary ventilation in an effort to exhale carbon dioxide and normalize the blood pH. Chemoreceptors in the carotid bodies located at the bifurcation of the right and left carotid arteries detect increased carbon dioxide levels and stimulate the respiratory center. When carbon dioxide levels decrease, the stimulus for ventilation is removed. A decreased blood oxygen level or blood pH is detected by carotid chemoreceptors and stimulates ventilation via the respiratory center.[44]

The first subtle sign of respiratory distress is increased respiratory rate. This is followed by a change in respiratory pattern, which is determined by the site of the injury or disease. Difficult or labored breathing is called *dyspnea.* As distress progresses, the patient assumes various postures in attempts to bring relief, followed by open-mouth and labored breathing. Cyanosis (bluish mucosae) is a late sign of respiratory distress and is often followed quickly by death.[2,18,22,30]

Respiratory patterns can suggest the anatomic site of disease and guide lifesaving intervention. *Stridor* (loud breathing heard without the aid of a stethoscope) indicates upper airway disease (nasal passages, larynx/pharynx, trachea). Inspiratory stridor should direct investigation to the extrathoracic airways, especially the larynx. Expiratory stridor is usually due to intrathoracic tracheal changes. Rapid, shallow breathing suggests infringement of the pleural space (e.g., by air or fluid). Labored breathing on both inspiration and expiration is most typical of lung parenchymal disease. Distress on expiration, with a short inspiration, directs attention to the small airways.[2,14,18,30]

Auscultation can help distinguish pleural disease from lung disease. Moist lung sounds suggest fluid in lung tissues. Dry, coarse sounds on inspiration and expiration suggest fibrosis of the lung. Absence of lung sounds indicates interruption of sound transmission by air or fluid in the pleural space.[2,14,18,30]

With increasing respiratory distress, the animal assumes a posture that aids the respiratory effort. Cats often crouch, with the sternum elevated. Dogs extend their necks, abduct their elbows, and arch their backs.[18]

In general, respiratory rates below 8 or above 30 per minute are considered abnormal (see Table 18-1). Low respiratory rates can be caused by trauma to the brain or spinal cord, diseases affecting respiratory drive (e.g., chronic obstructive pulmonary disease, low blood carbon dioxide level), and drugs (e.g., sedatives). Increased respiratory rates can be caused by fever, pain, anxiety, trauma to the brain or chest, metabolic alterations (e.g., alkalosis), pulmonary disease (e.g., pneumonia or edema of the lungs), and drugs (e.g., oxymorphone).[18,23]

Heart rate. Cardiac output (volume of blood pumped by the heart per unit of time) depends on the rate and force of contraction. The force of the contraction results from stretch of the myocardium from ventricular filling. The volume of blood returned to the heart *(venous return)* determines ventricular filling. Heart rate and contractility are affected by sympathetic stimulation of the heart and heart rate by parasympathetic stimulation.[12,15] If venous return is reduced by hemorrhage or fluid loss (e.g., into the gut, uterus, peritoneum), the heart responds by increasing both the heart rate *(tachycardia)* and force of contraction *(inotropy)* through sympathetic stimulation.[14] However, tachycardia and inotropy can occur with stress, pain, fever, and drug administration, unrelated to intravascular volume loss.[3,15,23]

An increase in heart rate and contractility increases the force and volume of blood flow to tissues. Tachycardia can be normal or may be associated with shock, stress, excitement, fever, or hyperthyroidism.[15,23] However, when the heart rate increases above a critical level, the heart muscle becomes exhausted and coronary perfusion decreases, causing myocardial hypoxia.[15] Cardiac arrhythmias and myocardial failure can result, leading to systemic hypoxia and organ failure.

A decreased heart rate *(bradycardia)* can decrease cardiac output. Causes of bradycardia include hypothermia, metabolic disorders (e.g., hyperkalemia, hypoglycemia, hypothyroidism), and parasympathetic (vagal) stimulation. Parasympathetic stimulation can occur with brain, pulmonary, and gastrointestinal diseases, or a diseased sinoatrial node. Heart rates below a critical level can lead to tissue hypoxia, organ failure, and death.[3,15,23]

Heart rhythm. The heart's conduction system regulates the heart rate. The rhythm of contractions depends upon the route of electrical impulses through the conduction system. A normal impulse starts at the sinoatrial node in the right atrium, travels through the atria to the atrioventricular node (at the junction of the atria and ventricles), and to the bundle of His and ventricular nerves (Purkinje fibers).[10,12,15]

An *arrhythmia* is an irregular heartbeat. Arrhythmias can be detected by auscultating the heart. An abnormal conduction system or diseased heart muscle causes an arrhythmia. When ventricular contraction does not forcefully propel blood to the periphery, a *pulse deficit* is detected.[16,25]

Not all arrhythmias are pathologic. When the ECG has a P wave associated with most QRS complexes and the QRS complexes are of normal width, the rhythm is termed *supraventricular. Sinus arrhythmia* is fluctuation of heart rate with respiration, decreasing with expiration and increasing with inspiration; this is normal in dogs.[29] *Ventricular rhythm* is characterized by QRS complexes that are wide and bizarre and not associated with P waves. Supraventricular and ventricular arrhythmias can be subdivided into bradyarrhythmias or tachyarrhythmias.[10,46]

Listen to the heart by placing the stethoscope over the left and right side of the animal's thorax at the fourth to sixth intercostal space, while palpating the pulse (Fig. 18-5).[4,42] Pericardial fluid, pleural air or fluid, severe hypovolemia, or herniated abdominal organs cause muffled heart sounds. Tachycardia, bradycardia, muffled heart sounds, and pulse deficits require immediate attention by the veterinary team.

Indications of perfusion. Mucous membrane color, capillary refill time, pulse strength and quality, and body temperature reflect perfusion of (blood flow to) peripheral tissues. Blood pumped into the aorta during ventricular contraction creates a fluid wave that travels from the heart to the peripheral arteries. This wave is called a *pulse.* The character of the pulse depends on stroke volume, heart rate, force of ejection, and vascu-

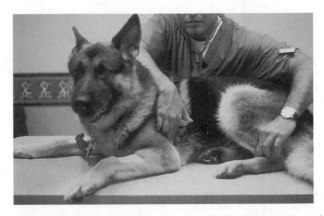

FIG. 18-5 The pulse can be evaluated while the thorax is auscultated. Any difference between heart and pulse is termed a *pulse deficit.*

lar tone (resistance). Evaluation of pulse strength is based on the difference between the systolic (heart contracting) and diastolic (heart filling) pressure, called the *pulse pressure.* With normal pulse pressure, the pulse is easily palpated and strong. When the difference is great, the pulse is bounding. Causes of a bounding pulse include fever, hyperthyroidism, patent ductus arteriosus, and early shock. When the difference is small or the time to maximum systolic pressure is prolonged, the pulse feels weak. Any condition that decreases cardiac output (e.g., late shock, heart failure, arrhythmias) causes a weak pulse.[16,29,39]

The pulse is palpated by lightly placing the tips of the index and middle fingers at a site where an artery crosses over bone or firm tissue. The most common pulse points assessed are the femoral and dorsal pedal arteries. In cats, both femoral pulses should be assessed simultaneously to detect caudal aortic obstruction, as seen with a saddle thrombus. In large animals, the pulse can be assessed where the facial artery crosses the ventral border of the mandible.

A bounding pulse may reflect pain, fever, or early shock, and it indicates the need for intervention with analgesics (pain relievers) and fluid replacement. A weak pulse is cause for immediate concern and warrants aggressive measures to improve cardiac output (e.g., IV fluids for shock, appropriate cardiac medications for heart failure).

Capillary refill time is the time required for blood to refill capillaries after displacement by finger pressure. Prompt refilling of capillaries depends upon cardiac output and vascular tone.[15,42]

To measure the capillary refill time, apply pressure with the index finger to an unpigmented area of mucous membrane and then release. The time for the color to return to the blanched area is the capillary refill time. Normal values are 1 to 2 seconds. A prolonged capillary refill time (more than 2 seconds) suggests poor peripher-

TABLE 18-2 Interpretation of mucous membrane color[23,36]

Membrane color	Interpretation	Causes
Pink	Normal	Adequate perfusion and oxygenation of peripheral tissues
Pale	Anemia, poor perfusion, vasoconstriction	Blood loss, shock, vasopressors
Blue	Cyanosis, inadequate oxygenation	Hypoxemia
Brick red	Hyperdynamic perfusion, vasodilation	Early shock, sepsis, fever, systemic inflammatory response syndrome
Icteric	Bilirubin accumulation	Hepatic/biliary disorder, hemolysis
Brown	Methemoglobinemia	Acetaminophen toxicity in cats
Petechiae or ecchymoses	Coagulation disorder	Platelet disorder, disseminated intravascular coagulation, coagulation factor deficiencies

temperature.[13,20] These chemicals may be *pyrogens* secreted by bacteria or *cytokines* associated with inflammation.[35] Brain disease (e.g., cerebral edema, neurosurgery, trauma, tumors) can reset the thermostat to a higher level.[1,5,13]

Hyperthermia (increased body temperature) increases tissue oxygen requirements. The body responds by increasing ventilation to release body heat. Cerebral vasoconstriction and brain hypoxia can develop if the blood carbon dioxide levels fall too low from hyperventilation. Cardiac work and oxygen demands increase. Peripheral vessels dilate in an effort to release heat. Damage to vascular cells can lead to disseminated intravascular coagulation, sloughing of the gastrointestinal mucosa, bacterial translocation, and hypovolemia.[1,5,26]

Hypothermia (subnormal body temperature) reduces the metabolic rate, enzyme functions, oxygen consumption, and the ability of hemoglobin to release oxygen to tissues. Hypothermia can cause peripheral vasoconstriction, decreased heart rate, and hypotension. Gastrointestinal motility is decreased, and ileus (lack of bowel motility) may occur.[1,20,22,23,26]

Body temperature should be monitored from a single site, usually the rectum (see Table 18-1). Serial readings are more informative than a single reading. Other sites include the axillary and inguinal regions. Readings in these areas generally are 1 to 2 degrees lower than the rectal temperature. Body temperatures can also be measured with an ear probe inserted carefully into the external ear canal. Serial temperatures taken from the same area are more important than single values.[22]

al perfusion (e.g., late shock, severe vasodilation or vasoconstriction, pericardial effusion, heart failure). A short capillary refill time (less than 1 second) can be related to anxiety, compensatory shock, fever, and pain.[15,42]

Although mucous membrane color is most commonly assessed by examining the gums, one can also use the conjunctiva of the eye and the membranes of the vulva and penis.[15,42] The normal pink color of unpigmented mucous membranes requires adequate blood hemoglobin concentration, tissue oxygen tension, and peripheral capillary blood flow (Table 18-2).[12,45] Pale gums with prolonged capillary refill time warrants oxygen administration and a rapid search for the underlying cause. Patients with these signs may require aggressive fluid therapy.

The body maintains its normal temperature by balancing heat production with heat loss through a thermostatic feedback mechanism in the hypothalamus.[1,5,13,20,26] This mechanism can be altered by disease of the central nervous system or other illness.[22] Chemical substances released in disease can reset the thermoregulatory center, increasing the metabolic rate, and producing and conserving heat, elevating the body

A SYSTEMATIC APPROACH TO PHYSICAL EXAMINATION

After the vitals are recorded, proceed to the physical examination, beginning at the tip of the nose and concluding at the tip of the tail. The examination can be divided into several areas: head and neck; trunk and forelimbs; thorax; abdomen; hind limbs; and external genitalia and perineum.[21,27,28,29]

Examination of the Head and Neck[6,19,21,25,28,29,36]

Observing the patient at arm's length allows comparison of the two sides of the face and head for symmetry. Look for unilateral (one-sided) facial paralysis and unilateral or bilateral (two-sided) nasal/ocular discharge, and note any irregularities in head shape or size.

Assess the eyes for size, position, and any discharge. Observe for ectropion (everted eyelids) or entropion (inverted eyelids). Assess pupil size and the response to light. Check the cornea for clarity and contour, looking for scars, ulcers, infiltrates, and pigmentation. Assess the color and condition of the sclera and conjunctiva. Note any signs of jaundice, hemorrhage, or increased vascularization.

Evaluate the nose and nares for symmetry and conformation, as well as evidence of nasal discharge. If there is swelling evident or a history of chronic nasal discharge, determine patency of the nares. If the patient allows it, close the mouth, cover one nostril first and then the other, and assess nasal air flow. Note any areas with increased malleability of facial bones.

Check the lips for areas of inflammation, swelling, masses, or lip-fold pyoderma. Retract the lips and assess the oral mucosa and gingivae (gums) for color, capillary refill time, inflammation, jaundice, and ulcers. Check for fractured, missing, or loose teeth and periodontal disease. Assess the soft and hard palates for tumors, ulcerations, and foreign bodies.

Evaluate the carriage and position of the ears, thickness and malleability of the pinnae, and cleanliness of the ear canals. Check for odors, fluid, or exudate in the ear canal. Patients exhibiting pain or discomfort during examination of the ear canal should have a more detailed otoscopic examination.

After examining the ears, palpate the cervical and mandibular lymph nodes, salivary glands, larynx, and thyroid gland. Palpate the trachea to determine if it is on the midline. In patients with inspiratory dyspnea, gently palpate the trachea to detect tracheal ring abnormalities. A sustained cough, retching, or gagging after gentle compression of the larynx and trachea is abnormal.

Examination of the Trunk and Forelimbs[6,19,21,25,28,29,36]

Palpate each forelimb, feeling for abnormalities in angulation, deformities, swelling, bleeding, bony protrusions, obvious fractures, or joint luxations. Assess both limbs in weight-bearing and non–weight-bearing positions. Assess for masses or lymph node abnormalities. Palpate for points of tenderness, stiffness, or crepitus at the joints. Note the condition of the feet, nails, or hooves; nail bed or hoof color may give an indication of perfusion. Palpate both brachial pulses for quality and strength.

Examine the haircoat for alopecia (hair loss), eruptions, parasites, dryness, or excessive oil. Palpate for any skin masses or lacerations. Assess the elasticity of the skin.

Examination of the Thorax

Observe the patient's respiratory rate, effort, and depth. Look for evidence of dyspnea, such as rapid open-mouth breathing, increased effort, an increased abdominal component, abnormal posture to assist in breathing, and cyanosis.

Observe and palpate the thorax for conformation, symmetry, and movement of the ribs, sternum, or vertebral column. Palpate for masses. Palpate the area between the fourth and sixth intercostal spaces on both sides of thorax for the point of maximum intensity of the heartbeat and cardiac thrills.[8,21,22,25,28,29,36,39,42]

Assess the respiratory tract. Listen for noisy breathing at the mouth and nares without the use of a stethoscope. Use a stethoscope to auscultate the lungs. Divide each side of the thorax (left and right) in four quadrants: craniodorsal, caudodorsal, cranioventral, and caudoventral. Begin by auscultating the right side at the craniodorsal quadrant and continue in a clockwise fashion, then do the same on the left side.

Normal respiratory sounds are described as *vesicular* or *bronchial,* depending on where they are auscultated. Vesicular sounds are heard over normal lung parenchyma and are produced by movement of air through small bronchi, bronchioles, and alveoli. Vesicular sounds are best heard on inspiration. They have been described as resembling the sound made by wind blowing through trees or the sound of rustling leaves.[21,29,39] Bronchial sounds are produced by movement of air through the trachea and large bronchi. They are usually heard over the area of the trachea and carina, most noticeably during expiration.[21,22,25,28,29,39,42]

Abnormal lung sounds include crackles (sometimes referred to as *rales*), wheezes, dull lung sounds, or muffled lung sounds. *Crackles* are usually caused by air movement through small airways within the lumen reduced by fluid, mucus, or thickened walls. *Dry crackles* are associated with passage of air through relatively solid material in the bronchi or trachea. *Moist crackles* are caused by passage of air through fluid material. Crackles are mostly heard in such conditions as pulmonary edema, bronchopneumonia, and pulmonary fibrosis. *Wheezes* are high-pitched, musical sounds heard mostly on expiration. They are associated with infectious or allergic bronchitis (e.g., asthma in cats). *Dull or muffled lung sounds* may be due to collapse or consolidation of a lung lobe, tension pneumothorax, pneumomediastinum, hydrothorax, pyothorax, a mass displacing the lung, or diaphragmatic hernia.[8,19,21,22,25,28,29,36,39]

Cardiac auscultation can detect murmurs, arrhythmias, and muffled heart sounds. When assessing murmurs, it is important to determine in which quadrant the murmur is the loudest; this helps identify the valvular area involved. Arrhythmias most commonly detected are sinus arrhythmia (normal), atrial fibrillation, heart block, premature ventricular contractions, and gallop rhythm. Muffled heart sounds can be due to obesity, pericardial effusion, pleural effusion, an intrathoracic mass, or diaphragmatic hernia.[8,19,21,22,25,28,29,39]

Examination of the Abdomen

The abdomen should be inspected for distention, deformity, displacement, symmetry, and bruising. In trauma patients, examine the umbilicus for red discoloration, suggestive of intraabdominal bleeding.[38] If the abdomen is distended, use percussion to determine if the distention is due to peritoneal effusion, gastric dilatation or volvulus, an intraabdominal mass, or obesity. Percussion that produces tympanic sounds suggests gastric or small intestinal obstruction and gas entrapment.[6,8,9,21,25,28]

Auscultate the abdomen to detect intestinal hypermotility (increased frequency or intensity of intestinal sounds) or hypomotility (decreased frequency or intensity of intestinal sounds). Absence of bowel sounds suggests ileus (lack of intestinal motility) or a fluid-filled abdomen.[6,8,9,21,28,29,38]

The abdomen of most small animals can be readily palpated, but this may not be feasible in patients with tense abdominal muscles. Abdominal palpation in large animals is more in the form of *ballottement,* in which the fist is rhythmically pressed into an area of the abdomen in an attempt to "bump" any large underlying masses or organs.

Palpate the abdomen in an orderly fashion. Divide the abdomen into three areas: cranial, middle, and caudal. Start the procedure at the cranial portion and conclude at the caudal portion. Palpate the cranial abdomen to assess the stomach, duodenum, biliary structures, liver, and the area of the pancreas (seeking pain on palpation). In the midabdominal area, assess the spleen, kidneys, adrenal glands, mesenteric lymph nodes, and intestines. Organs assessed upon caudal abdominal palpation are the urinary bladder, prostate, uterus (in the intact female if enlarged), and colon. A normal uterus is not ordinarily palpable.[6,9,19,21,25,29,38,39]

Examination of the Hind Limbs[6,19,21,25,28,29,39]

Palpate each hind limb, feeling for abnormalities in angulation, deformities, swelling, bleeding, bony protrusions, obvious fractures, or joint luxations. Assess both limbs in weight-bearing and non–weight-bearing positions. Assess for masses or lymph node abnormalities. Note the position of the patellas when assessing the stifle. Palpate the popliteal lymph nodes for size and consistency. Palpate for points of tenderness, stiffness, or crepitus at joints. Also evaluate muscle mass and tone.

Palpate the pelvic region for conformation and symmetry. Palpate the vertebral column to assess for deviations and pain.

Examination of External Genitalia and Perineum[6,19,21,25,28,29,39]

In males, inspect the prepuce and penis, noting any discharge. In dogs, expose the penis by retracting the preputial sheath. Look for masses and evidence of trauma, and note any color abnormalities (such as jaundiced or bruising). If the patient is intact (not castrated), inspect both testicles for symmetry, size, location (with-

in the scrotum), and conformation. If you detect only one testicle (cryptorchidism), palpate the inguinal area and caudal abdominal region for a retained testicle. A rectal examination to determine texture, size, and conformation of the prostate is done by the veterinarian.

Female genital examination includes inspection and palpation of the mammary glands for tumors or cysts. In the lactating bitch or female dogs in pseudopregnancy, determine if there is evidence of mastitis or milk. In lactating cows, palpate for excessive heat and areas of firmness (induration). A California mastitis test can quickly assess the milk of lactating cows. Inspect the vulva for any discharge (blood, pus), polyps, tumors, or structural defects.

Rectal examination is done with a finger in small animals and with the hand and arm in large animals. Assess the sublumbar lymph nodes in the dorsal aspect of the pelvic canal. Feel for evidence of pelvic fracture and note anal tone and fecal consistency. Check for masses in the pelvic canal and caudal abdomen. In large animals, feel for displaced or distended loops of bowel, and assess the kidneys, if within reach.

Inspect the perianal area for hair mats, hernias, feces, masses, and evidence of discharge. In dogs, palpate for impacted or abscessed anal sacs.

PHYSICAL EXAMINATION IN EMERGENCIES
Triage, Primary Survey, and Secondary Survey

The procedure called *triage* (French, "to sort") is used to classify patients according to the severity of illness or injury to determine their relative priority for treatment. In its original application in combat, triage was used by French military medical personnel to sort wounded soldiers into three categories: those that would survive without immediate treatment; those that would die despite immediate treatment; and those that would survive only if given immediate treatment. Emergency treatment of only the last group (those likely to survive) allowed them to salvage the most lives using limited resources.

In veterinary medicine, triage is used primarily in emergency situations. It can also be used in the critical care setting as a means of prioritization and assessment, and it guides the veterinary care team in efficient delivery of medical and patient care.[8,11] Using triage, the treatment team focuses initially on life-threatening conditions (e.g., an obstructed airway or massive external hemorrhage) and institutes immediate measures to correct them with the most efficient use of available manpower and skills. A *primary survey* is used to detect any life-threatening problems. A *secondary survey* is used to broaden the evaluation to include all organ systems in a progressive, detailed manner. In triage of multiple patients (e.g., after a barn fire or horse trailer accident, or in a busy emergency clinic), those with a compromised airway, breathing difficulties, and/or circulatory problems (ABCs) should be assessed and treated first.

Vital signs assessed during triage include level of consciousness, respiratory rate and effort, heart rate and rhythm, and indications of perfusion (pulse, mucous membrane color, capillary refill time, temperature). These vital signs can indicate trends of deterioration, warning the team of complications. Vital signs should be assessed at frequent, regular intervals to detect trends, using initial values as the baseline.[6,11,23,36]

In the emergency setting, no disease, injury, or physiologic abnormality should be considered as an isolated entity. The team should consider the current status, physiologic reserve, and potential for deterioration of each organ system or problem, rather than just the primary problem (e.g., fractured femur), and develop a plan of action.

During the primary survey and initial management, life-threatening conditions are addressed in the following order of priority:

1. Airway patency (open airway)
2. Breathing
3. Circulation
4. Neurologic deficit assessment

During the primary survey, neurologic status can be evaluated with the aid of the acronym *AVPU*: Is the patient *Alert* and aware of its surroundings? Is it *Voice* responsive? Is it *Pain* responsive? Is it *Unresponsive*?[37]

Such metabolic derangements as hypoxia (low blood oxygen levels), hypercapnia (high blood carbon dioxide levels), acidemia (low blood pH), alkalemia (high blood pH), hypoglycemia (low blood glucose level), hyperglycemia (high blood glucose level), hypocalcemia (low blood calcium level), hypercalcemia (high blood calcium level), hyperammonemia (high blood ammonia level), and drugs previously given must be considered in patients with altered mental status.[6,23,36]

After the ABC areas have been addressed and resuscitation measures have been initiated, the secondary survey is performed. Vital signs are reassessed and the patient is rapidly and thoroughly examined from head to tail. The thorax, abdomen, pelvis, and extremities are visually inspected, palpated, and auscultated where appropriate. Neurologic status is repeatedly assessed. Appropriate radiographic and laboratory studies are obtained.[8,11,23,37] Other diagnostic procedures that may be done at this time include, but are not limited to, an ECG, measurement of blood pressure and central venous pressure, and pulse oximetry.

Classification System for Triage. When dealing with more than one emergency or critically ill patient, the team can use a classification system based on the nature of the presenting complaint, as well as vital signs assessed during triage.[8,23,31]

Class I. Patients in class I must receive treatment immediately and are usually those suffering from acute trauma, respiratory or cardiorespiratory arrest or failure, or airway obstruction, or are unconscious. Class I patients may be dying before your eyes. They are usually in a decompensatory stage of shock. The decompensatory stage of shock is characterized by cyanosis, ashen white mucous membranes, prolonged capillary refill time or no capillary refill, cold skin, a decreased rectal temperature, weak or undetectable femoral pulses, and oliguria (reduced urine production). They may be unconscious, stuporous, or losing consciousness. The bleeding patient may have seizures as a result of low blood pressure if the hemorrhage is substantial.

Class II. Patients in class II are critically ill. These patients are suffering from multiple injuries, shock, or severe bleeding but have adequate respiratory function. They require treatment within minutes to an hour. They may be in a mild state of shock. Mild shock is characterized by pale or ashen mucous membranes, prolonged capillary refill time, cool skin, a decreased rectal temperature, and weak femoral pulses. Class II patients may show tachycardia, oliguria, and altered mentation (e.g., depression, seizures, excitation). Hemorrhage may be profuse or a slow trickle.

Class III. Patients in class III are seriously ill but not critically ill. These patients usually have severe open wounds or fractures, burns, penetrating wounds to the abdomen without active bleeding, or blunt trauma. They are not in shock or exhibiting an altered level of consciousness. They require treatment within a few hours.

Class IV. Patients in class IV are less seriously ill but are still of concern. This classification does not apply to most trauma patients. The mucous membranes may be red or pale pink and capillary refill time under 1 second. The skin and rectal temperatures are normal, and femoral pulses are normal or bounding. These patients often have normal respiration, tachycardia or a normal heart rate, normal urine output, and normal mentation, evidenced by alertness and awareness of their surroundings. Usually these patients are mildly depressed to slightly excited and generally are not actively hemorrhaging. Class IV patients require treatment within 24 hours.

REFERENCES

1. Ahn AH: *Approach to the hypothermic patient.* In Bonagura JD, Kirk RB, editors: *Kirk's current veterinary therapy XII, small animal practice,* Philadelphia, 1995, WB Saunders, pp 157-160.
2. Aldrich J, Haskins SC: *Monitoring the critically ill patient.* In Bonagura JD, Kirk RB, editors: *Kirk's current veterinary therapy XII, small animal practice,* Philadelphia, 1995, WB Saunders, pp 98-105.

3. Allen DG: *Special techniques.* In Allen DG, Kruth SA, Garvey MS, editors: *Small animal medicine,* Philadelphia, 1991, JB Lippincott, pp 1035-1093.

4. Atkins CE: *Abnormal heart sounds.* In Allen DG, Kruth SA, Garvey MS, editors: *Small animal medicine,* Philadelphia, 1991, JB Lippincott, pp 197-202.

5. Ayers SM, Keenan RL: *The hyperthermic syndromes.* In Ayers SM, et al, editors: *Textbook of critical care,* ed 3, Philadelphia, 1995, WB Saunders, pp 1520-1523.

6. Brace JJ, Bellhorn T: The history and physical examination of the trauma patient, *Vet Clin North Am Small Anim Pract* 10:533-538, 1980.

7. Chrisman C: *Coma and altered states of consciousness.* In Chrisman C: *Problems in small animal neurology,* ed 2, Philadelphia, 1991, Lea & Febiger, pp 219-233.

8. Crowe DT: *Triage and trauma management.* In Murtaugh RJ, Kaplan PM, editors: *Veterinary emergency and critical care,* St Louis, 1992, Mosby, pp 77-121.

9. Davenport DJ, Martin RA: *Acute abdomen.* In Murtaugh RJ, Kaplan PM, editors: *Veterinary emergency and critical care medicine,* St Louis, 1992, Mosby, pp 153-161.

10. Edwards NE: *Basic principles of electrocardiography: ECG manual for the veterinary technician,* Philadelphia, 1993, WB Saunders, pp 1-16.

11. Fagella A: First aid, transport, and triage, *Vet Clin North Am Small Anim Pract* 24:997-1014, 1994.

12. Ford PJ: *Cardiovascular pathophysiology.* In Price SA, Wilson LM, editors: *Pathophysiology: clinical concepts of disease processes,* ed 4, St Louis, 1992, Mosby, pp 369-508.

13. Guyton AC: *Body temperature, temperature regulation and fever.* In *Textbook of medical physiology,* ed 8, Philadelphia, 1991, WB Saunders, pp 797-808.

14. Guyton AC: *Cardiac output, venous return and their regulation.* In *Textbook of medical physiology,* ed 8, Philadelphia, 1991, WB Saunders, pp 221-232.

15. Guyton AC: *The heart muscle: the heart as a pump.* In *Textbook of medical physiology,* ed 8, Philadelphia, 1991, WB Saunders, pp 98-116.

16. Guyton AC: *Vascular distensibility and functions of the arterial and venous systems.* In *Textbook of medical physiology,* ed 8, Philadelphia, 1991, WB Saunders, pp 159-168.

17. Harkness JE, Wagner JE, editors: *Biology and husbandry.* In *The biology and medicine of rabbits and rodents,* ed 4, Baltimore, 1995, Williams & Wilkins, pp 13-73.

18. Hawkins EC: *Clinical manifestations of lower respiratory tract disorders.* In Allen DG, Kruth SA, Garvey MS, editors: *Small animal medicine,* Philadelphia, 1991, JB Lippincott, pp 180-213.

19. Holzworth J, Stein B: *The sick cat.* In Holzworth J, editor: *Diseases of the cat: medicine and surgery,* Philadelphia, 1986, WB Saunders, pp 1-14.

20. Hudi EH, Demling RH: *Hypothermia and cold-related injuries.* In Ayers SM, et al, editors: *Textbook of critical care,* ed 3, Philadelphia, 1995, WB Saunders, pp 1516-1520.

21. Jones D: *History and physical examination.* In Birchard SJ, Sherding RG, editors: *Saunders manual of small animal practice,* Philadelphia, 1994, WB Saunders, pp 1-12.

22. Kaplan PM: *Monitoring.* In Murtaugh RJ, Kaplan PM, editors: *Veterinary emergency and critical care medicine,* St Louis, 1992, Mosby, pp 21-36.

23. Kirby R: *Approach to the trauma patient.* Waltham Sympos Treatment Sm Anim Dis: Emerg Crit Care, 1990, pp 15-25.

24. Kozier B, Erb G, Olivieri R, editors: *Assessing health status.* In *Fundamentals of nursing: concepts, process, and practice,* ed 4, Redwood City, Cal, 1991, Addison-Wesley, pp 355-447.

25. Kruth SA: *History and physical examination of the dog and cat.* In Allen DG, Kruth SA, Garvey MS, editors: *Small animal medicine,* Philadelphia, 1991, JB Lippincott, pp 7-11.

26. Lee-Parritz DE, Pavletic MM: *Physical and chemical injuries: heatstroke, hypothermia, burns and frostbite.* In Murtaugh RJ, and Kaplam PM, editors: *Veterinary emergency and critical care medicine,* St Louis, 1992, Mosby, pp 194-211.

27. Lorenz MD: *The problem-oriented approach.* In Lorenz MD, Cornelius LM, editors: *Small animal medical diagnosis,* Philadelphia, 1987, JB Lippincott, pp 1-12.

28. Low DG: General examination of dogs, *Vet Clin North Am* 1:3-14, 1971.

29. Magne ML: *History and physical examination.* In McCurnin DM, editor: *Clinical textbook for veterinary technicians,* ed 2, Philadelphia, 1990, WB Saunders, pp 31-42.

30. McGee M, Spencer CL, Van Pelt DR: *Critical care nursing.* In Bonagura JD, Kirk RB, editors: *Kirk's current veterinary therapy XII, small animal practice,* Philadelphia, 1995, WB Saunders, pp 106-109.

31. McQuillan KA, Wiles CE III: *Initial management of traumatic shock.* In Cadona VD, et al, editors: *Trauma nursing, from resuscitation through rehabilitation.* Philadelphia, 1988, WB Saunders, pp 160-183.

32. *The Merck veterinary manual: clinical values and procedures,* Rahway, NJ, 1991, Merck, pp 933-976.

33. Oliver JE, Lorenz MD: *Neurologic history and examination.* In *Handbook of veterinary neurology,* ed 2, Philadelphia, 1993, WB Saunders, pp 3-45.

34. Potter PA, Perry AG, editors: *Health assessment and physical examination.* In *Basic nursing: theory and practice,* ed 2, St Louis, 1991, Mosby, pp 247-307.

35. Purvis D, Kirby R: Systemic inflammatory response syndrome: septic shock, *Vet Clin North Am Small Anim Pract* 24:1225-1248, 1994.

36. Rivera AM, Rudloff E, Kirby R: *Monitoring the ICU patient, Vet Technician* 17:27-43, 1996.

37. Rutherford WF, Panacek EA: *Principles of critical care medicine, resuscitation and stabilization.* In Hall JB, Schmidt GA, Wood LDH, editors: *Principles of critical care,* New York, 1992, McGraw-Hill, pp 559-567.

38. Saxon WD: The acute abdomen, *Vet Clin North Am Small Anim Pract* 24:1207-1224, 1994.

39. Shaer M: *The medical history, physical examination, and restraint.* In Sherding RG, editor: *The cat: diseases and clinical management,* ed 2, New York, 1994, Churchill Livingstone, pp 7-23.

40. Swartz MH: *The art of interviewing.* In *Textbook of physical diagnosis, history and examination,* ed 2, Philadelphia, 1994, WB Saunders, pp 3-44.

41. Swartz MH: *The science of physical examination.* In *Textbook of physical diagnosis, history and examination,* ed 2, Philadelphia, 1994, WB Saunders, pp 61-67.

42. Ware WA: *Disorders of the cardiovascular system.* In Nelson RW, Couto GC (editors): *Essentials of small animal internal medicine,* ed 1, St Louis, 1992, Mosby, pp 3-147.

43. West JB: *Mechanics of breathing.* In *Respiratory physiology: the essentials,* ed 5, Baltimore, 1995, Williams & Wilkins, pp 89-116.

44. West JB: *Control of ventilation.* In *Respiratory physiology: the essentials,* ed 5, Baltimore, 1995, Williams & Wilkins, pp 117-136.

45. West JB: *Gas transport to the periphery.* In *Respiratory physiology: the essentials,* ed 5, Baltimore, 1990, Williams & Wilkins, pp 71-88.

46. Wingfield WE: Recognition and management of serious cardiac dysrhythmias, *Proc Intl Vet Emerg Crit Care Symp,* pp 45-66, 1988.

CHAPTER 19

Diagnostic Imaging

C. Han
C. Hurd
C. Bretz

Learning Objectives

After reviewing this chapter, the reader should understand the following:

Anatomy and function of x-ray machines
Way in which x-rays are produced
Factors affecting radiographic quality
Techniques and devices used to optimize radiographic quality
Dangers of radiation and how to avoid radiation injury

Procedures used to develop radiographs
Positioning of animals for radiographs
Basic physics of ultrasound
Anatomy and function of ultrasound machines
Techniques used to produce high-quality sonograms
Types, uses, and maintenance of endoscopes
Procedures for endoscopic examination of the gastrointestinal and respiratory tracts

RADIOGRAPHY

C. HAN
C. HURD

X-RAY GENERATION

X-rays are a form of electromagnetic radiation. X-rays are similar to visible light, but they have a shorter wavelength. X-rays are generated when fast-moving electrons collide with any form of matter. The x-ray tube of an x-ray machine projects a stream of electrons toward a metal target. The energy of the electrons interacting with the atoms of the target is converted to heat (99%) and x-radiation (1%). Heat generation in the x-ray tube is a limiting factor in the production of x-rays. This is why higher-output x-ray machines have rotating anode x-ray tubes.

X-RAY TUBE ANATOMY

The x-ray tube contains a heated tungsten filament in the *cathode,* where the electrons are generated, and an *anode* containing a tungsten target where x-rays are generated. Both are enclosed in a vacuum-filled glass envelope. A beryllium window in the glass envelope allows x-rays to pass with minimal filtration. An aluminum filter is placed across the window to absorb the low-energy (soft) x-rays, while allowing the more energetic and useful x-rays to form the x-ray beam. The entire tube is surrounded by oil, which acts as an electrical barrier while absorbing heat generated by the tube. The tube and oil are encased in a metal housing to prevent damage to the glass envelope and to absorb stray radiation (Fig. 19-1). The tungsten filament is housed within a focusing cup to focus the beam of electrons on the focal spot of the anode. The focal spot is the tungsten metal plate where the x-rays are generated. The focal spot is oriented at an angle of 11 to 20 degrees.

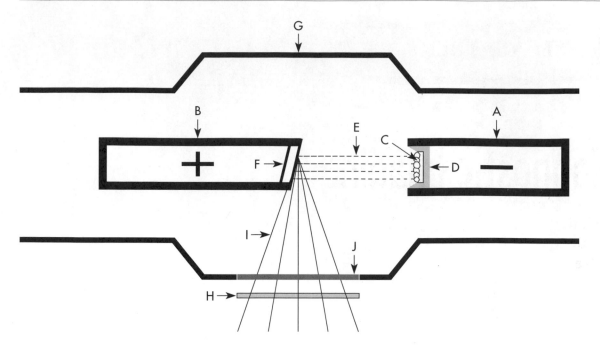

FIG. 19-1 Anatomy of an x-ray tube. **A,** Cathode. **B,** Anode. **C,** Tungsten filament. **D,** Focusing cup. **E,** Accelerating electrons. **F,** Tungsten target. **G,** Glass envelope. **H,** Aluminum filter. **I,** Generated x-rays. **J,** Beryllium window.

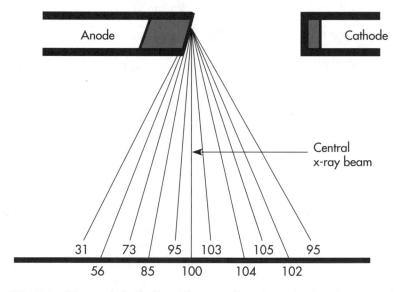

FIG. 19-2 The anode heel effect. The x-ray beam intensity decreases toward the anode side because of absorption by the target and anode material.

Anode Heel Effect. Anode heel effect is the unequal distribution of the x-ray beam intensity emitted from the x-ray tube. Tubes with lower target angles (e.g., 11 degrees) have a distribution of x-ray beam intensity that decreases rapidly on the anode side of the tube (Fig. 19-2). This is caused by absorption of the x-ray beam by the target and by anode material. This can be used to advantage when radiographing areas of unequal thickness, such as the thorax or abdomen. By placing the patient's head toward the anode side, the part of the x-ray beam with the higher intensity (cathode side) is directed to the thickest area. This produces a more even film density. The heel effect is most noticeable when large films and short focal-film distances are used.

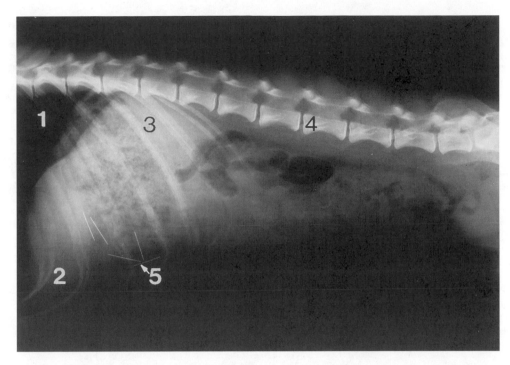

FIG. 19-3 Subject densities: *1,* Air. *2,* Fat. *3,* Water. *4,* Bone. *5,* Metal. Air is least dense, allowing x-rays to penetrate and expose the film. Metal is the most dense, absorbing most of the x-rays and allowing only a few to penetrate, exposing the film.

RADIOGRAPHIC QUALITY
Radiographic Density

Radiographic density is the degree of blackness on a radiograph. The dark areas are made up of black metallic silver deposits on the finished radiograph. These deposits occur in areas where x-rays have penetrated the patient and exposed the emulsion of the film. Radiographic density can be increased by increasing the mA or the exposure time. Either one increases the number of x-rays produced by increasing the number of electrons in the electron cloud or the time the electrons are allowed to travel from the cathode to the anode. A higher *kilovoltage peak (kVp)* yields more radiographic density by increasing the penetrating power of the x-ray beam.

Radiographic Contrast

Radiographic contrast is defined as the differences in radiographic density between adjacent areas on a radiographic image. Radiographs that show a *long scale of contrast* have a few black and white shades, with many shades of gray. A *short scale of contrast* has black and white shades, with only a few shades of gray in between. For most studies, a long scale of contrast is desirable. Obtaining a long scale of radiographic contrast depends on four factors: subject density, kVp level, film contrast, and film fogging.

Subject density is the ability of the different tissue densities to absorb x-rays. The extent to which x-rays penetrate the various tissues depends on the differences in atomic number and thickness. On radiographs, air is least radiodense, followed in increasing radiodensity by fat, water and muscle, bone and metal, the last being most radiodense (Fig. 19-3). Bone, containing mainly calcium and phosphorus, has a high average atomic number as compared with muscle, which contains mainly hydrogen and nitrogen. Bone absorbs more x-rays than muscle and appears whiter on the finished radiograph. The thickness of the area also affects the number of x-rays absorbed. If you radiograph an area that ranges from 5 to 20 cm in thickness, the 20-cm–thick area absorbs more x-rays than the 5-cm area.

The scale of radiographic contrast can be lengthened or shortened by increasing or decreasing the *kVp.* The higher the kVp, the longer the scale of contrast (the more grays that can be visualized). Radiographs made with a high kVp have more exposure latitude, allowing minor errors in technique without affecting the diagnostic quality of the radiograph.

Film contrast also affects radiographic contrast. Some types of film can produce a long scale of contrast or long latitude. *Long-latitude film* allows for more variation in technique while still producing a diagnostic radiograph. The scale of contrast can be shortened by

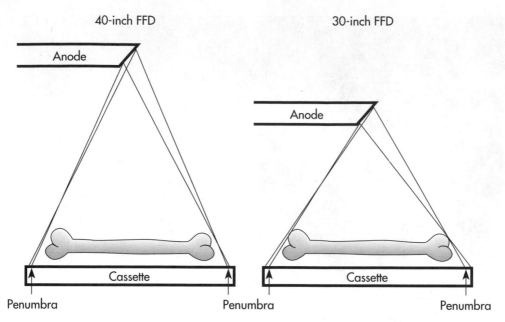

FIG. 19-4   Increasing the focal-film distance (FFD) decreases the amount of penumbra, increasing the radiographic detail.

changing the exposure technique when using long-latitude film. However, the scale of contrast cannot be lengthened when using contrast film (film that produces a short scale of contrast).

Film fogging can greatly decrease radiographic contrast by decreasing the differences in densities between two adjacent shadows. Care must be taken in the storage and handling of x-ray film to prevent fogging. Film can become fogged from low-grade light leaks in the darkroom, scatter radiation, heat, and improper processing.

Radiographic Detail

A diagnostic radiograph is one with good radiographic detail. Radiographic detail is considered to be good when the interfaces between tissues and organs are sharp. Many factors can affect the detail on a radiograph. The most common are patient motion and the penumbra effect.

Patient motion causes loss of detail because of blurred interfaces. A blurred image is generally a result of long exposure time combined with motion of the patient. This can be controlled by using the shortest possible exposure. If the image remains blurred, the patient should be sedated.

A loss of detail is also caused by the penumbra effect. Excessive penumbra causes blurring at the edges of the shadows cast by the x-ray exposure. Three main factors influence the amount of penumbra on a radiograph. Changes in these factors increase or decrease the radiographic detail. The first factor is the *size of the focal spot*. The larger the focal spot is, the more pronounced

the penumbra effect. Decreasing the focal spot size decreases the penumbra; however, this is not something that can be changed on most equipment. Manufacturers design the focal spot as small as possible while maintaining the ability to dissipate heat effectively.

Another factor that affects the amount of penumbra is the *focal-film distance (FFD)*. This is the distance from the target to the film. The penumbra effect can be decreased by increasing the focal-film distance (Fig. 19-4). There is a limit to which the FFD can be increased because of what is stated in the inverse square law. The intensity decreases at a rate inverse to the square of the distance. In simpler terms, if the FFD is doubled, the mAs must increase four times to maintain the same radiographic density. In most cases this is not practical, because the shortest possible exposure times are necessary to counteract patient motion. An FFD of 36 to 40 inches is sufficient to minimize the penumbra effect.

The third factor affecting penumbra is the *object-film distance* (OFD). This is the distance from the object being imaged to the film. The penumbra is decreased by keeping the OFD as short as possible (Fig. 19-5). Using a combination of these factors, the penumbra can be minimized and good radiographic detail achieved.

Distortion

Foreshortening occurs when the object is not parallel to the recording surface. This distorts size by shortening the length of the object. This occurs mainly when imaging the long bones, such as the humerus or femur. If one

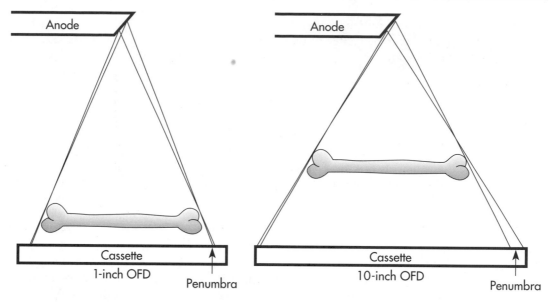

FIG. 19-5 Increasing the object-film distance (OFD) increases the amount of penumbra, decreasing the radiographic detail.

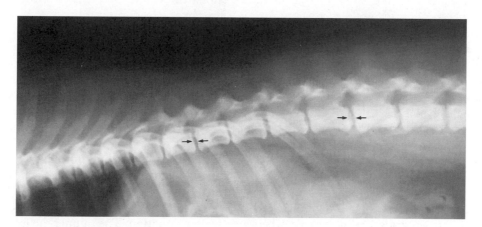

FIG. 19-6 The intervertebral spaces appear narrow toward the edges of the radiograph *(arrows)* as compared with the spaces in the center of the radiograph.

end of the bone is farther from the recording surface than the other, the bone appears shorter. The object being radiographed must be parallel to the recording surface and the OFD as short as possible. Increasing the OFD increases the penumbra and greatly magnifies the size of the object. The degree of magnification increases as the distance to the recording surface increases.

It is important to accurately project areas between a series of radiodense and radiolucent objects. The vertebral column is a good example. The vertebrae must be parallel to the recording surface. When radiographing the cervical vertebrae in lateral recumbency, if the patient is allowed to lie naturally, the midcervical vertebrae tend to sag. This produces false narrowing of the intervertebral spaces. A small amount of padding beneath the patient brings the vertebral column paral-

lel to the recording surface. Care must be taken not to use too much padding because this can elevate the spinal column, also producing false narrowing of the intervertebral spaces.

Distortion can also occur when the x-ray beam is not perpendicular to the recording surface. X-rays in the center of the primary beam penetrate perpendicular to the intervertebral spaces. As the distance from the center of the primary beam increases, the x-rays strike the intervertebral spaces at an increasing angle. False narrowing of the intervertebral space occurs because of this increase in distance from the center of the primary beam (Fig. 19-6). To combat such distortion, sometimes it is necessary to make multiple images of the vertebral column, centering the primary beam over multiple areas. This type of distortion is also apparent when radiographing complex joints, such as the stifle and elbow. When imaging these areas, make sure the center of the primary beam is directly over the joint.

Scatter Radiation

When an x-ray photon strikes an object, it can do one of three things. It can penetrate the object, be absorbed by the object, or produce scatter radiation. Scatter radiation fogs the film, greatly decreasing the contrast. It also is a safety hazard to patients and personnel. Scatter radiation is projected in all directions. Exposure techniques using a high kVp produces more scatter radiation. Body parts measuring 10 cm or more produce enough scatter radiation to significantly decrease detail on the radiograph.

Beam-limiting devices are commonly used to decrease scatter radiation by confining the primary beam to the area being examined. Several types of beam-limiting devices are available. *Cones* are lead cylinders placed over the collimator on the x-ray tube head. This restricts the primary beam to the size of cone used. *Diaphragms* are sheets of lead with a rectangular, square, or circular opening that limits the size of the primary beam to the size of diaphragm used. *Collimators* consist of adjustable lead shutters installed in the tube head of the x-ray machine. Finally, *filters* are used to absorb the less penetrating or soft x-rays as they leave the tube head. They are made of a thin sheet of aluminum and are placed over the tube window.

Grids. Grids are used to decrease scatter radiation and increase the contrast on the radiograph. As the thickness of the area being imaged increases, the amount of kVp required also increases. The higher the kVp is, the more scatter radiation that is produced. To minimize scatter radiation, grids are necessary when radiographing areas 10 cm or more in thickness.

A *grid* is a series of thin, linear strips made of alternating radiodense and radiolucent material. The radiodense strips are made of lead, whereas the radiolucent interspacers are plastic, aluminum, or fiber. The grid is placed between the patient and the cassette. X-rays that penetrate the patient and pass in perfect alignment between the lead strips expose the film. Scatter radiation diverges in all directions and is more likely to be absorbed by one of the lead strips.

The grid also absorbs a portion of the usable x-rays. To compensate for this loss, the number of x-rays generated must be increased by increasing the mAs. Depending on the type of grid used, the increase may be up to 6.6 times the mAs required for the table-top exposure.

Grids are manufactured with either parallel or focused lead strips arranged in crossed or linear configuration.

Parallel grids have the lead strips placed perpendicular to the grid surface. X-rays and scatter radiation that interact with the lead strips are absorbed, whereas the ones that interact with the interspacers pass through to expose the film. A disadvantage of a parallel grid is that the x-ray beam diverges at increasing angles and is absorbed at the periphery of the grid. This decreases the number of x-rays reaching the film near the grid edges, commonly called *grid cut-off.*

Focused grids have the lead strips placed at progressively increasing angles to match the divergence of the x-ray beam. By angling the lead strips, cut-off of the primary beam is eliminated and radiographic density is uniform. The grid manufacturer supplies a list of distances, called the *grid focal distance.* Setting the FFD out of the grid focal distance results in primary beam cut-off on the periphery of the radiograph. Cut-off of the primary beam also occurs if the grid is not perpendicular to or centered with the x-ray tube (Fig. 19-7).

Linear grids have the lead strips placed parallel to each other and parallel with the length of the table. With linear grids, the primary x-ray beam can be angled along the length of the grid without absorption of x-rays by the lead strips.

Crossed grids have two linear grids placed one on top of the other. The lead strips on the top grid cross those on the bottom grid. This type of grid removes more scatter radiation than the linear grid. However, the tube cannot be tilted without producing cut-off. Because crossed grids contain more lead, more x-rays are absorbed, requiring a higher mAs than used with linear grids.

Grids produce thin white lines on the finished radiograph. Visibility of the grid lines can be decreased in three ways. First, the lead strips can be made as thin as possible while retaining the ability to effectively absorb scatter radiation. The thinner the lead is, the thinner the white line is that it produces on the radiograph.

The second way is to increase the number of grid liner per inch, making the individual lines less visible. To increase the grid lines per inch and keep the thickness of the lead the same, the width of the radiolucent strips must be decreased. This produces a grid with more lead in it, which absorbs more of the primary beam and requires a higher mAs. A grid with 80 to 100 lines per inch is sufficient to make the grid lines less visible.

The third way is by using a *Potter-Bucky diaphragm,* also called a "Bucky." This device sets the grid in motion as the x-rays are generated, blurring the white grid lines on the radiograph. The Bucky is placed in a cabinet beneath the x-ray table, with a tray to hold the cassette. When using a grid in combination with a Bucky, fewer lines per inch are necessary. This allows for a lower mAs. One disadvantage of using a Bucky mechanism in veterinary medicine is the noise and vibration it produces. Some animals may object to this and struggle or move during the x-ray exposure.

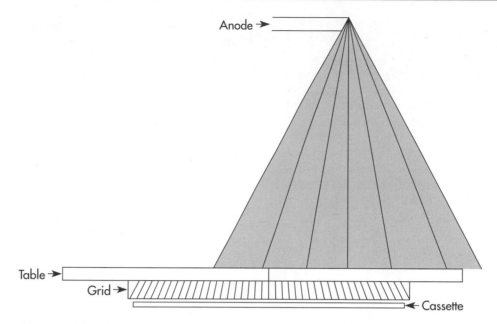

FIG. 19-7 When the grid is not centered with the x-ray tube, grid cut-off occurs. This produces visible grid lines more prominently on one end of the film and an overall decrease in radiographic density.

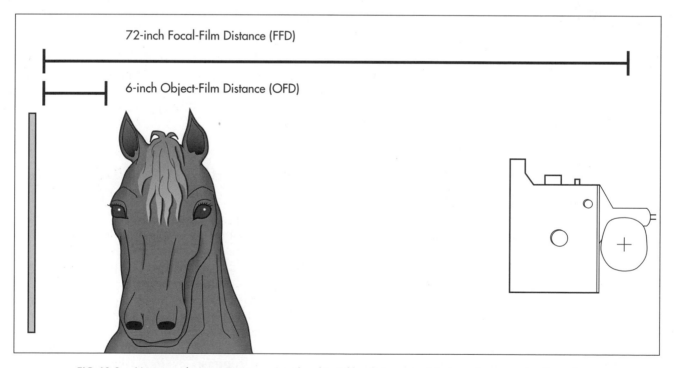

FIG. 19-8 Air gap technique. By increasing the object-film distance to 6 inches, the scatter is allowed to pass by the cassette, not affecting the film. Then, increasing the focal-film distance to 72 inches decreases the magnification and penumbra that occurred from increasing the object-film distance.

Air Gap Technique. Scatter radiation can also be reduced using the air gap technique. This method is most useful in large animal radiography, where use of a grid cassette may not be possible. With this technique, the FFD is increased to 6 feet and the OFD is increased to 6 inches.

By increasing the OFD, the amount of scatter radiation that reaches the cassette is decreased. Increasing the FFD decreases the penumbra and magnification produced by a greater OFD. The air gap acts somewhat like a grid, allowing the scatter radiation to pass by the cassette (Fig. 19-8).

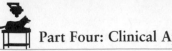

EXPOSURE VARIABLES

Four exposure factors control radiographic density, contrast, and detail. These are mAs, kVp, focal-film distance (FFD), and object-film distance (OFD). Changing one of these factors usually requires adjustments in another factor to maintain the same radiographic density.

mAs

The mAs is a product of the milliamperage and the exposure time. The milliamperage controls the number of electrons in the electron cloud generated at the filament of the cathode. This is done by controlling the temperature of the cathode filament. When the milliamperage (mA) is increased, the temperature of the filament is increased, producing more electrons to form the electron cloud. Increasing the mA increases the amount of radiographic density, because more x-rays are generated.

The other factor is the time during which the electrons are allowed to flow from the cathode to the anode. By varying the exposure time, the number of x-rays generated is controlled. Using a longer exposure time allows the electrons more time to cross from the cathode to the anode, generating more x-rays.

Exposure time and mA are inversely related. The higher the mA is, the shorter the exposure time required to maintain the desired number of x-rays generated. Many different combinations of mA and time can be used to produce the same mAs. For example:

300 mA at $\frac{1}{60}$ sec = 5 mAs

200 mA at $\frac{1}{40}$ sec = 5 mAs

100 mA at $\frac{1}{20}$ sec = 5 mAs

When faced with a choice of which mAs to use, always choose the one with the highest mA and the fastest exposure time. The mAs can be used to adjust the radiographic density by following these rules:

- *To double the radiographic density, double the mAs.*
- *To halve the radiographic density, halve the mAs.*

kVp

The kilovoltage peak (kVp) is the voltage applied between the cathode and the anode. It is used to accelerate electrons flowing from the cathode toward the anode side. Increasing the kVp increases the positive charge on the anode. This causes the electrons to move faster, increasing the force of the collision with the target. This produces an x-ray beam with a shorter wavelength and more penetrating power. The correct kVp setting is determined by the thickness of the part being imaged. The thicker the part, the higher the kVp setting because more penetration is needed. A higher kVp produces a longer scale of contrast and more exposure lat-

itude. A greater exposure latitude allows for more variation in exposure factors, which will still produce a diagnostic radiograph. As with mAs, there are rules when changing the radiographic density with kVp:

- *To double the radiographic density, increase the kVp by 20%.*
- *To halve the radiographic density, decrease the kVp by 16%.*

Focal-Film Distance

Focal-film distance (FFD) is the distance from the target to the recording surface (film). For most radiographic procedures, this distance is held constant, around 36 to 40 inches. In some situations the FFD must be changed. This requires changing one of the other factors to maintain radiographic density. The inverse square law states that the intensity of the x-ray beam is inversely proportional to the square of the distance from the source of the x-ray (see p. 328). If the FFD is doubled, the mAs must be increased four times to maintain radiographic density. The same number of x-rays must diverge to cover an area that is four times as large. Changing the FFD does not affect the penetrating power of the beam, so kVp remains constant.

Object-Film Distance

The object-film distance (OFD) is the distance from the object being imaged to the recording surface (film). This distance should be short as possible to minimize the penumbra effect and the magnification that occurs with a long OFD.

RADIOGRAPHIC FILM AND SCREENS
X-ray Film

X-ray film consists of three layers: a thin protective layer, an emulsion containing silver halide crystals, and a polyester film base. The first layer is a thin, clear gelatin that acts as a protective coating. This protective material helps protect the sensitive film emulsion. The second layer is the emulsion that contains finely precipitated silver halide crystals in a gelatin base.

The emulsion coats both sides of the film base. This gives the film greater sensitivity, increasing the speed, density, and contrast. By increasing the speed of the film, the exposure required to produce an image can be decreased, thus decreasing exposure of the patient and veterinary personnel. The silver halide emulsion is 90% to 99% silver bromide crystals and 1% to 10% silver iodide crystals. The gelatin that suspends the silver halide crystals is a colloid. It liquefies in high temperatures and remains solid in cool temperatures. When placed in the developing chemicals, the emulsion swells, allowing the chemicals to act on the exposed or sensitized crystals without actually losing the crystals. Once the emulsion is dry, it hardens again, trapping the black metallic silver. The film base is in the center of the film, giving it support. It does not produce a visible light pattern or absorb the light, although a blue tint has been added to ease eye strain.

When the silver halide crystals are exposed to electromagnetic radiation, they become more sensitive to chemical change. These sensitized crystals are what make up the *latent image*. When the film is placed into the developer, the latent image is reduced to black metallic silver. The remaining silver halide crystals are removed in the fixer. This produces varying shades of black metallic silver and the clear film base.

Film is sensitive to all types of electromagnetic radiation. These include gamma radiation, particulate radiation (alpha and beta), x-rays, heat, and light. Film is also sensitive to excessive pressure, so care must be taken when handling and storing radiographic film.

The two types of film used in veterinary radiography are *screen-type film* and *direct-exposure film*. Screen-type film is more sensitive to the light produced by intensifying screens. Two screen-type films are *blue-sensitive film* and *green-sensitive film*. Blue-sensitive film is more sensitive to light emitted from screens containing blue-light–emitting phosphors. Calcium tungstate and some rare-earth phosphors are the most common blue-light–emitting phosphors. They emit light in the ultraviolet, violet, and blue light range. Green-sensitive film is most sensitive to light from green-light–emitting phosphors. Rare-earth phosphors are the most common green-light–emitting phosphors.

Direct-exposure film is more sensitive to direct x-rays than it is to light. Because it does not use the intensifying effect of the screens, it requires a higher mAs than screen film. General anesthesia or heavy sedation may be necessary to prevent patient motion and blurring on the radiograph because of the higher mAs. Direct-exposure film is mainly used to image the extremities or rostral mandible or maxilla, where good detail is needed. It is packaged in a paper folder enclosed in a stout light-proof envelope. Take care when handling this film, because it is protected only by paper. Pressure artifacts can easily occur. Some direct-exposure film can only be manually processed because of the thickness of the emulsion. However, some types of direct-exposure film can be processed in an automatic developer.

Film speeds are rated as *high* (regular or fast), *average* (par), and *slow* (detail). The faster the film, the more sensitive it is and the less mAs it requires. High-speed film requires less exposure than slow-speed film to produce a given radiographic density. Film speed is changed by increasing the size of the silver halide crystals. High-speed film has larger silver halide crystals than average-speed or slow-speed film. The drawback

to using high-speed film is that, with the larger crystal size, the image has a more granular appearance. This decreases the detail considerably. Average-speed film should be used for most veterinary radiography.

Another important feature in x-ray film is *film latitude*. This is the film's inherent ability to produce shades of gray. Film with long or increased latitude can produce images with a long scale of contrast (many shades of gray). Longer-latitude film is desirable, because it allows for greater exposure errors but still produces a diagnostic radiograph.

Proper storage and handling of the film are important to ensure a good diagnostic radiograph. Unexposed film should be stored in a cool, dry place, away from strong chemical fumes. A base fog can develop if film is stored under adverse conditions over a long period. Film is pressure sensitive, so it should be stored on end and not laid flat on its side.

Intensifying Screens

Intensifying screens contain fluorescent crystals bound to a cardboard or plastic base. When exposed to x-rays, they emit foci of light. Placing radiographic film in direct contact with the screens accurately records any x-rays that penetrate the patient. Approximately 95% of the film's radiographic density is due to fluorescence of the intensifying screens and only 5% is due to direct x-ray exposure. For each x-ray photon the screen absorbs, it emits 1000 light photons, amplifying the photographic effect of the x-rays. The film is sandwiched between two screens mounted inside a light-proof cassette. The cassettes hold the film in close uniform contact with the screens (Fig. 19-9).

The screens are supported by a plastic or cardboard base. Next to the base is a thin reflecting layer, which reflects the light back toward the film side or front of the screen. The third is the phosphor layer. The two

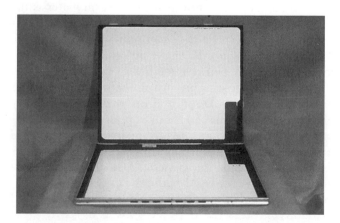

FIG. 19-9 Cassettes hold the film in close uniform contact with the screens.

most common phosphors used are calcium tungstate and compounds containing rare-earth elements. Calcium tungstate is a "blue light" emitter. Some of the rare-earth phosphors also emit blue light. Lanthanum oxybromide and gadolinium oxysulfide are rare-earth phosphors that emit green light. The rare-earth phosphors differ from calcium tungstate in their increased ability to absorb x-rays and convert them into light energy. Rare earth screens allow shorter exposure time compared with a calcium tungstate screen of the same thickness. Over the phosphor layer is a thin, waterproof protective coating that prevents static during cassette loading and unloading, provides physical protection, and provides a surface that can be cleaned.

Intensifying screens are available in three different speeds: high (regular), par (medium), and slow (detail or fine). High-speed screens require less exposure time as compared with the par or slow speeds, but detail is decreased. With shorter exposure times, high-speed screens are ideal for imaging soft tissues, such as the thorax and abdomen, that are accompanied by unavoidable movement. Better detail can be achieved with slow-speed screens requiring longer exposure time. When changing from a high-speed screen to a par-speed screen, the mAs must be increased two times. When changing from high speed to slow speed, the mAs must be increased four times to maintain radiographic density.

Proper care of intensifying screens is very important in veterinary radiography. Regular cleaning is necessary to ensure that the screens are free from dirt and foreign material. Such material can block the light emitted from the screens, leaving parts of the film unexposed. The result is a white area on the film in the likeness of the foreign material. Identifying the cassettes on the screens and on the outside of the cassette enables the dirty cassette to be retrieved and cleaned. Processing chemicals can cause permanent damage if the screen surface is not promptly cleaned. The screens should be cleaned with a soft, lint-free cloth and screen cleaning solution. If a commercial cleaner is not available, warm water is the next best thing. Do not use denatured alcohol or abrasive products, because they can damage the protective coating and phosphor layer. Be sure to allow the screen to completely dry before reloading.

Cassettes are precision instruments and should be handled that way. Do not drop them or set heavy objects on them. This can result in poor film-screen contact and blurring of one area of the image. To check the film-screen contact of your screens, place paper clips over the surface of the cassette. Use enough to completely cover every area. Expose the cassette using 50 to 60 kVp and half the mAs you would use for non-grid extremity. Process the film and view it dry. Any areas with poor film-screen contact are indicated by a blurred image of the paper clips.

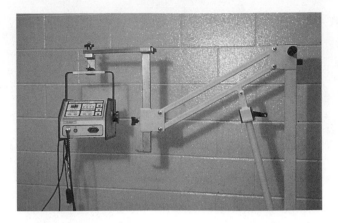

FIG. 19-10 Tempo Technology Laseray portable x-ray unit.

X-RAY EQUIPMENT

There are many factors to consider when choosing x-ray equipment. The needs of individual practices vary, depending upon the species majority, the case load, and the degree of technology desired.

There are three basic types of x-ray equipment to choose from: portable, mobile, and stationary units. A *portable unit* can be carried to the animal. These machines generally have a fixed mA set by the manufacturer at 15 to 30 mA, a variable kVp ranging from 40 to 90, and exposure times as short as $1/120$ seconds (Fig. 19-10). Portable units are ideal for large animal extremities but can be used to radiograph some small animals. Because the mA is fixed, the exposure time is changed to increase the radiographic density. For this reason, motion can be a problem for some exposures because of the prolonged exposure times.

The *mobile x-ray machine* can be transported to the patient; however, because of its large size, it is limited to in-hospital use, such as in the treatment room or perhaps in a driveway (Fig. 19-11). These units generally produce a maximum 300 mA, 125 kVp, and $1/120$ second exposure. The tube head on a mobile unit can be lowered to the ground for large animal radiography or suspended above a table for small animal radiography.

Stationary units are those that are installed in a room with proper shielding for radiography. These units have many different exposure capabilities, depending on the quality desired. A general small animal practice that does mainly routine radiographic examinations may be well served by a machine with 300 mA, 125 kVp, and at least $1/60$ second output (Fig. 19-12). However, practices that provide specialty services, such as internal medicine or surgery referrals, may require higher-output equipment.

Case load should be taken into account when choosing x-ray equipment. If a practice has an average of one to two cases requiring radiographs each week, with the

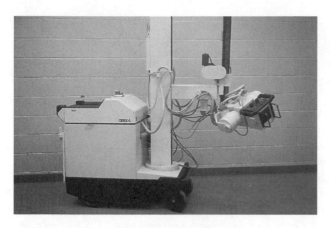

FIG. 19-11 AMX-4 mobile x-ray unit. This unit has been modified to allow the tube head to be lowered to the ground.

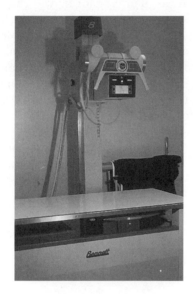

FIG. 19-12 Stationary Bennett x-ray machine.

majority of those being large animal extremities and an occasional small animal film, a portable unit might be considered. If a practice has an average of 3 to 15 radiography cases per week, with a mixture of large and small animals, a mobile unit might be considered. A high-volume practice that radiographs an average of more than 16 cases per week would benefit from a stationary unit.

Accessory equipment used depends on the type of x-ray machine needed. Basic equipment requirements for a stationary x-ray machine include the x-ray generating system, collimator, grid, table, tube stand, and positioning aids. Because most large animal extremity radiographs are made with portable or low-output x-ray machines, tube stands and cassette holders should be used. These pieces of accessory equipment allow the individuals to be positioned farther from the primary beam, thus decreasing personal exposure. The cassettes or x-ray tubes should never be hand held.

FLUOROSCOPY

Fluoroscopy uses a device called a *fluoroscope* to record an x-ray image on a fluorescent screen. Fluoroscopy differs from conventional radiography in several ways. With fluoroscopy, the x-ray tube is mounted beneath the table and a continual flow of x-rays is directed up toward a fluoroscopic screen. The image is then transferred to a monitor and can be recorded on spot film or videotape. Conventional radiography produces a single exposure from an x-ray tube suspended above the table. The image is captured on radiographic film. Fluoroscopy should never be used in place of radiography. Radiation risks greatly increase with constant x-ray production used in fluoroscopy. One method used to decrease the risk to personnel while using fluoroscopy is to depress the x-ray button intermittently instead of holding it down continuously.

RADIATION SAFETY

Ionizing radiation can be a difficult concept to grasp, because at diagnostic levels it cannot be seen, felt, or heard by the patient or operators. Why is radiation safety important? Radiation ionizes intracellular water. This releases toxic products, which can damage critical components of the cell, such as DNA. When radiation comes in contact with the cells of living tissue, it can:
- Pass through the cells with no effect
- Produce cell damage that is repairable
- Produce cell damage that is *not* repairable
- Kill the cells

Radiation damages the body in several ways. It may have *carcinogenic effects,* which means that cancer may develop in body tissues. Effects on the body may be *somatic,* occurring in future generations. Tissues that are most sensitive to ionizing radiation are those with rapidly growing or reproducing cells. The reproductive organs may suffer from temporary or permanent infertility, decreased hormone production, or mutations. The hematopoietic (blood-forming) cells are relatively sensitive to ionizing radiation. The lymphocytic series of blood cells is most sensitive. Damage to these cells can reduce resistance to infection and cause clotting disorders. The thyroid gland, intestinal epithelium, and lens of the eye are also radiosensitive. There may be an increased incidence of squamous-cell carcinoma with chronic, low-level skin exposure. Radiodermatitis (reddened, dry skin) can result from excessive, chronic, low-level radiation exposure.

The developing fetus is sensitive to the effects of ionizing radiation. The degree of sensitivity depends on the stage of pregnancy and the dose received. The preimplantation period (0 to 9 days) is the most critical time for the embryo regarding intrauterine lethality. The period of organogenesis (10 days to 6 weeks) carries the greatest risk of congenital malformation in the fetus, because this is the critical development period for fetal organs. The fetus may have skeletal or dental malformations. Other abnormalities include microphthalmia (small eyes) and overall growth retardation. A fetal dose greater than 25 rads (0.25 Gray) is recognized as the threshold for significant damage to the fetus (for an explanation of these units of measure, see following terminology section). The fetal period (6 weeks to term) is the least sensitive time for the fetus; however, growth and mental retardation may still occur. Irradiation after 30 weeks is less likely to cause abnormalities because the sensitivity of the fetus approaches that of the adult.

Terminology

REM stands for Roentgen Equivalent Man. REM is used to express the dose equivalent that results from exposure to ionizing radiation. REM takes into account the quality of radiation, so doses of different kinds of radiation can be compared. *Sievert (SV)* is the current terminology used to define a REM (1 SV = 100 REM). A *millirem (MREM)* is equal to 0.001 REM or 1/1000 REM. A *rad* is the Radiation Absorbed Dose. Current terminology is *Gray (GY) (1 GY = 100 rad)*. This chapter concerns x-rays only and not other types of radiation, so rads can be considered equivalent to REMs. Other types of radiation

must have a quality factor figured in to determine the dose. MPD is the Maximum Permissible Dose. This may be calculated by the following equation:

$$\text{MPD in REMs} = \text{current age (in years)}$$

The National Council on Radiation Protection and Measurements recommends that the dose for occupationally exposed persons not exceed 5 REM per year. An occupationally exposed individual is one who normally performs his or her work in a restricted access area and has duties that involve exposure to radiation. *ALARA* stands for As Low As Reasonably Attainable. The MPD for nonoccupational persons is 10% of the MPD for occupationally exposed persons, or 0.5 REM per year. This is known as the *ALARA MPD*. Also, a fetus should not receive more than 0.5 REM during the entire gestation period. A pregnant employee who chooses to continue working around radiation-producing devices should wear an additional badge at waist level, underneath the lead gown, to monitor the fetal dose. This badge should not exceed 0.05 REM per month.

There are three important ways to minimize occupational exposure to radiation. The first is *lead shielding*. Lead shielding should be a requirement for all personnel remaining in the room while an exposure is made. Lead gowns, gloves, and thyroid shields should all contain at least 0.5 mm of lead. Lead-based glasses can also be worn to protect the lens of the eye.

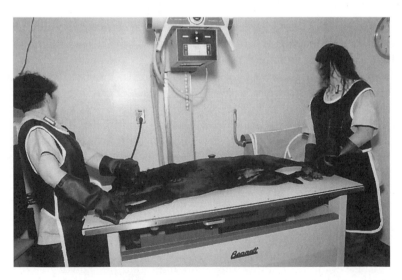

FIG. 19-13 Proper radiation safety practices. The restrainers have increased their distance from the primary beam by leaning back. They are also protecting the lenses of their eyes by looking away.

Lead apparel is very expensive, so it should be handled appropriately. Lead aprons should be draped over a rounded surface, without folds or wrinkles, to prevent cracks in the lead. Lead gloves can be stored with open-ended soup cans inserted to prevent cracks and to provide air circulation to the liners. Lead gloves should be radiographed every 6 months to check for damaged areas. Lead gowns should be checked every 12 months to screen for holes and cracks in the lead. A commonly used technique for this procedure is 5 mAs and 80 kVp. This can be adjusted as needed to attain the proper density in your radiographs.

Another method for decreasing personnel exposure is by *increasing the distance from the primary beam*. Personnel restraining the animal should try to remain as far as possible from the x-ray source during the exposure. During exposure, the restrainers should lean back and look away from the beam to protect the lenses of their eyes (Fig. 19-13). Employees should take care to wear lead apparel properly to obtain full protection, unlike the personnel in Fig. 19-14. Placing a glove on top of a hand for protection does not protect the hand from scatter radiation. The scatter can come from any direction, including from under the tabletop.

A third technique for reducing radiation exposure is *reduced exposure time*. Using the fastest film-screen combinations allows reduced exposure time for the patient and personnel. Proper darkroom practices and technique charts allow for consistent production of high-quality films, which reduces the number of repeated radiographs. It is very important to collimate the beam down to the area of interest, because this reduces exposure of personnel to scatter radiation. Cones and diaphragms may also be attached to the tube window to increase detail and reduce scatter radiation. A 2-mm aluminum filter is used at the tube window to filter out soft rays that are too weak to penetrate the patient. If these rays are not filtered out, they scatter about the room, fogging the film and striking personnel.

Each clinic should have a radiation protection supervisor. This role can be filled by a veterinary technician. Responsibilities include educating personnel on radiation safety, monitoring safety practices, and maintaining a radiologic badge system. The supervisor also maintains x-ray equipment, darkroom facilities, and radiographic records. A good radiation control program consists of safe x-ray equipment, low-exposure techniques, shielding, and monitoring personal radiation exposure (Box 19-1). The x-ray equipment is usually under control of the state government (e.g., State Board of Health). Regulations vary between states, so check with your state government about their policy regarding radiation-producing devices.

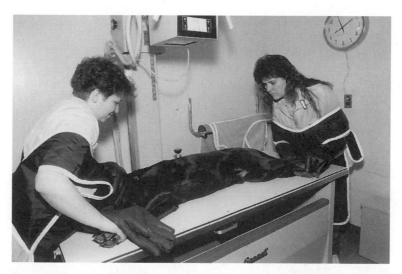

FIG. 19-14 Improper radiation safety practices. The restrainers are leaning in and looking at the patient. Also, one hand is not properly gloved.

DARKROOM TECHNIQUES

Along with a good technique chart, proper darkroom techniques should be followed to ensure consistent production of high-quality radiographs. Properly exposed radiographs can quickly become nondiagnostic with poor film handling and darkroom techniques.

Darkroom Setup

For most veterinary practices the darkroom does not need to be large or fancy, as long as the layout is designed for efficiency. The room must be just large enough to provide a "dry bench" area away from the "wet bench" area (Fig. 19-15). The dry bench area is for unloading and loading cassettes and film storage. The wet bench is for film processing and drying. These areas must be separated to prevent processing chemical splashes from damaging the dry films or sensitive intensifying screens. In a small room this can be achieved by placing a partition between the two areas. Sufficient electrical outlets should be available to power the safelights, viewboxes, and labeling equipment.

The most important feature of a darkroom is that it must be *light tight*. White light that leaks around the door, through a blackened window, or around ventilation fans can fog the film. Film is more sensitive after it has been exposed to x-rays, so even low-grade light leaks decrease the quality of the finished radiograph. When checking for light leaks, stand in the darkroom for

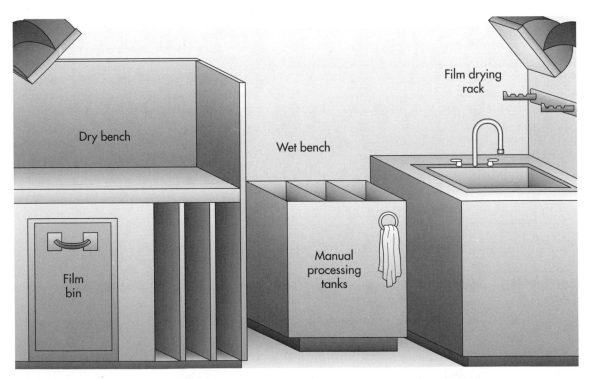

FIG. 19-15   Schematic drawing of a darkroom. Notice the dry bench has been separated from the wet bench by a partition.

at least 5 minutes to allow your eyes to adjust to the darkness. Look around the door frame, ventilation fan, or blackened windows for any signs of white light. When performing this test, vary the intensity of light outside the door. Because work in the darkroom is done with a limited amount of light, painting the walls and ceiling a light color that reflects the available light helps greatly.

The darkroom should have *adequate ventilation* to prevent volatile chemical fumes from accumulating in the room. These fumes can cause fogging of the film, damage to electrical equipment, and even health problems for personnel. A light-tight ventilation fan installed in the ceiling helps remove the fumes and also controls the temperature and humidity in the room. The exhaust from automatic processors and film dryers should also be vented away from the darkroom, because they contain volatile chemical fumes.

Cleanliness is important in the darkroom, because intensifying screens and the film are exposed to this area. Dirt and hair on countertops can fall into cassettes, causing white artifacts on subsequent radiographs from that cassette. Chemical spills also cause artifacts on the radiographs and damage the intensifying screens. Keeping both wet and dry areas of the darkroom clean prevents these problems. Film hangers for manual processing should also be cleaned regularly. Chemicals that remain on the hanger clips could drip down the next film to be processed, causing an artifact.

Film Identification

Permanent labeling is necessary for all radiographs. Each film must be identified before the film is processed for legal purposes and for certification organizations. The labeling can be done during the exposure or after the exposure, but it must be done before the film is processed. The label should include the clinic name, date, owner's name, address, patient's name, and some patient data, such as age and breed.

There are several methods for film identification. One method is the photo labeler. This uses a cassette containing a leaded window that protects the area during exposure. During identification, the window slides back from the protected area to expose the information on a card. This forms a latent image of the information on the film. Manual printers are similar to photo labelers, except they use a flash of light through an information card to produce a latent image on the film. The manual printer is placed in the darkroom and the film is taken out of the cassette to be identified. Another method uses lead letters or radiopaque tape. These are placed on the cassette during exposure of the radiograph.

Safelights

Safelight illuminators are important for darkroom processing. A safelight provides sufficient light to work in the room but does not cause fogging of the film. Safelights can be mounted to provide light directly or indirectly. With direct lighting, the safelight is mounted at least 48 inches above the workbench and directed toward the workbench. Indirect lighting has the safelight directed toward the ceiling and uses the reflected light to illuminate the room. With indirect lighting, the safelight can be mounted closer to the bench but should be as high as possible (Fig. 19-16).

Many types of safelight filters are available to filter out light in different areas of the light spectrum. The type of film used dictates which filter is necessary. Film that is "blue-light sensitive" requires a safelight that filters out blue and ultraviolet light. Film that is "green-light sensitive" requires a safelight to filter both green and blue light. This filter can also be used with blue-light–sensitive film. A red light bulb should never be used to replace a safelight filter. It does not filter the light; it only colors it. A white frosted 7 1/2- to 10-watt bulb is recommended for most safelight filters.

Periodically check the safelight filter. First, make a moderate exposure on a film using approximately 1 to 2 mAs and 40 to 50 kVp. Film that has been exposed to x-rays is more sensitive to low-grade light, producing an overall fogged appearance. Cover two thirds of the film with black paper or cardboard and allow the remaining one third to be exposed to the safelight for 30 seconds. This is a little longer than it should take to place the film in an automatic processor or to place the film on a hanger and into the manual tanks. After 30 seconds, uncover another one third of the film and wait 30 more seconds. Repeat the process for the final one third and develop the film. This test exposes portions of the film to the safelight for 30 seconds, 60 seconds, and 90 seconds. Once the film is dry, look for areas of increased film density. If an increase in density is detected, a close check of the darkroom is necessary. Improper safelight distance, a cracked safelight filter, and light leaking around the filter can all cause film fogging.

Manual Processing

Equipment. Manual processing tanks are usually made from stainless steel and are large enough to accept 14-inch × 17-inch film hangers. Tanks with 5-gallon capacity are sufficient. Plastic or wooden lids are needed to cover the developer and fixer tanks. This reduces the rate of evaporation and oxidation of the chemicals. Separate stirring rods for the developer and fixer are used to mix the chemicals before processing. Also, an accurate timer and a floating thermometer should be available.

Developer. The developer's main function is to convert the sensitized silver halide crystals into black metallic silver. Sensitized silver halide crystals are those that

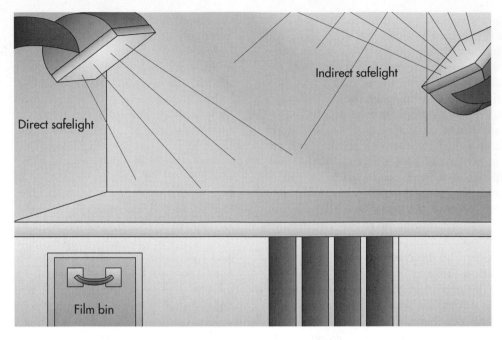

FIG. 19-16   Direct and indirect safelight illumination.

have been exposed to electromagnetic radiation, making them susceptible to chemical change. The developer contains five ingredients: a solvent, reducing agents, restrainer, activator, and a preservative.

Water is used as the *solvent* to keep all the ingredients in solution. It also causes the film emulsion to swell so that the reducing agents can penetrate the sensitized crystals.

The *reducing agents* change the sensitized silver halide crystals into black metallic silver. The most common reducing agents are a combination of hydroquinone and p-methylaminophenol.

The *restrainers* are used to protect the unexposed silver halide crystals by preventing the reducing agents from affecting the unsensitized crystals. Potassium bromide and potassium iodide are the most common restrainers. Bromide ions are produced during the exchange between the reducing agents and the sensitized crystals. In a fresh solution, the bromide ions are not available.

They are added as a starter solution but are not placed in replenishing solutions. Excessive bromide ions inhibit the reducing agents.

The *activator* helps to soften and swell the film's emulsion so that the reducing agents can work effectively. Reducing agents cannot function in an acidic or neutral solution. The activators, usually a carbonate or hydroxide of sodium or potassium, provide an alkaline pH in the range of 9.8 to 11.4.

The *preservative* prevents the solution from rapidly oxidizing. Sodium and potassium sulfite are the most commonly used preservatives.

Developing chemicals are manufactured in two forms: liquid and powder. The liquid form requires dilution with water. The powder form should never be mixed in the darkroom, because the chemical dust contaminates unprotected film, causing artifacts. Always mix the powder in a bucket outside the darkroom and then finish the dilution in the darkroom.

Developing x-ray film is a chemical process that depends on the duration of immersion in the chemicals and the temperature of the chemicals. The recommended time for development is 5 minutes. This allows just enough time for the reducing agents to convert the sensitized silver halide crystals. The temperature of the chemicals is also important. The warmer the temperature, the more the emulsion swells and the faster the chemicals work. Cold temperatures also affect the chemicals by decreasing their ability to penetrate the film emulsion. Manufacturers generally recommend a temperature for the chemicals they produce. Most use 68° F (20° C), with 5 minutes of developing time. For some cases this may not be possible, so the time can be adjusted to compensate for the increase or decrease in temperature. The time can be decreased by 30 seconds for every 2° increase in developer temperature. Also, the time can be increased by 30 seconds for every 2° decrease in developer temperature. This applies only between 65° F (18° C) and 74° F (23° C).

Rinse Bath.   The rinse bath removes developer from the film, preventing carryover into the fixer tank. Agitating the film in the running water bath for 30 seconds adequately removes the developer. The rinse water should be continually exchanged to prevent accumulation of developer. The temperature of the incoming rinse water can often be used to regulate the temperature of the developer and fixer tanks.

Fixer. The fixer removes the unchanged silver halide crystals from the film emulsion, leaving the black metallic silver. It also hardens the film emulsion, decreasing the susceptibility to scratches. The fixer contains five ingredients: a solvent, a fixing agent, an acidifier, a hardener, and a preservative.

As with the developer, the *solvent* for the fixer is water. It keeps the ingredients in solution and causes the film emulsion to swell, allowing the fixing agents to reach the unexposed crystals. The *fixing agent* is sodium or ammonium thiosulfate. This clears the remaining silver halide crystals from the film emulsion. The *acidifier* is acetic or sulfuric acid and is used to neutralize any alkaline developer remaining on the film. Ammonium chloride is used as a *hardener*. It hardens and prevents excessive swelling of the film emulsion, shortening the drying time. The final ingredient is the *preservative*. As with the developer, sodium sulfite is used to prevent decomposition of the fixing agents.

Fixer chemicals are manufactured in two forms: liquid and powder. The liquid form requires dilution with water. It is more expensive than the powder form but is more efficient. The powder form requires dissolving and mixing to get it into solution. It should never be mixed in the darkroom, because the chemical dust can contaminate unprotected film, causing artifacts. Always mix the powder in a bucket outside the darkroom and then finish the dilution in the darkroom. Also the powder requires a longer clearing time than the liquid form.

The fixing process is also dependent on immersion time and temperature of the chemicals. The standard temperature is 68° F (20° C), and the fixing time is double the developing time. The temperature affects the time the film is left in the fixer. The warmer the chemicals are, the shorter the fixing time is. The film can be removed from the fixer after 30 seconds and viewed with white light. However, it must be placed back into the fixer for the remainder of the time. The clearing time increases as the thickness of the emulsion increases. Direct-exposure film has a thicker emulsion and requires a longer time in the fixer.

Final Wash. The final wash rinses away the processing chemicals. Failure to rinse the film completely results in a film that eventually becomes faded and brown. This is due to oxidation of the chemicals remaining in the film emulsion. The wash tank should have fresh circulating water to decrease the time needed for the final wash. Generally, the wash time is at least 30 minutes.

Maintaining the Tanks. There are two methods for maintaining manual processing tanks. The first is the *exhausted method*. With this method, allow the chemicals to drain back into their respective tanks and not into the wash tank. This permits the exhausted chemi-

---

Box 19–2 Steps for manual processing

Daily items to check:
- Check chemical temperature (optimal chemical temperature is 68° F (20° C).
- Stir both of the chemicals.
- Check the chemical levels.
- Clean countertops.
- Turn on water to the wash tank.

Processing individual films:
1. Locate the proper size hanger(s).
2. Set the timer.
3. Turn on the safelight.
4. Turn off the white lights.
5. Unload the cassette and place the film on the hanger.
6. Immerse the film in the developer. The optimal time is 5 minutes at 68° F (20° C).
7. Gently agitate the film to dislodge any air bubbles that may cling the film's surface.
8. Reload the empty cassette.
9. After 5 minutes of developing time, place the film in the wash tank and agitate for 30 seconds.
10. Lift the film out of the wash tank, allowing the excess water to drain back into wash tank.
11. Place the film into the fixer tank and agitate gently to dislodge air bubbles that cling to the surface.
12. Turn on white lights without causing problems after 30 seconds clearing time in the fixer.
13. Place the film in the wash tank for 30 minutes or longer, depending on the amount of water replenishing.
14. After washing the film, let it hang until dry.

Every 3 months:
- Completely drain all three tanks.
- Clean the tanks with a 1:32 solution of laundry bleach and water.
- Rinse the tanks well.
- Refill the tanks with fresh chemicals.

---

cals to remain in the tank, maintaining the chemical levels. The second method is the *replenishing method*. Do not allow the chemicals to drain back into their respective tanks, but place them in the wash tank. The chemical levels are maintained with replenishing chemicals that are more concentrated than the initial solutions. In this way, the potency and levels of the chemicals can be preserved. With either method the chemicals should be changed every 3 months.

Box 19-2 details the steps for manual processing.

Automatic Processing. Use of an automatic processor has some advantages over manual processing. Automatic processors can develop film more quickly. They can process and dry a film in 90 to 120 seconds. Also, automatic processors consistently provide high-quality radiographs. This eliminates the need for repeat radiographs because of processing errors.

Automatic processors move the film through the developer, fixer wash bath, and dryers at a uniform rate of speed. Chemicals and film are specially manufactured to withstand the high temperatures involved in automatic processing. The chemicals are kept at temperatures around 95° F (35° C), depending on the type of film and equipment used. The emulsion on film designed for automatic processing is harder than on film designed for manual processing, preventing scratches from the roller. This film can also be manually processed in case of mechanical problems with the automatic processor.

Small tabletop automatic processors are easily maintained in most veterinary practices. The equipment should be completely cleaned every 3 months. This includes draining and cleaning the tanks. A 1:32 solution of laundry bleach (e.g., Clorox) helps to reduce algae and remove chemical buildup. The rollers can be cleaned with a mild detergent and soft sponge. When any cleaning solution is applied to the tanks or rollers, they should be rinsed thoroughly before replacing the chemicals. Also, check the springs and gears for signs of wear and replace if necessary. Wipe the feed tray and top rollers with a clean soft sponge every day. This helps to remove dirt, debris, and chemical residue between episodes of routine maintenance.

TABLE 19-1 Common radiographic artifacts that occur before processing

Artifacts	Possible causes
Fogged film (overall gray appearance)	Film exposed to excessive scatter radiation. A grid is necessary when radiographing areas measuring 10 cm or more. Film exposed to radiation during storage. Film stored in an area that was too hot or humid. Film exposed to a safelight filter that was cracked or inappropriate for type of film used. Film exposed to a low-grade light leak in darkroom. Film expired.
Black crescents or lines	Rough handling of film before or after exposure (Fig. 19-17). Static electricity caused by low humidity. Scratched film surface before or after exposure. Fingerprints from excessive pressure before of after exposure.
Black areas	Black irregular border on one end of film caused by light exposure while still in box or film bin. Black irregular border on multiple sides of film caused by felt damage in cassette.
White areas	Foreign material between film and screen (Fig. 19-18). Chemical spill on screen, causing permanent damage to phosphor layer. Contrast medium on patient, table, or cassette. White fingerprints on film from oil or fixer on fingers before processing.
Visible grid lines	Grid lines on entire film from focal-film distance outside the range of grid's focus. Grid lines more visible on one end of film and overall decrease in radiographic density caused by grid's not being centered in primary beam. Grid lines on entire film caused by grid not being perpendicular to center of primary beam. Grid lines more visible in some areas than others from grid damage.
Decreased detail	Patient motion. Poor film-screen contact. Increased object-film distance. Decreased focal-film distance.

Silver Recovery. When an exposed film is placed in the developer, the exposed silver halide crystals are converted to black metallic silver. The remaining silver halide crystals are removed from the film in the fixer. Over time, the fixer solution becomes rich with silver that can be reclaimed. Silver recovery systems can be attached to automatic processors to filter and store the silver that would normally be discarded down the drain. The black metallic silver in the radiographs can also be recovered.

The manual processing fixer solution, silver recovery systems, and old radiographs can be sold to companies that reclaim the silver. These companies are usually listed in the Yellow Pages under the headings of "Gold and Silver Refiners and Dealers."

RADIOGRAPHIC ARTIFACTS

An *artifact* is any unwanted density in the form of blemishes arising from improper handling, exposure, processing, or housekeeping. Artifacts can mimic or mask a disease process or distract from the overall quality of the film.

Before radiographing an animal, check for external changes on the animal. Remove any dirt or mats from the coat. If the coat is wet, try to dry it as much as possible. Remove any collars, leashes, or halters. Bandage material is visible on radiographs, so remove it if feasible. Tables 19-1 and 19-2 list common artifact problems.

TABLE 19-2 Common radiographic artifacts that occur during manual or automatic processing

Artifacts	Possible cause
Increased radiographic density, with poor contrast	Film overdeveloped (longer than manufacturer recommendation). Film developed in hot chemicals. Correct temperature for manual tanks is 68° F (20° C), for automatic processor is 95° F (35° C). Film overexposed.
Decreased radiographic density, with poor contrast	Film underdeveloped (shorter than manufacturer recommendation). Film developed in cold chemicals. Correct temperature for manual tanks is 68° F (20° C), for automatic processor is 95° F (35° C). Film processed in old or exhausted chemicals. Film underexposed.
Uneven development	Lack of stirring allows chemicals to settle to tank bottom. Repeated withdrawal of film from tank to check on development results. Uneven chemical levels.
Black areas, spots, or streaks	Identical black areas on two films processed together from films stuck to one another in the fixer and not cleared properly. Black area on only one film from film sticking to side of tank. Well-defined spots or streaks from developer splash before processing. Black lines along full length of film and equal distance apart from pressure of rollers in processor.
Defined areas of decreased radiographic density	Identical light areas on two films processed together from films sticking together in developer. Light area on one film from film sticking to side of tank during development (Fig. 19-19). Air bubbles clinging to film during development. Well-defined spots or streaks from fixer splash before processing.
Clear areas or spots	Streaks where emulsion scratched away. Large clear areas from leaving film in final wash too long and emulsion sliding off film base.
Entire film clear	No exposure. Film placed in fixer before developer.
Film turns a brown color	Improper final wash.

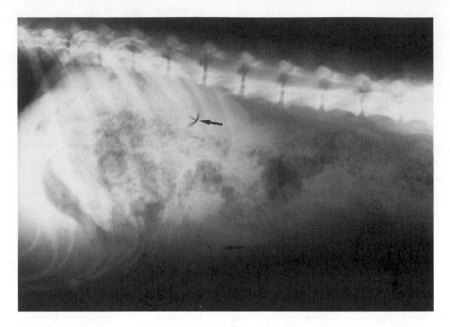

FIG. 19-17   Black crescent from rough handling of the film before or after the exposure.

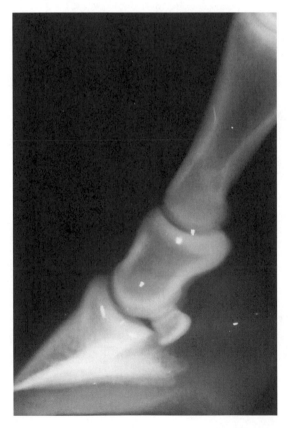

FIG. 19-18   Foreign material between the film and screen blocks light from exposing the film, creating white areas.

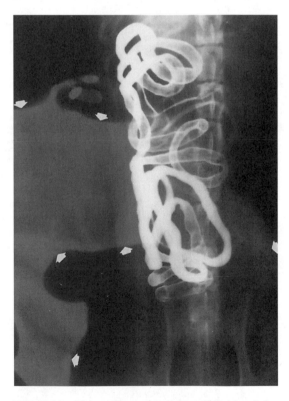

FIG. 19-19   This radiograph stuck to the side of the manual tank while in the developer. The arrows outline the artifact. A light image can still be seen because the film has emulsion on both sides of the film base. One side developed normally.

RADIOGRAPHIC POSITIONING AND TERMINOLOGY

Proper patient positioning is as important as the radiograph itself. Misinterpretations can result from inaccurate positioning. Following is a reference for radiographic procedures conducted in a veterinary hospital.

A basic knowledge of directional terminology is essential when describing radiographic projections. The American College of Veterinary Radiology (ACVR) has standardized the nomenclature for radiographic projections by using the currently accepted veterinary anatomic terms. The projections are described by the direction the central ray enters and exits the part being imaged (see Chapter 4, Fig. 4-1).

Ventral (V): Body area situated toward the underside of quadrupeds.

Dorsal (D): Body area situated toward the back or topline of quadrupeds. Opposite of ventral.

Medial (M): Body area situated toward the median plane or midline.

Lateral (L): Body area situated away from the median plane or midline.

Cranial (Cr): Structures or areas situated toward the head (formerly anterior).

Caudal (Cd): Structures or areas situated toward the tail (formerly posterior).

Rostral (R): Areas on the head situated toward the nose.

Palmar (Pa) Situated on the caudal aspect of the front limb, distal to the antebrachiocarpal joint.

Plantar (Pl): Situated on the caudal aspect of the rear limb, distal to the tarsocrural joint.

Proximal (Pr): Situated closer to the point of attachment or origin.

Distal (Di): Situated away from the point of attachment or origin.

Oblique Projections

Oblique projections are used to set off an area that normally would be superimposed over another area. Some rules should be followed when deciding what type of oblique projection is needed and how it is identified.

- *The area of interest should be as close to the cassette as possible.* This decreases magnification and increases detail.
- *Place a marker on the cassette during exposure to indicate the direction of entry and exit of the primary beam.*

Table 19-3 shows the landmarks used to produce radiographs of various body parts.

CONTRAST STUDIES

The purpose of a contrast study is to delineate an organ or area against surrounding soft tissues. They are useful in determining the size, shape, position, location, and function of an organ. The information obtained from a contrast study complements or confirms findings of the survey radiographs. A contrast study should never replace survey radiographs.

With contrast studies, tissues of interest appear either radiopaque or radiolucent on the finished radiograph. Areas that are radiopaque appear white. Positive-contrast agents are radiopaque on a radiograph. Radiolucent areas on the finished radiograph appear black. Negative-contrast agents produce radiolucencies on a radiograph.

Obtaining survey radiographs before doing a contrast study establishes proper exposure technique and proper patient preparation. In addition, a diagnosis may be achieved from survey radiographs, eliminating the need for the contrast study. Because most contrast studies require multiple images, it is very important to label each film with the time and sequence. Always record the amount, type, and administration route of the contrast agent.

Positive-Contrast Media

Positive-contrast media contain elements with a high atomic number. Elements with a high atomic number absorb more x-rays. Thus, fewer x-rays penetrate the patient and expose the film, making a white area on the radiograph. Two common types of positive-contrast agents are barium sulfate and water-soluble organic iodides.

Barium sulfate is commonly used for positive-contrast studies of the gastrointestinal tract. It is insoluble and not affected by gastric secretions. Therefore, it provides good mucosal detail on the radiograph. Barium sulfate preparations are relatively inexpensive and are manufactured in the form of powders, colloid suspensions, or pastes. One disadvantage of using barium sulfate is that it can take 3 or more hours to travel from the stomach to the colon. Also, it can be harmful to the peritoneum, so it should never be used when gastrointestinal perforations are suspected. Barium is insoluble and the body cannot eliminate it, resulting in granulomatous reactions in the abdominal cavity. While administering barium orally, take care to prevent the patient from aspirating barium into the lungs. Aspiration of large amounts could be fatal. Barium sulfate may also aggravate an already obstructed bowel by causing further impactions.

Water-soluble organic iodides in ionic form are also used for positive-contrast procedures. Different forms of the water-soluble organic iodides can be adminis-

TABLE 19-3 Landmarks used in producing radiographs of various body areas

Body part	Cranial or proximal landmark	Caudal or distal landmark	Center landmark	Comments
Thorax	Manubrium sterni	Halfway between xiphoid and last rib	Heart	Expose at peak inspiration
Abdomen	3 rib spaces cranial to xyphoid	Greater trochanter	Last rib	Expose at peak expiration
Shoulder	Midbody scapula	Midshaft humerus	Over joint space	
Humerus	Shoulder joint	Elbow joint	Midshaft	
Elbow	Midshaft humerus	Midshaft radius	Over joint space	
Radius/Ulna	Elbow joint	Carpal joint	Midshaft	
Carpus	Midshaft radius	Midshaft metacarpus	Over joint space	
Metacarpus	Carpal joint	Include digits	Midshaft	
Pelvis	Wings of ilium	Ischium		
Pelvis VD, flexed	Wings of ilium	Ischium		Pushes stifles cranially
Pelvis VD, extended	Wings of ilium	Stifle joint		Femora parallel to each other and table
Femur	Coxofemoral joint	Stifle joint	Midshaft	
Stifle	Midshaft femur	Midshaft tibia	Over joint space	
Tibia/fibula	Stifle joint	Tarsal joint	Midshaft	
Tarsus	Midshaft tibia	Midshaft metatarsal	Over joint space	
Metatarsus	Tarsal joint	Include digits	Midshaft	
Cervical vertebrae	Base of skull	Spine of scapula		Extend front limbs caudally, collimate width of beam to increase detail
Thoracic vertebrae	Spine of scapula	Halfway between xiphoid and last rib		Collimate width of beam to increase detail
Thoracolumbar vertebrae	Halfway between xiphoid and last rib		Halfway between xiphoid and last rib	Collimate width of beam to increase detail
Lumbar vertebrae	Halfway between xiphoid and last rib	Wings of ilium		Collimate width of beam to increase detail

tered intravenously, orally, or by infusion into a hollow viscus or into the subarachnoid space. Being water soluble, they are absorbed into the bloodstream and excreted by the kidneys.

A commonly used oral form of ionic water-soluble organic iodide is a solution of meglumine and sodium diatrizoate. It is used when performing contrast studies of the gastrointestinal tract when perforation is suspected. When this agent is administered orally, transit through the gastrointestinal system is rapid, usually within 48 to 60 minutes. However, the hypertonic solution draws fluid into the bowel lumen. Thus, the contrast medium is diluted, decreasing the quality of the study. Fluid loss may further complicate hypovolemia in a dehydrated animal. Water-soluble organic iodides should never be used in place of barium sulfate and should be used only when perforations are suspected.

Ionic water-soluble organic iodides for intravenous use are prepared in various combinations of meglumine and sodium diatrizoate. Diatrizoate can also be infused into hollow organs, such as the urinary bladder, or into fistulous tracts. Sodium diatrizoate is commonly used for excretory urography because it provides better opacification of the kidneys. Nausea, vomiting, or decreased blood pressure can occur when a large bolus of contrast medium is injected intravenously. Ionic water-soluble organic iodides cannot be used for myelography, because they are irritating to the brain and spinal cord.

Nonionic water-soluble organic iodides are used for myelography. Because of their low osmolarity and chemical nature, they cause fewer adverse effects when placed in the subarachnoid space. Three commonly used media are metrizamide, iopamidol, and iohexol. Nonionic water-soluble organic iodides are suitable for myelography and can also be used intravenously. However, they are approximately 10 times more expensive than the ionic media. Metrizamide is supplied as a powder because it cannot be heat sterilized and is unstable in solution. Before metrizamide is used, it must be reconstituted and filtered through a 0.22-μ bacteriostatic filter.

Negative-Contrast Media

Negative-contrast agents include air, oxygen, and carbon dioxide. They all have a low atomic number, appearing radiolucent on the finished radiograph. Oxygen and carbon dioxide are more soluble than water. Care must be taken not to overinflate the organs, such as the bladder. Air embolism can occur when air enters ulcerative lesions, causing cardiac arrest.

Double-Contrast Procedures

Double-contrast procedures use both positive- and negative-contrast media to image an organ or area. The most common organs imaged with double-contrast are the urinary bladder, stomach, and colon. In most cases, the negative-contrast medium is added first, then the positive-contrast medium. Mixing negative-contrast medium with positive-contrast medium can cause air bubbles to form, which might be misinterpreted as lesions.

DIAGNOSTIC ULTRASOUND

Diagnostic ultrasound (*ultrasonography*) is a noninvasive method of imaging soft tissues. A transducer sends low-intensity, high-frequency sound waves into the soft tissues, where they interact with tissue interfaces. Some of the sound waves are reflected back to the transducer and some are transmitted into deeper tissues. The sound waves that are reflected back to the transducer (*echoes*) are then analyzed by the computer to produce a gray-scale image. Use of ultrasound in conjunction with radiography gives the veterinarian an excellent diagnostic tool. Radiographs demonstrate the size, shape, and position of the organs. Ultrasound displays the findings found on the radiographs as well as the soft tissue textures and the dynamics of some organs (e.g., motility of the bowel).

Transducers

Ultrasound *transducers* emit a series of sound pulses and receive the returning echoes. A weak electrical current applied to the piezoelectric crystals incorporated in the transducer causes the crystals to vibrate and produce sound waves. After sending a series of pulses, the crystals are dampened to stop further vibrations. When struck by the returning echoes, the crystals vibrate again, and convert these echoes into electrical energy.

Transducers are available in different configurations, which are mechanical or electronic. The scan plane can either be a *sector scan* (pie-shaped image) or a *linear-array scan* (rectangular image). A mechanically driven sector scan can be produced by a belt and pulley used to wobble a single crystal or rotate multiple crystals across a scan plane. Another method of producing a sector scan is with use of phased-array or annular-array configurations. With *phased-array configuration*, the crystals are pulsed sequentially with a built-in delay to create a "pseudo-sector" scan plane. *Annular array* arranges the crystals in concentric rings. By using electronic phasing of the many crystals, annular-array transducers produce a two-dimensional image by steering the entire array through a sector arc.

Sector scanners are useful when imaging areas limited by ribs, gas-filled bowels, or lungs. The narrow near field and wide far field enable the transducer scan plane to be positioned between or around these structures. Linear-array scanners produce a scan plane by alternately firing groups of crystals in sequence. The pulsing of each group of crystals occurs so rapidly that individual pulses cannot be observed by the human eye. Linear-array scanners are useful in areas with unrestricted window size. The rectangular scan plane is ideal for equine tendons or large or small animal transrectal imaging.

The frequency of the transducer determines the amount of detail or resolution of the image. The higher the frequency is, the shorter the wavelength. The shorter the wavelength is, the better the resolution of the image.

Transducers are expensive and the most fragile part of ultrasound equipment. Care must be taken when handling them. Avoid hard impacts that can severely damage the sensitive crystals. Prevent exposure to extreme temperature changes. Some transducers are sensitive to certain types of cleaning agents. Always refer to manufacturer's instructions for appropriate cleaning products.

Display Modes

There are three different display modes: A-mode (amplitude mode), B-mode (brightness mode), and M-mode (motion mode).

A-mode. A-mode is the earliest form of ultrasound and is the simplest as far as computer software. With A-mode, the returning echoes are displayed as a series of peaks on a graph. The higher the intensity of the returning sound is, the higher the peak at that tissue depth. A-mode is not used to show tissue motion or anatomy. The main use in veterinary medicine was to measure the amount of subcutaneous fat in pigs.

B-mode. B-mode uses bright pixels or dots on a screen, whereas A-mode uses peaks on a graph. A dot on the monitor screen corresponds to the depth at which the echo was formed. The degree of brightness is proportional to the intensity of the returning echo. The higher the intensity is, the brighter the dot. The image that is generated is a two-dimensional anatomic slice that is continually updated. This mode is currently used for diagnostic applications.

M-mode. M-mode is the continuous display of a thin slice of an organ over time. M-mode projects the echoes from a thin beam of sound over a time-oriented baseline. The main use is with echocardiography to assess the size of the heart chambers and the motion of the heart valves and walls.

Terminology Describing Echotexture

The terminology used to describe tissue texture within an ultrasound image is simple. *Echogenic* or *echoic* means that most of the sound is reflected back to the transducer. Echogenic areas appear white on the screen. *Sonolucent* means that most of the sound is transmitted to the deeper tissues, with only a few echoes reflected back to the transducer. Sonolucent areas appear dark on the screen. *Anechoic* is used to describe tissue that

FIG. 19-20 An area within an organ or the whole organ that is brighter than the surrounding tissue is described as hyperechoic. Areas that are darker than the surrounding tissue are described as hypoechoic. Areas that are the same as the surrounding tissue are described as isoechoic.

transmits all of the sound through to deeper tissues, reflecting none of the sound back to the transducer. Anechoic areas appear black on the screen and are generally fluid-filled structures.

Soft tissues are represented not only as black or white but also as many shades of gray. Additional terminology has been established to describe these areas. *Hyperechoic* is used to describe tissues that reflect more sound back to the transducer than surrounding tissues. Hyperechoic areas appear brighter than surrounding tissues. *Hypoechoic* is used to describe tissues that reflect less sound back to the transducer than surrounding tissues. Hypoechoic areas appear darker than surrounding tissues. *Isoechoic* is used to describe tissue that appears to have the same echotexture on the screen as surrounding tissues (Fig. 19-20).

Terminology has been established to describe areas displayed on the monitor screen. The screen is divided into nine zones, with each zone having its own label. In this way the sonographer can verbally indicate the area of interest, such as mid field right or near field left.

Patient Preparation

To achieve an optimal acoustic window and produce the best-quality image, the transducer head must be placed in close contact with the skin. The animal's hair must be clipped and in some cases shaved before the study. Occasionally, thin-coated animals can be imaged with minimal preparation. An acoustic coupling gel is used to eliminate the air interface and to improve the acoustic window. Before applying the acoustic coupling gel, wipe the area with alcohol or generous amounts of soapy water to remove any loose hairs, dirt, and skin oils.

Fasting of small animals before abdominal ultrasound examination is recommended. Ingesta and gas in the bowel decrease the amount of the abdomen that can be visualized.

Instrument Controls

Ultrasound equipment has many controls for adjusting the quality of the image. Improper adjustment of any of these can greatly decrease the quality of the image.

Brightness and Contrast. The monitor has controls to adjust the brightness and contrast for the image being displayed. If the brightness has been adjusted too high or too low on the monitor, compensating with any other control cannot correct the brightness or darkness. Most machines have a gray bar that displays the gray-scale capability. This capability varies from 16 to 128 shades of gray. The brightness and contrast should be adjusted so that black, white, and all the intermediate shades of gray can be seen.

Depth. The depth control allows for adjustment of the amount of tissue being displayed on the monitor. The depth from the surface of the transducer is measured in centimeters. The area of interest (e.g., kidney, heart) should cover at least two thirds of the screen. Decreasing the amount of depth being displayed causes the area in the near field to become larger.

Gain and Power. The gain (overall) and power (output) controls can affect the overall brightness of the image. Gain and power compensate for attenuation of the sound beam as it travels through the tissues. Increasing the gain increases the sensitivity of the transducer to receiving the returning echoes. This can be compared with the volume on a hearing aid. Turning the volume up increases the hearing aid's ability to hear incoming sounds. The power controls the intensity of the sound generated by the transducer. Increasing the power increases the intensity of the sound wave leaving the transducer. The sound is attenuated at the same rate, but a higher-intensity sound wave transmitted into the tissues produces a higher-intensity echo returning to the transducer.

Time Gain Compensation. The controls that make up the time gain compensation (TGC) are the most important and most often improperly set. The purpose of the TGC is to make like tissues look alike. The intensity of the sound decreases progressively as it returns from deeper tissues. For example, when imaging the liver, three similar reflectors located at 4 cm, 6 cm, and 8 cm of depth should have the same brightness on the monitor. However, because of the attenuation of the echoes returning from the deeper tissues, the brightness gradually decreases. To compensate for the loss of energy, TGC adds increasing amounts of electronic gain to the returning echoes. The three echoes returning from different depths then have the same brightness on the monitor.

Three typical controls that make up the TGC are *near field gain, far field gain,* and *delay.* The near field gain controls the amount of electronic gain added to the sound returning from the near field. This should be set so that the echoes blend uniformly with those displayed in the mid field. The far field gain controls the amount of electronic gain added to the echoes returning from the far field. Delay (also called *break point* or *starting point*) controls the depth at which the gain is first applied. This control is used only when imaging areas contain fluid in the near field (e.g., ascites, pleural fluid). Because sound is not attenuated much when traversing fluid, deeper structures appear too bright. Delaying the point at which the electronic gain is started compensates for lack of attenuation through the fluid. When scanning normal tissues, there is no need to apply any delay in the TGC.

If proper brightness cannot be achieved, verify the following items. First, check the brightness and contrast controls on the monitor. If the brightness and contrast controls are incorrectly set, changing the TGC cannot compensate for this error. Next, check the power setting to make sure it is not too low. If all the controls are set correctly, the next step is to attempt to improve the acoustic contact with the skin. This can be done by applying more coupling gel or shaving the clipped area with a razor. If none of these adjustments are productive, change to a lower-frequency transducer. Some resolution is lost, but it is a necessary trade-off when brightness cannot be achieved.

Artifacts

Artifacts can occur during any ultrasound study. Proper identification of these artifacts is important to prevent confusion or misinterpretation. Some artifacts are beneficial in making a diagnosis. Two such artifacts include acoustic shadowing and distant enhancement. Others, if not readily identified, can be confused as part of the anatomy or a disease process.

Acoustic shadowing occurs when the sound is attenuated or reflected at an acoustic interface (Fig. 19-21). This prevents the sound from being transmitted to the deeper tissues, resulting in no echoes or fewer echoes returning from those areas. Structures that can cause acoustic shadowing include bone, calculi, mineralized tissues, and occasionally fat. For acoustic shadowing to occur, the interface must be in the focal zone of the transducer. If not, the shadowed area may be in with echoes from surrounding tissues as the sound beam diverges. This artifact is more pronounced with higher-frequency transducers.

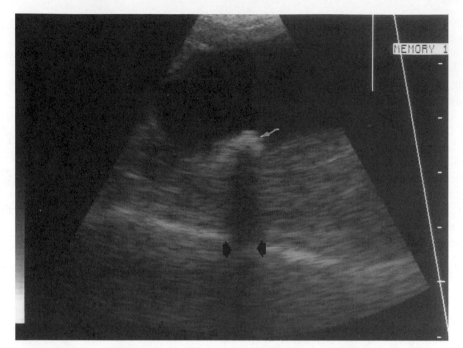

FIG. 19-21 Acoustic shadowing from a calculus in the urinary bladder. The white arrow indicates the highly reflective surface of the calculus. The black arrows indicate shadowing caused by the calculus.

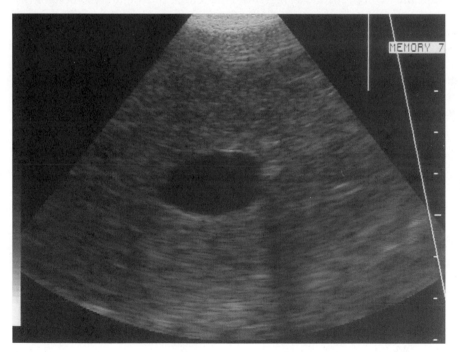

FIG. 19-22 Distance enhancement in the liver is caused by sound waves passing through the fluid-filled gallbladder.

Distant enhancement occurs when the sound beam traverses a cystic structure (Fig. 19-22). Tissues deep to the cystic structure appear brighter than surrounding tissues. The enhancement occurs because the sound that travels through the fluid-filled areas is less attenuated than in surrounding tissues. This artifact is useful in establishing that an anechoic or hypoechoic structure is in fact fluid-filled.

Many artifacts have no diagnostic use, though if not identified as artifacts they can lead to confusion. One of these includes the *slice thickness* artifact. This artifact occurs when imaging an anechoic or hypoechoic structure. Echoes are added when the transducer receives echoes with different amplitudes from the same area at the same depth. The computer then averages these amplitudes and incorporates them in the two-dimensional

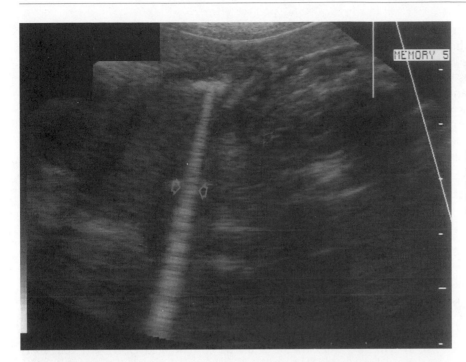

FIG. 19-23 Reverberation artifact caused by gas in the small intestines of a dog. Notice the equally spaced echoic lines (*white arrows*) trailing from the highly reflective interface created by the gas.

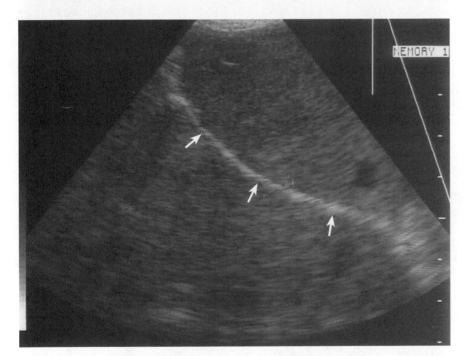

FIG. 19-24 Mirror-image artifact. The arrows indicate the liver/diaphragm to lung interface. In the near field *(top right)* is the actual liver. The far field *(bottom left)* represents the mirror image of the liver.

image. This artifact can be minimized by decreasing the overall gain; however, it does not totally eliminate it.

Reverberation occurs when sound is reflected off a highly reflective interface (e.g., soft tissues to air or soft tissues to bone/metal) and then reflected back into the tissues by the surface of the transducer (Fig. 19-23). This bouncing back and forth can continue until the sound energy has completely attenuated. Each time the sound returns to the transducer, it produces an image at a location on the screen that is proportional to the time of travel between the transducer and the reflective interface. This creates a series of lines per equal distance apart on the screen.

The *mirror-image* artifact creates the illusion of liver on the thoracic side of the diaphragm or the appearance of a second heart beyond the lung interface (Fig. 19-24). This artifact can be produced in areas with strongly reflective interfaces. Sound transmitted into the liver is reflected off the diaphragm. Some of those echoes are not reflected directly toward the transducer but back into the liver. In the liver, some of the misdirected echoes are reflected back to the diaphragm and then to the transducer. The computer sees the misdirected echoes as being reflected from the other side of the diaphragm. One way this artifact can be minimized is by decreasing the depth to include only the area of interest.

ENDOSCOPY

C. BRETZ

Veterinary teams are finding that endoscopes are essential tools for diagnosing many conditions and diseases. The opportunity to examine and obtain tissue samples without the invasiveness of surgery makes endoscopy one of the best methods of evaluating the digestive system. Responsibilities of veterinary technicians assisting with endoscopy include selection, care, and maintenance of the endoscopes, and care and positioning of the patient.

Types of Endoscopes

Rigid endoscopes are commonly used for rhinoscopy, cystoscopy, laparoscopy, arthroscopy, vaginoscopy, colonoscopy, and thoroscopy. *Flexible endoscopes* are used for gastrointestinal endoscopy, duodenoscopy, colonoscopy, and bronchoscopy. Flexible endoscopes are also used for percutaneous placement of gastrostomy tubes in small animals.

Rigid Endoscopes. Rigid endoscopes are composed of a metal tube, lenses, and glass rods (Fig. 19-25). They vary in sizes and characteristics; however, all are composed of a hollow tube containing no fiber bundles. Rigid endoscopes tend to be less expensive than flexible endoscopes, but their uses tend to be limited to that for which they were designed.

Rigid endoscopes should be held by the eyepiece and *not* by the rod. Even slight bending of the rod section could change the angle of deflection, decreasing the degree of visualization. Rigid endoscopes should never be handled in bunches or piled on top of one another.

Flexible Endoscopes. There are two types of flexible endoscopes: fiberoptic and video. *Fiberoptic endoscopes* use glass fiber bundles for transmission of images. These bundles transmit light from the light source to the distal tip of the endoscope. Fiberoptic glass fiber bundles are very fragile and can be damaged easily. Broken fibers show up on the monitor screen as black dots. Too many of these black dots (many broken fiber bundles) can significantly reduce the endoscopist's field of view. For this reason, fiberoptic endoscopes must be handled very carefully and never bent at a sharp angle.

The most recent development in veterinary endoscopy is *video endoscopes*. A microchip located at the distal end of the endoscope records and transmits the image to a computer and then to a monitor screen. The image can

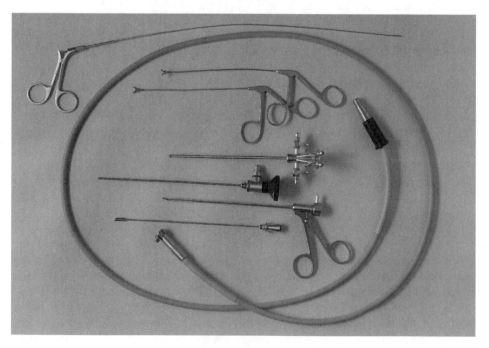

FIG. 19-25 Example of a rigid endoscope. This endoscope is used for cystoscopy and rhinoscopy. The light source cable and several biopsy forceps are also shown.

be recorded on a VCR, and pictures can be recorded to show the owner and be included in the patient's record. Many operators find the video endoscope more ergonomically pleasing, because the controls are held at the waist and not up near the face. Eventually, video endoscopes will replace fiberoptic endoscopes.

Purchasing an Endoscope

Although the cost of an endoscope may be a substantial initial investment, many years of use and its value as a diagnostic tool will make the endoscope more than just a convenience to the veterinary hospital. The endoscope should pay for itself in the first year. The endoscope's life expectancy is 5 to 10 years.

Commonly associated costs include the intravenous catheter, preprocedure enemas, preanesthetic blood studies and evaluation, the endoscopist's time, anesthesia, and laboratory fees. Skilled technical time involved in the preparation and cleaning of the endoscope must be also be considered.

An endoscope of poor quality will rarely be used, so the veterinary team must decide which endoscope is appropriate for the hospital. A good-quality fiberoptic endoscope can be used for many purposes. Reproductive and gastrointestinal endoscopy, colonoscopy, and respiratory procedures can all be performed with one properly functioning endoscope. For most small animal practice situations, a 110-cm gastroscope/duodenal flexible endoscope should provide sufficient length for dogs and cats.

The diameter of the endoscope is also an important factor. Most human endoscopes are appropriate for endoscopic examination of large dogs; however, a human pediatric endoscope (insertion tube diameter 7.9 to 9 mm) is ideal. The larger endoscopes are difficult to pass into the pyloric canal to the duodenum in small dogs and cats.

Some important characteristics that an endoscope should possess include four-way deflection capability, 180-degree upward deflection tip, water flush, air insufflation, and suction. Many models can be completely immersed, allowing thorough cleaning and disinfection.

One can easily locate a good-quality, lower-cost, used endoscope through a human hospital. These hospitals are constantly updating their equipment and are often willing to sell their relatively new equipment at a reduced price. If you are considering a used endoscope, be sure to check for holes, cracks, or scratches on the insertion tube that might promote leakage of fluids into the endoscope. Look through the eyepiece and check for broken fibers, which appear as small black dots. A few fiber bundles can be expected to break over time, but an excessive number of broken bundles inhibits visualization. Also check the intensity of the light by attaching the endoscope to the light source. If you purchase a used endoscope from a human hospi-

tal, be sure to ask for the operator's manual or other information that accompanies the endoscope. If no information is available, call the manufacturer of the endoscope and request a new operator's manual.

The Endoscopy Room

In an ideal situation, all endoscopic examinations are performed in the same room. This room should preferably be out of the way of hospital traffic. Because the lights are usually dimmed during endoscopic examination to reduce glare on the viewing monitor, a room with curtains or shades is ideal. The room should never be so dark, however, that proper anesthetic monitoring is inhibited.

A sturdy cart with three or four shelves can conveniently store the light source, suction unit, endoscope, and any accessory equipment until ready for use. All necessary equipment should be located near this endoscopy unit so that it can be reached quickly if needed during endoscopy. These items should be meticulously organized. The assisting staff must be able to locate any necessary equipment quickly during a procedure.

To avoid complications and delays, the procedure room should be well stocked before the endoscopic examination begins. All anesthetic equipment must be ready before the procedure begins. Procedure cards or checklists are excellent ways to ensure that each type of endoscopic examinations starts with the proper equipment.

Accessory Instruments

Accessory instruments can be passed through the working channel of the flexible endoscope and directed to a specific area. The most basic instruments include biopsy forceps, foreign body removal forceps, and a cytology brush (Fig. 19-26).

Endoscopes are fragile and expensive, so personnel must be instructed in their proper care, use, and maintenance before endoscope use. Before each endoscopic examination, make sure each piece of ancillary equipment is functioning properly, and anticipate the need for these pieces of equipment. They should be cleaned as soon as possible after use or the jaws of the forceps may become locked in the closed position. If this occurs, soaking the tip of the biopsy forceps in warm water for 10 to 15 minutes helps to loosen the debris around the jaws.

All personnel involved with endoscopic procedures should wear latex examination gloves. This protects the animal from contamination and also protects the clinician and technician. The endoscope should not be allowed to directly contact the video accessories or any other potentially conductive object; wearing latex gloves offers an added protection against electrical shock.

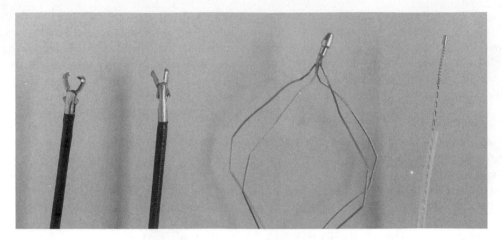

FIG. 19-26 Accessory equipment. *From left to right:* Rat-toothed forceps, biopsy (cup) forceps, basket foreign-body retrieval forceps, and cytology brush.

CLEANING A FLEXIBLE ENDOSCOPE

All endoscopy equipment should be thoroughly cleaned as soon as possible after the procedure. The manufacturer's specific cleaning instructions should be carefully followed. Endoscopes must be handled carefully during cleaning and never placed where they could fall or be bumped. It is also a good idea for the person cleaning the endoscope to wear latex examination gloves.

Gather the necessary supplies:
- Latex examination gloves
- Cleaning solution
- Two large basins for cleaning solution and distilled water
- Distilled water
- Methyl alcohol
- Lint-free gauze pads
- Cotton-tipped applicators
- Channel cleaning brush

Immediately after the procedure, flush water and then air through the air-water channel of the flexible endoscope. Gently wipe off the insertion tube with a soft gauze or cloth that has been soaked in an approved detergent solution. Do not squeeze the flexible section. Place the distal end of the endoscope in detergent water and suction a small amount through. Alternately suction water and then air a few times. Remove the air-water valve, suction valve, and biopsy cap, and place them in a small amount of cleaning solution to soak. Pass the channel cleaning brush through the biopsy channel and suction channel repeatedly until the brush comes out clean. Clean off the brush each time it is passed through the channel.

If the endoscope has a suction cleaning tube, this should then be placed on the biopsy port. Place the end of the suction cleaning tube and the end of the endoscope into a mixture of detergent and water. Cover the suction valve hole with your finger and suction soapy water, then distilled water, and then air to dry the endoscope. Remove the suction cleaning tube and carefully clean the valve holes with a cotton-tipped swab. Clean and rinse the air-water valve, suction valve, and biopsy cap, and replace them on the endoscope.

It is a good preventive measure to lightly lubricate the air-water and suction valves periodically to prevent cracking. Wipe off the outside of the endoscope with an alcohol-soaked gauze pad. Clean the lenses with an approved lens cleaner by applying some lens cleaner onto a soft gauze pad and rubbing the lens; then rub with a clean gauze pad. Replace any lens caps, light source insertion bar covers, and ETO caps before placing the endoscope back into the cabinet. For proper drying of the biopsy channel, leave the biopsy port in an open position.

Biopsy instruments should be immersed in soapy water, brushed carefully with a cleaning brush, and then rinsed. Check to make sure that the jaws of biopsy instruments are not sticking by carefully opening and then closing them.

STORING THE ENDOSCOPE

The ideal way to store a flexible endoscope is in a hanging position in a well-ventilated cabinet. This allows the endoscope to drain completely after cleaning and permits better air movement through the channels. The padded case in which the endoscope was supplied by the manufacturer is another possible storage area; however, little air circulates in these containers and moisture in the channels of the endoscope offers an environment for bacterial growth. Rigid endoscopes are best stored in their original carrying case.

GASTROINTESTINAL ENDOSCOPY

Flexible endoscopes are most commonly used to examine the gastrointestinal tract, including the esophagus. Gastrointestinal endoscopy allows visualization of the upper and lower digestive tract, including its contents.

Patient Preparation

The patient should be fasted for 12 to 24 hours. A longer period of fasting may be required in patients with delayed gastric emptying. An intravenous catheter should be placed and fluid administration started. There are various opinions as to which drugs may impair passage of the endoscope into the duodenum; however, a combination of atropine and morphine is known to make endoscope passage more difficult. Use of these drugs together should be avoided for gastrointestinal endoscopy. Endotracheal intubation and proper endotracheal tube cuff inflation are needed to avoid aspiration of gastric contents in the event of regurgitation.

Place the patient in left lateral recumbency, with a mouth speculum placed to prevent damage to the endoscope from biting. Raise the table to a height that does not require excessive bending of the endoscope near the handpiece (Fig. 19-27). Lubricate the insertion tube with a water-soluble lubricant, such as K-Y Jelly, avoiding the distal end of the endoscope. Use of petroleum-based lubricants, such as Vasoline, is not advised because over time they cause stretching and deterioration of the rubber components of the endoscope. As the endoscope is introduced into the patient's mouth, avoid scraping the endoscope against the teeth in the back of the mouth. Air insufflation is usually needed to facilitate visualization; however, overinsufflation may cause overdistention of the stomach or abdomen and can interfere with ventilation.

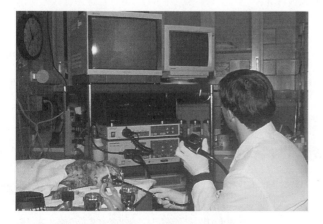

FIG. 19-27 Patient in left lateral recumbency, with a mouth speculum in place. Note that the table is positioned at a height convenient for the endoscopist.

Obtaining Samples

Tissue samples are obtained by grasping the mucosa with biopsy forceps. The biopsy forceps are passed down the operating channel of the endoscope with the forceps jaws in a closed position. Care must be taken to not open or close the forceps too forcefully, as they can become locked or broken. Also, make sure the jaws of the biopsy forceps are in the closed position before bringing them back out through the biopsy channel of the endoscope; otherwise the accessory equipment and the endoscope may be damaged.

Once a tissue sample is obtained, the specimen is gently teased out of the forceps with a 25-gauge needle or shaken directly from the biopsy forceps into the vial of preservative. If the latter technique is used, the biopsy forceps must be rinsed with water before reinsertion into the endoscope channel.

Upon completion of the gastroscopic examination, the stomach and esophagus are suctioned with the endoscope, using gentle external pressure on the abdomen to remove fluids, debris, and excess air.

The endotracheal tube cuff should remain partially inflated when extubating to bring out any remaining material.

COLONOSCOPY

Two types of colonoscopes are available: a rigid colonoscope (Fig. 19-28) and a flexible endoscope. Each requires different protocols for patient preparation and sedation. *Rigid colonoscopy* allows direct examination of the rectum and descending colon. *Flexible colonoscopy* allows examination of the transverse and ascending colon, cecum, ileocolic valve, and ileum.

Ideally, all feces should be removed from the colon before endoscopic examination; however, this is not always possible. Food should be withheld from the patient for at least 36 hours. Several different colonic cleansing protocols can be used, depending upon how cooperative the patient is and the amount of help available. For rigid colonoscopy, a warm-water enema (10 to 20 ml/kg) the evening before the procedure, another enema the following morning, and a final enema 1 hour before the examination usually provide enough cleansing.

To successfully observe the entire colon with a flexible endoscope, the bowel must be completely cleansed before the examination. Colon electrolyte lavage solutions, such as Golytely (Braintree Laboratories, Braintree, MA) or Colyte (Endlaw Preparations, Farmingdale, NY), are administered orally by stomach tube, usually the day before the procedure. Often a repeat dose is given the morning of the examination. These commercial solutions are superior to traditional soapy water enemas. Rigid colonoscopy can be performed using heavy sedation, but

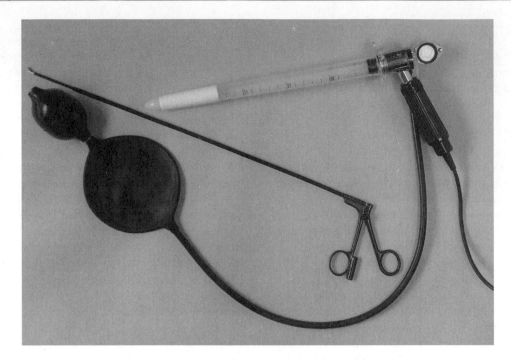

FIG. 19-28   Reusable procto/sigmoidoscope.

a light plane of anesthesia is usually preferred. The patient is placed in right lateral recumbency, with the table slightly tilted so that any residual material drains away from the endoscopist.

Anesthesia is necessary for flexible colonoscopy. The patient is placed in left lateral recumbency to assist passage of the endoscope into the transverse and ascending colon. Colonic insufflation is used to facilitate passage of the endoscope, and often air escapes through the anal sphincter. If this occurs, manual pressure around the anus by a gloved assistant helps to prevent this escape of air.

AIRWAY ENDOSCOPY

Airway endoscopy allows visualization of the trachea and bronchi. It is most useful when diagnosing collapsed trachea, airway parasitism, and foreign bodies. Tissue samples may also be obtained through the endoscope for histopathologic, cytologic, and microbiologic examinations.

The most common endoscope used for medium-size or large dogs is a small-diameter gastrointestinal endoscope. For smaller dogs and cats, a flexible human pediatric bronchoscope is required. Because bronchoscopes have a smaller working channel, any biopsies obtained are smaller. Before use for lower airway endoscopy, the endoscope must be sterilized according to the manufacturer's guidelines.

General anesthesia is required for lower airway endoscopy. In medium-size to large dogs, the endoscope is passed through a shortened sterile endotracheal tube. Oxygen and/or anesthetic gases can also be delivered to the patient using a bronchoscope tube adapter. The patient must be closely monitored for proper oxygenation and anesthetic depth. A mouth speculum is necessary to prevent damage to the endoscope.

In cats and small dogs, the bronchoscope is passed down the trachea without an endotracheal tube in place. Great care must be taken to evaluate the patient before the procedure, because the patient's airway is occluded by the endoscope. It may become necessary to stop the endoscopy for some time while the patient is oxygenated. Oxygen can also be delivered through the suction channel of the bronchoscope to help prevent hypoxemia.

RECOMMENDED READING

Barr F: *Diagnostic ultrasound in the dog and cat,* London, 1990, Blackwell Scientific.

Brearley MJ et al: *A colour atlas of small animal endoscopy,* St Louis, 1991, Mosby.

Burk RL, Ackerman N: *Small animal radiology and ultrasonography,* ed 2, Philadelphia, 1996, WB Saunders.

Curry TS, et al: *Christensen's physics of diagnostic radiology,* ed 4, Philadelphia, 1990, Lea & Febiger.

Han CM, Hurd CD: *Practical guide to diagnostic imaging: radiography and ultrasonography,* St Louis, 1994, Mosby.

Nyland TG, Mattoon JS: *Veterinary diagnostic ultrasound,* Philadelphia, 1995, WB Saunders.

Tams T: *Small animal endoscopy,* St Louis, 1990, Mosby.

Thrall DE: *Textbook of veterinary diagnostic radiology,* ed 2, Philadelphia, 1994, WB Saunders.

Traub-Dargatz JL, Brown CM: *Equine endoscopy,* ed 2, St Louis, 1997, Mosby.

CHAPTER 20

Anesthesia, Analgesia, and Anesthetic Nursing

C.L. Tyner
S.W. Rundell

Learning Objectives

After reviewing this chapter, the reader should understand the following:

Goals and fundamentals of anesthesia
Types of anesthetic agents and their effects, advantages, and disadvantages

Steps involved in anesthetizing animals
Equipment used for anesthetizing animals
Procedures used in medicating and monitoring animals before, during, and after anesthesia

General anesthesia is the purposeful derangement of the patients' normal physiologic processes to produce a state of unconsciousness, analgesia, and amnesia. This altered physiologic state may become progressively deranged until it is incompatible with life. Vigilance at all stages of the anesthetic procedure can warn of an impending crisis, usually with adequate time to take preventive or corrective actions.

Perfusion (Latin *perfundere,* to pour over) refers to the passage of oxygenated blood through body tissues. Poor perfusion may imply poor blood flow and/or poor blood oxygenation. It can be said that death is a late sign of poor perfusion; patients are not normally perfused one minute and dead the next. Common complications of poor perfusion, sometimes referred to as the "five hypos," are hypoxemia, hypoventilation/hypercapnia, hypotension, hypovolemia, and hypothermia.

Hypoxemia is insufficient oxygenation of the blood (PaO_2 less than 60 mm Hg). Hypoxia is a common sign of pulmonary compromise during anesthesia and is the reason for oxygen enrichment of inspired air.

Hypoventilation is reduced rate and depth of ventilation as determined by increased arterial carbon dioxide levels (hypercarbia or hypercapnia) ($PaCO_2$ above 45 mm Hg). Hypercarbia is an early sign of pulmonary compromise.

Hypotension is inadequate arterial blood pressure. Hypotension is the most common sign of cardiovascular depression. *Hypovolemia* is insufficient circulating blood volume. Hypovolemia is a common cause of hypotension. For this reason, fluid administration is one of the most valuable supportive measures one can provide during anesthesia. *Hypothermia* is abnormally low body temperature (2° to 3° C below normal). Hypothermia is a sign of central nervous system and cardiovascular depression.

THE GOALS OF AN ANESTHETIC PLAN

The goals of every anesthetic plan are to predict complications, prevent complications, recognize complications if and when they occur, and correct those complications. Complications can be prevented by using the correct apparatus, avoiding drugs that enhance a preexisting condition, and supporting the specific needs of the patient. Supporting respiration with oxygen enrichment and supporting perfusion with appropriate fluids may be adequate to prevent common arrhythmias or hypotension. Promptly recognizing anesthetic complications requires close, continuous monitoring. Specific attention should be paid to the "five hypos" and other predicted complications.

THE FUNDAMENTALS OF ANESTHESIA

The fundamentals of anesthesia can be summarized as follows:

1. Carefully evaluate the medical history, physical examination findings, and laboratory data.
2. Prepare for the expected and unexpected. Work with adequately trained personnel.
3. Minimize anesthesia time by planning ahead (e.g., prepare the surgical site before anesthesia).
4. Carefully select and use the correct dose of anesthetic drugs, based on the patient's health status, species, and breed. Avoid drugs that can enhance preexisting health problems.
5. Avoid administration of induction agents until calming agents have taken effect.
6. Reevaluate and stabilize (if necessary) vital signs before induction.
7. Maintain a patent airway and monitor ventilation; support with supplemental oxygen and assisted ventilation.
8. Monitor cardiovascular function; support with fluids and oxygen.
9. Monitor body temperature; support by preventing heat loss and providing external sources of heat.
10. Continually monitor and support all body systems from premedication through recovery.
11. Use analgesics to minimize pain and discomfort. Use calming agents to reduce excitement.
12. Keep an accurate record of the anesthetic procedure, monitoring efforts, and all major anesthetic events.

STEPS OF ANESTHESIA
Step 1: Patient Evaluation and Preparation

Patient evaluation means to "carefully judge" the patient's medical history and physical condition to determine health status and predict potential complications. This is the most important step, because all anes-

thetic decisions are based on health status. The medical history and physical examination are absolutely critical before anesthesia. All abnormalities discovered should be pursued to determine their potential effect on anesthetic outcome. Patient evaluation includes consideration of patient characteristics, medical history, physical examination, and laboratory data.

- *Patient characteristics:* Species, breed, age, and sex may prompt special considerations
- *Medical history:* Injuries, diseases, past anesthetic complications, concurrent medication
- *Physical examination:* Emphasis on cardiovascular, respiratory, hepatic, renal, and central nervous systems
- *Laboratory data:* PCV, total plasma protein level, liver function, kidney function, acid-base balance, electrolyte levels, blood gas values, blood clotting

Preanesthetic Patient Preparation. Patient preparation requirements vary, depending upon the performed procedure. Standard practice is to withhold food for 8 to 12 hours and water for 2 to 4 hours before anesthetic induction. However, special preparation may be required in complex procedures. Pediatric or smaller patients should have food withheld for only 2 hours before anesthesia. Chronically compromised patients should have their condition stabilized, when possible, before induction. For example, anemic patients (PCV below 20%) should have a transfusion to ensure adequate red blood cells and hemoglobin to oxygenate tissue. Dehydrated patients should receive sufficient intravenous fluids to restore hydration status. Patients with low total plasma protein levels (less than 3 g/dl) may benefit from administration of plasma.

Clipping the surgical site and placing an intravenous catheter before induction minimize anesthesia time. Efforts to maintain patient calmness reduce stress and may lower anesthetic induction requirements. Avoid unnecessary handling and noisy personnel or equipment. Provide an environment free of excitement or anxiety. Oxygenation before and during induction may improve PaO_2 in patients with cardiopulmonary compromise, especially during mask or chamber induction.

Preanesthetic checklists should be completed before all procedures to ensure that appropriate items are readily available, important health issues have been addressed, and all involved persons have communicated. This is especially important in high-volume clinics, when several people are involved in patient evaluation and preparation. Anesthetic induction must not be initiated until the checklist is completed (Boxes 20-1 and 20-2).

Box 20-1 Preanesthesia checklist

Personnel

- ☐ Select personnel and identify roles.
- ☐ Review procedure.
- ☐ Review emergency procedures.

Patient

- ☐ Identify patient properly.
- ☐ Verify patient was fasted (as appropriate).
- ☐ Perform special prep (as needed, e.g., bowel prep).
- ☐ Perform preanesthetic examination (health, sex confirmed).

Drugs

- ☐ Select drugs; confirm they are available.
- ☐ Review routes of drug administration.
- ☐ Check crash cart inventory.

Fluid administration

- ☐ Select IV fluids; maintain at proper temperature.
- ☐ Confirm sufficient fluids available for adverse events.
- ☐ Gather necessary equipment:
  - IV catheters (20 gauge for < 10 kg, 18 gauge for > 10 kg)
  - Injection caps
  - Materials for securing IV catheter (tape, adhesive)
  - Heparinized saline (2-4 IU/ml), in syringe with needle
  - Fluid delivery sets (60 drops/ml for < 10 kg, 15 drops/ml for 11-40 kg, 10 drops/ml for > 40 kg)

Endotracheal intubation

- ☐ Select and inspect three sizes of endotracheal tube.
- ☐ Gather necessary equipment:
  - Lubricating gel
  - Rolled gauze for securing
  - Laryngoscope and appropriate blades
  - Stylets
  - Lidocaine spray

Equipment

- ☐ Review anesthetic machine checklist (see Box 20-2).
- ☐ Select and inspect monitoring equipment.

Miscellaneous supplies

- ☐ Ophthalmic ointment
- ☐ Circulating warm-water blanket, table padding or insulation
- ☐ Face mask

Box 20-2 Checklist for daily inspection of anesthetic equipment

- ☐ Sufficient oxygen available
- ☐ Vaporizer filled
- ☐ All gas lines correctly connected
- ☐ Attach breathing circuit, tubes, reservoir bag
- ☐ Scavenger system properly connected and operational
- ☐ Check for leaks:
  - Close pop-off valve
  - Occlude patient end of breathing circuit at Y-piece
  - Fill circuit with oxygen to a pressure of 30 to 40 cm H_2O
  - Turn on oxygen flow to 100 ml/min
  - If the pressure increases, any leaks are within acceptable limits
  - If the pressure drops, increase the flow until the pressure remains stable
  - Leaks exceeding 200 ml/min should be corrected via machine maintenance
  - Open the pop-off valve while occluding Y-piece; pressure should drop to 0 cm H_2O

Step 2: Equipment and Supplies

More anesthetic mishaps are attributed to poor planning and preparation than to improper use of drugs. Correct selection, preparation, and use of anesthetic equipment are essential to patient safety. All equipment should be prepared and checked to be in good working order before administration of anesthetic compounds; the need for intubation and oxygenation may occur unexpectedly.

Supplies for Intravenous Fluid Administration. Placement of an intravenous catheter is essential for patient safety during anesthesia. Intravenous catheters provide immediate access for intravenous injection and administration of fluids. Catheters should be placed before induction of anesthesia, when possible, because most anesthetic agents produce hypotension or vasoconstriction and may complicate catheter placement. Appropriately sized catheters, infusion sets, needles, syringes, and other supplies necessary for aseptic catheterization should be arranged for easy access. The correct catheter size is that large enough to deliver large volumes of intravenous fluids (90 ml/kg/hr).

Infusion sets are available as vented or non-vented sets. *Vented administration sets* are required when using non-vented bottles. *Non-vented administration sets* can be used with plastic fluid bags or vented bottles. Delivery rates of 10 drops/ml, 12 drops/ml, 15 drops/ml, and 60 drops/ml are commonly used in veterinary medicine. Smaller drop sizes improve the accuracy of delivery in

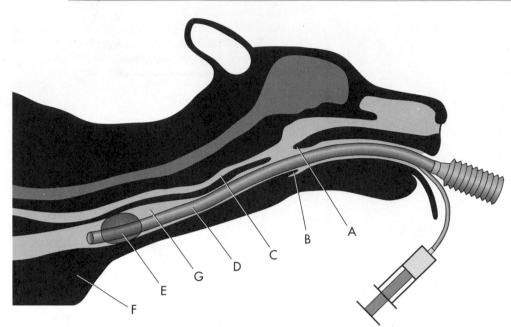

FIG. 20-1 Correct placement of an endotracheal tube. The connector is located near the incisor teeth, minimizing mechanical dead space. The cuffed end is in the cervical trachea, near the thoracic inlet. **A,** Soft palate. **B,** Epiglottis. **C,** Esophagus. **D,** Endotracheal tube. **E,** Inflated cuff. **F,** Thoracic inlet. **G,** Cervical trachea.

TABLE 20-1 Guide to selection of intravenous fluid delivery sets

$$\frac{\text{body weight in kg} \times \text{ml/kg/hr} \times \text{drops/ml}}{60 \text{ min/hr}} = \text{drops/min}$$

Weight (kg)	ml/hr (10 ml/kg/hr)	60 drops/ml	Drops/minute 15 drops/ml	10 drops/ml
5	50	50	—	—
10	100	—	25	—
15	150	—	38	—
20	200	—	50	—
30	300	—	—	50
40	400	—	—	66
60	600	—	—	100

Small animals: Select a drip set that delivers approximately 50 to 60 drops/min, to provide the desired flow rate (ml/hr); this allows for adjusting the rate as needed.
Large animals: Select a drip set that delivers approximately 10 drops/min.

smaller patients. Generally, patients weighing less than 10 kg should receive fluids through a "microdrip" (60 drops/ml) infusion set to increase accuracy of fluid delivery. Patients requiring large fluid volumes (e.g., horses) need 10 drops/ml sets. Routine fluid delivery rates during anesthesia should be 5 to 10 ml/kg/hr for larger animals and 10 to 20 ml/kg/hr for smaller animals (Table 20-1).

Endotracheal Tubes. Endotracheal intubation ensures a patent airway, facilitates patient ventilation, and provides easy delivery of volatile anesthetics. Endotracheal intubation is not necessarily indicated for general anesthesia; however, be prepared for immediate intubation if any respiratory complications arise. It is *rarely* a mistake to place an endotracheal tube.

Endotracheal tube positioning and length are important. The inserted tip of the tube should not extend beyond (caudal to) the thoracic inlet, because right bronchial intubation may occur. The adapter end of the tube should not extend more than 1 or 2 inches beyond (rostral to) the mouth to limit the increase of mechanical dead space (Fig. 20-1). Stylets may be used to facili-

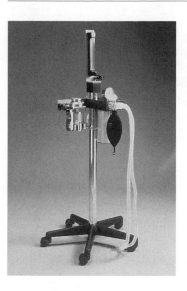

FIG. 20-2 Typical compact small animal anesthesia machine with pediatric circle breathing circuit. Components include precision vaporizer, flow meter, pressure manometer, oxygen flush valve, CO$_2$ absorber, common gas outlet, and waste gas scavenging device. *(Courtesy of Anesco, Inc., Georgetown, KY.)*

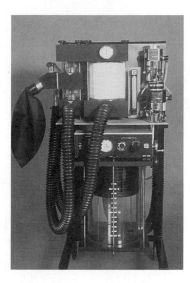

FIG. 20-3 Typical large animal anesthesia machine and ventilator, with large animal breathing circuit, two precision vaporizers, and standard anesthetic machine components. *(Courtesy of Anesco, Inc., Georgetown, KY.)*

tate intubation with small-diameter or very flexible tubes. When using a stylet, the tip of the stylet should not extend beyond (caudal to) the tip of the endotracheal tube to prevent damage to or penetration of the trachea. Secure the endotracheal tube to the maxilla, mandible, or head with gauze or tape to prevent dislodgment or excessive movement during the procedure.

Laryngoscopes. The laryngoscope facilitates visualization of the endotracheal tube as it passes through the upper airway and between the vocal cords. Laryngoscopes consist of a handle and detachable blades in a variety of sizes and shapes.

Medical Gas Supply. Medical gases may be delivered from compressed gas cylinders by central pipeline or by direct attachment to the anesthetic machine. Medical-grade oxygen and nitrous oxide are the commonly used gases in veterinary medicine, although the benefits of nitrous oxide in veterinary practice are limited. The nitrous oxide source must be independent of the oxygen source; nitrous oxide is mixed with oxygen just before passing through the vaporizer.

The most commonly used sizes of compressed medical gas cylinders are the *E cylinder* (4.25 × 26 inches) and the *H cylinder* (9.25 × 51 inches). All medical gas cylinders are color coded; oxygen cylinders are green and nitrous oxide cylinders are blue. E cylinders attached to the anesthetic machine for backup should be kept in the *off* position until in use to ensure that they remain full until needed.

Pressure regulators attached to the cylinder valve on H cylinders and near the hanger yokes for E cylinders reduce oxygen pressure to the normal working pressure of the anesthetic machine, 50 pounds per square inch gauge (PSIG). Pressure reduction is necessary to prevent damage to the anesthetic machine and allows a constant rate of oxygen delivery to the flow meter. Cylinder pres-

sure gauges are associated with the pressure regulator and may be used to estimate the relative volume of gas remaining in a cylinder. Oxygen cylinders contain only compressed oxygen vapors and the pressure is proportional to content. The pressure in a fully charged oxygen cylinder, regardless of size, is near 2,200 PSIG. A fully charged H cylinder contains 7,000 liters of oxygen and fully charged E cylinders contain 700 liters. A fully charged cylinder of nitrous oxide is 95% liquid; therefore, cylinder contents are not directly proportional to cylinder pressure. Pressure begins to drop only after the liquid is completely vaporized and about 75% of the contents have been used. The remaining gas can be estimated after pressure begins to fall. Fully charged nitrous oxide cylinders have a pressure of 750 PSIG. An H cylinder contains about 16,000 L and an E cylinder about 1,600 L.

Anesthesia Machines. Several companies manufacture anesthesia machines for small and large animal use (Figs. 20-2 and 20-3). Anesthetic machines deliver a mixture of oxygen and inhalation anesthetic to the breathing circuit. The components of an anesthetic machine are the oxygen source, pressure regulator, oxygen pressure valve, flow meter, vaporizer, and oxygen flush valve (Fig. 20-4).

Flow meters. Flow meters receive medical gases from the pressure regulator. Their purpose is to measure and deliver a constant gas flow to the vaporizer, the common gas outlet, and the breathing circuit. Oxygen enters the flow meter near the bottom and travels upward through a tapered, transparent flow tube. A floating indicator, either a ball or plumb-bob, inside the flow tube indicates the amount of gas passing through the control valve. The flow rate is indicated on a scale associated with the flow tube. When the control valve is open, oxygen enters the tube, pushing the floating indicator upward.

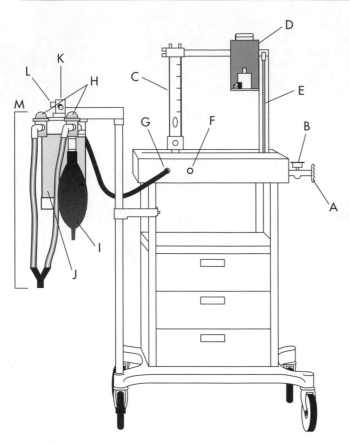

FIG. 20-4 Basic small animal anesthesia machine.
A, Oxygen hanger yoke. **B,** Oxygen pressure gauge.
C, Oxygen flow meter. **D,** Precision vaporizer.
E, Common gas line. **F,** Oxygen flush valve.
G, Common gas outlet. **H,** Unidirectional dome
valves. **I,** Reservoir bag. **J,** Carbon dioxide absorbent
canister. **K,** Pressure-relief valve. **L,** Scavenger inter-
face. **M,** Patient rebreathing circuit.

Where the indicator hovers in equilibrium, the rate of
flow is determined by reading the calibrated scale from
the center of the ball or the top of the plumb-bob.

Flow meters are gas specific and must not be inter-
changed; an oxygen flow meter cannot safely be replaced
with a nitrous oxide flow meter. Control knobs to regulate flow of medical gases must be distinguishable from
each other. Specifically, the oxygen control knob must be
green and permanently marked with the word or symbol
for oxygen. The valve should be fluted, project beyond
other knobs, and be larger in diameter than other knobs.

Flow meters are common sources of leaks and should
be checked at regular intervals for cracks in the flow
tube. Dirt or static electricity may cause a float to stick,
causing flows to be higher or lower than indicated.
Control knobs are easily damaged by excessive tightening, a bad habit leading to expensive repair. Overtight-
ening may prevent the flow meter from closing completely, causing significant leaking in the off position.
Leaking may lead to unexpected shortage of medical
gases and exhaustion (saturation) of carbon dioxide
absorbent from constant flow of gas through the
absorbent. Exhausted carbon dioxide absorbent may
produce carbon monoxide when exposed to inhalation
anesthetics, producing carbon monoxide toxicity manifested as tissue hypoxia.

Vaporizers. Inhalation anesthetic agents are volatile
liquids that vaporize at room temperature. The primary
function of a vaporizer is controlled enhancement of anesthetic vaporization. Vaporizers in common use are of two
general types: precision vaporizers (for use with halothane
or isoflurane) and non-precision vaporizers (used for
methoxyflurane). Their functional differences apply to the
administration of volatile anesthetics (Box 20-3).

Precision vaporizers, designed for a specific anesthetic
agent, deliver a constant concentration (%) that is automatically maintained with changing oxygen flow rates
and temperature. The percent setting on the control dial
approximates delivery to the breathing circuit. Precision
vaporizers are designed to function out of the breathing
circuit; that is, between the flow meter and the breathing
circuit. The inherent safety attributed to precision vaporizers is that the anesthetic concentration delivered to the
breathing circuit and patient cannot increase above the
vaporizer setting. Precision vaporizers may deliver less
than dial settings when flows are very low (250 ml/min
or lower) or very high (15 L/min or higher). Examples of
precision vaporizers for delivery of halothane and isoflurane are the Fluotec Mark III (Ohmeda) and the Ohio
Calibrated Vaporizer (Ohmeda), respectively (Figs. 20-5
and 20-6). Precision vaporizers are more expensive than
non-precision vaporizers.

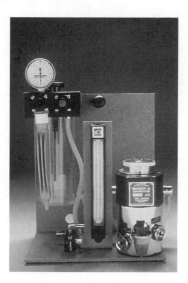

FIG. 20-5 Ohio calibrated vaporizer for vaporization of halothane or isoflurane, with output calibrated in volume % *(left)*. Manometer used to monitor breathing circuit pressure and to check tracheal tube inflation pressure *(center)*. *(Courtesy of Sensor Devices, Inc., Waukesha, WI.)*

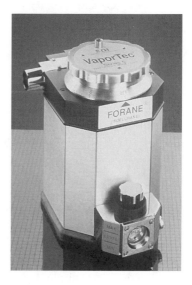

FIG. 20-6 VaporTec Series 5 precision vaporizer, calibrated for volume % delivery of halothane or isoflurane. *(Courtesy of Sensor Devices, Inc., Waukesha, WI.)*

Box 20-3 Factors affecting anesthetic output of vaporizers

Non-precision, in-circle vaporizers
- Vaporizer setting: Does not equate to a known concentration
- Fresh gas flow: High flows dilute the circuit concentration; low flows allow increase of the circuit concentration
- Patient minute ventilation: Increased ventilation increases vaporizer output
- Temperature of anesthetic agent: Increased temperature increases vaporizer output

Precision, out-of-circle vaporizers
- Vaporizing setting: Generates a known anesthetic concentration; increased setting increases vaporizer output
- Fresh gas flow: No effect on vaporizer output
- Patient minute ventilation: No effect on vaporizer output
- Temperature of anesthetic agent: No effect on vaporizer output

---

Non-precision vaporizers are rudimentary, allowing some control of vaporization, but delivering an unknown concentration. The dial scale is not a percent concentration, but rather a relative number indicating the amount of fresh gas diverted through the chamber. A lever setting of 0 on the Ohio #8 vaporizer indicates that no gas flows through the chamber, with no anesthetic delivered to the patient. When the lever is set on 10, all of the circuit gases are diverted through the chamber, increasing the anesthetic concentration delivered to the patient. The approximate percent of anesthetic delivered varies with the agent's vapor pressure and temperature, and the patient's minute ventilation. Knowing the precise concentration delivered to the patient is advantageous. However, if one monitors the patient's anesthetic depth and health status, simply increasing or decreasing the dial setting in response to observations allows relatively safe delivery of the agent.

Anesthetic concentrations could exceed 12% when administering isoflurane or halothane through a non-precision vaporizer (Ohio or Stephens type) located in the breathing circuit. Concentrations of this magnitude greatly increase the potential for overdosing; this risk outweighs the economy gained by purchase of jar-type vaporizers. There are sufficient concerns with administration of anesthetic agents without the added worry of gross anesthetic overdose.

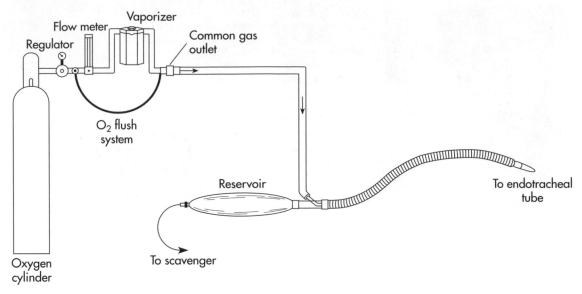

FIG. 20-7 Anesthetic delivery system with attached non-rebreathing system. *(Courtesy of R. Spangler, Morehead State University.)*

Non-precision vaporizers are designed to function in the breathing circuit ("in the circle"). Location of the vaporizer in the circle has disadvantages. The anesthetic concentration may increase over time without change in setting because of positive-pressure ventilation, increased minute ventilation, increased room temperature, and/or low fresh gas flow. High fresh gas flow decreases the anesthetic concentration by dilution of anesthetic in the breathing circuit.

Several hazards are associated with vaporizers. Filling with the incorrect agent can lead to delivery of an excessively high or low concentration of vapor to the patient. Delivering an unknown agent may present varied cardiovascular effects. Tipping the vaporizer may allow liquid agent to enter the fresh gas line, increasing the anesthetic concentration. Overfilling the chamber decreases the volume of vapor available to mix with fresh gas and may allow liquid anesthetic to reach the common gas outlet line. Leaks are also common at the inlet fitting, outlet fitting, filling port, and drain port. Vaporizers incorrectly located in the common gas outlet can deliver excessive anesthetic concentrations when the oxygen flush is activated. The additional flow through the vaporizer (35 to 75 L/min) increases the volume of vapor delivered to the breathing circuit.

Breathing circuits. Medical gases pass from the anesthetic machine to the patient through tubing known as a *breathing circuit.* Breathing circuits deliver "fresh gases" (oxygen and anesthetic vapor) to the patient and transport exhaled gases from the patient. Carbon dioxide is eliminated from the circuit by "wash out" using high gas flow rates and/or soda lime absorption.

Non-rebreathing circuits do not have a carbon dioxide absorber (Fig. 20-7). Removal of carbon dioxide depends on fresh gas flow rates. Properly used, non-rebreathing circuits allow no significant rebreathing of exhaled gases. The point of entry into the circuit, the flow rate, and the expiratory port location determine the amount of carbon dioxide rebreathed. Ultimately, the composition of the inspired gas mixture depends upon the fresh gas flow rate. Flow rates near two to three times the patient's minute ventilation are required to prevent rebreathing. Flow rates below two times minute ventilation allow some rebreathing and warrant monitoring for signs of hypoxemia and hypercarbia.

The most frequently used non-rebreathing circuits in veterinary medicine are the *Bain circuit* and the *Norman mask elbow.* Advantages of non-rebreathing circuits include decreased resistance to breathing, rapid change of inspired anesthetic concentration, light weight, and ease of cleaning and use. Disadvantages are primarily associated with the required high fresh gas flow rates and include increased use of oxygen and anesthetic, enhanced risk of hypothermia, and dehydration.

The term *rebreathing* literally means "to breathe again" and refers to exhaled gases (carbon dioxide, oxygen, anesthetic). Rebreathing circuits ("circle system") are most commonly used in veterinary practice. The amount of carbon dioxide rebreathed depends on the degree of carbon dioxide absorption and the fresh gas flow rate. The components of the circle system include the absorber, absorbent, fresh gas inlet, unidirectional dome valves, positive-pressure-relief valve (pop-off valve), manometer, reservoir bag, and a remov-

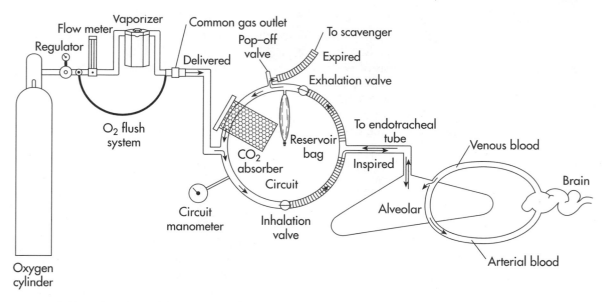

FIG. 20-8 Anesthetic delivery system showing the pathway traveled by anesthetic, from the vaporizer to the brain. *(Courtesy of R. Spangler, Morehead State University.)*

able set of breathing tubes (Fig. 20-8). Some circuits also have a negative-pressure-relief valve.

Standard breathing tubes are 22 mm in diameter and 1 m long for small animal patients weighing 7 to 135 kg. Shorter 15-mm–diameter tubes are preferred for patients weighing less than 7 kg. Large animal tubes are 500 mm in diameter and 1.7 m long. The classic setup uses separate inhalation and exhalation tubes connected via a Y-piece to the endotracheal tube adapter. Recently, the Universal-F circuit was developed to place the inhalation tube inside of the exhalation tube. The advantages of this arrangement include warming of inhaled gases by exhaled gases (Fig. 20-9).

Advantages of the rebreathing circuit include conservation of body heat and fluids, reuse of exhaled oxygen and anesthetic gases, and cost-efficient lower flow rates. Disadvantages of rebreathing circuits include the danger of hypercarbia resulting from malfunction of the carbon dioxide absorbent, particularly at flow rates low enough to produce a closed system. There also exists a potential for increased work of breathing because of added resistance from faulty unidirectional valves, carbon dioxide absorbent, or faulty pop-off valves. Additionally, there is a slow change in the inspired anesthetic concentration at lower flows.

The *reservoir bag* provides a gas volume sufficient for the patient to inhale maximally without creating negative pressure in the circuit. It is also used for positive-pressure ventilation or to inflate the lungs when needed. Reservoir bag sizes of 0.5 to 5 L are used for small animals and 15 to 30 L for large animals. The ideal reservoir bag is five times the patient's normal tidal volume of 10 ml/kg.

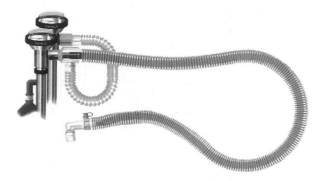

FIG. 20-9 Universal F circuit. This circle breathing system is modified to promote heat exchange between exhaled and inhaled gases and minimize patient heat loss. *(Courtesy of Anesco, Inc., Georgetown, KY.)*

The *circuit manometer* is useful to monitor circuit pressure. Excessive circuit pressure (above 4 cm H_2O) may prevent normal respiration and increase intrathoracic pressure, resulting in decreased venous return and a subsequent drop in cardiac output. During positive-pressure ventilation ("bagging"), the manometer allows delivery of the correct circuit pressure. *Barotrauma* (respiratory tract injury from excessive circuit pressures) decreases oxygenation of blood. Typically, healthy dogs and cats are ventilated to pressures of 15 to 20 cm H_2O to ensure adequate tidal volume. Horses may require positive-pressure ventilation pressures of 30 to 40 cm H_2O to achieve adequate tidal volume. Ventilation rates should not exceed one third of the heart rate to avoid significant cardiac output decrease.

The *positive-pressure-relief (pop-off) valve* prevents excessive pressure in the rebreathing circuit and allows removal of excess waste gases. A common cause of anesthetic mishap is leaving the pop-off valve closed after performing positive-pressure ventilation. The pop-off valve is equipped with a scavenger interface, permitting connection to a waste gas removal system to prevent waste gas discharge into the operating room air.

The *carbon dioxide absorbent* (soda lime or Baralyme) removes carbon dioxide from the breathing circuit by chemical reaction. Inadequate absorbent function may lead to hypercarbia (excessive carbon dioxide in the blood), with resultant increased respiratory rate and initially increased heart rate, followed by cardiovascular depression. The absorbent should be changed after 6 to 8 hours of use, depending upon gas flow rates and patient size. Desiccated carbon dioxide absorbents may react with volatile anesthetics, producing carbon monoxide sufficient to cause carbon monoxide toxicity. This has not been reported in veterinary medicine; however, take precautionary measures to ensure that the absorbent is reasonably fresh.

The *unidirectional dome valves* maintain one-way flow of gases within the breathing circuit. This ensures that exhaled gases pass through the carbon dioxide absorbent before reaching the patient again.

Anesthetic Systems. Taken together, all of the components of the anesthetic machine and breathing circuit make up an *anesthetic system*. There are several types of anesthetic systems: semi-closed, closed, and open.

The terms *semi-closed* and *closed* refer to operation of rebreathing circuits. A given circuit may be operated as semi-closed or closed. A circuit is semi-closed if oxygen flow is greater than patient oxygen uptake. The circuit is closed if oxygen flow is equal to patient oxygen uptake (4 to 7 ml/kg/min for small animals and 2 to 3 ml/kg/min for large animals). Regardless of the position of the pop-off valve (open or closed), the circuit may be semi-closed or closed. With a closed system, elimination of carbon dioxide is solely dependent on functional carbon dioxide absorbent.

The term *open system* describes delivery of anesthetic gases via face mask, insufflation, or induction chamber (Fig. 20-10). Open systems are advantageous for very small or aggressive patients. They permit induction by inhalation anesthetics when injectable techniques are contraindicated or impractical. Disadvantages may include prolonged induction time, passage through a stressful excitement phase, inability to monitor the patient, air pollution from waste anesthetics, and increased expense because of high flow. Excitement during inhalation induction, by mask or chamber, increases the anesthetic risk in compromised patients.

Chambers used for induction should be large enough to permit recumbency without compromising respiration. With mask or chamber induction, patients should breathe oxygen-enriched air for several minutes before induction to optimize alveolar oxygen concentration. Chamber induction allows large amounts of waste anesthetic gases to escape into the surgery area. Serious effort to minimize human exposure is prudent. A safety tip is to switch to the face mask as soon as the patient is manageable. This conserves anesthetic and allows greater control and better monitoring of the patient. Patients should be intubated when sufficiently relaxed to avoid maintenance by mask except in very short procedures. The inhalation agent of choice for open induction is isoflurane.

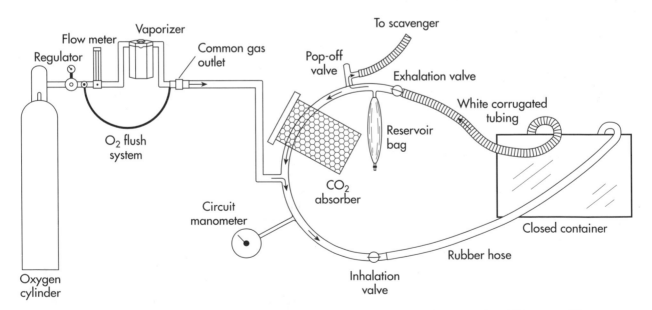

FIG. 20-10 Anesthetic machine with rebreathing circuit attached to induction chamber. (*Courtesy of R. Spangler, Morehead State University.*)

Step 3: Preanesthetic Medication

Benefits of Preanesthetic Medication. Preanesthetic medication is usually beneficial to the patient and should be considered for all patients. The need is based entirely on patient health status and temperament and drugs selected for induction and maintenance. Selection of preanesthetics is based on the patient's health status, not on the surgical procedure. Various drugs are used for premedication, including calming agents, analgesics, and anticholingerics (Box 20-4). Benefits of preanesthetic medication include the following:

- Reduces patient stress and minimizes sympathetic effects, which improves handling during preparation for procedures
- Usually decreases the required dose of more potent induction and maintenance agents
- Facilitates anesthetic induction and maintenance, dampening the sudden changes in anesthetic depth associated with surgical stimulation
- Allows a smoother recovery and reduces pain

Anticholinergics. Anticholinergics block the action of the neurotransmitter acetylcholine at cholinergic recep-

---

Box 20-4 Summary of characteristics of drugs used in veterinary anesthesia

Atropine

- Concentration: 0.54 mg/ml
- Dosage: 0.04 mg/kg IV, IM, or SC
- Duration of action: 60–90 minutes
- Anticholinergic; use only when indicated
- Prevents vagal effects, bradycardia, heart block, excessive salivation
- Avoid of tachycardia present (dogs > 140/min, cats > 200/min)
- May increase myocardial oxygen consumption
- Indications: before use of narcotics and alpha-2 agonists, muscle relaxant reversal, combat bradycardia or bradyarrhythmia

Glycopyrrolate (Robinul-V: Robins)

- Concentration: 0.2 mg/ml
- Dosage: 0.01 mg/kg IV, IM, or SC
- Duration of action: 2–4 hours
- Anticholinergic; use only when indicated
- Prevents vagal effects, bradycardia, heart block, excessive salivation
- Does not cross blood-brain barrier; may be less effective in CPR
- Longer duration of action and fewer side effects than atropine
- Indications: before use of narcotics and alpha-2 agonists, muscle relaxant reversal, combat bradycardia or bradyarrhythmia

Acepromazine (Promace: Fort Dodge)

- Concentration: 10 mg/ml; dilute to 1 mg/ml for small animal use
- Dosage 0.05–0.1 mg/kg IV, IM or SC (3 mg maximum total dose)
- Avoid in cardiovascular compromise
- Decreases vascular resistance
- May protect against arrhythmias, good antiemetic
- May prolong recovery in animals with liver disease
- May lower seizure threshold
- Avoid concurrent use with organophosphates
- Tachycardia may develop with associated hypotension

Diazepam (Valium: Roche)

- Concentration: 5 mg/ml
- Dosage 0.2–1.0 mg/kg IM
- Avoid rapid IV injection; may produce pain and hypotension
- Anxiolytic, amnesic, muscle relaxant, anticonvulsant
- Useful in central nervous system and cardiac patients
- Little sedative effect in healthy animals; may cause profound depression in compromised patients
- Do not mix with other agents in same syringe
- Administer cautiously in aggressive patients
- Effects may be prolonged effects in hepatic dysfunction
- Propylene glycol base may cause arrhythmias
- Flumazenil (Romazicon: Roche) is an effective antagonist (0.1 mg/kg IV)

Midazolam (Versed: Roche)

- Concentration: 1 mg/ml
- Dosage: 0.2–0.4 mg/kg IV
- Effects similar to those of diazepam
- Water soluble
- More potent, more rapid onset of action, shorter duration of action than diazepam
- Excellent choice in critically ill patients
- May cause excitement and pain if rapidly administered
- Flumazenil is an effective antagonist (0.1 mg/kg IV)

Xylazine (Rompun: Miles)

- Concentration: 20 mg/ml
- Dosage: 0.2–0.4 mg/kg IV, IM, or SC (5 mg maximum total dose)
- Precede xylazine injection with anticholinergic injection
- Alpha-2 agonist, lowers sympathetic tone
- Excellent preanesthetic in healthy animals, but a poor anesthetic
- Avoid in animals with cardiovascular compromise (decreases myocardial contractility, produces bradycardia and heart block, sensitizes myocardium to catecholamine-induced arrhythmias)

Continued.

Xylazine—cont'd

- Limit use to healthy, aggressive, or convulsing patients
- Effects antagonized by yohimbine (Yobine: Lloyd, 0.1 mg/kg IV slowly to effect) or atipamazole (Antisedan: Pfizer)

Opiates and opioids

- Include opioid agonists, opioid agonist-antagonists, and opioid antagonists
- Opioid portion may be reversed
- Generally sparing to cardiovascular system
- Depress respiration; assisted ventilation may be necessary
- May cause excitement and panting
- Repeated or large doses may produce bradycardia
- Indicated for relief of postoperative pain; more effective if administered before pain develops

Oxymorphone (Numorphan: DuPont)

- Concentration: 1.5 mg/ml
- 10–15 times more potent than morphine
- Dosage: 0.05–0.2 mg/kg IV, IM, or SC (3 mg maximum total dose)
- Reliable relief of pain for 2–4 hours

Butorphanol (Torbugesic: Fort Dodge)

- Concentration: 10 mg/ml; dilute to 1 mg/ml for small animal use
- 2–5 times more potent than morphine
- Dosage: 0.2–0.5 mg/kg IV, IM, or SC
- Decreases cough reflex
- Somewhat reliable for relief of pain; combine with a sedative for best results
- Provides 2–4 hours of analgesia

Buprenorphine (Buprenex: Norwich-Eaton)

- 3–5 times more potent than morphine
- Dosage: 0.005–0.01 mg/kg IV or IM
- Somewhat reliable for relief of pain
- Provides 4–12 hours of analgesia
- May cause excitement; combine with a sedative for best results

Morphine (Astramorph: Astra)

- Dosage: dogs 0.1–0.2 mg/kg IV, IM, or SC; cats 0.05–0.1 mg/kg IV, IM, or SC
- Duration of action: reliable pain relief for up to 4 hours
- May cause histamine release or panting; combine with a sedative for best results
- Epidural administration: 0.1 mg/kg; onset of action within 30 minutes; duration 10–24 hours

Naloxone (Narcan: DuPont)

- Pure narcotic antagonist
- Dosage: 0.002–0.02 mg/kg IM or slowly IV to effect
- Dilute to 0.4 mg/ml of sterile distilled water and administer to effect
- Observe for return of effects

Fentanyl and droperidol (Innovar-Vet: Mallinckrodt)

- Concentration: each ml contains 0.4 mg fentanyl and 20 mg droperidol
- Dosage: 1 ml/10 kg IM or 1 ml/20 kg IV
- 50-100 times more potent than morphine
- Used as preanesthetic and for chemical restraint
- May cause respiratory depression, bradycardia, aggression, altered behavior, defecation, and flatulence
- Provides 30–60 minutes of analgesia

Acepromazine and butorphanol

- Dosage: glycopyrrolate IM at 0.01 mg/kg with acepromazine IM at 0.1 mg/kg (3 mg maximum total dose)
- Wait 10 minutes, then give butorphanol IM at 0.1–0.4 mg/kg
- Reduce dosage for IV use; administer to effect
- Used as preanesthetic and for chemical restraint

Acepromazine and oxymorphone

- Dosage: glycopyrrolate IM at 0.01 mg/kg with acepromazine IM at 0.1 mg/kg (3 mg maximum total dose)
- Wait 10 minutes, then give oxymorphone IM at 0.05-0.2 mg/kg (3 mg maximum total dose)
- Reduce oxymorphone dosage for IV use; administer to effect
- Used as preanesthetic and for chemical restraint

Xylazine and butorphanol

- Dosage: glycopyrrolate IM at 0.01 mg/kg with xylazine IM at 0.2 mg/kg (5 mg maximum total dose)
- Wait 10 minutes, then give butorphanol IM at 0.1–0.4 mg/kg
- Reduce dosage for IV use; administer to effect
- Used as preanesthetic and for chemical restraint

Thiopental (Pentothal: Abbott)

- Ultra-short–acting barbiturate (thiobarbiturate)
- Concentration: 2%–5%
- Dosage: 5–10 mg/kg slowly IV to effect
- Is safe as induction agent; redistribution enhances recovery
- Use small dose in patients with cardiopulmonary, hepatic, or renal compromise
- May produce arrhythmias and apnea (pre-oxygenation beneficial)
- Use dilute concentrations for small or debilitated patients
- Support ventilation during apnea to reduce risk of cardiopulmonary arrest
- Administer fluids and oxygen to improve outcome
- Provides smooth transition to unconsciousness; no excitement if preanesthetic used
- Use with caution in sighthounds

Ketamine (Ketaset: Fort Dodge)

- Concentration: 100 mg/ml
- Do not use without calming agent
- Dosage: 5–30 mg/kg IM or 1–6 mg/kg IV
- Provides only limited analgesia, poor muscle relaxation
- Causes apnea, enhancing hypoxia and hypercarbia
- Increases heart rate and blood pressure, increasing myocardial oxygen demand
- Usually maintains cardiac output and blood pressure better than barbiturates
- May increase intracranial and ocular pressure
- Avoid in patients with renal, hepatic, or cardiac disease, ocular surgery, and epileptics
- Transition to inhalation anesthesia may be rougher than with barbiturates
- Apnea reduces uptake of inhalation agent; animal awakens abruptly when ketamine wears off

Ketamine and diazepam

- Useful combination for induction
- Dosage: ketamine at 5 mg/kg and diazepam at 0.25 mg/kg, both slowly IV
- Alternative dosage: mix equal volumes of ketamine (100 mg/ml) and diazepam (5 mg/ml) and give IV at 1 ml/10 kg

Zolazepam and tiletamine (Telazol: Fort Dodge)

- Concentration: zolazepam 50 mg/ml and tiletamine 50 mg/ml
- Dosage: 2–6 mg/kg IV or IM
- Rapidly induces surgical plane of anesthesia for 10–20 minutes; recovery period varies
- Provides analgesia superior to that provided by ketamine
- Large doses can produce apnea, leading to hypoxia and hypercarbia
- Excitement may occur during recovery if zolazepam is eliminated from tissues before tiletamine; administer an additional sedative IV
- Recovery may be prolonged with use of large doses if zolazepam is not completely metabolized; reverse with flumazenil
- In cats, tiletamine is often metabolized first; in dogs, zolazepam usually metabolized first
- Very effective in exotic and aggressive patients

Xylazine, zolazepam, and tiletamine

- Useful combination for anesthesia in healthy patients
- Give glycopyrrolate 0.01 mg/kg IV, IM, or SC as preanesthetic, then xylazine IM or SC at 0.2 mg/kg (5 mg maximum total dose)
- Wait 15 minutes, then give zolazepam and tiletamine (Telazol) IM at 6 mg/kg
- Provides surgical plane of anesthesia for 20–40 minutes; recovery varies

Acepromazine, zolazepam, and tiletamine

- Useful combination for anesthesia in healthy patients
- Give acepromazine IM or SC at 0.05–0.1 mg/kg
- Wait 15 minutes, then give zolazepam and tiletamine (Telazol) IM at 6 mg/kg
- Provides surgical plane of anesthesia for 20–40 minutes; recovery varies

Propofol (Diprivan: Zeneca)

- Concentration: 10 mg/ml
- Dosage: 2–6 mg/kg IV to effect
- Highly lipid soluble; can produce the "five hypos"
- Only advantage over barbiturate is rapid recovery and absence of drowsiness
- Not recommended for pregnant or nursing females
- Provide cardiovascular and pulmonary support
- Does not store well; sterility is critical
- Highly overrated and overpriced anesthetic

Halothane (Fluothane: Ayerst)

- Inhalant agent
- Moderately rapid induction and recovery
- Hepatotoxic, arrhythmogenic
- Thymol preservative contaminates equipment

Methoxyflurane (Metofane: Abbott)

- Inhalant agent
- Slow induction and prolonged recovery
- Less arrhythmogenic than halothane but more so than isoflurane
- Can produce nephrotoxicity
- Avoid concurrent use with tetracyclines or aminoglycosides; do not use on unhealthy animals
- Effects not reversed by doxapram

Isoflurane (Aerrane: Ohmeda)

- Inhalant agent
- Provides greatest margin of safety of all currently used gas anesthetics
- Excellent anesthetic for high-risk patients
- Indications: liver disease, renal failure, trauma, arrhythmias, cesarean section, old animals, obese animals, hypersensitivity to other anesthetics

tors in the heart, salivary glands, and smooth muscle fibers throughout the body. Effects may include increased heart rate (with concomitant increase in myocardial oxygen demand), decreased salivation and bronchial secretions, mydriasis (dilated pupils), bronchodilation, decreased gastric and intestinal motility, reduced tear formation, and blocking of vagus-mediated reflexes. Central effects (e.g., sedation or excitement) may occur with anticholinergics that cross the blood-brain barrier.

Atropine and glycopyrrolate (Robinul-V) are the anticholinergics most commonly used in veterinary anesthesia. Anticholinergics are indicated when vagus-mediated reflexes, bradycardia, second-degree heart block, or excessive salivation exist or are anticipated. Because of the expected cardiovascular effects of opioid or alpha-2 agonists (e.g., xylazine) or before reversing the effects of muscle relaxants, an anticholinergic may be indicated. Anticholinergics are used during cardiopulmonary resuscitation (CPR) to alleviate bradyarrhythmias. They are contraindicated in the presence of tachycardia (above 140 beats/min in dogs, above 200 beats/min in cats) or ventricular fibrillation. Routine preanesthetic use of anticholinergics was once common but is now considered inappropriate by many anesthesiologists.

Calming and Analgesic Agents. Tranquilizers, sedatives, and analgesics (pain relievers) are useful adjuncts to general anesthesia, if given before (preanesthetic), during (maintenance), or after anesthesia (postanesthetic). Patients that are calm, sedated, and free of pain generally require less anesthesia for induction and maintenance. Excited patients or those in pain have higher levels of circulating catecholamines that may increase the likelihood of adverse cardiovascular effects, such as cardiac arrhythmias. Sedation or analgesia may improve recovery from anesthesia. Each of these agents has beneficial as well as adverse effects on physiology.

Drug combinations may have additive, synergistic, complementary, or antagonistic interactions. If the effects are additive or synergistic, less of each drug is needed to produce the desired effect. Complementary effects are useful when a drug lacks a particular effect (e.g., xylazine complements the poor muscle relaxation of ketamine). Drugs commonly used for this purpose fall into several drug categories: phenothiazine derivatives, benzodiazepines, thiazine derivatives, barbiturates, and opioids. Chapter 13 presents detailed information on the effects and use of these agents.

Step 4: Induction

When gas anesthesia is to be performed, *anesthetic induction* is the transition from the conscious, preanesthetic state to the level of anesthesia at which the patient may be intubated. The ideal induction agent provides a smooth and calm transition from consciousness to unconsciousness, abolishes oropharyngeal and tracheal reflexes, has a brief duration of effect, produces minimal or no toxicity, and requires minimal metabolism for recovery. Recognize that induction is short-term general anesthesia and that induction agents are frequently used alone to perform short surgical or diagnostic procedures. Balanced anesthesia should be used for procedures lasting longer than approximately 45 minutes or performed in patients with organ dysfunction.

Drugs for Anesthetic Induction. Several methods are used for induction before inhalation anesthesia, each having advantages and disadvantages. Intravenous administration is preferred in most cases. Intravenous injection of a thiobarbiturate is a standard induction method before inhalation anesthesia in dogs. Thiopental sodium (Pentothal) is a commonly used thiobarbiturate in veterinary anesthesia. Thiobarbiturates provide rapid, smooth induction of anesthesia, with abolition of oropharyngeal and tracheal reflexes lasting several minutes.

Dissociative anesthetics (e.g., ketamine, tiletamine) may be used in combination with acepromazine, xylazine, or diazepam to induce anesthesia in a wide variety of species. Dissociative agents administered alone may cause extreme excitement or seizures. The effects of dissociative combinations last longer than those of thiobarbiturates, affecting the patient well beyond the induction period.

Induction with an *inhalant agent* (e.g., halothane, isoflurane) via face mask or induction chamber (tank), with or without preanesthetic medication, is occasionally desirable. Advantages of inhalation induction include avoidance of multiple drugs in the blood and tissues (important for some research protocols), rapid recovery, and ease of induction of very small animals (e.g., rats, mice, cats) that are difficult to handle. Disadvantages include slower induction with passage through an excitement phase that may be quite stressful to the patient, difficulty restraining and monitoring the patient, high potential for pollution of room air with inhalation anesthetics, and the expense of the high flow rates and anesthetic levels needed. The excitement of inhalation induction increases the risk of anesthetic complications in compromised patients predisposed to cardiac or respiratory insufficiency. In healthy patients, stress-induced catecholamine release may produce cardiopulmonary compromise. If struggling occurs, chamber induction is as stressful as mask induction. The animal may also contort itself into a position that compromises respiration.

Mask or chamber induction requires several minutes of pre-oxygenation to increase the margin of safety. With chamber induction, large amounts of anesthetic vapor escape into the room air when the chamber is opened. The procedure should ideally be performed under a hood that removes effluent gases. Once anesthesia is induced, the patient should be masked or intubated and maintained on the inhalant anesthetic. When direct inhalant induction is indicated, the agent of choice is isoflurane.

Step 5: Maintenance

Following induction, the patient must be maintained in the anesthetized state until the procedure is completed. A common misconception is that maintenance involves only keeping the patient from moving during the procedure, regardless of the patient's needs. Maintenance is the management period of the anesthetic procedure. Monitoring and support of organ function are essential during anesthetic maintenance. An anesthetic record provides important documentation of your vigilance, and it notes adverse trends and important events occurring in the perioperative period (Fig. 20-11). A well-organized anesthetic record serves as legal documentation of anesthetic events, drug dosages used, and patient values during anesthesia, and it guides the actions of the anesthetist by tracking trends in cardiopulmonary function.

General Considerations. Drugs used for maintenance of anesthesia include inhalant agents and a variety of injectable drugs. Surgical or diagnostic procedures requiring more than 30 to 45 minutes are best performed with inhalation anesthesia. Injectable anesthetics are not recommended for long-term maintenance of anesthesia. Repeated injections of the induction agent to maintain anesthesia cause tissue accumulation, with increased risk of adverse events and greater dependence upon metabolism for recovery. Steady states of anesthesia and a consistent depth of anesthesia are easier to maintain with inhalants.

The amount of anesthetic needed to maintain an appropriate level of anesthesia is not a constant. Anesthetic depth is a product of the amount of drug reaching the brain, degree of painful stimulus applied, and patient health status. In a typical abdominal surgical procedure, minimal anesthesia is needed during the surgical preparation, moderate anesthesia during the skin incision, maximal anesthesia during the intraabdominal phase, and moderate anesthesia during skin suturing. Hypothermia and hypotension reduce anesthetic requirements. If anesthetic administration is not reduced in the presence of hypothermia or hypotension, patients may become too deeply anesthetized, with further compromise of tissue perfusion.

Inhalant Anesthetics. Among the inhalant anesthetics commonly used in veterinary medicine are nitrous oxide, methoxyflurane, halothane, and isoflurane. When mixed with oxygen and inhaled by the patient, they diffuse rapidly into the bloodstream and are then distributed to all body tissues. As the concentration of drug in the brain rises, the CNS becomes progressively depressed. With the loss of consciousness and response to painful stimuli, the patient enters the *plane of surgical anesthesia*. Further rise of anesthetic concentrations in the brain continues to depress the CNS until vital functions cease and death ensues. The degree of anesthetic depth required by a patient during a particular procedure and the amount of inhalation anesthetic required to achieve and maintain that depth are unpredictable and variable.

Advantages of using inhalant agents include the ease and speed of controlling anesthetic depth, good muscle relaxation, rapid recovery with minimal dependence upon metabolism of the agent, and delivery of high levels of oxygen with the agent through an endotracheal tube. Placement of an endotracheal tube provides a patent airway and the ability to support ventilation as needed.

Disadvantages of inhalant agents include the relatively expensive equipment and the knowledge and skill required for their use. Also, halothane sensitizes the myocardium to epinephrine-induced arrhythmias and produces liver damage in some patients. Methoxyflurane produces renal tubular damage. Isoflurane is the least toxic of these agents, partially because of its small degree of biotransformation in the body.

A drug's *potency* is a measure of how much of the drug is needed to produce a standard effect, as compared with similar agents. For inhalant agents, potency is determined largely by the lipid solubility of the agent and is reflected by the minimum alveolar concentration (MAC). The MAC is defined as the lowest alveolar concentration of anesthetic required to prevent gross, purposeful movement in response to a painful stimulus. The MAC varies with species and individuals. The higher the MAC is, the less potent the agent.

Anesthetic Delivery, Uptake, Distribution, and Elimination. The relationship between the vaporizer setting and the time required to achieve effective brain levels of anesthetic is fundamental to inhalation anesthesia. Anesthetic delivery, uptake, and distribution are the processes by which the anesthetic reaches its intended site of action, the brain. The process of getting anesthetic to the pulmonary alveoli is known as *anesthetic delivery*. *Anesthetic uptake* is the movement of anesthetic molecules from the pulmonary alveoli into the bloodstream. It is analogous to the absorption phase of injectable agents. *Anesthetic distribution* is the movement of anesthetic molecules throughout the body via the bloodstream and diffusion into the tissues. Movement of gas molecules from the blood into the tissues is also called *tissue uptake*. Gas molecules must pass sequentially through these phases to reach the brain and produce anesthesia. If any one phase is altered, the chain of events leading to anesthesia is altered.

Anesthetic delivery to the alveoli is determined by the inspired concentration and alveolar minute ventilation. Increased anesthetic concentration in the breathing circuit increases the inspired concentration. The primary

MONITORING	"EARLY WARNING"				RECOVERY PERIOD
Time:	10 20 30 40 50	10 20 30 40 50	10 20 30 40 50	10 20 30 40 50	
AGENTS:	ml/hr	ml/hr	ml/hr	ml/hr	**TOTALS**
Fluids:					Fluids:
Blood:					Blood:
Plasma:					Plasma:
Meds:					Meds:
Oxygen Flow:					Vaporizer Off:
Vaporizer Setting:					ETT Removed:
End Tidal Conc:					Sternal:
Light					Standing

PLANE: Light — Deep

Anesthesia	A	250	
		240	
Operation	⊙	230	
		220	
End ⊙⊗		210	
		200	
End A	A	190	
		180	
Systolic P	V	170	
		160	
Diastolic P	Λ	150	
		140	
Mean P	X	130	
		120	
Heart Rate	•	110	
		100	
Resp. Rate	O	90	
		80	
Spont.	S	70	
		60	
Assist.	A	50	
		40	
Ventil.	V	30	
		20	
		10	
		0	

SUPPORT
1. None
2. Heating
3. Fluids
4. Oxygen
5. ICU
6. Other

COMPLICATIONS
1. None
2. Arrhythmias
3. Aspiration
4. Cardiac Arrest
5. Convulsions
6. Cyanosis
7. Death
8. Excitement
9. Hypothermia
10. Injury
11. Laryngospasm
12. Panting
13. Regurgitation
14. Resp. Arrest
15. Resp. Depression
16. Resp. Obstruction
17. Salivation
18. Other

Temperature (°F)	
E.C.G.	
pH	
Pco_2	
Po_2	
HCO_3	
Base Balance	
Event	

Complications:

1. None	5. Cardiac Arrest	9. Hyperthermia	13. Panting	17. Resp. Obstruct.
2. Apnea	6. Cyanosis	10. Hypotension	14. Regurgitation	18. Salivation
3. Arrythmias	7. Death	11. Hypothermia	15. Resp. Arrest	19. Tympany
4. Aspiration	8. Hemorrhage	12. Inadequate Relaxation	16. Resp. Depression	20. Variable Depth

Assigned to Student Clinician at:_____

Student Anesthetist:

Student Clinician:

FIG. 20-11 Typical anesthetic record for recording information related to an anesthetic procedure.

means of accomplishing this is by increasing the vaporizer setting. Anesthetic uptake (removal of anesthetic from the alveoli by the blood) is determined by solubility of the agent in blood, cardiac output, and the difference between alveolar and venous partial pressure of anesthetic. Uptake by the blood continually removes anesthetic from the alveoli. The more soluble the agent is in blood, the greater is this effect and the longer it takes to produce anesthesia. This is why less soluble agents like isoflurane induce anesthesia rapidly.

Vessel-rich tissues include the brain, heart, liver, kidney, lungs, and gastrointestinal tract. These organs make up less than 10% of the body weight but receive 75% of cardiac output. Because of this large volume of blood flow, anesthetic is rapidly distributed to these vessel-rich tissues. Muscle makes up about 50% of body mass and receives nearly 20% of cardiac output. This large tissue group is significant in that, during induction, most of the anesthetic delivered to muscle is removed from the blood. Fat makes up nearly 20% of total body mass but only receives about 4% of cardiac output. Although anesthetics are highly lipid soluble, low blood flow to this group limits anesthetic uptake, with little effect on induction rate. However, fat continually takes up anesthetic over time, and this must be released upon recovery. Prolonged procedures allow fat to accumulate enough anesthetic to significantly delay recovery. Vessel-poor tissues, such as fascia and ligaments, make up 20% of body mass and receive approximately 1% of the cardiac output. This tissue group has an insignificant effect on anesthetic induction or recovery despite the fact that it is significant in proportion.

In summary, anesthesia does not occur until the brain concentration of anesthetic is sufficient to induce loss of consciousness. The more soluble the anesthetic in the blood, the slower the induction time. Increasing the inspired anesthetic concentration and patient minute ventilation shortens the induction time.

Anesthetic elimination is the reverse of uptake and distribution, wherein anesthetic molecules move from the tissues into the blood, and then into the pulmonary alveoli to be exhaled.

The speed of uptake and elimination is important in inhalation anesthesia, because this determines how rapidly one may alter anesthetic depth. Major factors that determine the speed of uptake are the inhaled concentration of anesthetic, minute ventilation, alveolar diffusion area, the agent's solubility coefficient and molecular weight, pulmonary blood flow, and the anesthetic partial pressure gradient between alveolar gas and plasma.

Specific Inhalant Agents. Three halogenated hydrocarbon anesthetic agents have been used extensively for veterinary anesthesia: methoxyflurane (Metofane), halothane (Fluothane), and isoflurane (Aerrane). Although

methoxyflurane is still in clinical use, halothane and isoflurane account for the largest proportion of inhalation procedures.

Halothane and isoflurane concentrations may rise to lethal levels very easily if they are not strictly controlled. For this reason, halothane and isoflurane are used in precision vaporizers positioned *out of the breathing circle*. With methoxyflurane, maximal vaporization is more difficult to achieve and it may be used in a nonprecision vaporizer in the breathing circuit. Although methoxyflurane has gained a reputation for ease of use and relative safety, its significant disadvantages make halothane or isoflurane the better choices.

Methoxyflurane provides the slowest induction (10 to 15 minutes) and recovery rates (30 minutes to several hours) of these agents because of its high blood-gas solubility coefficient. Isoflurane, in contrast, has the lowest blood solubility and the fastest induction (3 to 5 minutes) and recovery rates (less than 5 minutes). Halothane induction lies between isoflurane and methoxyflurane, with induction requiring 3 to 5 minutes and recovery 5 to 20 minutes.

The degree of metabolism required for elimination of these agents also varies. As much as 50% of methoxyflurane is metabolized by the liver, with 20% of halothane and 0.2% of isoflurane; this partially explains the rapid recovery and low toxicity of isoflurane. Methoxyflurane has a direct nephrotoxic effect. Halothane has some potential for causing hepatitis. Isoflurane has no significant toxicity. Methoxyflurane produces the best muscle relaxation of these three agents. Halothane and isoflurane produce adequate muscle relaxation.

Nitrous oxide is occasionally used in veterinary anesthesia as an adjunct to other agents. Its very low blood solubility allows very rapid uptake, distribution, and elimination. Addition of nitrous oxide to an inhalation protocol speeds uptake of the anesthetic gas (a second gas) into the blood, decreasing the time required for induction by inhalant anesthetics. This phenomenon is called the *second gas effect*. Unfortunately, nitrous oxide is not potent enough to produce general anesthesia alone. It is most commonly used with halothane, permitting a reduction in the amount of halothane required and therefore less occurrence of myocardial depression. There is little to be gained by use of nitrous oxide with isoflurane.

Use of nitrous oxide requires some caution, because it can diffuse into gas-filled body spaces, causing them to expand. Nitrous oxide is contraindicated in patients with pneumothorax or a diaphragmatic hernia with bowel in the thorax. Diffusion hypoxia may occur during recovery. Rapid movement of nitrous oxide from the blood to alveoli may cause hypoxia by displacing oxygen or by diluting alveolar carbon dioxide, which may decrease respiratory stimulation and ventilation. Adequate ventilation should be maintained and a high flow rate of 100% oxygen used for the first 5 to 10 minutes of recovery after nitrous oxide use.

Step 6: Recovery

Recovery means "to restore to a normal state." This reminds us that, during anesthesia, patients are in an abnormal state. Vigilance and support of organ function should continue until the patient is satisfactorily recovered from anesthesia. Pain relief and maintenance of a patent airway are important during recovery. The critical period has passed when the body temperature is normal, sternal recumbency is achieved, and oropharyngeal reflexes are restored. However, observation should continue until the patient can stand and is free of all drug effects.

ANESTHETIC MONITORING

Comprehensive monitoring of the anesthetized patient involves observing anesthetic equipment and evaluating the central nervous system, pulmonary function, and cardiovascular function. Early detection of equipment failure and/or depression of vital organ function allows execution of corrective measures, which are more effective than treating complications. Corrective actions to maintain or restore tissue perfusion are determined by integrating information from all body systems.

Monitoring of Anesthetic Equipment

Monitoring of anesthetic equipment is the most neglected portion of anesthetic monitoring. The functionality of anesthetic equipment should be carefully tested before and continuously throughout anesthetic procedures. The most common anesthetic complications by far are hypoxemia and inadequate depth. The oxygen source, anesthetic machine, and breathing circuit must be observed for leaks and carbon dioxide absorbent should be checked to ensure that it is not exhausted.

All anesthetic equipment should be clean, calibrated, and maintained in good working order. During anesthesia, frequently check connections to the patient or anesthetic circuit. Power sources to monitoring equipment and heat sources should be verified throughout the procedure. Be skeptical of sudden changes or erroneous monitoring device readings. Verify monitoring device readings with quick, simple observations, such as mucous membrane color, capillary refill time, pulse rate, and pulse quality. If the blood pressure reads zero but the mucous membranes are pink and well perfused, common sense dictates that the blood pressure reading is probably erroneous.

Monitoring Anesthetic Depth

Monitoring of the CNS includes estimation of anesthetic depth. Anesthetic depth refers to the degree of CNS depression. Typically, as the CNS becomes progressively more depressed, one can observe progressive changes in patient response and condition. For the standard anesthetics, these observable signs have been grouped into stages of anesthesia (with some of the stages being subdivided into planes). Clinically, it is common to refer to anesthetic depth as "light" if the degree of CNS depression is minimal and "deep" if it is profound (Box 20-5 and Table 20-2). In reality this assessment is very subjective and requires integration of numerous factors, such as muscle tone, ocular reflexes, heart rate, respiratory rate and depth, and blood pressure. The progressive signs of anesthetic depth vary with the anesthetic drugs used, the species, and the individual patient. One cannot rely on a single sign but must use all available information to evaluate anesthetic depth.

Anesthetic depth is not a steady state, but rather a product of the anesthetic drugs on board and surgical or physical stimulation applied to the patient at a particular time. If the anesthetic dose is constant, increased surgical stimulation may quickly result in movement or awakening. Increasing the anesthetic dose to compensate for periods of extreme surgical stimulation may precipitate sudden overdose in the absence of stimulation. In summary, anesthetic depth is dose dependent; more drug produces more CNS depression. However, the degree to which a given anesthetic dose produces CNS depression (general anesthesia) is quite variable.

Anesthetic depth is sufficient when gross patient movement does not interfere with the procedure being performed. Anesthetic depth is estimated by assessing skeletal muscle tone and selected reflexes. Jaw muscle tone and eye reflexes are useful signs of anesthetic depth and diminish with progression toward deeper planes of anesthesia.

Box 20–5 Progression of anesthetic depth

1. Analgesia and amnesia
2. Loss of consciousness and motor coordination
3. Reduced protective reflexes
4. Blockade of afferent stimuli
5. Muscle relaxation
6. Respiratory and cardiovascular depression
7. Depression of cardiovascular and respiratory reflexes
8. Apnea
9. Cardiac arrest

Eye reflexes are frequently used to assess anesthetic depth. Nystagmus and active palpebral reflexes indicate light anesthesia, which is inadequate for most surgical procedures. Absence of the palpebral reflex and presence of the corneal reflex are considered signs of a medium level of anesthesia, at which routine surgical procedures may be performed. Absence of corneal reflex or drying of the cornea indicates deep anesthesia, in which the patient should be monitored closely for adequate cardiopulmonary function and the anesthetic level lightened if possible. Direct response to surgical stimulation is the most reliable sign of light anesthesia. In many patients, movement is often preceded by other signs, such as increased rate and depth of respiration.

Monitoring Respiratory Function

Respiratory function is monitored to ensure adequate oxygenation and removal of carbon dioxide from the blood. Respiratory function may be evaluated by respiratory rate, tidal volume, breathing patterns, hemoglobin saturation, end-tidal carbon dioxide, and arterial blood gases. Arterial blood gas analysis, the most reliable method by which to assess respiratory function, is not possible in all clinical settings because it requires an arterial blood sample and special equipment. Equipment useful for monitoring respiratory function includes a blood gas machine, pulse oximeter, end-tidal carbon dioxide analyzer (capnometer), rate monitor, and ventilometer. However, the most essential monitor is a well-prepared, highly skilled individual performing continuous monitoring.

Hearing, vision, and touch can be used to monitor the respiratory system and airway. Good indicators that air is moving in and out of the lungs are auscultation of breathing and lung sounds with a standard or esophageal stethoscope, observation of the chest wall and of the reservoir bag for movement, and feeling the reservoir bag for resistance (Box 20-6). However, air movement does not ensure adequate exchange of oxygen and carbon dioxide between the alveoli and blood. Observation of bright red arterial blood at the surgical site and observing mucous membranes for pinkness are reasonably reliable for determining blood oxygenation. Color changes are not evident until severe hypoxemia exists, however.

Monitoring Cardiovascular Function

Cardiovascular function is monitored to ensure that cardiac output and forward movement of blood are contributing to tissue perfusion. Cardiovascular function is evaluated by the heart rate, heart sounds, pulse quality and rate, mucous membrane color, and capillary refill time. Electrocardiography is recommended for evaluation of rhythm and conduction disturbances. Comparison of heart rate and pulse rate enables detection of pulse

---

Box 20-6 Informative auscultatory sounds

Respiratory sounds

- Partial airway obstruction: increased or decreased sound volume, harshness
- Severe narrowing of airways: stridor, snoring, squeaking, whistling
- Fluid: crepitation
- Excessive fluid: bubbling

Cardiac sounds

- Loudness indicates contractile strength and cardiac output
- Murmurs may mean decreased forward movement of blood
- Simultaneous pulse palpation can reveal arrhythmias

TABLE 20-2 Signs of anesthetic depth

	Anesthetic depth		
	Light	Surgical	Deep
Spontaneous movement	Possible	None	None
Reflex movement	Possible	None	None
Anesthetic concentration	1 MAC	1.1 to 1.5 MAC	1.5 to 2 MAC
Jaw muscle tone	Tense	Moderate	Relaxed
Palpebral reflex	Present	None or slight	None
Globe position	Central	Ventromedial	Central
Corneal moisture	Moist	Moist	Dry
Pupil size	Medium	Reduced	Dilated

deficits. Blood pressure, urine output, and body temperature are also indicators of cardiovascular function.

All anesthetic drugs used today have dose-dependent cardiovascular depressant effects, such as arrhythmias, decreased contractility, vasodilation, or vasoconstriction. Monitoring the cardiovascular system does not require a grand display of electronic instrumentation. Although mechanical devices are appealing, the senses of touch, hearing, and vision are extremely useful for evaluation of cardiovascular function. Pulse palpation, capillary refill, blood color, and heart sounds may be determined with simple instrumentation. The stethoscope provides much information useful to estimate cardiovascular status. Monitoring equipment can be used to enhance evaluation of cardiovascular function but can never replace what you observe, feel, or hear (Table 20-3).

Heart rates are easily determined with a simple stethoscope, esophageal stethoscope, or ECG. Counting the rate of the peripheral pulse and the heart rate simultaneously is very useful. Although heart rates vary significantly with patient size and species, the pulse rate and the heart rate should be equal. The presence of a heart sound with an absent or extremely weak pulse indicates a pulse deficit and should be investigated before anesthesia proceeds. Ordinarily, smaller patients have faster heart rates than larger patients of the same species. Memorizing "normal" heart rates (above which is termed *tachycardia* and below which is termed *bradycardia*) is of limited value in estimating cardiac output. Changes in heart rate may indicate adverse anesthetic effects, pain, or vagal reflex stimulation.

Auscultation. Auscultation of the heart with a standard or esophageal stethoscope can provide valuable information, in addition to the heart rate. The rhythm and loudness of the heart beat reflect overall cardiovascular function. Heart sounds are easily amplified by inexpensive monitoring devices. These small amplifiers provide the convenience of easily audible heart sounds

TABLE 20-3 Normal physiologic values in dogs, cats, horses, and cattle

	Dogs	Cats	Horses	Cattle
Heart rate	60-160/min	80-200/min	24-50/min	60-120/min
Respiratory rate	20-40/min	20-40/min	8-20/min	20-40/min
Tidal volume	10-20 ml/kg	10-20 ml/kg	10-20 ml/kg	10-20 ml/kg
Minute volume (resp rate × tidal vol)	200-800 ml/kg/min	200-800 ml/kg/min	200-800 ml/kg/min	200-800 ml/kg/min
Blood pH	7.35-7.45	7.35-7.45	7.35-7.45	7.35-7.45
PaO$_2$	80-110 mm Hg	80-110 mm Hg	80-110 mm Hg	80-110 mm Hg
PaCO$_2$	35-45 mm Hg	35-45 mm Hg	35-45 mm Hg	35-45 mm Hg
HCO$_3$	22-27 mm Hg	22-27 mm Hg	22-27 mm Hg	22-27 mm Hg
Total CO$_2$	38-54 mm Hg	38-54 mm Hg	54-72 mm Hg	47-72 mm Hg
Base excess	−4 to +4	−4 to +4 (correct if −5 to −10)	−4 to +4	−4 to +4
Central venous pressure (standing)	3-4 cm H$_2$O	3-4 cm H$_2$O	3-4 cm H$_2$O	3-4 cm H$_2$O
Central venous pressure (anesthetized and recumbent)	2-7 cm H$_2$O	15-25 cm H$_2$O	——	——

while freeing the surgeon or technician to move around within the surgical area. Abnormal heart rates, irregular rhythm, and weak or muffled heart sounds may indicate diminished cardiac function. Altered heart rate and irregular rhythm suggest arrhythmias, whereas diminished heart sounds may indicate low cardiac output from myocardial hypoxemia or hypotension. Integrating this information with mucous membrane color, pulse quality, and capillary refill time provides usable information. However, it is a mistake to simply assume that because there is an audible beep or heart sound, everything is fine.

Electrocardiogram. The electrocardiogram (ECG) provides reliable information concerning heart rate and rhythm. The ECG is valuable for diagnosis of specific cardiac arrhythmias. Remember that the ECG is only an indicator of the electrical activity of the heart muscle and alone is a poor indicator of normal contraction or blood flow. Normal contraction requires normal electrical conduction of activating electrical impulses through cardiac muscle tissue. Abnormal or skipped contractions resulting from abnormal electrical activity (ECG) may diminish blood flow, consequently producing pulse deficit. If sufficient skipped beats occur (10 to 12 per min), perfusion may be significantly affected, requiring organ support. The sequence of adverse events is abnormal ECG, abnormal or skipped beats, decreased blood flow, weak or absent pulse, and finally cardiac arrest.

Pulse. Although the pulse is not produced by passage of blood itself, palpation of peripheral pulse strength is a useful indicator of stroke volume. Normal pulse rate and adequate pulse quality are indicators of adequate blood flow. The peripheral pulse rate is not necessarily the heart rate. Pulse rate is easily determined by palpation or pulse oximetry. Auscultation of the heart while simultaneously palpating peripheral pulse is an excellent method of recognizing pulse deficits that may be due to cardiac arrhythmias. Significant arrhythmias produce skipped beats. Pulse deficits occurring at a rate of 10 to 12 times per min or more may significantly diminish coronary and peripheral perfusion and require immediate attention. Anesthetics produce dose-related decreases in pulse quality. Frequent causes of decreased pulse quality during anesthesia include hypovolemia, hypotension, hypoxia, hypothermia, and decreased cardiac output. If the pulse weakens, decrease the anesthetic concentration, increase the infusion rate of fluids, determine the underlying cause, and make appropriate corrections.

Mucous Membrane Color. Mucous membrane color can be used to estimate tissue perfusion and oxygenation. Mucous membranes are normally pink, indicating adequate respiratory and cardiovascular function. Cherry red mucous membranes may be seen with carbon monoxide poisoning. However, in severe carbon monoxide poisoning, cyanosis may mask the cherry red color. Hemoglobin has 200 times the affinity for carbon monoxide than oxygen and its presence reduces the oxygen-transporting capability of hemoglobin, resulting in hypoxemia. Carbon monoxide poisoning has occurred during anesthesia of people using halogenated hydrocarbons. There is reason for the same concern in veterinary anesthesia, although it has not yet been reported. Apparently, desiccated soda lime and Baralyme react with halogenated inhalation anesthetics to produce toxic concentrations of carbon monoxide. The tendency for veterinary clinics to delay changing of carbon dioxide absorbent must be seriously addressed.

Pale mucous membranes indicate vasoconstriction or a decrease in circulating red blood cells. Pale mucous membranes are not always a sign of poor hemodynamic status or shock. Cyanosis is a sign of respiratory insufficiency and an indication of hypoxemia. Absence of blueness does not ensure adequate blood oxygenation. Anemic patients may not have sufficient hemoglobin to produce blueness, even when hypoxia is severe.

Capillary Refill Time. Capillary refill time (CRT) provides another way to estimate tissue perfusion and oxygenation. It is an indication of cardiovascular tone; it suggests that blood is filling the capillary beds. CRT of less than 2 seconds in small animals and less than 3 seconds in large animals is considered normal. However, in a head-down position or in the presence of vasodilation, patients may have normal or reduced CRT in the presence of severely compromised blood flow. This is especially true in horses, cattle, and other very large patients. Vasoconstriction prolongs the CRT. In summary, the presence of shortened or normal CRT may not be a reliable sign of adequate perfusion, but a prolonged CRT is significant.

Arterial Blood Pressure. Arterial blood pressure is an indicator of perfusion and cardiac output but not a true measure of blood flow. Anesthetics produce dose-dependent decreases in blood pressure; therefore, monitoring blood pressure during anesthesia is useful for depth determination and evaluation of patient health status. Blood pressure may be determined by direct or indirect methods. Direct or invasive monitoring requires special equipment and placement of an arterial catheter. Indirect or noninvasive methods require special equipment but do not require an invasive arterial catheter to measure blood pressure. Doppler and oscillometric methods are indirect and noninvasive and are frequently used to determine blood pressure in clinical settings. The equipment used to measure blood pressure by noninvasive methods is priced within range of most veterinary facilities.

Low arterial blood pressure may be due to hypovolemia, cardiac depression, or vasodilation. The awake or lightly anesthetized, healthy patient rapidly compensates for hypotension by increasing cardiac output or by increasing vascular tone. However, patients anesthetized to surgical planes of anesthesia may be unable to compensate or maintain acceptable blood pressure because of dose-dependent autonomic nervous system depression produced by anesthetic drugs. In most anesthetized patients, intravenous administration of crystalloid fluids at 10 to 20 ml/kg/hr, along with careful monitoring of tissue perfusion and anesthetic depth, prevents hypotension.

Monitoring Body Temperature

Monitoring body temperature during anesthesia provides an indication of CNS function and cardiovascular function. Depression of thermoregulatory centers in the brain and decreased blood flow produced by anesthetic agents lead to *hypothermia* (low body temperature). It may be produced in response to various drug combinations, specifically halothane, isoflurane, succinylcholine, and ketamine. Continuous measurement of core temperature with a rectal or esophageal thermometer warns of significant temperature change.

It is much easier to prevent heat loss than to restore heat. Minimizing potential heat loss requires planning. Minimizing anesthesia time and depth, avoiding cold surfaces and cold scrub solutions, using a circulating-water blanket or hot-water bottles, and warming intravenous fluids help prevent hypothermia. It is also useful to warm and moisturize inspired air, use warm blankets, keep body cavities closed when possible, and use warm irrigation solutions. Fluids, hot-water bottles, or warming blankets should not be warmed to temperatures greater than 40° C or body surfaces may be burned.

Responding to Adverse Events

Hypothermia. If the body temperature drops below 35° C, decrease the anesthetic concentration, ensure adequate circulation, insulate from cold surfaces, dry the body surface, apply warm blankets and/or hot packs, warm inspired air, and decrease fresh gas flow to minimum requirements.

Tachycardia. If the patient is not moving (anesthetic depth is adequate), decrease the anesthetic concentration, increase oxygen flow, increase the rate of intravenous fluid delivery, and support ventilation. If tachycardia persists, prepare for cardiac arrest.

Bradycardia. Bradycardia caused by alpha agonists may be treated with anticholinergics or a specific alpha antagonist. Opioid-induced bradycardia can be managed with anticholinergics. Bradycardia resulting from excessive anesthetic depth usually responds to a decreased anesthetic concentration and support with oxygen and fluids. Vagus-mediated bradycardia is usually transient and diminishes as vagal stimulation is discontinued. If bradycardia worsens or persists, administration of an anticholinergic may be required, along with fluid administration. Hypothermic patients exhibiting bradycardia must be warmed and may require intravenous fluid administration to correct bradycardia. Anticholinergics should be avoided in hypothermic patients because of the increased risk of cardiac arrhythmia.

Pain. Pain should be treated with an analgesic that produces less cardiovascular depressant effect than additional general anesthetic. Hypotension is usually controlled by appropriate fluid administration and lowering the anesthetic concentration.

Hypercarbia. Hypercarbia is managed by increasing ventilation ("bagging") to remove carbon dioxide from the patient.

Hypoxemia. Hypoxemia is initially treated by increasing inspired oxygen concentration and ensuring adequate ventilation.

Excessive Depth. Excessive anesthetic depth is reversed by decreasing the vaporizer setting, increasing the oxygen flow rate, and ensuring adequate ventilation and circulatory support.

INHALATION ANESTHETIC TECHNIQUES
Goals of Proper Technique

A primary goal of proper anesthetic technique is to provide maximum safety for the patient and personnel. Of paramount importance is to minimize or avoid personnel exposure to anesthetic waste gases (Box 20-7). Anesthetic techniques have evolved to avoid specific problems encountered in the past. Although the consequences of error or mishap in any one step of a procedure may seem negligible, the cumulative effects of marginal technique may produce serious consequences. The following selected procedural guidelines should be followed routinely.

Induction Technique

Anesthetic induction may proceed after a vein is catheterized, the equipment is readied, and the surgeon is available. Administration of the induction or maintenance agent should provide a smooth and safe transition to unconsciousness (see Box 20-4 for specific information on induction agents). When jaw muscle tone and orolaryngeal reflexes are lost, intubate the patient.

Endotracheal Intubation

Dogs and Cats. Dogs and cats are placed in sternal position, with the head and neck extended in a straight line to aid visualization of the larynx. If an assistant is available, have him or her position the head while the anesthetist places the endotracheal tube. A laryngoscope

---

Box 20-7 Techniques for minimizing exposure to waste anesthetic gases

- Check for and correct leaks in the anesthesia machine and breathing circuit.
- Use a cuffed endotracheal tube of the proper size; inflate the cuff if needed.
- Do not disconnect patient from breathing circuit immediately after anesthesia; if possible, wait several minutes for gases to dissipate.
- Connect the pop-off valve to a scavenger system, preferably one that discharges outdoors.
- Connect non-rebreathing systems to a scavenger system.
- Avoid use of chamber or mask induction techniques.
- Avoid spilling liquid anesthetic while filling the vaporizer; recap the bottle and vaporizer immediately.
- Maintain adequate ventilation of the area.

---

aids intubation. Place the largest tube that will enter the airway without causing trauma or undue stimulation of vagal reflexes, which may induce cardiac arrhythmias. Applying lidocaine to the larynx by spray or with a cotton-tipped swab, especially in cats and swine, facilitates intubation. Cetacaine (benzocaine) spray should not be used because it can cause methemoglobinemia. Lubrication of the cuff with sterile water-soluble lubricant facilitates intubation and protects the tracheal mucosa from drying where the inflated cuff contacts the mucosa. Proper positioning of the endotracheal tube may be confirmed by condensation of respiratory gases on the inside of the tube with expiration, ability to palpate only one tubular structure in the neck (trachea), auscultation of lung sounds when bagging the patient, and the carbon dioxide reading on the capnometer.

Attach the Y-piece to the endotracheal tube adapter before inflating the cuff (see discussion of cuff inflation below). Open the oxygen flow meter to deliver 3 L/min and set the vaporizer to the appropriate delivery concentration (1% to 3%). Secure the tube with gauze or tape to the mandible or maxilla and begin cardiopulmonary observations. Once the tube is in place and secured, and the system is free of leaks, apply ophthalmic ointment to protect the cornea (if not previously done) and proceed with preparation for the procedure. When moving the patient is required, it is prudent to disconnect the Y-piece from the endotracheal tube to avoid trauma or dislodgment.

Horses. Horses are intubated similar to small animals, except the horse is placed in lateral recumbency. The oral cavity must be flushed thoroughly with water to remove food and debris before induction and intubation. It is necessary to place an oral speculum between the incisor teeth to prevent biting the tube, causing obstruction of the airway. A tube of the largest diameter that will pass without excessive force is selected. The endotracheal tube is lubricated with copious amounts of water-soluble sterile lubricant and passed through the pre-inserted speculum, avoiding the sharp edges of the check teeth. Although the glottis cannot be visualized, the tube enters with little difficulty. If difficulty is encountered while blindly intubating, rotating the tube while applying slight pressure usually facilitates tube passage. Box 20-8 presents a summary of techniques used in equine anesthesia.

Endotracheal Cuff Inflation. The endotracheal tube cuff is inflated to allow positive-pressure ventilation and prevent aspiration in the event of regurgitation. A pressure of 20 to 25 cm H_2O is sufficient for both purposes. *Do not inflate the cuff until the need has been determined.* To determine the need for cuff inflation, perform the following steps:

1. Close the pressure-relief valve and squeeze the reservoir bag while observing the manometer and listening for leakage of gas around the endotracheal tube.
2. If circuit pressure reaches 25 cm H_2O without leaking around the tube, do not inflate the cuff.
3. If leakage occurs below 25 cm H_2O, inflate the cuff just enough to prevent this leakage. Should the cuff be inflated beyond 25 cm H_2O, the excessive pressure may damage the tracheal mucosa.

Tissue damage from traumatic intubation or an over-inflated cuff is often manifested as coughing a few days after anesthesia.

Maintenance of Anesthesia

After intubation and stabilization, the anesthetized patient is considered in the stage of maintenance. The anesthetist's attention now focuses on monitoring and support of vital organ function. Connect all monitoring instruments and begin recording all pertinent information on the patient's anesthetic record. Monitoring should be continuous and data should be recorded every 5 to 10 minutes or whenever significant changes occur.

The oxygen flow rate may be reduced to maintenance levels at this time, depending on the type of breathing circuit used. Non-rebreathing circuits require high flows throughout maintenance, whereas rebreathing circuits may use reduced flows for semi-closed or closed operation. The typical flow rate for semi-closed operation is 1 L/min. It should be recognized that lower flow rates increase the time it takes to change the anesthetic concentration of the breathing circuit.

Box 20-8 Quick reference guide for equine anesthesia

Preparation

1. Withhold food for 24 hours and water for 6 to 12 hours, when possible. Telephone the client to remind about food and water restriction.
2. Obtain the horse's body weight by weighing or chest girth tape measurement for estimation.
3. Avoid or delay elective procedures in horses that are not healthy. Perform a physical examination before administration of any drug. Minimum data should include heart rate, respiratory rate, mucous membrane color, pulse quality, ocular or nasal discharge, lymph nodes, PCV, and total plasma protein assay.
4. Administer fluids to debilitated horses or horses to be anesthetized for long procedures.
5. Use an IV set with a drip chamber. Do not use a simplex.
6. Place an IV catheter.
7. Use a trained technician (rather than a client or barn staff) to assist, monitor vital organ function, and administer drugs.
8. Avoid stress, such as from extreme heat or long trailer rides, before induction of anesthesia.
9. Keep the horse calm before induction of anesthesia.

Sedation and analgesia in standing horses

Xylazine and butorphanol

Give xylazine IM or IV at 4 to 7 mg/kg.
Wait 10 minutes.
Give butorphanol IV at 2 to 5 mg/kg.
Monitor sedation and heart rate.
Give small IV doses of xylazine and butorphanol as needed.
  Give xylazine in IV boluses of 50 to 100 mg (maximum of 500 mg/hr).
  Give butorphanol in IV boluses of 5 to 10 mg (maximum of 50 mg/hr).
If the patient has difficulty standing, do not administer more drug.

Detomidine and butorphanol

Give detomidine IV at 0.02 mg/kg or IM at 0.04 mg/kg.
Wait 10 minutes.
Give butorphanol IV at 2 to 5 mg/kg.
Monitor sedation and heart rate.
Give small IV doses of detomidine and butorphanol as needed.
  Give detomidine in IV boluses of 2 mg (maximum of 20 mg/hr).
  Give butorphanol in IV boluses of 5 to 10 mg (maximum of 50 mg/hr).
If the patient has difficulty standing, do not administer more drug.

Anesthetic induction and maintenance

Xylazine and ketamine

Give xylazine IV at 1.1 mg/kg. If the horse is not sedated by xylazine, administer 10 to 20 mg (total dose) of diazepam or butorphanol IV, rather than additional xylazine.
Give ketamine as an IV bolus at 2.2 mg/kg.
Anticipate 8 to 12 minutes of anesthesia.
Anesthesia may be prolonged with "Triple Drip" (see below) or with up to two additional doses of xylazine and ketamine, using half the original dosage. Do not give more than two additional doses.

Diazepam with xylazine and ketamine

Give diazepam IM or slowly IV at 0.05 mg/kg.
Wait 20 to 40 minutes for maximum effect.
Give xylazine IV at 1.1 mg/kg.
When the horse is sedated (may occur rapidly), give ketamine as an IV bolus at 2.2 mg/kg.
Provides smooth induction, 12 to 20 minutes of anesthesia, and smooth recovery.
Anesthesia may be prolonged with "Triple Drip" (see below).

Butorphanol with xylazine and ketamine

Give butorphanol IM or slowly IV at 0.05 mg/kg.
Wait 20 minutes.
Give xylazine IV at 1.1 mg/kg.
When the horse is sedated, give ketamine as an IV bolus at 2.2 mg/kg.
Anticipate 12 to 20 minutes of anesthesia and analgesia.
Anesthesia may be prolonged with "Triple Drip" (see below) or guaifenesin.

"Triple Drip"

Add 1,000 to 2,000 mg of ketamine (1 to 2 mg/ml) and 500 mg of xylazine (0.05 mg/ml) to 1 liter of 5% guaifenesin (50 mg/ml).
Infuse IV at a constant drip rate of approximately 1 to 2 ml/kg/hr.
"Triple Drip" is useful for maintenance following induction with xylazine and dissociative anesthetics.

Adjust the vaporizer to provide the desired depth. The correct setting provides just enough anesthesia to perform the procedure. Excessive concentrations should be avoided. Begin administration of intravenous fluids as soon as possible (10 to 20 ml/kg/hr).

Throughout maintenance, the patient should be ventilated twice per minute or as needed to maintain a $PaCO_2$ of 40 to 45 mm Hg. This is accomplished by closing the pop-off valve and squeezing the reservoir bag to inflate the lungs to a pressure of 15 to 20 cm H_2O. This artificial "breath" should mimic a normal breath in terms of inspiratory time (do not hold pressure; just inflate and release).

Recovery from Anesthesia

Recovery begins when administration of anesthetic is discontinued. The patient should be maintained on 100% oxygen to ensure oxygenation and allow exhaled anesthetic gases to enter the scavenger system, rather than the room air. As the patient begins to awaken, the endotracheal tube cuff should be deflated and the tie undone. When the patient exhibits swallowing reflexes, the tube should be gently removed. Close observation is essential immediately after extubation, as the patient may regurgitate or have difficulty breathing. Brachycephalic dogs are especially notorious for developing breathing difficulties after extubation.

Fluid administration should continue until recovery is adequate. Recovery is considered adequate (but not complete) when the body temperature is normal, the patient's vital signs are stable, and sternal recumbency is maintained. Observation should continue until the patient can stand and walk without assistance.

RECOMMENDED READING

Anon: Commentary and recommendations on control of waste anesthetic gases in the workplace, *J Am Vet Med Assoc* 209:75-77, 1996.

Muir WW et al: *Handbook of veterinary anesthesia,* ed 2, St Louis, 1995, Mosby.

Riebold TW et al: *Large animal anesthesia: principles and techniques,* ed 2, Ames, Iowa, 1995, Iowa State University Press.

Short CE: *Principles and practice of veterinary anesthesia,* Baltimore, 1987, Williams & Wilkins.

Thurmon JC, Tranquilli WJ: *Lamb and Jones' veterinary anesthesia,* ed 3, Baltimore, 1996, Williams & Wilkins.

CHAPTER 21

Principles of Surgical Nursing

T.W. Fossum
H.B. Seim
T.P. Colville

Learning Objectives

After reviewing this chapter, the reader should understand the following:

Terminology used in surgery
Principles of aseptic technique
Methods used to disinfect and sterilize surgical instruments and supplies

Method used to prepare and components of surgical packs
Procedure for preparing the surgical site
Types of surgical instruments and their uses and maintenance
Principles of wound closure and hemostasis
Types of suture needles and suture materials

GENERAL SURGICAL PRINCIPLES

T.P. COLVILLE

The roles of veterinary technicians in surgical procedures can be many and varied. During the presurgical period, veterinary technicians are usually responsible for preparation of the patient, the surgical instruments and equipment, and the surgical environment. During surgery, the veterinary technician may be responsible for anesthesia of the patient. The veterinary technician will probably assist the surgeon, either directly, by actually scrubbing in, or indirectly, by properly opening surgical packs, suture materials, or other supplies and by knowing how to function in a sterile surgical environment without causing contamination. In the postsurgical period, the veterinary technician is frequently responsible for postoperative patient care and monitoring, instructing clients on proper patient care during the recovery period, and removing sutures.

BASIC SURGICAL TERMINOLOGY
Combining Forms

Six suffixes are commonly combined with anatomic terms to produce words describing surgical procedures.

-ectomy = to remove (to excise). For example, a splenec*tomy* is a surgical procedure to remove the spleen.

-otomy = to cut into. For example, a cysto*tomy* (incision into the urinary bladder) is often performed to remove urinary calculi (bladder stones).

-ostomy = surgical creation of an artificial opening. For example, a perineal urethro*stomy* is a surgical procedure often performed on male cats for relief of urethral obstruction. It involves excision of the penis (pen*ectomy)* and creation of a widened new urethral opening.

-rrhaphy = surgical repair by suturing. For example, abdominal hernio*rrhaphy* is the surgical repair of an abdominal hernia by suturing the defect in the abdominal musculature.

-pexy = surgical fixation. For example, gastro*pexy* (suturing of the stomach to the abdominal wall to fix it in place) is often performed in cases of gastric torsion.

-plasty = surgical alteration of shape or form. For example, pyloro*plasty* enlarges the pyloric orifice of the stomach to facilitate gastric emptying.

Abdominal Incisions

Abdominal surgery is commonly performed in animal species. Entry into the abdomen is usually gained by any of four common abdominal incisions. Named according to its location, each incision offers different advantages and a different exposure of the abdomen.

A *ventral midline incision* is located on the ventral midline of the animal. It offers excellent exposure of the entire abdominal cavity. Because the abdominal cavity is entered through the linea alba, where the abdominal muscles on each side are joined, the abdominal wall can be closed with a single layer of sutures in the linea alba. Closure of a ventral midline incision must be very secure, because the weight of the abdominal organs exerts tension on the incision when the animal stands. Also, any exertion by the animal can create tension on the suture line.

A *paramedian incision* is located lateral and parallel to the ventral midline of the animal. It is usually used when exposure of only one side of the abdomen is needed, such as for removal of a cryptorchid (retained) testis. The muscles of the abdominal wall are individually incised, so closure of the abdominal wall usually requires multiple layers of sutures.

A *flank incision* is generally performed on either a standing animal or one in lateral recumbency. It is oriented perpendicular to the long axis of the body, caudal to the last rib. A flank incision provides good exposure of the organ(s) immediately deep to (beneath) the incision but does not allow exploration of much of the remainder of the abdomen. It is, therefore, useful for such procedures as rumenotomy and nephrectomy, in which the organ in question lies directly beneath the incision. The muscles of the abdominal wall usually require a multiple-layer closure. In contrast to tension exerted on a ventral midline incision, the weight of the abdominal organs generally tends to keep a flank incision closed rather than pulling it apart.

A *paracostal incision* is oriented parallel to the last rib and offers good exposure of the stomach and spleen in monogastric animals. The muscles of the abdominal wall are usually closed in multiple layers.

Common Surgical Procedures

Soft Tissue Procedures. *Ovariohysterectomy,* commonly referred to as a "spay," involves removal of the ovaries and uterus.

Cesarean section is a method of delivering newborn animals in cases of dystocia (difficult labor). It consists of an abdominal incision (flank or ventral midline) and then an incision into the uterus through which the newborn(s) is (are) delivered.

Orchiectomy (castration) is the surgical removal of the testes.

Lateral ear resection is often performed in animals with chronic external ear infection. It involves removal of the lateral wall of the vertical portion of the external ear canal to allow improved ventilation and to establish drainage for exudates.

Laparotomy is an incision into the abdominal cavity, often through the flank. *Celiotomy* is another term for laparotomy.

Cystotomy is an incision into the urinary bladder, frequently for removal of urinary calculi (bladder stones).

Gastrotomy is an incision into a simple stomach, whereas a *rumenotomy* is an incision into a rumen.

Gastropexy involves suturing of the stomach to the abdominal wall to fix it in place. This procedure is frequently done in cases of gastric torsion.

Splenectomy is the removal of the spleen.

Thoracotomy is an incision into the thoracic cavity (chest).

Herniorrhaphy is the surgical repair of a hernia by suturing the abnormal opening(s) closed.

Enterotomy is an incision into the intestine, often for removal of a foreign body.

Intestinal resection and anastomosis involves removal of a portion of the intestine (resection) and suturing the cut ends together to restore the continuity of the intestinal tube (anastomosis).

Urethrostomy involves incision into the urethra and suturing of the splayed urethral edges to the skin to create a larger urethral orifice. This procedure is frequently performed on male cats with recurrent urethral obstruction.

Mastectomy involves removal of part or all of one or more mammary glands.

Orthopedic (Bone) Procedures. *Onychectomy* is the surgical removal of a claw, commonly called *declawing.*

Intervertebral disk fenestration is done to remove prolapsed intervertebral disk material causing pressure on the spinal cord.

Intramedullary bone pinning involves insertion of a metal rod (bone pin) into the medullary cavity of a long bone to fix fracture fragments in place.

Cranial cruciate ligament repair is performed when that stifle joint ligament has ruptured. Lack of an intact cranial cruciate ligament creates instability in the stifle, causing abnormal movement. This can damage the joint surfaces of the distal femur and proximal tibia.

Femoral head ostectomy involves amputation of the head of the femur. It is usually performed in animals with severe damage to the femoral head or neck, or with a damaged acetabulum.

PREOPERATIVE AND POSTOPERATIVE CONSIDERATIONS

Preoperative Evaluation

Anesthesia and surgery are very stressful events that put an animal's life at risk. The role of a proper preoperative evaluation is to gather enough pertinent information to minimize that risk. That information can be gathered through a patient history, a physical examination, and appropriate laboratory tests.

Postoperative Evaluation

After a flawlessly executed surgical procedure, a patient receiving poor postoperative care can suffer devastating consequences. The postoperative period should be considered critical for all patients. Because of the possibility of unforeseen complications, it is essential that patients be continually monitored after any type of surgery.

Body Temperature. After surgery, every patient should have its rectal temperature measured at least once a day, and preferably two to three times a day. A 1° or 2° increase in rectal temperature for the first few postoperative days is a normal physiologic response to the trauma of major surgery. A higher or more prolonged temperature increase may indicate infection.

Body Weight. Daily monitoring of a surgical patient's body weight gives a measure of the animal's nutritional status and general body condition. One of the most frequently neglected aspects of postoperative patient care is provision of adequate nutrition. The healing process after surgery increases an animal's nutritional needs, particularly for protein. Those needs must be met so that healing can proceed without delay.

Attitude. An animal's behavior during the immediate postoperative period can give important information about the amount of pain it is enduring and possible complications that might be developing. If a patient is very depressed, the reasons for that state must be determined and appropriate treatment instituted quickly.

Appetite and Thirst. Surgical patients must receive adequate nutrition and fluid intake. Animals should begin eating and drinking as soon as possible after surgery. Lack of interest in food and/or water indicates problems that should be investigated without delay.

Urination and Defecation. Elimination patterns give important information about kidney and GI tract function in patients recovering from surgery. Assuming adequate fluid and food intake, urination and defecation should proceed normally.

Appearance of the Surgical Wound. The surgical incision should be examined at least daily during the immediate postoperative period. It should be evaluated by visual inspection as well as gentle palpation. Such abnormalities as fluid accumulation, inflammation, and impending dehiscence (opening) of the surgical wound can be detected and corrected early if the incision is carefully evaluated.

Postoperative Complications

Hemorrhage. If not quickly corrected, postoperative hemorrhage can lead to serious consequences for an animal, even death from shock. External hemorrhage is usually relatively easy to evaluate and control because it is easily visible. Internal hemorrhage is not readily apparent and, therefore, often more serious. An animal can bleed to death through hemorrhage into the abdominal cavity or thoracic cavity. The status of an animal's cardiovascular system should be frequently monitored during the immediate postoperative period for signs that might indicate hemorrhage. Pulse rate, capillary refill time, temperature of the extremities, and color of the mucous membranes can give valuable information on cardiovascular function.

Seroma. Seromas (accumulations of serum) and hematomas (accumulations of blood) beneath the surgical incision are usually caused by "dead space" left in the incision that the body naturally fills with fluid. Though unsightly, small seromas and hematomas are usually of cosmetic importance only, unless the skin sutures tear out. Treatment usually involves drainage of the fluid via needle and syringe and application of a pressure bandage, or resuturing of the incision to eliminate the dead space. Seromas and hematomas can be prevented with adequate suturing.

Infection. A persistently or drastically elevated rectal temperature, depressed attitude, poor appetite, or a swollen, inflamed incision are all signs of possible postoperative infection.

Postoperative infections can be superficial, subcutaneous, within a body cavity, or spread throughout the body. Superficial infection often results in a draining wound that does not heal well. Subcutaneous infections frequently progress to abscess formation. Infection in the abdominal cavity (peritonitis) or thoracic cavity (pleuritis) often results from a penetrating injury or damage to organs in that body cavity. Septicemia is a generalized infection that spreads via the bloodstream. Fortunately, septicemia is not common after surgery.

When the danger of postoperative infection is high, as with long or potentially contaminated procedures, begin administration of a broad-spectrum antibacterial 24 hours before surgery to achieve an effective blood level. Continue drug use for at least 5 consecutive days after surgery.

Wound Dehiscence. Wound dehiscence (disruption of the surgical wound) is one of the most serious postoperative complications that can occur. Possible causes of wound dehiscence include the following:

- Suture failure (loosening, untying, breakage)
- Infection

- Tissue weakness (old or debilitated animals, hyper-adrenocorticism, prolonged corticosteroid use)
- Mechanical stress (stormy anesthetic recovery, chronic vomiting, chronic cough, excessive activity)
- Poor nutrition

Early signs of surgical wound dehiscence are frequently seen within the first 3 or 4 days after surgery. They may include a serosanguineous discharge from the incision, firm or fluctuant swelling deep to (under) the suture line, and palpation of a hernial ring or loop of bowel beneath the skin.

If only the muscle layer of an abdominal incision breaks down and the skin sutures remain intact, a doughy swelling can be palpated under the skin. This is a serious situation but is not an acute emergency. A bandage should be applied for support, and the suture line should be repaired as soon as possible.

If both the muscle layer and the skin sutures of an abdominal incision break down, the animal can eviscerate (abdominal organs protrude through suture line). If evisceration occurs, the involved organs can become bruised and grossly contaminated, and may even be mutilated by the animal itself. This is an acute emergency that must be attended to immediately. Carefully gather the exteriorized viscera in a moist towel and hold them in place near the incision while others are preparing the animal and operating room for the repair.

PRINCIPLES OF SURGICAL ASEPSIS

H.B. SEIM
T.W. FOSSUM

ASEPTIC TECHNIQUE

Aseptic technique is the term used to describe all of the precautions taken to prevent contamination, and ultimately infection, of a surgical wound. Its purpose is to minimize contamination so that postoperative healing is not delayed.

Contamination vs Infection

Contamination of an object or a wound implies the *presence* of microorganisms within or on it. Contamination of a wound can, but does not necessarily, lead to infection.

With *infection*, microorganisms in the body or a wound *multiply and cause harmful effects*. Four main factors determine if infection occurs:

- *Number of microorganisms:* There must be sufficient microorganisms to overcome the defenses of the animal
- *Virulence of the microorganisms:* Their ability to cause disease

- *Susceptibility of the animal:* Some individuals have a greater natural resistance to infection than others
- *Route of exposure to the microorganisms:* Some routes of exposure are more likely to result in infection than others

Veterinary professionals have little or no influence over the virulence of microorganisms in the environment or the susceptibility of the patient. The route of exposure to microorganisms during surgery is determined by the surgical procedure. The factor that can be most significantly influenced is the *number of microorganisms that enter the surgical wound*, by application of strict aseptic technique before and during surgery.

Rules of Aseptic Technique

During surgery, aseptic technique protects the exposed tissues of the patient from four main sources of potential contamination: the operative personnel, the surgical instruments and equipment, the patient itself, and the surgical environment.

Surgical Instruments and Equipment
- Only sterile items should touch patient tissues.
- Only sterile items should touch other sterile items.
- Any sterile item touching a nonsterile item becomes nonsterile.
- If the sterility of an item is in doubt, consider it nonsterile.

Surgical Personnel
- Only scrubbed personnel should touch sterile items.
- Nonscrubbed personnel should touch only nonsterile items.

Table 21-1 presents a more detailed list of rules of aseptic technique and their underlying logic.

Sterilization and Disinfection

Sterilization refers to the destruction of all microorganisms (bacteria, viruses, spores) on a surface or object. It usually refers to objects that come in contact with sterile tissue or enter the vascular system (e.g., instruments, drapes, catheters, needles). *Disinfection* is the destruction of most pathogenic microorganisms on inanimate (nonliving) objects; *antisepsis* is the destruction of most pathogenic microorganisms on animate (living) objects. Antiseptics are used to kill microorganisms during patient skin preparation and surgical scrubbing; however, the skin cannot be sterilized. Common disinfectants and their uses, properties, and disadvantages are listed in Table 21-2.

Steam Sterilization. Pressurized steam is the most common method of sterilization used in hospitals. Steam destroys microbes via coagulation and cellular protein denaturation. To destroy all living microorganisms, the correct relationship among temperature, pressure, and exposure time is critical. If steam is contained in a closed compartment under increased pressure, the

TABLE 21-1 Rules of aseptic technique

Rule	Underlying logic
Surgical team members remain within the sterile area	Movement out of the sterile area may encourage cross-contamination
Talking is kept to a minimum	Talking releases moisture droplets laden with bacteria
Movement in the operating room by all personnel is kept to a minimum; only necessary personnel should enter the operating room	Movement in the operating room may cause turbulent air flow and result in cross-contamination
Nonscrubbed personnel do not reach over sterile fields	Dust, lint, or other vehicles of bacterial contamination may fall on the sterile field
Scrubbed team members face each other and the sterile field at all times	A team member's back is not considered sterile, even if she is wearing a wrap-around gown
Equipment used during surgery must be sterilized	Nonsterile instruments may be a source of cross-contamination
Scrubbed personnel handle only sterile items; nonscrubbed personnel handle only nonsterile items	Nonscrubbed personnel may be a source of cross-contamination
If the sterility of an item is questioned, it is considered contaminated	Nonsterile, contaminated equipment may be a source of cross-contamination
Sterile tables are sterile only at table height	Items hanging over the table edge are considered nonsterile because they are out of the surgeon's vision
Gowns are sterile from mid-chest to waist and from the gloved hand to 2 inches above the elbow	The back of the gown is not considered sterile, even if it is a wrap-around gown
Drapes covering instrument tables or the patient should be moisture-proof	Moisture carries bacteria from a nonsterile surface to a sterile surface (strike-through contamination)
During pouch opening, if a sterile object touches the sealing edge of the pouch, it is considered contaminated	Once a pouch is opened, the sealed edges of the pouch are not sterile
Sterile items within a wrapper that is damaged or wet are considered contaminated	Contamination can occur from perforated wrappers or strike-through from moisture transport
Do not fold hands into the axillary region; rather, clasp the hands in front of the body and hold above the waist	The axillary region of the gown is not considered sterile
If the surgical team begins the surgery sitting, they should remain seated until the surgery is completed	The surgical field is sterile only from table height to the chest; movement from sitting to standing during surgery may increase cross-contamination

TABLE 21-2 Commonly used disinfectants

Agent	Practical uses	Disinfectant properties	Antiseptic properties	Disadvantages
Alcohol: 70-90% isopropyl and ethyl	Spot cleaning; injection site prep	Good	Very good	Corrosive to stainless steel, steel, volatile
Chlorine compounds: hypochlorite	Cleaning floors and countertops	Good	Fair	Inactivated by organic debris; corrosive to metal
Iodine compounds: iodophors	Cleaning dark-colored floors and countertops	Good	Good	Stains fabric and tissue
Glutaraldehyde: 2% solution	Disinfecting lenses, delicate instruments	Good	None	Tissue reaction; odor; rinse instruments well before using

temperature increases as long as the volume of the compartment remains the same. If items are exposed long enough to steam at a specified temperature and pressure, they become sterile. The unit used to create this environment of high-temperature, pressurized steam is called an *autoclave*.

Gas Sterilization. Ethylene oxide is a flammable, explosive liquid that becomes an effective sterilizing agent when mixed with carbon dioxide or freon. Equipment that cannot withstand the extreme temperature and pressures of steam sterilization (e.g., endoscopes, cameras, plastics, power cables) can be safely sterilized with ethylene oxide. Environmental and safety hazards associated with ethylene oxide are numerous and severe. It is critical to the safety of the patient and hospital personnel that all materials sterilized with ethylene oxide be aerated in a well-ventilated area for a minimum of 7 days or 12 to 18 hours in an aerator.

Items should be clean and dry before ethylene oxide sterilization; moisture and organic material bond with ethylene oxide and leave a toxic residue. If an item cannot be disassembled and all surfaces cleaned, it cannot be sterilized. Items are packed and loaded loosely to allow gas circulation. Complex items (e.g., power equipment) are disassembled before processing. Items that cannot be sterilized with ethylene oxide include acrylics, some pharmaceutical items, and solutions.

Cold Chemical Sterilization. Liquid chemicals used for sterilization must be noncorrosive to the items being sterilized. Glutaraldehyde solution is noncorrosive and provides a safe means of sterilizing delicate, lensed instruments (endoscopes, cystoscopes, bronchoscopes). Most equipment that can be safely immersed in water can be safely immersed in 3% glutaraldehyde. Items for sterilization should be clean and dry; organic matter (e.g., blood, pus, saliva) may prevent penetration of instrument crevices or joints. Residual water causes chemical dilution. Complex instruments should be disassembled before immersion. Immersion times suggested by the manufacturer should be followed (e.g., for sterilization in 3% glutaraldehyde, 10 hours at 20° to 25° C; for disinfection, 10 minutes at 20° to 25° C). After the appropriate immersion time, instruments should be rinsed thoroughly with sterile water and dried with sterile towels to avoid damaging the patients' tissues.

Sterilization Indicators. Simply placing an item in a sterilizer and initiating the sterilization process does not ensure sterility. Failure to achieve sterility may be caused by improper cleaning (if an item cannot be disassembled and all surfaces cleaned, it cannot be sterilized), mechanical failure of the sterilizing system, improper use of sterilizing equipment, improper wrap-

ping, poor loading technique, and/or failure to understand the underlying concepts of sterilization processes.

Sterilization indicators allow monitoring of the effectiveness of sterilization. Indicators undergo either a chemical or biologic change in response to some combination of time and temperature. *Chemical indicators* are generally paper strips or tape impregnated with a material that changes color when a certain temperature is reached. The chemical responds when a certain heat, pressure, or humidity has been attained, but the response does not indicate the duration of exposure, which is critical to the sterilizaiton process. Therefore, it is important to remember that *chemical indicators do not indicate sterility. Their response indicates only that certain conditions for sterility have been met.*

Preparation of Surgical Packs

Regardless of the technique used for sterilization, instruments and linens (e.g., towels, gowns, and drapes) must be cleaned of gross contamination. Instruments should be cleaned manually or with ultrasonic cleaning equipment and appropriate disinfectants as soon after surgery as possible; linens should be laundered. Items sterilized by pressurized steam or other methods (e.g., ethylene oxide) must be wrapped in the manner described below. The procedure for wrapping items is based on enhancing the ease of sterilization and preserving sterility of the item, not for convenience or personal preference.

Before they are packed, instruments are separated and placed in order of their intended use. If steam or gas sterilization is used, the selected wrap should be penetrable by steam/gas, impermeable to microbes, durable, and flexible.

Specific guidelines should be followed when preparing packs for steam and gas sterilization to allow maximal penetration. A presterilization wrap for steam sterilization consists of two thicknesses of two-layer muslin or nonwoven (paper) barrier materials. The poststerilization wrap (after sterilization and proper cool down period) consists of a waterproof, heat-sealable plastic dust cover; this wrap is not necessary if the item is used within 24 hours of sterilization. Small items may be wrapped, sterilized, and stored in heat-sealable paper/plastic peel pouches. Items to be gas sterilized are wrapped in heat-sealable plastic peel pouches or tubing or muslin wrap.

For steam and gas sterilization, instruments should be organized on a lint-free (huck) towel placed on the bottom of a perforated metal instrument tray (Fig. 21-1). Instruments with boxlocks should be autoclaved opened. A 3- to 5-mm space between instruments is recommended for proper steam/gas circulation. Complex instruments should be disassembled when possible and power equipment should be lubricated before steriliza-

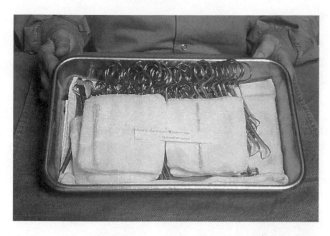

FIG. 21-1 Organize instruments on a lint-free (huck) towel placed on the bottom of a perforated metal instrument tray. Be sure that boxlocks are open. Place a standard count of radiopaque surgical sponges and a sterilization indicator in each pack before wrapping. *(From Fossum TW: Small animal surgery, St Louis, 1997, Mosby.)*

tion. Items with a lumen should have a small amount of water flushed through them immediately before steam sterilization, because water vaporizes and forces air out of the lumen. Conversely, moisture left in tubing placed in a gas sterilizer may decrease the sterilization efficacy below the lethal point. Containers (e.g., saline bowl) should be placed with the open end facing up or horizontally; containers with lids should have the lid slightly ajar. Multiple basins should be stacked with a towel between each. A standard count of radiopaque surgical sponges should be included in each pack (see Fig. 21-1). A sterilization indicator is placed in the center of each pack before wrapping (see Fig. 21-1). Solutions should be steam sterilized separately from instruments using the slow exhaust phase. Linens may be steam sterilized. The maximum size and weight of linen packs that can be effectively steam sterilized is $12 \times 12 \times 20$ inches and 6 kg, respectively. Closely woven table drapes should be packed separately. Layers of linen are alternated in their orientation to permit steam penetration. A sterilization indicator should be placed in the center of each pack.

Wrapping Instrument Packs

Wrap the instrument pack in a clean huck towel (Fig. 21-2, A). Place a large unfolded wrap diagonally in front of you. Place the instrument tray in the center of the wrap so that an imaginary line drawn from one corner of the wrap to the opposite corner is perpendicular to the two sides of the instrument tray. Fold the corner of the wrap that is closest to you over the instrument tray and to its far edge (Fig. 21-2, B). Fold the right corner over the pack as illustrated in Fig. 21-2, C.

Then, fold the left corner similarly (Fig. 21-2, D). Turn the pack around and fold the final corner of the wrap over the tray, tucking it tightly under the previous two folds (Fig. 21-2, E). Fold the tip of the final fold so that it is exposed for easy unwrapping. Wrap the pack in a second layer of cloth or paper in a similar manner. Secure the last corner of the outer wrap with masking tape; fold one end of the tape on itself so that it can be easily grasped and removed. Place a small piece of heat-sensitive indicator tape over the masking tape (Fig. 21-2, F). Label the tape with the current date, date of expiration (optional), contents, and whether it is to be gas or steam sterilized.

Packs may not be completely sterilized if they are wrapped too tightly or improperly loaded in the autoclave or gas sterilizer container. Instrument packs should be positioned vertically (on edge) and longitudinally in an autoclave. Heavy packs should be placed at the periphery, where steam enters the chamber. Allow a small amount of air space between each pack to facilitate steam flow (1 to 2 inches between each pack and surrounding walls). Load linen packs so that the fabric layers are oriented vertically (on edge). Do not stack linen packs on top of one another, because the increased thickness decreases steam penetration. Careful attention to exact standards for preparing, packaging, and loading of supplies is necessary for effective steam and gas sterilization.

Folding and Wrapping Gowns

Gowns must be folded so that they can be easily donned without breaking sterile technique. Place the gown on a clean, flat surface with the front of the gown facing up. Fold the sleeves neatly toward the center of the gown with the cuffs of the sleeves facing the bottom hem (Fig. 21-3, A). Fold the sides to the center so that the side seams are aligned with the sleeve seams (Fig. 21-3, B). Then, fold the gown in half longitudinally (sleeves inside the gown) (Fig. 21-3, C). Ties should be placed so that they can be touched without contaminating the gown. Starting with the bottom hem of the gown, fanfold it toward the neck (Fig. 21-3, D). Fanfolding allows compact storage and simple unfolding. Fold a hand towel in half horizontally and fanfold it into about four folds. Place it on top of the folded gown, leaving one corner turned back to allow it to be easily grasped (Fig. 21-3, E). Wrap the gown and towel in two layers of paper or cloth wrap as described above (Fig. 21-3, F).

Folding and Wrapping Drapes

Drapes should be folded so that the fenestration can be properly positioned over the surgical site without contaminating the drape. Lay the drape out flat with the

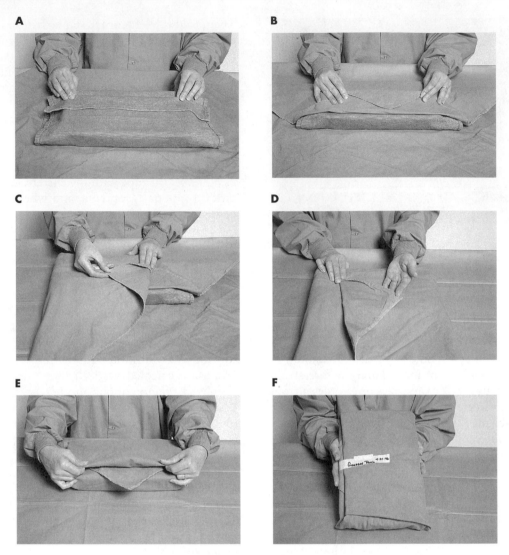

FIG. 21-2 Wrapping an instrument pack. Wrap the instrument pack in a clean huck towel, **A.** Place a large unfolded wrap in front of you and position the instrument tray in the center of the wrap so that an imaginary line drawn from one corner of the wrap to the opposite corner is perpendicular to the two sides of the instrument tray. Fold the corner of the wrap that is closest to you over the instrument tray and to its far edge, **B.** Fold the tip of the wrap over so that it is exposed for easy unwrapping. **C.** Fold the right corner over the pack; then fold the left corner similarly, **D.** Turn the pack around and fold the final corner of the wrap over the tray, tucking it tightly under the previous two folds, **E.** Wrap the pack in a second layer of cloth or paper in a similar manner. Secure the last corner of the outer wrap with masking tape and a piece of heat-sensitive indicator tape, **F.** *(From Fossum TW:* Small animal surgery, *St Louis, 1997, Mosby.)*

ends of the fenestration perpendicular and the sides of the fenestration parallel to you (Fig. 21-4, *A*). Grasp the end of the drape closest to you and fanfold one half of the drape toward the center. Make sure the edge of the drape is on top to allow it to be easily grasped during unfolding (Fig. 21-4, *B*). Then, turn the drape around and fanfold the other half toward the center,

similarly (Fig. 21-4, *C*). Next, fanfold one end of the drape to the center; repeat with the other end (Fig. 21-4, *D*). Note that when the drape is properly folded, the fenestration is on the ventral outermost aspect of the drape (Fig. 21-4, *E*). Fold the drape in half (Fig. 21-4, *F*) and wrap it in two layers of paper or cloth wrap as described above.

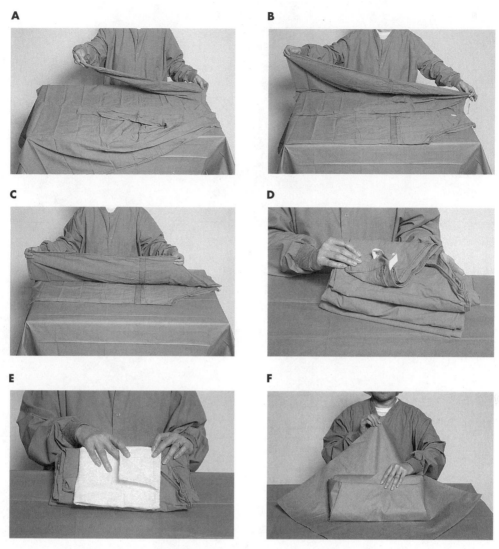

FIG. 21-3 Folding and wrapping surgical gowns. Place the gown on a clean, flat surface with the front of the gown facing up. Fold the sleeves neatly toward the center of the gown with the cuffs of the sleeves facing the bottom hem, **A.** Fold the sides to the center so that the side seams are aligned with the sleeve seams, **B.** Then fold the gown in half longitudinally (sleeves inside the gown), **C.** Starting with the bottom hem of the gown, fanfold it toward the neck, **D.** Fold a hand towel in half horizontally and fanfold it into about four folds. Place it on top of the folded gown, leaving one corner turned back to allow it to be easily grasped, **E.** Wrap the gown and towel in two layers of paper or cloth wrap as described in Fig. 21-2, **F.** *(From Fossum TW: Small animal surgery, St Louis, 1997, Mosby.)*

Storing Sterilized Items

Packs are allowed to cool and dry individually on racks when removed from the autoclave; placing instrument packs on top of each other during cooling may promote condensation of moisture, resulting in contamination via strike-through (wick action). After sterile packs are completely dry, they should be stored in waterproof dust covers in closed cabinets (rather than uncovered on open shelves) to protect them from moisture or exposure to particulate matter, such as dust-borne bacteria. Sterile packs are labeled with the date on which the item was sterilized and a control lot number to trace an unsterile item. Heat-sealed waterproof dust covers are placed on items not routinely used. Sterile shelf life varies with the type of outer wrap (Table 21-3).

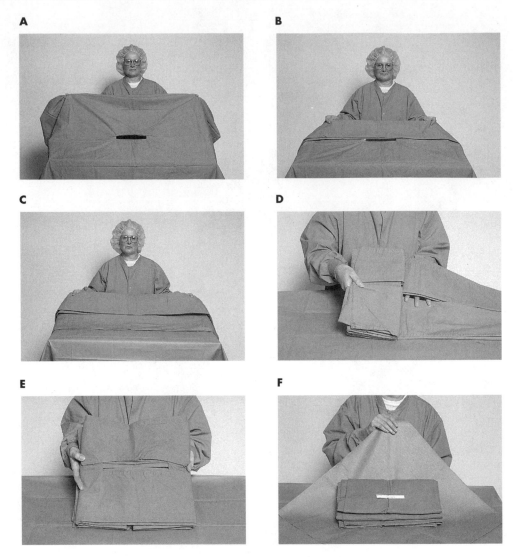

FIG. 21-4 Folding and wrapping drapes. Lay the drape out flat, with the ends of the fenestration parallel and the sides of the fenestration perpendicular to you, **A.** Grasp the edges of the drape nearest you and fanfold the drape to the center, **B.** The edge of the drape should be exposed (dorsal) to allow it to be easily grasped during unfolding. Turn the drape around and fanfold the other half similarly, **C.** Next, fanfold one end of the drape to the center; repeat with the other end, **D.** Note that when the drape is properly folded, the fenestration is on the ventral outermost aspect of the drape, **E.** Fold the drape in half, **F,** and wrap it in two layers of paper or cloth wrap as described in Fig. 21-2. *(From Fossum TW: Small animal surgery, St Louis, 1997, Mosby.)*

TABLE 21-3 Recommended storage times for sterilized packs*

Wrapper	Shelf life
Double-wrapped, two-layer muslin	4 weeks
Double-wrapped, two-layer muslin, heat-sealed in dust covers after sterilization	6 months
Double-wrapped, two-layer muslin, tape-sealed in dust covers after sterilization	2 months
Double-wrapped nonwoven barrier materials (paper)	6 months
Paper/plastic-peel pouches, heat-sealed	1 year
Plastic peel pouches, heat-sealed	1 year

*Note that sterilized items from hospitals adopting event-related sterility assurance have an indefinite shelf life.

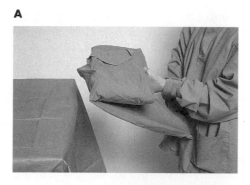

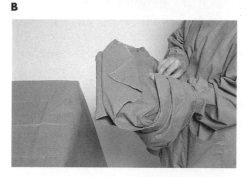

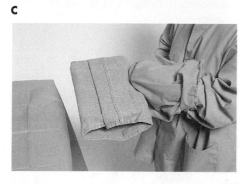

FIG. 21-5 To unwrap a sterile linen or paper pack that can be held during distribution, hold the pack in your right hand if you are left-handed (and vice versa), **A.** Using your right hand, unfold one corner of the wrap at a time, **B,** being careful to secure each corner in the palm of your left hand to keep them from recoiling and contaminating the contents, **C.** Hold the final corner with your right hand; your hand should be completely covered by the wrap. When the pack is fully exposed and all corners of the wrap secured, gently drop it onto the sterile field, being careful not to allow your hand and arm to reach across or over the sterile field. *(From Fossum TW: Small animal surgery, St Louis, 1997, Mosby.)*

Unwrapping or Opening Sterile Items

Unwrapping Sterile Linen or Paper Packs. If you are right-handed, hold the pack in your left hand (and vice versa). Using the right hand, unfold one corner of the outside wrap at a time (Fig. 21-5, *A*), being careful to secure each corner in the palm of the left hand to keep them from recoiling and contaminating the contents (Fig. 21-5, *B*). Hold the final corner with your right hand. When the pack is fully exposed and all corners of the wrap secured (Fig. 21-5, *C*), gently drop the pack

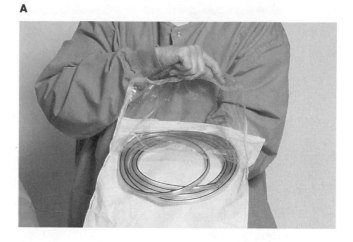

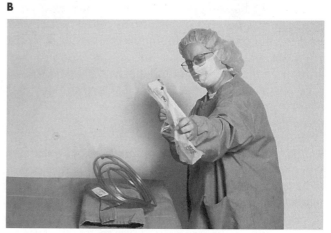

FIG. 21-6 To unwrap a sterile item in a plastic peel-back pouch, identify the edges of the peel-back wrapper and carefully separate them, **A.** Peel the edges of the wrapper back slowly and symmetrically to ensure the sterile item does not contact the torn edge of the wrapper, which is nonsterile. Do not lean over the table when placing the item on the sterile table, **B.** *(From Fossum TW: Small animal surgery, St Louis, 1997, Mosby.)*

onto the sterile field, being careful to not allow your hand and arm to reach across or over the sterile field. Or, have a sterile team member grasp the item and place it on the instrument table.

Unwrapping Sterile Items in Paper or Plastic or Plastic Peel-back Pouches. Identify the edges of the peel-back wrapper and carefully separate them. Peel the edges of the wrapper back slowly and symmetrically to ensure the sterile item does not contact the torn edge of the wrapper, which is nonsterile (Fig. 21-6, *A*). If the item is small, place it on the sterile area as described above, being careful not to lean across the sterile table (Fig. 21-6, *B*). If the item is long or cumbersome, have a sterile team member grasp it and gently pull it from the peel-back wrapper, taking care not to brush the item against the peeled edge of the wrapper. Packages containing scalpel blades and suture material are opened similarly.

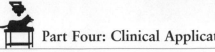

PREPARATION OF THE OPERATIVE SITE AND SURGICAL TEAM

T.W. FOSSUM
H.B. SEIM

PREPARATION OF THE OPERATIVE SITE

Surgery puts a patient at risk for *nosocomial infections* (hospital acquired). Because most surgical infections develop from bacteria that enter the incision during surgery, proper preparation of the surgical site is crucial to reduce the likelihood of infection. Resident skin flora (particularly *Staphylococcus aureus* and *Streptococcus* spp.) are the most common source of surgical wound contaminants. Although it is impossible to sterilize skin without impairing its natural protective function and interfering with wound healing, proper preoperative preparation reduces the likelihood of infection.

Hair Removal and Skin Scrubbing

Before preparing the patient for surgery, verify the patient's identity, surgical procedure being performed, and surgical site. It is useful to bathe the animal the day before the surgical procedure to remove loose hair, debris, and external parasites. Hair should be liberally clipped around the proposed incision site so that the incision can be extended within a sterile field. A general guideline is to clip 20 cm on each side of the incision. The hair can be removed most effectively with an Oster-type clipper and a #40 clipper blade. Patients with a dense haircoat may be clipped first with a more coarse blade (#10). The higher the blade number is, the shorter the remaining hair. Clippers should be held using a "pencil grip" and initial clipping should be done with the grain of the hair growth pattern. Subsequent clipping should be against the pattern of hair growth to obtain a closer clip. Depilatory creams are less traumatic than other hair removal methods, but they induce a mild dermal lymphocytic reaction. They are most useful in irregular areas where adequate hair clipping is difficult. Razors are occasionally used for hair removal (e.g., around the eye), but they cause microlacerations in skin that may increase irritation and promote infection.

After hair has been clipped from the site, loose hair is removed with a vacuum. For limb procedures, if exposure of the foot is not necessary, the foot can be excluded from the surgical area by placing a glove over the distal extremity and securing it to the limb with tape (Fig. 21-7). The glove should be covered with tape or Vetrap. The foot is then draped out of the sterile field (see p. 396). To enhance manipulation of limbs during surgery, a "hang-leg" preparation may be done. This requires that the limb be circumferentially clipped; the limb is hung from an intravenous pole during preparation to allow the sides of the limb to be scrubbed.

Before transporting the animal to the surgical site, the incision is given a general cleansing scrub and ophthalmic antibiotic ointment or lubricant is placed on the cornea and conjunctiva. In male dogs undergoing abdominal procedures, the prepuce should be flushed with an antiseptic solution. The skin is scrubbed with germicidal soap to remove debris and reduce bacterial populations in preparation for surgery. The area is lathered well until all dirt and oils are removed. This is a generous scrub that often encompasses the hair surrounding the operation site to remove unattached hair and dander that may be disturbed during draping.

Commonly used scrubbing solutions include iodophors, chlorhexidine, alcohols, hexachlorophene, and quaternary ammonium salts (see Table 21-2). Alcohol is not effective against spores, but it rapidly kills bacteria and acts as a defatting agent. Using alcohol by itself is not recommended, but it is commonly used in conjunction with povidone-iodine. Hexachlorophene and quaternary ammonium salts are less effective than other available agents.

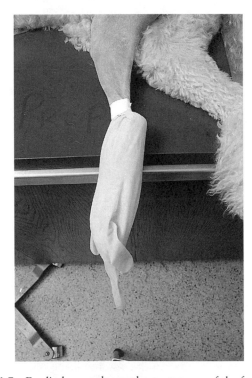

FIG. 21-7   For limb procedures where exposure of the foot is not required, exclude the foot from the surgical area by placing a glove over the distal extremity and securing it to the limb with tape. Wrap the glove with tape or Vetrap (see Fig. 21-8). *(From Fossum TW: Small animal surgery, St Louis, 1997, Mosby.)*

Positioning

Before sterile application of the epidermal germicide, the animal is moved to the operating room and positioned so that the operative site is accessible to the surgeon and secured with ropes, sandbags, troughs, or tape. The animal is generally placed on a water circulating heating pad; if electrocautery is being used, the ground plate should be positioned under the patient. If a "hanging-leg" preparation is used, the limb should be carefully suspended from an intravenous pole with tape (Fig. 21-8).

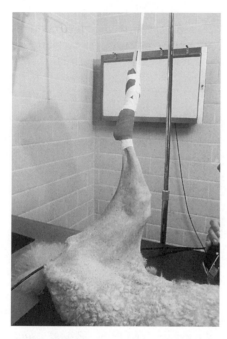

FIG. 21-8 Manipulation of the limb during orthopedic procedures may be facilitated with a "hanging-leg" preparation. The limb is clipped circumferentially and carefully suspended from an intravenous pole with tape. *(From Fossum TW: Small animal surgery, St Louis, 1997, Mosby.)*

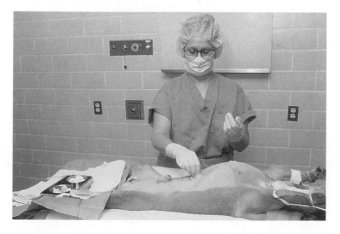

FIG. 21-9 Start the sterile preparation near the center of the clipped area using a circular scrubbing motion and moving from the center to the periphery. *(From Fossum TW: Small animal surgery, St Louis, 1997, Mosby.)*

Sterile Skin Preparation

Sterile preparation of the surgical site begins after transporting and positioning the animal on the operating table. Gauze sponges are sterilized in a pack, along with bowls into which the germicides can be poured. Sponges are handled with sterile sponge forceps or the gloved hand, using aseptic technique. The dominant hand should be used to perform the sterile preparation, while the less dominant hand is used to retrieve sponges from the prep bowl. Transferring the sterile sponges to the dominant hand before scrubbing the site helps ensure that the hand picking up the sponges remains sterile during the procedure.

Scrubbing is started at the incision site, usually near the center of the clipped area. A circular scrubbing motion is used, moving from the center to the periphery (Fig. 21-9). Sponges should not be moved from the periphery to the center lest bacteria be transferred onto the incision site. Sponges are discarded after reaching the periphery. Frequently, when using povidone-iodine and alcohol, the site is scrubbed alternatively with each solution three times to allow for 5 minutes of contact time. However, using alcohol between the povidone-iodine scrubs decreases contact time of povidone-iodine with skin and may decrease its efficacy. Excess solution on the table or accumulated in body "pockets" should be blotted with a sterile towel or sponges. When the final povidone-iodine scrub is completed, a 10% povidone-iodine solution should be sprayed or painted on the site. If chlorhexidine is the preparation solution, it remains in contact with the skin at the end of the preparation procedure or may be rinsed with saline. Because chlorhexidine binds to keratin, contact time is less critical than with povidone-iodine. Two 30-second applications are considered adequate for antimicrobial activity.

Draping

Once the animal has been positioned and the skin prepared, the animal is ready to be draped. The drapes maintain a sterile field around the operative site. If electrocautery is being used, sufficient time should elapse between skin preparation and application of drapes to permit complete evaporation of flammable substances (e.g., alcohol) from the skin. If an abdominal incision extends to the pubis in males, the prepuce should be clamped to one side with a sterile towel clamp.

Draping is performed by a gowned and gloved surgical team member and begins with placement of field drapes (quarter drapes) to isolate the unprepared portion of the animal. These towels should be placed one at a time at the periphery of the prepared area. Field (quarter) drapes may be huck towels or disposable, nonabsorbent towels. Drapes should not be flipped, fanned, or shaken, because rapid movement of drapes creates air currents on which dust, lint, and droplet nuclei can migrate. Drapes, supplies, and equipment extending over or dropping below the table level should be considered nonsterile because they are not within the surgeon's visual field and their sterility cannot be verified.

Once the towels are placed, they should not be readjusted toward the incision site, because this carries bacteria onto the prepared skin. Towels are secured at the corners with Bachhaus towel clamps (Fig. 21-10). *The tips of the towel clamps, once placed through the skin, are considered nonsterile and should be handled appropriately.* Generally, field towels do not cover the edges of the table; do not brush a sterile gown against this nonsterile field. When the animal and incision site are protected by field drapes, final draping can be performed (Fig. 21-11 and 21-12). A large drape is placed over the animal and entire surgical table to provide a continuous sterile field. Cloth drapes should have an appropriately sized and

positioned opening that can be placed over the incision site, while the drape covers the remaining surfaces.

To drape a limb, place field drapes and secure them as described above to isolate the surgical site or the proximal aspect of the limb, if the leg is hung (Fig. 21-13). A nonsterile member of the surgical team holds the nonprepared area of the limb, and the tape holding the elevated limb is cut. The limb is presented to the sterile surgical member so that it may be taken with a hand in a sterile stockinette or towel. The limb should not be turned loose until it is securely held by the sterile surgical team member. If a stockinette is used, it should be carefully unrolled down the limb and secured with towel clamps (Fig. 21-14). If a sterile towel is used, the limb should be carefully wrapped with the towel before securing it to skin with a towel clamp. Water-impermeable (disposable) towels (plus the

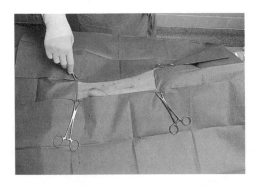

FIG. 21-10 Secure field drapes at the corners with sterile Bachhaus towel clamps. The tips of the towel clamps, once placed through the skin, are considered nonsterile and should be handled appropriately. *(From Fossum TW: Small animal surgery, St Louis, 1997, Mosby.)*

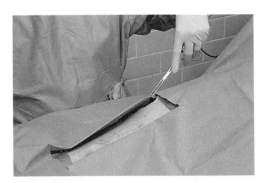

FIG. 21-12 If the drape does not have a fenestration, cut an appropriately sized hole. The edges of the drape can be secured to the field drapes with Allis tissue forceps (not towel clamps). Do not cut holes through the outer drape. *(From Fossum TW: Small animal surgery, St Louis, 1997, Mosby.)*

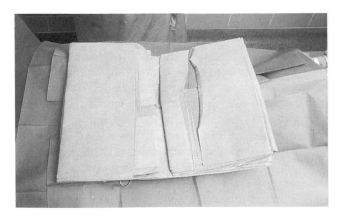

FIG. 21-11 When the animal and incision site are protected by field drapes, final draping can be performed. Place the large drape with the center (or fenestration) over the surgical site and unfold it. To avoid contaminating the drape, do not hold it in the air while unfolding it. *(From Fossum TW: Small animal surgery, St Louis, 1997, Mosby.)*

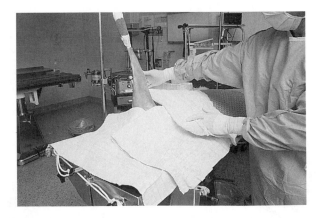

FIG. 21-13 When performing a "hanging-leg" preparation, place field drapes around the limb as illustrated and secure them with towel clamps. *(From Fossum TW: Small animal surgery, St Louis, 1997, Mosby.)*

towel clamp) should then be covered with sterile Kling. If a cloth towel is used, it (and the towel clamp) should be covered with sterile Vetrap. The limb is now ready to be placed through a fenestration of a lap or fanfold drape and the drape secured (Fig. 21-15). The end of the stockinette is wrapped with sterile Vetrap.

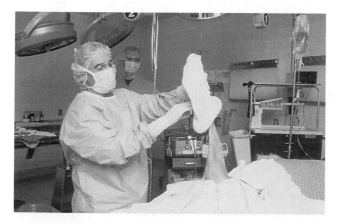

FIG. 21-14 The prepared limb may be grasped by the surgeon with a hand covered by a sterile stockinette. The stockinette is carefully unrolled down the limb and secured with towel clamps. *(From Fossum TW: Small animal surgery, St Louis, 1997, Mosby.)*

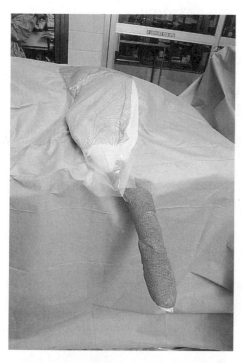

FIG. 21-15 The limb is placed through a fenestration of a lap or fanfold drape and the drape secured. A plastic adhesive drape has been applied to the skin and surrounding drapes. *(From Fossum TW: Small animal surgery, St Louis, 1997, Mosby.)*

PREPARATION OF THE SURGICAL TEAM
Surgical Attire

All persons entering the operating room suite, regardless of whether a surgery is in progress or not, should be appropriately clothed. To minimize microbial contamination from operating room personnel, wear scrub clothes rather than street clothes in the operating suite. With two-piece pant suits, tuck loose-fitting tops into the trousers. Tunic tops that fit close to the body may be worn outside the trousers. The sleeves of the top should be short enough to allow the hands and arms to be scrubbed. Pants should have an elastic waist or drawstring closure. Nonscrubbed personnel should wear longsleeved jackets over their scrub clothes. Jackets should be buttoned or snapped closed during use to minimize the risk of the edges' inadvertently contaminating sterile surfaces. Scrub clothes should be laundered between wearings and changed if they are visibly soiled or wet to prevent transfer of microorganisms to the environment. Wearing scrub clothes outside the surgical environment increases microbial contamination. If a scrub suit must be worn outside the surgery room, a laboratory coat or single-use gowns should be used to cover it.

Other surgical attire includes hair coverings, masks, shoecovers, gowns, and gloves. Hair is a significant carrier of bacteria; when left uncovered, it collects bacteria. Because bacterial shedding from hair increases surgical wound infection rates, complete hair coverage is necessary. Even when surgery is not in progress, caps and masks should be worn in the surgical suite. Caps should completely cover all scalp and facial hair, and masks should cover the mouth and nostrils (Fig. 21-16). Sideburns and/or beards necessitate a hood for complete coverage. Skullcaps that fail to cover the side hair above the ears and hair at the nape of the neck should not be worn.

Any footwear that is comfortable can be worn in the surgery area. Shoecovers should be donned when first entering the surgical area and should be worn when leaving it to keep shoes clean. New shoecovers are donned when returning to the surgical area. Shoecovers are generally made of reusable or disposable materials that are water-repellent and resist tearing.

Masks, constructed from lint-free material containing a hydrophilic filter web sandwiched between two outer layers, should be worn whenever entering a sterile area (see Fig. 21-16). Their major function is to filter and contain droplets of microorganisms expelled from the mouth and nasopharynx during talking, sneezing, and coughing. Masks must be fitted over the mouth and nose and secured in a manner that prevents venting (see Fig. 21-16). The dorsal aspect of the mask is secured by shaping the reinforcing top edge tightly around the nose.

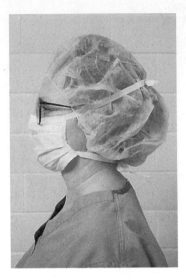

FIG. 21-16 Hair should be covered by a bouffant-style surgical cap. This is the correct way to tie a surgical mask. *(From Fossum TW: Small animal surgery, St Louis, 1997, Mosby.)*

Surgical gowns may be reusable and made of woven materials (usually cotton), or disposable. Disposable (single-use) gowns are nonwoven and made directly from fibers rather than yarn. Loosely woven cotton is commonly used for reusable gowns. This fabric is instantly permeable to bacteria when it becomes wet. Fewer microorganisms contaminate the surgical environment when disposable (single-use) nonwoven materials are used.

The Surgical Scrub

Surgical scrubbing cleans the hands and forearms to reduce the numbers of bacteria that come in contact with the wound from scrubbed personnel during surgery. All sterile surgical team members must perform a hand and arm scrub before entering the surgical suite. Objectives of a surgical scrub include mechanical removal of dirt and oil, reduction of the transient bacterial population (bacteria deposited from the environment), and reduction of the skin's resident bacterial population. Relying on latex gloves alone (without a surgical scrub) to prevent microbial contamination is not recommended; up to 50% of surgical gloves contain holes at the completion of surgery. This proportion may increase with long or difficult surgeries.

Antimicrobial soaps or detergents used for scrubbing should be rapid acting, broad-spectrum, and nonirritating, and they should inhibit rapid rebound microbial growth. They should not depend on accumulation for activity. The most commonly used surgical scrub solutions are chlorhexidine gluconate, povidone-iodine, and hexachlorophene.

Surgical scrubs physically separate microbes from skin and inactivate them via contact with the antimicrobial solution. Two accepted methods of performing a surgical scrub are the *anatomic timed scrub* (5-minute scrub) and the *counted brush stroke method* (strokes per surface area of skin) (Box 21-1). Recommendations regarding the number of times one should lather and rinse during the scrub, number of strokes per surface area, and time spent on each surface vary. However, both methods ensure sufficient exposure of all skin surfaces to friction and antimicrobial solutions.

If the hands and arms are grossly soiled, lengthen scrub time or increase brush counts; however, avoid skin irritation or abrasion because this causes bacteria residing in deeper tissues (e.g., around base of hair follicles) to become more superficial, increasing the number of potentially infective organisms on the skin surface. Contact time between the antimicrobial soap or detergent should be based on documentation of product efficacy in the scientific literature. An initial 5- to 7-minute scrub for the first case of the day, followed by a 2- to 3-minute scrub between additional surgical operations is generally adequate.

Before scrubbing, remove all jewelry (including watches) from your hands and forearms, because they are reservoirs for bacteria. Fingernails should be free of polish and trimmed short, and cuticles should be in good condition. Artificial nails (bondings, tips, wrappings, tapes) should never be worn. More gram-negative bacteria have been cultured from the fingertips of personnel wearing artificial nails than from personnel with natural nails, both before and after handwashing. Fungi residing between an artificial nail and the natural nail can contaminate the surgical wound. Hands and forearms should be free of open lesions and breaks in skin integrity, because such skin infections may contaminate surgical wounds.

Once the scrub has been started, nonsterile items cannot be handled without breaking sterility. If your hands or arms inadvertently touch a nonsterile object (including surgical personnel), repeat the scrub. During and after scrubbing, keep the hands higher than the elbows. This allows water and soap to flow from the cleanest area (hands) to a less clean area (elbow). A single scrub brush can generally be used for the entire procedure. No difference has been documented in the effectiveness of a sterilized reusable brush and disposable polyurethane brush/sponge combination.

When the scrub has been completed, dry the hands and arms with a sterile towel. When picking up the sterile towel from the table, take care not to drip water on the gown beneath it and step back from the sterile table. Hold the towel lengthwise and dry one hand and arm, working from hand to elbow with one end of the towel; use a blotting motion. Bend over at the waist when drying the arms so that the end of the towel will not brush against your scrub suit. After one hand and arm are dry, move the dry hand to the opposite end of the towel. Dry the other hand and arm in a similar manner. Drop the towel into the proper receptacle or on the floor if a receptacle is not provided. Do not lower your hands below waist level.

Gowning

Gowns are another barrier between the skin of the surgical team and the patient. They should be constructed of a material that prevents passage of microorganisms between sterile and nonsterile areas. Gowns should be resistant to fluid, lint accumulation, stretching, and tearing (especially at the forearm, elbow, and abdominal areas) and should be comfortable, economical, and fire resistant. Reusable or single-use disposable gowns are available.

Gowning and gloving should occur away from the surgical table and the patient to avoid dripping water onto the sterile field and contaminating it. Gowns are folded so that the inside of the gown faces outward (see Fig. 21-3). Grasp the gown firmly and gently lift it away from the table. Step back from the sterile table to allow room for gowning. Hold the gown at the shoulders and allow it to gently unfold. Do not shake the gown, because this increases the risk of contamination. Once the gown is opened, locate the armholes and guide each arm through the sleeves. Keep your hands within the cuffs of the gown. Have another person pull the gown up over your shoulders and secure it by closing the neck fasteners and tying the inside waist tie. If a sterile-back gown is used, do not secure the front tie until you have donned sterile gloves.

Box 21-1 Surgical scrub procedure

- Locate scrub brushes, antibacterial soap, nail cleaners.
- Remove watches, bracelets, and rings.
- Wet hands and forearms thoroughly.
- Apply 2-3 pumps of antimicrobial soap to hands, and wash hands and forearms.
- Clean nails and beneath nails with a nail cleaner under running water.
- Rinse arms and forearms.
- Apply 2-3 pumps of antimicrobial soap to hand and forearms.
- Apply 2-3 pumps of antimicrobial soap to sterile scrub brush.

Anatomic timed method	Counted brush stroke method
• Start timing; scrub each side of each finger, between fingers, and back and front to the hand for 2 minutes. • Proceed to scrub the arms, keeping the hand higher than the arm. • Scrub each side of the arm to 3 inches above the elbow for 1 minute. • Total scrub time is 2 to 3 minutes per hand and arm.	• Apply 30 strokes (one stroke consists of up and down or back and forth motion) to the very tips of your fingers and thumb. • Divide each finger and thumb into 4 parts and apply 20 strokes to each of the 4 surfaces, including the finger webs. • Scrub from the tip of the finger to the wrist when scrubbing the thumb, index, and small fingers. • Divide your forearm into 4 planes and apply 20 strokes to each surface.

- Rinse the scrub brush well under running water and transfer the brush to your scrubbed hand. Do not rinse the scrubbed hand and arm at this time.
- Repeat the process on your other hand and arm.
- When both hands and arms have been scrubbed, drop the scrub brush in the sink.
- Starting with the fingertips of one hand, rinse under running water by moving your fingertips up and out of the water stream and allowing the rest of your arm to be rinsed off on the way out of the stream.
- Allow the water to run from fingertips to elbows
- Never allow fingertips to fall below the level of your elbow.
- Never shake your hands to shed excess water, allow the water to drip from your elbows.
- Rinse off your other hand similarly.
- Hold your hands upright and in front of you so that they can be seen, and proceed to the gowning and gloving area.

Gloving

Latex rubber gloves are another barrier between the surgical team and the patient; however, they are not a substitute for proper scrubbing methods. If the glove of a properly scrubbed hand is perforated during a surgical procedure, bacteria are rarely cultured from the punctured glove. Lubricating agents for latex gloves, such as magnesium silicate (talcum) or cornstarch, allow gloves to slide more easily onto the hand. Unfortunately, these agents cause considerable irritation to various tissues, even if gloves are vigorously rinsed in sterile saline before surgery. Therefore, the surgeon should use gloves in which the inner surfaces are lubricated with an adherent coating of hydrogel.

Closed Gloving. This method ensures that the hand never comes in contact with the outside of the gown or glove. Working through the gown sleeve (your bare hand must not be allowed to touch the cuff of the gown or outside surface of the glove), pick up one glove from the wrapper. Lay the glove palm down over the cuff of the gown, with the thumb and fingers of the glove facing your elbow (Fig. 21-17, *A*). Working though the cuff of the gown, grasp the cuff of the glove with your index finger and thumb. With your other hand still inside the cuff of the gown, take hold of the opposite side of the edge of the glove between your index finger and thumb. Lift the cuff of the glove up and over the gown cuff and hand, bringing the glove cuff below your knuckles. Release and come to the palm side of the glove and take hold of the gown and glove, pulling them toward your elbow while pushing your hand through the gown cuff and into the glove (Fig. 21-17, *B*). Proceed with the opposite hand, using the same technique. Do not allow the bare hand being gloved to contact the gown cuff edge or sterile glove on the opposite hand.

Open Gloving. The open method of gloving is used when only the hands must be covered (e.g., as for urinary catheterization, bone marrow biopsy, sterile patient preparation) or during surgery when one glove becomes contaminated and must be changed. It should not be used routinely for gowning and gloving. If one hand is contaminated during surgery, have the glove removed as described below. Open the glove wrapper and pick up the correct glove at the folded edge with your sterile hand. Gently insert your hand into the glove until your fingers are in the fingers of the glove. Do not allow the glove to roll up over the back of your hand. Place your thumb inside the thumb of the glove and hook the cuff of the glove over your thumb (Fig. 21-18, *A*). Release the glove. Place the fingers of your sterile hand under the cuff at the palm of the glove (Fig. 21-18, *B*) and bend the wrist of the hand being gloved 90 degrees, pointing the fingers down (Fig. 21-18, *C*).

Gently walk your fingers around to the front of the cuff (Fig. 21-18, *C*) while pulling the cuff up and over your gown (Fig. 21-18, *D*).

If both gloves are being donned, pick up one glove by its inner cuff with the opposite hand (Fig. 21-19, *A*). Do not touch the glove wrapper with your bare hand. Slide the glove onto the opposite hand; leave the cuff down. Using the partially gloved hand, slide your fingers into the outer side of the opposite glove cuff (Fig. 21-19, *B*). Slide your hand into the glove and unfold the cuff; do not touch the bare arm as the cuff is unfolded. With your gloved hand, slide the fingers under the outside edge of the opposite cuff and unfold it.

A

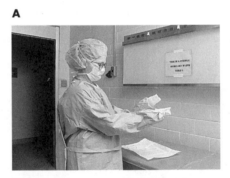

B

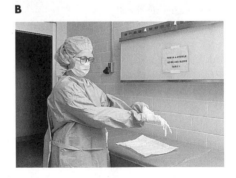

FIG. 21-17 Closed gloving. Working through the gown sleeve, pick up one glove from the wrapper. Lay the glove palm down over the cuff of the gown, with the thumb and fingers of the glove facing your elbows, **A.** Grasp the cuff of the glove with your index finger and thumb. With the index finger and thumb of the other hand (within the cuff), grasp the opposite side of the edge of the glove. Lift the cuff of the glove up and over the gown cuff and hand. Release, move to the palm side of the glove, and grasp the gown and glove, pulling them toward the elbow while pushing the hand through the cuff and into the glove, **B.** Proceed with the opposite hand using the same technique. *(From Fossum TW: Small animal surgery, St Louis, 1997, Mosby.)*

Assisted Gloving. When gloving another person, the person assisting with the gloving should have on a sterile gown and/or gloves. The assistant's hands should not touch the nonsterile surface of the person being gloved. If *both* gloves are being replaced, have the assistant pick up one glove and place his or her fingers and thumb under the cuff of the glove (Fig. 21-20, *A*). With the thumb of the glove facing you, have the assistant hold the glove open for you to slip your hand into (Fig. 21-20, *B*). The assistant then brings the cuff of the glove up and over the cuff of your gown and gently lets it go. The assistant picks up the other glove. Assist him or her by holding the cuff of the glove open with the fingers of your sterile hand, while putting your ungloved hand into the open glove (Fig. 21-20, *C*). The assistant keeps his or her thumbs under the cuff while you thrust your hand into it. Ensure that the glove cuff is above your gown cuff before the assistant gently releases it (he or she should not let the cuff snap sharply). If only *one* glove is being replaced, the assistant picks up the glove with the palm facing away from you. Assist the gloving process as described above for the second hand by placing your sterile hand under the cuff.

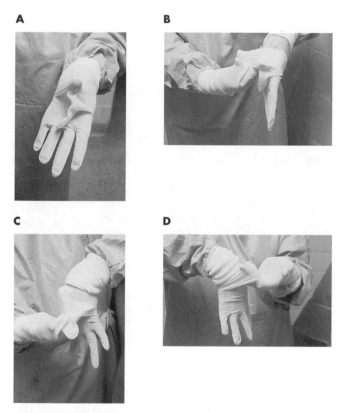

FIG. 21-18 Open gloving when one hand is sterile. Open the glove wrapper and pick up the correct glove at the folded edge with your sterile hand. Gently insert your hand into the glove until your fingers are in the fingers of the glove. Place your thumb inside the thumb of the glove and hook the cuff of the glove over your thumb, **A.** Release the glove. Place the fingers of your sterile hand under the cuff at the palm of the glove, **B,** and bend the wrist of the hand being gloved 90 degrees, **C.** Gently walk your fingers to the front of the cuff while pulling the cuff up and over your gown, **D.** *(From Fossum TW: Small animal surgery, St Louis, 1997, Mosby.)*

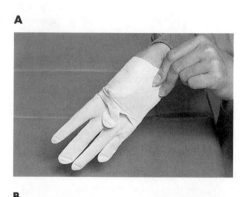

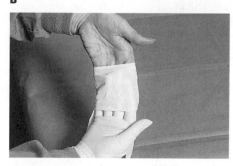

FIG. 21-19 Open gloving when neither hand is sterile. Pick up one glove by its inner cuff with the opposite hand, **A.** Slide the glove onto the opposite hand; leave the cuff down. Using the partially gloved hand, slide your fingers into the outer side of the opposite glove cuff, **B.** Slide your hand into the glove and unfold the cuff; do not touch your bare arm as the cuff is unfolded. With the gloved hand, slide your fingers under the outside edge of the opposite cuff and unfold it. *(From Fossum TW: Small animal surgery, St Louis, 1997, Mosby.)*

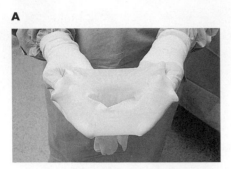

A

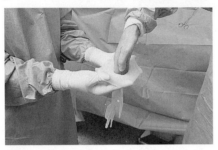

B

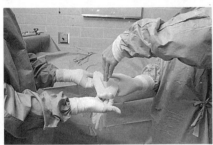

C

FIG. 21-20 Assisted gloving. Have the assistant pick up one glove and place his or her fingers and thumb under the cuff of the glove, **A.** With the thumb of the glove facing you, slip your hand into the glove, **B.** Then, have the assistant bring the cuff of the glove up and over the cuff of your gown and gently let it go. Have the assistant pick up the other glove. Assist him or her by holding the cuff of the glove open with the fingers of your sterile hand, while inserting your ungloved hand into the open glove, **C.** The assistant keeps her thumbs under the cuff while you thrust your hand into it. *(From Fossum TW: Small animal surgery, St Louis, 1997, Mosby.)*

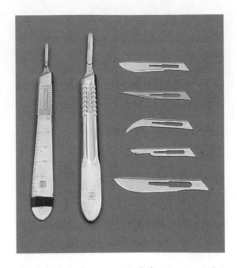

FIG. 21-21 Scalpel handles (No. 3, *left;* No. 4, *right*) and blades *(top to bottom):* No. 10, 11, 12, 15, and 20. *(From Fossum TW: Small animal surgery, St Louis, 1997, Mosby.)*

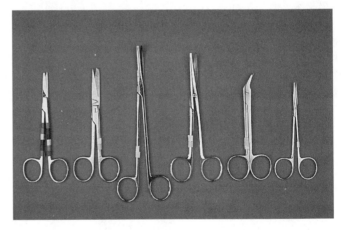

FIG. 21-22 Scissors *(left to right):* stitch (suture removal), sharp/blunt, Metzenbaum, Mayo, wire, tenotomy. *(From Fossum TW: Small animal surgery, St Louis, 1997, Mosby.)*

SURGICAL INSTRUMENTS

T.W. FOSSUM

TYPES OF SURGICAL INSTRUMENTS
Scalpels and Blades

Scalpels are the primary cutting instrument used to incise tissue (Fig. 21-21). Reusable scalpel handles (Nos. 3 and 4) with detachable blades are most commonly used in veterinary medicine; disposable handles and blades are also available. Blades are available in various sizes and shapes, depending on the task for which they are used (see Fig. 21-21). Scalpels are usually used in a "slide cutting" fashion, with pressure applied to the knife blade at a right angle to the direction of scalpel pressure.

Scissors

Scissors are available in a variety of shapes, sizes, and weights, and are generally classified according to the type of points (blunt-blunt, sharp-sharp, sharp-blunt), blade shape (straight, curved), or cutting edge (plain, serrated) (Fig. 21-22). Curved scissors offer greater

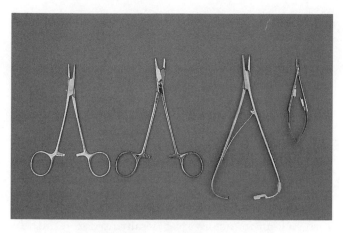

FIG. 21-23 Needle holders *(left to right)*: Mayo-Hegar, Olsen-Hegar, Mathieu, Castroviejo. *(From Fossum TW: Small animal surgery, St Louis, 1997, Mosby.)*

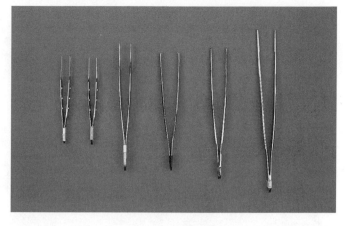

FIG. 21-24 Tissue forceps *(left to right):* Bishop-Harmon (smooth tip), Bishop-Harmon (toothed), Brown-Adson, 1 × 2 tissue, serrated, DeBakey. *(From Fossum TW: Small animal surgery, St Louis, 1997, Mosby.)*

maneuverability and visibility, whereas straight scissors provide the greatest mechanical advantage for cutting tough or thick tissue. *Metzenbaum* or *Mayo scissors* are most commonly used in surgery. Metzenbaum scissors are more delicate and should be reserved for fine, thin tissues. Mayo scissors are used for cutting heavy tissues, such as fascia. Tissue scissors should not be used to cut suture material; suture scissors should be used. *Suture scissors* used in the operating room are different from *suture removal scissors*. The latter have a concavity at the top of one blade that prevents the suture from being lifted excesively during removal. Delicate scissors, such as *tenotomy scissors* or *iris scissors,* are often used in ophthalmic procedures and other surgeries, where fine, precise cuts are necessary. *Bandage scissors* have a blunt tip that, when introduced under the bandage edge, reduces the risk of cutting the underlying skin.

Needle Holders

Needle holders are used to grasp and manipulate curved needles (Fig. 21-23). *Mayo-Hegar* and *Olsen-Hegar needle holders* have a ratchet lock just distal to the thumb. *Castroviejo needle holders* have a spring and latch mechanism for locking. *Mathieu needle holders* have a ratchet lock at the proximal end of the handles of the holder, permitting locking and unlocking simply by a progressive squeezing together of the needle holder handles.

Tissue Forceps

Tissue (thumb) forceps are tweezer-like, nonlocking instruments that are used to grasp tissue (Fig. 21-24). The proximal ends are joined to allow the grasping ends to spring open or to be squeezed together. They are available in a variety of shapes and sizes; tips (grasping ends) may be pointed, flattened, rounded,

smooth, or serrated, or have small or large teeth. Tissue forceps with large teeth should not be used to handle tissue that is easily traumatized; smooth tips are recommended with delicate tissue (e.g., blood vessels). The most commonly used tissue forceps, *Brown-Adson,* have small serrations on the tips that cause minimal trauma but hold tissue securely.

Hemostatic Forceps

Hemostatic forceps, commonly called "hemostats," are crushing instruments used to clamp blood vessels (Fig. 21-25). They are available with straight or curved tips and vary in size from smaller (3-inch) *mosquito hemostats* with transverse jaw serrations, to larger (9-inch) *angiotribes*. Serrations on the jaws of larger hemostatic forceps may be transverse, longitudinal, or diagonal, or a combination of these. Longitudinal serrations are generally gentler on tissue than cross serrations. Serrations usually extend from the tips of the jaws to the boxlocks, but in *Kelly forceps,* transverse (horizontal) serrations extend over only the distal portion of the jaws. Similarly sized *Crile forceps* have transverse serrations that extend the entire jaw length. Kelly and Crile forceps are used on larger vessels. *Rochester-Carmalt forceps* are larger crushing forceps, often used to control large tissue bundles (e.g., during ovariohysterectomy). They have longitudinal grooves with cross grooves at the tip ends to prevent tissue slippage.

Curved hemostats should be placed on tissue with the curve facing up. The smallest hemostatic forceps that will accomplish the job should be used to grasp as little tissue as possible to minimize trauma. To avoid having fingers momentarily trapped within the rings of hemostats, fingertips should be placed on the forceps finger rings or your fingers should be inserted into the rings only as far as the first joint.

A

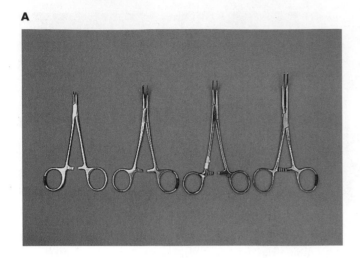

B

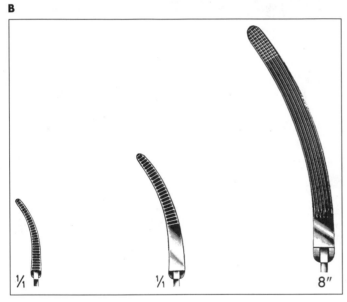

FIG. 21-25 Hemostatic forceps *(left to right)*: mosquito hemostats, Kelly, Crile, Carmalt. The insert shows tip detail. *(From Fossum TW: Small animal surgery, St Louis, 1997, Mosby.)*

Retractors

Retractors are used to retract tissue and improve exposure. The ends of hand-held retractors may be hooked, curved, spatula-shaped, or toothed. Some hand-held retractors may be bent (i.e., malleable) to conform to the structure being retracted or area of the body in which retraction is being performed. *Senn (rake) retractors* are double-ended retractors. One end has three finger-like, curved prongs; the other end is a flat, curved blade. Self-retaining retractors maintain tension on tissues and are held open with a boxlock (e.g., *Gelpi, Weitlaner*) or other device (e.g., set-screw). Examples of the latter are *Balfour retractors* and *Finochietto retractors*. Balfour retractors are generally used to retract the abdominal wall, whereas Finochietto retractors are commonly used during thoracotomies.

Miscellaneous Instruments

Instruments are available to suction fluid, clamp drapes or tissues, cut and remove bone pieces *(rongeurs)*, hold bones during fracture repair, scrape surfaces of dense tissue *(currettes)*, remove periosteum *(periosteal elevators)*, cut or shape bone and cartilage *(osteotomes and chisels)*, and bore holes in bone *(trephines)*.

Instruments for Large Animal Surgery

Dehorning Instruments. Various instruments, including gouges and saws, are used to remove horns from cattle (Fig. 21-26). The smaller instruments are used on calves. Saws are generally used to remove the horns of adult cattle.

Castrating Instruments. An *emasculator* is used in open castrations to crush and sever the spermatic cord (Fig. 21-27). An *emasculatome* (see Fig. 21-27) is used to accomplish the same thing through the intact skin during closed castrations, particularly when fly infestation is likely to be a problem.

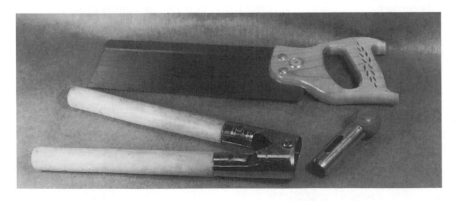

FIG. 21-26 Dehorning instruments: dehorning saw *(top)*: Barnes dehorner *(bottom left)*, horn gouge *(bottom right)*. *(From Pratt PW: Medical surgical and anesthetic nursing for veterinary technicians, St Louis, 1994, Mosby.)*

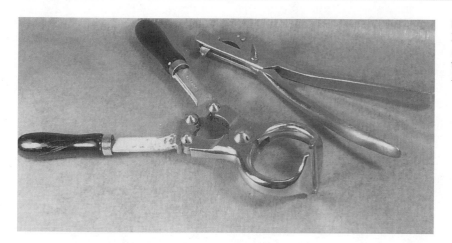

FIG. 21-27 Castration instruments: emasculatome *(bottom left)* and emasculator *(top right)*. *(From Pratt PW: Medical, surgical and anesthetic nursing for veterinary technicians, St Louis, 1994, Mosby.)*

CARE AND MAINTENANCE OF SURGICAL INSTRUMENTS

Good surgical instruments are a valuable investment and must be used and maintained properly to prevent corrosion, pitting, and/or discoloration. Instruments should be rinsed in cool water as soon after the surgical procedure as possible to avoid drying of blood, tissue, saline, or other foreign matter on them. Many manufacturers recommend that instruments be rinsed, cleaned, and sterilized in distilled or deionized water, because tap water contains minerals that may cause discoloration and staining. If tap water is used for rinsing, instruments should be dried thoroughly to avoid staining. Instruments with multiple components should be disassembled before cleaning. Delicate instruments should be cleaned and sterilized separately.

Instrument Cleaning

Ultrasonic and enzymatic methods of cleaning are effective and efficient. Before putting soiled instruments in an ultrasonic cleaner, they should be washed in cleaning solution to remove all visible debris. Dissimilar metals (e.g., chrome and stainless steel) should not be mixed in the same cycle. All instruments should be placed in the ultrasonic cleaner with their ratchets and boxlocks open. Instruments should not be piled on top of each other to avoid damaging delicate instruments. They should be removed from the cleaner and rinsed and dried at the completion of the cycle.

If an ultrasonic cleaner is not available, instruments should be manually cleaned as thoroughly as possible, paying particular attention to boxlocks, serrations, and hinges. Nylon brushes and cool cleaning solution may be used for most instruments. Rasps and serrated parts of instruments may require a wire brush. A cleaning solution with a neutral pH should be used to avoid staining. Cleaning solutions should be prepared as instructed by the manufacturer and changed frequently. Enzymatic solutions may be used to remove proteinaceous materials from general surgical instruments and endoscopic equipment.

Instrument Lubricating and Autoclaving

Autoclaving is not a substitute for proper instrument cleaning. Before they are autoclaved, instruments with boxlocks and hinges and power equipment should be lubricated with instrument milk or surgical lubricants. Do not use industrial oils to lubricate instruments because they interfere with steam sterilization. Instruments are generally grouped into packs or kits according to their use (Tables 21-4 and 21-5). Before instruments are autoclaved, wrap them in cloth or place them on a cloth inside a fenestrated pan to absorb moisture. Instruments should be sterilized with the boxlocks or hinges open. The autoclave chamber should not be overloaded. Avoid stacking of instruments to prevent damage to delicate instruments. Kits should be double-wrapped and sealed with tape (e.g., Auto Clave Tape: 3M), and a monitor (e.g., Steam Clox) should be added before autoclaving. Avoid rapid cooling of instruments to prevent condensation.

DRAPING AND ORGANIZING THE INSTRUMENT TABLE

Instrument tables should be height adjustable to allow them to be positioned within reach of surgical personnel. The instrument table should not be opened until the animal has been positioned on the surgical table and draped. Large, water-impermeable table drapes should be used to cover the entire instrument table. To open these drapes, the drape and outer wrap are positioned on the instrument table, the exposed undersurface of the drape is gently grasped, and the ends and then the sides

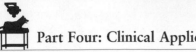
TABLE 21-4 Common components of a basic soft tissue pack, such as for ovariohysterectomy, laparotomy, and wound repair

Instrument	Quantity
Halsted-Mosquito hemostats, curved, 5 inch	2
Halsted-Mosquito hemostats, straight, 5 inch	2
Kelly hemostats, curved, 5.5 inch	2
Crile forceps, straight, 5.5 inch	2
Rochester-Carmalt hemostats, curved, 7.25 inch	4
Mayo-Hegar or Olsen-Hegar needle holders, 7 inch	1
Brown-Adson tissue forceps	1
Allis tissue forceps, 6 inch, 5 × 6 teeth	4
Bachhaus towel clamps, 5.25 inch	4
Metzenbaum scissors, 8 inch, curved	1
Suture scissors, sharp/blunt, straight, 5 inch	1
Instrument tray	1
Senn retractors	2
Blade handle, No. 3	1
Ovariohysterectomy (spay) hook	1
Saline bowl	1
Radiopaque sponges (4 × 4 inches)	20

TABLE 21-5 Common components of a basic orthopedic pack*

Instrument	Quantity
Jacobs chuck and key	1
Spoon Holmann retractor	2
Army-Navy retractor	2
Periosteal elevator	1
Wire twister	1
Medium pin cutter	1
Kern or Lane bone-holding forceps	2
Reduction forceps	1
Orthopedic wire (18, 20, 22 gauge)	1 each size
Kirschner wires	2 each size
Intramedullary pins	2 each size

*Augmented with the general pack described in Table 21-4.

are unfolded. Once the drape has been opened, nonsterile personnel should not reach over it. *Mayo stands* are often used in procedures that require additional instruments (e.g., bone plating); specially designed Mayo stand covers are available to cover these tables. When the instrument pack has been opened, instruments should be positioned so that they can be readily retrieved. The instrument layout is generally determined by the surgeon's preference, but grouping similar instruments (e.g., scissors, retractors) facilitates their use.

When a body cavity is to be opened, sponges should be counted at the beginning of the procedure (before the first incision) and before closure to ensure that none have been inadvertently left in the body cavity. Contaminated instruments or soiled sponges should not be placed back on the instrument table.

WOUND CLOSURE AND HEMOSTASIS

T.W. FOSSUM

SUTURE MATERIALS
Suture Characteristics

The word *suture* refers to any strand of material that is used to approximate tissues or ligate blood vessels. The ideal suture material is easy to handle, reacts minimally in tissue, inhibits bacterial growth, holds securely when knotted, resists shrinking in tissues, is noncapillary, nonallergenic, noncarcinogenic, and nonferromagnetic, and is absorbed with minimal reaction after the tissue has healed. Such an ideal suture material does not exist; therefore, surgeons must choose one that most closely approximates the ideal for a given procedure and/or tissue to be sutured.

Monofilament sutures are made of a single strand of material. They create less tissue drag than multifilament suture material and do not have interstitial spaces that may harbor bacteria. Care should be used in handling monofilament sutures because nicking or damaging them with forceps or needle holders weakens them and predisposes to breakage. *Multifilament sutures* consist of several strands that are twisted or braided together. Multifilament sutures are generally more pliable and flexible than monofilament sutures. They may be coated to decrease tissue drag and enhance handling characteristics.

The most commonly used standard for suture size is the U.S.P. (United States Pharmacopeia), which denotes suture diameters from fine to coarse according to a numeric scale; size 10-O material has the smallest diameter (finest) and size 7 has the largest diameter (most coarse). U.S.P. uses different size notations for various suture materials (Table 21-6). The smaller the suture diameter is, the lower its tensile strength. Stainless-steel wire is usually sized according to the metric or U.S.P. scale or by the Brown and Sharpe wire gauge (see Table 21-6).

Absorbable Suture Materials

Absorbable suture materials lose most of their tensile strength within 60 days after placement in tissue and eventually are absorbed from the site (Table 21-7).

Surgical Gut. Surgical gut is commonly called "catgut." Surgical gut is made from the submucosa of sheep intestine or the serosa of bovine intestine. It comprises approximately 90% collagen. *Plain surgical gut* is broken down by phagocytosis and elicits a marked inflammatory reaction, as compared with other materials. "Tanning," by exposure to chrome or aldehyde, slows absorption. Surgical gut so treated is called *chromic surgical gut.* Surgical gut is rapidly absorbed from infected sites or where it is exposed to digestive enzymes. Knots in surgical gut may loosen when wet.

Synthetic Absorbable Materials. Synthetic absorbable

TABLE 21-6 Systems used to indicate suture sizes

Diameter (mm)	Metric gauge	Synthetic suture materials (U.S.P.)	Surgical gut (U.S.P.)	Wire gauge (Brown and Sharpe)
0.02	0.2	10 - O		
0.03	0.3	9 - O		
0.04	0.4	8 - O		
0.05	0.5	7 - O	8 - O	41
0.07	0.7	6 - O	7 - O	38 - 40
0.1	1	5 - O	6 - O	35
0.15	1.5	4 - O	5 - O	32 - 34
0.2	2	3 - O	4 - O	30
0.3	3	2 - O	3 - O	28
0.35	3.5	O	2 - O	26
0.4	4	1	O	25
0.5	5	2	1	24
0.6	6	3, 4	2	22
0.7	7	5	3	20
0.8	8	6	4	19
0.9	9	7		18

TABLE 21-7 Characteristics of suture materials commonly used in veterinary medicine

Generic name	Trade name	Manufacturer	Characteristics	Reduction in tensile strength*	Complete absorption	Knot security†	Tissue reaction‡
Chromic surgical gut (catgut)	—		Absorbable Multifilament	33% at 7 days 67% at 28 days	60 days	wet: − dry: +	+++
Polyglactin 910	Vicryl	Ethicon	Absorbable Multifilament	35% at 14 days 60% at 21 days	60 days	++	+
Polyglycolic acid	Dexon S (uncoated) Dexon II (coated)	Davis & Geck	Absorbable Multifilament	35% at 14 days 65% at 21 days	60-90 days	++	+
Polydioxanone	PDS II	Ethicon	Absorbable Monofilament	14% at 14 days 31% at 42 days	180 days	++	+
Polyglyconate	Maxon	Davis & Geck	Absorbable Monofilament	30% at 14 days 45% at 21 days	180 days	++	+++
Silk	—	—	Nonabsorbable Multifilament	30% at 14 days 50% at 1 year	2 years	−	+++
Polyester	Mersilene (uncoated) Ethibond (coated) Dacron (uncoated) Ticron (coated)	Ethicon Ethicon Davis & Geck Davis & Geck	Nonabsorbable Multifilament	—	—	−	++
Nylon	Ethilon (monofilament) Nurolon (multifilament) Dermalon (monofilament) Surgilon (multifilament)	Ethicon Ethicon Davis & Geck Davis & Geck	Nonabsorbable Monofilament or multifilament	Mono: 30% at 2 years Multi: 75% at 180 days	—	−	−
Polypropylene	Prolene Surgilene Fluorofil	Ethicon Davis & Geck Mallinckrodt	Nonabsorbable Monofilament	—	—	+++	−
Polybutester	Novafil	Davis & Geck	Nonabsorbable Monofilament	—	—	++	−
Polymerized caprolactam	Supramid Braunamid	S. Jackson B. Braun Melsungen Ag Mallinckrodt	Nonabsorbable Multifilament	—	—	++	++ (if coating damaged)
Stainless-steel wire	Vetcassette II	Davis & Geck Ethicon	Nonabsorbable Monofilament or multifilament	—	—	+++	−

*Values given are approximate. Actual loss of tensile strength may vary, depending on suture material and tissue.
†(−) = Poor (<60%); (+) = fair (60-70%); (++) = good (70-85%); (+++) = excellent (>85%).
‡(−) = Minimal to none; (+) = mild; (++) = moderate; (+++) = severe.

materials (e.g., polyglycolic acid, polyglactin 910, poly-dioxanone, polyglyconate) are generally broken down by hydrolysis (Table 21-7). There is minimal tissue reaction to synthetic absorbable suture materials. The rate of tensile strength loss and rate of absorption are fairly constant in different tissues. Infection or exposure to digestive enzymes does not significantly influence their rates of absorption.

Nonabsorbable Suture Materials

Organic Nonabsorbable Materials. *Silk* is the most common organic nonabsorbable suture material, used as a braided multifilament suture that is uncoated or coated (see Table 21-8). Silk has excellent handling characteristics and is often used in cardiovascular procedures; however, it does not maintain significant tensile strength after 6 months in tissues and is therefore contraindicated for use with vascular grafts. It should also be avoided in contaminated sites, because it increases the likelihood of wound infection.

Synthetic Nonabsorbable Materials. Synthetic nonabsorbable suture materials (see Table 21-7) are available as braided multifilament (e.g., polyester, coated caprolactam) or monofilament (e.g., polypropylene, polyamide, polyolefins, polybutester) threads. They are typically strong and induce minimal tissue reaction. Nonabsorbable suture materials consisting of an inner core and an outer sheath (e.g., Supramid) should not be buried in tissues, because the outer sheath tends to degenerate, allowing bacteria to migrate to the inner core. This predisposes to infection and fistula formation.

Metallic Sutures. Stainless steel is the most commonly used metallic suture. It is available as monofilament wire or twisted multifilament wire. The tissue reaction to stainless steel is generally minimal; however, the knot ends evoke an inflammatory reaction. Wire tends to cut tissue and may fragment. It is stable in contaminated wounds and is the standard for judging knot security and tissue reaction to suture materials.

Suture Needles

Suture needles are available in a wide variety of shapes and sizes. The type of suture needle used depends on the characteristics of the tissue to be sutured (penetrability, density, elasticity, thickness), wound topography (deep, narrow), and characteristics of the needle (type of eye, length, diameter). Most surgical needles are made from stainless steel because it is strong and corrosion free and does not harbor bacteria.

The three basic components of a suture needle are the attachment end (swaged or eyed), body, and point (Fig. 21-28, *A*). Suture material must be threaded onto *eyed needles*. Because a double-strand of suture is pulled through the tissue, a larger hole is created than when a swaged needle is used. Eyed needles may be closed (round, oblong, or square) or French (with a slit from the inside of the eye to the end of the needle for ease of threading) (Fig. 21-28, *B*). Eyed needles are threaded from the inside curvature. With *swaged needles,* the needle and suture are joined in a continuous unit, minimizing tissue trauma and increasing ease of use.

The needle body comes in a variety of shapes (Fig. 21-28, *C*); tissue type and depth and size of the wound determine the appropriate needle shape. *Straight (Keith) needles* are generally used in accessible places where the needle can be manipulated directly with the fingers (e.g., placement of pursestring sutures in the rectum). *Curved needles* are manipulated with needle holders. The depth and diameter of the wound are important when selecting the most appropriate curved needle. One-fourth (¼) circle needles are primarily used in ophthalmic procedures. Three-eighths (⅜) and one-half (½) circle needles are the most commonly used surgical needles in veterinary medicine (e.g., abdominal closure). Three-eighths circle needles are more easily manipulated than one-half circle needles because they require less manipulation of the wrist. However, because of the larger arc of manipulation required, they are awkward to use in deep or inaccessible locations. A one-half circle or five-eighths (⅝) circle needle, despite requiring more wrist manipulation, is easier to use in confined locations.

The needle point (cutting, taper, reverse-cutting; Fig. 21-28, *D*) determines the sharpness of a needle and type of tissue in which the needle is used. *Cutting needles* generally have two or three opposing cutting edges. They are used in tissues that are difficult to penetrate (e.g., skin). With conventional cutting needles, the third cutting edge is on the inside (concave) curvature of the needle. The location of the inside cutting edge may promote "cut-out" of tissue because it cuts toward the edges of the wound or incision. Reverse-cutting needles have a third cutting edge located on the outer (convex) curvature of the needle. This makes them stronger than similarly sized conventional cutting needles, and reduces the risk of tissue cut-out. Side-cutting needles (spatula needles) are flat on the top and bottom. They are generally used in ophthalmic procedures.

Tapered needles (round needles) have a sharp tip that pierces and spreads tissues without cutting them. They are generally used in easily penetrated tissues (e.g., intestine, subcutaneous tissues, fascia). Tapercut (Ethicon) needles have a reverse-cutting edge tip and a taper-point body. They are generally used for suturing dense, tough fibrous tissue (e.g., tendon) and for some cardiovascular procedures (e.g., vascular grafts). *Blunt-point needles* have a rounded, blunt point that can dissect through friable tissue without cutting. They are occasionally used for suturing soft, parenchymal organs (e.g., liver, kidney).

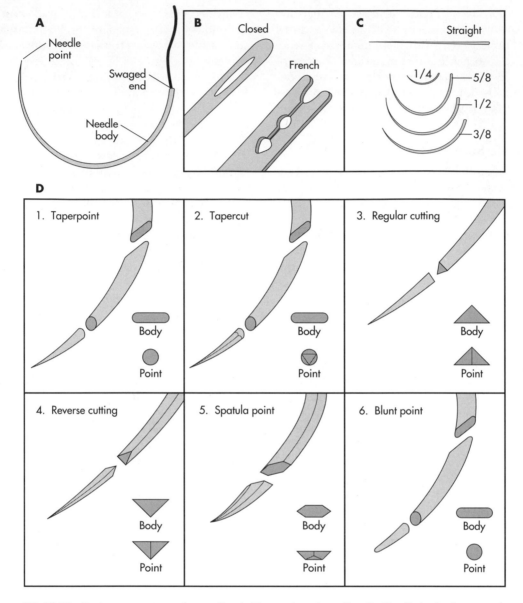

FIG. 21-28 Basic components of a needle, **A.** Types of eyed needles, **B.** Needle body shapes and sizes, **C** and **D.** *(From Fossum TW: Small animal surgery, St Louis, 1997, Mosby.)*

OTHER MATERIALS USED IN WOUND CLOSURE

Tissue Adhesives

Cyanoacrylates ("super glue") are commonly used for tissue adhesion during some procedures (e.g., declawing, tail docking, ear cropping). Products advocated for use in veterinary patients include Tissueglue (GRX Medical), Vetbond (3M Co), and Nexabond (Tri-Point Medical). These adhesives rapidly polymerize in the presence of moisture and produce a strong flexible bond. Adhesion of tissue edges generally takes less than

15 seconds but may be delayed by excessive hemorrhage. Persistence of the glue in the dermis may result in granuloma formation or wound dehiscence, and placement in an infected site may cause fistulation.

Ligating Clips and Staples

Metal *clips* (Hemoclips, Ligaclips) may be used for vessel ligation. They are particularly useful when the vessel is difficult to reach or when multiple vessels must be ligated. Use of ligating clips on vessels more than 11 mm in diameter is not recommended. The vessel should be dissected free of surrounding tissue before the clip is applied and 2 to 3 mm of vessel should extend beyond the clip to prevent slippage. The vessel should be one third to two thirds the size of the clip.

Metal *staples* (e.g., Michel clips) are used to appose wound edges or attach drapes to the skin. Care must be used to ensure that the staple is appropriately bent so that, when staples are used for skin closure, they cannot be easily removed by the animal. A special "staple-remover" facilitates clip removal after healing.

Surgical Mesh

Surgical mesh may be used to repair hernias (e.g., perineal hernias) or reinforce traumatized or devitalized tissues (abdominal hernias). Occasionally it is used to replace excised traumatized or neoplastic tissues. Surgical mesh is available in nonabsorbable (Mersilene, Prolone) or absorbable (Vicryl, Dexon) forms.

SUTURE REMOVAL

Skin incisions are usually closed with nonabsorbable suture material. Because they are not absorbed, nonabsorbable sutures are removed once healing is sufficient to prevent wound dehiscence, usually after 10 to 14 days. However, delayed healing, as in very debili-

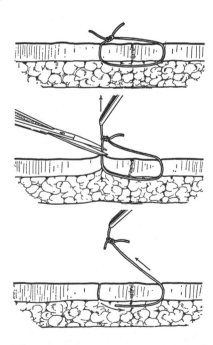

FIG. 21-29 When removing a suture, grasp one or both free ends of the suture, elevate the knot, cut the suture at the skin surface, and pull the suture out. *(From Pratt PW: Medical, surgical and anesthetic nursing for veterinary technicians, St Louis, 1997, Mosby.)*

tated animals, may require that sutures be left in place for longer periods. Additionally, if fibrosis is desired (e.g., aural hematoma), delayed suture removal may be considered.

Skin suture removal is begun by grasping one or both of the suture ends, which were deliberately left long for that purpose, and pulling the knot away from the skin (Fig. 21-29). Using suture removal scissors, cut one of the two strands of suture beneath the knot at the skin surface, and pull the suture out. It is important that only one of the strands is cut to avoid leaving some of the suture material buried beneath the skin, where it could act as an irritant.

HEMOSTATIC TECHNIQUES AND MATERIALS

Hemostasis, or the arrest of bleeding, allows visualization of the surgical site and prevents life-threatening hemorrhage. Low-pressure hemorrhage from small vessels can be controlled by applying pressure to the bleeding points with a gauze sponge. Once a thrombus has formed, the sponge should be gently removed to avoid disrupting clots. Large vessels must be ligated (tied off). Hemostatic agents used to control hemorrhage during surgery include bone wax and hemostatic materials made of gelatin or cellulose (e.g., Surgicel, Gelfoam).

Electrocoagulation can be used to achieve hemostasis in vessels less than 2 mm in diameter; larger vessels should be ligated. The term *electrocautery* is often erroneously used in place of *electrocoagulation*. With electrocautery, the needle tip or scalpel is heated before it is applied to the tissue; with electrocoagulation, heat is generated in the tissue as a high-frequency current is passed through it. Excessive use of electrocautery or electrocoagulation retards healing.

RECOMMENDED READING

Auer JA: *Equine surgery,* Philadelphia, 1992, WB Saunders.
Bojrab MJ: *Current techniques in small animal surgery,* ed 4, Malvern, Penn, 1997, Williams & Wilkins.
Colahan PT et al: *Equine medicine and surgery,* ed 5, St Louis, 1998, Mosby.
Colville TP: The veterinary technician's guide to surgery room conduct, *Vet Technician* 7:392-396, 1986.
Fossum TW: *Small animal surgery,* St Louis, 1997, Mosby.
Heath MM: Scrubbing procedures and surgical attire, *Vet Technician* 9:345-350, 1988.
Kagan KG: Aseptic technique, *Vet Technician,* 13:65-80, 1992.
Pratt PW: *Medical, surgical, and anesthetic nursing for veterinary technicians,* St Louis, 1994, Mosby.
Slatter D: *Textbook of small animal surgery,* ed 2, Philadelphia, 1993, WB Saunders.
Tracy DL: *Small animal surgical nursing,* ed 2, St Louis, 1994, Mosby.

CHAPTER 22

Emergency and Critical Care

H. Davis, Jr.

Learning Objectives

After reviewing this chapter, the reader should understand the following:

Considerations in rendering first aid to injured or critically ill animals

Steps in initially evaluating injured or critically ill animals

Procedures used to support vital functions in injured or critically ill patients

Methods used to monitor the condition of critically ill patients

Placement and care of catheters, chest drains, and tracheostomy tubes

Considerations for blood transfusions and fluid therapy in injured or critically ill patients

Procedures used in maintaining recumbent patients

Emergency care is action directed toward assessment, treatment, and stabilization of a patient with an urgent medical problem. *Critical care* is the ongoing treatment of a patient with a life-threatening or potentially life-threatening illness or injury whose condition is likely to change on a moment-to-moment or hour-to-hour basis. Such patients require intense and often constant monitoring, reassessment, and treatment.

The clinic facilities should be set up and organized to handle any emergency likely to be presented. This may be an area in the clinic designated for emergency management of patients or a mobile "crash cart" system (Fig. 22-1). An oxygen source should be readily available. Good lighting facilitates examination of the patient, endotracheal intubation, visualization of veins, and completion of minor surgical procedures. The designated area should be centralized and stocked with key emergency supplies and equipment (e.g., ECG, defibrillator, and suction). The supplies should be organized for easy location and use. Crash carts/kits make the resus-

citation endeavor more efficient. The emergency area should be checked at the beginning of each shift and restocked immediately after each use.

PREHOSPITAL CARE
Telephone Contact

Often, the first contact the animal owner has with the veterinary clinic is via telephone. The technician should be capable of recognizing what constitutes an emergency, giving basic first-aid advice, and providing clear directions to the hospital. If possible, talk directly to the owner or the person caring for the animal, rather than obtaining secondhand information from a well-intentioned person. Basic information should be obtained from the owner or handler:

- *What is the nature of the illness/injury?* Has the animal been traumatized or been exposed to a toxin, or does it have a chronic illness?

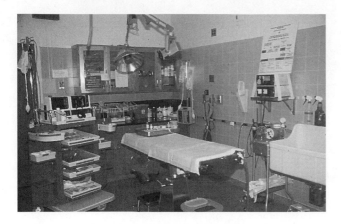

FIG. 22-1 Emergency receiving room. The room is large enough for the emergency team and has good lighting. Emergency equipment (ECG machine, defibrillator, crash cart, suction, and oxygen) is in close proximity to the patient.

- *What is the condition of the animal?* Is the animal alert and responsive or unconscious? Is it able to breathe freely? Is there any bleeding? If so, where? Is it otherwise injured?
- *How long ago did the injury occur, or when was the illness first noticed?* Has the animal's condition improved or deteriorated, and over what period?
- *Does the animal have a preexisting illness?* Is it receiving any medications?
- *What are the animal's age, sex, breed, and weight?*

With this information, basic first-aid advice may be given and/or the client told to bring the animal immediately to the hospital. This information can also be used to prepare for the arrival of the patient. The technician could set up oxygen, IV catheters, fluids, or other equipment and supplies that might be needed.

First Aid

Trauma is perhaps the number one reason for the need of prehospital first aid. Clients should be instructed to survey the scene of the accident before rendering aid. This ensures that neither the people rendering aid nor the animal will be placed in further danger (e.g., animal found in the middle of a busy highway). Clients should exercise caution when approaching an injured animal. Most owners do not understand that their pet might bite them when it is injured. Clients should be instructed on how to make a muzzle using a leash, belt, tie, rope, or strips of cloth. If the animal is experiencing breathing difficulty, a muzzle should not be applied.

The acronym *ABC* (airway, breathing, circulation) applies to field emergencies as well as hospital emergencies.

Airway. Owners should make sure the airway is free of blood, mucus, vomitus, and dirt. If the animal is unconscious, the tongue should be pulled out and the head and neck gently extended to provide an airway or access to it (unless head or neck injuries are possible). If the animal is conscious and fluid is evident in the mouth, the animal should be placed in a head-down position to minimize aspiration of fluid into the airway. If an airway obstruction is suspected (ball, bone, chew toy), the owner can use the *Heimlich maneuver* to dislodge the obstruction as follows: Place the animal in lateral recumbency and place the hands caudal to the animal's ribs. With the hands, deliver quick, short compressions toward the animal's diaphragm. The maneuver can also be performed as for people, with the animal held in a vertical position with its back to the rescuer. Place the hands on the cranial abdomen, caudal to the rib cage, and direct the compressing force dorsally and cranially.

Breathing. Owners should note if the animal is breathing. If not, the open airway should be verified as outlined above and then mouth-to-nose breathing instituted (Fig. 22-2). With the animal's head and neck extended, the person's mouth should be placed over the animal's nostrils (nostrils and mouth in small dogs and cats) and the lips held closed to prevent escape of air. The owner should blow into the nostrils every 3 to 5 seconds, making the chest rise with each breath. Artificial ventilation should be continued until spontaneous ventilation resumes or until the animal is under professional care.

If the animal has difficulty breathing, the handler should try to minimize stress. If practical and safe, the animal should be carried. The owner should be told to avoid placing a leash around the neck of dogs. If a leash is needed, it should be placed loosely around the chest, caudal to the front legs.

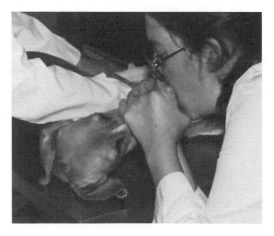

FIG. 22-2 Artificial respiration is given by cupping the hands around the muzzle and blowing into the nares. *(From Pratt PW: Medical, surgical and anesthetic nursing for veterinary technicians, St Louis, 1994, Mosby.)*

Circulation. The patient's heartbeat should be checked by placing a hand over the chest, just caudal to the elbow. If the animal is not breathing and a heartbeat is not palpable, chest compressions should be performed. The animal's chest should be compressed directly over the heart, with the animal in lateral recumbency. The rate of compression is 80 to 120 per minute. If cardiopulmonary resuscitation (CPR) is performed by one person, the ventilation to chest compression ratio is 2:15. If CPR is done by two people, the ratio is 1:5.

If the animal is bleeding externally, pressure should be applied directly to the wound with bandage material or a clean cloth. Owners should be warned that this may be painful to the animal, and so it may need to be muzzled. Bite wounds often are more serious than they first appear. The owners should be told this and instructed to bring the animal in for an examination. Large wounds should be bandaged with a clean cloth or towel to prevent further contamination. If an object, such as a stick or arrow, is protruding from the body, the owner should be told *not* to remove it. If the object is long, it may be cut 2 to 3 cm outside the body wall so as not to create a fulcrum that can lead to further damage.

If the animal has an open fracture (bone penetrating through the skin), the exposed bone should be covered with moist, clean cloths. If the owner notices that the leg is in an abnormal position, attempts should be made to prevent movement of the limb. Distal extremity fractures can be stabilized with materials found around the home, such as rolled newspaper, cardboard, or wood. The splint is tied to the leg in several locations, being sure to avoid the fracture site. Immobilization should include the joint proximal and distal to the fracture.

The client must be instructed in proper transport of an injured animal. In the nonambulatory animal, spinal trauma should be assumed until proven otherwise. The animal should be immobilized in lateral recumbency on a flat, rigid surface, in a neutral in-line position. The principles of fracture stabilization apply here as well. The joint proximal and distal to the injury should be immobilized. This means that the head and pelvis should be secured to the rigid surface. Various aids can be found around the home for transport, such as boards, blankets, boxes, or carriers.

Immediate professional care should be sought if an animal exhibits acute ocular pain or vision loss, deformity of the globe, or sudden change in the appearance of the eye. The owner should be instructed to approach the animal gently and carefully, because eye injuries may be painful. If a foreign body is protruding from the eye, it should be left alone until professional help is obtained. If the eye was exposed to an irritant, flush the eye with water for at least 5 minutes. If the globe is proptosed (prolapsed from the socket), it should be kept moist if the patient will tolerate it.

If an animal is thought to have ingested a toxin, instruct the owner to come to the hospital immediately. The owner should be instructed to bring the product container so that the active ingredient can be determined and the poison control center can be consulted. Should the animal vomit, have the owner bring in a sample of the vomitus for possible toxicologic analysis. Although some people advocate having the owner induce the animal to vomit before bringing the animal to the clinic, time is wasted trying to do this at home and rarely is it successful. If the animal cannot reach professional help within 30 to 40 minutes, one might consider inducing the animal to vomit at home. Concentrated salt water, 3% hydrogen peroxide solution, and syrup of ipecac are potential inducers. The veterinarian should be consulted before recommending this to the owner. Vomiting should *not* be induced if the animal ingested a caustic substance or petroleum distillates. Induced vomiting is not without risk. One of the major risks is aspiration of the material, which often causes pneumonia.

HOSPITAL CARE
Initial Evaluation

Initial management of the emergency patient requires immediate assessment and therapy. Attention must be focused on seeing that the needs of the patient are met in a timely fashion. This can be done by dividing the initial management into three phases: primary survey and resuscitation; secondary survey; and definitive management.

Primary Survey and Resuscitation. The primary survey is the initial, brief assessment which involves A-B-C-D-Es: *A* for airway, *B* for breathing, *C* for circulation, *D* for dysfunction or disability of the central nervous system, and *E* for examination. When a life-threatening problem is identified during the primary survey, resuscitative action should be instituted immediately.

Airway/Breathing. First, airway and adequacy of ventilation should be assessed. This is done by visualization, palpation, and auscultation. Life-threatening airway/breathing problems may be due to apnea, airway obstruction, open chest wounds, tension pneumothorax, or hemopneumothorax. Clinical signs (Table 22-1) associated with inadequate ventilation vary, depending on the severity of respiratory compromise.

Normally, the animal should have a free, easy, and regular ventilatory pattern. It should not be exerting an extraordinary amount of effort to breathe. The tidal volume should be adequate. The mucous membrane color should be pink. Cyanotic or blue mucous mem-

---

TABLE 22-1 Signs of inadequate ventilation
Stridor
Intercostal retraction
Decreased breath sounds
Restlessness and/or anxiety
Minimal or absent chest wall motion
Cyanosis (late sign)
Absence of air exchange from the nose or mouth
Labored use of accessory muscles of respiration

branes indicate hypoxemia, which is a decrease of the arterial oxygen concentration. Cyanosis is not a reliable indicator of hypoxia; it is not always present in hypoxia. It is always a late sign and does not occur in severe anemia. Normal lungs should sound clear over a large area of the lung fields.

Management of life-threatening airway/breathing problems may include a variety of techniques. In the case of suspected airway obstruction, the mouth and pharynx should be examined for easily removable foreign bodies. If the mouth cannot be examined or the foreign body removed, preoxygenation and rapid safe anesthetic induction is in order. If the obstruction cannot be removed, the patient should be intubated (oral or tracheostomy) in an attempt to bypass the obstruction. If the patient is apneic, mechanical or manual ventilation will be required. Initial ventilatory requirements are 10 to 15 breaths/minute; inspiratory time of approximately 1 second; and a proximal airway pressure of 15 to 20 cm H_2O or a tidal volume of 10 to 20 ml/kg. If the animal has an open chest wound, this can be temporarily closed by placing a "glob" of ointment and a sterile dressing over the wound. Thoracentesis or thoracostomy tube placement should be performed to relieve respiratory distress resulting from pleural filling defects.

Circulation. Circulation is assessed by visualization, palpation, and auscultation. Shock is inadequate tissue perfusion resulting in inadequate oxygen delivery. Signs of shock are indicative of decreased tissue perfusion and sympathetic autonomic responses. The signs of shock include increased heart rate (an effort to increase cardiac output), poor pulse quality (indicates poor pulse pressure or stroke volume), pale mucous membranes, prolonged capillary refill time, and decreased appendage temperature (indicators of poor peripheral perfusion). Shock may be due to pump failure (intrinsic heart failure, arrhythmias, cardiac tamponade) or hypovolemia as a result of external or concealed blood loss (loss into body cavity or limb). Hypovolemic shock is a sequel to a variety of problems, such as trauma, sepsis, and gastric dilatation/volvulus.

Fluid therapy is the cornerstone of shock therapy. Intravenous fluid therapy must be initiated to return heart rate, blood pressure, cardiac output, and oxygen delivery to normal. Fluid options for fluid resuscitation include crystalloids (solutions with electrolytes similar to plasma, e.g., lactated Ringer's, Normasol R, Plasmalyte 148, and normal saline), and colloids (plasma, Dextran 70, 6% Gentran: Baxter, 6% Hetastarch : Abbott, and whole blood). Initially, crystalloids are used in treatment of shock. The shock dosage of a crystalloid is 80 to 90 ml/kg and 50 to 55 ml/kg in the dog and cat, respectively (equivalent to one blood volume). It may be necessary to administer 0.5 to 1.5 times the blood volume to resuscitate the patient. Approximately 75% of the crystalloids shift from the intravascular space into the interstitial space in about 30 minutes. Colloids are better blood volume expanders; 50% to 80% of the infused volume remains in the intravascular space. Colloids should be administered when crystalloids are not improving or maintaining blood volume restoration. Blood and/or plasma are given in sufficient quantities to maintain the packed cell volume above 25% and a total plasma protein level above 4.0 mg/dl. Colloids are given IV at 10 to 40 ml/kg and 5 to 20 ml/kg in the dog and cat, respectively.

Hypertonic saline (7.0% sodium chloride injection USP : Sanofi Animal Health) has been recommended for use in shock therapy in cases where it is difficult to administer large volumes of fluids rapidly enough to resuscitate the patient. Hypertonic saline causes fluid shifts from the intracellular space to the extracellular (including intravascular) space, resulting in improved venous return and cardiac output. Hypertonic saline may have other beneficial cardiovascular effects as well. The recommended dosage is 4 to 6 ml/kg infused during 5 minutes. Dextran 70 has been added to hypertonic saline to potentiate and sustain vascular augmentation.

Use of corticosteroids in the treatment of hypovolemic shock has been controversial for many years. Some studies show that corticosteroids are beneficial in septic shock, while other studies show no beneficial effect in reversing shock or reducing mortality. It is thought that corticosteroids stabilize lysosomal membranes, inhibit vasoactive peptides, and improve oxygen delivery to the tissues. If corticosteroids are to be administered, it should be done early. Suggested shock dosages are dexamethasone sodium phospate (Vedco) at 4 to 8 mg/kg and prednisolone sodium succinate (Solu Delta Cortef : Upjohn) at 10 to 30 mg/kg.

Sympathomimetics, such as dopamine (Dopamine HCl Injection : Solopak) and dobutamine (Dobutrex : Lilly) are indicated when the patient is unresponsive to vigorous fluid therapy, and arterial blood pressure, vasomotor tone, and tissue perfusion have not returned to acceptable levels. These drugs support myocardial contractility and blood pressure with minimal vasoconstriction. If these drugs are used, blood pressure monitoring is necessary. Sympathomimetics should not be a substitute for adequate volume restoration.

Dysfunction/Disability. Dysfunction/disability refers to the neurologic status of the patient. This may be assessed through visualization and palpation. A cursory neurologic examination is performed, focusing on the patient's level of consciousness, pupillary light reflex, posture, and response to pain (superficial and/or deep).

The terms *normal, obtuned, stupor,* and *comatose* are used to characterize the level of consciousness but are not specific for a particular type of neural lesion. Pupils are normally equal in size and respond quickly to light. Progressive constriction, dilation, or anisocoria with diminished pupillary light reflex in the absence of ocular trauma indicate neurologic deterioration. Abnormal postures, such as decerebrate rigidity, decerebellate rigidity, and Schiff-Sherrington, should be noted. Decerebrate and decerebellate rigidity are characterized by extensor rigidity in the front limbs and opisthotonos. The rear limbs are in extensor rigidity in the decerebrate posture and flexed or extended decerebellate. The decerebrate patient is unconscious, while the decerebellate patient has varying levels of obtundation. If decerebellate progresses to decerebrate rigidity, it indicates progression of brainstem damage. Schiff-Sherrington posture consists of extensor rigidity of the forelimbs and flaccid hind limbs. This posture indicates a lesion at T2-L4. It is a poor prognostic sign when a patient doses not perceive pain. Superficial pain is tested by pricking or pinching the skin. Deep pain is tested by applying noxious stimuli to the toes or joint. The patient should show some visible response.

Nonambulatory traumatized patients should be treated as spinal trauma patients until proven otherwise.

Examination. During this final phase of the primary survey, a rapid whole-body examination is performed. Major lacerations may be uncovered and areas of bruising noted. Areas of bruising that appear to be worsening could indicate active bleeding. Abdominal girth should also be measured if abnormal bleeding is anticipated.

Secondary Survey. The secondary survey is the timely, systematic, and directed evaluation of each body system for injury. Injuries of a lower priority are addressed following initial stabilization. The A-B-C-D-Es are quickly reviewed to ensure that no new problems have developed. A thorough head-to-tail physical examination and history are completed. Finally, a comprehensive plan of diagnostics and monitoring is developed.

Definitive Management. A review is made of the initial ancillary diagnostics that were performed (e.g., radiographs, ECG, laboratory data), and a management plan is developed. This plan might result in emergency surgery or temporary stabilization of fractures and continued monitoring.

Emergency Procedures

Endotracheal Intubation. Endotracheal intubation ensures a patent airway in an unconscious patient and may be used to provide ventilatory support, to administer inhalational anesthetics, and to administer oxygen (Box 22-1).

Box 22-1 Technique for endotracheal intubation

1. Gather the necessary equipment.
   - Endotracheal tubes (various sizes)
   - Laryngoscope or other light source
   - 0.5% lidocaine
   - Sterile lubricating jelly (water-soluble)
   - Gauze strip, 12-15 inches long
   - 12-ml syringe
2. Check the endotracheal tube cuffs for leaks.
3. Pre-measure the tube against the patient's neck (plan to insert the tube to a level so that the tip and cuff are about midway in the cervical trachea).
4. Apply a small amount of lubricating jelly to the distal end of tube (do not get any in the lumen).
5. Have the assistant place the patient in sternal or lateral recumbency. The assistant should extend the head and neck, open the mouth wide, and pull the tongue rostrally.
6. Using a laryngoscope to visualize the larynx, depress the epiglottis with the laryngoscope or the endotracheal tube (if a laryngoscope is not available); pass the endotracheal tube caudally through the glottis and into the trachea with a gentle rotating action.
7. Check the endotracheal tube for proper placement by visualization, palpation, and gentle chest compression.
8. Tie the gauze tightly to the tube and loosely around the muzzle.
9. Listen for air passage around the tube while applying positive pressure to the rebreathing bag. Inflate the cuff to just stop air escaping around the tube.

Complications: Cats are prone to laryngospasm. It is helpful to apply a few drops of 0.5% lidocaine to the larynx of cats before intubation. The vagus nerve is stimulated during intubation, causing bradycardia and sometimes asystole. The intubation procedure should be smooth and atraumatic. Pre-atropinization minimizes this reflex. Pressure necrosis can result from an overinflated cuff. Endobronchial intubation may lead to collapse of one lung and hypoxemia. The tube may become occluded or kinked.

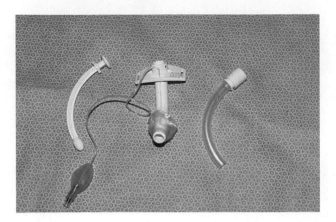

FIG. 22-3 Shiley tracheostomy tube *(center)* with obturator *(left)* and inner cannula *(right)*. The inner cannula fits into the tracheostomy tube.

Tracheostomy Tube Placement. Tracheostomy is indicated with airway obstruction and to facilitate long-term access to the airway and positive-pressure ventilation. Usually an endotracheal tube can be placed first, while preparation is made to place a tracheostomy tube (Figs. 22-4 and 22-5) under aseptic conditions (Box 22-2). The veterinary technician should set up for the procedure, prepare the patient, assist in tube placement, and provide pre- and posttracheostomy wound and tube care.

Thoracentesis. Thoracentesis is useful for collection of pleural fluid to obtain samples for laboratory evaluation or to alleviate respiratory distress (Box 22-3). This procedure might be used in patients with respiratory distress from pneumothorax and decreased or inaudible lung sounds from pleural effusion or hemothorax.

Chest Tube Placement. Chest tubes are placed to relieve progressive pneumothorax and to relieve progressive pleural effusion (Box 22-4).

Equipment. Commercial chest tubes are available in a variety of sizes, with and without trocars. Sizes of 14 to 16 French (Fr) may be used in cats and very small dogs; 18 to 22 Fr, for small dogs; 22 to 28 Fr, for medium-sized to large dogs; and 28 to 36 Fr, for very large dogs. If necessary, red rubber or Foley catheters may be used. It may be beneficial to cut a few more holes in the chest tube.

Oxygen Therapy. Oxygen should be given to patients with hypoxemia (PaO_2 <60 mm Hg) or dyspnea. High inspired oxygen concentrations can be achieved with a properly fitted face mask. Unfortunately, patients often fight the face mask, thereby increasing oxygen consumption and canceling the effects of oxygen therapy.

An alternative to the face mask is a clear plastic bag or hood placed over the head of a patient, with an oxygen hose placed near the animal's nose. The bag remains open along the animal's neck to allow gas to

---

Box 22-2 Tracheostomy tube placement

1. Gather the necessary supplies:
   - Various tracheostomy tubes (including one size smaller and one larger than the estimated size tube)
   - Surgical kit
   - Sterile drapes
   - Bandage material
   - Sandbags (for patient positioning)
2. Sedate patient if necessary; place it in dorsal recumbency and position as straight as possible. Place sandbag or a roll of towels beneath the neck to cause dorsiflexion in the cervical region. This helps to keep the trachea near the skin surface and the site accessible. Clip the hair over the region of the incision site and antiseptically prepare the skin.
3. The clinician will make a midline skin incision from approximately the first to the fourth tracheal ring (Fig. 22-4). Blunt dissection is continued until the trachea is clearly exposed. Three types of tracheal incisions have been used: transverse, tracheal flap, and vertical. It may be helpful to place sutures around the tracheal ring, cranial and caudal to the opening (in the transverse incision). The sutures are left in place for the duration of the tracheostomy. The sutures help to manipulate the tracheal rings during intubation and reintubation if the tube becomes dislodged.
4. Clean the trachea of blood and mucus before intubation.
5. Insert the tracheostomy tube and inflate the cuff.
6. Close the skin incision but not tightly around the tube and tie the tube securely around the patient's neck with umbilical tape or some other material.
7. Drape a sterile 4 × 4-inch piece of gauze around the tube to absorb serum and secretions from the ostomy site.

Complications: Complications include tube obstruction with mucus (Fig. 22-5), tube dislodgement from the trachea, infection of the incision site, and tracheal stenosis as a result of an oversized tracheostomy tube, torqued tube positioning, excessive tracheal tube movement, or cuff overinflation.

---

escape. A flow rate of 5 to 8 L per minute is used. Animals that resist the oxygen mask are more likely to tolerate the hood.

An oxygen cage must have a system for eliminating carbon dioxide, must deliver a known amount of oxy-

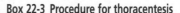

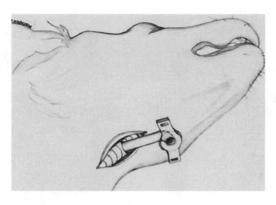

FIG. 22-4 After the skin is incised on the ventral midline of the neck, the ligament between two tracheal rings is incised and the tracheostomy tube is inserted. *(From Pratt PW: Medical, surgical and anesthetic nursing for veterinary technicians, St Louis, 1994, Mosby.)*

Box 22-3 Procedure for thoracentesis

1. Gather the necessary equipment:
   - Butterfly catheter, hypodermic needle, or peripheral venous catheter
   - Three-way stopcock
   - 3-ml syringe (to obtain a fluid sample)
   - 35- or 60-ml syringe (to remove a substantial volume of fluid)
   - IV extension set
   - Surgical prep solution and scrub
2. Clip and prepare the site on the lateral or ventral thorax (dorsally for collection of air, ventrally for fluid).
3. After putting on sterile gloves, assemble the needle or butterfly, stopcock, and syringe (Fig. 22-6). Palpate the cranial edge of the rib. Insert the needle into the pleural space so the needle comes to lie on the pleural surface of the palpated rib. Direct the bevel away from the rib.
4. Aspirate using gentle pressure.

Complications: Complications include iatrogenic lung trauma, pneumothorax, and hemothorax.

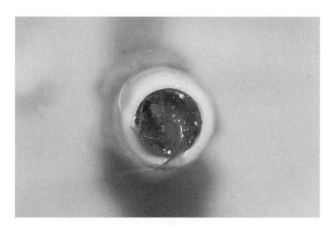

FIG. 22-5 Partial obstruction of tracheostomy tube with dried airway secretions and mucus.

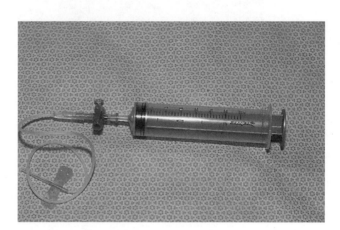

FIG. 22-6 Thoracentesis equipment. A syringe is attached to a stopcock and butterfly catheter. If the butterfly catheter is too small, IV extension tubing attached to a needle or an over-the-needle IV catheter may be used.

gen in a concentration beneficial to the patient (40% to 50%), and must have a mechanism for controlling temperature (70° F) and humidity (50%). The disadvantages of oxygen cages are that they are expensive to purchase and operate, they provide care givers with limited access to the patient, and they may be unable to accommodate large patients.

Nasal insufflation is an excellent way to provide oxygen therapy (Box 22-5). Nasal insufflation does not require an expensive oxygen cage, you can use supplies found in your clinic, you have direct access to the patient at all times, and it is well tolerated by most patients.

Jugular Catheterization. Jugular catheters can be used to administer fluids and medications, to measure central venous pressure, and to facilitate blood sample collection (Box 22-6).

Box 22-4 Chest tube placement

1. Gather the necessary supplies:
   - Chest tube
   - 2% lidocaine
   - Surgical kit
   - Suture material
   - Sterile gloves
   - Sterile drapes
   - Bandaging material
2. Clip the hair over the caudal dorsal quadrant of the chest wall and prepare the area for surgery.
3. Have an assistant grasp the skin along the entire lateral chest wall just caudal to the elbow and pull it cranioventrally.
4. Locate an intercostal space (eighth or ninth) dorsally on the chest wall (near the junction of the most dorsal 1/3 and ventral 2/3 of the chest wall).
5. Inject lidocaine along the path of the skin and intercostal muscle incision.
6. Make a skin incision the length of which is 1½ times the tube diameter.
7. Make an intercostal relief incision but do not penetrate the pleura.
8. Insert the chest tube through the chest wall and into the pleural space (Fig. 22-7). Guide the tube in a cranioventral direction at about a 45-degree angle. If a trocar is used, pull it back from the tip of the chest tube as soon as the pleura is penetrated. When the tube is in the desired location, remove the trocar and clamp the tube.
9. Have the assistant release the skin, creating a tunnel that prevents air from entering the pleural space.
10. Verify the position of the chest tube with the trocar on the outside of the chest.
11. Secure the chest tube to the chest wall and apply a triple antibiotic dressing.

Complications: Complications include infection, laceration of an intercostal artery, lung trauma with pneumothorax, trauma to heart and great vessels with hemorrhage, and subcutaneous emphysema.

Critical Care

Once the patient has made the transition from the crisis or emergency-care phase, critical-care nursing may be required. Critical-care patients require intensive monitoring and nursing care on a moment-to-moment basis. The technician should be able to monitor and reassess the

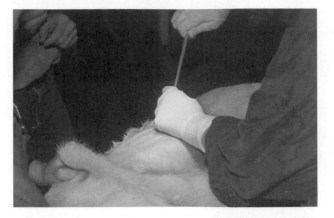

FIG. 22-7 Insertion of a chest tube. Note that the skin is pulled cranially by the assistant to facilitate creation of a subcutaneous tunnel.

patient's condition and respond to the patient's needs in an appropriate manner as the condition changes. In addition, the veterinary technician should be knowledgeable in fluid therapy and critical-care nursing protocols.

Patient Assessment and Monitoring. A great deal of the veterinary technician's responsibility lies with patient monitoring. The heart rate (dog 100 to 140/min, cat 110 to 140/min) is a nonspecific measurement; there are various causes of tachycardia and bradycardia. If arrhythmias are detected, an electrocardiogram (ECG) is indicated. The ECG measures electrical activity in the heart; it does not measure mechanical activity. Indicators of peripheral perfusion include mucous membrane color, capillary refill time (normal 1 to 2 seconds), urine output, and appendage temperature. A full, strong pulse indicates good pulse pressure and stroke volume.

Normal systolic, diastolic, and mean blood pressures are approximately 100 to 160, 60 to 100, and 80 to 120 mm Hg, respectively. Noninvasive methods of measuring blood pressure include ultrasonic Doppler and oscillometric devices.

The ultrasonic Doppler device detects flow of blood through an artery and converts this to an audible signal. When an occlusive cuff is applied to a limb and inflated, flow is occluded. The cuff pressure is slowly decreased while looking at a sphygmomanometer. With the first sound of blood flow, the pressure reading from the sphygmomanometer is noted; this approximates systolic pressure. The Vet/BP 6000 (Sensor Devices) and Dinamap (Criticon) blood pressure units use the oscillometric technique. A cuff is applied to a limb and automatically inflated; the cuff detects oscillations in the underlying artery. As the cuff is gradually deflated, oscillations are detected. The first detected pulsation is the *systolic pressure.* The point at which the maximum pulsation is detected is the *mean blood pressure.* The point where oscillations disappear is the *diastolic pressure.*

Box 22-5 Nasal oxygen insufflation

1. Gather the necessary supplies:
   - Red rubber urinary catheter or infant feeding tube (5 Fr for cats or small dogs, 8 Fr for medium-sized to large dogs)
   - 2% lidocaine
   - Lubricating jelly (water-soluble)
   - Suture material
   - ½-inch tape
   - Cold bubble humidifier
   - Extension tubing
   - O_2 source
2. Place a few drops of 2% lidocaine in a nostril, wait 30 to 60 seconds, and repeat.
3. Select a catheter of appropriate size. Measure the distance from the tip of the nose to the medial canthus of the eye. Mark the catheter at the tip of the nostril.
4. Lubricate the catheter with sterile water-soluble lubricating jelly. Insert and direct the catheter ventromedially and caudally into the nostril until you reach the catheter mark.
5. Bend the uninserted portion out around the alar notch and suture the catheter to the skin at that point. Position the catheter back over the head and suture it to the top of the head.
6. Fill a bubble-through humidifier with sterile water and attach it to an oxygen source. Attach this to the nasal catheter. Flow rates of 50 to 200 ml/kg/minute seem to be effective in increasing inspired oxygen concentration to 40% or greater. The goal is to improve mucous membrane color, decrease anxiety, decrease breathing and/or heart rate, decrease the magnitude of respiratory distress, and improve PaO_2 to an acceptable level.

Complications: Complications of oxygen administration may include gastric distention, epistaxis, serous or mucoid nasal discharge, decreased mucus clearance without humidification, and patient discomfort.

Box 22-6 Jugular catheter placement

1. Gather the necessary supplies:
   - Through-the-needle catheter and T-port
   - Heparinized saline and 6-ml syringe
   - Sterile gloves, drapes, suture material, and surgical set
   - Antimicrobial ointment and bandaging material
2. Place the patient in lateral recumbency with a sandbag or roll of towels under the shoulder and neck area. Extend the patient's neck and head and have an assistant pull its forelimbs caudally. The patient must be positioned properly and the vein immobilized. If the vein is not immobilized properly, it may roll laterally or wrinkle longitudinally.
3. Clip a wide area of hair over the catheterization site. The area should be wide enough to prevent contamination during the catheterization procedure. Prepare the catheterization site as you would a surgical site. Wear sterile gloves to prevent contamination of the catheter and catheter site. Use sterile drapes to widen the sterile field.
4. Have the assistant hold off the vein by pressing into the thoracic inlet with one or two fingers; this causes the vein to engorge and bulge.
5. Introduce the needle subcutaneously. Position the needle tip over the vein and align it as closely as possible to the longitudinal axis of the vein. Insert the needle tip into the vein; this may require that you angle the needle slightly to penetrate the vein wall. Once the needle tip is in the vein, thread the catheter through the needle into the vein. Once the catheter is threaded, apply pressure over the catheter site and back the needle out. Once the bleeding has stopped, secure a needle guard around the needle. Aspirate the catheter to confirm proper placement and to clear the catheter of air; then flush with heparinized saline. If blood cannot be aspirated, withdraw the catheter slowly until blood can be aspirated.
6. Cap the catheter with an injection cap or T-port and again flush with heparinized saline. Suture or staple the catheter close to the insertion site. Cover the insertion site with antimicrobial ointment and a sterile 2 × 2 gauze pad. Secure the catheter with an occlusive bandage.

Complications: Complications of jugular catheters include sepsis (cellulitis, septicemia), phlebitis, thrombosis (vein, catheter lumen), bleeding, and catheter dislodgement.

Respiratory System. Several questions are asked when monitoring the respiratory system. Are the rate (8 to 30/min) and tidal volume (10 to 20 ml/kg) adequate? Is the breathing effort smooth and easy, or labored? Is the breathing pattern regular? Can you auscultate normal breath sounds? Abnormal breath sounds may be described as crackles, wheezes, squeaks, muffled, or quiet. Can the patient meet its ventilation and oxygenation requirements?

Central Nervous System. What is the patient's mental status: conscious, unconscious, or somewhere in between? Patients that are conscious on presentation should be monitored to ensure that their level of consciousness does not change for the worse. Pupils should be equal in size and reactive to light. Pupils are considered abnormal if they show any combination of unresponsiveness, dilation, constriction, or asymmetry in the absence of ocular trauma. Irregular breathing patterns indicate brainstem disease. The patient should be observed for abnormal postures, such as opisthotonos.

Fluid Balance. Urine output is an excellent reflection of tissue perfusion. If the kidneys are producing urine, then the other organs are probably being perfused adequately. Normal urine output is 1 to 2 ml/kg/hour.

In addition to quantitation of urine, it is also helpful to quantitate defecation and emesis. This can provide a more accurate assessment of total fluid balance. Weight gains and losses should be monitored daily. Acute changes in weight are usually a result of fluid balance, as opposed to muscle mass.

Fluid losses should be compared with fluid intake; they should approximately balance. Any large discrepancy may be significant.

Temperature. Core temperature may be monitored by placing a deep rectal or esophageal thermometer. Early recognition of hypothermia or hyperthermia is important. Causes of *hypothermia* (<38.3° C) include prolonged exposure to a cold environment and central thermoregulation impairment. Causes of *hyperthermia* include a hot environment with poor ventilation, infection or inflammation, and thermoregulatory dysfunction.

Critical-Care Nursing Procedures. A basic physical examination should be performed by the technician on each patient as soon as possible at the start of the day or shift. This provides a baseline for comparison of the patient's status throughout the day. In addition to taking temperature, pulse, and respiration measurements, auscultate the lungs, palpate the bladder, and note mentation. Also check operation of all IV and urinary catheters and other monitoring apparatus, and cleanliness of the patient and bedding.

Check emergency supplies and equipment to be sure that all the emergency drugs are present, their shelf life has not expired, and the equipment is functional. Pay special attention to endotracheal tubes and cuffs and oxygen supply.

IV catheter care. IV catheters should be inspected every 48 hours or as needed. The catheter dressing should be removed and the site inspected. Signs of phlebitis (inflammation of a vein) may include erythema, a thickened sensitive vein, and an apparent increase in skin temperature over the vein. Signs of thrombosis include a vein that appears engorged without occlusion and feels like a thick cord. When signs of phlebitis or thrombosis are apparent, the catheter should be removed and a new one placed at a different site. If the catheter site looks normal, the site should be cleaned and rebandaged routinely.

Urinary catheter care. Urinary catheters should be inspected and cleaned every 8 hours. This entails cleaning the prepuce or vulva and surrounding area with povidone-iodine scrub and a water rinse. Then flush the sheath or vestibule with a solution of 2 parts povidone-iodine solution and 5 parts water. Apply povidone-iodine ointment to the sheath or vulvar opening with cotton swabs. The urinary catheter itself should be kept clean, especially in the female patient, where the vulva is in close proximity to the rectum. Use of the closed urinary collection system helps to minimize the risk of urinary tract infection.

Chest drain/gastrostomy tube care. The procedure for chest drain and gastrostomy tube care is much like IV catheter care. Remove the bandage and inspect the insertion site every 24 hours. Clean the site and rebandage.

Tracheostomy tube care. Patients with indwelling tracheostomy tubes require observation 24 hours a day. It is important to provide airway humidity, clear airway secretions, and prevent infection. Because the artificial airway bypasses the patient's natural system to warm and humidify inspired air, it is important to provide humidity. Humidification may be accomplished by nebulization or by instilling saline down the tracheostomy tube.

Coupage may be used in conjunction with nebulization to promote removal of respiratory secretions. The patient is allowed to stand, sit sternal, or lie in lateral recumbency. Place your hands cupped and facing downward, with the fingers and thumbs together, on the patient's chest wall, clapping the chest wall over the involved lung. Coupage is delivered by flexion and extension of the wrist while keeping the shoulders and elbows relaxed. Coupage should be administered for 3 to 5 minutes in a steady, consistent fashion.

Suction should be applied to the tracheostomy tube or tracheal tube at regular intervals. Suctioning clears secretions from the trachea down to the primary bronchi. The airway should be nebulized before suctioning to liquefy secretions. Administer oxygen before suctioning to prevent hypoxemia. Pass the suction catheter down the trachea (without suction) until resistance is met, then withdraw the catheter a few millimeters and apply suction. As the catheter is withdrawn, apply a rotating or winding motion. Suction should be applied no longer than 10 to 15 seconds to minimize hypoxemia and small airway collapse. Then administer 100% oxygen for a short time. If the secretions are minimal or thick, inject saline into the trachea at 0.2 ml/kg, again hyperinflate the lungs several times with oxygen, and repeat the suctioning. If the secretions are readily withdrawn, there is no need to inject saline. Repeat the suction procedure several times, especially if it is very productive. It is important to oxygenate and hyperinflate the patient immediately before and immediately after each suctioning attempt. The suctioning procedure should be stopped immediately if the patient displays excessive discomfort, restlessness, or changes in cardiac or respiratory rhythm.

Inspect the site around the tracheostomy tube every 8 hours for signs of infection. Clean the site with hydrogen peroxide and cover with a gauze square.

Blood Transfusion. Transfusions with whole blood or its components is indicated in acute blood loss, chronic anemia, thrombocytopenia, hypoproteinemia, and coagulopathies. Chapter 24 contains detailed information on blood transfusion.

Fluid Therapy. The basic components of a fluid therapy plan include determination, calculation, and replacement of the volume deficit (percent dehydration), compensating for abnormal ongoing losses, and providing maintenance fluid needs. Types of fluids used and the rates are determined by the veterinarian. In addition to the previously mentioned components, potassium and sodium bicarbonate supplementation must be taken into consideration. Chapter 24 presents detailed information on fluid therapy.

Care of Recumbent Patients. Recumbent patients should be turned every 2 to 4 hours. Turning the patient prevents formation of decubital ulcers and atelectasis of the lungs. Decubital ulcers develop over bony prominences as a result of continuous pressure and ischemic damage to the skin. Atelectasis is small airway and alveolar collapse and lung consolidation.

Bedding is an important factor in prevention of decubital ulcers. Air mattresses, fleece pads, a waterbed mattress, or a deep bed of clean straw work well. Disposable diapers are excellent for absorbing urine and keeping the patient dry, and they also allow quantitation of urine production (weigh the diapers before and after urination). If an animal becomes urine soaked, it should be bathed immediately to prevent urine scalding. Once the skin has been dried, apply a protective ointment or absorbent powder to help protect the skin.

If exercise is not contraindicated, passive exercise and massage should be instituted. Passive exercise involves moving the limbs back and forth and flexing the joints. Passive exercise may help to improve muscle tone. If peripheral edema is present, massage may help reduce edema.

Nosocomial Infection. *Nosocomial infections* are hospital-acquired infections. Factors that predispose to nosocomial infections include age (geriatric or neonatal), immunosuppression, diagnostic and therapeutic invasive procedures, antimicrobial therapy, and long-term hospitalization. Organisms commonly involved in nosocomial infection include *Escherichia coli, Klebsiella, Salmonella,* canine parvovirus, and feline panleukopenia virus.

Ways to help reduce the chance of hospital-acquired infection include diligent hand washing by staff before handling medications, fluids, IV lines, and patients; swabbing injection ports with alcohol before administering IV medication; use of diposable thermometer sheaths; disinfection of patient-care equipment (clipper blades, ECG leads and clips, endotracheal tubes, and breathing circuits); disinfection of environmental surfaces; use of aseptic technique in catheter/tube placements (IV, urinary, chest); and treating patients with known infection last when doing treatment rounds.

Patient's Mental Well-Being. Before treating a patient (poking, sticking, and prodding), take the time to make friends with patient. This may set the tone for further encounters. You may find it helpful to talk to and pet them when treatments are not due so that they do not assume that every time you open the cage or stall door it means more poking and prodding.

Taking a patient for a walk can do a lot to lift its spirits. Because many dogs do not like to urinate in a cage, this gives them the opportunity to urinate outdoors. With cats, try to position their cage near a window so that they can get a little sun and look outside.

It is important for patients to have time to rest. In a 24-hour intensive-care unit, a patient may have treatments every hour. If possible, treatments should be grouped so that the patient has some time to rest.

If a patient refuses to eat, it may be helpful to find out from the owner what the patient likes to eat normally. Also find out what time it eats when at home. When a patient enters the hospital, its normal routine is disrupted. Try to adhere to its normal routine as much as possible so that it may feel a little better.

RECOMMENDED READING

Kirby R et al: Critical care, *Vet Clin North Am Small Anim Pract* 19(6), 1989.

Kirby R et al: Emergency medicine, *Vet Clin North Am Small Anim Pract* 24(6), 1994.

Murtaugh RJ et al: *Veterinary emergency and critical care medicine,* St Louis, 1992, Mosby.

Plunkett SJ: *Emergency procedures for the small animal veterinarian,* Philadelphia, 1993, WB Saunders.

Smith B: *Large animal internal medicine,* ed 2, St Louis, 1996, Mosby.

Thelan LA et al: *Critical care nursing: diagnosis and management,* ed 2, St Louis, 1994, Mosby.

CHAPTER 23

Management of Wounds, Fractures, and Other Injuries

S.M. Fassig

Learning Objectives

After reviewing this chapter, the reader should understand the following:

Phases of wound healing
Categories of wounds

Principles of first-aid treatment of wounds
Principles of wound closure
Types and application of bandages
Types and application of splints and casts
Ways in which specific types of wounds are managed

A *wound* is a disruption of cellular and anatomic functional continuity. *Wound healing* is the restoration of this continuity. *Acute wounds* are those induced by surgery or trauma that heal normally, with healing time determined by the depth and size of the lesion. Examples of acute wounds include surgical incisions, blunt trauma, bite wounds, burns, gunshots, and avulsion injuries. *Chronic wounds* have various causes and, as determined by their underlying pathology, may take months or years to heal completely. Decubital ulcers (pressure sores), diabetic ulcers, and vascular ulcers are examples of chronic wounds.

WOUND HEALING
Phases of Wound Healing

Most healing of soft tissue occurs as a result of epithelial regeneration and fibroplasia, both of which occur simultaneously. The epidermis serves as a barrier from the environment and is necessary for optimal appear-

ance, function, and protection. A bed of granulation tissue is required for migration of epithelium across the defect. The three phases of soft tissue wound healing are the exudative-inflammatory-debridement phase, the proliferative-collagen phase, and the maturation phase. The phases of wound healing are overlapping events; a wound may have more than one phase occurring at the same time. The phases of wound healing are summarized in Table 23-1. Details on tissue response to injury are presented in Chapter 8.

Types of Wound Healing

Relatively clean, minor wounds, such as small lacerations, heal by *primary* or *first-intention healing*. The tissues can be pulled together with sutures and healing progresses without complication. Wounds that are larger, more complicated, or infected may need to heal by *second intention*. In this case, the wound is left open and allowed to heal from the inner areas to the outer surface. Although sometimes necessary, second-intention healing is a less desirable method of healing.

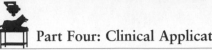

TABLE 23-1 Events in the three phases of wound healing

Exudative-inflammatory-debridement phase	Proliferation-collagen phase	Remodeling-maturation phase
Inflammation starts immediately and predominates for up to 6 hours	Starts at 12 to 36 hours after injury	Starts after about 2 weeks
	Fibroblasts and endothelial cells proliferate	Lasts 2 to 3 weeks in rapidly healing tissues (viscera)
This phase can last for several weeks	Neutrophils decrease while macrophages increase	Can last for years in slowly healing tissues (bone, tendon, ligament)
Acute vasoconstriction followed by vasodilation	Collagen synthesis starts after 4 to 6 days	Slow increase in tensile strength
Plasma proteins leak from vessels into interstitial space	Components of granulation tissue become engaged in healing; endothelial buds grow into damaged or intact blood vessels; mesenchymal cells follow the budding endothelium, secreting ground substance	Equilibrium of collagen synthesis and breakdown
Leukocytes (neutrophils, monocytes, macrophages) exit blood vessels		Collagen cross-linking slowly increases tissue strength
Fibroblasts differentiate		
Endothelial cells begin to proliferate		

Some very large or grossly contaminated wounds are allowed to heal initially by second intention and then are closed with sutures. After a healthy granulation bed is formed and infection is no longer present, the granulation bed is closed with sutures. This is described as *third-intention healing.* Very large wounds treated with third-intention methods may heal more rapidly than if allowed to heal by second intention.

First-intention healing of fractures is primary bone healing, with rigid internal fixation (e.g., pins, plates). Second-intention ("normal") healing of fractures is by callus formation, using no internal fixation.

Wound healing is impaired by numerous factors, including infection, debris and necrotic tissue, old age, malnutrition, poor perfusion, drugs (e.g., corticosteroids), and hypothermia.

WOUND CONTAMINATION AND INFECTION

Wound *contamination* is not the same as wound *infection.* All wounds, even those created during surgery using strict aseptic technique, are *contaminated* by microorganisms in the environment. Initially these organisms are loosely attached to tissues and do not invade adjacent tissue; there is no host immune response to these organisms. With time, the microorganisms multiply. *Infection* is the process by which organisms bind to tissue, multiply, and then invade viable tissue, eliciting an immune response. Tissue infection depends on the number and pathogenicity (or virulence) of the microorganisms. In general, a wound is infected when the number of microorganisms reaches 100,000 per gram of tissue or milliliter of fluid. At these numbers, the microoganisms have exceeded the host's defense mechanisms to control them. If the animal is presented for treatment more than 12 hours after injury, any wounds should be considered *infected.* Infection is characterized by erythema, edema, pus, fever, elevated neutrophil count, pain, change in color of exudate, or uncharacteristic odor.

Contaminated wounds may become infected when foreign bodies are present (e.g., organic material, bone fragments, suture material, glove powder, bone plates and screws), excessive necrotic tissue is left in the wound, excessive bleeding results in higher levels of ferric ion (necessary for bacterial replication), local tissue defenses are impeded (e.g., excessive hemoglobin in burn patients or patients receiving immunosuppressive drugs), the vascular supply is altered, and dirt and debris are present. Appropriate treatment soon after injury is important to avoid infection.

Wound Categories

Open traumatic wounds can be categorized according to the degree of contamination present (Table 23-2). Management of these wounds varies according to the severity of the injury and the patient's condition. In general, wounds that are grossly contaminated and/or dirty may not be good candidates for primary closure. Until contamination and infection can be eliminated, open wound management is necessary. Dead and dying tissues must be excised (debrided) to minimize the potential for bacterial infection and create a viable wound bed.

Use of Antibacterials

The decision to use antibacterials systemically or topically in a surgical wound depends on several preoperative factors, including the patient's condition and immune status, the nature of the surgery (emergency versus elective), the location of the wound (orthopedic versus abdominal), the predicted duration of the surgical procedure, the surgeon's experience, and the environment in which the procedure is performed.

It is generally thought that antibacterials are not needed for patients in good health, with an adequate immune status, undergoing a relatively short (less than 90 minutes) elective orthopedic or soft tissue surgical procedure (not abdominal), performed by an experienced surgeon, in a clean surgical facility using aseptic technique.

In clean surgical wounds, preoperative antibacterials should be considered in cases of shock, severe systemic trauma, long procedures, traumatic procedures, poor blood supply, foreign bodies, dead space (seromas, hematomas), malnutrition, obesity, or other factors altering host defense mechanisms. When systemic (injected) antibacterials are used, they are most effective if administered just before surgery or shortly after surgery is begun.

Traumatic wounds, as opposed to "clean" surgical wounds, may contain devitalized tissue and/or foreign material and are contaminated by microorganisms. Traumatized tissue provides a suitable environment for bacterial multiplication and provides a route of entry for penetration of pathogens into adjacent viable tissue. Chronic (long-standing) wounds offer an ideal environment for bacterial proliferation, with copious wound fluid, necrotic tissue, and deep cracks and crevices on the wound surface. In such cases, antibacterials with a broad spectrum of antimicrobial activity are given systemically.

It is likely that we often do more harm than good by applying topical medications to wounds. The adverse effect of these products on wound healing is independent

---

TABLE 23-2 Categories of wounds

Type of Wound	Description
Clean	Surgical wounds Elective incisions Highly vascular tissues not predisposed to infection
Clean-Contaminated	Minor contamination evident Surgical wounds with minor break in aseptic technique Elective surgery in tissues with normal resident bacterial flora (e.g., gastrointestinal tract, respiratory tract, or genitourinary tract) No spillage of organ contents
Contaminated	Moderate contamination evident Fresh traumatic injuries, open fractures, penetrating wounds Surgery with gross spillage of organ contents Presence of bile or infected urine Surgical wounds with major break in aseptic technique
Dirty	Grossly contaminated or infected Contaminated traumatic wounds more than 4 hours old Perforated viscera, abscess, necrotic tissue, foreign material

of their antimicrobial action. Generally, water-soluble antibacterial products tend to impede wound healing more than do ointments or creams. Solutions tend to evaporate, contributing to drying of the wound surface. Ointments and creams remain in contact with the wound longer than solutions, preventing drying of the wound surface. A clean wound in a healthy patient can heal optimally without application of ointments, salves, etc. Certain topical products may be beneficial at times; however, a focus on aseptic technique and appropriate "clean" management of wounds is more appropriate.

WOUND MANAGEMENT
First Aid

In the field and/or before transport to a treatment facility, the would should be protected with some sort of bandage. An occlusive bandage is preferred. This type of bandage controls hemorrhage, prevents additional contamination, and provides immobilization of an extremity. Open fractures should be splinted. In open or compound fractures, exposed bone should not be forced into position below the skin. This avoids additional soft tissue trauma and reduces chances of deep tissue contamination. At the treatment facility, the wound is evaluated for antimicrobial therapy. The wound should be protected during preparation of the surrounding area (e.g., clipping and scrubbing).

Wound Assessment

Wound assessment includes evaluation of the wound's location, size, and depth; exudate (drainage); tissue in the wound bed; and any signs of infection. Wound management revolves around three considerations: cleansing, closing, and covering. Control of hemorrhage is usually the first step in wound management. After initial hemostasis, it is important to evaluate the wound for bacterial contamination and the potential for bacterial growth. To avoid introduction of microorganisms, the wound should be cleaned under aseptic or at least sanitary conditions.

Clipping

In initial wound treatment, the wound must be protected while areas around the wound are clipped and cleaned. It is often helpful to cover the wound with a water-soluble sterile ointment (e.g., K-Y Lubricating Jelly, Johnson & Johnson, New Brunswick, NJ) or moistened sterile gauze sponges before the area around the wound is clipped and cleaned. This helps to prevent loose hair from further contaminating the wound. The wound can also be temporarily closed with towel clamps or a continuous suture. This may require analgesia. Before clipping and shaving areas around head or face wounds, an ophthalmic ointment should be instilled in the conjunctival sac to protect the cornea and conjunctiva.

If the animal is covered with dirt and debris (and is not in critical condition), it should be bathed before clipping. This reduces further contamination. (Clipper blades also stay sharper longer when cutting clean hair.) Clipping removes sources of contamination (e.g., hair, dirt, and debris) and allows better visualization of the wound. An electric clipper with a No. 40 blade attached to a vacuum suction system is preferred. Two pairs of clipper blades are advantageous; the second set of blades is disinfected for use in areas of elective surgical sites. Hair at wound edges may be trimmed with scissors or a handheld No. 10 scalpel blade dipped in mineral oil, K-Y Jelly, or water so that the hair sticks to the blade and does not enter the wound.

Scrubbing

After the area around the wound has been clipped, replace the gauze sponges or gel over the wound. Gently scrub the surrounding intact skin, not the wound itself. The most commonly used surgical scrubs for skin preparation contain an antimicrobial agent plus a detergent/surfactant, such as chlorhexidine (Nolvasan, Fort Dodge) or povidone-iodine (Betadine, Purdue Frederick). Rinsing with saline or 70% isopropyl alcohol does not seem to influence the antimicrobial effect.

Wound Lavage

Cleansing and debridement of the wound begins after the surrounding area has been cleaned. Obvious foreign bodies and gross contamination must be removed. Usually, a noncaustic solution is used to clean the wound without creating further irritation. Lavaging with a sterile solution and gentle scrubbing are the primary methods used for cleaning the wound. Care should be taken not to use forceful lavage and not to scrub too vigorously, because this may force bacteria into the wound and spread contamination. Often more than one session of lavage and additional debridement may be necessary to remove debris and necrotic tissue. Bandaging with wet wound dressing can facilitate this process. As a general rule, wound lavage should be discontinued before the tissues take on a "water-logged" appearance.

Lavage solutions are most effective when delivered with a fluid jet impacting the wound with a pressure of at least 7 pounds per square inch (psi). This can be achieved by forcefully expelling solution from a 35- to 60-ml syringe through an 18-gauge needle. Lavage solutions can also be delivered using a spray bottle or "Water Pik." The Water Pik should be used with care, as it can deliver fluids at up to 70 psi. Adequate fluid pressure cannot be achieved with gravity flow, bulb syringe, or turkey baster.

Isotonic ("normal") saline, lactated Ringer's solution, or *plain Ringer's solution* may be used for lavage. These physiologic (isotonic, isosmotic, and sterile) solutions do not damage tissue but have no antibacterial properties.

Povidone-iodine solution is commonly used to lavage wounds because of its broad antimicrobial spectrum. Dilutions of povidone-iodine in the range of 1% to 2% are more potent and more rapidly bactericidal than commercial 10% povidone-iodine solution because dilution makes more "free iodine" available. A 1% solution can be prepared by diluting 1 part of commercial 10% povidone-iodine with 9 parts of sterile water or electrolyte solution. The bactericidal effect of povidone-iodine lasts only 4 to 6 hours. It is inactivated by blood, exudate, and organic soil, reducing the period of residual action. The detergent form of povidone-iodine (scrub) is deleterious to wound tissues, causing irritation and potentiation of wound infection.

Chlorhexidine diacetate solution has a broad antimicrobial spectrum and is commonly used on small animals. In dogs, it is more effective against *Staphylococcus aureus* than is povidone-iodine. When chlorhexidine is applied to intact skin, the antimicrobial effect is immediate, with a lasting residual effect. Prolonged tissue contact with solutions of 0.5% or more concentrated solutions may be harmful. Currently, 0.05% chlorhexidine solutions are recommended for use in wound lavage. A 0.05% solution can be prepared by diluting 1 part of a 2% stock solution with 40 parts of water. Chlorhexidine has sustained residual activity. Systemic absorption, toxicosis, and inactivation by organic material do not seem to be problematic.

Hydrogen peroxide is commonly used as a foaming wound irrigant. It has little antimicrobial effect, except on some anaerobes. It is more effective as a sporicide. In concentrations of 3% and more, hydrogen peroxide is damaging to tissues. It also causes thrombosis in the microvasculature adjacent to the wound margins, impairing proliferation of blood vessels. Hydrogen peroxide should be reserved for one-time initial irrigation of dirty wounds. It should not be delivered to wounds under pressure, because its foaming action forces debris between tissue planes, enlarging the wound and allowing accumulation of air in tissues.

Anesthesia and Analgesia

After preparation of the surrounding area, the wound is prepared for analgesia and debridement. Local, regional, or general anesthesia may be used for wound management. General anesthesia is preferred if the patient can tolerate it. Tranquilizers or sedatives (e.g., xylaxine, acepromazine, diazepam) are often used in conjunction with local and regional anesthesia.

Local anesthetics, such as lidocaine and bupivacaine, are used for pain control if the animal is not a candidate for general anesthesia. It may be beneficial to lavage a wound initially with 2% lidocaine for 1 or 2 minutes before irrigating to make removal of foreign bodies less painful. Local anesthetics do not usually offer analgesia sufficient for surgical debridement.

Epinephrine is included in some local anesthetic products. It causes vasoconstriction and helps reduce hemorrhage and prolong the anesthetic effect. Epinephrine may cause tissue necrosis along the wound edge, adversely affect tissue defenses, and potentiate infection. In general, local anesthetics containing epinephrine should not be used in wound care.

Debridement

Debridement is the removal of devitalized or necrotic tissue. Necrotic tissue must be removed, as epithelium will not migrate over nonviable tissue, a wound will not contract without debridement, and necrotic tissue may act as a growth medium for bacteria. Debridement also removes sources of contamination, infection, and mechanical obstructions to healing.

Debridement is complete when the wound bed consists of only healthy tissue, commonly referred to as a "clean wound." However, this does not mean the wound is free of bacteria. Acute traumatic wounds are usually debrided to facilitate surgical closure, whereas chronic wounds are usually debrided to reduce the risk of infection and facilitate second-intention healing.

Wounds are usually debrided by mechanical means, such as with surgical instruments, irrigation, or dry-to-dry or wet-to-dry dressings. Nonmechanical debridement techniques include application of enzymatic agents or chemicals. In many cases, a combination of techniques is used.

Debridement should be performed as an aseptic procedure. To protect the wound from further contamination, sterile surgical gloves and mask should be worn and the area draped. Ideally, several sets of sterile instruments should be used to prevent reintroducing contaminated instruments into the wound.

After a wound is cleansed and free of devitalized tissue, the surgeon explores the wound using sterile techniques. Other diagnostic procedures, such as radiographic studies using contrast materials, collection and assessment of fluid samples, and cytologic examination, may be performed to assist in the overall evaluation. Once this process is completed, a decision is made regarding how the wound will be managed, including if drainage is required. If primary closure is elected, decisions concerning anesthesia, antibacterials, nonsteroidal antiinflammatory drugs, tetanus status (if the injured animal is a horse), and bandaging (if required) are made. The wound is then prepared for suturing.

Drainage

Drains implanted in a wound provide an escape path for unwanted air and/or wound fluids, thus preventing or reducing seroma or hematoma formation in tissue pockets or dead space.

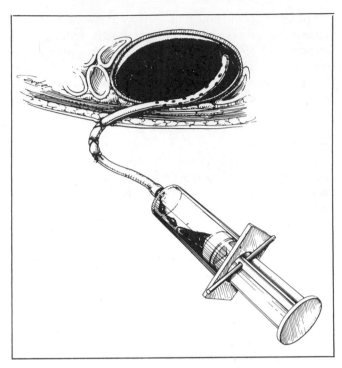

FIG. 23-1 Fluids can be drained by periodic aspiration with a syringe attached to the drain.

Accumulation of exudate in a wound favors infection. Excessive fluid prevents phagocytic cells from reaching bacteria within a wound and provides a medium for bacterial growth. Drains are needed when wounds produce fluids and exudates for several days after initial treatment. They are indicated as follows:

- For treatment of an abscess cavity
- When foreign material and nonviable tissue are present and cannot be excised
- When contamination is inevitable (e.g., wounds near anal area)
- To obliterate dead space
- As a prophylaxis against anticipated fluid or air collection after a surgical procedure

Penrose drains are made of soft latex rubber. Their sizes range from ¼ to 1 inch in diameter and 12 to 18 inches long. They provide a simple conduit for gravity flow. If the drain is covered by a bandage, there may be some capillary action. Fluid flows through the drain's lumen and around the tube and is related to the surface area of the tubing. The fenestrations (holes) in the drain decrease the surface area and reduce its effectiveness. Cutting the Penrose drain in half lengthwise increases the surface area by 100%. Penrose drains should not be left in place for more than 3 to 5 days, because most gravitational drainage has subsided by that time.

Closed-suction drains provide drainage with a vacuum applied to the drain lumen with no air vent. Closed-suction drains allow wounds and dressings to

---

Box 23-1 Guidelines for and complications of drain use

Guidelines for drain use

Provide adequate drainage, using the fewest possible drains with the least number of drain holes.

Clip a generous area of skin around the drain to prevent contamination of the drain end by hair.

Do not tunnel the drain too far subcutaneously before entering the wound pocket, because this may collapse the drain and prevent proper drainage.

To minimize the chance of misplaced drains, record the number and size of drains used in the patient, and count them again when the drains are removed.

Make the stab incision for the drain exit large enough to allow adequate drainage.

Make the drain exit through a separate stab incision; drains that exit the primary wound/incision may cause dehiscence.

Place the drain dorsoventrally to allow drainage through the dependent opening.

Bandage the drain, if possible, to increase drainage by capillary action and prevent ascending infection, self-mutilation, and premature drain removal.

Use radiopaque drains (evident on radiographs).

Suture the drain to the skin at the point of exit.

Complications of drain use

Infection from bacteria ascending the drain

Drain obstruction

Retention of the drain if the exposed portion of the drain retracts under the skin, requiring surgical removal

Foreign-body reaction

Damage to surrounding tissues

Pain

Premature loss and/or removal by the patient

Delayed healing, with increased possibility of wound dehiscence or formation of a fistulous tract

---

stay dry, prevent bacterial movement through and around the drain, afford continuous drainage, and eliminate the need for irrigation.

These drains help hold the skin grafts in contact with the granulating wound bed to enhance revascularization. Excessively high negative pressure in the drain system can injure tissue. The vacuum for these drain systems can be generated by glass vacuum bottles, a compressible plastic canister (Hemovac), a compressible plastic canister with two one-way valves (Drevac), or a simple syringe (usually a modified 60-ml syringe) (Fig. 23-1).

Gauze or umbilical tape "setons" may be passed into a wound opening to keep the wound from closing before all exudates have drained. They are unsatisfactory for drainage purposes because they do not promote drainage once the gauze is saturated. They act as wicks, retaining bacterial contaminants, and can be mechanically irritating.

Box 23-1 presents guidelines for and complications of drain use.

WOUND CLOSURE

The patient's ability to tolerate anesthesia influences initial wound management. It is usually best to close fresh wounds as quickly as possible, when the risk of infection and complications is very low. Wounds with minor contamination may be cleaned, debrided, and closed. Sometimes a drain is installed to facilitate removal of tissue fluids associated with significant soft tissue trauma. Wounds that require optimal wound drainage because of gross contamination, tissue necrosis, and/or infection are managed as open wounds until they can be closed at a later time. Table 23-3 summarizes the types of closure used with different types of wounds.

A wound should be closed only when the veterinarian is certain that all devitalized and contaminated tissue has been removed and there is adequate skin to appose the wound edges. Covering the wound and allowing it to heal by second intention or delayed closure should perhaps be considered more often by veterinarians. Unfortunately, wounds are often closed prematurely, resulting in dehiscence (opening) and infection a few days later. If there is any doubt about the advisability of a surgical closure, the clinician should cover the wound with a proper dressing and manage the wound with frequent dressing changes (at least daily), lavage, debridement, and reassessment as required.

Closure with Sutures

When wound closures requires suturing, certain fundamental considerations apply:

- Potential tissue reaction to the suture material must be acceptable.
- The suture material need not be stronger than the tissue in which it is placed.
- The sutures must retain their strength until healing keeps the wound edges together.
- Suture patterns should not impair blood supply to the wound.
- Knots must be tied securely with sufficient but not excessive "throws."

In selecting suture material, considerations include suture construction (monofilament, braided), suture material (absorbable, nonabsorbable), suture size (diameter), suture pattern, knot type, and needle type. Chapter 21 presents detailed information on suture materials.

Nonclosure

In second-intention healing (nonclosure), the wound is not sutured but heals by contraction and epithelialization. Second-intention healing is selected for wounds involving significant tissue loss. In horses, it is especially useful for wounds of the neck, body, and proximal limbs. Although these wounds are prepared with the same care as for primary closure and delayed primary closure, wounds of the extremities in horses are often left uncovered or managed with a pressure bandage or a cast. If left open to heal by second intention, the wound should be cleaned daily at first to remove accumulated exudate. Skin distal to the wound is also cleaned and protected with petroleum jelly or a similar product to prevent skin maceration ("serum burns").

Second-Intention Healing in Horses. Wounds of the distal limbs of horses (carpus and distally) with large tissue deficits present a special problem, mainly the formation of excessive granulation tissue (Fig. 23-2). With newly formed moist granulation tissue protruding slightly above the skin edges, application of a corticosteroid-antibacterial combination ointment with an overlying pressure bandage can control granulation tissue growth. The topical corticosteroids seem to have little effect on wound healing and epithelialization at this early stage. If the granulation tissue is mature and protrudes well above the skin surface to form a fibrogranuloma, sharp excision is preferred. If excessive granulation tissue must be excised with a scalpel, a pressure bandage is applied immediately after excision to control the considerable hemorrhage. Several hours after surgery, this bandage must be changed.

Topical application of caustics (e.g., silver nitrate or triple dye) and astringents can remove and prevent formation of granulation tissue by chemically destroying it. This destructive chemical action is indiscriminate, however, and also harms migrating epithelial cells. Often

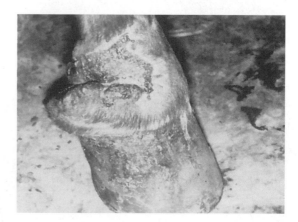

FIG. 23-2 Large granulating wound on the pastern of a horse. *(From Colahan PT et al: Equine medicine and surgery, ed 4, St Louis, 1991, Mosby.)*

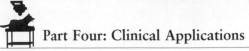

TABLE 23-3 Types of wound closures

Type of closure	Type of wound healing	Conditions of use
Primary closure	First-intention healing	Wound closed with sutures or staples Full-thickness apposition of wound edges Tissues in direct apposition Minimal edema No local infection No serious discharge Minimal scar formation Rapid healing
Nonclosure	Second-intention healing	Wound left open because of infection, extensive trauma, tissue loss, or incorrect apposition of tissues Healing by contraction and epithelialization, from inner layers to outer surface Contraction starts after around 72 hours and stops when wound edges meet or tension exceeds strength of contraction Epithelialization starts within 24 hours after injury and requires a moist, oxygen-rich environment Delayed by healing
Delayed primary closure	Form of third-intention healing	Closure 3 to 5 days after cleaning and debridement, but before granulation tissue forms Wound strength and rate of healing not affected by delaying primary closure
Secondary closure	Form of third-intention healing	Closure after more than 3 to 5 days after granulation tissue has formed in the wound bed
	Third-intention healing	Safe method for repair of dirty, contaminated, or infected wounds with extensive tissue damage Allows for management of infection or necrosis before closure Surgeon debrides damaged tissue and wound is closed, with accurate apposition of tissues
Adnexal reepithelialization	Second-intention healing	Partial-thickness skin loss with epitheliazation primarily from compound hair follicles ("road burns")

this prolongs healing and produces more scarring than sharp resection, bandaging, and casting. Large wounds of the distal extremities with skin deficits tend to heal very slowly due to reduced blood supply, increased movement, and excessive contamination. They heal by formation of scar tissue covered with a thin layer of easily damaged epithelial cells. Skin grafting is often recommended in these cases.

COVERING WOUNDS

Nature provides "natural bandages" as a part of normal healing. A partial-thickness wound that forms a blister rarely becomes infected and heals more rapidly if the blister is not broken. The scab of a full-thickness wound and the eschar of a burn also serve as natural bandages. The scab protects from external contamination, maintains internal homeostasis, and provides a surface beneath which cell migration and movement of skin edges occur. The eschar of large burn wounds serves as a biologic dressing that is protective and is considered by many surgeons superior to artificial bandaging materials.

Principles of Bandage Application

In veterinary application, bandages have the following functions:

- Protect wounds
- Hold clean or sterile dressings in place
- Absorb exudate and debride a wound
- Serve as a vehicle for therapeutic agents
- Serve as an indicator of wound secretions
- Pack the wound
- Provide support for bony anatomic structures
- Support and stabilize soft tissue
- Secure splints
- Prevent weight bearing
- Provide compression to control hemorrhage, dead space, and tissue edema
- Discourage self-grooming
- Restrict motion to eliminate stress of the wound edges
- Provide patient comfort
- Provide an aesthetic appearance

The basic principles of bandage application are as follows:

1. *Properly prepare the area before application of a bandage.* This may require clipping of the hair, wound debridement, and/or cleaning of surrounding skin.
2. *Use porous materials where possible.* This allows circulation of air and escape of excessive moisture.
3. *Use absorbent materials where exudates may be a problem.* Change absorbent dressings when they become saturated and before saturation is evident externally ("strike through").
4. *Use appropriate materials of adequate width* to avoid producing a tourniquet effect.
5. *Apply bandage materials as smoothly as possible.* Ridges and lumps lead to skin irritation and necrosis.
6. *Secure protective wound pads to the skin* so that they do not shift from the site.
7. *Check bandages frequently* to determine if there is persistent swelling, skin discoloration, or coolness. A bandage applied too tightly can impair circulation, resulting in serious damage to soft tissues.
8. *Instruct owners on basic care of bandages and signs of bandage failure.* This includes the physical appearance of the bandage, as well as behavior of the animal.

Ideally, materials used for bandaging should have the following properties:

- Permeable to oxygen and other gases
- Conform to body contours
- Acceptable appearance
- Inert
- Long storage life
- Inexpensive
- Easily sterilized
- Unaffected by disinfecting and cleaning solutions
- Nonflammable
- Will not shred, with particles contaminating the wound
- Compatible with topical therapeutic agents
- Do not adhere to the wound but can remove exudate and debris from the wound
- Maintains a moist wound surface but free from exudate

Bandage Components

In most situations, bandages are generally composed of three layers, each with its own properties and function. The *primary layer* rests on the wound and may or may not be adherent. The *secondary layer* provides absorbency and padding. The *tertiary layer* is the outer layer that holds the underlying layers in place. This is usually the only layer the owner sees. Clients often judge the quality of treatment solely on the appearance of this outer bandage layer.

Primary Layer. The primary layer is in contact with the wound itself. When debridement is the goal, an adherent layer is used for the primary bandage. Once the wound is in the proliferation phase and granulation tissue has formed, a nonadherent dressing should be used to avoid disruption of this new tissue. The primary layer should be sterile, be comfortable, allow fluids to pass to the secondary layer, protect the wound from exogenous contamination, and be nontoxic and nonirritating to tissue.

Adherent bandaging material, such as sterile gauze sponges with wide mesh openings and noncotton filler, can be used to provide debridement during the early stage of wound healing. This layer removes devitalized tissue and wound exudate when it is taken off during a bandage change. Adherent dressings may be wet or dry, depending upon the nature of the wound. Some bandages are applied wet and then allowed to dry. Use of an adherent primary layer should be discontinued after the wound has been cleared of necrotic debris and heavy exudate.

If loose necrotic tissue or foreign material is present on the surface of the wound, a *dry-to-dry dressing* may be the best type to use. Dry gauze with a large mesh is placed directly on the wound. An absorbent layer is placed over this primary layer and fluid is absorbed from the wound and allowed to dry. Necrotic material adheres to the gauze and is removed with the bandage. Although this type of bandage removes tissue debris, bandage removal is very painful and may also remove viable tissue. For this reason, dry-to-dry dressings should be used only when necessary.

If the exudate is especially viscous or if dried foreign matter must be removed, a *wet-to-dry dressing* may be appropriate. The bandage is applied wet, which dilutes the exudate for absorption. As the bandage dries, the foreign material adheres to the bandage and is later removed with the bandage. Solutions used to wet the primary layer include physiologic (0.9%) saline or a water-soluble bacteriostatic or bactericidal compound, such as 0.05% chlorhexidine diacetate solution (Nolvasan, Fort Dodge, Wilmington, OH).

For wounds with copious exudate or transudate, a *wet-to-dry dressing* may be best. Wet dressings absorb fluid more rapidly than dry dressings. They may be used to transport heat to a wound and/or enhance capillary action to promote wound drainage. A water-soluble bacteriostatic or bactericidal solution can be used to wet the dressings to help control microorganisms. The primary layer is applied wet and kept wet after the secondary and tertiary layers have been applied. This bandage is also removed wet. Wet-to-wet dressings cause less pain than dry dressings when removed; by using a warm solution, patient comfort is increased. A disadvantage is that these bandages tend to cause tissue maceration and have little debriding capacity.

A nonadherent primary layer is indicated during the reparative stage of wound healing, with formation of granulation tissue and production of a more serosanguineous exudate. In the early repair stage, petrolatum-impregnated products can be used in the presence of exudate and when little or no epithelialization has taken place. Later, when there is little fluid and during epithelialization, nonadherent dressings are indicated. Nonadherent dressings are used to cover lacerations, skin graft donor sites, minor burns, abrasions, and surgical incisions. The main goal is to minimize tissue injury upon removal. They do not absorb much fluid; draining wounds usually require a secondary dressing. Examples of nonadherent dressing materials include Adaptic (Johnson & Johnson), Release (Johnson & Johnson), and Telfa adhesive pads (Kendall/Curity). These semiocclusive, nonadherent materials leave the granulation bed undisturbed yet still move fluid away from the wound.

Secondary Layer. The secondary (intermediate) layer provides support and moves exudate or transudate away from the wound. Materials used in this layer include gauze bandaging material (e.g., Sof-Band, Kling, Sof-Kling, Johnson & Johnson), cast padding, and bandaging cotton.

The secondary layer should be thick enough to absorb moisture, pad the wound from trauma, and inhibit wound movement. If the bandage allows evaporation of fluid from absorbed exudate, this partially dry environment retards bacterial growth. With wounds producing copious fluids, evaporation does not keep the bandage dry. If such a moist bandage is not changed frequently, the wound fluids serve as a growth medium for bacteria.

Tertiary Layer. The tertiary (outer) layer holds the underlying bandage layers in place. Materials used in this layer include adhesive tapes (e.g., Zonas, Johnson & Johnson), elastic bandages (Elastikon, Johnson & Johnson, New Brunswick, NJ); Vetrap, 3M; Conform, Kendall; Medi-Rip, CoNco Medical), and conforming stretch gauze. This layer should be applied carefully to provide support without constricting.

Porous adhesive tape allows evaporation of fluid from the bandage. It can also allow movement of fluid (e.g., saliva, rainwater) into the wound, which may be undesirable. Waterproof adhesive tape repels water but also prevents evaporation. If the wound is producing considerable exudate, the tissues may become macerated from retained fluids. The resultant damp environment favors bacterial growth.

Elastic adhesive tape is compliant and applies continuous, dynamic pressure to the wound as the patient moves. Elastic tape products should be wrapped over the underlying bandage materials carefully to apply even but not excessive pressure. Elastic adhesive tapes tend to adhere to themselves, so minimal external taping is needed. Self-adherent products (e.g., Vetrap, MediRip) have no adhesive undercoat. Although these products tend to adhere to themselves, in veterinary practice, some external tape is usually required at the ends to keep the bandage from coming apart during movement.

ORTHOPEDIC BANDAGES AND SPLINTS
Robert Jones Compression Bandage

The Robert Jones compression bandage is illustrated in Fig. 23-3.

Indications. The Robert Jones bandage is generally used in large and small animals to temporarily immobi-

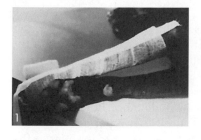

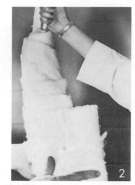

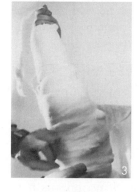

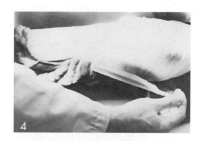

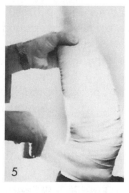

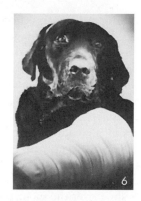

FIG. 23-3 The Robert Jones bandage. *1,* Porous tape stirrups are applied to the dorsal and palmar aspects of the leg, extending from the elbow or knee to well beyond the toes. A layer of stretch Sof-Kling is applied over the stirrups. *2,* With the limb suspended, roll cotton is applied, beginning at the foot and moving proximally up the limb to the axilla or groin, overlapping each pass. *3,* Wide Sof-Kling is stretched as tightly as possible over the cotton, overlapping each pass. *4,* Each stirrup is reflected proximally. *5,* Elastikon tape is applied, starting at the foot and working proximally, stretching the tape as tightly as possible. *6,* The completed bandage should be firm. *(Courtesy of Mallinckrodt Veterinary.)*

lize fractures distal to the elbow or tarsus, support injured soft and bony tissues, and prevent excessive swelling. It may be modified to incorporate the thorax or pelvis to provide additional stabilization of more proximal limb fractures. It absorbs exudates, decreases or prevents edema and swelling through compression, and reduces (but does not totally inhibit) movement of fracture fragments. It is an excellent emergency treat-

ment for distal limb injuries, reduces or prevents limb swelling postoperatively, and absorbs drainage before or after surgery. In horses, the Robert Jones bandage is used as an emergency method for treating fractures and tendon and ligament disruptions until repair can be made. It is used to immobilize a limb to protect from further damage through weight bearing or motion.

Materials. 1-inch adhesive tape, dressing for primary layer if needed, "pound cotton" rolls (1 lb cotton/10 kg body weight in small animals), 4- to 8-inch Kling or roll gauze, 4- to 8-inch elastic or Ace-type bandage.

Technique. In small animals, suspend the limb vertically if possible; this allows gravity to work for you. Dress any wounds. Apply porous tape stirrups, extending to the elbow or knee and considerably past the toes. Apply a snug layer of Sof-Kling to prevent slippage. Unroll rolled cotton to remove the separation paper, then reroll before application. Apply cotton to the limb, starting at the foot and extending to the groin or axilla, overlapping one quarter to one half the width of the roll. An assistant should hold the limb in extreme abduction to facilitate this process. Wrap the cotton as tightly as possible, with no wrinkles or twists. The object is to make the limb into a straight cylinder. Wrap the cotton with Kling or Sof-Kling gauze as tightly as possible, again overlapping half the width of the roll. Separate the tape stirrups to the sides of the bulky bandage. This provides a small opening to assess blood flow to the toes. Apply self-adherent elastic adhesive tape or an Ace-type bandage, starting at the toes and working proximally, overlapping by about half the width. The completed bandage should be very firm and should produce a sound similar to a ripe watermelon when thumped.

Stirrups are not used in horses. Apply rolls of cotton to the limb, from the distal limb proximally, in gradual spirals to the proximal forearm, with the proximal edge of the bandage extending as far proximally as possible. Apply five to eight consecutive rolls of cotton with firm pressure. When the final layer of cotton has been applied, the bandage should be of even thickness throughout its length. Secure the bandage in place with one or two layers of 6-inch gauze. The tertiary layer consists of an elastic bandage that will be covered with a 4-inch elastic adhesive tape as the final wrap. Apply the elastic adhesive tape, overlapping by about half, in several layers, depending on the strength and durability of the bandage desired. Then apply the adhesive bandage layer. This bandage requires six to eight rolls of Ace elastic bandage, six or seven rolls of Elastikon, four to six rolls of Sof-Kling, Kling or other conforming bandage, and a roll of porous tape to secure the ends of each roll of Ace elastic bandage used.

Precautions. The Robert Jones bandage may act as a heavy pendulum if used for injuries proximal to the

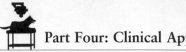

elbow or stifle unless modified. It should never be used as a definitive fracture treatment for any type of fracture.

Soft Padded and Coaptation Bandages

Indications. These bandages include the Schanz soft padded bandage, the Mesa-Meta Splint, and the coaptation bandage made with a thermoplastic splint (Orthoplast, Johnson & Johnson), fiberglass strips (C-Splint, Johnson & Johnson), or other casting materials. The Schanz soft padded bandage is the most commonly used limb bandage. It is designed to cover abrasions and lacerations, and to provide light support following long bone or joint surgery.

Materials. 1- or 2-inch porous adhesive tape, wound dressing for the primary layer, Kling, a splint of appropriate size (width, curvature, length), cast padding or soft bandage (e.g., Sof-Band bulky bandage), and elastic self-adherent tertiary layer (e.g., Elastikon, Vetrap).

Technique. Apply a primary dressing to the wound area. Form stirrups of porous tape to prevent bandage slippage. Apply the stirrups on the medial and lateral surfaces of the limb, leaving a tab on the distal end, if possible, to be pulled apart later. Apply cast padding snugly to the limb, starting at the foot and moving proximally, overlapping one quarter to one half the roll width, to a point proximal the elbow joint. Apply a layer of Sof-Kling or other conforming bandage in the same manner. Separate the tape stirrups and attach them to their respective sides. Apply adherent elastic bandage tape, being careful not to pull the tape too tightly. Pulling the tape to its elastic limits can compromise the circulation of the limb. Leave the toes exposed to allow assessment of circulation.

The soft padded bandage may be modified to provide additional support of a limb by incorporating splint materials. The resultant bandages can support the limb distally to the elbow or hock. They are generally used to provide additional support for fractures or other orthopedic injuries after surgical intervention. For some types of fractures, they may be used as the primary means of stabilization.

Precautions. Bandages in this category should not be used for fractures near the elbow or tibiotarsal joint, severely comminuted or collapsing fractures, or as definitive treatment for ligament or tendon ruptures.

Spica Splint

The spica splint is a semirigid splint bandage. It is usually brought over the trunk to immobolize the elbow or shoulder. It is made from casting material or a thermoplastic splint fitted to the lateral portion of the limb, incorporated into a padded bandage, and fixed to the limb with conforming gauze and surgical porous or elastic adherent tape.

Schroeder-Thomas Splint

The Schroeder-Thomas splint is an external weight-bearing device. It is best used for closed fractures of the radius/ulna or tibia/fibula in young dogs. These fractures heal rapidly with moderate stabilization. It is also of value in elbow dislocations, because the elbow can be held in position following reduction. Fractures proximal to the elbow or stifle are better repaired by internal fixation than with the Schroeder-Thomas splint. After surgical bone or joint repair, this device can provide additional stabilization and restrict movement of the limb. It is best if the aluminum splint rod is custom made for each individual patient.

Ehmer Sling

Indications. An Ehmer sling is applied after reduction of hip luxation. It maintains the hip joint in flexion, abduction, and internal rotation; the sling provides limited abduction. The Ehmer sling helps keep the femoral head deeply seated within the acetabulum by internally rotating and abducting the hip.

Materials. 4-inch Elastikon, 2-inch nonporous bandage.

Technique. The traditional Ehmer sling is based on a modified figure-8 bandage. Wrap Elastikon around the abdomen just cranial to the affected rear leg (just cranial to the prepuce in males). This tape anchors the tapes used to hold the leg in abduction. Apply a figure-8 sling to the limb first, applying tape just proximocaudal to the paw, passing it medial to the stifle. Pass the tape over the stifle and medially, to the hock, creating a figure-8 pattern. Repeat several times. Cover the limb completely with several more wraps of tape. Abduct the limb by attaching tape strips from the medial surface of the figure-8 sling over the metartarsals, passing it dorsally over the back and fully around the body, onto the tape previously placed as a "belly band" around the abdomen. Monitor for swelling resulting from impaired circulation.

Modified Ehmer Sling

Indications. The modified version maintains hip flexion and abduction but no internal rotation. The modified Ehmer sling can be adjusted to ensure abduction and relieve swelling by simply cutting the tape, repositioning it, and retaping. These adjustments cannot be made easily with the traditional Ehmer sling.

Materials. 4-inch Elastikon, 2-inch nonporous tape.

Technique. Place the elastic wrap around the metartarsals, from medial to lateral, *without encircling the limb,* and adhere the tape to itself. Carry the tape dorsally and cranially to encircle the trunk at the level of the caudal thorax and anchor it to the body around the caudal ribs. This location avoids compression of the abdomen and avoids the prepuce in male dogs. Applying tension to the wrap before encircling the trunk provides both hip joint flexion and abduction. Before encircling the trunk, pull the skin from the dorsal back toward the affected limb to prevent the limb from dropping into an abducted position. Once the elastic wrap is secured, apply 2-inch waterproof tape, covering the elastic wrap and eliminating any stretch of the elastic material. Apply the waterproof tape, fanning outward from the metatarsal area to the trunk. This ensures that the stifle joint remains covered and medial to the bandage.

Velpeau Sling

Indications. The Velpeau sling prevents weight bearing on the forelimb by cradling the forelimb against the shoulder and chest wall. It is indicated for scapular fractures not requiring open reduction and internal fixation, postoperative splintage of scapular fractures and shoulder dislocations, and ligament and joint capsule injuries of the shoulder joint.

Materials. 6-inch Kling gauze, Elastikon, Ace bandage, or Vetrap.

Technique. Slightly flex the carpus and metacarpus to a comfortable position and wrap them. Comfortably flex the antebrachium across the cranial chest wall (with paw pointing toward the opposite scapulohumeral joint). Apply additional wraps around the chest and flexed limb. This bandage is well tolerated for prolonged periods.

Precautions. The Velpeau sling should not be used in patients with internal or external thoracic trauma or disease; respiratory compromise; limbs with swelling, edema, or cellulitis; lateral luxation of the scapulohumeral joint; scapular neck fractures; or fractures involving the scapulohumeral joint.

CASTS

Indications. Casts are simple and very effective devices for providing support for some fractures in companion animals. Indications include external fixation of noncollapsing fractures of the radius, ulna, tibia, metacarpals, and digits; as an adjunct to internal fixation, including arthrodesis; immobilization of a limb after tendon repair or surgery; protection from self-mutilation; and restriction of motion after plastic or reconstructive surgery.

Bending forces, primarily transmitted perpendicularly to the long axis of a bone are well neutralized by a cast. Rotational, compressive, shearing, and tensile forces transmitted parallel to the long axis of a bone are poorly neutralized by a cast. Incomplete or minimally displaced, transverse, or short oblique diaphyseal fractures of the radius/ulna and tibia/fibula, especially in younger animals, are ideally suited for cast fixation.

Materials. For many years plaster was the only cast material available. Disadvantages of plaster casts included heavy weight, permeability to water, and susceptibility to breakage and mutilation.

Fiberglass casting material is now widely used because of its light weight, rigidity, ventilation, and waterproof characteristics. In small animals, fiberglass casts are highly effective for external fracture fixation and as an adjunct to internal fixation techniques (e.g., pinning, plating). Equine practitioners use fiberglass casts to protect heel bulb and flexor tendon lacerations, protect granulation tissue beds in wounds, and treat laminitis. Casts are also used after surgical fracture repair and in management of midbody sesamoid fractures following a bone graft, by keeping the leg in a flexed position. In neonatal calves, fiberglass casts have proven to be of value for external fixation of forelimb fractures caused by assisted deliveries in dystocia.

Technique. Proper application of a fiberglass cast requires practice and experience (Fig. 23-4). Patient movement during application can create pressure points. General anesthesia is required for cast application. The skin of the affected area should be clean and dry before casting. If a hoof is to be covered with fiberglass casting material, it should be cleaned and disinfected to prevent foot rot and thrush. Surgical incisions, lacerations, or wounds should be debrided and, if indicated, sutured and covered with a sterile nonadherent primary dressing. Cast padding should be kept to a minimum and applied only at pressure points. Cast padding is used infrequently in equine and bovine patients.

The cast should be of sufficient length to immobolize the joints proximal and distal to the lesion. Assistants should be advised to use the flat portion of the hand to support the limb during cast application to prevent indentations that may cause pressure sores. Any sharp edges at proximal and distal ends of the cast should be well padded. For horses and cattle, tape should be placed around the proximal rim of the cast to prevent foreign material from entering between cast and skin. If horses or cattle are to be kept outside after casting, the hoof should be covered with a rubber boot to prevent excessive moisture from entering the cast. Owners must be instructed about observing the cast, cast care, adverse clinical signs, and limiting the animal's activity.

MAINTAINING BANDAGES, SPLINTS, AND CASTS

Every bandage, splint, cast, or orthopedic appliance should be examined by a trained staff member every 6 to 8 hours during the first day after application. The

A

B

C

D

E

F

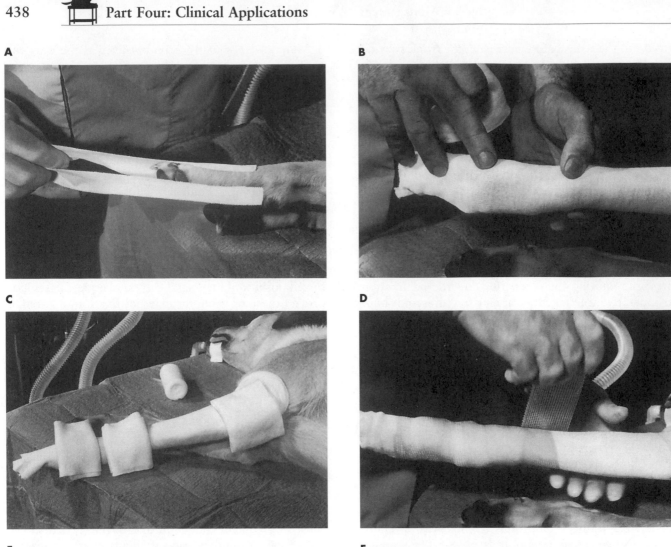
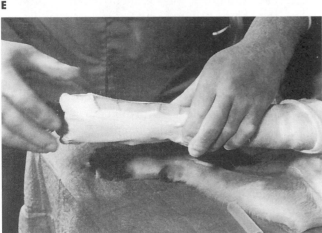
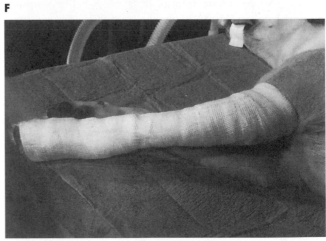

FIG. 23-4 Application of a fiberglass cast. **A,** Stirrups of porous taper applied to the dorsal and palmar aspects of the limb, extending well beyond the toes. **B,** A stockinette is applied over the limb, with excess material at the proximal and distal ends. **C,** Padding material is applied to cover bony protuberances. **D,** After the rolled fiberglass casting material has been soaked in warm water and excess water squeezed out, the material is rolled onto the limb, beginning at the toes and working proximally, overlapping each pass. **E,** The stockinette ends and the tape stirrups are reflected onto the limb and are incorporated into the case by two or three more overlying layers of fiberglass. **F,** The completed cast can be molded by hand during the last few minutes before setting. *(Courtesy of Mallinckrodt Veterinary.)*

device should be removed immediately if evidence of constriction is detected.

Home Care of Bandages

It is important to involve owners in wound management, especially for outpatients. Clients play a significant role in detection of adverse conditions affecting the bandage. Many problems can be avoided by taking the time to instruct owners on care of the bandage, splint, or cast placed on their animal. An information sheet with home care instructions is often helpful (e.g., Erlewein and Kuhns: *Instructions for veterinary clients,* St Louis, 1996, Mosby). However, an instruction sheet cannot replace face-to-face communications between the animal's owner and veterinary staff. Before leaving the clinic, the owner must be shown how to check the bandage or orthopedic appliance. It is often a good idea to telephone the client the next day to inquire about any problems.

Bandage, Cast, and Splint Removal

To remove the bandages, it is often easiest and safest to *carefully* cut the outer layer with scissors or a scalpel blade and then tear the cotton material from distal to proximal along the lateral aspect of the extremity, rather than trying to cut the cotton with bandage scissors. Casts are typically removed with an oscillating saw (e.g., Stryker). Splints can be removed with bandage scissors. With bandages or casts around any body part, be sure to determine the exact location of underlying structures *before* cutting the bandage. It is very easy to cut off the tip of an ear, toe, foot pad, or the tail if the area is not identified before cutting.

MANAGEMENT OF SPECIFIC WOUND TYPES
Penetrating Wounds

Gunshot wounds. High-velocity rifles and the more powerful handguns generate tremendous explosive kinetic energy that can shatter bone, cause massive tissue destruction, and propel fragments of metal and bone into surrounding soft tissue. High-velocity projectiles also destroy tissue by shock waves or "cavitation." Large exit wounds are common. Treatment of high-velocity missile wounds generally requires extensive debridement that creates a considerable tissue defect. This prolongs the healing time and usually requires more elaborate reconstructive procedures than low-velocity wounds.

Bullets from most handguns are considered low-velocity projectiles; however, they can inflict serious injuries at close range. Handgun bullets produce an entry wound, with or without an exit wound. As these missiles travel through tissues, they create a tract via crushing and laceration, damaging only tissues contacted by the projectile. When these wounds are confined to soft tissues, they may require little or no exploration or debridement, unless vital or important structures are involved. The tract is considered contaminated by bacteria. Clipping of hair around the wound, local wound cleaning, lavage, and application of topical dressings may suffice. Easily accessible projectiles may be removed. Retention of projectiles in the hypodermis, fascia, or muscle poses little health threat to the patient. If perforation or penetration involves the abdomen, surgical exploration is required. Missile fragments in joints should be removed.

Shotguns fire multiple small pellets or a single large slug. At close range, shotguns are among the most lethal and traumatic of weapons, causing massive tissue destruction. At extremely close range, the wadding of the explosive charge may be driven into the tissues.

Arrow Wounds. Broad-head arrows, used for hunting, have razor-sharp blades to lacerate vessels and vascular visceral tissues. Field-point arrows, usually used for target practice, have a rounded point about the size of the arrow shaft. They can penetrate deeply but do not lacerate tissues like broad-head hunting arrows.

Deeply embedded arrows, especially broad-heads, are best removed surgically by the veterinarian, not the owner. Shafts of arrows may be cut short by owners with a bolt cutter for transport of the animal to the veterinary facility. The owner should be discouraged from pulling the arrow out before transport to the clinic. The shaft end of some arrows is threaded for changing heads. If the arrow's head is accessible to the clinician, it can be grasped with a forceps and unthreaded from the shaft to facilitate removal.

Thorough examination is essential to identification and management of injuries caused by projectiles. This includes radiographs of the involved body region. Abdominal cavity wounds require surgical exploration to prevent bacterial peritonitis resulting from perforation of the bowel. Penetrating thoracic wounds generally do not require exploration unless there is significant hemorrhage, pneumothorax, or esophageal involvement.

Snakebites

Treatment of snakebite is directed toward preventing and controlling shock, neutralizing venom, minimizing necrosis, and preventing secondary infection. Fatal snakebites are more common in dogs than in any other domestic animal. Dogs are typically bitten in the head region. Because of their size, horses and cattle rarely die from snakebites; however, swelling on the muzzle, head, or neck can produce dyspnea and then death. Domestic animals vary in their sensitivity to the venom of pit vipers.

In North America, venomous snakes of the Crotalidae group, sometimes listed as a subfamily of Viperidae, are most commonly encountered in bite cases. These include the copperhead, cottonmouth, and rattlesnake. Owners should be instructed to bring the *dead* snake along with the bitten animal when possible, without mutilating the snake's head, because it may be needed for identification.

Systemic effects of envenomation include hypotension, shock, lethargy, salivation, lymph node pain, weakness, muscle fasciculations, and possible respiratory depression. Venomous snakebites often produce tissue necrosis and require reconstructive surgery. Tissue damage varies with the depth of bite and amount of venom injected. Local signs include fang puncture wounds (one or two), bleeding, swelling, tissue discoloration, and pain. The severity of envenomation cannot be judged by local signs alone.

Diphenhydramine hydrochloride (Benedryl, Parke-Davis) is often given as a pretreatment (10 mg for small dogs and cats, 25 mg for large dogs). Half the dose is given subcutaneously and the remainder intravenously after an intravenous catheter has been placed and fluid administration (lactated Ringer's solution, physiologic saline, colloids) has commenced.

Antivenin (polyvalent for Crotalidae, Fort Dodge Laboratories) should be given, as soon as possible, according to package insert recommendations. Antivenin can prevent systemic reactions and limits tissue necrosis. Although antivenin is expensive, it helps prevent large necrotic sloughs and may reduce costs associated with reconstructive surgery.

Necrotic snakebite wounds should be managed as an open infected wound during sloughing. Broad-spectrum antibacterial therapy is warranted to help prevent wound infection; tetanus antitoxin should be given. When sloughing is complete and healthy granulation tissue has formed, the wound should be assessed for possible reconstruction, grafting, or management as an open wound.

Burns

Thermal Burns. Thermal burns caused by exposure to excessive heat are classified according to their depth. *First-degree burns* are superficial and involve only the epidermis. Except in pigs, first-degree burns in animals do not form vesicles or blisters, as commonly seen in people. *Third-degree burns* destroy the full thickness of the skin. They form a dark brown, insensitive, leathery covering called an *eschar. Second-degree burns* fall between these two classifications.

Burn patients may be sedated to relieve pain and provide restraint if cardiovascular function is stable. Fluid therapy with a balanced electrolyte solution or lactated Ringer's solution should be used to treat shock associated with burns.

If started soon after injury, application of ice/cold water compresses or submersion in icewater may relieve pain and arrest progression of the burn. Hair should be clipped or removed from the burned surface and the area washed gently with a detergent antiseptic. The antiprostaglandin effects of topical aloe vera products may reduce the severity of burns.

Burns should be carefully debrided. In first-degree and second-degree burns, cleaning the burn may constitute debridement. A third-degree eschar may retain infection under it and prevent wound contraction. As the eschar separates from underlying tissue during healing, it should be removed with scissors. This is painful and the animal's pain tolerance should be considered. After the eschar has been removed from second-degree and third-degree burns, topical antibacterial medication (e.g., silver sulfadiazine or bacitracin cream) and light bandages are applied. Bandages are changed at least twice daily. Occlusive dressings and ointments are usually contraindicated. The prognosis depends on the total area of the burn, depth of penetration, location, and age and condition of the animal.

Electrical Burns. Electrical burns occur most often when animals chew on electrical cords. The most common signs are tissue damage with necrosis, cardiac dysrhythmias, and acute pulmonary edema. Often, there is charring of tissue at the point of contact (e.g., lips or mouth). Because the electrical current may flow along blood vessels to tissues, ischemic demarcation and sloughing often occur 2 or 3 weeks later. Managing lip and mouth injuries associated with electrical burns requires debridement and possibly reconstructive surgery.

Chemical Burns. Chemical burns cause denaturation and coagulation of tissue protein. They often produce hard and soft eschars, with underlying ulcers. They may also be deeper and more extensive than they initially appear. Chemical burns are managed in much the same manner as thermal burns, with reconstruction or open wound healing.

Bite Wounds

Bite wounds usually appear as punctures, lacerations, or avulsions of skin flaps. Massive subcutaneous and muscle contamination, maceration, dead space, serum accumulation, and infection leading to abscess formation (especially in cats) may develop in underlying tissues. Bite wounds in cats commonly form abscesses and draining sinuses. These should be surgically explored, lavaged, and initially managed as a dirty wound. Systemic antibacterials should be used in bite wound patients.

Decubital Ulcers

Decubital ulcers ("pressure sores") are open wounds that develop over bony prominences as a result of pressure in animals recumbent for long periods. Pressure sores can also develop over bony prominences covered by a cast or bandage as a result of insufficient or loose padding or overly tight application of the cast or bandage.

Decubital ulcers should be cleaned thoroughly with a surgical scrub and debrided when necessary.

Following cleaning, the area should be completely dried. Astringents (e.g., Burrow's solution) can be used to help dry the lesion. The decubital ulcer should be padded to prevent further pressure injury by use of a soft padded bandage held in the shape of a donut, with the ulcer in the center. These protective bandages leave the ulcer open to the air and relieve pressure. Use of antibacterial agents may be considered; however, decubital ulcers heal best if kept clean and dry.

In recumbent patients, decubital ulcers can be prevented using the following measures:

1. Provide sufficient soft padding or bedding material. This can include water pads, air mattresses, artificial fleece, rubber grids, straw, and towels. The material should be disposable or washable.
2. Change the animal's position frequently. Turn from side to side. Intermittent use of slings or carts may be considered.
3. Periodically check the skin over bony prominences for signs of ulcer formation. These include hyperemia, moisture, and easily epilated hair.
4. Keep the skin clean and dry. Bathe the animal frequently.
5. Provide a well-balanced, high-protein diet.
6. Apply casts and bandages correctly. Safeguard bony prominences with adequate padding.

RECOMMENDED READING

Bojrab MJ: *A handbook on veterinary wound management,* Ashland, Ohio, 1994, KenVet.

Fossum TW: *Small animal surgery,* St Louis, 1997, Mosby.

Gfeller RW, Crowe DT: Emergency care of traumatic wounds, *Vet Clin North Am Small Anim Prac* 24:1249-1274, 1994.

Pavletic MM: The clinician's guide to basic wound management, *Proc North Am Vet Conf* 1996, pp 512-513.

Stashak TS: *Equine wound management,* Philadelphia, 1991, Lea & Febiger.

Swaim SF, Henderson RA: *Small animal wound management,* Philadelphia, 1990, Lea & Febiger.

CHAPTER 24

Fluid Therapy and Blood Transfusions

D.A. Oakley

Learning Objectives

After reviewing this chapter, the reader should understand the following:

Indications for fluid therapy
Ways of assessing hydration status
Types of fluids used in fluid therapy
Ways of assessing bleeding patients
Types of blood products used in transfusion medicine
Blood groups of dogs, cats, and horses
Techniques used in blood collection, crossmatching, and transfusion
Signs of adverse reactions to blood transfusion

FLUID THERAPY

In a normal animal, fluid (water) and electrolyte balance is closely regulated. Good health, proper nutrition, and a readily available supply of clean drinking water are essential in maintaining this balance. In sick animals unable to regulate their own fluid balance, it is necessary to supplement them to varying degrees with fluid therapy. Fluid therapy is used primarily to correct fluid deficits, electrolyte disturbances, and acid-base imbalances.[25,33]

Fluid Physiology

Fluid Distribution. Approximately 60% of the body is composed of fluid, often referred to as *total body water (TBW)*. About two thirds of TBW lies within the cells and is called *intracellular fluid (ICF)*. The remaining third is *extracellular fluid (ECF)*, which lies outside the cells. About 75% of ECF is *interstitial fluid*, which surrounds the cells and is outside the blood vessels. In addition to the fluid surrounding the cells, the intersti-

tial fluid also includes *transcellular fluid*, such as cerebrospinal fluid, synovial fluid, lymph fluid, intraocular fluid, and the serous fluid in the visceral spaces (i.e., pericardial, pleural, and peritoneal spaces). The remaining 25% of ECF is *intravascular fluid*, which is contained within the blood vessels. Intravascular fluid is also referred to as *plasma* (Fig. 24-1).[34,51,72,100]

The ability of a solution to initiate water movement is referred to as *tonicity*. The tonicity of a fluid is dependent on its solutes and their ability to pass through a membrane. For example, if cells are placed in a fluid that is less concentrated than the contents of the cell, water moves into the cell by osmosis, causing the cell to swell. A fluid into which normal body cells can be placed without causing either shrinkage or swelling of the cells (i.e., similar concentration) is said to be *isotonic* (e.g., 0.9% sodium chloride). A solution that causes cells to swell is said to be *hypotonic* (e.g., 0.45% sodium chloride with 2.5% dextrose). A solution that causes cells to shrink is said to be *hypertonic* (e.g., 7% sodium chloride).[51,68]

Electrolytes. Sodium is the most abundant and important extracellular ion. The distribution of body water is influenced by sodium more than by any other electrolyte. Because sodium attracts water, it is the primary factor responsible for determining extracellular fluid volume. When animals become dehydrated, their losses may include sodium. This fluid and electrolyte depletion commonly occurs through urinary losses, gastrointestinal losses (e.g., vomiting, diarrhea), third-space losses (e.g., peritonitis, pleural effusion), and cutaneous losses (e.g., open wounds, burns). [24,76]

Potassium is the primary intracellular ion. It is necessary for maintenance of several body functions, most importantly the generation of electrical potentials in muscles and nerves. Relatively small changes in plasma potassium concentration can seriously alter nervous and cardiac functions. Thus, serum levels of potassium must be maintained within very close limits.[26,65,76,83]

The dosage and route (e.g., oral, subcutaneous, intravenous) of potassium supplementation depend on the cause and severity of the deficiency. Intravenous administration can be used to correct severe potassium defi-

ciencies. The rate of potassium-augmented fluid infusion depends on the amount of potassium added to the fluid (Table 24-1). The maximum rate of potassium supplementation in fluids is 0.5 mEq/kg/hr.[74] Potassium should never be administered in an undiluted form directly into the circulation because of the potential risk of cardiac arrest. Fluid with potassium in concentrations up to 30 to 35 mEq/L can be administered subcutaneously without discomfort or irritation.[33,74]

Acid-Base Balance. Acid-base balance is the regulation of hydrogen ion concentration in body fluid. Hydrogen ion concentration is expressed as *pH*. A low pH corresponds with a high hydrogen ion concentration and is referred to as *acidosis*. A high pH corresponds with a low hydrogen ion concentration and is referred to as *alkalosis*. The normal pH of arterial blood is 7.4; the pH of venous blood and interstitial fluid is approximately 7.35. There are major complications in life support if the pH falls below 7.2 or rises above 7.6 for more than a few hours.[34,83]

Clinical Aspects of Fluid Therapy

Maintenance Fluid Requirements. In healthy animals at rest, the daily intake of water, nutrients, and minerals matches the daily excretion of these substances. *Sensible water loss* refers to that lost through the urine and feces. *Insensible water loss* includes water lost through the respiratory tract (e.g., panting). Normal fluid losses are approximately 40 to 60 ml/kg/day. Urinary losses are approximately 20 ml/kg/day, fecal losses are 5 ml/kg/day, and respiratory and transcutaneous losses are 15 ml/kg/day.[68,74]

These losses are balanced daily through intake of consumed water, water in food, and metabolic breakdown of fat, carbohydrate, and protein. To maintain body fluid volume, an animal's daily intake of fluid must equal the sum of sensible and insensible losses.[68] This is defined as the daily *maintenance fluid requirement*. Maintenance fluid requirements may be calculated from charts that relate body weight to basal metabolic rate (Fig. 24-2).[7,33,74]

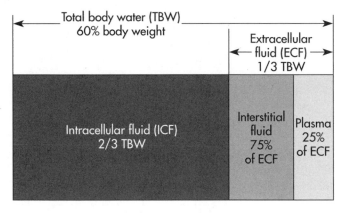

FIG. 24-1 Fluid compartments of the body. *(Adapted from Vander: Human physiology: the mechanisms of body function, ed 4, New York, 1985, McGraw-Hill.)*

TABLE 24-1 Guidelines for intravenous potassium (K) supplementation*

Serum potassium level	KCl safely added to 250 ml of fluid	Maximal rate of infusion
<2.0 mEq/L	20 mEq	6 ml/kg/hr
2.1 to 2.5 mEq/L	15 mEq	8 ml/kg/hr
2.6 to 3.0 mEq/L	10 mEq	12 ml/kg/hr
3.1 to 3.5 mEq/L	7 mEq	16 ml/kg/hr

*The infusion rate should not exceed 0.5 mEq/kg/hr. (From Muir WW, DiBartola SP: *Fluid therapy.* In Kirk RW: *Current veterinary therapy VIII,* Philadelphia, 1983, WB Saunders.)

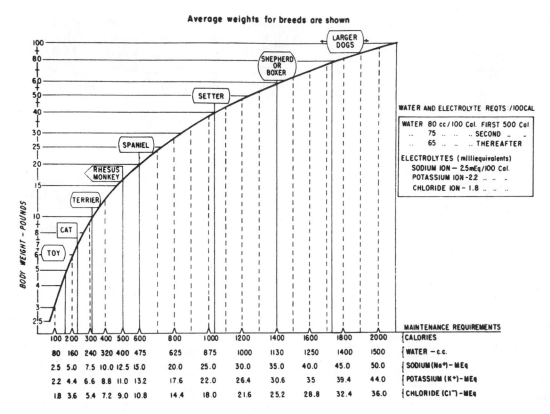

FIG. 24-2 Daily water, calorie, and electrolyte requirements for dogs and cats. *(From Harrison JB et al: Fluid and electrolyte therapy in small animals,* J Am Vet Med Assoc *137:638, 1960.)*

Indications for Fluid Therapy. Dehydration and hypovolemia are the two most common indications for fluid therapy. The degree of dehydration can be roughly estimated by clinical assessment (Table 24-2). Animals can be dehydrated and have normal intravascular volume, or they can have normal hydration but hypovolemia. A good example of this is a dog that has been hit by a car. The patient has a weak, rapid pulse as a result of intraabdominal hemorrhage. This patient is not dehydrated but has hypovolemia. *Dehydration* is reduced total body water with preservation of the vascular volume. *Hypovolemia* is reduced intravascular volume, which can impair cardiac output. Although dehydration should be corrected slowly so as not to overexpand the vascular space, hypovolemia requires rapid reexpansion of intravascular volume. Short-term fluid therapy is used in emergency situations to rapidly replace plasma volume in animals with hypovolemia. Long-term fluid therapy is used to replace fluid deficits (dehydration), provide maintenance requirements, and compensate for ongoing losses.[61]

Emergency fluid therapy. Aggressive fluid therapy is indicated for hypovolemic animals. These patients require fluid administration rates that sometimes exceed those used in treating shock at 60 to 90 ml/kg/hr. The volume and rate of fluid administered are adjusted according to the animal's response to therapy.[19,25,28,33,61,72,85]

Maintenance fluid therapy. After the initial intravascular volume expansion, one must attempt to quantitate the amount of fluid lost before presentation, daily maintenance requirements, and ongoing fluid losses in addition to normal losses.[19,28,61,65,72,74,85]

$$\text{Daily fluid requirement} = \text{Replacement} + \text{Maintenance} + \text{Ongoing losses}$$

The history and physical examination findings are used to estimate fluid deficits when an animal is first presented. Increased losses are usually due to vomiting, diarrhea, or polyuria. Deficits are more severe when coupled with decreased water intake. Physical examination can provide a rough estimate of dehydration (see Table 24-2). The fluid deficit can be calculated using the degree of dehydration and body weight:

$$\text{Fluid deficit (ml)} = \% \text{ dehydration} \times \text{body weight (kg)} \times 10$$

Most fluid deficits can be replaced with fluid administration over 12 to 24 hours, depending upon the underlying disease process and the severity and duration of the dehydration. In general, it is better to overestimate rather than underestimate the replacement volume, unless the patient has some underlying restrictive condition (e.g., cardiac or renal disease). Preexisting

TABLE 24-2 Clinical estimation of degree of dehydration

Degree of dehydration	Clinical signs
< 5%	Not clinically detectable
5% to 6%	Subtle loss of skin elasticity
6% to 8%	Obvious delay in return of tented skin to normal position Slightly prolonged capillary refill time Eyes possibly sunken in orbits Possibly dry mucous membranes
10% to 12%	Skin remains tented Very prolonged capillary refill time Eyes sunken in orbits Dry mucous membranes Possibly signs of shock (tachycardia, cool extremities, rapid, weak pulse)
12% to 15%	Obvious signs of shock Death imminent

From Muir WW, DiBartola SP: *Fluid therapy*. In Kirk RW: *Current veterinary therapy VIII*, Philadelphia, 1983, WB Saunders.

fluid deficits are usually replaced with intravenous fluid formulated for replacement (e.g., Normosol-R or lactated Ringer's solution).

Maintenance requirements are estimated by body weight and are 40 to 60 ml/kg/day.[74] Maintenance requirements should be provided with a solution intended for maintenance therapy (e.g., Normosol-M or 0.45% NaCl with KCl). This is especially important for animals receiving maintenance therapy only, given that their potassium needs will not be met with a replacement solution. Once the animal is rehydrated, maintenance fluids can be administered PO, SC, IV, or intraosseously.

Ongoing losses should be estimated from the daily volume of urine, diarrhea, vomiting, tube drainage, etc. The calculated amount should be divided over 24 hours and added to the maintenance fluid dose. Replacement fluids are given to compensate for ongoing losses. Box 24-1 shows calculations of fluid requirements for a hypothetical case.

Correcting electrolyte imbalances. Dehydration and certain diseases can cause electrolyte changes in the body. These imbalances are most often corrected through fluid therapy. The fluid choice, additive solutions, and administration route and rate are dependent on the disease, patient status, and laboratory values.

Diuresis. Certain diseases (e.g., kidney disease) and treatments (e.g., chemotherapy) require diuresis (increased fluid loss through the kidneys) as part of the therapeutic plan. Intravenous catheters are placed and aggressive fluid therapy is instituted. Patients undergoing diuresis should be monitored closely for signs of overhydration, in addition to urine production. If there is some question as to adequate renal function, an indwelling urinary catheter should be placed and maintained so urine output can be measured and fluid therapy adjusted accordingly.

Determining the Need for Fluid Therapy. Determining the need for fluid administration requires assessment of the animal's state of hydration (see Table 24-2) and estimation of fluid deficits through subjective patient evaluation. Formulation of a fluid therapy regimen is based on information gathered from an accurate history, a thorough physical examination, and laboratory tests.[20]

History. A complete history helps to establish the presence of dehydration. The history should include information on the animal's food and water intake, routinely and currently. Any information regarding urination, defecation (including diarrhea), and vomiting is useful. Ensure that there is no history of trauma or evidence of hemorrhage. To help assess the degree of dehydration, consider exposure to extreme environmental heat, excessive exercise, fever, panting, and the period over which losses have occurred.[74] Information pertaining to medication the animal has been or is currently taking can be useful. Some medications can have potentially harmful or complicating side effects.

Physical examination. A complete physical examination can help to define the avenue of fluid loss. Dehydration and hypoperfusion are the most frequently encountered conditions. Remember, not all patients that are dehydrated are hypovolemic and not all hypovolemic patients are dehydrated.

Certain physical signs can help estimate hydration status, including dry, tacky mucous membranes, skin turgor, position of the eye in the orbit, body temperature, evidence of decreased peripheral circulation, and changes in body weight (see Table 24-2).[25,74,85] Skin turgor is not the most accurate way to detect or estimate dehydration. Skin turgor is affected by the amount of subcutaneous fat and elastic tissue, in addition to tissue hydration.[25,72] The most commonly tested area is over the trunk; avoid the loose skin of the neck region and the top of the head. The skin is lifted a short distance (tented) and then released, monitoring its return to the initial position. Normal skin returns to its position immediately. The skin of dehydrated animals may show varying degrees of slow return to the initial position. The skin turgor of obese animals may appear normal in light of dehydration because of

---

Box 24-1 Calculating daily fluid requirements in a hypothetical case

Patient	5-month-old, 20-kg Rottweiler
History	3 days anorexia, lethargy 2 days of vomiting and diarrhea, 5-6 times/day, becoming bloody No vaccinations
Physical examination findings	Depression Heart rate: 140 beats/minute Pulse: weak to moderate Capillary refill time: 1-2 seconds Tented skin slowly returns to normal position
Replacement requirements	Fluid deficit = % dehydration × body weight × 10 8 × 20 × 10 = 1,600 ml
Maintenance requirements	Maintenance requirement = 40-60 ml/kg/day 50 × 20 = 1,000 ml/day
Ongoing losses	Ongoing losses = losses in diarrhea and vomitus Estimated diarrhea volume/episode = 100 ml 5 episodes/day = 500 ml Estimated vomitus volume/episode = 50 ml 5 episodes/day = 250 ml Ongoing losses 500 + 250 = 750 ml/day
Daily fluid requirement	Daily fluid requirement = fluid deficit + maintenance + ongoing losses = 1,600 + 1,000 + 750 = 3,350 ml/day = 3,350 ml over 24 hr/day Infusion rate = 140 ml/hr

excessive stores of subcutaneous fat. Likewise, the skin of emaciated animals lacks subcutaneous fat and elastic tissue, and, therefore, may lead to an overestimation of dehydration.[25] In addition, skin turgor is harder to evaluate in long-haired animals.

Body weight decreases with fluid loss. Dehydration can be more accurately assessed if the patient's current body weight can be compared with a weight obtained before the current episode. A change in body weight of 1 kg represents a gain or loss of 1 L of fluid.[72,100] Frequent, serial body weight measurement is a good monitoring tool for continued fluid loss during treatment. Keep in mind that fluid loss can occur from the ECF into the gastrointestinal tract and thoracic or peri-toneal cavities without creating a change in body weight. These areas are referred to as the "third space."[72] Auscultation and abdominal palpation may help determine the presence of third-space losses.

The cardiovascular and respiratory system should be carefully evaluated. Assessment of perfusion is based on mucous membrane color, capillary refill time, heart rate, and pulse rate, strength, and character. Most of these assessments are subjective. For this reason, monitoring is more accurate when serial examinations are performed consistently by an experienced member of the health care team.

Mucous membrane color. Normal mucous membranes are pink and moist to the touch but can range in color from pale to cyanotic to muddy or injected. Mucous membrane color can be used to detect problems or to monitor the patient's response to therapy.[78] Dry oral mucous membranes may result from panting and should be evaluated in addition to other values or mucous membranes. The degree of dehydration in patients that are vomiting and salivating could be underestimated if one relies solely on mucous membrane assessment.

Capillary refill time. Capillary refill time (CRT) provides an indication of peripheral perfusion.[78] Pressure is applied to the pink mucosa of the gum or the inner lip and then released. The time required for the blanched area to return to pink should be 1 to 2 seconds. Prolonged refill time is suggestive of compromised tissue perfusion and shock. Rapid refill time of less than 1 second is usually associated with tachycardia as a result of the heart's attempt to increase cardiac output in compensating for hypovolemia.[67,78]

Peripheral pulses. Mucous membrane color, CRT, and pulse intensity should be evaluated with respect to cardiac and pulmonary function. Pulse rate and intensity provide information regarding heart rate and perfusion pressure. Technicians should become proficient at assessment, accurate interpretation, and monitoring of pulse intensity. Most easily accessible and palpable are the femoral, dorsal metatarsal, and ulnar arteries. A skilled technician can learn to use pulse pressure in estimating blood pressure when more advanced equipment is not available. A weak, rapid pulse often suggests severe dehydration and poor perfusion; a bounding pulse suggests hypovolemia.[28,67,78]

The heart and lungs should be auscultated before the onset of fluid therapy and frequently throughout treatment. Cardiac auscultation allows detection of heart murmurs and arrhythmias. Palpation of a peripheral pulse while auscultating the heart helps detect pulse deficits. If a compromise in cardiac function is suspected, the approach to fluid therapy may require adjustment. On pulmonary auscultation, crackling sounds indicate fluid accumulation in the alveoli or bronchioles, suggesting edema or overhydration.[78] Wheezing sounds are usually a result of some degree of airway obstruction. When wheezing sounds are detected during auscultation, the stethoscope should always be placed over the trachea to determine if the same sounds can be heard in this area as those heard over the lung fields. If present, these sounds most likely can be classified as *referred upper respiratory noise*. Absence of lung sounds is abnormal and may suggest consolidation of lung tissue, as in pneumonia. The depth of respiration, along with the rate and effort, should also be noted. Dyspneic animals have an increased respiratory rate with a marked abdominal component.

Body temperature. Hypothermic and hyperthermic patients require adjustments in fluid therapy and close monitoring. Environmental temperature, cardiac function, renal function, respiratory character, and neurologic status should be immediately evaluated.

Laboratory tests. Laboratory tests may be vital in establishing the nature and extent of fluid imbalances and in monitoring treatment. Serial determinations of the *hematocrit* (packed cell volume) and total plasma protein level are important for establishing a trend and adjusting therapy. A decreasing hematocrit and total plasma protein level can suggest acute or chronic bleeding or hemodilution. Patients with a low serum protein level (hypoproteinemia) are in danger of losing fluid from the intravascular space into the interstitium because of low intravascular oncotic pressure. Once the protein level falls below 3.5 g/dl or the albumin level below 2.0 g/dl, natural or synthetic colloid administration should be considered.[66,67] An increasing hematocrit and total plasma protein level can indicate fluid loss from the intravascular space, ultimately resulting in dehydration. These two values should routinely be evaluated together to avoid misleading information that could be obtained from evaluation of either value alone.[25]

Urine output is a reflection of cardiac function, circulating blood volume, perfusion, and function of the kidneys and lower urinary tract. The normal urine output in an animal is 1 to 2 ml/kg/hr. Urine production should be monitored in patients when abnormalities of these factors are suspected or confirmed.

Evaluation of hydration status is necessary before proper assessment of urine production. Dehydrated patients require fluid replacement before oliguria (urine production of less than 1 ml/kg/hr) is confirmed. Oliguria associated with adequate hydration and normal blood pressure could suggest renal failure. Patients receiving aggressive fluid therapy or unintentional fluid overload are likely to become polyuric (increased urine output).[19,25,67]

Urine specific gravity is a measurement of solids in solution and indicates the kidney's ability to concentrate urine. In a normal animal, the specific gravity depends on fluid intake and urine output. An increased urine specific gravity is most likely in animals with decreased water intake. Upon rehydration, the urine specific gravity should decrease.[19] Urine specific gravity should be measured before and during fluid therapy to help evaluate renal function.[74]

Types of Fluids Used. The goal of fluid therapy is to restore the body fluid losses and reestablish normal blood volume. The choice of fluid is based on the composition of fluid lost, abnormalities requiring correction, and the severity and type of dehydrating process.[19,72,74] The choice, composition, and volume of fluid being administered typically require adjustment throughout the course of treatment.

Crystalloid solutions (e.g., lactated Ringer's solution, 0.9% NaCl, Normosol-R) contain small molecules that, when in solution, can pass through a semipermeable membrane and enter all body compartments. Crystalloid solutions can be categorized as *balanced* if similar in composition to plasma (e.g., lactated Ringer's solution, Normosol-R), or *unbalanced* if electrolyte composition differs from that of plasma (e.g., 5% dextrose in water, 0.9% NaCl).[25] For example, lactated Ringer's solution and Normosol-R contain sodium, chloride, potassium, calcium, and lactate in the same concentrations as in plasma. Although these solutions are comparable with plasma in regard to electrolyte composition, they do not contain phosphorus, proteins, or other substances. These solutions are, however, identical in tonicity to plasma and are referred to as *isotonic*. Unbalanced crystalloid solutions can have electrolyte compositions that differ from those found in plasma. These solutions vary in osmolality (solute concentration) and tonicity. They are classified as *isotonic* if they have an osmolality of approximately 300 mOsm/L (used most frequently), *hypotonic* with an osmolality of less than 300 mOsm/L, or *hypertonic* with an osmolality of greater than 300 mOsm/L.[74]

Crystalloid solutions can also be classified as to whether they meet maintenance or replacement needs. *Maintenance solutions* differ from plasma in that they contain less sodium and more potassium (e.g., Normosol-M, 0.45% NaCl with KCl). *Replacement solutions* have a composition similar to that of plasma, with high sodium and low potassium (e.g., lactated Ringer's solution, Normosol-R).[25]

Most animals requiring fluid therapy can be treated with crystalloid solutions containing certain additives. The most commonly used crystalloid solutions are balanced replacement solutions (e.g., lactated Ringer's solution, Normosol-R). When used for maintenance therapy or in animals with conditions causing loss of potassium, supplementation may be necessary. If additives of any type are incorporated into the main fluid source, the fluid bag should be labeled to note the additive, its concentration and amount, and the date and time of addition, and it should then be initialed by the person adding the solution.

When using isotonic crystalloid fluid solutions, remember that they pass readily through the blood vessel wall. By 30 minutes after infusion, only about 25% of the fluid remains in the vasculature, with the remaining 75% being redistributed to the interstitium. Although volume replacement can be achieved with crystalloid solutions, the effect may be short lived. In some cases, it is difficult, if not impossible, to administer adequate volumes of crystalloid fluids to reverse hypovolemia. If volume depletion does not resolve or if it recurs, administration of colloid solutions may be necessary. Hemodilution is a common concern when using crystalloid therapy only. Addition of a synthetic colloid solution decreases the volume of additional fluids required.[53,54]

Colloid solutions (e.g., whole blood, plasma, Dextran 70, Hetastarch, hypertonic saline) contain large molecules that do not readily pass through a semipermeable membrane. When colloid solutions are administered intravenously, their distribution is limited to the intravascular compartment, making them more effective than crystalloids at expanding blood volume. Ultimately, these solutions increase osmotic pressure, and, therefore, are used in conditions in which the vascular space cannot retain an adequate fluid volume (e.g., hypoproteinemia). Although more expensive, they are more cost effective—they promote better tissue perfusion and colloid oncotic pressure at a lower infusion volume.[30,86] Selection is based on the patient's needs. As a rule of thumb, colloids should be used in combination with crystalloid solutions to support the fluid shift from the extravascular to the intravascular compartment.[25,67] One limitation with synthetic colloid solutions is their potential to cause or aggravate coagulopathies.[30,67,90] Patients receiving these solutions should be monitored accordingly.

Routes of Fluid Administration. Fluids can be given by various routes. An appropriate route is chosen after careful evaluation of the route of fluid loss, volume of fluid loss, rate of fluid loss (acute vs. chronic), fluid selected, volume and rate of administration, and patient status. In veterinary medicine, medical, practical, and economic considerations may affect the fluid and route used. Complications related to fluid administration include phlebitis, osteomyelitis, hematomas, and tissue sloughing from extravasation of irritating products.[25,74]

Oral. "If the gut works, use it!" Oral fluid therapy can be used if the gastrointestinal tract is working properly (no vomiting, diarrhea, or gastrointestinal obstruction). Unfortunately, this route cannot be used to rapidly correct severe fluid deficits in critically ill patients in need of rapid fluid and electrolyte delivery. If the patient is only mildly dehydrated and will eat and drink, and there is no evidence of vomiting, the oral route is an ideal choice for fluid delivery. It should also be the route of choice for animals with maintenance needs only and not requiring replacement fluids or sustaining ongoing losses.

Animals sometimes voluntarily drink any of several commercially available human electrolyte products. If the patient does not drink the fluid, it can be administered via syringe into the mouth, nasogastric tube, pharyngostomy tube, percutaneous gastrostomy tube, or jejunostomy tube.[69] Consideration must be given to the amount of stress imposed on the patient.

Subcutaneous. Subcutaneous fluid administration is frequently employed. Advantages of this method include ease of administration, reduced cost, and avoidance of problems potentially encountered with intravenous administration. The subcutaneous route is the delivery method of choice when small volumes are needed, such as maintenance requirements in small animals. When animals are being weaned from intravenous fluid therapy and would recuperate much more quickly at home, owners can be instructed on how to administer subcutaneous fluids.

Subcutaneous fluid administration cannot be used in animals that require large replacement volumes, nor in animals that are severely dehydrated or hypothermic. These conditions cause peripheral vasoconstriction, ultimately reducing the fluid absorption rate. Absorption may also be prolonged in animals that are hypotensive. The most effective approach to rehydrate the patient is by initially using the intravenous route to improve circulation to the subcutaneous tissues. There are also limitations as to the volume that can be mechanically infused under the skin. The volume that can be administered via injection or gravity flow varies from animal to animal. Usually 50 to 150 ml can be infused at each SC site, depending on the elasticity of the skin.[84] If larger volumes are required, multiple sites may be used and treatment repeated every few hours.

Subcutaneous infusion can be given anywhere over the trunk area of the animal. Fluids are usually administered in subcutaneous space over the dorsal neck and cranial trunk, where loose connective tissue is abundant. The areas where the limbs join the trunk should be avoided, because fluid can gravitate into the limbs and cause discomfort. Warming the fluids before infusion encourages absorption and benefits hypothermic animals.

To avoid skin sloughing, administer only nonirritating, isotonic fluids subcutaneously. A solution of 5% dextrose in water (D5W) should not be given SC. This fluid is devoid of electrolytes; when the fluid is not immediately absorbed, electrolytes from the body can equilibrate into this pooled fluid and potentially initiate or aggravate electrolyte imbalances.[25]

Intravenous. The intravenous route of fluid administration is preferable when treating animals that are critically ill, severely dehydrated, or hypovolemic, or are experiencing some electrolyte or metabolic disorder. Fluid administered intravenously has the most rapid effect on blood volume. If fluid loss is acute, it is important to replace deficits rapidly. If fluid losses have occurred over an extended period, the body has had time to adjust, and slow fluid replacement is generally all that is required. Intravenous delivery allows titration of fluids to meet requirements of the patient. Complications of IV infusion are more numerous than with other routes (e.g., infection, phlebitis, hematoma formation, thrombosis).[25,28,61]

Isotonic and hypotonic solutions can be easily administered through any vein, but hypertonic solutions (e.g., solutions for total parenteral nutrition) must be delivered through large veins, such as the jugular vein. These vessels have higher blood flow, and, therefore, any hemolytic effects of the fluid can be minimized by dilution with the blood.

Central venous pressure (CVP) reflects the heart's ability to accommodate fluid administration. It is regulated by a balance between the ability of the right heart to pump blood to the lungs and the tendency for blood to flow from peripheral vessels back into the right atrium. Valuable information regarding the relationship among intravascular volume, venous return, and right heart function can indirectly be provided with these measurements. CVP monitoring can be useful as a clinical guide for determining rate of fluid administration, but not as an indication of fluid volume to be replaced.[7,55,56,74,77]

In small animals, the most frequently used superficial veins include the cephalic, medial femoral, and the lateral saphenous veins. In large animals, the jugular vein is most commonly used. Central vein (jugular or medial femoral vein) catheterization is preferred in patients that require long-term fluid administration or parenteral nutrition, administration of hypertonic solutions or irritating drugs, frequent blood sampling, or CVP monitoring.

Intraperitoneal. The intraperitoneal route is seldom used, because other routes are superior. Although fluid given IP is eventually absorbed, large volumes of fluid should not be infused IP. In addition, this method of administration can be painful, has a potential degree of injury or perforation of an abdominal organ, and creates the risk of peritonitis.

Intraosseous. Intraosseous catheters provide excellent access to the peripheral circulation, with absorption equivalent to that of intravenous infusion. Fluids can be administered via a needle or catheter introduced into the intramedullary space. The bones of choice for placement include the femur, humerus, and wing of the ilium. This is an excellent method for fluid delivery in young animals or in animals where vascular access is a problem. Fluids administered through the intramedullary space are almost immediately available to the general circulation and all solutions can be given, regardless of their composition. One limitation is the rate at which fluids can be delivered. Also, a major complication associated with this route is the potential for introduction of infection, resulting in osteomyelitis.[36,79] Secure placement of the intraosseous catheter can be a challenge but is of utmost importance to maintain vascular access and decrease infection risk.

Rate of Fluid Administration. The disease process, rate of fluid loss, severity of clinical signs, fluid composition and delivery route, and cardiac and renal function influence the rate of fluid administration.[25,28,61]

Patients with poor perfusion because of severe dehydration or hypovolemia must be given immediate and rapid intravenous fluid replacements. The goal is to restore intravascular fluid volume and improve tissue perfusion as quickly as possible, as long as the cardiopulmonary and renal systems can handle the fluid load. Animals with marginal cardiovascular function cannot tolerate rapid fluid infusion, so their deficits must be restored with greater care. These patients are excellent candidates for CVP monitoring. Improved perfusion is manifested by improved mucous membrane color and capillary refill time, stronger peripheral pulses, and resolution of tachycardia.

Critically ill, shocky, severely dehydrated, or poorly perfused patients may require infusion rates of 60 to 90 ml/kg/hr, to a volume equivalent to 1 total blood volume. Flow rates even higher than this may be required in some instances. The maximum rate of fluid administration is usually limited by mechanical ability to administer fluids. In a life-threatening situation, two or more catheters may be used simultaneously to administer large volumes of fluid. In addition, a commercially available pressure infusion cuff allows rapid delivery of fluid. Pressure should not exceed 300 mm Hg. Care should be taken to not introduce air into the system and risk infection or air emboli.

Replacement fluids can be given over 12 to 24 hours.[28,61] This decision is usually dictated by the animal's presenting condition and response to therapy. Patients with lesser deficits require less aggressive fluid therapy. After replacement needs have been managed and ongoing losses no longer exist, normal maintenance fluid requirements are 40 to 60 ml/kg/day or 1 ml/lb/hr. These fluid volumes can be given intravenously as bolus infusions or at a constant rate throughout the day, or subcutaneously, divided into three or four doses over a 24-hour period.

In hypoproteinemic animals, caution should be exercised with the rate of administration, even when the animal is severely dehydrated or poorly perfused. Diminished colloid in the vascular space results in less retention of fluid in the circulation, ultimately risking development of edema and respiratory compromise.[67]

Many sick animals have ongoing fluid losses (e.g., vomiting, diarrhea, excessive panting, exudates and effusions, polyuria). In these animals, sufficient fluid should be provided to replace both the water and electrolyte losses incurred.[25] It is helpful to record fluid volumes given and compare this with urine output.

Patients receiving fluid support should be closely monitored for signs of overhydration. These include restlessness, shivering, tachycardia, serous nasal or ocular discharge, respiratory distress, pulmonary crackles or rales, coughing as a result of pulmonary edema, vomiting, and diarrhea.[21,25] Fluid administration must then be slowed or stopped, depending on the severity of clinical signs.

TOTAL PARENTERAL NUTRITION

Fluid therapy should be considered as the first supportive measure in reestablishing nutritional balance. Only after the primary goals of rehydration, replacement of electrolytes, and normalization of acid-base balance should parenteral feeding be introduced. As a rule of thumb, animals that have been off food for 3 to 5 days should be considered candidates for total parenteral nutrition (TPN).[69]

Parenteral nutrition is indicated for patients that are severely malnourished and cannot meet nutritional needs adequately using the oral or enteral route. Ideally, nutrition should be maintained via the gastrointestinal tract. If any part of the alimentary tract is nonfunctional, nutrients can be infused IV for some time. Total parenteral nutrition is not an innocuous treatment. Complicating factors associated with TPN include placement and use of a central catheter dedicated solely to administration of TPN solution, potential septic and mechanical problems if the catheter not placed and maintained properly, possible metabolic disturbances as a result of TPN solution composition, concentration, and administration, and expense.[12,57,69,70]

The three main ingredients of a TPN solution are dextrose, amino acids, and lipids. Dextrose supplies the calories; amino acids supply protein, nitrogen, and electrolytes; and lipid emulsions serve as a concentrated energy source. Because TPN solutions are hypertonic, they must be infused into a central vein (e.g., jugular, medial femoral) to allow for rapid dilution of the fluid. Because of the high level of nutrients in TPN solutions, they should be infused slowly to prevent possible rebound hypoglycemia.[12,57,69,70]

TRANSFUSION MEDICINE

Proficiency in transfusion therapy and blood banking techniques is an invaluable skill for veterinary technicians. Blood products are used in treatment of many patients with hematologic disorders. Administration of blood products in private veterinary practices has always been hampered by the limited availability of blood.

Clinical Evaluation of Bleeding

An accurate history, thorough physical examination, and certain laboratory tests are used to evaluate bleeding patients, determine a diagnosis, and define a therapeutic plan.

History. Gather all pertinent information regarding patient history from the owners. Questions should be very clear and thought-provoking. Devising a list of questions for owners to review could help stimulate them to think of some very important, most likely not obvious, facts.

It is vital to evaluate the current bleeding episode. Determine whether the bleeding is localized to one site or is multifocal. Is this the animal's first bleeding episode, or is there a history of bleeding tendency? These facts can help characterize the bleeding as either an acquired or a hereditary disorder. The breed may suggest specific coagulopathies. Any information the owner may have regarding breed history could provide helpful clues. Many breeders are becoming educated in regard to bleeding disorders that affect their breed, and, specifically, their family line.

The animal's environmental history may suggest exposure to toxic substances, such as anticoagulant rodenticides or lead. Tick exposure should also be considered. Is the animal currently receiving any medication? Many drugs have a toxic effect on platelets, white blood cells, and red blood cells.[23] Also, many organic and other substances (e.g., onions, zinc) can cause hemolytic conditions. Does the animal have any previously diagnosed diseases? For example, animals with liver failure may have compromised clotting, because most clotting factors are produced by the liver.

Physical Examination. Small surface hemorrhages (e.g., petechiation, ecchymoses) and other minor bleeding (epistaxis, hematuria) suggest platelet or vascular abnormalities. Larger hemorrhages or bleeding into body cavities (e.g., hematoma formation, hemarthrosis, hemoperitoneum) suggest clotting factor deficiencies. A combination of these clinical signs is not uncommon. Mucous membrane color, capillary refill time, pulse rate and quality, and respiratory rate and effort can help provide useful information.

Laboratory Tests. Serial hematocrit determinations can determine progression or stabilization of bleeding. Red blood cell indices and morphology can help characterize an anemia.[98] A reticulocyte count helps classify the anemia as *regenerative* or *nonregenerative*. Keep in mind, however, that reticulocytosis (high reticulocyte numbers) is usually not evident until several days from the onset of anemia. A platelet count can help detect thrombocytopenia (low platelet count). Normal platelet numbers are 150,000 to 400,000/μl. Abnormal bleeding tends to occur with platelet counts below 40,000/μl. Some animals with a platelet count of 2,000/μl, however, do not exhibit abnormal bleeding.

Prothrombin time (PT) assesses the extrinsic and common clotting pathway, whereas the *activated partial thromboplastin time (APTT)* assesses the intrinsic and common clotting pathway.[46,97] The PT and APTT are prolonged when clotting factors are depleted to less than 30% of normal factor activity.[29] Increased levels of fibrin degradation products (FDP) in the blood indicate excessive bleeding and fibrinolysis and are also seen in animals with severe liver dysfunction.[97] If interpreted in conjunction with the PT,

APTT, and platelet count, the FDP level is used to diagnose disseminated intravascular coagulation.

Practical Hemostatic Tests

Estimated platelet count. An estimate of platelet number from a stained blood smear is much quicker than an actual platelet count. With some practice, platelet estimation can be reasonably accurate.[99] After routine preparation and staining, the blood smear is first scanned to ensure that platelets are evenly distributed on the smear and there is no platelet clumping. The average number of platelets in 5 to 10 oil-immersion fields is determined to estimate platelet numbers. This should be adequate to categorize platelet numbers as very low, low, normal, or high.[98] One platelet per oil-immersion field represents approximately 20,000 platelets.[46] Approximately 8 to 12 platelets should be seen per oil-immersion field. An estimated platelet count can quickly detect thrombocytopenia in an emergency situation, but a true platelet count is necessary to classify the severity of the depletion.

Bleeding time. Bleeding time is the time it takes for bleeding to stop after a minor vessel is punctured. *Buccal mucosa bleeding time* assesses the platelet and vascular portion of hemostasis. A disposable spring-loaded device is used to produce small, standardized incisions in the mucosal surface of the upper lip.[62] The duration of bleeding from these incisions is monitored.

The buccal mucosa bleeding time is a screening test. As with any screening test, it is not 100% sensitive, and, therefore, not all primary hemostatic defects can be detected. This test also does not differentiate between vascular defects and platelet function defects. Buccal mucosa bleeding time is prolonged with thrombocytopenia/thrombopathy, von Willebrand's disease, uremia, and aspirin therapy.[8,62] Do not perform this test on any patient that is known to be thrombocytopenic.

Cuticle bleeding time is useful for evaluating overall hemostasis. It is sensitive to defects in vascular integrity, platelet function, and coagulation.[45] The tip of a nail is cut, just into the quick, using a guillotine-type nail clipper (e.g., Resco). The nail is allowed to bleed freely, *undisturbed*, and the time until bleeding stops is noted. Normal bleeding time in dogs is less than 5 minutes and in cats is less than 3 minutes. If the nail resumes bleeding after it has stopped, clotting is considered abnormal.

Cuticle bleeding time is prolonged with primary or secondary hemostatic defects. The cuticle bleeding time is even less specific than the buccal mucosa bleeding time, in that it does not differentiate between primary and secondary hemostatic compromise. It is difficult to standardize, but it can be done consistently with practice. It can be painful, because it transects a richly innervated and highly vascular area of the nail. For this reason, the cuticle bleeding time is best performed on anesthetized patients. It is a good test to use for presurgical assessment of bleeding potential in patients at risk based on their history and physical examination.[27,97]

Activated clotting time. Activated clotting time (ACT) is a simple, inexpensive screening test for severe abnormalities in the intrinsic and common pathways of the clotting cascade. It evaluates the same pathways as the APTT.[46] Some argue that the ACT is less sensitive in detecting factor deficiencies in that factor levels must be decreased to less than 5% of normal before the ACT is prolonged, whereas the APTT is prolonged with a factor deficiency of less than 30% of normal.[97] Normal ACT in dogs is 60 to 110 seconds and 50 to 75 seconds in cats.

The ACT is prolonged with severe factor deficiency in the intrinsic and/or common clotting pathway (e.g., hemophilia), in the presence of inhibitors (e.g., heparin, warfarin), or in cases of severe thrombocytopenia resulting from lack of platelet phospholipid (mild prolongation of 10 to 20 seconds).[46,97] The ACT is inexpensive, easily learned, quick to perform, and reproducible, and it provides immediate results. It is a very useful measurement of coagulation in emergency situations. In most situations, the ACT should be followed up with an APTT.

Whole Blood and Blood Components

Initial collection yields fresh whole blood. However, a transfusion of fresh whole blood is not always indicated. The trend in veterinary transfusion medicine is to use blood components in transfusion therapy when possible, rather than whole blood. With the availability of variable-speed, temperature-controlled centrifuges and plastic storage bags with integral tubing for collection, processing, and administration, specific blood component therapy is possible. Whole blood can be stored or separated into packed red blood cells, fresh plasma, stored plasma, cryoprecipitate, or platelet-rich plasma/platelet concentrates. Blood components permit specific replacement therapy for specific disorders, reduce the number of transfusion reactions as a result of diminished exposure to foreign material, decrease the time needed for transfusion, and extend the use of one unit of whole blood.[89]

Blood comprises of two portions: the cellular portion (red blood cells, white blood cells, platelets) and plasma, which acts as a carrier medium for the cells, proteins, gases, nutrients, and waste products. Each component of blood has a specific function. Certain diseases necessitate replacement of one or any combination of these components.

Fresh Whole Blood. Whole blood is considered *fresh* for up to 6 hours after collection.[101] Fresh whole blood provides red blood cells (RBCs), white blood cells (WBCs), platelets, plasma proteins, and coagulation factors. Certain components in blood are more fragile

than others, and these become less effective over time and with changes in ambient temperature. Platelet and coagulation factor efficacy becomes questionable once whole blood is refrigerated.[101] Therefore, to achieve the full benefit of all components, administer fresh blood immediately after collection.

Fresh whole blood is transfused into actively bleeding, anemic animals with thrombocytopenia/thrombopathy, anemia with coagulopathies, disseminated intravascular coagulation, and massive hemorrhage. Massive transfusion is defined as infusion of a volume of blood, within a 24-hour period, approaching or exceeding replacement of the recipient's total blood volume.[101]

Stored Whole Blood. A unit of whole blood more than 6 hours old is termed *stored whole blood;* this provides RBCs and plasma proteins. The time a unit of whole blood can be stored under refrigeration depends on the anticoagulant-preservative solution used in collection. With the advantages of use of blood components and the wider availability of these products as a result of commercial blood banks, use of stored whole blood is no longer considered the treatment of choice.[14] Although it seems logical that blood loss should be replaced with whole blood, most blood loss is adequately treated by replacing the circulating volume with packed RBCs and crystalloid or colloid solutions. This is perfectly adequate therapy for most acutely bleeding patients. However, stored whole blood can be used in patients that require intravascular volume expansion, as well as improved oxygen-carrying capabilities.

Packed Red Blood Cells. *Packed RBCs* can be harvested from whole blood (fresh or stored) by centrifuging the unit at 5000 G at 4° C for 5 minutes.[101] If a refrigerated centrifuge is not available, RBCs can be harvested by allowing whole blood to separate by sedimentation over 1 to 2 days. After sedimentation, the plasma is removed, ideally with a plasma extractor, and placed in a sterile transfer pack. If a plasma extractor is unavailable, a syringe and needle or two heavy books can be used to create the same force as the plasma extractor. Ideally, packed RBCs should be reconstituted with a nutrient solution before storage to maintain the cells in a healthier environment. This extends storage time; also, reconstitution of the RBCs reduces viscosity during administration. Packed RBCs can be refrigerated at 1° to 6° C, with storage time determined by the anticoagulant-preservative or additive solution used in collection and processing.[82,103,104] If a nutrient solution is not used at the time of processing, packed RBCs can be reconstituted with 100 ml of 0.9% NaCl before administration to reduce viscosity. Reconstitution with nonisotonic fluids may cause RBC damage.

Packed RBCs are the component of choice for treating most anemias (e.g., hemolytic anemia, symptomatic oxygen-carrying deficiencies).[14] In human medicine, more than 80% of all transfusions performed incorporate packed RBCs.[64,95]

Fresh or Fresh-Frozen Plasma. *Fresh plasma* is the by-product of the harvesting of packed RBCs from fresh whole blood. Fresh plasma provides plasma proteins and coagulation factors but does not contain viable platelets. The same value is retained for up to 1 year if fresh plasma is frozen at a minimum of -20° C within 6 hours after the time of collection.[101] If natural separation is used in preparing plasma, clotting factor efficacy is compromised. *Fresh-frozen plasma* is used in animals with coagulation factor deficiencies (e.g., liver disease, disseminated intravascular coagulation, anticoagulant rodenticide toxicity).

Stored Plasma. Stored plasma is the by-product of harvesting packed blood cells from stored whole blood. Stored plasma provides plasma proteins only; it contains no functional platelets or coagulation factors. Stored plasma can be administered after refrigeration at 1° to 6° C for up to 35 days, depending on the anticoagulant preservative solution used in collection, or after freezing at -20° C or colder for up to 5 years.

Stored plasma can be used in cases of acute hypoproteinemia (e.g., parvoviral enteritis). If the animal is severely or chronically protein deficient, stored plasma must be administered in large volumes to have a measurable impact on pulmonary edema, pleural effusion, and oncotic pressure. In such cases, use of synthetic colloid solutions should be considered, because they are more effective and more readily available.

Cryoprecipitate. Cryoprecipitate is harvested from fresh-frozen plasma that has been thawed at 1° to 6° C until it is of slushy consistency (approximately 12 to 18 hours). The slurried plasma is then centrifuged at 5000 G at 4° C for 7 minutes.[101] Plasma is expressed using a plasma extractor, leaving behind a white, foamy precipitate (mostly adhered to the bag) in approximately 50 to 100 ml of liquid plasma. This precipitate provides von Willebrand's factor, factor VIII:C, fibrinogen, and fibronectin. Cryoprecipitate can be frozen at -20° C or colder and has a shelf life of 1 year from the date of collection. Cryoprecipitate can be used in patients with von Willebrand's disease, hemophilia A, and hypofibrinogenemia.

Platelet-Rich Plasma. Platelet-rich plasma is harvested by centrifuging fresh whole blood at 1200 G at 22° to 24° C for 2 minutes.[16] After centrifugation, the bag is allowed to sit undisturbed for 30 minutes and the platelet-rich plasma is removed. This product may then be stored at room temperature for up to 72 hours with intermittent agitation. Refrigerated platelets do not maintain function or viability as well as platelets stored at room temperature.[101]

The major indication for platelet transfusion is to stop bleeding in patients with low platelet numbers and/or impaired function. A significant volume is needed to measurably increase platelet numbers in larger patients. In some patients, however, bleeding stops after platelet transfusion without a measurable increase in platelet number. Because of the impracticality associated with production of this component, in veterinary medicine we routinely treat thrombocytopenia/thrombopathy accompanied by active bleeding with fresh whole blood, through which the patient receives both platelets and RBCs. In conditions causing platelet destruction, such as idiopathic thrombocytopenic purpura, transfused platelets survive only minutes rather than days.[75] If the patient is acutely bleeding into a vital structure (e.g., brain, myocardium, pleural cavity), platelet transfusion may be warranted. In most instances, however, medical management is most often the treatment of choice.

Blood Groups

Blood Groups of Dogs. Fourteen specific antigens, or *blood types,* have been identified on the surface of canine RBCs.[1,6,18,87,91,92,93,94] These include dog erythrocyte antigen (DEA) 1.1, 1.2, 1.3, and 3 to 13. Because of the limited availability and inadequacies associated with typing reagents, limited work has been done to determine the prevalence of these blood types and their significance in transfusion.

The canine "universal donor" blood type is DEA 1.1 negative, and, ideally, also should be DEA 1.2 and DEA 7 negative.[42] The most severe antigen-antibody reaction is seen after transfusion with these antigens, most specifically DEA 1.1.[42] Significant naturally occurring alloantibodies do not occur in dogs; therefore, antigen-antibody reactions are not likely to occur after an initial transfusion. However, dogs that are DEA 1.1, 1.2, and 7 negative can develop alloantibodies to DEA 1.1, 1.2, and 7 from a mismatched transfusion. This can occur within 4 to 14 days after an initial transfusion.[6,87,106,107] These antibodies can destroy the donor's RBCs (delayed hemolytic transfusion reaction), ultimately minimizing the benefits of the transfusion. Because of the absence of clinically significant naturally occurring alloantibodies in dogs, the initial crossmatch performed on a dog that has not previously been transfused should yield a compatible result. However, crossmatching is important with subsequent transfusions.

Ideally, all blood donors and all recipients should be blood typed and crossmatched before transfusion. Blood that is DEA 1.1 positive should be administered only to dogs that are DEA 1.1 positive. A commercial card blood typing kit allows veterinary practices to easily and economically test for this antigen (Fig. 24-3).[1,52] If typing is unavailable or in an emergency situation, recipients should be crossmatched with "universal donors" before transfusion to avoid sensitization.

Blood Groups of Cats. One blood group system, the AB system, has been recognized in cats. It contains three blood types: A, B, and the extremely rare AB.[2,59] These

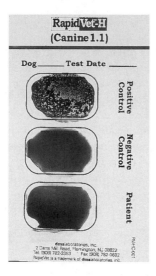

FIG. 24-3 Commercial canine blood typing card using DEA 1.1. *(Available from dms Laboratories, Flemington, NJ.)*

blood type	red blood cell agglutination with	
	anti-A serum	anti-B reagent
type A	strong	none
type B	none	strong
type AB	strong	strong

FIG. 24-4 Feline blood typing using a simple whole blood test. Anti-A serum is collected from any type B cat. The anti-B reagent is lectin triticum vulgaris. *(Available from Dr. Urs Giger, Veterinary Hospital of the University of Pennsylvania, Philadelphia, PA.)*

blood types represent antigens, or protein markers, on the RBC surface.[50] Nearly all domestic shorthair and domestic longhair cats have type A blood, the most common. Many purebred cats (and some domestic shorthairs) have type B blood.[2,41,44] The proportion of A and B types varies among cat breeds and also nationally and internationally.[2,43,44]

Cats differ from dogs in that they have significant, naturally occurring alloantibodies against the other blood type.[2,11,41,44,49] Cats with type B blood appear to have very strong naturally occurring anti-A alloantibodies, whereas type A cats have relatively weak anti-B alloantibodies.[2,11] These alloantibodies can cause two serious problems.[99] Cats with relatively rare type B blood can experience potentially fatal transfusion reactions if they are transfused with the common type A blood. Cellular components of mismatched transfusions have short half-lives and are ineffective.[3,4,39,40] If a queen with type B blood is bred to a type A tom and the mating produces kittens with type A blood, the antibodies in the colostrum of the queen destroy the RBCs in the kittens, a condition called *neonatal isoerythrolysis*.[13,38]

After administering type B blood to a type A cat, there may not be any obvious clinical reaction, but the transfused red cells have a half-life of only approximately 2 days.[40] Ultimately, this is of no benefit to the patient. With transfusion of type A blood to a type B cat, the type A RBCs survive only minutes to hours and clinical signs are severe, sometimes fatal.[40] Administration of a small amount of blood to test for incompatibility is no longer an acceptable procedure. Life-threatening acute hemolytic transfusion reactions can be observed with administration of as little as 1 ml of AB-incompatible

blood.[49] These reactions can be avoided by typing and crossmatching the blood of donors and patients. A simple test using whole blood and blood typing reagents is available (Fig. 24-4).[49] Blood typing cards similar to those used in dogs are also commercially available, yielding accurate results in minutes.[1]

Blood Groups of Horses. Seven blood groups have been recognized in horses: A, C, D, K, P, Q, and U.[73,105] None of these types is considered a "universal donor," and even a single transfusion of cross-matched blood can elicit alloantibody production. These alloantibodies can cause serious problems if a second transfusion is given or if a brood mare is given the transfusion, because the mare's foal could develop neonatal isoerythrolysis. Alloantigens Aa and Qa are most prevalent and immunogenic. Transfusion of Aa- or Qa-positive blood into an Aa- or Qa-negative horse elicits alloantibody production, and subsequent transfusion can cause a severe hemolytic reaction.[73,105]

Sources of Donor Blood

Historically, veterinarians have relied on donors living within the hospital facility as a source of blood for transfusion purposes. The cost of an in-house donor is quite often overlooked, and the charges for a unit of blood are severely underestimated.[60] In the past few years, several commercial blood banks have been established to help meet blood transfusion needs in primarily small animal medicine. Purchasing products from these banks and maintaining an inventory within your facility are much more efficient and cost-effective than maintaining a donor colony within your hospital. Using employee-owned personal pets and healthy client-owned animals as blood donors is a good alternative to maintaining in-house donors. For reasons to be discussed, this type of program is more practical for dogs than cats.[49]

Canine Blood Donors. Blood donors can be recruited through employee personal pets, client-owned animals, breeders, and organized dog clubs.[10,32] Many owners are happy to volunteer their animal for periodic blood donation (e.g., 3 to 4 times yearly) once they understand the need for blood products in veterinary medicine.

Donors must be at least 1 year of age and weigh at least 25 kg.[10,14,32] Dogs can safely donate up to 22 ml/kg body weight every 21 days without need for nutritional supplementation.[81] They should have current vaccination status for distemper, hepatitis, leptospirosis, parainfluenza, parvovirus, and rabies, not be on medication at the time of donation (excluding heartworm and flea preventive), and be in good health. Good temperament is a must for successful donation.

A history, physical examination, and hematocrit (above 40%) or hemoglobin concentration (above 13.5 g/dl) should be obtained before each donation. A complete blood count, blood chemistry profile, and testing for infectious agents (e.g., *Ehrlichia canis, Babesia canis*) should be performed annually. Donors should be negative for DEA 1.1, and preferably, DEA 1.2 and 7.[42] Dogs that are positive for these antigens can be accepted into the donor pool, as long as recipients are typed before transfusion. DEA 1.1 positive blood should be given only to patients positive for DEA 1.1. Donors can be screened for von Willebrand's factor antigen levels to identify the population of the donor pool with the highest concentration of this adhesive protein for use in patients with such deficiencies.

Feline Blood Donors. At present, there are few commercial feline blood banks. In addition, volunteer programs for cats hold many risks. Although blood can be collected from dogs with minimum restraint, most donor cats must be sedated for blood collection. There are legal ramifications associated with sedating employees' personal pets for blood donation. Another concern is that cats can harbor infectious agents more readily than dogs.[49] Because of this, only totally indoor cats should be used.

Feline blood donors should be large, good-natured, lean, young adults weighing at least 5 kg.[9,64] Blood collection is easier in cats with short hair. Good health can be verified through history, physical exam, and routine laboratory testing. Donors should have current vaccination status for rhinotracheitis, calicivirus, panleukopenia, and rabies. Annual laboratory screening should include a complete blood count, serum biochemistry profile, and screening for feline leukemia virus, feline immunodeficiency virus, feline infectious peritonitis virus, and *Hemobartonella felis*.[9,37,64] Before each

donation, the hematocrit (above 35%) or hemoglobin (above 11 g/dl) should be checked.[49] A well-balanced, high-performance diet should be fed, with iron supplementation if donors are used on a monthly basis.

Because of the presence of naturally occurring alloantibodies, there is no "universal donor" type in cats. All feline blood donors and recipients must be blood typed, and only typed, matched blood should be administered. The extremely rare blood type AB cat can be safely transfused with type A blood.[48]

Equine Blood Donors. Donor horses should be healthy geldings, screened for equine infectious anemia, and ideally have blood free of Aa, Qa, and Ca antigens, as well as alloantibodies.[73,105] Quarter Horses and Standardbreds are most likely to be suitable, as these breeds have a lower prevalence of Aa and Qa antigens. Donor horses should never have received a blood transfusion and should be regularly screened for alloantibodies.

Blood Collection

Anticoagulants. Several anticoagulants, anticoagulant-preservatives, and additive solutions are available for collection of blood for transfusion.[82,102,104,105] These solutions maintain blood cell viability during blood storage. Storage time varies with the anticoagulant preservative solution used.

Citrate-phosphate-dextrose-adenine (CPDA-1) is considered the best anticoagulant-preservative solution. Whole blood remains viable for 35 days and blood cells for 21 days. It is used at a ratio of 1 ml of CPDA-1 to 7 ml of blood. With *citrate-phosphate-dextrose* (CPD), cells remain viable for 21 days. It is used at a ratio of 1 ml of CPD to 7 ml of blood. In *acid-citrate-dextrose* (ACD), cells remain viable for 21 days in dogs and 28 days in cats.[71,88] It is used at a ratio of 1 ml of ACD to 7 ml of blood.

Sodium citrate (3.8%) has no preservative properties and citrated blood must be used within 24 to 48 hours. It is used at a ratio of 1 ml of sodium citrate to 9 ml of blood. Heparin is not recommended for transfusion purposes. It has no preservative properties and heparinized blood must be used within 24 to 48 hours. It is used at a ratio of 5 to 10 units of heparin to 1 ml of blood. Additive solutions (e.g., Adsol, Fenwal Laboratories; Nutricell, Miles) are protein-free solutions added to RBCs after plasma removal from whole blood. Red blood cells remain viable for approximately 37 days.

Blood Collection Systems. Whole blood is most often collected into commercially available plastic bags (available from Baxter Healthcare and Miles). These sterile bags are considered "closed" collection systems in that they allow for collection, preparation, and storage of blood and blood components without exposure to the environment.[101] A single bag is used for collection of blood to be administered as whole blood. It consists of a main collection bag containing anticoagulant preservative solution and integral tubing with an attached 16-gauge needle. This system is not recommended for component preparation in that the bag must be entered to harvest components, risking bacterial contamination. If the bag is entered, the product must be used within 24 hours.[101]

Other collection systems consist of a primary collection bag containing anticoagulant preservative solution, usually CPD, and one, two, or three satellite bags intended for component preparation. One satellite bag may contain 100 ml of an additive solution used for RBC reconstitution after plasma removal (Fig. 24-5). Additive solutions (e.g., saline, dextrose, adenine) extend storage time by enhancing packed RBC survival and function.[102,103,104] All bags are attached via integral tubing, allowing for collection, processing, and storage of products within a closed system.

Vacuum-filled glass bottles containing ACD anticoagulant-preservative have been the most popular collection system used in veterinary medicine.[32] Although blood collection is much easier with this system, it has many limitations and disadvantages. This is considered an "open" collection system subject to contamination. The glass activates platelets and certain clotting factors. The foam created during collection causes hemolysis, and component preparation is not possible.[35,80]

Blood collection using a sterile syringe containing an anticoagulant is effective but is considered an "open" system. Blood can be transferred from the syringe into an empty sterile bag or transfer pack, making delivery more efficient.[63] Products collected via syringe should not be stored.

Blood Collection. The recommended collection site is the jugular vein. Because of this vein's size and increased blood flow, RBC trauma is minimized during collection. Blood should be collected via a single venipuncture to avoid cell damage and excessive activation of coagulation factors. Strict aseptic technique and use of sterile equipment minimize the possibility of bacterial contamination.

In dogs and horses, blood can be collected using a commercial collection bag containing a sterile anticoagulant-preservative solution or with a large (e.g., 60 ml) syringe containing sterile anticoagulant (Box 24-2).

Because of the difficulties associated with collection, component preparation, and limited storage time with an "open" system, most cats in need of transfusions receive fresh whole blood collected with a syringe. A 19- or 21-gauge butterfly catheter or 20-gauge needle attached to a three-way stopcock and sterile 10- to 30-ml syringes containing anticoagulant may be used.[49] Donor cats are typically sedated. During collection, the syringes should be gently inverted to allow for mixing of blood and anticoagulant, preventing clot formation. Blood should be

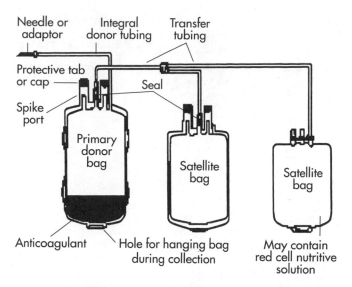

FIG. 24-5 Triple blood collection bag for use in preparing blood components. *(From Hohenhaus AE: Transfusion medicine,* Prob Vet Med 4, 1992).

transferred to a transfer pack after collection.[63] This is considered an "open" system with risk of bacterial contamination, so feline blood collected in this way should not be stored.

Blood Administration

Blood Typing and Crossmatching. Ideally, patients should be blood-typed and crossmatched before any blood transfusion. If blood typing reagents or cards are not available, at the very least a blood crossmatch test should be done. Blood typing determines the blood group antigens on the surface of RBCs. A blood crossmatch test is used to identify antibodies in donor or recipient plasma against recipient or donor RBCs. The *major blood crossmatch test* detects alloantibodies in the recipient's plasma against donor RBCs, whereas the *minor blood crossmatch test* detects alloantibodies in the donor plasma against recipient RBCs (Box 24-3). If there is evidence of macroscopic agglutination of the patient's blood (rarely seen in cats) or severe hemolysis of the patient's blood sample, a blood crossmatch test cannot be performed.[49,98]

Dogs being transfused for the first time (not sensitized) can have a compatible crossmatch, despite differing blood types, because they often do not have significant, naturally occurring alloantibody. Even if type-specific blood components are used for the first transfusion, crossmatching is advised because all RBC antigen groups have not been fully characterized. Although the blood crossmatch test can detect many incompatibilities, it does not guarantee against future sensitization. A blood crossmatch test should always be performed in dogs that were previously transfused. If neither crossmatching nor typing is available, or it is an emergency situation with no time

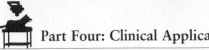

Box 24-2 Canine and equine blood collection using commercial bags

Materials:

commercial blood collection bag (450 ml) with 16-gauge needle

tube stripper

heat sealer, sealer clips/crimper

Procedure:

1. Clip the hair over the jugular groove and surgically prepare the area.

2. Restrain the donor securely but comfortably (dogs in right lateral recumbency, horses standing).

3. Apply pressure at the thoracic inlet to facilitate visualization and palpation of the jugular vein.

4. Perform venipuncture using the 16-gauge needle attached to the main collection bag. The bag should be positioned lower than the animal to aid gravitational flow.

5. Periodically invert the bag gently to mix the blood with anticoagulant solution. The collection bag should be weighed intermittently to ensure that an appropriate volume of blood is collected (1 ml of blood weighs approximately 1 g). One unit of

blood should contain 450 ml of blood ± 10% (i.e., weighs 405 to 495 g). If lesser amounts are collected (300-405 ml), only the RBCs can be used after plasma removal because of concern for excessive citrate in plasma and possible resultant hypocalcemia in certain patients (e.g., liver disease, severe hypothermia).[101]

6. When the bag is full, remove the needle from the jugular vein and apply pressure over the venipuncture site to prevent hematoma formation. The donor should remain recumbent (dogs) or quietly restrained (horses) until clotting has occurred.

7. Strip remaining blood from the tubing into the bag and mix it with anticoagulant solution (Fig. 24-6, A).

8. Allow the tubing to refill with anticoagulated blood and clamp the distal end with a heat sealer clip (Fig. 24-6, B and 24-6 C).

9. Section the entire length of the collection tubing into 3- or 4-inch segments to be used for subsequent crossmatches (Fig. 24-6 D).

10. Label the bag with donor identification, date of collection, date of expiration, blood type, unit volume, and anticoagulant used.

---

for crossmatching, universal donor blood (DEA 1.1, 1.2, and 7 negative) should be given to the dog. All feline patients with unknown blood type should be crossmatched. It is possible to predict the blood type of a cat based on the blood crossmatch test results because of the presence of naturally occurring alloantibodies (excluding the rare blood type AB).[49] Crossmatching of equine blood is done in commercial veterinary laboratories. Most horses not previously transfused can tolerate transfusion of whole blood.

Preparing Blood for Transfusion. Refrigerated blood may be gently warmed by allowing it to sit at room temperature for approximately 30 minutes. Properly administered cold blood will not increase the chance of a transfusion reaction, but large amounts of cold blood infused rapidly can induce hypothermia and cardiac arrhythmias. Warming of RBC products is recommended for neonates and patients that require large-volume transfusion.[101] In an emergency situation, the tubing of the administration set can be immersed in a warm-water bath (not to exceed 37° C) so that the blood is warmed as it passes through the tubing. The entire unit should not be warmed at one time. Frozen products should be thawed in a 37° C warm-water bath. Blood products should not be exposed

to temperatures exceeding 50° C, because this results in hemolysis and protein denaturation. Warming RBC products or thawing plasma products in a microwave oven is not recommended.

Transfusion Volume. The aim of transfusion in anemic patients is to correct the clinical signs rather than return the packed cell volume (PCV, hematocrit) to normal. One generally aims to raise the PCV by approximately 10%. The volume of whole blood or plasma needed can be calculated as follows:[47,105]

whole blood volume required (ml) in dogs and cats =

body weight in lb × (40 in dogs, 30 in cats) × desired

$$\frac{PCV - recipient's}{PCV \ donor's \ PCV}$$

whole blood volume required (L) in horses =

(0.08 × recipient's body weight in kg) ×

$$\frac{30 - recipient's \ PCV}{donor's \ PCV}$$

plasma volume required (ml) = 3 to 5 ml/lb up to 4 times daily (repeat as needed)

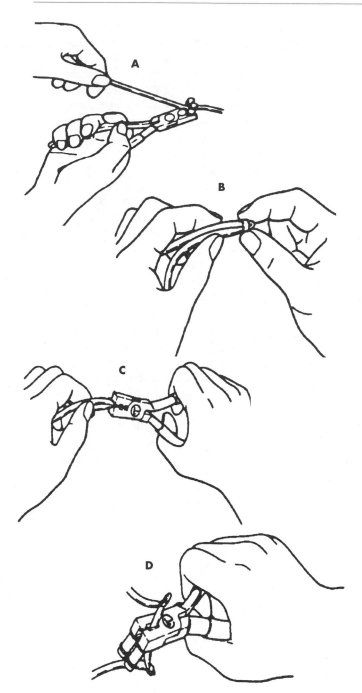

FIG. 24-6   **A,** Using the roller part of the stripper, strip the blood from the distal end of the tubing into the blood collection bag and allow it to mix with the anticoagulated blood. **B,** To seal the donor bag and tubing, fold the tubing and place a sealer clip over the folded tubing. **C,** Crimp the sealing clip. Repeat this for as many tubing segments as needed. **D,** Cut the tubing between each sealed segment to obtain samples for crossmatching. *(From Hohenhaus AE: Transfusion medicine,* Prob Vet Med 4, 1992).

Box 24-3 Blood crossmatching

Materials:

anticoagulated blood from donor and recipient

centrifuge

test tubes

0.9% sodium chloride

microscope slides

Procedure:

1. Collect 2 ml of EDTA-anticoagulated blood each from the donor and recipient.

2. Centrifuge the blood samples for 1 minute at 3000 G. Remove the plasma to prelabeled tubes.

3. Make a 2% RBC suspension by mixing 0.1 ml of the RBCs and 5 ml of 0.9% saline solution. Mix the suspension.

4. Centrifuge the suspension for 1 minute and discard the supernatant. Resuspend the RBCs in another 5 ml of 0.9% saline and centrifuge. Repeat this washing procedure three times.

5. Place two drops of the recipient's plasma and two drops of the donor's RBC suspension in a 3-ml test tube; this is the *major* part of the crossmatch. Then place two drops of the recipient's RBCs and two drops of the donor's plasma in another 3-ml test tube; this is the *minor* part of the crossmatch. Mix well and incubate the tubes for 30 minutes at room temperature.

6. For controls, use the donor's and recipient's own cells and plasma following the same procedure as above. Centrifuge for 1 minute at 3000 G. You now have a total of four tubes.

7. *Reading the crossmatch:* Grossly check for agglutination and hemolysis, and then place a drop on a slide and examine microscopically at 40× agglutination.

Administration Routes. Blood and blood components are best administered intravenously, making the infused RBCs or plasma products immediately available to the general circulation. Intraosseous infusion is used in puppies or kittens when vascular access is difficult or unsuccessful. Blood cells and proteins are available to the general circulation within 5 minutes after intraosseous infusion.[79,96] The most common sites for intraosseous catheter placement are the trochanteric fossa of the femur, the wing of the ilium, and the shaft of the humerus.[96] Care should be taken in placement of these catheters because of the risk of osteomyelitis.

Intraperitoneal infusion of blood products is not recommended. Transfusion by this route can be painful and there is danger of causing peritonitis. Absorption of blood cells is delayed; only approximately 50% of infused RBCs and proteins reach the circulation after 24 hours.[96]

Administration Rates. Administration rates vary. For example, a patient with massive hemorrhage may require a more rapid transfusion than a normovolemic patient with chronic anemia. Blood should not be administered at a rate exceeding 22 ml/kg/hr.[47,105] However, the infusion rate is less critical in a hypovolemic animal than in a normovolemic animal, where circulatory overload is a potential problem. Animals with cardiovascular compromise cannot tolerate infusion rates above 4 ml/kg/hr.[47]

Initially in all patients, blood should be delivered slowly (0.5 to 1.0 ml/lb during the first 15 to 20 minutes) while monitoring for signs of an acute transfusion reaction.[49] Infusion of a single unit of blood or blood component should not take longer than 4 hours.[101] Before infusion, baseline values of attitude, rectal temperature, pulse rate and quality, respiratory rate and character, mucous membrane color, capillary refill time, hematocrit, total plasma protein, and plasma and urine color should be recorded.[42] Patients should be monitored closely during transfusion. Blood values should be checked after transfusion to ensure that the desired effect has been achieved.

Transfusion Reactions

Patients should be carefully monitored for any adverse reactions during and for several weeks following transfusion. Transfusion reactions can be immune-mediated or nonimmune-mediated in origin.[15,47,58,64,96] Immune-mediated hemolytic reactions can occur within minutes or up to 21 days after transfusion.[80,96] Hemolytic transfusion reactions are the most serious but are rare. In acute situations, intravascular hemolysis is due to pre-existing antibodies, as seen in the mismatched transfusion of feline type A blood to a cat with type B blood, or in previously sensitized DEA 1.1 negative dogs receiving DEA 1.1 positive blood.[42,49] Clinical signs include fever, tachycardia, weakness, tremors, vomiting, collapse, hemoglobinemia, and hemoglobinuria. Hemolytic transfusion reactions can eventually lead to renal failure as a result of damage caused by clearance of RBC debris.[15,22] The most common hemolytic transfusion reaction is delayed in presentation. Sensitization can occur as a result of a mismatched transfusion, resulting in hemolysis. This phenomenon can occur for up to 21 days as antibodies are produced.

Nonhemolytic transfusion reactions are a result of antibodies to white blood cells, platelets, or plasma proteins.[96] These reactions are most often transient in nature and do not cause life-threatening situations. Clinical signs include anaphylaxis, urticaria, pruritus, fever, and neurologic signs. Vomiting can be noted with any type of transfusion reaction. Patients receiving blood products should be fasted before administration to avoid this potential complication.[37,49]

Various factors can cause nonimmune-mediated transfusion reactions. Any type of trauma to the RBCs can cause hemolysis (e.g., overheating, freezing, warming and then rechilling, mixing RBC products with nonisotonic solutions, and collecting or infusing blood through small needles or catheters). Bacterial pyrogens and sepsis can be a complication of improperly collected and stored blood. Dark brown to black supernatant plasma in stored blood indicates digested hemoglobin from bacterial growth.[5,47,96] Any blood with discolored supernatant should be immediately discarded. Patients given such blood typically develop a febrile response 15 to 20 minutes after the start of infusion; the response usually subsides within 2 to 4 hours of transfusion completion.

Citrate intoxication may occur when the citrate/blood volume ratio is disproportionate or in massively transfused patients, particularly in patients with liver dysfunction.[5,58,96] Common signs include tremors, cardiac arrhythmias, and decreased cardiac output. This compromised state can be confirmed by obtaining an ionized serum calcium level. If citrate toxicity if suspected, blood administration should be discontinued and calcium gluconate administered IV.

Because blood is a colloid solution, vascular overload is a potential complication of transfusion. Clinical signs include coughing (as a result of pulmonary edema), dyspnea, cyanosis, tachycardia, and vomiting.[5,22] If volume overload is of concern, blood administration should be temporarily discontinued and supportive care instituted. Pulmonary microembolism can occur with massive transfusion as a result of microaggregates of platelets, white blood cells, red blood cells, or fibrin strands.[5,22] This can be prevented by using a commercially made blood infusion set with an in-line filter system (e.g., 170μ). All blood products should be filtered to help prevent thromboembolic complications.

REFERENCES

1. Andrews GA, Chavey PS, Smith JE: Production, characterization, and applications of a murine monoclonal antibody to dog erythrocyte antigen 1.1, *J Am Vet Med Assoc* 201:1549-1552, 1992.
2. Auer L, Bell K: The AB blood group system in cats, *Anim Genet* 12:287-297, 1981.
3. Auer L, Bell K: Transfusion reactions in cats due to AB blood group incompatibility, *Res Vet Sci* 35:145-152, 1983.
4. Auer L, Bell K, Coates S: Blood transfusion reactions in the cat, *J Am Vet Med Assoc* 180:729-730, 1982.

5. Authement JM, Wolfsheimer KJ, Catchings S: Canine blood component therapy: product preparation, storage, and administration, *J Am Anim Hosp Assoc* 23:483, 1986.

6. Bell K: *The blood groups of domestic animals.* In Agar AS, Board PG, editors: *Red blood cells of domestic animals,* Amsterdam, 1983, Elsevier Science Publishers.

7. Bell FW, Osborne CA: *Maintenance fluid therapy.* In Kirk RW, editor: *Current veterinary therapy X, small animal practice,* Philadelphia, 1989, WB Saunders.

8. Brassard JA, Meyers KM: Evaluation of the buccal bleeding time and platelet glass bead retention assays of hemostasis in the dog, *Thromb Haemos* 62:191-195, 1990.

9. Brooks M: Transfusion medicine, part I, *Proc Am College Vet Int Med* 8:77-80, 1990.

10. Bucheler J, Cotter SM: *Outpatient blood donor program.* In Hohenhaus AE, editor: *Transfusion medicine, problems in veterinary medicine,* Philadelphia, 1992, JB Lippincott.

11. Bucheler J, Giger U: Alloantibodies against A and B blood types in cats, *Vet Immunol Immunopathol* 38:283-295, 1993.

12. Buffington CAT: *Nutritional management of critical care patients.* In *14th Kal Kan Waltham symposium: emergency medicine and critical care medicine,* Vernon, Cal, 1991, Kal Kan Foods.

13. Cain GR, Suzuki Y: Presumptive neonatal isoerythrolysis in cats, *J Am Vet Med Assoc* 187:46-48, 1985.

14. Callan MB et al: Canine red blood cell transfusion practice, *J Am Anim Hosp Assoc* 32:303-311, 1996.

15. Capon SM, Sacher RA: Hemolytic transfusion reactions: a review of mechanisms, sequelae, and management, *J Intensive Care Med* 4:100, 1989.

16. Clemmons RM et al: Platelet function, size and yield in whole blood and in platelet-rich plasma prepared using differing centrifugation force and time in domestic and food producing animals, *Thromb Haemost* 50:838-843, 1983.

17. Coles EH: *Kidney function.* In *Veterinary clinical pathology,* ed 4, Philadelphia, 1986, WB Saunders.

18. Colling DT, Saison R: Canine blood groups: I. Description of new erythrocyte specificities, *Anim Blood Groups Biochem Gen* 11:1-12, 1980.

19. Cornelius LM: *Fluid, electrolyte, and acid-base therapy.* In Lorenz MD et al: *Small animal medical therapeutics,* Philadelphia, 1992, JB Lippincott.

20. Cornelius LM: Fluid therapy in small animal practice, *J Am Vet Med Assoc* 176:110-114, 1980.

21. Cornelius LM et al: Physiologic effects of rapid infusion of Ringer's lactate solution into dogs, *Am J Vet Res* 39:1185-1190, 1978.

22. Cotter SM: *Clinical transfusion medicine.* In Cotter SM, editor: *Comparitive transfusion medicine: advances in veterinary science and comparative Medicine,* vol 36, San Diego, 1991, Academic Press.

23. Davenport DJ, Carakostas MC: Platelet disorders in the dog and cat: Part I: physiology and pathogenesis, *Comp Cont Educ Pract Vet* 4:762-797, 1982.

24. DiBartola SP: *Disorders of sodium and water: hypernatremia and hyponatremia.* In DiBartola: *Fluid therapy in small animal practice,* Philadelphia, 1992, WB Saunders.

25. DiBartola SP: *Introduction to fluid therapy.* In DiBartola SP: *Fluid therapy in small animal practice,* Philadelphia, 1992, WB Saunders.

26. DiBartola SP, de Morais A: Disorders of potassium and water: hyperkalemia and hypokalemia. In DiBartola SP: *Fluid therapy in small animal practice,* Philadelphia, 1992, WB Saunders.

27. Dodds JW: Personal communication, 1996.

28. Drobatz K: Personal communication, 1996.

29. Duncan JR, Prasse KW: *Veterinary laboratory medicine: clinical pathology,* ed 2, Ames, Iowa, 1986, Iowa State University Press.

30. Duval D: Use of hypertonic saline solutions in hypovolemic shock, *Comp Cont Educ Pract Vet* 17:1228-1231, 1995.

31. Eisenbrandt DL, Smith JE: Evaluation of preservatives and containers for storage of canine blood, *J Am Vet Med Assoc* 163:988, 1973.

32. Feldman BF, Kristensen AT: Modern veterinary blood banking practices and their applications in companion animal practice. In Kristensen AT, Feldman BF, editors: *The veterinary clinics of North America, small animal practice: canine and feline transfusion medicine,* Philadelphia, 1995, WB Saunders.

33. Finco DR: *Fluid therapy.* In Kirk RW, editor: *Current veterinary therapy VI.* Philadelphia, 1977, WB Saunders.

34. Frandson RD: *Anatomy and physiology of farm animals,* ed 3, Philadelphia, 1981, Lea & Febiger.

35. Gabrio VW, Finch CA, Huennekens FM: Erythrocyte preservation: a topic in molecular biochemistry, *Blood* 11:103, 1956.

36. Garvey MS: Fluid and electrolyte balance in critical patients, *Vet Clin North Am* 19:1021-1057, 1989.

37. Giger U: *Feline transfusion medicine.* In Hohenhaus AE, editor: *Transfusion medicine, problems in veterinary medicine,* Philadelphia, 1992, JB Lippincott.

38. Giger U: *The feline AB blood group system and incompatibility reactions.* In Kirk RW, editor: *Current veterinary therapy XI.* Philadelphia, 1992, WB Saunders.

39. Giger U, Akol KG: Acute hemolytic transfusion reaction in an Abyssinian cat with blood type B, *J Vet Intern Med* 4: 315-316, 1990.

40. Giger U, Bucheler J: Transfusion of type-A and type-B blood to cats, *J Am Vet Med Assoc* 198: 411-418, 1991.

41. Giger U, Buchelor J, Patterson DF: Frequency and inheritance of A and B blood types in feline breeds of the United States, *J Hered* 82:15-20, 1991.

42. Giger U et al: An acute hemolytic transfusion reaction caused by dog erythrocyte antigen 1.1 incompatibility in a previously sensitized dog, *J Am Vet Med Assoc* 206:1358-1362, 1995.

43. Giger U et al: Geographical variation of the feline blood type frequencies in the United States, *Feline Prac* 19:21-27, 1991.

44. Giger U et al: Frequencies of feline blood groups in the United States, *J Am Vet Med Assoc* 195:1230-1232, 1989.

45. Giles AR, Tinlin S, Greenwood R: A canine model of hemophilic (factor VIII:C deficiency) bleeding, *Blood* 60:727-730, 1982.

46. Green RA: Hemostatic disorders: coagulopathies and thrombotic disorders. In Ettinger SJ: *Textbook of veterinary internal medicine,* ed 2, Philadelphia, 1989, WB Saunders.

47. Greene CE: Practical considerations of blood transfusion therapy, *AAHA 47th Annu Meet Proc* 187-191, 1980.

48. Griot-Wenk M, Giger U: Cats with type AB blood in the United States, *J Vet Intern Med* 5:139, 1991.

49. Griot-Wenk M, Giger U: *Feline transfusion medicine: blood types and their clinical importance.* In Kristensen AT, Feldman BF, editors: *The veterinary clinics of North America, small animal practice: canine and feline transfusion medicine,* Philadelphia, 1995, WB Saunders.

50. Griot-Wenk M et al: Biochemical characterization of the feline AB blood group system, *Anim Genet* 24:401-407, 1993.

51. Guyton AC: *Human physiology of mechanisms and disease,* ed 4, Philadelphia, 1987, WB Saunders.

52. Hale AS: *Canine blood groups and their importance in veterinary transfusion medicine.* In Kristensen AT, Feldman BF, editors: *The veterinary clinics of North America, small animal practice: canine and feline transfusion medicine,* Philadelphia, 1995, WB Saunders.

53. Haljamae H: Rationale for the use of colloids in the treatment of shock and hypovolemia, *Acta Anaesthesiol Scand* 29:48-54, 1985.

54. Haskins SC: Management of septic shock, *J Am Vet Med Assoc* 200(12): 1915-1922, 1992.

55. Haskins SC: *Shock.* In Kirk RW, editor: *Current veterinary therapy VIII,* Philadelphia, 1983, WB Saunders.

56. Haskins SC: *Standards and techniques of equipment utilization.* In Sattler FP, Knowles RP, Whittick WG, editors: *Veterinary critical care,* Philadelphia, 1981, Lea & Febiger.

57. Hill RC: *Critical care nutrition.* In Wills JM, Simpson KW, editors: *The Waltham book of clinical nutrition of the dog and cat,* Tarrytown, NY, 1994, Elsevier Science.

58. Hohenhaus AE: *Transfusions, infusions and other solutions.* In *Proc 12th Annu Memb Meet, Am Coll Vet Intern Med Forum,* 158, 1994.

59. Holmes R: The occurrence of blood groups in cats, *J Exp Biol* 30:350-357, 1953.

60. Howard A et al: Transfusion practices and costs in dogs, *J Am Vet Med Assoc* 201:1697-1701, 1992.

61. Hughes D: Personal communication, 1996.

62. Jergens AE et al: Buccal mucosal bleeding items of healthy dogs in various pathologic states, including thrombocytopenia, uremia, and von Willebrand's disease, *Am J Vet Res* 48:1337-1342, 1987.

63. Kaufman PM: *Supplies for blood transfusions in dogs and cats.* In Hohenhaus AE, editor: *Transfusion medicine, problems in veterinary medicine,* Philadelphia, 1992, JB Lippincott.

64. Killingsworth C: Use of blood and blood components for feline and canine patients, *J Vet Crit Care* 7:6-10, 1984.

65. King L: Personal communication.

66. Kirby R: Colloids - those magic fluids, *Proc IVECCS IV,* 648-654, 1994.

67. Kirby R: Minimizing the bone pile: the rule of 20. In *Proc IVECCS IV,* 665-672, 1994.

68. Kohn CW, DiBartola SP: *Composition and distribution of body fluids in dogs and cats.* In DiBartola SP: *Fluid therapy in small animal practice,* Philadelphia, 1992, WB Saunders.

69. Lewis LD, Morris ML, Hand MS: *Anorexia, inanition, and critical care nutrition.* In *small animal clinical nutrition III,* Topeka, Kan, 1992, Mark Morris Associates.

70. Lippert AC, Buffington CAT: *Parenteral nutrition.* In DiBartola SP: *Fluid therapy in small animal practice,* Philadelphia, 1992, WB Saunders.

71. Marion RS, Smith JE: Posttransfusion viability of feline erythrocytes stored in acid-citrate-dextrose solution, *J Am Vet Med Assoc* 183:1459, 1983.

72. Miller MW, Schertel ER, DiBartola SP: *Conventional and hypertonic fluid therapy: concepts and applications.* In Murtaugh et al, editors: *Veterinary emergency & critical care medicine,* St Louis, 1992, Mosby.

73. Morris DD: *Therapy in hemolymphatic diseases.* In Colahan PT et al: *Equine medicine and surgery,* ed 4, St Louis, 1991, Mosby.

74. Muir WM, DiBartola SP: *Fluid therapy.* In Kirk RW, editor: *Current veterinary therapy VIII,* Philadelphia, 1983, WB Saunders.

75. Myers K, Wardrop KJ: *Platelets and coagulation.* In Cotter SM, editor: *Comparative transfusion medicine, advances in veterinary science and comparative medicine,* San Diego, 1991, Academic Press.

76. Nelson RW: *Electrolyte imbalances.* In Nelson et al, editors: *Essentials of small animal medicine,* St Louis, 1992, Mosby.

77. Oakley D: Establishing and monitoring central venous pressure in the critical patient, *Vet Tech* 1:40-46, 1987.

78. Otto C: *Monitoring emergency patients.* In Lorenz MD et al: *Small animal medical therapeutics,* Philadelphia, 1992, JB Lippincott.

79. Otto CM, McCall-Kaufman G, Crowe DT: Intraosseous infusion of fluids and therapeutics, *Comp Cont Educ Pract Vet* 11:421-430, 1989.

80. Pichler ME, Turnwald GH: Blood transfusion in the dog and cat, *Comp Cont Educ Pract Vet* 7:66-71, 1985.

81. Potkay S, Zinn RD: Effect of collection interval, body weight, and season on the hemograms of canine blood donors, *Lab Anim Sci* 19:192-197, 1969.

82. Price GS et al: Evaluation of citrate-phosphate-dextrose-adenine as a storage medium for packed canine erythrocytes, *J Vet Intern Med* 2:126-131, 1988.

83. Rose BD: *Clinical physiology of acid-base and electrolyte disorders,* ed 3, New York, 1989, McGraw-Hill.

84. Schaer M: General principles of fluid therapy in small animal medicine, *Vet Clin North Am* 19:203-213, 1989.

85. Senior DF: *Fluid therapy, electrolyte, and acid-base control.* In: Ettinger SJ, editor: *Textbook of veterinary internal medicine,* Philadelphia, 1989, WB Saunders.

86. Smiley LE, Garvey MS: The use of Hetastarch as adjunct therapy in 26 dogs with hypoalbuminemia: a phase two clinical trail, *J Am Vet Med Assoc* 8(3): 195-202, 1994.

87. Smith JE: Erythrocytes, *Adv Vet Sci Comp Med* 36:9-55, 1991.

88. Smith JE, Mahaffey E, Board P: A New storage medium for canine blood, *J Am Vet Med Assoc* 172:701, 1978.

89. Stone E, Badner D, Cotter SM: Trends in transfusion medicine in dogs at a veterinary school clinic, *J Am Vet Med Assoc* 200:1000-1003, 1992.

90. Stump DC et al: Effects of hydroxyethel starch on blood coagulation, particularly factor VIII, *Transfusion* 25(4):349-354, 1985.

91. Swisher SN, Bull R, Bowdler J: Canine erythrocyte antigens, *Tissue Antigens* 3:164-165, 1973.

92. Swisher SN, Young LE: The blood group system of dogs, *Phys Rev* 41:495-520, 1961.

93. Symons M, Bell K: Canine blood groups: description of 20 specificities, *Anim Genet* 23:509-515, 1992.

94. Symons M, Bell K: Expansion of the canine A blood group system, *Anim Genet* 22:227-235, 1991.

95. Tangner CH: Transfusion therapy for the dog and cat, *Comp Cont Educ Pract Vet* 4:521-527, 1982.

96. Turnwald GH: Blood transfusion in dogs and cats. Part II: Administration, adverse effects, and component therapy, *Comp Cont Educ Pract Vet* 7:115-122, 1985.

97. Tvedten HW: *Hemostatic abnormalities.* In Willard MD et al, editors: *Small animal clinical diagnosis by laboratory methods,* ed 2, Philadelphia, 1994, WB Saunders.

98. Tvedten HW: *The complete blood count and bone marrow examination: general comments and selected techniques.* In Willard MD et al, editor: *Small animal clinical diagnosis by laboratory methods,* ed 2, Philadelphia, 1994, WB Saunders.

99. Tvedten HW, Grabski S, Frame L: Estimating platelets and leukocytes on canine blood smears, *Vet Clin Pathol* 17:4-6, 1988.

100. Vander AJ, Sherman J, Luciano D: *Human physiology: the mechanisms of body function,* ed 4, Philadelphia, 1985, WB Saunders.

101. Walker RH, editor: *Technical manual of the American Association of Blood Banks,* ed 10, Arlington, Va, 1990, American Association of Blood Banks.

102. Wardrop KJ: *Selection of anticoagulant-preservatives for canine and feline blood storage.* In Kristensen AT, Feldman BF, editors: *The veterinary clinics of North America, small animal practice: canine and feline transfusion medicine,* Philadelphia, 1995, WB Saunders.

103. Wardrop KF, Owen TJ, Meyers KM: Evaluation of an additive solution for preservation of canine red blood cells, *J Vet Intern Med* 8:253-257, 1994.

104. Wardrop KJ, Young J, Wilson E: An in vitro evaluation of storage media for the preservation of canine packed red blood cells, *Vet Clin Pathol* 23:83-88, 1992.

105. Williamson L: *Blood and plasma therapy.* In Robinson E: *Current therapy in equine medicine,* ed 3, Philadelphia, 1992, WB Saunders.

106. Young LE, Ervin DM, Yuile CL: Hemolytic reactions produced in dogs by transfusion of incompatible dog blood and plasma, *Blood* 4:1218-1231, 1949.

107. Young LE et al: Blood groups in dogs - their significance to the veterinarian, *Am J Vet Res* 13:207-213, 1952.

CHAPTER 25

Dentistry

H.B. Lobprise

Learning Objectives

After reviewing this chapter, the reader should understand the following:

Anatomy of teeth
Terms used to describe teeth and their surfaces

Dental formulas of companion animals
Instruments used in dentistry
Procedures used in dental prophylaxis
Treatments for common dental problems

As much as in probably any other field in veterinary medicine, the role a technician can play in dentistry can be extremely important. In many practices, the technician provides the majority of hands-on care that the patients' teeth receive, particularly in performing dental prophylaxis or teeth cleaning. It may also be the technician who takes the history, performs the initial examination, and informs the clinician of any pertinent facts. The health of the oral cavity and the whole patient may depend greatly on the technician's ability to assess the situation sufficiently to call attention to any specific problems and to provide quality care. The technician may also discuss with the animal owner dental hygiene and home care. Depending on the "dental I.Q." and skills of the technician, the service provided could be of great benefit or detriment to the patient.

Although the oral cavity may not seem like one of the more important areas of the body, its role in the overall health of the individual can be quite significant. Oral and dental disease not only affects local structures but also can contribute to many systemic problems, particularly when bacteremia originating from the mouth may have profound effects on other organs.[1] A patient with oral problems may not eat well or groom itself, and halitosis could make the patient an unwelcome guest. A high proportion of veterinary patients have dental problems; up to 80% of dogs show some indication of active periodontal inflammation.[2] If even half of those owners sought professional help or were informed that help was available, it would have a tremendous impact on practice income.

The importance of dentistry in a practice should never be minimized, nor should the importance of patients' health be minimized. Veterinary commitment is to provide the best care possible for patients, and this goal certainly includes the care of the oral cavity.

ORAL ANATOMY

As with every other body system, it is essential to know the normal anatomic structures of the oral cavity, and how they are to function. Knowing this, one can determine whether a certain condition is abnormal and if further assessment is necessary.

Teeth

Teeth are the primary functional structures of the oral cavity. A mature tooth can be divided into the exposed crown and "submerged" root portions that join at the neck (cementoenamel junction, or CEJ) of the tooth (Fig. 25-1). The enamel covering of the crown is the hardest substance in the body (96% inorganic) and is made of hydroxyapatite crystals. The root is covered by a layer of cementum, which is closer in composition (45% to 50% inorganic) to bone than enamel. Cementum also has capabilitites of regeneration, unlike enamel, because of the presence of cementoblasts that also participate in the initial formation of cementum. Underlying the enamel and cementum for the entire length of the tooth is a layer of dentin (70% inorganic, 30% organic collagen fibers and water). Although the dentin layer is initially very thin in immature teeth, odontoblasts from pulpal tissue continue to manufacture dentin in a tubular pattern throughout the life of the tooth. This makes the dentinal walls progressively thicker and the canal space of the tooth more narrow as the tooth matures.

The internal canal space surrounded and protected by the dentin is called the *pulp cavity* for the entire tooth; the *pulp chamber*, including pulpal horns, for the crown; and the *root canal* for the root. This internal space, or pulp cavity, houses the blood vessels, nerves, and connective tissue that serve the tooth. These pulpal structures enter the tooth in small animals at the apical, or root tip end, often through the delta foramina, a formation with many small openings. These pulpal tissues provide oxygen and nutrients through the blood vessels, contain cells instrumental in laying down and removing dentin (odontoblasts and odontoclasts), and have nerves to conduct impulses in response to various stimuli.

Though teeth can "sense" a variety of stimuli from cold to heat (depending on the health or sensitivity of the teeth) and pressure, the only perception the animal feels is one of pain. This is a good defense mechanism because if a tooth is compromised to the extent that it is sensitive to cold or heat, the resulting pain may alert an owner to the animal's denture problem.

The teeth, both *deciduous* (primary) and *permanent* (adult), arise from a ridge of dental laminar epithelium. In a young animal with deciduous teeth, the permanent tooth buds are located adjacent to them underneath the gingiva (gum). Any stimulus, from generalized infection

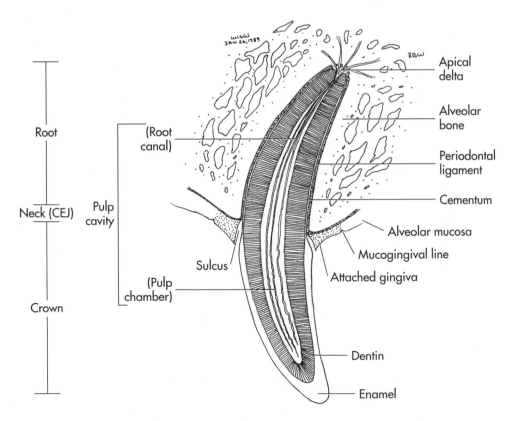

FIG. 25-1 Anatomy of a tooth and supporting structures.

(distemper) or fever to a local infection from an abscessed deciduous tooth, can affect development of the permanent tooth, much like a developing fetus in the uterus. Deciduous teeth are often shed in sequence as the permanent teeth erupt. This sequence can be influenced by many factors, including genetics, nutrition, and trauma. If a deciduous tooth is still present when a permanent tooth is erupting, the deciduous tooth should be carefully extracted to avoid deflection of the adult tooth into an abnormal position. (See orthodontic section on p. 475.)

Dental Formulas. A *dental formula* (Box 25-1) is a way of expressing the normal number and arrangement of deciduous and permanent teeth in a species. By knowing the dental formula for a species, you can determine when there is an inappropriate number of teeth or a variation in tooth eruption times.

Although some breeds have specific tooth numbers and placement (see Orthodontic Assessment), in most animals the important thing to note is the presence of healthy, functional dentition. A few missing teeth may not pose a problem, as long as they are not embedded, and a few extra teeth can sometimes fit in nicely, as long as overcrowding does not predispose the area to food accumulation and periodontal disease. Tooth form and structure may also vary at times, from reduced crown

size to extra roots. As long as the root canal (pulp cavity) system is intact and viable, however, the tooth should remain functional.

Directional Terms. It is important to be able to describe where on a tooth or in the oral cavity that a lesion exists. Directional terms may be helpful in noting lesions in the patient's record. In addition, certain dental abnormalities may also be defined (Box 25-2). Fig. 25-2 shows directional terms pertaining to teeth.

Periodontium

The supporting structure around the teeth, or *periodontium,* maintains the stability of the teeth in the oral cavity. The periodontium includes the gingiva, the cementum of the root, the periodontal ligament (goes from the cementum to the alveolar socket) and the alveolar bone or socket (see Fig. 25-1). The mandible and maxilla have a series of depressions, or sockets, in the alveolar ridge to house the root structures. The periodontal ligament stablizes the tooth within the socket and absorbs some of the shock of the occlusal forces generated during chewing. The cementum must remain healthy to maintain attachment of the periodontal ligament to the tooth. Covering all of these structures is the gingival mucosa.

The specialized tissue of the attached gingiva immediately adjacent to the tooth structure provides the first line of defense against bacteria for the rest of the periodontium. The attached gingiva is histologically different from

---

Box 25-1 Dental formulas for cats and dogs

Cats

Deciduous: 2 × (Id 3/3; Cd 1/1; Pd 3/2) = 26

Permanent: 2 × (I 3/3; C 1/1; P 3/2; M 1/1) = 30

	Time of Eruption	
	Deciduous	Permanent
Incisors	2-3 weeks	3-4 months
Canines	3-4 weeks	4-5 months
Premolars	3-6 weeks	4-6 months
Molars	—	4-6 months

Dogs

Deciduous: 2 × (Id 3/3; Cd 1/1; Pd 3/3) = 28

Permanent: 2 × (I 3/3; C 1/1; P 4/4; M 2/3) = 42

	Time of Eruption	
	Deciduous	Permanent
Incisors	3-5 weeks	3-5 months
Canines	3-6 weeks	3.5-6 months
Premolars	4-10 weeks	3.5-6 months
Molars	—	3.5-7 months

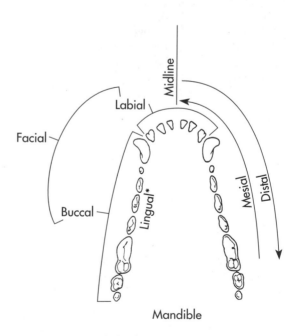

*Or palatal in the maxilla

FIG. 25-2 Directional terms used in dentistry.

Box 25-2 Dental terminology

Dental directional terms

Mesial: surface of tooth toward the rostral midline

Distal: surface of tooth away from the rostral midline

Palatal: surface of tooth toward the palate (maxillary arcade)

Lingual: surface of tooth toward the tongue (mandibular arcade)

Labial: surface of tooth toward the lips

Buccal: surface of tooth toward the cheeks

Facial: labial and/or buccal surface

Occlusal: surface of tooth facing a tooth in opposite jaw

Interproximal: surface between two teeth

Apical: toward the apex (root)

Coronal: toward the crown

Dental abnormalities

Macrodontia: crown oversized

Microdontia: crown reduced

Dilacerated: crown or root distortion (twist)

Dens-in-dente: enamel layer "folds" into itself/tooth

Enamel pearls: beads of enamel at CEJ, furcation

Fusion tooth: fusion of two tooth buds during formation

Gemination: complete tooth duplication but incomplete split

Twinning: complete tooth duplication and split

Enamel hypocalcification ("hypoplasia"): enamel pitting/discoloration

Hypodontia: some teeth missing

Oligodontia: most teeth missing

Anodontia: all teeth missing

Supernumerary: extra tooth/teeth

---

the more loose alveolar mucosa. Interdigitations of connective tissue (rete pegs) provide firm attachment to the underlying periosteum of the alveolar bone. Without this specialized keratinized epithelium, bacteria could readily attack the underlying periodontal ligament and bone. A minimum of 1 to 2 mm of attached gingiva is necessary to provide this protection and can be measured from the mucogingival line that delineates its connection to the alveolar mucosa. This mucogingival line is most readily apparent on the facial or buccal surfaces of the teeth.

The free edge, or gingival margin, of this epithelial collar is often not directly attached to the tooth itself, although it can be very close to the teeth in a cat's mouth. The space between the tooth and the free gingiva is termed the *gingival sulcus.* At the depth of the sulcus, the junctional epithelium attaches to the tooth. A sulcus depth of up to about 3 to 4 mm is considered normal in dogs (depending on patient size); sulcus depth should not be more than 0.5 to 1.0 mm in cats without a concurrent disease process. Any variation in sulcus pocket depth should alert the technician to potential problems (see Periodontal Disease).

PERIODONTAL DISEASE

Periodontal disease is the most common oral disease in pets and is probably the most common infectious process in the body. Bacteria are normally found in the oral cavity as a component of plaque. Plaque is a soft mixture of bacteria and mucopolysaccharides that adheres to the tooth. The bacteria and associated endotoxins in the plaque initiate the inflammatory process in the gingival tissue (gingivitis). The inflammation may start as a mild gingivitis with edema and redness of the free gingival margin. If the inflammation is limited to this region and there is no attachment loss, it can be reversible with appropriate therapy (stage I periodontal disease: gingivitis). A slight increase in sulcus depth is typically attributable to swollen gingival margins and usually resolves when the edema subsides.

More extensive involvement of the periodontal ligament without intervention leads to periodontitis and subsequent attachment loss, as evidenced by an increased pocket depth and bone loss (stage II periodontal disease: periodontitis). Stage II periodontal disease consists of pockets up to 5 mm deep in dogs (1 mm in cats) or up to approximately 25% attachment loss. Pockets up to 9 mm deep (1.5 mm in cats) and 50% attachment loss is characteristic of stage III periodontal disease. Stage IV periodontal disease shows greater than 9 mm pocket depth and over 50% attachment loss. Often there are different stages of periodontal disease in different areas of a patient's mouth.

The bacteria associated with reversible gingivitis are generally located above the gumline (supragingivally) and tend to be aerobic, gram-positive, nonmotile cocci. As the disease progresses, the periodontal pockets enlarge, and bacteria work their way into the deeper structures. The bacterial flora in these deeper tissues tends to be more anaerobic, gram-negative, motile bacilli. The damage from bacteria and associated toxins can be significant, but the body's response with influx of many neutrophils, lymphocytes, and plasma cells can cause as much or more tissue destruction than the bacteria. Therefore, the primary goals of treating periodontal disease are controlling bacterial populations while minimizing pocket depth and maintaining healthy attached gingiva.

Dental Instruments

Although antibiotics and antiinflammatories have their place in treating periodontal disease, mechanical removal of plaque, calculus, bacteria, and abnormal tissue with dental instruments is the focus of treatment. A wide variety of equipment is available to help manage periodontal disease.

Power Scaling Units. The most commonly used scaling unit in veterinary dentistry is the ultrasonic scaler. The magnetostrictive scaler works through vibrations of the metal stacks that cause the tip at around 45,000 Hz, with continuous emission of an aerosolizing water spray. This vibration helps to remove the tartar or calculus from the teeth. Piezoelectric ultrasonic scalers use the vibrations generated from electrical current running through a quartz crystal. Newer ceramic models show promise with potentially less damage, but these are fairly expensive. Ultrasonic scalers produce heat, and a constant water flow is essential to keep the instrument cool.

Sonic scalers vibrate at 16,000 to 20,000 Hz generated from the pressurized air of a high-speed handpiece. Although sonic scalers do not produce excessive heat, the water spray is helpful to flush debris from the tooth surface. A soft steel rotary bur with six cutting flutes rotating at 300,000 rpm on a high-speed handpiece produces a frequency similar to that of an ultrasonic unit, but it is potentially very damaging to the tooth. Although power scaling units can quickly remove tartar, if improperly used they can generate excessive heat, even with adequate water flow, and can damage the tooth structure inadvertently.

Hand Scaling Instruments. Although power equipment is certainly faster, at times hand scaling instruments may be the better choice. Hand instruments used for scaling include scalers and curettes. Although hand scaling instruments are available in various types, the most typical form is a *sickle scaler*. These instruments, with their sharp tip and triangular cross-section (Fig. 25-3), can be used to scale calculus off the crown of the tooth. Sickle scalers should never be used subgingivally because of the potential for gum damage.

The instrument of choice in removing subgingival deposits is the curette, with rounded toe and back (see Fig. 25-3). With small to moderate subgingival pockets less than 5 mm deep, the curette can be gently introduced into the pocket and used to scale the root surface and debride the lining of the soft tissue.

The working end of scalers and curettes must be sharpened at least after every use; dull instruments only burnish the calculus instead of removing it. Although the face of the instrument can be sharpened with a conical sharpening stone, it is usually best to use an oiled flat stone, drawing the working edge across at a 110-degree angle to approximate the angle of the head.

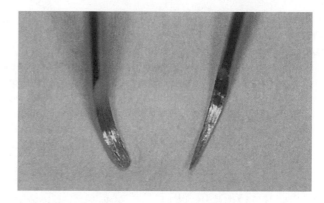

FIG. 25-3 Curette *(left)* and scaler *(right)*. *(From Harvey CE, Emily PP: Small animal dentistry, St Louis, 1993, Mosby.)*

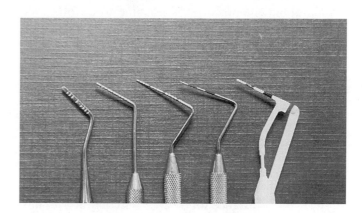

FIG. 25-4 Various types of periodontal probes.

Other hand instruments that are essential in evaluation of periodontal disease are periodontal explorers and probes. A *periodontal explorer* has a sharp, thin tip, often curved into a "shepherd's crook." This fine instrument is used in human dentistry to detect softened areas of enamel that are starting to decay. Because carious lesions are not as common in pets, this tactile instrument can be used to detect roughened areas or residual calculus on the tooth surface, resorptive areas (feline neck lesions), and open canals in broken teeth.

The *periodontal probe* is an even more important tool in assessment of periodontal disease. Probes are marked in varying millimeter increments, with either notches or color changes on the working end, which can be round or flat (Fig. 25-4). A probe can be gently introduced into the gingival sulcus to determine the depth of any pocket. Measurements at up to six sites around a tooth's circumference give an indication of any increased pocket depth, which can then be noted on the record.

Polishing Equipment

Polishing equipment is another essential tool in treatment of periodontal disease. Scaling roughens the enamel surface of a tooth; this must be polished to produce a smooth surface that slows accumulation of plaque. Battery-operated polishing instruments can be used, but these typically do not last long. Rotary hand tools (Dremel-type) can be used to power the polishing handpiece, but rotational speed must be controllable and maintained at less than 3000 rpm. Micromotor units often have the option of using a prophy angle, or the slow-speed handpiece of an air-driven unit can be used.

ORAL RADIOGRAPHY

Radiographic equipment is essential for a quality dental practice. Although one may purchase expensive dental radiographic equipment, it is possible to do oral radiography using standard equipment with intraoral films and rapid developer/fixer solutions.

Extraoral films and oblique projections can be used for survey films, but these generally produce some degree of superimposition of other oral structures over the area to be viewed. Small, flexible intraoral films can be used with the standard radiographic unit with few variations. Intraoral films provide excellent detail, and superimposition of other oral structures is rarely a problem, unless positioning was incorrect. The unit can be used with the radiographic head positioned at a 36- to 40-inch focal distance for ⅖ to ⅗ second at 100 mA. It is preferable if the radiographic head is mobile, however, to decrease the focal distance to 12 inches and the exposure time to 1/10 to 1/15 second to minimize distortion and exposure. Depending on the equipment, the kVp may vary from 65 for a small dog or cat up to 85 for a giant breed.

The intraoral films come in a variety of small sizes (0,1, 2, 3, 4); No. 2 film *(periapical)* is most commonly used (Fig. 25-5). No. 4 film *(occlusal)* measures 2 by 3 inches and can be used to view a larger area of the incisors and canines or the nasal cavity (also for small rodents, birds, and cat feet). These nonscreened, double-emulsion films are encased in a black paper sleeve with a lead foil back sheet that helps prevent back scatter produced by x-rays bouncing back off the table. A paper or plastic covering protects the films until after exposure, when they are removed before developing.

Dental films can be developed in standard tanks or automatic processors (taped to the lead end of a larger film.) They take the same amount of time and volume of developing solutions as for a larger film. These smaller films can sometimes be lost in standard developing tanks. As an option, rapid dental developer and fixer solutions can be used in individual containers, either in the existing darkroom or in a chairside developer at the dental station. After rehydrating the emulsification of the film in water for 3 to 5 seconds, devel-

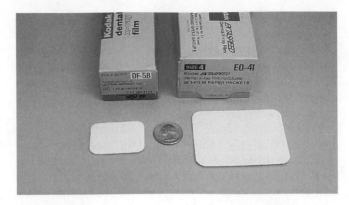

FIG. 25-5 Intraoral films: size 2 *(left)* and size 4 *(right)*.

oping time ranges from 15 to 30 seconds, using fresh developing solutions. After a water rinse, fixing time is in the same range, so a film can be developed in less than a minute. This makes use of dental films very convenient. Rapid development time is particularly important when multiple films must be made.

The difficulty of oral radiography lies in positioning the film and the patient to obtain an image with the least distortion. A *parallel technique* is used only with the mandibular premolars/molars, when the film can be placed parallel to the teeth, with a corner pressing down into the intermandibular space. With the film so positioned, the x-ray head can then be aimed perpendicular to the parallel items. Elsewhere in the oral cavity, the film cannot be positioned directly against the object to be viewed, particularly in the maxilla. To accommodate for this obstacle, the *bisecting angle technique* can be used to minimize distortion that is inherent when the film cannot be placed parallel to the tooth.

If the x-ray beam were to be aimed perpendicular to the film, the tooth image would be shortened; if aimed perpendicular to the long axis of the tooth, the image would be elongated. Therefore, if the beam is aimed midway between the two positions, the image should approximate the size of the tooth itself. One way to visualize this is to imagine an angle formed by the line of the film and the line of the long axis of the tooth or its root. Once this angle is assessed, a line that would bisect this angle is determined. By aiming the beam perpendicular to this bisecting line, the image will closely approximate the tooth size.

A dental radiographic unit with mobile head is optimal to attain these positions, but a standard radiographic unit can sometimes be adjusted accordingly. If the unit is not mobile, the animal's head can be positioned so that the determined bisecting line is parallel to the table, thus becoming perpendicular to the beam. Once exposed and developed, these films reveal many problems that otherwise might not have been grossly visible, particularly during routine prophylaxis.

PROPHYLAXIS AND PERIODONTAL THERAPY

Because periodontal disease is the most common oral problem in pets, it is safe to say that periodontal treatment is the most frequent oral/dental procedure performed in a practice. The primary goals of periodontal therapy include removing any accumulations of plaque, calculus, and diseased tissue, and trying to minimize gingival pocket depth while maintaining at least 1 to 2 mm of attached gingiva.

The term *prophylaxis* is often used to describe the process of cleaning the teeth by removing plaque and calculus. The true meaning of the word is "prevention"; there are relatively few patients to which this term applies. When there is merely accumulation of plaque and calculus with reversible gingivitis, a thorough cleaning helps to prevent further periodontal disease at that time. If there is any indication of extended periodontitis, particularly with any attachment loss, the more appropriate terminology is *periodontal therapy*. Not only is this term more correct, it also helps impress upon clients the level of care necessary for their pet. The term *prophylaxis* will be used here to avoid confusion.

Procedure

The steps of a "complete prophylaxis" should be followed in a systematic manner to avoid missing any particular step. The first step is removal of any grossly visible plaque and calculus on the crowns of the teeth. After this process, the animal's mouth may look greatly improved, but this is only the beginning of adequate treatment. One must remember that most of the periodontal disease process is occurring below the gingiva, in the sulcus or pocket. A concentrated effort should be made to thoroughly evaluate the oral cavity for any periodontal pockets, no matter how slight, and to adequately clean each area.

The legal definition of oral surgery and how much a technician is legally able to perform subgingivally vary among states. In some areas, any work that is to be done under the gumline is considered oral surgery, and legally must be performed by the veterinarian. In other locales, areas of slightly increased sulcus depth can be gently cleaned by a technician, using curettes to remove any subgingival debris.

Smaller curettes can be used in pockets up to 5 mm in depth in a process known as *closed root planing*. In this technique, the curette is gently introduced into the sulcus down to the depth of the junctional epithelial attachment. The cutting edge of the curette is then adjusted to engage the surface of the root, and the curette is withdrawn from the pocket in a pulling action. Repeating the process in varying directions in a cross-hatched pattern (horizontal, vertical, oblique) on the tooth surface ensures thorough cleaning of the root surface. The goal is to remove all calculus, debris, and diseased tissue without removing excessive amounts of normal cementum. The term *periodontal debridement* is sometimes used, instead of *root planing*, to denote a more controlled therapy. The curette can also be used in the pocket by changing the position of the working head to gently debride the inner lining of the soft tissue with slight digital pressure from the outside. This subgingival curettage removes infected or necrotic pieces of gingiva lining the sulcus, and any associated debris.

Once the pocket area has been adequately cleaned, it should be gently irrigated with sterile saline or dilute chlorhexidine or fluoride to remove any remnants of calculus or tissue that could cause a periodontal abscess if left in the pocket. It is best to use a blunt, side-slot needle for irrigation to minimize damage to the soft tissue and avoid forceful extrusion of fluids into the junctional epithelium. A gentle air blast or flow can open up the pocket slightly to allow better visualization of the root surface. At that time, remaining areas of calculus deposition show up as a chalky white residue.

POLISHING

All scaled tooth surfaces should be polished to minimize any roughening of the enamel that would predispose the area to accelerated plaque accumulation. Generally, a medium to fine prophy paste can be used, applying enough pressure to gently splay the foot of the prophy cup against the tooth. Lack of sufficient paste and use of excessive pressure or time spent on the tooth should be avoided, because this can cause overheating and enamel damage. The speed of the prophy angle should be at around 1500 rpm, not to exceed 3000 rpm. After polishing, a final irrigation should be performed to flush out any remaining debris or prophy paste.

FLUORIDE APPLICATION

Although there is some difference of opinion on use of fluoride in the oral cavity, its antibacterial properties and use on sensitive teeth because of enamel wear or after root planing are some considerations. It is best to limit any possibility of fluoride ingestion; in an anesthetized animal, more control is possible. After the final irrigation, the tooth surfaces should be dried, particularly when using sodium fluoride. The fluoride should be placed on the tooth with a small brush (if a gel) to avoid excessive application. It may be more difficult to control the exact amount when using a form, but an attempt should be made not to leave excessive material in the oral cavity. After the appropriate time, the fluoride should be blown off the teeth with air or wiped off—never rinsed away, because this would inactivate the effects of the fluoride. If there is an indication for home use of fluoride, the owner should be instructed to apply it carefully and therefore limit the amount of fluoride that could be ingested by the pet.

DENTAL RECORDS

Throughout the process of the prophylaxis, the mouth is continuously evaluated for any abnormalities. Although notations can be made at any time during the procedure, it is often best to review the entire oral cavity after prophylaxis and made sure that all items are noted on the record. Recording observations in the dental chart should follow a systematic order to avoid missing any details. Many forms of dental records are available, including complete record sheets, stickers to affix to the records, and even ink stamps. Any variations in tooth appearance, pocket depth, or other abnormalities should be recorded, along with the appropriate treatment. Individual teeth can be described using several different techniques, but be sure to use a consistent style. In longhand terms, the tooth should be described as *deciduous* or *permanent,* which quadrant (right or left, mandibular or maxillary), and number and type (first, second, etc.; incisor, canine, premolar, or molar).

A shorthand method uses the abbreviation for the tooth (I, C, P, M) and its numbered position around the tooth, depending on quadrant. For example, the upper left second incisor is noted as ^{2}I. Canine teeth can be designated with the number *1* and deciduous teeth can be designated with a lower case letter (which can be hard to distinguish from an upper case letter) or by using the letter *d* (e.g., Id, Cd, Pd, Md).

The triadan system can also be used, particularly when using a computer system, as it relies on a three-digit "code." The first digit (hundreds) signifies the quadrant (upper right 100; upper left 200; lower left 300; lower right 400) and the last two digits indicate the tooth number, starting with 01 to 03 for incisors, 04 for canines, 05 to 08 for premolars, and 09 to 11 for molars. Dogs and cats do not have 11 teeth in each quadrant (pigs do), so some variation will be seen in the numbering systems for various species. Deciduous teeth can be identified with the triadan system using 500 for the upper right quadrant, 600 for the upper left, 700 for the lower left, 800 for the lower right. Further delineations of tooth number are less obvious. Current anatomic guidelines state that there are no "deciduous molars," so all deciduous teeth caudal to the canines are considered premolars.

Examples of triadan numbering are as follows:
104 - C^1: right maxillary canine

> ### Box 25-3 Common dental abbreviations and symbols
>
> X: extracted
> O: missing
> FE: furcation exposure
> RE: root exposure
> \: tooth fracture
> CLL, CNL, FRL: cervical line lesion, cervical neck lesion, feline resorptive lesion (stage 1 to 4)
> EH: enamel hypocalcification (hypoplasia)
> S: supernumerary tooth
> GR: gingival recession
> GH: gingival hyperplasia

307 - $_3$P: left mandibular third premolar
802 - Id$_2$: deciduous right mandibular second incisor

On the dental chart, many different symbols can be used to designate specific problems observed. Any system can be used, as long as it is consistent and the information can be readily interpreted. Some commonly used abbreviations and symbols are listed in Box 25-3.

The depth of periodontal sulci or pockets should be measured at six sites around the tooth, taking particular care to evaluate the palatal aspect of the maxillary canines. Often pockets can exist with no external sign of a problem, so the examination should be thorough.

RADIOGRAPHS

Radiographs should always be made in animals with periodontal disease to evaluate bone loss, with "neck lesions" to evaluate root integrity, with crown fracture or discoloration to look for apical problems, and any time a problem is suspected. Extensive lesions not apparent grossly can be hidden subgingivally, so radiographs can be very useful.

HOME DENTAL CARE

Routine home care is an important part of maintaining oral health. The technician is often responsible for instructing the owner on the type and frequency of recommended home dental care. *Brushing* is the best way to remove plaque from the tooth surface before it calcifies into calculus. A soft-bristle, disposable toothbrush is ideal for most patients. Many fine brushes for pets are on the market, particularly some of the smaller brushes for cats, but even children's toothbrushes are useful for some pets. It may take some training to accustom an animal (and owner) to routine brushing, so a gradual, gentle beginning is recommended.

The owner can begin by touching the pet more around the mouth and head, gently keeping the mouth closed with one hand and lifting the lips with the other. A soft washcloth or gauze can be used to carefully wipe the outer surface of the teeth. In dogs, garlic powder or canned meat can be used on the cloth to make the experience more pleasant; the liquid from water-packed canned tuna can be used with cats. Once the patient accepts the initial attempts, a soft toothbrush can be introduced to the regimen.

Depending on the individual, the animal may immediately accept a flavored toothpaste or it may have to become accustomed to toothpaste. Human toothpastes should not be used because of their fluoride and detergent content. Most pets do not spit out the excess but swallow it instead. Baking soda products should be avoided in older or cardiac patients because of the potential for sodium overload. Daily brushing is ideal for good oral hygiene, but even two to three times a week can make a big difference.

Other oral products include solutions and gels, such as chlorhexidine and fluorides, to reduce bacterial populations in the mouth. Chlorhexidine products work best when retained in the mouth for a minute or more, so the more viscous gels or gingival patches are more efficient. Though fluoride helps control oral bacteria and helps prevent carious lesions, it should not be overused, because excessive ingestion can cause toxicity. Zinc ascorbate liquids and gels can aid healing of soft tissue after oral surgery and can be useful in animals that will not tolerate tooth brushing.

FOOD AND CHEW TOYS

Different food products vary in efficacy in controlling plaque and tartar. There does seem to be some benefit of hard foods over soft, though the result of studies may conflict. Newer products have a specialized fiber composition to help clean the teeth as the food is eaten, or contain substances that discourage mineralization of plaque.

Chew toys can also help reduce accumulation of plaque and calculus, especially the more fibrous, "chewy" objects. Extremely hard objects, such as cattle hooves and bones and ice, can cause severe wear and even fractures of teeth. It is sometimes difficult to find the right balance for an animal that is a heavy chewer; a product may not break the teeth, but it often does not last long. Finding the right chew toy can sometimes be a challenge for the owner. For dogs that continue to chew harder objects, the carnassial teeth (upper fourth premolar, lower first molar) should be regularly inspected for fractures.

TREATMENT OF COMMON ORAL PROBLEMS

As discussed previously, the periodontal examination should be quite thorough. At the time of pocket evaluation, the amount of exposed root should be noted, because the combined degree of root exposure and pocket depth gives the most accurate assessment of total attachment loss. In other words, if the gingival margin starts 2 mm below the neck of the tooth and there is an additional 4 mm in pocket depth, the attachment is a total of 6 mm below the normal placement. These measurements should consider the size of the animal to determine the percentage of attachment loss in comparison with the normal degree of attachment for that size of animal.

PERIODONTAL SURGERY

In cases of gingival hyperplasia, there can be increased pocket depth without any attachment loss because of falsely "elevated" gingival margins. Typically, resection of the excessive tissue using periodontal probes to determine the normal extent of the sulcus can restore a more normal amount of attached gingiva without excessive pocket depth that could predispose to periodontal disease.

If pockets more than 5 mm deep are associated with attachment loss and extensive periodontal disease, closed-root planing is typically not helpful, as the curettes cannot effectively reach those depths. Some form of periodontal surgery, including releasing gingival flaps to expose the area and provide access for proper therapy, should be performed by the veterinarian. Specialized procedures can be performed to graft or move (pedicle flap) healthy attached gingiva to replace areas with less than 2 mm of tissue. In areas with sufficient gingiva and moderately deep pockets, some gingiva can be excised to reduce pocket depths, as seen with gingival hyperplasia. If the amount of attached gingiva is barely sufficient but a significant pocket is present, releasing and then suturing the gingiva back at a lower position on the tooth after cleaning the roots and bone (apically repositioned flap) can be done to preserve the remaining gingiva while reducing the pocket depth.

Procedures can be done to stimulate formation of bone or periodontal ligament. With deep pockets, a gingival flap can be performed to expose the site for cleaning. Barrier material or a membrane is placed to keep soft tissue from growing into the site. The palatal area of the upper canine teeth (Fig. 25-6) is especially important, because extensive bone loss on the palatal surface can expose the nasal cavity, causing an oronasal fistula. If a fistula is suspected in a deep pocket here, a gentle stream of water can be flushed into the region to see if there is communication with the nasal passages. If bone

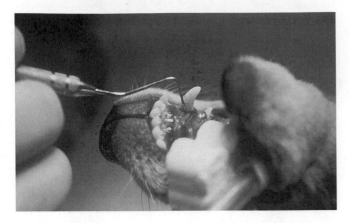

FIG. 25-6 Periodontal probe inserted into a palatal pocket of an upper canine tooth.

loss is extensive enough for fistulation, periodontal ligament regeneration is not possible and the tooth must be extracted.

Simple closure of the area is not adequate because of the tension placed on the sutures every time the animal breathes. A mucoperiosteal flap from the remaining gingiva and alveolar mucosa may be elevated from the underlying attachment to prevent tension and the defect sutured. With chronic or large openings, a flap can be harvested from the palate for additional repair.

TOOTH EXTRACTION

If attachment loss or accompanying infection are too advanced to warrant additional therapy, the tooth can be extracted. The decision to extract a tooth should consider several factors, particularly in "borderline" cases. If the client is committed to perform home care, some periodontal procedures can be performed to save a tooth that would otherwise be sacrificed. Furcation exposure is not always a criterion for extraction if the client can regularly clean the area and keep it free of debris. On the other hand, specialized procedures, particularly flaps and regenerative ones, should not be performed if the commitment to home care is lacking. Selection of the teeth to be extracted may also depend on the function of the tooth itself. Some teeth are considered more "strategic" than others, such as the canines and carnassial teeth (upper fourth premolars and lower first molars in dogs and cats). These teeth tend to be more vital in function or structure than small teeth and may warrant additional effort in their preservation. In addition, early periodontal disease of smaller teeth that could end up affecting adjacent strategic teeth may lead a practitioner to decide on extraction of the "nonstrategic" teeth.

Retained deciduous teeth should be extracted. There should *never* be two teeth (deciduous or permanent) trying to be in the same place at the same time. Clients should be instructed to monitor the progress of eruption of permanent teeth. If a deciduous tooth has not been exfoliated (shed), it should be extracted. If it remains in the mouth during eruption of that permanent tooth, the permanent tooth will be deflected to an abnormal position. Most permanent teeth erupt in a more lingual position when a deciduous tooth is retained, including the incisors and the lower canines. These displaced permanent teeth can be malpositioned enough to impinge on the palate (base narrow). The permanent upper canines, however, erupt more mesial (rostral) to their normal position, sometimes even pointing straight forward and often impinging on the space that the lower canine would normally occupy, thereby displacing that tooth.

Another indication for deciduous tooth removal is when a deciduous malocclusion would impede normal growth of the jaws. Examples include base-narrow mandibular deciduous canines hitting the palate, or upper incisors located lingual to the corresponding lower incisors. If these situations can be discovered in young animals (8 to 12 weeks of age), careful extraction of the teeth can often resolve the malocclusion and allow the jaws to grow to their proper length. If there is a genetic predisposition for the jaw to be abnormal, however, this procedure will not change the eventual outcome.

Deciduous teeth should also be extracted if they are broken or discolored and abscessed. The close proximity of the permanent tooth bud under the gingival surface makes it very susceptible to infection from the deciduous tooth. The position of the permanent tooth bud close to the deciduous tooth necessitates careful extraction of deciduous teeth. Even with careful elevation of the deciduous tooth during extraction, the permanent tooth structure and position can be altered.

Permanent teeth should also be extracted with care. Extractions can be challenging and even frustrating, so most cases should be handled by the veterinarian, depending on state laws. Certainly, a loose single-rooted tooth poses no problem; however, solidly anchored multi-rooted teeth often require gingival flaps, sectioning the tooth into single-root fragments, and good elevation technique to adequately remove the tooth without damaging surrounding tissue.

ROOT CANAL THERAPY

Any permanent tooth with nonvital or compromised pulp (fracture with open canal) and that will not receive endodontic (root canal) therapy should be extracted. Except for a tooth that has been recently fractured, especially in a young animal that can have vital pulpotomy/pulp capping performed to preserve the rest of the pulp, any tooth with an open canal or gray to purple discoloration should be considered nonvital. Nonvital pulp provides substrate for bacterial growth, which could allow bacteria to enter the bloodstream. If a root canal will not be performed to remove the infected pulp and seal the canal, the tooth must be extracted. Such a tooth should never be ignored because it does not seem to be bothering the animal. Animal patients may tolerate pain and discomfort much better than we do, but this does not excuse ignoring a potentially dangerous situation. Once such teeth are treated, the animal often shows improvement (eating or feeling better), even though the client noticed no abnormal signs previously. A root canal procedure can preserve the structure of the tooth by removing the potential for ongoing infection. Also, metal or metal and porcelain crowns can be placed on the tooth to provide additional strength.

Excessive tooth wear can expose the pulp canal, necessitating some form of treatment. If the wear is gradual, odontoblasts in the pulp tissue manufacture additional dentin to protect the pulp as it "retreats." A dark spot on a worn tooth that is smooth, hard, and solid is most likely reparative dentin and the pulp is probably still protected. Radiographs should be made in these cases and in cases with minor fractures without pulpal exposure, because even if the pulp cavity is not open, the pulp tissue still could be compromised and eventually die, necessitating treatment. Radiographic signs of a nonvital pulp with extension of infection into the bone around the root include a periapical lucency or halo around the apex.

CARIES

The teeth can also be compromised by carious lesions or cavities, though caries are not as common in pets as in people. Occasionally a carious lesion is seen on the occlusal surface of the upper first molar. The sharp tip of the explorer tends to penetrate this region of dark, soft enamel. Very shallow lesions that do not extend into the pulp cavity can be debrided and restored with amalgam or composites. By the time most carious lesions are detected, however, there is extensive damage to the tooth and extraction may be the only option.

RESORPTIVE LESIONS IN CATS

The teeth of cats can develop resorptive lesions, known as *cervical line lesions*, or feline odontoclastic resorptive lesions. Although these lesions can be found in various areas of the teeth, the most typical presentation is a loss of tooth structure at or near the neck or cervical

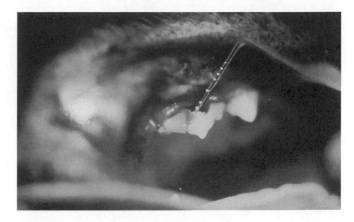

FIG. 25-7 Erosive lesion on the buccal aspect of an upper fourth premolar.

region of the tooth, frequently on the buccal surface (Fig. 25-7), but sometimes on the lingual or palatal surface. These may be grossly apparent or may be hidden by overlying calculus or an area of hyperplastic, reddened gingiva that grows into the space created. They often become apparent during prophylaxis, as the patient "twitches" when the area is touched by the scaler, even under general anesthesia. The cause of these painful lesions is unknown, but they tend to be progressive, even with attempts at treatment. Restoration of an affected tooth, generally with a glass ionomer, should be performed only with very early lesions that affect just the enamel and some of the dentin. Even lesions that appear shallow often exhibit radiographic signs of root resorption, which is an indication for extraction of the tooth. Affected teeth are often ankylosed (joined) to the underlying bone and are difficult to remove intact. In cats with an inflamed mouth (stomatitis), every effort should be made to remove the entire tooth structure.

Even without resorptive lesions, sometimes tooth extraction is the only effective treatment for cats with severe stomatitis. In less severe cases, regular prophylaxis and home care, combined with use of antibiotics and antiinflammatories as indicated, can often help control the inflammation. In cats that eventually become nonresponsive to such conservative treatment, removal of all of the teeth (and therefore the surfaces that plaque can adhere to) may substantially decrease the amount of inflammation. Extraction of the caudal teeth (molars and premolars) is sometimes sufficient, particularly when the cat will no longer be chewing on the inflamed tissue. Some affected cats, however, require extraction of all of their teeth. Certain breeds, such as Abyssinians, Maine coon cats, and some of the Oriental breeds, are predisposed to stomatitis, but it can occur in any cat. Cats with stomatitis should be checked for infection with feline leukemia virus or feline immunodeficiency virus before any treatment is given, particularly with antiinflammatories.

CONGENITAL PROBLEMS

Animals may be born with oral defects, because of either a genetic influence or stimuli during fetal development. Some of these lesions may be quite obvious, as with a puppy that cannot nurse or has milk coming out of its nose after nursing due to a cleft palate. The genetic defect called *microglossia*, or "bird tongue," may not be readily apparent (Fig. 25-8). Affected animals have a small tongue and cannot adequately nurse; they often weaken quickly. Unless microglossia is diagnosed, failure of these puppies to thrive may be attributed to the "fading puppy" syndrome. Other congenital abnormalities include a variation in tooth number, certain developmental tumors, and other inherited defects of the oral cavity, as in gray Collie syndrome.

ORAL TRAUMA

Trauma to the head can cause significant damage to the oral cavity. With any trauma, the patient's condition must be stabilized before any corrective oral work can be attempted. Fractured teeth are one of the most common results of trauma. Teeth can be fractured by external sources of trauma, but more commonly they are fractured by chewing on hard objects, such as bones, cattle hooves, or even ice. External trauma frequently damages other tissues in the mouth, so the soft tissue and bones of the head and mouth should be carefully examined.

A tooth can also be avulsed (lost or ejected) from the socket. If handled correctly and in a timely fashion,

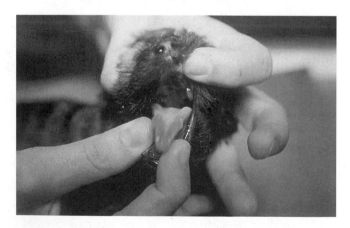

FIG. 25-8 Microglossia (bird tongue) in a puppy.

these avulsed teeth can be reimplanted into the socket to preserve the tooth. An avulsed tooth should immediately be placed in sterile saline and the reimplantation procedure performed as quickly as possible. If saline is not available, the client can place the tooth in cold milk until reaching the clinic. After reimplantation, the tooth will also need endodontic treatment. If the previous presence of the tooth must be documented for legal or breed registry reasons (i.e., some working breeds, Schutzen dogs), a preoperative radiograph can demonstrate the empty alveolus or a retained root if the crown has broken off.

Mandibular or maxillary fractures often occur with severe head trauma. Many basic techniques of fracture reduction have been attempted in the oral cavity, but certain long bone fracture repair techniques do not adapt well to this region. The mandibular canal is not suitable for intramedullary pinning. External fixators, screws, plates, and pins often damage root structures when placed improperly. In addition, fracture reduction and stabilization are not the only considerations. Restoring normal occlusion must also be addressed when repairing these fractures. Interdental or transosseous wiring, with or without use of acrylics, is often employed for stabilization. Additional injuries, such as palate separation or temporomandibular joint luxation, must be addressed accordingly.

Soft tissue trauma should be thoroughly evaluated and addressed in conjunction with any bony or dental injuries. Depending on the degree of damage, the region should be flushed and cleaned of debris and nonvital tissue, and tissues sutured in their proper position if possible, without interfering with occlusion or mastication. All attempts should be made to preserve as much attached gingiva as possible when it is involved.

A degloving type of injury to the rostral portion of the mandibular (lower) lip can occur as it is nearly scraped off the mandible. Often the soft tissue must be sutured by securing it around the mandibular canine teeth. Soft tissue injury in the sublingual area can go undetected. By gently pressing a finger up into the intermandibular area while opening the animal's mouth, the tongue can be elevated and the area beneath can be better visualized. Lacerations, ulcerations, foreign bodies, and even tumors can be better assessed using this method.

The oral cavity can be a common location for foreign bodies, particularly in young animals that indiscriminately chew on objects. Foreign bodies can lodge anywhere in the mouth, such as rib bones lodged against the palate, round bones stuck behind the canines or around the mandible, fish hooks, needles, or tacks penetrating the lips or palate, or string or fishing line caught around the base of the tongue. With smaller foreign bodies, such as burrs or plant awns, the object may not be visible because it is embedded in granulomatous tissue, sometimes coalescing into a large lesion if multiple burrs are embedded, such as in the tongue.

Chewing on electric cords can cause significant damage and burns in the oral cavity, not to mention serious damage to internal organs and severe pulmonary edema. Conservative debridement of necrotic tissue can help to preserve as much normal oral tissue as possible. Burns and ulcerations from ingestion of caustic chemicals can be moderate to severe, depending on the compound and degree of exposure. As with any other oral injuries, supportive care must be provided until the animal can comfortably eat and drink.

ORAL TUMORS

As both veterinary staff and animal owners continue to improve their dental "I.Q." and as pets are living longer lives, oral tumors are more likely to be detected. Unless the owner is doing regular home care or examining the pet often, oral tumors often have grown to a large size before they are detected. Considering the aggressive biologic nature of malignant oral tumors, by the time the tumor is diagnosed, it may have already metastasized (spread to other body areas).

The most common oral malignancy of dogs is *melanosarcoma* (Fig. 25-9). Melanosarcoma is more prevalent in older (more than 10 years of age), male dogs with dark pigmentation of the skin and mucosae, and in certain breeds (e.g., Cocker Spaniels). These tumors grow rapidly and can be found on the gingiva, palate, tongue, or lips. By the time of detection, they have most likely metastasized throughout the lymphatics or to the lungs, so thoracic radiographs should be made. Although aggressive resection combined with chemotherapy and/or radiation therapy can increase the anticipated survival rates, melanosarcoma still warrants a guarded prognosis.

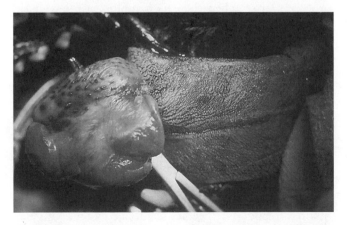

FIG. 25-9 Melanosarcoma on the tongue of a 10-year-old male Chow Chow.

Another common oral tumor in dogs is the *fibrosarcoma*, which can be seen in larger dogs, often on the palate. These are typically firm, and sometimes flat and ulcerated. Fibrosarcomas are locally invasive but slow to metastasize, and they tend to recur after resection. *Squamous-cell carcinoma* in dogs shows variable biologic characteristics, depending on its site in the oral cavity. Tonsillar forms are extremely invasive, often metastasize, and warrant a grave prognosis. Nontonsillar squamous-cell carcinomas are often found on the buccal mucosa or tongue. If found in the rostral oral cavity, these tumors tend to be less aggressive than tumors found in the caudal portion of the mouth. Squamous-cell carcinoma is the most common oral tumor seen in cats. They have a variable presentation in cats, depending on the site. Cats can also have fibrosarcomas, but melanosarcomas are rare in cats.

Of the benign tumors found, the *epulis* is probably the most frequently seen. The fibromatous epulis and the ossifying epulis can often be treated adequately with excision and extraction of the associated teeth (they arise from the periodontal ligament). The acanthomatous epulis tends to be a more locally invasive tumor, requiring more radical surgery to address the problem. *Viral papillomatosis* may also be seen in dogs, as can some developmental tumors (e.g., odontoma, dentigerous cyst).

ORTHODONTICS

Orthodontics is the branch of dentistry concerned with prevention or correction of malocclusion (improper bite). In veterinary dentistry, orthodontics involves assessment of an animal's occlusion to determine if orthodontic measures can help alleviate pain and discomfort and provide a more normal bite.

The relationship between the upper and lower incisors is usually evaluated. The relationship between the upper and lower arcades is better assessed by looking at the premolars. Ideally, the upper and lower incisors should meet in a *scissors* fashion, with the upper incisors slightly rostral to the lower incisors. The American Kennel Club permits many breeds to have a *level bite*, with the incisal edges of the incisors contacting; this can be an uncomfortable situation. Brachycephalic (pug-nosed) breeds have a *reverse scissors bite*, with the lower incisors rostral to the upper incisors. This is considered "normal" within certain limits for these breeds.

When the relationship of the maxilla and mandible is correct, the lower canine tooth is positioned directly between the upper canine and upper corner incisor, with equal spacing on either side (mesial and distal aspects) of the lower canine. The premolars should also be positioned in an "interdigitation" with the cusp tip of the rostral mandibular premolars, like a pair of pinking shears.

Animals with properly aligned upper and lower arcades (premolar interdigitation, canine placement) may have misplaced individual incisor teeth, as from retained deciduous teeth, that cause a maxillary incisor to erupt palatal to its normal position. Such *anterior crossbites* can sometimes be uncomfortable and result in abnormal wear to the teeth, even causing them to be sensitive.

Retention of deciduous teeth can also influence another malocclusion, when the mandibular canines are deflected lingually, often to the extent that they contact the palate. If the soft tissue contact is at the edge of the palate, excision of the gingival "groove" that is formed may be sufficient to relieve the problem. When teeth contact the palate with full force, some form of correction is necessary to relieve pain. The offending teeth can be extracted, the coronal height can be reduced (with vital pulpotomy and pulp capping), or orthodontic movement with incline planes can be considered. Any extensive work requires specialized training, as well as owner commitment to home care while the orthodontic appliance is in place.

Rostral or mesial deviation of an upper canine tooth can occur as a result of retention of its deciduous counterpart. The prevalence tends to be higher in certain breeds, such as Shelties and Italian Greyhounds (lance tooth), indicating possible genetic involvement. Rostral positioning of this tooth can also result in lateral or buccal displacement of the lower canine. Orthodontic movement can help resolve these problems.

With any malocclusion or orthodontic case, the genetic implications should always be thoroughly discussed with the owner. It must be stressed that correction is done only to relieve any pain or discomfort the animal might be experiencing. If the abnormality appears to be an inherited one, the owner should be counseled against breeding that animal. In addition to the forms of malocclusion previously discussed, many other inherited problems warrant serious consideration of that animal's breeding potential. For example, consider an animal with what appears to be a normal scissors bite, with the lower canine positioned tightly against the upper corner incisor. This indicates a mandible that is relatively longer than the maxilla, but held in place by the canines' position. Such an individual may produce offspring with a distinct malocclusion. Orthodontic correction should never be done to conceal or camouflage an abnormality.

SYSTEMIC PROBLEMS AFFECTING THE ORAL CAVITY

The mouth is sometimes the first, or the most noticeable, place where certain systemic diseases or conditions become apparent. The gingival mucosa, with its high vascularity, shows distinct changes when anemia (pale), lack of oxygen (cyanotic), toxicity (chocolate brown), or bleeding abnormalities (petechiation) are present.

Gingival ulcerations may be present with renal disease (e.g., uremia), during certain infections (e.g., calicivirus), or as a sequel to immunodeficiency (e.g., feline immunodeficiency virus). Hyperparathyroidism, either primary or secondary to severe renal disease, causes "rubber jaw" when the calcium in the bones is depleted. The bones of affected animals are less radiodense, and the teeth appear to be "floating" without jaw contact. There may be swelling and softening of the maxilla and mandible. Autoimmune diseases (e.g., pemphigus vulgaris, bullous pemphigoid) often have oral signs. Recognizing abnormalities in the oral cavity alerts the veterinary staff to potential problems elsewhere in the body.

DENTISTRY IN OTHER SPECIES
Rabbits and Rodents

Animals other than dogs and cats are occasionally presented for specific oral problems. Rodents and rabbits have specific oral and dental needs related to the structure and function of the teeth and mouth. Rodents and rabbits have four prominent incisor teeth for gnawing. Rabbits also have two additional small maxillary incisors, peg teeth, caudal to the large ones. These incisor teeth have very long "root" structures, and grow continuously for the life of the animal. They are termed *aradicular hypsodont teeth*, because the apex never closes into a distinct root structure. As the animal chews on rough or abrasive objects, the teeth wear down but continue to erupt. In rabbits and some rodents (e.g., chinchillas, guinea pigs), the cheek teeth (premolars and molars) also grow continuously.

Continuous growth of the incisors poses no problems when the animal has a normal occlusion; however, problems arise when there is a malocclusion and the upper and lower teeth do not meet correctly. If this is the case, particularly with the incisors, the teeth do not wear down in the proper manner, and they overgrow, often causing a worse malocclusion. These teeth must be trimmed every 6 to 8 weeks to prevent additional problems of cheek teeth overgrowth.

These teeth are best cut with a bur on a high-speed handpiece; such instruments as nail trimmers can break or split a tooth, exposing the pulp cavity. Another alternative to frequent trimmings can be extraction of all four incisors, which can be challenging with their long, curved roots. The use of small instruments and even blunted hypodermic needles (25 to 18 gauge) with gentle elevation around the tooth can often successfully remove these teeth.

TABLE 25-1 Dental procedures performed on horses of various ages

Age	Examine for necessary dentistry	Dental procedure
2-3 years	1. 1st premolar vestige (wolf teeth) 2. 1st deciduous premolar (upper and lower) 3. Hard swelling on ventral surface of mandible beneath 1st premolar. 4. Cuts or abrasions on inside of cheek in region of the 2nd premolars and molars. 5. Sharp protuberances on all premolars and molars.	1. Remove wolf teeth if present. 2. Remove deciduous teeth if ready. If not, file off corners and points of premolars. 3. Make radiographs. Extract retained temporary premolar if present. 4. Lightly float or dress all molars and premolars if necessary. 5. Rasp protuberances down to level of other teeth in the arcade.
3-4 years	1. 1, 2, 3, and 5 above 2. 2nd deciduous premolar (upper and lower)	1. 1, 2, 4, and 5 above. 2. Remove if present and ready.
4-5 years	1. 1, 4, and 5 above. 2. 3rd deciduous premolar.	1. 1, 4, and 5 above. 2. Remove if present and ready.
5 years and older	1. 1, 4, and 5 above. 2. Uneven growth and "wavy" arcade. 3. Unusually long molars and premolars.	1. 1, 4, and 5 above 2. 1, 4, and 5 above. 3. Unusually long molars and premolars may have to be cut if they cannot be filed down.

From Baker GJ: *Diseases of the teeth.* In Colahan PT et al: *Equine Medicine and Surgery,* ed 4, St Louis, 1991, Mosby.

Other oral problems, such as periodontal disease, can occur in these small pets. This can be quite challenging, particularly if the problem is in the caudal portion of the oral cavity, because the mouth opening is quite restrictive in rabbits and rodents.

Horses

It should be noted that the continually growing teeth of rabbits and rodents are different from the teeth found in horses and some other herbivores. In horses, the teeth are considered to be continually erupting but not continually growing. These teeth continue to erupt, but without further growth at the root. Tooth length diminishes as the animal ages and the erupted tooth is worn away. These can be described as *radicular hypsodont teeth* (long crowned, with a root), in comparison with the teeth of rodents and lagomorphs *(aradicular hypsodont)* or dogs and cats *(brachyodont,* short crowned).

Horses can also experience overgrowth of incisors and cheek teeth, particularly when the teeth wear unevenly. This uneven wear forms sharp hooks or ridges that must be periodically filed down *(floated)*. Table 25-1 lists the dental procedures performed on horses at various ages.

REFERENCES

1. DeBowes L: Systemic effects of oral disease, *AVDC/AVD Proceed* 65, 1992.
2. Wiggs RB et al: Gingival crevicular fluid aspartate aminotransferase as a marker of naturally occurring periodontal disease in the dog, Manuscript submitted for publication, 1977.

RECOMMENDED READING

Crossley CA Penman S: *Manual of small animal dentistry,* Gloucestershire, UK, 1995, Brit Small Anim Vet Assoc.
Harvey CE, Emily PP: *Small animal dentistry,* St Louis, 1993, Mosby.
Holmstrom SE, Front P, Gammon RL: *Veterinary dental techniques,* Philadelphia, 1992, WB Saunders.
Wiggs RB, Lobprise HB: *Oral disease (33): Dental disease (52).* In Norsworthy GD: *Feline practice,* Philadelphia, 1993, JB Lippincott.
Wiggs RB, Lobprise HB: *Veterinary dentistry: principles and practice,* Philadelphia, 1997, JB Lippincott.

PART FIVE

Nursing Care

CHAPTER 26

Nursing Care of Dogs and Cats

C. Winters

Learning Objectives

After reviewing this chapter, the reader should understand the following:

Methods of sample collection for laboratory analysis
Routes of administration of medication
Types of catheters and how they are placed

Techniques used in general nursing care of dogs and cats
Procedures used in providing respiratory support
Procedures used in providing nutritional support
Procedures used in grooming and skin, nail, and ear care
Procedures used in caring for recumbent patients
Procedures used in rehabilitative therapy

SAMPLE COLLECTION

Veterinary technicians often are required to collect samples from patients for diagnostic testing. These may include blood samples by venipuncture or arterial puncture, or fluid samples by centesis.

Venipuncture

Venipuncture can be performed using either a syringe and needle or a vacuum tube system (e.g., Vacutainer, Becton-Dickinson). The syringe and needle technique (Box 26-1) is the method of choice for blood gas analysis and can be used to collect blood for almost all tests except for coagulation profiles, von Willebrand's factor, and activated clotting times. Large volumes of blood must be collected from a large vessel using the Vacutainer system; otherwise, clots may form before all of the blood is removed by syringe and needle.

Following are some tips to facilitate venipuncture:

- The vessels of cats are usually very superficial and fragile.

- Wet the skin with alcohol before occluding the vessel. Occlude the vessel and watch it fill with blood.
- If unable to visualize the vessel, palpate while occluding the vessel. It feels more spongy than surrounding tissue.
- The jugular vein runs in a line from the point of the mandibular ramus to the thoracic inlet.
- For jugular venipuncture, do not overextend the neck, because this tends to flatten the vessel.
- The jugular vein of brachycephalic (short-nosed) breeds is more lateral than in other breeds.
- In patients with limb edema, wrap the limb (not too tightly) with Vetwrap from the toes to just proximal to the venipuncture site and attempt venipuncture after 5 or 10 minutes; discard the sample if the needle did not directly penetrate the vessel.
- Animals with some endocrine disorders (e.g., hyperadrenocorticism) have very thin skin and friable vessels.

The Vacutainer is useful when collecting blood in multiple tubes and can be used for all tests except for

Box 26–1 Syringe venipuncture

1. Choose the appropriate needle (20 gauge for most patients, 22 gauge for pediatric patients) and syringe for the amount of blood needed. A 25-gauge needle on a tuberculin syringe is good for small-volume samples.
2. The jugular vein (Fig. 26-1) is used in almost all situations except in patients with suspected von Willebrand's disease, coagulopathy, or anticoagulant toxicity (e.g., warfarin). The saphenous vein can be used in patients with bleeding disorders.
3. Occlude the vessel (usually with the left hand, if right-handed) while restraining the patient in sternal recumbency.
4. Swab the skin with alcohol and part the hair to visualize the vessel.
5. With the bevel of the needle directed up, penetrate the skin and vessel wall in one smooth motion at a 15- to 30-degree angle (Fig. 26-2).
6. Aspirate blood in a continuous draw. If blood flow stops, aspirate more slowly and gently or withdraw and redirect the needle.
7. Once the syringe is filled, release the vessel and negative pressure on the syringe, and withdraw the needle.
8. Apply slight pressure over the venipuncture site to prevent hematoma formation. A light bandage may be applied if needed.

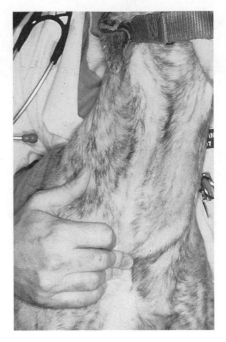

FIG. 26-1 With the dog restrained in sternal recumbency, the jugular vein is occluded for venipuncture.

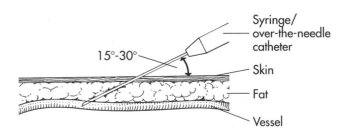

FIG. 26-2 Technique for venipuncture. The bevel of the needle is directed up and the needle is inserted at a 15- to 30-degree angle.

blood gas analysis. It is, however, difficult to use on cats, because the vacuum in the tube collapses the vessel. A steady hand and good patient restraint are necessary when changing tubes with the needle in place.

The technique is the same as for syringe/needle venipuncture, except that the first few drops of blood should be allowed to drip through the needle if the venipuncture did not cleanly penetrate the vessel. For an activated clotting time (ACT), the first five drops should be allowed to drip from the needle before the tube is attached. A pediatric Vacutainer holder can be used for 3-ml or smaller tubes. Always fill a clot (serum) tube first to ensure good positioning of the needle and free flow of blood through the needle. Remove the last tube from the needle before removing the needle from the vessel. Apply pressure at the sampling site.

Arterial Puncture

The arteries most commonly used for arterial puncture are the femoral artery and the dorsal pedal artery (Box 26-2). Under anesthesia, other arteries may be used. Usually the blood is drawn for arterial blood gas analysis to measure the oxygen content of the blood and to

monitor acid-base status. If more than one blood gas may be needed, an arterial catheter should be considered.

Catheterization

A central catheter can be placed via the jugular vein or the saphenous vein to the cranial or caudal vena cava, respectively. Central vein catheterization allows fluid administration and repeated blood sampling. An extension set (e.g., Minivolume, Baxter; Microbore, Abbott) is attached to the catheter. The extension set allows blood collection without getting near aggressive patients. A syringe or a Vacutainer system may be used to retrieve a blood sample. Using a catheter for blood sampling usually does not require an additional person to restrain the patient.

Centesis

Centesis involves inserting a needle or catheter into a body cavity for removal of fluid or gas. *Gastrocentesis*

Box 26–2 Arterial puncture

Materials:

3-ml syringe or Smooth-E arterial blood sampler (Radiometer America)

25- or 22-gauge needle

heparin (if syringe used)

rubber stopper

ice bath

Procedure:

1. If using the Smooth-E syringe, withdraw the plunger to the volume of sample required and attach the needle. If using a standard syringe, attach the needle and then aspirate heparin into the syringe and expel it.

2. Choose the arterial site with the strongest pulse. Palpate the pulse with two fingers of your dominant hand (Fig. 26-3). Holding the arterial blood sampler like a pencil, insert at a 45- to 90-degree angle into the artery. An artery feels thicker and more firm than a vein. In a normal animal the blood should flow easily and is brighter red than venous blood. If using a syringe, insert the needle into the artery and manually aspirate 1 ml of blood. The blood should flow in with very little aspiration.

3. Remove the needle from the artery and apply pressure on the insertion point for 5 minutes.

4. Expel air bubbles from the syringe and stick the needle into the stopper. Place the syringe and needle or the arterial blood sampler into the ice water bath and immediately have the sample analyzed.

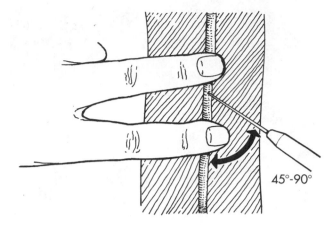

FIG. 26-3 Technique for arterial puncture. After the artery is located by palpation, the needle, attached to a syringe, is inserted at a 45- to 90-degree angle to the skin. The syringe is held between thumb and forefinger like a pencil.

Cystocentesis is removal of urine from the bladder with a syringe and needle. This technique prevents lower urinary tract contamination of the urine sample and is ideal for collecting urine samples for culture. Syringe size is dictated by the volume of urine needed for a standard urinalysis, specific gravity, and culture. A 22-gauge, 1¼-inch or 21-gauge, 2-inch needle is used. Restraint is crucial to the success of cystocentesis and patient safety. Cats are usually restrained in dorsal or lateral recumbency; in dogs, the procedure may also be done with the patient standing.

With the animal in dorsal recumbency, the "pooling" technique may help locate the best place for cystocentesis. A small amount of alcohol is poured onto the abdomen; the area on ventral midline where it pools is best for cystocentesis. In male dogs, move the prepuce to one side to allow insertion of the needle.

Immobilize the bladder by lightly holding it between thumb and fingers; do not squeeze the bladder during cystocentesis. Direct the needle (attached to the syringe) in a caudodorsal direction on the midline, just cranial to the pubis. The needle should penetrate at the neck of the bladder or trigone area in the ventral abdomen, just cranial to the pubis (Fig. 26-4). Once the needle is in the abdomen, never redirect the needle or withdraw and reinsert it, because this could contaminate the bladder or abdominal cavity. When the needle is in the lumen of the bladder, aspirate gently until urine flows into the syringe. Discontinue aspiration before removing the needle from the bladder. If the first attempt is unsuccessful, change needles and try one more time. If unsuccessful on the second attempt, wait an hour before attempting again. If the patient is struggling, discontinue attempts at cystocentesis unless the animal is sedated.

Cystocentesis is contraindicated in patients with bleeding disorders, suspected pyometra, or a bladder tumor.

involves insertion of a needle or catheter through the abdominal wall into the stomach to remove accumulated gas or fluid. This procedure is most commonly performed on dogs with gastric dilatation/volvulus, in which orogastric decompression fails. *Pericardiocentesis* involves insertion of a needle or catheter into the pericardial sac surrounding the heart to remove accumulated fluid. *Thoracentesis* involves insertion of a needle or catheter into the thoracic cavity to remove fluid or air. Chylous fluid (lymph) is removed with chylothorax; pus with pyothorax; air with pneumothorax; blood with hemothorax; and an effusion with hydrothorax.

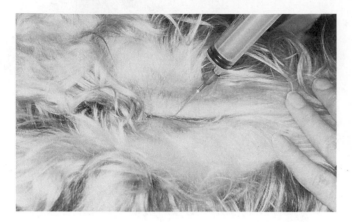

FIG. 26-4   Cystocentesis in a female dog restrained in dorsal recumbency.

Cystocentesis should also be avoided in patients recovering from recent abdominal surgery or trauma. Possible complications of cystocentesis include contamination of the bladder with fecal material from accidental intestinal penetration, bladder rupture, and puncture of a blood vessel in the skin, bladder, or abdominal wall.

ROUTES OF ADMINISTRATION
Oral Administration

Oral administration is the route most commonly used to administer medications. Medications given orally are metabolized slowly; another route of administration is necessary if more rapid absorption of medication is required. The patient must be able to swallow and have normal digestive function if medication is given per os (PO, by mouth).

Oral medications are available in tablet, capsule, and liquid form. If necessary, tablets can be crushed or capsule contents dissolved in water and given with a syringe or feeding tube. If the patient has a good appetite, the medication may be placed in a meatball of canned food (this does not work well with sick cats). If the oral cavity is damaged, it can be bypassed and medications, crushed and mixed with water, or the medication can be given directly into the gastrointestinal tract via nasogastric or gastrostomy tube.

A pilling device (e.g., Pet Piller, H-Bar-S Manufacturing) can be used to avoid being bitten. This is a plastic rod with a rubber-tipped plunger to hold the medication. Hemostats should not be used to administer medication, because they can damage the teeth or soft palate. Teach animal owners how to correctly administer oral medication and how to check the animal's mouth to ensure that all medications have been swallowed.

Place small patients at waist level and large dogs on the floor. Medicate cats by grasping the upper jaw over

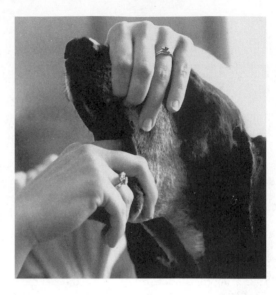

FIG. 26-5   Oral administration of a tablet or pill. *(From Pratt: Medical, surgical and anesthetic nursing for veterinary technicians, ed 2, St Louis, 1994, Mosby.)*

the top of the head and tipping the head back. The lower jaw will drop open, or it may need to be pried open slightly with the middle finger of the dominant hand, with the pill held between the thumb and forefinger of that hand. Place the pill in the center groove of the tongue, at the back of the throat. Do not scratch the soft palate with your fingers. With aggressive cats, a towel or cat bag may be necessary (see Chapter 17).

In dogs, grasp the muzzle using the fingers and thumb to press the skin against the teeth (Fig. 26-5). Slip the thumb of the left hand into the mouth and press up on the hard palate, keeping the lips against the teeth. Place the pill on the base of the tongue at the back of the throat. Keep the head slightly elevated, close the mouth, and hold it shut, while rubbing the throat until the patient swallows. Swallowing can be facilitated by blowing into its nose. After administering medication, always examine the patient's mouth for complete swallowing of the medication.

To administer liquid medication in a syringe, tilt the head back slightly and pull the lips outward slightly to form a pocket (Fig. 26-6). Place the syringe between the lips and back teeth so that the liquid flows between the molars, to the throat, and administer slowly in small boluses to allow the patient to swallow and not aspirate.

Orogastric Intubation

Orogastric tubes are inserted through the mouth to the stomach and used for administering liquid medication and fluids and flushing the stomach (gastric lavage). The animal must have a swallowing reflex to prevent

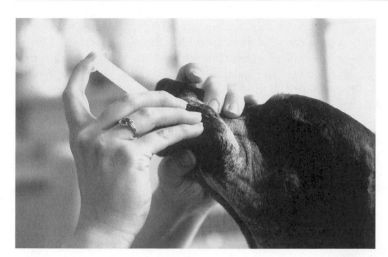

FIG. 26-6 Oral administration of a liquid. *(From Pratt:* Medical, surgical and anesthetic nursing for veterinary technicians, *ed 2, St Louis, 1994, Mosby.)*

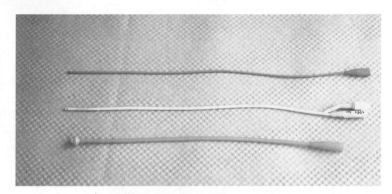

FIG. 26-7 A sample of the various feeding tubes available: soft red rubber feeding tube *(top),* used for orogastric feeding; Foley catheter *(center),* with inflatable balloon tip deflated, used for gastrostomy or jejunostomy feeding; and de Pezzer mushroom-tipped catheter *(bottom),* used for gastrostomy or jejunostomy feeding.

aspiration if the patient regurgitates. Another cause of aspiration is passing the orogastric tube into the trachea, instead of the esophagus, and administering the medication.

A soft, flexible feeding tube is used, of appropriate diameter and length and with a slightly rounded tip (Fig. 26-7). A speculum is needed to keep the mouth slightly open, to allow for passage of the tube. The speculum can be a roll of tape, syringe casing, or a piece of PVC pipe large enough to allow the tube to pass (Fig. 26-8).

Measure the distance from the tip of the nose to just caudal to the last rib. Mark the tube with a piece of tape or permanent marker. Lubricate the tube with water-soluble lubricating jelly. Place the patient in sternal recumbency or sitting, with the speculum in place. Two people may need to restrain the patient if chemical restraint is not used. Elevate the head slightly and extend the neck, while passing the tube slowly and gently into the esophagus (Fig. 26-8). Palpate the neck to ensure esophageal placement. Inadvertent passage of the tube and subsequent administration of medication into the trachea may result in severe lung damage and possibly death. Once the tube reaches the line marked, inject air through the tube and auscultate for air bubbling in the stomach or inject a small amount of sterile saline and listen for a

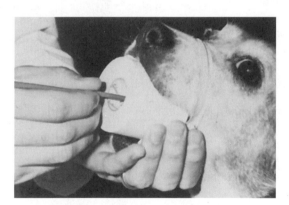

FIG. 26-8 Passage of a red rubber catheter for orogastric administration of medication. A roll of adhesive tape can be used as a speculum to hold the mouth open for tube passage. *(From Pratt P:* Medical, surgical and anesthetic nursing for veterinary technicians, *ed 2, St Louis, 1994, Mosby.)*

cough. Gas may be smelled as it exits the tube. If the tube cannot be passed to the line marked on the tube, withdraw it and try again. Administer the fluid with a syringe and flush the tube with a small amount of water or air to empty the tube of medication. Occlude or kink the end of the tubing to prevent spilling of liquid into mouth or trachea while the tube is being removed.

Rectal Administration

An enema introduces fluids into the rectum and colon to stimulate bowel activity, evacuate the large intestine for diagnostic procedures, and irrigate the colon (Box 26-3). Enemas soften feces and stimulate colonic motility. Tap water or saline adds bulk, whereas petrolatum oils soften, lubricate, and promote evacuation of hardened feces. Glycerin and water, mild soap and water, or commercial enema preparations can also be used for enema solutions. However, phosphate enemas (e.g., Fleet) should not be administered to cats or small dogs. Large volumes of warm water are administered with a bucket elevated above the patient and attached to soft red rubber tubing. Smaller volumes can be administered with a 60-ml syringe attached to the tubing. The solution should be at room temperature or tepid.

Box 26-3 Giving an enema

1. For an evacuation enema, place the animal in a tub, run, or large cage. Lubricate the tubing with water-soluble lubricating jelly.
2. Wearing gloves and with the animal restrained in a standing position, insert the lubricated tube into the rectum, at least 5 cm cranial to the anal sphincter, and administer the solution slowly. Water enemas to evacuate the bowel are safely given at 10 to 20 ml/kg of body weight. Rapid administration may cause the patient to vomit.
3. Remove the tubing from the rectum and allow the animal to evacuate in a large area. This may take minutes to hours.

Enemas are contraindicated if the bowel is perforated or recent colon surgery has been performed. Complications of enema administration include perforating the colon and leakage of fluid into the peritoneal cavity, vomiting if fluid is administered too quickly, and hemorrhage if the colon is irritated.

Nasal Administration

Some medications may be administered into the nasal cavity to be absorbed through the nasal mucosa. Occasionally, nasal insufflation tubes are inserted through the nares to administer oxygen and humidified air to the lungs; nasoesophageal and nasogastric tubes are inserted to provide nutrition. Respiratory vaccines and local anesthetics also may be placed into the nasal passages. Nasal administration, via syringe or dropper, is usually not stressful and most dogs tolerate it very well.

Have all medications and materials ready and within reach before starting. With the patient in sternal recumbency or sitting, tip the animal's head back so that the nose is slightly elevated, and instill the medication into the nares (Fig. 26-9). Once the medication is administered, keep the nose elevated until the medication is absorbed through the mucosa.

Endotracheal Administration

Oxygen, inhalant anesthetics, medication, and small volumes of fluid can be administered through the trachea for direct absorption through the mucosa or for diagnostic evaluation of tracheal/bronchial secretions (tracheal wash). Placement of an endotracheal tube allows direct administration of oxygen or anesthetics. Humidification and nebulization for respiratory therapy can be administered through an oxygen mask, nasal insufflation tube, tracheostomy tube, or endotracheal tube. Medications may be placed into the humidifier/nebulizer for direct

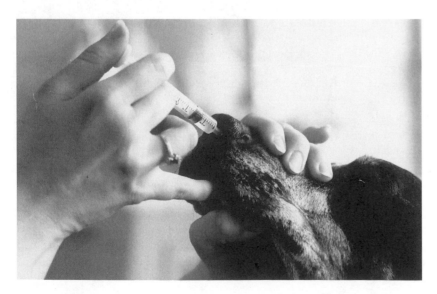

FIG. 26-9 Intranasal administration of medication or vaccines. Note that the head is elevated to allow flow of the medication into the nasal passages. *(From Pratt P: Medical, surgical and anesthetic nursing for veterinary technicians, ed 2, St Louis, 1994, Mosby.)*

administration, by aerosolization, to the bronchioles. For diagnostic evaluations of bronchial secretions, a sterile polypropylene catheter can be inserted through the skin and tracheal rings (transtracheal wash). To avoid respiratory distress, fluid volumes injected depend on the animal's size.

Ophthalmic Application

Medication can be applied topically onto the eye to treat the cornea, conjunctiva, and anterior chamber. Ophthalmic medications are available in liquid and ointment forms. Most eye conditions are very painful and may require restraint for application. Before applying the medication, the eye must be cleaned of any exudates. An ophthalmic irrigating solution and cottonballs are used to clean the surrounding area. Have all materials and medications ready and within reach before restraining the patient.

Restrain the patient in a sternal position or sitting, with the head tipped back and the nose pointed toward the ceiling. Grasp the muzzle to prevent the patient from moving its head. Gently clean the eye area with wet cottonballs. Flush the cornea and conjunctival sac by everting the eyelids and applying a gentle stream of irrigating solution from medial to lateral. If excessive ocular discharge has caused irritation of surrounding skin, apply a thin layer of petrolatum-based ointment onto the skin.

Ophthalmic solutions are easier to administer but may need to be administered more frequently than ointments. Most solutions are applied every few hours to maintain their effect. With the dropper or bottle held 1 or 2 inches above the eye and the upper eyelid pulled up, apply the solution directly onto the sclera; then release the eyelid (Fig. 26-10). To avoid contaminating the dropper bottle or tube, do not touch the eye or eyelid with it. If more than one solution is to be applied, wait a few minutes between applications. If both a solution and an ointment are to be used, apply the solution several minutes before the ointment.

Ointment is slightly more difficult to apply. Ointments are usually applied every 4 to 6 hours; they do not wash out but may soil the skin around the eye. The ointment tube must be held close to, but not in contact with, the eye. Evert the eyelid and place a ⅛- or ¼-inch strip of ointment medial to lateral onto the cornea or lower border of the eyelid, making sure not to touch the tube to the eye or eyelid (Fig. 26-11).

Otic Application

Liquids can be instilled into the ear canal to medicate or clean the ear. The ear should be cleaned before instilling medication to ensure that the medication is absorbed and fully dispersed. Otoscopic examination is necessary to ensure that the tympanic membrane is intact before ear

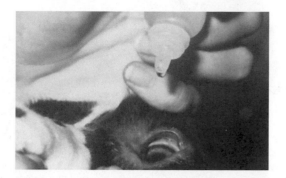

FIG. 26-10 Instillation of ophthalmic drops to the eye. Note that the container does not touch the eye. *(From Pratt P: Medical, surgical and anesthetic nursing for veterinary technicians, ed 2, St Louis, 1994, Mosby.)*

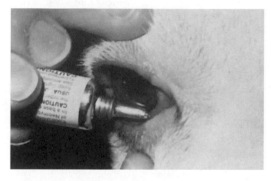

FIG. 26-11 Application of ophthalmic ointment to the eye. *(From Pratt P: Medical, surgical and anesthetic nursing for veterinary technicians, ed 2, St Louis, 1994, Mosby.)*

cleaning or applying medication. Obtain culture or cytologic samples, if necessary, before the ears are cleaned.

Most patients tolerate medication of the ear with minimal restraint. Start with the less affected ear first, to avoid contaminating the other ear. To straighten the ear canal, apply lateral tension on the pinna (ear flap). Instill the medication into the external ear canal and massage the base of the ear to disperse it (Fig. 26-12).

Topical Application

Medication applied to the skin provides a local effect and is also absorbed through the skin. Shaving and cleaning the area or parting the hair before application facilitates absorption of the medication. Wear latex gloves and/or plastic aprons when giving a medicated bath or applying topical medication. Topical medications include insecticidal shampoos for parasite infestation, fentanyl transdermal patches for analgesia, flea adulticides for once-a-month flea control, topical anesthetics, and nitroglycerin ointment.

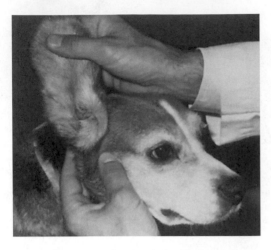

FIG. 26-12 After otic medication is instilled in the external ear canal, the base of the ear is massaged to distribute the medication. *(From Pratt P: Medical, surgical and anesthetic nursing for veterinary technicians,* ed 2, St Louis, 1994, Mosby.)

Parenteral Administration

Fluids and medications administered parenterally are injected via sterile syringe and needle or through a catheter. Parenteral routes include intradermal (ID), subcutaneous (SC), intramuscular (IM), intravenous (IV), intraosseous (IO), epidural, and intraperitoneal (IP). Local inflammation, infection, nerve damage, anaphylactic or allergic reactions, and necrosis at the injection site are possible complications of parenteral administration.

Before aspirating medications into a syringe, swab the rubber stopper of the medication vial with alcohol. Select the appropriate syringe and needle size for the dose and route chosen (22- to 25-gauge for ID, 18- to 22-gauge for SC, 22-gauge for IM, 20- to 22-gauge for IV, and 20- to 22-gauge for IP). Aspirate the medication into the syringe, hold the syringe vertically, and tap it to expel any air bubbles. Keep the needle covered while preparing the site for injection.

Intradermal (ID) injections are used primarily for skin testing and local anesthesia. Skin testing may require sedating the patient before placing in lateral recumbency; local anesthesia may or may not require sedation.

Prepare the skin for skin testing by shaving a large area over the lateral thorax or abdomen, being careful to prevent "clipper burn." Do not use antiseptics to clean the area. For local anesthesia of wounds, skin biopsies, and excision of small lesions, shave and prepare the area as for surgery.

Hold the skin taut between the thumb and forefinger of the left hand and insert the needle (bevel up) into the skin at an angle of approximately 10 degrees. The bevel of the needle should be within the dermis and not visible. Inject a small amount of allergen or local anesthetic intradermally to form a bleb at the site. If no bleb forms, the injection may have been subcutaneous and not intradermal.

Subcutaneous (SC) administration is used for sustained absorption of fluids and medications and administration of some vaccines. Medication and fluids are absorbed slowly over 20 or 30 minutes, or longer for larger volumes of fluids. Clients can easily be taught to give SC injections of medication (e.g., insulin) and fluids to patients at home.

Fluids are not readily absorbed when injected SC in severely dehydrated, "shocky," or debilitated patients. The IV route should be used in such cases. Hypertonic, caustic, or irritating solutions (e.g., some chemotherapeutic agents, dirofilaricides, thiopental) administered SC can cause damage and sloughing of the skin and should not be administered by this route. Read the drug's package insert before administering medications subcutaneously.

Large volumes of room-temperature fluids may be administered by gravity flow via fluid bag and administration set with a needle attached. This allows for patient comfort during the long process of administering larger volumes of fluid. The needle should be changed with each injection site change to prevent abscessation. The patient should be restrained in a comfortable sitting, standing, or sternal position. Most cats and dogs tolerate SC administration well. Carefully part the hair, clean the skin if excessively dirty, and apply a skin antiseptic, such as 70% alcohol.

Grasp the skin between thumb and forefinger along the dorsal aspect of the neck or back and lift gently to form a tent (Fig. 26-13). Insert the needle into the skin fold and aspirate. If blood is aspirated, withdraw the needle and use another injection site. If no blood is aspirated, inject the medication or fluids slowly.

Multiple injection sites can be used along the dorsum and lateral to the spine. Between 50 and 100 ml of fluid may be safely injected at each site without discomfort. Remove the needle, gently pinch the injection site, and

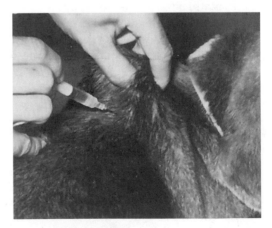

FIG. 26-13 Subcutaneous injections can be given at the back of the neck, with the skin grasped to form a tent. *(From Pratt P: Medical, surgical and anesthetic nursing for veterinary technicians,* ed 2, St Louis, 1994, Mosby.)

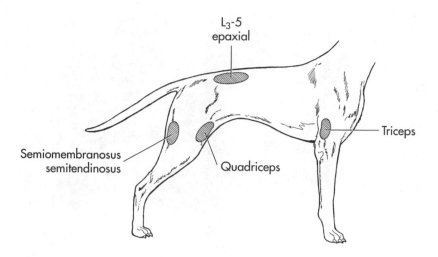

FIG. 26-14 Sites for intramuscular injection. The preferred site is the epaxial muscles lateral to the third to fifth lumbar vertebrae.

massage the area. This prevents leakage and facilitates dispersal and absorption of fluid or medication. Large volumes of fluid may gradually migrate ventrally before being absorbed completely.

Muscles are more vascular than subcutaneous tissue and medication is more readily absorbed after *intramuscular (IM) administration* than if given SC. However, muscle tissue cannot accommodate more than 2 to 5 ml of medication at any one site, and IM injections can be painful. Slow to moderate rates of administration with small-gauge (22- to 25-gauge) needles may be less painful than rapid injections. Intramuscular administration is never used for fluid therapy. Some medications that are poorly soluble and mildly irritating can be administered IM but not SC or IV.

Large muscle groups are used for IM injections, such as the epaxial muscles lateral to the dorsal spinous process of lumbar vertebrae 3 to 5, quadriceps muscles of the cranial thigh, and triceps muscles caudal to the humerus (Fig. 26-14). The epaxial muscles are the best site for IM injections in small patients. The semimembranosus/semitendinosus muscles on the caudal thigh should be avoided because of possible sciatic nerve damage from incorrect IM injection. If that muscle group must be used, insert the needle at a 45-degree angle directed caudally to avoid the sciatic nerve. Repeated IM injections should be alternated between muscle groups and given on different sides of the body.

Proper patient restraint is necessary to avoid painful injections. Restrain the patient's head and body during IM administration (see Chapter 17). After locating the muscle group by palpation, swab the injection site with a disinfectant. With the needle attached to the syringe, quickly insert the needle 1 to 2 cm at a 45- to 90-degree angle. Aspirate the syringe to ensure the needle is not placed in a blood vessel. If blood is aspirated, withdraw the needle and insert into a different site. This step is crucial when injecting potent medications, oil-based drugs, or microcrystalline suspensions. If no blood is aspirated, inject the medication at a slow to moderate rate. Remove the needle and massage the muscle to disperse the medication.

Medications and fluids administered *intravenously (IV)* are rapidly absorbed and reach a higher blood level faster than by other routes. Large volumes of solutions may be given in a short time. Caustic, irritating, or hypertonic medications can be given IV with fewer problems than with other routes. IV injections typically do not produce a lasting effect unless a continual infusion is given. A general rule is that if the solution is opaque, it cannot be safely given IV, except for parenteral nutrient solutions and propofol. Vaccines are never administered IV.

Drugs can be given IV with a syringe and needle, winged infusion set, or catheter (Box 26-4). The most commonly used veins for IV administration using a syringe and needle are the cephalic vein and the saphenous vein. The patient should be restrained sitting or in sternal recumbency if the cephalic vessel is being used, and in lateral recumbency if the saphenous vessel is used.

Patient restraint is very important if using a syringe and needle for administration of medication. The limb being used must remain immobile during administration. Any movement of the patient may lacerate the vessel with the needle and/or result in extravascular administration of medication. When injecting a caustic or irritating solution, an IV catheter should be placed to prevent extravascular injection.

Always attempt venipuncture at a distal point on the limb. If the needle lacerates the vessel, moving more proximally or using another vein may be indicated. Pressure should be applied at all venipuncture sites to prevent hematoma formation. To place a needle into small, rolling vessels or vessels surrounded by fat (i.e., in obese patients), insert the needle into the skin lateral to the vessel and then puncture the vessel.

Intraosseous (IO) administration is used to inject medication and fluids in small patients in which an IV

Box 26-4 Intravenous injection

1. The assistant restrains the patient, immobilizes the limb, and occludes the vessel proximal to the administration site to distend the vein. The venipuncture site may be shaved to visualize the vessel easier. The site can be prepared using 70% alcohol swabs to moisten the hair, clean the skin, and aid visualization of the vein (Fig. 26-15). Surgical preparation of the site is not necessary for IV administration with a syringe and needle, unlike catheter placement.
2. Grasp the metacarpal/metatarsal area and straighten the leg.
3. Using a 20- to 22-gauge needle attached to a syringe full of medication, direct the bevel of the needle up and insert the needle at a 30-degree angle through the skin and into the vessel lumen. Aspirate blood into the syringe to ensure venipuncture. Redirect the needle into the vessel if necessary.
4. Once the needle is in the vessel, have the veterinary technician's assistant release pressure on the vein while still holding the limb immobile.
5. Inject the medication slowly or rapidly, depending on the drug (e.g., thiopental is injected fairly rapidly, chemotherapeutic agents are given slowly).
6. After the medication is administered, withdraw the needle and apply pressure at the venipuncture site. A light compression bandage can minimize hematoma formation.

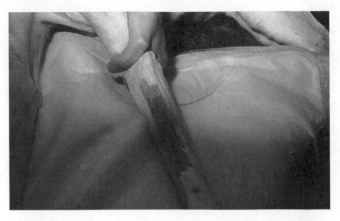

FIG. 26-15 Cephalic vein shaved and prepared for venipuncture.

and needle or standard IV catheter placed into the peritoneal space. To avoid hypothermia in neonates and critically ill animals, fluids should always be slightly warmer than room temperature. Cool fluids may be given IP to combat hyperthermia in adult animals. Complications of IP injection include peritonitis and perforation of the intestines, bladder, or other abdominal organs. A flexible catheter is less likely to cause damage than a needle. Aseptic technique must be used to avoid contamination of the abdomen.

Have all materials ready before placing the patient in lateral or dorsal recumbency. Shave and prepare the ventral abdominal midline caudal to the umbilicus, using triple applications of surgical soap and alcohol. Using a 22- to 25-gauge needle attached to a syringe, or a 22-gauge IV catheter, insert the needle or catheter into the abdominal cavity in a caudal direction. Aspirate; if fluid or bowel contents are aspirated, withdraw and use a new needle and syringe. If nothing is aspirated, inject the fluid slowly and then withdraw the needle or catheter.

CATHETER PLACEMENT

Catheters are flexible tubes used to administer or remove fluid or air. Typically they are made of polyethylene, metal, Vialon, Teflon, polyurethane, silicone, or polyvinyl chloride. Catheters may be placed in various parts of the body, such as the nasal passage, esophagus, stomach, thorax, pericardium, abdomen, veins, arteries, bone, and bladder.

Intravenous Catheterization

Intravenous catheters provide access to circulating blood for administration of medication, fluids, nutrients, and blood products, as well as monitoring blood pressure and collecting blood samples. Catheters are available in a wide variety of lengths and diameters (Fig. 26-16). Types

cannot be placed. It is performed with a needle or catheter inserted into the trochanteric fossa of the femur or the tibial tuberosity.

Epidural administration is used for injection of analgesics and anesthetics. Injection of local anesthetics or analgesics into the lumbosacral junction (L7-S1) provides complete analgesia and muscle relaxation caudal to the block.

Intraperitoneal (IP) administration provides faster but sustained absorption of fluids and medications than with SC administration. Medication or fluids may be administered into the peritoneal space in neonates with vessels too small for IV catheterization, or in patients needing peritoneal lavage (e.g., with pancreatitis). Irritating medications cannot be given intraperitoneally but blood transfusions may be given IP if an IV catheter cannot be placed. Debilitated or hypovolemic patients do not absorb IP fluids or medication readily.

Peritoneal lavage is performed with a peritoneal catheter set; IP fluids can be administered with a syringe of catheters include winged infusion needles (butterfly catheters), over-the-needle catheters, and through-the-needle catheters (e.g., Intracath, Becton-Dickinson). Common insertion sites are the cephalic vein, the saphenous vein, and the jugular vein. The medial or lateral auricular (ear) vein may be used in some patients (Fig. 26-17).

The longer the catheter, the more stable it is in the vessel and the less likely it is to cause mechanical irritation with resulting phlebitis. A short, peripheral over-the-needle catheter may be inserted distal to an area of flexion, such as in a cephalic vein distal to the elbow. A central catheter placed in a large vessel, such as the jugular vein, is less likely to cause mechanical or chemical irritation. The length of central catheters needed to reach the cranial or caudal vena cava depends on the size of the patient. For jugular insertion, measure from the insertion point to the third intercostal space; for a saphenous insertion, measure from the insertion point to the seventh lumbar vertebra.

The diameter (gauge) of the catheter depends on the diameter of the vessel. Large-diameter catheters placed in small vessels can compromise venous return and cause phlebitis. Small-diameter catheters decrease the flow rate of fluid delivery but do not compromise venous return. A fluid pump can facilitate delivery of fluids through a small catheter. Small-diameter catheters are easily occluded with fibrin clots and blood sample collection may be difficult.

Winged infusion (butterfly) catheters are for patients that need numerous IV infusions of medications (e.g., chemotherapeutic agents) but not long-term fluid therapy. Several medications can be given if the catheter is flushed with 0.9% saline between infusions of each medication. These catheters are simple to insert and cause fewest local infections; however, they can cause irritation and may perforate the vessel. Winged infusion catheters require constant monitoring while in place; stabilization of the catheter can be difficult.

Over-the-needle peripheral catheters are quick and relatively atraumatic to place, inexpensive, and easily stabilized with a light bandage (Box 26-5). They are used for infusion of fluids, medication, anesthetics, and blood products. They can be left in place for 72 hours before changing to another vessel. Unless care is taken during placement, the catheter can easily be contaminated. These catheters usually cannot be used for blood sampling. Easy removal by patients and subcutaneous infusion of fluids are complications of short over-the-needle catheters.

Central catheters are long catheters made of an inert material that causes little tissue reaction and can be left in for extended periods. Placement in the cranial or caudal vena cava does not compromise venous return and decreases the possibility of phlebitis from mechanical irri-

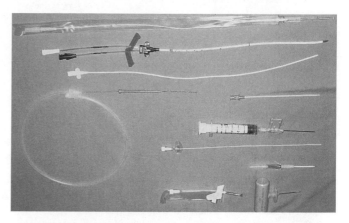

FIG. 26-16 Variety of catheters for administration of fluids and liquid medication. *From top to bottom:* through-the-needle catheter (Intracath, Becton Dickinson); over-the-guidewire double-lumen catheter (Double-Lumen Arrow, Arrow International); over-the-guidewire single-lumen catheter (Single-Lumen Arrow, Arrow International) with the vessel dilator directly below and the guidewire to the left; breakaway needle introducer with syringe attached for the L-Cath (Luther Medical Products); through-the-needle catheter with a breakaway needle (L-Cath, Luther Medical Products); over-the-needle catheter (Insyte, Becton Dickinson); pediatric through-the-needle catheter with a breakaway needle (Pediatric L-Cath, Luther Medical Products) on the lower left; and an intraosseous catheter.

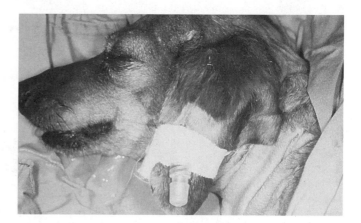

FIG. 26-17 Catheter in the medial auricular vein of a Dachshund.

tation. Two types of central catheters are the *over-the-guidewire catheter* and the *through-the-needle catheter*. Placement in large vessels allows greater dilution of hypertonic fluids, rapid infusion rates, administration of blood products, blood sampling, and central venous pressure monitoring. However, the cost of these catheters may be prohibitive for short-term (less than 3 days) fluid therapy.

Patients receiving hyperalimentation require a central catheter for nutritional support and an additional peripheral catheter for medication and fluid therapy.

Another central catheter is also necessary if central venous pressure (CVP) monitoring or blood sampling is required. Placement of one multi-lumen central catheter for CVP monitoring, blood sampling, nutritional support, fluid therapy, and medication administration reduces the need for a second catheter and can be maintained for long periods.

The catheter should be inserted in a long, straight vessel with no nearby infection, scars, lesions, wounds, or fractures, and little chance of the patient's contaminating the catheter insertion site. The catheter should be placed in the distal part of the vessel, away from any area of flexion and inserted toward the heart.

Proper skin preparation before catheter placement is essential to prevent phlebitis and infection. Strict aseptic technique must be followed during catheterization to avoid sepsis. All materials should be collected and placed within reach before skin preparation and catheter placement is begun. All catheters must be secured with tape or sutures and covered with a light bandage to protect the insertion site. Winged infusion catheters require only taping.

The selected vessel is occluded to raise the pressure in the vessel and allow for easier visualization and palpation. For jugular catheterization, the handler immobilizes the patient's head while placing one finger in the thoracic inlet and applying pressure on the vessel. For the cephalic vein, the patient's elbow is supported with the handler's fingers, while the thumb is placed over the vessel on the medial side and rotated laterally. The lat-

---

Box 26-5 Peripheral intravenous catheter insertion

Materials:

catheter of appropriate type, length, and diameter

clippers with a #40 blade

cottonballs or gauze sponges soaked in povidone-iodine (Betadine, Purdue Frederick) or chlorhexidine gluconate (Solvahex, Solvay)

cottonballs or gauze sponges soaked in 70% isopropyl alcohol

dry, sterile gauze sponges

two pieces of ½-inch-wide porous adhesive tape long enough to go around patient's limb two times or a ½-inch-wide roll of tape that has been unrolled and then loosely rerolled

two pieces of 1-inch porous adhesive tape long enough to go around patient's limb two times or a 1-inch-wide roll of tape that has been unrolled and then loosely rerolled

povidone-iodine ointment

2- or 3-inch roll of Kling (Johnson & Johnson)

2- or 4-inch roll of Vetwrap (3M)

extension set primed with heparinized saline (2 I.U. of heparin/1 ml of 0.9% saline) or the fluids to be administered

injection cap

Procedure:

1. Shave approximately 1 clipper blade width on each side of the vessel, with the shaved length (proximal to distal) approximately twice that of the width. This allows a second attempt at catheterization more proximal than the first.

2. Prepare the insertion site using a surgical soap and antiseptic.

3. While the handler occludes the vessel, grasp the limb with the left hand while the right hand holds the catheter with the bevel directed up.

4. With over-the-needle catheters, direct venipuncture is performed by holding the catheter at a 15- to 30-degree angle over the vein, puncturing the skin, and advancing the catheter needle into the vessel in a single, quick, smooth motion. Indirect venipuncture is performed by holding the catheter needle at a 45-degree angle slightly distal and to one side of the desired site of catheter entry into the vessel. Once the catheter needle is inserted into the skin, decrease the angle of the needle, advance the catheter needle into the vein, and slide the catheter into the vessel. If the catheter does not advance into the vessel, replace the catheter and attempt catheterization more proximal than the first attempt. With a winged infusion catheter, grasp the wings between thumb and forefinger and advance directly into the vessel, keeping the vessel steady until the catheter is stabilized. Tape the catheter in place using ½-inch tape attached to the wings and wrapped around the limb.

5. Once the catheter is advanced to the hub, remove the catheter needle and hold the catheter in place while attaching the injection cap or primed extension set. Flush a small amount of fluid or heparinized saline into the vessel to ensure catheter patency. For very small, pediatric patients, monitor the amount of fluid used to flush the catheter.

eral saphenous vein is occluded by placing one hand on top of and around the stifle, medial to lateral; the medial saphenous is occluded by applying pressure on the vessel in the inguinal area and stabilizing the stifle.

With butterfly catheters, once the blood starts flowing into the catheter tubing, attach the heparinized saline-filled syringe, aspirate the air out of the tubing, and flush to ensure catheter patency before administering medications. Administer the medication while holding the leg and the catheter steady. Occasionally aspirate to check catheter patency while administering medications. Once the medication has been administered, flush the tubing and the catheter with heparinized saline before removing the catheter. If multiple drugs are to be administered, flush between medications with heparinized saline. If any type of catheter is being used for fluid administration, the catheter end must be capped with an injection cap and flushed with heparinized saline solution four times daily to prevent clot formation.

Securing the catheter reduces movement of the catheter in the vessel and can decrease the likelihood of phlebitis (Figs. 26-18 and 26-19). Anchor a piece of 1/2-inch tape around the catheter hub and loosely wrap around the limb. For an over-the-needle jugular catheter in a pediatric patient, wrap the rerolled 1/2-inch tape around the catheter hub and secure loosely around the neck. Place a second piece of tape, sticky side down, underneath the catheter hub and wrap around the limb (not necessary for around the neck). If the tape is wrapped too tightly, the foot will swell and become painful, and the patient will chew at the catheter. If the tape is not placed immediately distal to the catheter insertion point and stuck to the hair, the catheter may back out of the vessel.

Conscientious nursing care of the catheter is necessary to maintain a catheter and prevent complications from catheterization. Catheter management can prevent sepsis, the most serious complication associated with catheters. Phlebitis, or local venous inflammation, can be caused by contamination of the catheter during placement, or chemical or mechanical irritation. Signs of phlebitis include swelling at the catheter site, redness, pain, thickening, or irritation of the vessel. Septicemia, thrombosis, or bacterial endocarditis can be caused by indwelling catheters. Signs of septicemia and bacterial endocarditis include cardiac arrhythmias, injected mucous membranes, fever, and leukocytosis.

The catheter bandage must be kept clean and dry, the catheter and extension set clear of any blood clots, and a closed administration system established to prevent contamination. The patient's body temperature should be measured at least once daily, the site proximal to the catheter monitored for any signs of phlebitis or subcutaneous fluid accumulation, and the toes checked for swelling. The catheter should be removed at the first

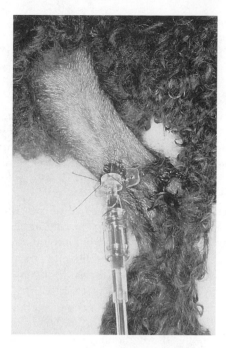

FIG. 26-18 Placement of a through-the-needle catheter (L-Cath) in the lateral saphenous vessel. The catheter has been secured with sutures, and an extension set has been attached.

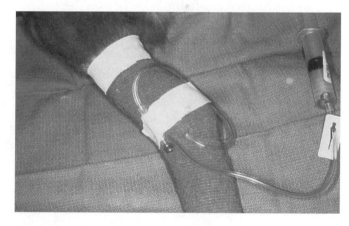

FIG. 26-19 The lateral saphenous catheter is bandaged. Note the security loop in the extension set.

sign of phlebitis, sepsis, or catheter malfunction. Routine changing of the catheter depends on hospital policy for the type of catheter placed.

When the catheter bandage becomes wet or soiled with organic material, it must be changed and the catheter evaluated for problems. The catheter may need to be covered with plastic to keep clean in incontinent patients. Swabbing the injection port with alcohol or a disinfectant before flushing or injecting medications can help decrease the chance of sepsis. Kinked or malfunctioning catheters and extension tubing with blood clots occluding the ports must be replaced.

The amount of time a catheter can be safely left in place is controversial. Depending on the established hospital policy, a short peripheral catheter is usually moved to another vessel (new catheter inserted) every 72 hours. Leaving it in place longer can contribute to instances of phlebitis. Continuous rotation of the veins used allows indefinite IV catheterization for therapy. Central catheters may be left in place for an extended period, with routine catheter bandage changes, provided the catheter is still functional.

Intraarterial Catheterization

Intraarterial catheters are placed to allow collection of multiple arterial blood gas samples, and for direct blood pressure monitoring in critically ill patients. Medication and fluids are not administered through an intraarterial catheter. The catheter is used for sampling and pressures only. Intraarterial catheters are more difficult to place than intravenous catheters and are not recommended in patients with a severe bleeding disorder.

An over-the-needle catheter may be placed into the artery, or a catheter manufactured specifically for arterial catheterization may be used. The area over and around the artery is clipped and prepared as for intravenous catheterization. With one finger over the artery, palpating the pulse, insert the catheter through the skin (see Fig. 26-3) as if placing an intravenous catheter. Once blood enters the catheter, advance the guidewire into the vessel, then advance the catheter over the guidewire to the hub of the catheter. Remove the guidewire and place an injection cap. Immediately flush with heparinized saline. Secure the catheter in place. Apply a light wrap to secure the catheter. Complications of intraarterial catheters are as for intravenous catheters. Intraarterial catheters must be flushed hourly unless direct blood pressure measurements are being taken. The catheter is automatically flushed while pressures are being measured.

Intraosseous Catheterization

Intraosseous catheterization is the placement of a special intraosseous catheter, spinal needle, or hypodermic needle into the trochanteric fossa of the femur or the tibial tuberosity for administration of fluids and medication, most commonly in neonates. Site preparation and catheter maintenance are similar to those for intravenous catheters. Intraosseous catheters, which are inserted through the skin into the bone, can be painful and should be replaced every 72 hours. In neonates, a jugular catheter is easier to place and maintain, is less painful, and can safely remain in the vessel longer than an intraosseous catheter.

Urinary Tract Catheterization

Urinary catheters provide access to the urinary bladder via the urethra to administer radiographic contrast material directly into the bladder, collect urine for urinalysis, relieve urethral obstruction, maintain urine flow, and provide a closed urinary collection system for precise monitoring of urine output, collection of contaminated urine, and patient cleanliness. Rarely, a percutaneous (suprapubic) catheter is inserted to keep the bladder empty before surgery. Percutaneous catheters are temporary and only for emergency catheterization of the bladder when a catheter cannot be passed through the urethra.

Urinary catheters are available in a variety of materials, diameters, and lengths (Fig. 26-20). Metal urethral catheters can be used to temporarily catheterize a female dog but can cause hematuria and injury to the urethra and bladder. Olive-tipped metal catheters can be used to relieve an obstruction at the tip of a male cat's penis. Polyethylene catheters (e.g., Sovereign, Sherwood Medical) are semirigid, made as small as a 3½ French, and used to bypass strictures or backflush urethral calculi. This catheter is recommended for temporary use because it can be irritating to the urethra and bladder.

Flexible rubber or silicone catheters for temporary or long-term use can prevent urethral trauma. Placement is slightly more difficult with flexible catheters but can be managed by first freezing the catheter to stiffen it, or by using a metal or plastic stylet or guidewire. Foley catheters are flexible catheters with an inflatable bulb at the tip to prevent the catheter from slipping out of the bladder. These catheters come in sizes as small as 5 French.

Careful placement of the most flexible, smallest-diameter catheter minimizes trauma to the urethra and bladder. However, an overly small catheter diameter may allow leakage of urine around the catheter. Always

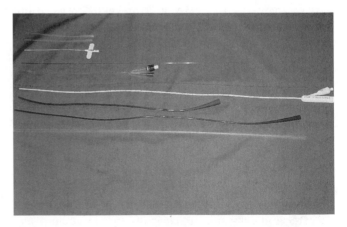

FIG. 26-20 Types of urinary catheters. From top to bottom: tomcat catheters with open and closed ends; flexible silicone tomcat catheter (Cook Veterinary Products) with stylet; metal stylet for Foley catheters; Foley urinary catheter; flexible guidewire for Foley catheter; long Foley catheter for placement in male dogs; two lengths of red rubber catheters; and a rigid polyethylene urinary catheter.

examine the catheter for defects and test the bulb of Foley catheters by gently inflating with sterile water or saline before placement.

Measure the distance from the tip of the penis or vulva to the neck of the bladder before placing the catheter. Catheters that are too rigid or long can traumatize the wall of the bladder (Fig. 26-21). Flexible catheters that are too long or advanced too far into the bladder can become kinked, knotted, or folded within the bladder and may require surgical removal. Foley catheters that are too short or inflated in the urethra and not in the bladder can damage the urethra.

In patients with a possible ruptured bladder, urethral stricture, or urolithiasis (bladder stones), air or radiographic contrast material may be administered through a urethral catheter to evaluate the bladder and urethra. When percutaneous cystocentesis is difficult or impossible, a urinary catheter may be passed aseptically to collect urine. Once the catheter is placed, a syringe is attached to the catheter, the sample is aspi-

rated, and the urinary catheter is removed. Patients with lower urinary tract disease, urolithiasis, or urethral stricture require a more rigid urinary catheter placed initially to pass the problem area in the urethra, then a softer, more flexible urinary catheter placed for continuous urine collection. Patients with bladder atony need a urinary catheter to keep the bladder small and to prevent urine retention. Large, nonambulatory patients with leg, pelvic, or spinal fractures or recent spinal surgery require a urinary catheter collection system to avoid moving the patient excessively for nursing care (Fig. 26-22).

Complications of urethral catheterization include iatrogenic ascending urinary tract infections, catheter breakage, and trauma to the urethra or bladder. Urinary catheters must be placed aseptically and a closed collection system used. Leaving the catheter open and exposed to the air can lead to infection. Remove urine from the collection system without disconnecting the lines. Changing the collection system (and, only if pos-

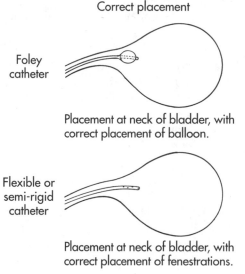

Correct placement   Incorrect placement

Foley catheter

Placement at neck of bladder, with correct placement of balloon.

Placement in urethra: balloon is dilating urethra.

Flexible or semi-rigid catheter

Placement at neck of bladder, with correct placement of fenestrations.

Placement in bladder: catheter irritating wall and could bend or form a knot.

FIG. 26-21 Correct and incorrect positioning of a urinary catheter. Top: The balloon of the Foley catheter should be placed in the neck of the bladder (*left*), rather than in the urethra (*right*). The tip of a flexible or semirigid catheter should be placed at the neck of the bladder (*left*), rather than against the bladder wall (*right*), where it could bend or cause irritation.

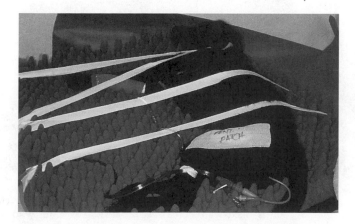

FIG. 26-22 Patient with a fractured spine, strapped to a board, with a urinary catheter in place for cleanliness and maintenance of bladder function. Note that the board is padded with rubber egg crates and the patient is taped to the board.

sible to replace easily, the urinary catheter) every 72 hours also helps prevent infection.

Most healthy cats require sedation or general anesthesia to place a urinary catheter, but very sick cats may not require chemical restraint. Most dogs do not require any chemical restraint and can be physically restrained. All patients should be placed in lateral recumbency for urinary catheterization. However, female dogs may also remain standing or be placed in sternal recumbency, with the vulva and pelvic limbs over the edge of the table for ease of placement. Male cats may also be placed in dorsal or lateral recumbency.

In female dogs, urinary catheters can be placed by visualization of the urethral orifice or by palpation. Palpation is usually better tolerated in canine patients and allows the catheter to be placed as quickly and easily as the visual method. The vagina of cats and small dogs may be too small for palpation, but a small, sterile, slit otoscope can be used with a light source to visualize the papilla for placement of a flexible urinary catheter with or without a stylet. A semirigid urinary catheter may be placed with the "blind" technique but can cause trauma to the tissues. Usually a Foley catheter is placed in females. The smallest Foley (5 Fr) can be placed in female cats.

Before placing a urinary catheter, gather all of the materials needed (Box 26-6). Clip any long hair around the prepuce or vulva and clean the immediate area. Wear sterile gloves when handling the catheter and use sterile water-soluble lubricant to prevent contamination of the catheter. Use of sterile 2% lidocaine jelly on the gloves, speculum, and urinary catheter minimizes patient discomfort.

For urinary catheters without suture wings or balloons, make a butterfly wing with elastic tape around the catheter approximately 0.5 cm from the tip of the prepuce. Suture the tape wings on each side of the prepuce. Attach the urinary catheter collection system aseptically. Depending on the patient and the type of catheter placed, a light abdominal wrap may be necessary. For male dogs, place an abdominal bandage (not necessary for Foley catheters) to keep the urinary catheter straight and clean. Place gauze sponges between the prepuce and abdomen for padding. Secure 1-inch tape around the catheter and wrap loosely around the abdomen. Cover the prepuce and urinary catheter connections with Kling wrapped around the abdomen. Create a security loop by looping the catheter extension tubing and taping it to the patient's abdomen. The extension is then attached to one of the rear legs. For male dogs with Foley catheters, attach 1-inch porous tape around the distal end of the catheter and loosely wrap around the abdomen with a security loop in the catheter extension.

Female dogs have the extension attached to the rear leg, with enough slack to prevent tension on the catheter during movement (Fig. 26-26). Cats have the extension tubing looped and attached to the tail or rear leg. Place the collection bag below the level of the patient to prevent backflow of urine into the bladder.

GENERAL NURSING CARE
Interacting with Patients

When interacting with the patient, place yourself on the patient's level by sitting on the cage edge or squatting down to pet and stroke the chest or chin, and talk quietly to the patient. Repeat this at every opportunity. Establish a rapport with the patient. At treatment times, double the amount of positive interaction, especially when the procedure or treatment involves pain or discomfort. Patients respond positively to gentle reassurance and support. Always call the patient by name during interaction. If the patient's condition permits, provide special snacks or food. Make the patient's hospitalization as positive as possible.

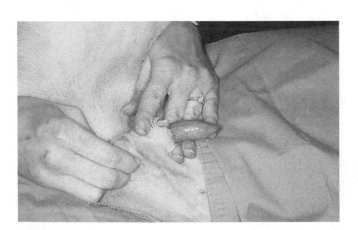

FIG. 26-23 Extrusion of the canine penis from the prepuce for urinary catheterization.

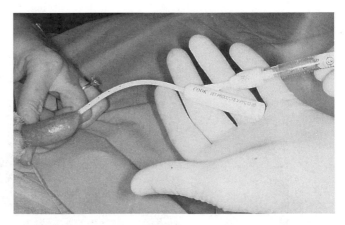

FIG. 26-24 Placement of a Foley catheter in a male dog. The balloon is filled with sterile saline. Sterile gloves are worn during placement.

Box 26-6 Urinary catheterization

Materials:

clippers with a #40 blade

gauze sponges for cleaning skin

cleaning solution (Nolvasan, Fort Dodge; pHisoHex, Winthrop)

sterile water-soluble lubricating jelly (K-Y, Johnson & Johnson; Surgilube, Fougera) or lidocaine jelly (Xylocaine, Astra)

sterile latex gloves

urinary catheter of appropriate type and size

20- or 22-gauge wire, flexible wire stylet, or plastic stylet for very flexible catheters

light source and sterile speculum for female patients

urinary collection system and connecting tubes

material to stabilize the urinary catheter in place (1-inch tape, suture material, gauze sponges, Kling, 3-inch elastic tape)

Catheter placement in male dogs

1. Shave the hair around the prepuce and apply thumb pressure caudally where the prepuce attaches to the abdomen. Retract the prepuce to expose the distal glans penis (Fig. 26-23). Clean away exudates with the gauze sponges and cleaning solution. The veterinary technician's assistant continues to hold the penis in this manner during catheterization.

2. With gloves on, place lubricating jelly onto the tip of the urinary catheter and insert the catheter into the distal urethral orifice. Advance the catheter into the bladder until urine flows out continuously, then advance 1 to 2 cm farther to place all catheter fenestrations in the bladder.

3. For Foley catheters, advance the catheter 4 or 5 cm farther to ensure the balloon is in the bladder. Inflate the balloon slowly with saline so that it does not burst (Fig. 26-24). To minimize the length of catheter in the bladder, gently withdraw the Foley catheter until the balloon halts withdrawal.

4. To place urinary catheters aseptically, without gloves, keep the catheter in its sterile package while advancing the tip of the catheter into the urethra. A paper tab can be made with the package and used to advance the catheter without directly touching the catheter. Avoid touching the penis with the paper tab. Advance the catheter as directed above.

5. Once the catheter is placed and urine is flowing freely, release the os penis and allow the prepuce to retract over the glans penis. Secure the catheter as described in the text.

Catheter placement in male cats

1. Clean the perineal area without saturating the fur. The assistant extrudes the penis from the prepuce by placing the thumb and index finger on each side of the prepuce and applying gentle pressure toward the ischium.

2. With gloves on, place lubricating jelly on the catheter tip and insert it into the penis. The catheter will not be able to advance beyond 1 or 2 cm because of the curve of the penile urethra. To straighten the penile urethra, allow the penis to retract into the prepuce, then gently pull the prepuce distally while advancing the catheter through the urethra into the bladder. Continue to advance the catheter until urine flows freely.

3. Allow the prepuce to cover the penis with the catheter in place. Attach elastic tape to the catheter if no suture wings are available on the catheter. Suture the urinary catheter to the prepuce and then attach the collection system. Always have a security loop attached to the patient to avoid excessive pressure on the catheter. Apply an Elizabethan collar before the patient awakens.

Catheter placement in female dogs

1. Shave the excess hair away from the vulva and clean the perineal area.

2. For placement of the urinary catheter by visualization, lubricate a sterile speculum, the catheter tip, and the stylet tip. Insert the stylet into the catheter. A slight bend in the stylet approximately 1 cm from the tip may help direct the catheter ventrally into the urethral orifice.

3. Gently place the speculum into the vagina and direct it dorsally and then cranially until the angle becomes more horizontal. The speculum is not inserted very far in female cats. Look through the speculum while slowly backing out of the vagina. The urethral orifice is on the ventral aspect of the vagina, cranial to the vulva.

4. Holding the speculum and light source steady, guide the urinary catheter and stylet gently through the speculum into the urethral orifice (Fig. 26-25). Gently advance the catheter through the urethral orifice into the bladder. Once the catheter is placed into the bladder, and urine is freely flowing through the catheter, advance the catheter 1 or 2 cm farther to ensure that the fenestrations or the entire balloon is in the bladder and inflate the balloon if using a Foley catheter.

Continued.

Box 26-6 Urinary catheterization—cont'd

5. Remove the speculum from the vagina and back the Foley catheter out until the balloon stops at the neck of the bladder. If using the sterile slit otoscope cone, remove the cone from the catheter by sliding the catheter through the slit. If using a red rubber or non-Foley catheter in a cat, the catheter will need butterfly wings attached to the catheter before suturing to the perineal area. Attach the extension of the collection system to the leg of the patient (Fig. 26-26). Place an Elizabethan collar if necessary.

6. For placement of a urinary catheter in a female by palpation, apply sterile lubricating jelly to the gloved finger tip, catheter tip, and, if using a stylet, the tip of the stylet. If the patient is small, using the smallest digit to palpate is least painful for the patient. Bending the stylet tip, once it is inserted into the catheter, may facilitate placement of the catheter but is not necessary, because the catheter is

directed into the orifice with the tip of the finger. A stylet may or may not be used, depending on the preference of the person placing the catheter.

7. Identify the urethral papilla; it is a firm, round mass on the ventral aspect of the vagina 3 to 5 cm cranial to the vulva in dogs. Bend the tip of the finger just cranial to the papilla to guide the catheter into the urethral orifice. Insert the catheter into the vagina and ventrally into the urethra and on into the bladder.

8. Once the catheter is advanced into the bladder, remove the finger and inflate the balloon of the Foley catheter. Back the urinary catheter out gently until the balloon stops at the neck of the bladder. Attach the urinary system to the catheter and tape to the patient.

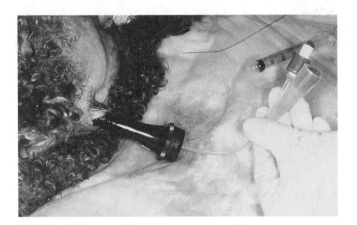

FIG. 26-25 Placement of a Foley catheter in the bladder of a female dog, using a sterile split otoscope cone for a speculum. The balloon is inflated with sterile saline. The metal stylet used can be seen at the upper right. Note the slight bend at the tip to direct the catheter into the urethral orifice.

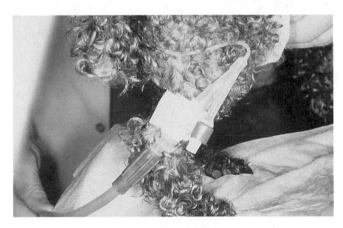

FIG. 26-26 Urinary collection system for a female dog. The system is attached to a rear leg with enough slack to allow leg movement without dislodging the catheter.

Weight

Weigh each patient daily, at the same time and on the same scale, to help monitor hydration and nutrition status.

Attitude or Mentation

Assessment of the patients' attitude can give important information on their care and treatment. Is the patient alert, depressed, sedated (recovering from anesthesia), agitated, quiet, or comatose?

Body Temperature

Body temperature can be monitored rectally with a standard mercury thermometer, a digital thermometer (battery operated), or an electronic probe for continuous monitoring rectally or in the ear canal. Leave the thermometer in the rectum for 2 or 3 minutes (count the pulse and respiratory rates while waiting) and record the temperature.

Maintenance of normal body temperature (normothermia) involves regulating the external environment as well as the internal environment of the patient. *Hypothermia* (subnormal body temperature) can occur with shock, after anesthesia or surgery, and with low environmental temperatures. Hypothermia can be combated with circulating warm-water blankets (*not* electric heating pads), warm-water bottles, warmed towels or blankets, a warm bath, blow dryer, heat lamp, or incubator. Fluids may be warmed to 37° C and slowly infused IV.

Monitor the rectal temperature at least hourly. Discontinue warming when the rectal temperature approaches the normal range. *Do not overheat the patient.* Most water blankets can be adjusted (lowered) to normal body temperature to maintain normothermia and not overheat patients. Always have a towel or pad between the water blanket and the patient. Electric heating pads are *not* recommended because of the possibility of electric shock, overheating, and burns. If a heat lamp is used, the patient must be able to move away from the heat source. When using an incubator, extreme care must be taken to avoid overheating the patient.

Hyperthermia (abnormally high body temperature) may occur with infection, inflammation, brain lesions (loss of thermoregulation), heat stroke, seizures, stress, and excitation. Patients with extreme and persistent hyperthermia require constant monitoring. Hyperthermia can be controlled with ice wrapped in towels, fans, alcohol application, cool-water enemas, and cool drinking water. Discontinue cooling when the rectal temperature reaches 40° C. *Do not overcool the patient.*

Pulse

Assessment of the pulse quality and rate can help determine the patient's medical status and guide the course of treatment. Auscultate the heart while palpating the pulse. A pulse deficit (more heartbeats than pulse beats) indicates an arrhythmia. Pulses can be described as weak and thready, strong and steady, bounding, or irregular.

If there is any question about the heart rate or pulse quality, monitor the patient with an electrocardiogram (ECG). Place the patient in right lateral recumbency and attach the alligator clips to the skin caudal to the elbows and on the stifles. If the clips are color coded, the right front is white, the left front is black, the right rear is green, and the left rear is red. Assess the ECG to determine if continuous monitoring is advisable. For continuous monitoring, apply adhesive ECG pads (Ultratrace, Conmed Andover Medical). Attach to shaved areas that have been cleaned with alcohol.

Blood Pressure

Blood pressure monitoring is also used in assessment of critically ill patients. Blood pressure is the pressure exerted by the blood on the wall of the vessel. The *systolic pressure* is the maximum force caused by contraction of the left ventricle of the heart. *Diastolic pressure* is the minimum force during the relaxation phase, when the aortic and pulmonic valves are closed. The *mean arterial pressure* (MAP) is the average pressure between systolic and diastolic.

Direct blood pressure monitoring requires an arterial catheter connected via IV extension tubing to an external monitor. For intermittent, indirect blood pressure monitoring by Doppler, the ultrasound probe is placed over a peripheral artery and the pressure cuff is placed proximal to the probe. Manually inflate the cuff until the sound of the blood flow stops, then deflate the cuff until the first sound is heard. The systolic pressure is read from the manometer when the first sound is heard. The diastolic pressure is read when the sound changes. It can be difficult to detect this change; therefore, the diastolic pressure reading may not be possible with this method. For continuous, indirect pressure monitoring with a Dinamap oscillometric unit, the cuff, placed distal to the elbow or tarsus, can affect the accuracy of the reading if an inappropriate size is used.

Central Venous Pressure

Central venous pressure (CVP) is the pressure within the cranial vena cava. It reflects the condition of the cardiovascular system and is influenced by many factors, including blood volume and cardiac function. The CVP is monitored in patients receiving large volumes of IV fluids, with poor cardiac or renal function, or with encephalopathies. It is monitored by catheterization of the cranial vena cava via the jugular vein. The catheter is connected to a fluid-filled column (manometer) and a source of fluid (syringe or bag). Normal central venous pressure is less than 5 cm water; however, the trend of CVP changes is more important than a single reading.

Respiration

Auscultate the patient's lungs, starting at the cranial thorax and working toward the caudal thorax. Normal respiration is quiet. The respiratory rate can be increased by nervousness, heat, pain, hypoxia, lung disease, or heart problems. A decreased rate may be caused by metabolic alkalosis. Increased respiratory sounds or short, shallow, rapid breathing can indicate pulmonary or bronchial disease. Dyspnea (labored breathing) may be manifested as extension of the neck, refusal to lie down, and open-mouthed breathing.

Urine Production

Urine production and composition reflect renal function, hydration status, bladder function, and endocrine function. Analysis of the urine, collected with a urinary catheter, by cystocentesis, by free catch during micturition, or by manual expression of the bladder, can aid diagnosis and monitor the response to treatment. Urinalysis includes measurement of the urine specific gravity, and analysis of urine components and sediment. Culture and sensitivity testing of aseptically collected urine (cystocentesis is preferred) guide treatment of urinary tract infections.

Urinary catheterization permits accurate measurement of urine output for comparison with fluid consumption or administration, facilitates collection of urine for analysis, promotes cleanliness of recumbent patients, and reduces exposure of other patients or personnel to contaminated urine (e.g., leptospirosis, chemotherapy). A urinary catheter and collection system also keeps the bladder empty in patients with bladder dysfunction.

In cats with lower urinary tract disease, urinary catheters prevent reobstruction. After catheter removal, the bladder should be palpated at intervals to ensure that the urethra has not been obstructed again. Cats without urinary catheters can have their urine output quantitated by using an empty litter pan, paper litter, or diapers. The paper litter and the litter pan should be weighed before placing in the cage. After a patient urinates on the diapers, remove them and weigh. Subtract the initial weight of the paper or diaper; the remainder is the weight of the urine. Convert that into milliliters to determine the approximate urine output.

Dogs can be taken outside to urinate if no urinary catheter is in place to collect and measure urine. Walk ambulatory canine patients outside every 4 hours during the day to eliminate. A bedpan works well for catching the urine; then pour the urine into a graduated container to measure. For dogs that are not housetrained or that urinate more frequently, preweighed underpads (Durasorb Underpads, Professional Medical Products) can be placed in the cage and then weighed when urinated upon.

Patients that cannot completely empty the bladder may need to have the bladder manually expressed to keep the bladder empty, improve bladder tone, and decrease the chance of urinary tract infection. Nonambulatory patients may be carefully taken outside on a gurney, assisted to stand, and, if necessary, have the bladder expressed to stimulate urination. Bladder expression keeps the patient much cleaner and reduces the chance of urine scalding.

Gastrointestinal Monitoring

Monitor all excretions (urine, feces, vomit, saliva) from the patient and record a description (including estimated quantity) on the patient's chart. The color and content of feces (e.g., yellow, green, coffee-ground, black, red with frank blood, mucoid, partially digested food, undigested food, watery, voluminous, projectile, foul-smelling) can aid diagnosis. Regurgitation must be differentiated from vomiting. In patients that do not or cannot drink water, calculated fluid losses may be replaced with IV fluids.

The patient's body must be kept clean and free of body waste and excretions. Cleaning and flushing the oral cavity with saline can help prevent or heal oral ulcers. Flushing any vomitus out of the mouth also makes the patient feel better. The mouth of patients that cannot take food or water per os may be moistened with a gauze sponge and water. The skin around the mouth should be kept clean of vomitus and saliva to prevent scalding and secondary bacterial infections.

Patients with diarrhea must be kept as clean and dry as possible. Clean the cage or run thoroughly and replace any soiled bedding. If a recumbent patient must be turned every few hours, be sure to place the patient down on the correct side. Face the recumbent patient with its head toward the cage door. The patient should be able to see activity and not be forced to face the wall. Also, the technician must be able to see the patient's head to monitor attitude, mucous membrane color, and respiration. Frequent walks outside to eliminate help the patient feel better and reduce cage cleanup.

Patients that have not had a bowel movement in the past 2 days but are still eating should be closely monitored and encouraged to eliminate (e.g., take outside on a long leash, place in an outdoor run, provide a larger litterbox or different litter). Diet changes may be necessary (e.g., canned food, addition of fiber). Enemas may be indicated if constipation is diagnosed. Any tenesmus (straining to defecate) should be reported to the veterinarian.

Pain Control

Analgesia (pain relief) can speed recovery and improve the patient's mental status. Pain can cause cardiovascular and respiratory irregularities, aggression, and hysteria. The ability to recognize a patient in pain and provide pain relief can prevent the patient from harming itself or the handler, improve patient health, and shorten the length of hospitalization.

Individual animals react differently to pain. If the patient is resting quietly in the cage, signs of pain may not be detected unless a physical examination is performed. Signs may include anorexia, depression, mydriasis (dilated pupils), partially closed eyes, third eyelid protrusion, tachypnea (increased respiratory rate), tachycardia (increased heart rate), pale mucous membranes, and ptyalism (excessive salivation). Other signs include whimpering or crying, sharp yiping when moved or touched, growling when approached, anxiety, avoidance behavior, restlessness, frequent repositioning in the cage, reluctance to lie down, arching of the spine, limping or non–weight-bearing on a limb, and chewing at a specific area.

Attempt to determine the location and severity of the pain, and, if possible, eliminate the cause or factors contributing to the pain. Application of heat or cold to the affected area, additional padding or bedding, massage, quietly speaking to the patient while stroking, and handfeeding highly palatable food may be of some comfort to the patient. Monitor the patient at regular intervals for change in the degree of pain.

When using medication to control pain, consult the package insert for the onset of analgesic effect. The route used may alter the onset and duration of action. For example, pain may be relieved immediately with IV analgesia, but the duration of action is short.

The common practice of waiting until a specified time has elapsed between doses of analgesic medication is not humane. Giving an analgesic before the onset of pain is more effective than giving the drug after the pain is present. At the conclusion of surgery, systemic, regional, epidural, or local analgesia can be administered before the animal is removed from inhalation anesthesia. A fentanyl citrate skin patch (Duragesic) can be applied for pain relief. Other analgesics can be administered systemically or locally (see Chapter 13).

RESPIRATORY SUPPORT

Respiration supplies body cells with oxygen and eliminates carbon dioxide from the body. Dyspnea is difficult or labored breathing resulting from airway obstruction (e.g., infection, neoplasia, laryngeal paralysis, asthma), changes in the lungs or thorax (i.e., metastasis, pneumothorax, diaphragmatic hernia, pneumonia, pleural effusion), or cardiovascular or hematologic abnormalities (e.g., anemia, heart failure, heartworm disease).

Respiratory therapy can improve or maintain pulmonary function and tissue oxygenation. The therapeutic objective is to maintain alveolar ventilation (with oxygen, ventilator therapy, or chest tube placement), control secretions (by decreasing production and increasing clearance), and normalize pulmonary reflexes.

Respiratory support may involve placement of an oxygen mask, nasal insufflation tube, tracheostomy tube, or endotracheal tube, or placing the patient in an oxygen cage or on a ventilator to provide oxygen to the lungs and prevent hypoxia. It may also involve placement of a chest tube to remove fluid or air surrounding the lungs and allow expansion of the lungs.

Oxygen Mask

An oxygen mask placed over the mouth and nose provides the patient with 100% oxygen. This is for temporary use only. Some patients may not tolerate the mask but may tolerate a hood made from an Elizabethan collar covered with clear plastic. Oxygen can be delivered through a hole in the collar. A clear plastic bag may also be placed loosely over the patient's head with oxygen tubing entering the hood near the patient's nose or mouth. Use caution with this method. Make sure oxygen is always flowing into the hood.

Oxygen Cage

Patients in acute respiratory distress can be placed in an incubator or oxygen cage. The cage provides an environment with stable temperature, humidity, and oxygen. The temperature should be adjusted to make the patient comfortable and the humidity kept at 40% to 60%, while oxygen is delivered to provide 40% oxygen in the environment (normal room air contains 20.9% oxygen). A major drawback to using the oxygen cage is limited access to the patient. If the cage is opened, the percentage of oxygen in the air immediately drops and the patient may become dyspneic. Use pillows to prop the patient in sternal recumbency in the oxygen cage.

Nasal insufflation is an easy way to provide oxygen without causing undue stress to the patient (Fig. 26-27). An oxygen flow rate of 100 ml/kg/minute provides approximately 40% oxygen to the patient. Nasal insufflation allows full access to the patient without decreasing or stopping the flow of oxygen during treatment procedures. Some patients may not tolerate a nasal insufflation tube and require an Elizabethan collar to prevent removal of the tube. Oxygen administered through a tube placed in the nasal cavity must be humidified to prevent drying of the respiratory mucosa. A humidification unit can be attached to the flow meter.

If a tracheostomy tube is placed in a patient, the tube, airway, and insertion site must be maintained. Intermittent nebulization through the tracheostomy tube humidifies the airway and helps liquefy secretions

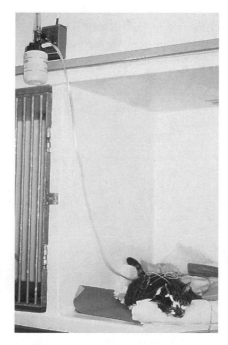

FIG. 26-27 Cat in sternal recumbency for nasal insufflation of oxygen. Note that the head is elevated to aid ventilation. The tubing is connected to a humidification unit attached to a flow meter.

(Fig. 26-28). If a nebulizer is unavailable, injecting 2 to 5 ml of sterile saline into the tracheostomy tube may help loosen secretions. Physical therapy can further mobilize secretions. The inner cannula should be periodically removed, examined for excessive secretions, cleaned with 0.025% chlorhexidine solution (Fig. 26-29), and rinsed with sterile saline. Aspiration (suctioning) of the tracheostomy tube, with the inner cannula removed, is necessary to prevent obstruction of the tracheostomy tube. The cannula is reinserted into the cleaned tracheostomy tube.

The tracheostomy site must be kept dry and free of exudates. Clean the area with normal saline and apply a sterile dressing. The tracheostomy tube itself is held in place by the inflated cuff and umbilical tape around the neck. Additional bandaging with a light wrap around the neck keeps the tube secure. When taking the patient outside on frigid days, a gauze sponge may be placed over the tracheostomy site only if the patient can breathe through the single layer of gauze. The tracheostomy tube should be removed by the veterinarian when the patient can breathe on its own.

Use of a Ventilator

In some patients, the trachea is intubated and attached to a ventilator. The cuff of the endotracheal tube must be inflated with a minimal volume of air for optimal sealing of the airway without producing excessive pressure on the tracheal wall. An overinflated cuff may cause tracheal necrosis. Periodic deflation of the cuff is not recommended due to the instability of the patient on controlled ventilation.

Endotracheal tube care is similar to tracheostomy tube care, except the patient cannot breathe while the tube is being suctioned. Suctioning should be done only if there is evidence of tracheal secretions. Patients attached to a ventilator should be oxygenated with 100% oxygen before suctioning of the tube. Once suctioning is completed (within 15 to 20 seconds), the patient is oxygenated again and placed reattached to the ventilator. The patient's tongue and mouth should be cleaned and moistened with a damp sponge and the eyes lubricated with ointment. The patient should be kept on thick pads or bedding and turned every 2 hours. The head should be placed slightly lower than the body for postural drainage (see Fig. 26-28).

Chest Tube

Chest tubes are placed through the chest wall into the pleural space to remove fluid or air from around the lungs, allowing the lungs to expand maximally. The chest tube must be securely attached (sutured) to the patient to prevent inadvertent leakage of air into the chest by accidental removal of the chest tube. More than one clamp (e.g., hemostats with padded jaws) and a three-way stopcock should be placed on the chest tube to prevent leakage of air into the pleural cavity between aspirations (Fig. 26-30). Aseptic removal of fluid or air from the chest prevents secondary infections.

The bandage securing the chest tube in place should be tight enough (or attached to the patient with tape) to prevent slippage but loose enough to allow the patient to breathe. Always cover the jaws of the hemostat and the three-way stopcock with an easily removed layer of tape (see Fig. 26-30). This will prevent the hemostats or the stopcock from catching on anything and becoming dislodged. If the patient is left unattended with a chest tube in place, an Elizabethan collar should be placed to

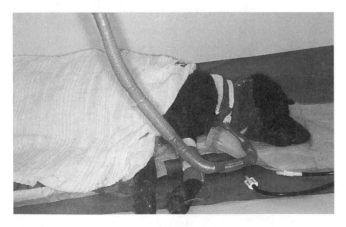

FIG. 26-28 Dog in lateral recumbency, with the hindquarters elevated and the head and chest lowered for postural drainage during and after nebulization. This dog is on a circulating warm-water blanket and covered with a blanket to maintain body temperature.

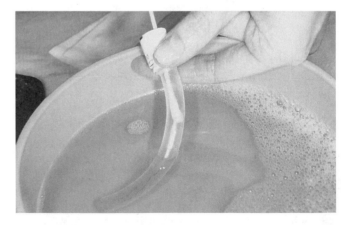

FIG. 26-29 Cleaning the cannula of a tracheostomy tube using sterile swabs and 0.025% chlorhexidine (Nolvasan, Fort Dodge).

prevent tube removal by the patient. Always check the bandage and the chest tube for security when aspirating.

Chest tubes may be aspirated intermittently or continuously with a Heimlich valve (pneumothorax only) or suction unit. To aspirate the tube intermittently, swab the injection port on the stopcock with alcohol or a disinfectant before aspirating. Using a large syringe with a 16- to 18-gauge needle, insert the needle into the stopcock, open the stopcock, and release the jaws of the hemostat. Aspirate gently with less than 5 ml of negative pressure. Excessive negative pressure may occlude the holes in the chest tube. Once the fluid or air has stopped flowing through the syringe easily, move the patient to a different position (e.g., lift the hindquarters, lift the front end, have the patient sit, walk, or lie down) and aspirate again. Once the syringe is full, replace the hemostats on the chest tube, turn the stopcock to the closed position, and remove the needle and syringe from the injection port. Record the amount of air or fluid removed from the chest tube.

Use another sterile needle and syringe and reswab the port when aspirating each time. Never reuse the same needle and syringe. Aseptically replace the injection caps once daily. Always double-check the clamps before leaving the patient. Tighten all connections once more.

A Heimlich valve continuously removes air from the chest tube only if the tube does not become occluded with blood or fluid. The valve must be monitored to ensure that it is working properly. Air or fluid can also be evacuated with a Pleurevac or Thoradrain. The quantity of fluid removed from the pleural cavity can be monitored but the amount of air removed cannot be measured. Follow the directions for setup of the unit. Attach the unit to the patient and turn the vacuum on

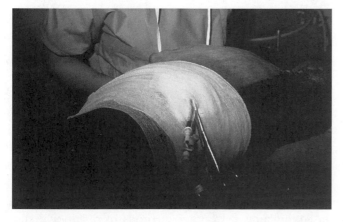

FIG. 26-30 Chest tube placed in a dog. The tube is occluded with hemostats and a three-way stopcock. *(Courtesy of Dr. Nancy Poy, Michigan State University.)*

to the desired level of suction. Make sure all connections are tightly sealed. If the patient must be disconnected for any reason, use two clamps on the chest tube before removing the tubing from the suction unit.

Control of Respiratory Secretions

Nasal and pulmonary secretions may be decreased with systemic or topical administration of antibiotics, antifungals, or corticosteroids. Patients with pulmonary edema are treated during nebulization with antifoaming agents. Dried secretions may be rehydrated and loosened by aerosolization/nebulization with saline and cleared by coupage or physical therapy.

Ultrasonic nebulization provides humidification of inspired gases and promotes mobilization of the mucous layer to aid removal of secretions. In conjunction with percussion and vibration, postural drainage (using gravity) moves secretions from small airways into the bronchi, where they can be coughed up. Exercise and stimulation of the cough reflex (e.g., by tracheal manipulation) also improves clearance of secretions.

Ultrasonic nebulizers produce a dense mist of microdroplets. They are used to administer medication (e.g., bronchodilators, antibiotics, detergents, mucolytics) directly to the lungs, humidify air inhaled by the patient, hydrate and loosen dried bronchial secretions, restore the epithelium in the lungs, and promote coughing. Effective nebulization must also be accompanied by other physical therapy techniques (e.g., coupage, postural drainage, exercise, cough stimulation) to be effective in clearing the lungs. Nebulization for 15 to 30 minutes every 4 to 6 hours, with additional respiratory therapy, is more effective than continuous ultrasonic aerosolization.

The nebulizer equipment should be cleaned and all removable parts sterilized before use on each patient. Each patient should have its own sterile fluid reservoir and hoses leading from the nebulizer. Sterile fluids should be used whenever possible. Complications can also occur if the dried secretions are not suctioned immediately after nebulization therapy. The patient can become more dyspneic from swelling of the rehydrated secretions. The patient should never be left unattended once ultrasonic nebulization therapy has begun. Fluid overload may occur in pediatric patients on continuous therapy; therefore, always use intermittent nebulization therapy.

The nebulizer hose may be attached to an oxygen mask for direct administration to the patient. Patients that do not tolerate a face mask may allow an Elizabethan collar to be placed and covered with plastic to form a tent over the head. The nebulizer hose can be attached to the tent to permit aerosolization of the patient. Another method of administration is by covering the cage door with plastic and nebulizing the cage. A cage specifically for nebulization may be used, but this can cause cross-contamination between patients if the unit is not thoroughly cleaned between uses.

Respiratory Physiotherapy

Immediately after nebulization, the rehydrated, loosened secretions must be mobilized and cleared out of the lungs using physiotherapy. Coupage (percussion and vibration) and tracheal manipulation to stimulate the cough reflex, postural drainage, and mild exercise (improves tidal ventilation) are methods of physiotherapy.

Percussion is the creation of waves of air to loosen secretions in the lungs. *Vibration* is high-frequency compression of the chest wall. For manual percussion, the cupped hands are clapped against each side of the chest, trapping air between the hands and the chest wall, starting with the caudal lung lobes and working cranially to move the secretions out of the tract. A mechanical vibrator/percussor (Puritan-Bennett) produces continuous percussion and vibration. Care must be taken to strike the chest wall without causing discomfort or bruising. Percussion may be contraindicated in patients with a bleeding disorder, fractured ribs, or fragile bones. Rhythmic percussion loosens and mobilizes secretions; postural drainage, exercise, and coughing help expel the secretions.

Recumbent patients may be turned to the other side or placed sternally, with the head lower than the chest to augment gravitational drainage of secretions. After nebulization and coupage, dogs may be walked outside to help increase drainage of secretions. Cats may be placed in a large cage to encourage physical activity, which increases clearance of secretions.

NUTRITIONAL SUPPORT

Proper nutritional support is an important aspect of therapy for hospitalized patients. Sick or injured patients need good nutritional support to counteract the immunosuppressive effects of sepsis, neoplasia, chemotherapy, anesthesia, and surgery. This support enhances wound healing and minimizes the length of hospitalization without significant weight loss and muscle atrophy. Initiation of nutritional support early in the course of hospitalization is crucial for a successful outcome.

Nutritional status should be assessed when the patient is admitted into the hospital and daily during hospitalization. During the physical examination, the patient's weight is recorded and compared with that of previous visits. A history from the owners regarding type of food, quantity fed, and frequency of feeding is helpful. During hospitalization, the patient is a candidate for nutritional support if the patient loses more than 10% of body weight; has a decreased appetite or anorexia; loses body condition from vomiting, diarrhea,

trauma, or wounds; and has increased needs because of fever, sepsis, wounds, surgery, low serum albumin, organ dysfunction or chronic disease.

Unfortunately, nutritional support in hospitalized patients is often delayed because the patient is not reassessed daily for nutritional needs, the amount of food a patient consumes is not recorded, the patient is not weighed daily, and dextrose and electrolyte solutions are erroneously thought to provide adequate nutritional support. Most previously healthy dogs can go approximately 1 week without nutritional support and suffer few ill effects. Cats, however, especially overweight cats, can go only a few days without nutritional support before ill effects develop, such as hepatic lipidosis.

Nutritional support is often the last consideration when evaluating the patient's daily treatment regimen, until the patient does not recover as quickly as expected. The goal of nutritional support is to provide the patient's nutritional requirements while it is recovering from its disease process and/or anorexia, trauma, or surgery, until the patient is able to eat enough on a regular basis to accommodate any ongoing losses. With nutritional support, patients can gain weight and have an improved response to medical or surgical therapy.

The route of nutritional support administration can be enteral, parenteral, or a combination of both. Enteral feeding may be accomplished with orogastric, nasogastric, nasoesophageal, pharyngostomy, gastrostomy, and jejunostomy tubes. Parenteral nutrition is administered via a catheter placed in the cranial or caudal vena cava.

The route selected depends upon such factors as function of the gastrointestinal (GI) tract, the disease process, duration of support, equipment and personnel available to provide the necessary support, and cost of the chosen method. Enteral support is chosen most often because it is physiologically sound, easy, relatively free of complications, and inexpensive. If the gastrointestinal tract is functional and the patient can swallow, use as much as possible. Parenteral support should be used if the patient has a medical or surgical condition that prevents ingestion or digestion of nutrients (e.g., vomiting, diarrhea, ileus, pancreatitis, malabsorption, reconstructive surgery, coma), and as adjunctive therapy for patients with organ failure or when malnutrition is severe.

Enteral Nutritional Support

Handfeeding favorite foods and tempting with warm, odoriferous foods in multiple, small meals, can be used in conjunction with other methods of nutritional support. Forced feeding can be stressful to the patient and may deliver only a portion of the nutrition required for recovery.

Orogastric intubation is excellent for rapid administration but can cause aspiration and trauma and is very stressful in patients other than neonates. This method is for short-term use only.

Placement of a nasoesophageal or nasogastric tube is an easy, simple, and relatively inexpensive procedure that allows liquid nutritional support for an extended time and can be easily administered by the owner at home for continued convalescence.

A nasoesophageal or nasogastric tube is placed through the nasal cavity into the distal esophagus or stomach to bypass the oral cavity. Placement is contraindicated in patients with nasal masses, esophageal disorders (e.g., megaesophagus), or no gag reflex. A nasoesophageal or nasogastric tube can usually be placed without chemical restraint (ideal for animals unable to tolerate general anesthesia). It is tolerated by most patients and used when the animal is anorexic, too stressed for forced feeding, and not receiving enough nutrition through handfeeding. The tube can remain in place for a week or longer, until the patient's appetite increases or the oral cavity can be used again. Feedings through the tube can start immediately after placement, unlike pharyngostomy or gastrostomy tubes. Have the patient in a sitting position when tube feeding. Common problems with nasoesophageal or nasogastric tubes include epistaxis (nosebleed) when the tube is first placed, accidental placement in the trachea, patient intolerance of the tube, and tube obstruction by medications or diet.

Soft, flexible pediatric feeding tubes, red rubber tubes, and polyurethane tubes (Seamless), in a variety of lengths and diameters, are used for cats and dogs. Animals weighing less than 5 kg require a 5-French feeding tube, whereas some cats and all dogs weighing 5 to 15 kg can accept an 8-French tube. In larger dogs, the larger-diameter feeding tubes require a guidewire for placement in the esophagus or stomach.

For nasoesophageal placement with the tube tip at the level of the midthoracic esophagus, measure from the tip of the nose to the eighth or ninth rib (Fig. 26-31). For nasogastric placement, measure from the tip of the nose to the thirteenth rib. Occasionally, tubes placed in the stomach may cause gastroesophageal reflux and irritation, but this is usually not a problem with a small-diameter tube. Mark the premeasured length on the tube with a permanent marker (Box 26-7).

For nasoesophageal tube feeding, aspirate the tube before each feeding. If air is aspirated, do not feed. During aspiration, there should be negative pressure on the syringe if the tube is correctly placed. Accidental tracheal intubation can cause aspiration pneumonia. Before each feeding, also assess tube location by injecting 3 ml of sterile water through the tube and listening for coughing or gagging. If this occurs, do not administer the feeding; remove the tube.

A pharyngostomy tube is placed through the wall of the pharynx into the esophagus or stomach, bypassing the oral cavity. Placement requires general anesthesia

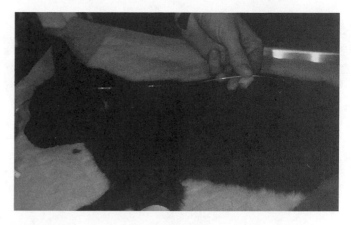

FIG. 26-31 Measurement of the tube before nasoesophageal placement.

and surgery. The many possible complications (e.g., esophagitis, pharyngitis, laryngitis, vomiting, regurgitation, aspiration pneumonia) and the difficulty of pharyngostomy tube placement outweigh the benefits.

A jejunostomy tube is a feeding tube surgically placed in the mid- to distal duodenum or proximal jejunum, bypassing the stomach. Continuous feeding of easily digestible diets through the jejunostomy tube requires prolonged hospitalization, without the benefits of home care. This procedure is rarely used because of the cost of placement and maintenance and possible complications.

A gastrostomy tube is placed through the body wall into the lumen of the stomach, bypassing the mouth and esophagus (Fig. 26-33). A gastrostomy tube is used for patients requiring long-term nutritional supplementation because of orofacial neoplasia, surgery or trauma, esophageal disorders, or liver disease. The diet can be easily prepared and administered by the owner, increasing owner compliance. The tube's bulb or mushroom tip helps retain the tube in the desired location. Gastrostomy tubes can be placed with use of endoscopic equipment (i.e., percutaneous endoscopic gastrostomy) or without endoscopic equipment (i.e., blind percutaneous gastrostomy). Placement requires general anesthesia and trained personnel.

Enteral Nutrition Daily Caloric Requirements

Diet selection is based on caloric density, diameter of the feeding tube, and daily caloric needs of the patient. Each illness is assigned a factor to increase the calculated estimate of the patient's basal energy requirements by 25% to 75% (Figs. 26-34 and 26-35). The volume and consistency of the diet are limited by the size of the animal's stomach and diameter of the feeding tube, but total caloric requirements can usually be delivered when using a calorically dense diet. Stomach volume is approximately 20 ml/kg body weight. Daily water requirement is 12 ml/kg.

Patients with a nasoesophageal or nasogastric tube require a liquid diet (because of small tube diameter).

Box 26-7 Nasoesophageal tube placement

1. Restrain the animal in sternal recumbency or sitting, with the head held level or slightly elevated. Anesthetize the nostril with a few drops of topical ophthalmic anesthetic. While waiting for the topical anesthetic to take effect, lubricate the tip of the feeding tube with a water-soluble lubricant or 5% lidocaine jelly.
2. Place the tip of the tube in the nares and direct the tube dorsomedial to the alar fold. After the tip has been inserted 1 or 2 cm into the nostril, direct the tube caudoventrally into the esophagus.
3. When the tube is inserted to the premeasured line, infuse a small amount of sterile saline into the tube. If coughing occurs, the tube is probably in the trachea. Remove and reinsert the tube. If no coughing occurs, aspirate the syringe. If air is removed from the tube, the tube could be in the trachea. If negative pressure is evident, the tube is in the esophagus. If fluid is aspirated, the tube is in the stomach. If there
is any question of tube location, make a lateral radiograph to determine placement.
4. Move the proximal end of the tube laterally alongside the nares, place a small strip of elastic tape around the tube, and either suture or glue it alongside the nares. The tube may be sutured without tape using a series of handties around the tube. Move the tube caudally between the eyes (alongside the dorsal nasal midline) and suture or glue (Fig. 26-32). Cap the end of the tube to prevent air from entering.
5. Apply an Elizabethan collar to prevent the patient from removing the feeding tube (see Fig. 26-32). Evaluate the sutures or glue at each feeding to ensure that the tube is stable and not malpositioned.
6. To remove the tube, flush the tube with air to clear fluid out of the tube. Remove the sutures or gently pull the glued tube away from the skin, and pull the tube out of the nose.

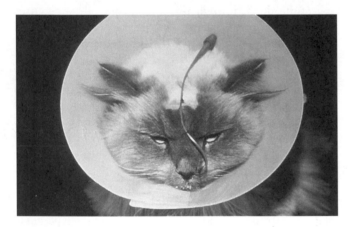

FIG. 26-32 Cat with a nasoesophageal tube sutured in place. An Elizabethan collar has been applied to prevent dislodgment of the tube. *(Courtesy of Dr. Nancy Poy, Michigan State University.)*

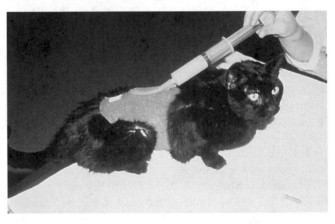

FIG. 26-33 Feeding through a gastrostomy tube. *(Courtesy of Dr. Nancy Poy, Michigan State University.)*

Human enteral feeding products are easily administered through these tubes but are not developed for veterinary patients and may need supplementation with additional nutrients. Hyperosmolar diets can cause diarrhea. Liquid veterinary products, such as CliniCare Canine and Clini-Care Feline, are available. Also, canned diets, such as Hill's a/d and Eukanuba Nutritional Recovery Formula, can be delivered through a feeding tube as small as 8 French.

Select the appropriate diet of canned food and calculate the caloric density (kcal/ml) of the diet based on information on the label or supplied by the manufacturer. The total volume (ml) to be delivered per day is calculated by using the maintenance energy requirement (MER) and caloric density:

$$\text{volume/day (ml)} = \frac{\text{MER (kcal/day)}}{\text{energy density (kcal/ml)}}$$

$$\text{volume/feeding (ml)} = \frac{\text{volume/day (ml)}}{\text{feedings/day (usually 4-6 a day)}}$$

For anorexic patients, after placement of the tube, the volume fed is gradually increased over 3 days, with 5 ml of water administered through the tube every 2 hours

MICHIGAN STATE
U N I V E R S I T Y

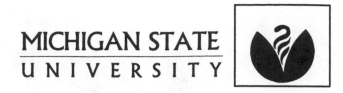

Veterinary Teaching Hospital
East Lansing, Michigan 48824-1314

TPN WORKSHEET FOR DOGS

Date:_____

Body weight_____ kg.

1. Basal energy requirement (BER)
   BER = (30 × body weight in kg) + 70 = _____ kcal/day (for >2 kg)
   or 70 (body weight in kg)$^{0.75}$ = _____ kcal/day (for animals <2 kg)

2. Maintenance energy requirement (MER)
   • cage rest: MER = 1.25 × BER
   • post surgery: MER = 1.35 × BER
   • major trauma, neoplasia: MER = 1.5 × BER
   • sepsis, major burn: MER = 1.75 × BER

   MER = _____ × _____ (BER) = _____ Kcal/day (provided as non-protein calories)

3. Protein requirement (renal failure see below)
   • Adult dogs =   4 gm/100 Kcal/day
   • Dogs with extra protein losses = 6 gm/100 Kcal/day
   _____ (4-6 gm) × _____ (Kcal from step 2) divided by 100 = _____ gm/day

4. Volume of solutions needed****
   • Dextrose 50% = 1.7 Kcal/ml (to provide 50% of Kcal/day from step 2)
          _____ Kcal/day ÷ 2 = _____ Kcal ÷ 1.7 = _____ ml Dextrose 50%
     (On day 1 use ½ of dextrose increase day 2 if blood glucose <200 mg/dl)
   • Lipid 20% = 2 Kcal/ml (to provide 50% of Kcal/day from step 2)
          _____ Kcal/day ÷ 2 = _____ Kcal ÷ 2 = _____ ml Lipid 20%
   • Amino Acid 8.5% with electrolytes = 0.085 gm/ml
                          _____ gm/day ÷ 0.085 = _____ ml A.A. 8.5%
   • Additional fluids (LRS)   = _____ ml LRS
                                    Total Volume = _____ ml
                        Rate = total volume ÷ 24 = _____ ml/hr
   • Add multivitamin (MVC) 3 ml/1000 ml total volume = _____ ml MVC

****Note: For volumes >300 ml round off volume to nearest 100 ml
              For volumes <300 ml round off volume to nearest 10 ml

Renal Failure Patients: 1. Use Amino Acid without Electrolytes 2 gm/100 Kcal
                           2. Add 20 ml TPN electrolytes II/1000 ml total volume

References:
   • Remillard RL, Thatcher CD: Parenteral nutrition support in the small animal patient. Vet. Clin. North Am. Sm. Animal Pract. 19:1287,1989.
   • Lippert AC, Armstrong PJ: Parenteral nutrition support. CVT X, 1989, pp 25-30.
   • Lewis LD, Morris ML, Hand MS: Small animal clinical nutrition III, 1990, Ch 5, pp 2-43.
   • Remillard RL, Martin RA: Nutritional support in the surgical patient. Semin. Vet. Surg. 5:197, 1990.

FIG. 26-34 Worksheet to calculate fluid requirements for total parenteral nutrition in dogs. *(Courtesy of Michigan State University Veterinary Teaching Hospital.)*

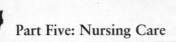

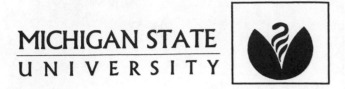

MICHIGAN STATE
U N I V E R S I T Y

Veterinary Teaching Hospital
East Lansing, Michigan 48824-1314

TPN WORKSHEET FOR CATS

Date:_____

Body weight_____ kg.

1. Basal energy requirement (BER)
   BER = (30 × body weight in kg) + 70 = _____ kcal/day (for cats >2 kg)
   or 70 (body weight in kg)$^{0.75}$ = _____ kcal/day (for cats <2 kg)

2. Maintenance energy requirement (MER)
   - cage rest: MER = 1.25 × BER
   - post surgery: MER = 1.35 × BER
   - major trauma, neoplasia: MER = 1.5 × BER
   - sepsis, major burn: MER = 1.75 × BER

   MER = _____ × _____ (BER) = _____ Kcal/day (protein and non-protein calories)

3. Protein requirement (renal failure see below) 6 gm/100 Kcal/day
   6 gm × _____ (Kcal/day from step 2) divided by 100 = _____ gm/day

4. _____ gm/day of protein × 4 Kcal/gm = _____ Kcal from protein
   MER - Kcal from protein = _____ Kcal to be provided by non-protein (Dextrose & Lipid)

5. Volume of solutions needed****
   - Dextrose 50% = 1.7 Kcal/ml (to provide 50% of non-protein Kcal/day from step 4)
     _____ Kcal/day ÷ 2 = _____ Kcal ÷ 1.7 = _____ ml Dextrose 50%
     (On day 1 use ½ of dextrose increase day 2 if blood glucose <200 mg/dl)
   - Lipid 20% = 2 Kcal/ml (to provide 50% of non-protein Kcal/day from step 4)
     _____ Kcal/day ÷ 2 = _____ Kcal ÷ 2 = _____ ml Lipid 20%
   - Amino Acid 8.5% with electrolytes = 0.085 gm/ml
     _____ gm/day ÷ 0.085 = _____ ml A.A. 8.5%
   - Additional fluids (LRS)   = _____ ml LRS
                                Total Volume = _____ ml
                  Rate = total volume ÷ 24 = _____ ml/hr
   - Add multivitamin (MVC) 3 ml/1000 ml total volume   = _____ ml MVC

****Note: For volumes >300 ml round off volume to nearest 100 ml
             For volumes <300 ml round off volume to nearest 10 ml

Renal Failure Patients: 1. Use Amino Acid without Electrolytes 2 gm/100 Kcal
                           2. Add 20 ml TPN electrolytes II/1000 ml total volume

References:
   - Remillard RL, Thatcher CD: Parenteral nutrition support in the small animal patient. Vet. Clin. North Am. Sm. Animal Pract. 19:1287,1989.
   - Lippert AC, Armstrong PJ: Parenteral nutrition support. CVT X, 1989, pp 25-30.
   - Lewis LD, Morris ML, Hand MS: Small animal clinical nutrition III, 1990, Ch 5, pp 2-43.
   - Remillard RL, Martin RA: Nutritional support in the surgical patient. Semin. Vet. Surg. 5:197, 1990.

FIG. 26-35 Worksheet to calculate fluid requirements for total parenteral nutrition in cats. *(Courtesy of Michigan State University Veterinary Teaching Hospital.)*

for 12 hours. Change to the selected diet and double the volume to 10 ml every 2 hours for 12 to 24 hours. Gradually increase the volume to achieve full caloric intake, divided into four to six feedings a day, by the third day. For patients with delayed or inadequate gastric emptying, a meal may need to be skipped, or smaller, more frequent feedings administered if too much food remains in the stomach. If the patient vomits, skip the next scheduled feeding and adjust the amount, rate, and frequency of the feeding.

To prepare the diet using canned food, place one can of food in a blender and add enough water to achieve a consistency that will pass through a large-bore nasogastric tube or a gastrostomy tube. Dry food can also be used by allowing the food to soak thoroughly in water before blending. The mixture must be blended well and then strained twice to remove any large chunks that would occlude the feeding tube. All food should be able to pass through a syringe without occluding the tip. For example, one can of Hill's Feline p/d mixed with 340 ml of warm water is of the consistency to pass through the feeding tube; it has a caloric density of 0.8 kcal/ml.

The volume of water added to the canned food when blended is usually adequate for the patient's water requirement. All feedings should be administered slowly, at room temperature. Hill's a/d and Eukanuba Nutritional Recovery Formula can be given straight out of the can through an 8-French feeding tube, at room temperature or slightly warmed, with no premixing with water. The a/d provides 1.2 kcal/ml and Nutritional Recovery Formula provides 2.1 kcal/ml. If a smaller-diameter tube is used, mixing two 5.5-oz. cans of a/d with 50 ml of water provides a caloric density of 1.0 kcal/ml. Flush the tube with 5 or 10 ml of water after each feeding to prevent tube occlusion.

Animals with feeding tubes in place should be offered fresh food before each feeding once the oral cavity and esophagus can be used. Most animals begin to eat with the feeding tube still in place. When the animal begins to voluntarily eat at least half of its maintenance energy requirement daily, the amount of food given through the feeding tube can be decreased until the patient is consuming its full caloric intake per os. The change from enteral feedings to the normal diet should be gradual over 3 to 5 days if the patient's normal diet is not used for enteral feedings.

Clients can be instructed on how to feed their animal through the tube at home, if necessary. Ease of administration, minimal maintenance, and owner compliance makes this method of nutritional support a viable alternative for patient care in a nonhospital situation.

Parenteral Nutritional Support

Patients that cannot receive enteral nutrients must be supported by total parenteral nutrition (TPN), which involves intravenous infusion of nutrient solutions. This is a practical alternative for patients that cannot absorb nutrients through the GI tract (e.g., malabsorption), require rest of the GI tract (e.g., vomiting due to severe pancreatitis), cannot swallow (e.g., comatose patients), or are so debilitated that additional nutrition must be administered by another route.

Carbohydrates are administered in the form of dextrose. The most common concentration used is 50% dextrose, which provides 1.7 kcal/ml. Dextrose is used to provide 50% of the canine patient's daily MER. Lipids provide the other 50% of the canine MER. Dextrose and lipids are used in a 1:1 ratio to meet the MER (see Figs. 26-34 and 26-35).

Gradual introduction of dextrose is necessary to avoid hyperglycemia. On the first day of TPN, only half of the calculated amount of dextrose is administered. If the patient's urine glucose remains negative and the blood glucose level is below 200 mg/dl, the entire calculated dose of dextrose can be administered on day two. Occasionally a patient requires addition of insulin to the TPN solution. This should be added immediately before administration of the parenteral nutrition.

Lipids (including essential fatty acids) provide the fat required by the patient. These are available in 10% and 20% solutions, with 20% more commonly used. Made of soybean or safflower oil, egg yolk phospholipids, and glycerol, they provide a concentrated energy source that supplies 50% of the patient's energy requirements. Visually checking the patient's plasma for lipemia on a daily basis can help decrease hyperlipidemia. Patients with hepatic, pancreatic, or endocrine disease may develop hyperlipidemia. For patients with severe hyperlipidemia, decrease the rate of infusion or the concentration of the lipids, or discontinue use of lipids altogether.

Proteins are supplied in the form of crystalline amino acids, made of essential and nonessential amino acids, available in a variety of concentrations, with or without electrolytes. The most common concentration used is 8.5% with electrolytes. The basic solutions of amino acids contain all of the essential amino acids required by dogs and cats, except taurine (see Chapter 14). If TPN is to be continued for longer than 1 week, supplementation of taurine is essential in cats. For patients with renal or hepatic insufficiency, reduced amounts of amino acids or specially formulated amino acid products should be administered.

Electrolytes can be included in the amino acid solutions. This is usually sufficient to maintain a normal electrolyte balance. Hypokalemia is the most common electrolyte abnormality. For patients with ongoing potassium losses (e.g., vomiting), additional supplementation may be necessary. If the patient is in renal failure, amino acids are administered without electrolytes.

Vitamins are administered as a multivitamin supplement. B-complex vitamins should be added daily to the feeding solution. Vitamin K is incompatible with parenteral solutions and should be administered SC or IM only if parenteral nutrition is continued longer than 1 week.

Trace elements only need to be supplemented if long-term (more than 1 week) parenteral nutritional support is needed. Zinc may need to be supplemented after 1 week in patients with GI disease. Phosphorus may be added for diabetics.

Figs. 26-34 and 26-35 show how to calculate daily TPN feeding requirements for dogs and cats. The total daily fluid volume for maintenance TPN is 30 ml/lb of body weight. If the total volume of TPN is less than the calculated required amount, add an additional amount of balanced electrolyte solution or sterile water to equal the calculated fluid requirements. If the patient is experiencing ongoing fluid losses, a second catheter or an additional lumen on a central catheter can be used to deliver the fluids.

When mixing the appropriate solutions, strict asepsis is essential. Using a laminar flow hood, an automatic mixing pump, or an "all-in-one" bag will help keep contamination to a minimum. Add the dextrose and amino acids before the lipids to prevent lipid destabilization. Add the water or electrolyte solutions next, and any vitamins last.

Parenteral nutrition is administered via a catheter in the cranial or caudal vena cava. A double-lumen catheter is of benefit if additional medication, fluids, blood products, or blood sampling are needed. Administration by a fluid pump is the most accurate method of delivering parenteral nutrition.

Many complications of parenteral nutrition involve problems with the catheter. Sepsis is another complication of parenteral nutrition. Nutrient solutions are an excellent growth medium for bacteria. Contamination of the solutions, lines, or catheters can cause such signs as fever, depression, and pain or swelling at the catheter insertion site. Daily patient monitoring can help eliminate or minimize this complication. Administering TPN through a "dedicated" IV line can decrease the likelihood of sepsis. The catheter should be used for parenteral nutrition only, and not for blood sampling, medication administration, or CVP monitoring. New bags of TPN solution should be made daily for the patient and hung at room temperature for a maximum of 24 hours before changing to another bag. All of the administration lines should be changed every 48 hours when the bag is changed. The catheter bandage should be replaced whenever it is soiled, as well as every 48 hours, when the administration lines are changed.

Gradually tapering off of TPN can prevent hypoglycemia. If TPN must be discontinued abruptly, use a 5% dextrose solution to maintain blood glucose levels.

Patients on TPN longer than 1 week may develop intestinal villus atrophy. Partial parenteral nutrition in conjunction with enteral nutrition may be advised when parenteral nutrition is being withdrawn. Care must be taken when changing from one diet to another; the transition should be gradual.

GROOMING AND SKIN CARE

Some hospitalized patients develop skin problems (e.g., decubital ulcers, pyoderma, urine scald, dry scaly skin) because of recumbency, urinary or fecal incontinence, and general lack of appropriate care. Others have been healthy until admitted for trauma. Regardless of the reason for admittance to the hospital, all patients require routine grooming and skin care. Patients also feel better when kept clean and dry.

When a patient is admitted and its condition has been stabilized, any vomit, diarrhea, urine, or blood should be removed from the skin to prevent secondary infections. Skin care of the hospitalized patient involves bathing to remove body fluids, skin oil, or exudates, brushing to prevent mat formation, padding to prevent decubital ulcer formation, and medicating affected areas of skin. Before the patient is discharged from the hospital, such routine procedures as toenail trimming, anal sac expression, and ear cleaning should be performed before a final bath.

Skin Care

Many critically ill patients are too weak or unable to get up to relieve themselves. Urine and fecal scalding develops if these patients are not cleaned after each occurrence. However, use good judgment before partially or completely bathing a critically ill patient. For example, if a dyspneic animal in an oxygen cage urinates on itself, remove the soiled bedding and spot clean the patient. Do not jeopardize the patient's overall health to completely bathe the animal; also, do not let the patient continue to lie in body waste without attempting to clean it.

Any long hair should be trimmed to prevent moisture from being trapped and causing a secondary infection. Carefully shave the hair around the perianal and inguinal areas for ease of cleaning. Avoid nicking or cutting the patient with the clippers. Apply a light tail wrap on long-haired patients with diarrhea to help keep the tail clean and prevent scalding. Wrap the tail loosely and incorporate some of the hair to keep the wrap in place. Change the wrap after each episode of diarrhea.

Patients with minor soiling can be spot cleaned with mild solutions (e.g., Peri-Wash, Sween). Continuous diarrhea can cause perineal irritation and ulceration and ascending urinary tract infections. A complete bath is recommended when large areas are soiled. Clean contaminated incision areas gently with water and a washcloth. Soak off any dried organic material. Pat the incision dry. Remove as much organic material from the patient as possible before placing in a bathtub and bathing. Apply a light layer of triple antibiotic ointment to the incision to prevent contact with water and shampoo.

Recumbent patients can be kept cleaner and drier if a urinary catheter is placed to prevent urine scald. If the patient is large, transfer the patient on a gurney to a tub with a grate placed over it, or slide the patient out of the cage onto a rack elevated above a floor drain. Have shampoo, several buckets of warm water, and towels ready before starting. If the patient does not have a urinary catheter, encourage urination before bathing. Express the bladder if the patient is incontinent. If the patient has not defecated in days, enemas or digital removal of feces may be necessary. Use this opportunity to make the patient more comfortable *before* bathing. Cover any clean and dry bandages with plastic to reduce the need for bandaging after the bath. Change any contaminated bandages.

Wet the patient on the exposed side, apply shampoo, and scrub gently with the hands. Rinse thoroughly and turn the patient to the other side. Repeat the shampooing. Remove all wet and soiled bandages at this time. Clean and completely dry the areas under the bandages before replacing. Squeeze excess water from the fur and towel dry. Use a blow dryer to dry the exposed side; then turn the patient over and repeat on the other side. Completely dry the patient with a hand-held dryer or cage dryer.

Using a comb or brush while drying the patient decreases drying time. Use care when brushing thin-skinned patients with a slicker brush. The wire bristles can scratch the skin easily. Remove mats with scissors or electric clippers while the hair is dry, preferably before bathing. Before replacing the patient back in the cage, make sure the patient is completely dry and all irritated areas on the skin are examined, shaved if necessary, cleaned, and treated appropriately. Ointments, creams, lotions, drying solutions, or powders can be reapplied at this time. For recumbent patients, place clean towels or padding placed between the patient's legs to aerate the skin, make the patient more comfortable, and prevent scrotal edema. Roll stockinette into a donut-shape to pad any decubital ulcers.

Vomiting patients should have the hair on the face and front legs kept clean or trimmed and their mouth rinsed of vomit.

Bathing

Baths are given to clean the entire patient. Any coat conditioners are applied after shampooing and towel drying. Trim the toenails, express the anal sacs (dogs), and clean the ears (dogs) before bathing. Wear a gown or apron for bathing. Have all supplies ready and within reach before placing the patient in the tub: shampoo, bucket, washcloth, towels, conditioning spray, clippers or scissors if necessary, brush and comb, blow dryer, and cologne. Dilute the cleansing shampoo with water for easier application and lathering.

Dogs and cats can be placed directly into a tub. Some cats will not tolerate a sprayer hose and do better if placed in a tub already partially filled with water. Use a cup to pour water over the body, starting at the neck (not over the head). Allow the patient to move around in the tub unless it becomes too frantic. Holding the cat gently by the scruff is usually all of the restraint necessary. A second person may be needed for restraint if the animal becomes agitated or fractious. Never leave the patient unattended in the tub.

Starting at the base of the head, soak the patient with warm water before applying shampoo. In cats, some medicated shampoos can cause toxicity. Always read the directions before applying any shampoo. Any cleaning needed for the head can be done with a wet cloth after the body is bathed. If shampoo inadvertently gets into the eyes, rinse with sterile saline. Rub in the shampoo gently down to the skin and work into a lather. Rinse thoroughly and remove excess water from the patient before towel drying. Medicated dips can be applied at this time. Place the patient on a table at waist level to blow dry and brush out. If using a cage dryer to dry the patient, place the setting on low or warm. Patients can become overheated quickly if left unattended with the dryer on a high setting. Monitor patients frequently during drying. Insecticidal sprays, powders, or mousses may be applied after drying.

Medicated shampoos may be antiseptic, moisturizing, degreasing (keratolytic and keratoplastic), antipruritic, antifungal, or insecticidal. Patients with bacterial dermatitis may need to be carefully shaved before shampooing. Avoid clipper burns and irritating the skin when shaving with a No. 40 blade. The goal for bathing patients with seborrhea is to remove the scales and crusts while decreasing oiliness. Massaging the shampoo into the coat disperses the medication while loosening any scales and crusts.

External parasites (e.g., fleas, ticks) may be treated by bathing with an insecticidal shampoo, application of a dip solution after bathing, or application of sprays, powders, or mousses. Pay strict attention to the package insert. Insecticides may cause toxicities in cats and certain dog breeds, such as Collies, Shelties, and Old English Sheepdogs. Signs of toxicity include vomiting, diarrhea, excessive salivation, bradycardia, miosis, ataxia, and seizures; these need immediate medical attention. Mildly affected animals can be treated by rebathing with a non-medicated shampoo to remove any remaining insecticide on the fur. Rinse and dry thoroughly.

Insecticidal Applications

Insecticidal dips are used after bathing the animal and before drying. Careful application of the properly diluted dip is extremely important. Mix the dip according to the package insert and apply to the patient with a sponge, avoiding the eyes. Discard any used sponges to prevent contamination of other patients and personnel. Do not towel dry the patient, because this removes much of the dip. Allow the animal to air dry naturally or use a blow dryer.

Insecticidal sprays, powders, or mousses can be applied after the patient is dried. The animal does not necessarily have to be bathed before application. Most patients tolerate application of a spray, but some cats do not like the sound of sprays and are more cooperative when powders or mousses are applied. Spray the haircoat or apply the powder or mousse lightly while ruffling the hair against the direction of growth to work the product down to the skin. Avoid inhaling the spray or powder. Rub into the hair to evenly disperse the insecticide.

NAIL CARE

The claws or nails of cats and dogs are regularly trimmed to prevent ingrown nails, injury from traumatic nail fractures, and impaired walking from overlong nails that impinge on the footpads. Trimming also minimizes damage to the environment (e.g., bedding and padding) and injury to handlers and other animals. The nail should not extend beyond the level of the footpad and should be trimmed accordingly. However, animals that do not have their nails trimmed routinely can have an overlong "quick" or ungual blood vessel that bleeds with trimming; this vessel will gradually regress

with frequent nail trimming. To avoid injury of veterinary staff, cats should have their claws trimmed before starting any procedure.

Purposely "quicking" the nails (cutting the nail short, causing bleeding) is unnecessarily cruel and painful. "Quicking" is viewed unfavorably by clients and causes the animal to resist subsequent nail trimming. Unless the patient has a history of painful nail trims, most animals do not resent nail trimming.

Nail trimmers are available in a variety of styles and sizes (Fig. 26-36). Guillotine-type trimmers (e.g., Resco) are available in regular and large sizes. The blade can be replaced when it becomes dull. Scissors-type trimmers work well for nails that are ingrown, for the nails of puppies and kittens, and for cat claws. Human nail trimmers can also be used to trim cats' nails. Always make sure the chosen trimmers are clean and sharp.

The patient should be in lateral or sternal recumbency or sitting. An assistant may be necessary to help restrain the animal. Hold the toe between thumb and forefinger, with the foot grasped firmly in that hand. Push the toe distally to extend the nail and allow the guillotine trimmer to slide over the tip of the nail (Fig. 26-37). Position all types of trimmer blades to within 2 mm from the end of the quick. With a swift, smooth motion, cut the nail just distal to the quick. In patients with white toenails, the quick is visible and easy to avoid. In those with dark nails, pare the end of the nail down a bit at a time until a clearer or lighter color appears in the cross-section of the nail. This is the tip of the quick. Compare the remaining untrimmed dark nails with the trimmed nail for proper length of trim.

The nail should be cut cleanly, with no frayed edges; smooth off any rough edges with nail file or emery board. After trimming, examine each nail for bleeding before going on to the next nail. Examine each foot to

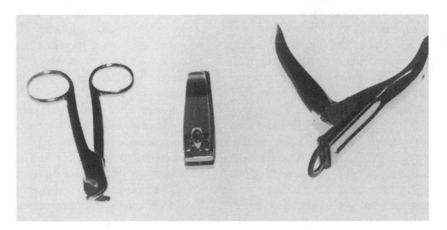

FIG. 26-36 Instruments for trimming claws or nails: scissors type (*left*); human toenail type (*center*); guillotine type (*right*).

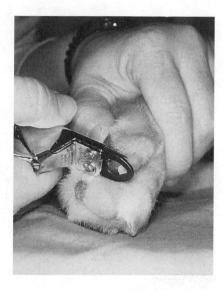

FIG. 26-37 Trimming toenails using a guillotine-type trimmer.

ensure that all nails, including the dewclaws, have been trimmed cleanly and are not frayed.

If the quick is accidentally cut, apply a cauterizing agent, such as silver nitrate applicators. Place the tip of the applicator directly on the quick and apply pressure. If no cauterizing agent is available, apply pressure with a cottonball or gauze sponge directly on the quick to gradually stop the bleeding. Silver nitrate application may cause some discomfort in patients, so be prepared for the patient to attempt to withdraw the foot.

ANAL SAC CARE

The anal sacs are paired sacs located beneath the skin on either side of the anus at the 4 o'clock and 8 o'clock positions, each with a duct opening directly into the terminal rectum. The anal sacs normally empty their malodorous secretions during defecation. Occasionally, animals (rarely cats) may not be able to empty the anal sacs naturally and develop painful distention or impaction of the anal sacs. Signs include "scooting" on the hindquarters and licking of the anal area. The anal sacs of dogs can be expressed (emptied manually) as a routine part of grooming, as part of the physical examination, and before bathing. The anal sacs are emptied with the dog restrained in the standing position. Anal sac expression may cause discomfort and a muzzle may be necessary.

For internal anal sac expression, wear latex gloves, well-lubricated with a water-soluble lubricant or 2% lidocaine jelly. With the handler holding the tail dorsally or laterally, insert the first joint of the index finger into the rectum and gently palpate the anal sac between thumb (externally) and forefinger. Gently massage with light to moderate pressure, milking the secretions medi-

ally into the anal opening; repeat on the other side. Notify the veterinarian of any unusual secretions. Clean the perineum with a deodorizer or spot cleaner if not bathing immediately after expression.

For external anal sac expression, place a gauze sponge or paper towel over the anus while applying gentle, firm pressure craniomedially against the perineum. Examine the secretions and repeat on the opposite side. External expression does not completely empty the anal sacs but may cause less discomfort than internal expression.

Anal sac abscesses may need to be treated with hot packs to the perineum, instilling medication into the anal sacs, drains, or surgical intervention. Patients with recent rectal surgery should not have the anal sacs expressed.

EAR CARE

Before cleaning ears, visually examine the external ear canal and tympanic membrane for any irregularity. Cleaning the ears and instilling medication without examination may cause further damage to the tympanic membrane and result in loss of hearing, loss of vestibular function, or facial nerve paralysis. The tympanic membrane must be intact before any products other than saline or water are instilled into the ear (Box 26-8). Look for any redness, discharge, ulceration, excessive tissue formation, narrowing (stenosis) of the canal, abnormal odor, or debris in the outer ear and on the pinna. These could indicate a bacterial or yeast infection, ear mite infestation, or tumors. Thickening of the pinna could indicate an aural hematoma. Signs of ear disease include excessive shaking of the head, scratching at the ears, head tilt, and ataxia.

If the animal has an ear problem, examine the less affected ear first. Most patients tolerate ear examination with minimal restraint while sitting or in sternal recumbency. Patients with painful ears or chronic ear disease require general anesthesia for ear examination and cleaning. Use a separate clean otoscope cone for each ear to avoid contaminating a normal ear with organisms from an infected ear.

Grasp the pinna and carefully insert the otoscope cone into the ear canal. Straighten the ear canal by gently pulling the pinna laterally, while advancing the otoscope cone into the canal to visualize the tympanic membrane. Occasionally, the ear canal is occluded with debris and must be cleaned and flushed with saline to visualize the tympanic membrane. If cultures or cytologic samples are required, obtain the samples before cleaning the ears.

Some dog breeds, such as Poodles, have hair growth in the ear canal. This hair traps moisture and debris and increases the likelihood of infection. Hair in the ear canal

---

Box 26-8 Cleaning dogs' ears

Materials:

basin

bulb syringe

cottonballs or cotton swabs

hemostats

ceruminolytic agents, saline solution, cleansing solution, or dilute vinegar

Procedure:

1. Tip the head and ear slightly ventrally, grasp the pinna, and place the solution into the ear canal, with the bulb syringe directed ventromedially into the canal. Have the basin ready below the ear to catch the excess.

2. Massage the base of the ear to distribute the cleansing solution and loosen any debris. Flush the ear again. Use cottonballs on a hemostat to clean the debris in the ear canal. Never insert cotton-tipped swabs into the canal of an inadequately restrained patient. These cotton swabs should be used for the external ear canal and interior of the pinna only. Allow the patient to shake its head occasionally to loosen more debris. Flush and clean the ears until debris is no longer visible. Dry the ear canal with cottonballs.

3. Examine the ears with an otoscope and apply any medications necessary. Massage the ear canal to distribute the medication evenly and thoroughly.

---

should be plucked out with hemostats or the fingertips, a few strands at a time. This procedure may be painful, so appropriate restraint of the head is necessary. Sedation or tranquilization may be necessary. Grasp a few hairs at a time with the hemostats and quickly pluck the hair out. Grasping too much hair in the hemostats is painful and may cause more inflammation.

Ensure the tympanic membrane is intact before any cleaning. Most cleaning solutions are ototoxic if the tympanic membrane is not intact. If the membrane is not intact, use a saline solution to clean the ears. Antimicrobial agents, such as a povidone-iodine solution (e.g., Xenodine, Solvay), may be used. If the membrane is intact, various ceruminolytic agents (e.g., Clear X, DVM

Pharmaceuticals; Oti-Clens, SmithKline Beecham) are available for breaking up debris and cleansing. Cleansing products with a drying agent (e.g., Epi-Otic, Allerderm) are good for cleaning the ears of dogs with long, droopy ears, such as Poodles and Cocker Spaniels.

It is good public relations to have the patient looking better (as well as feeling better) upon discharge than when it was admitted. Examine every patient before discharge to ensure that all extraneous bandages are removed, it is bathed, groomed, de-matted, and smelling good, and the nails are trimmed, ears cleaned, and anal sacs expressed. Brush one last time and spray with a lightly scented spray. Educating clients on proper skin care and grooming can prevent many problems and will keep the animal in better health.

Acknowledgment. The author is grateful to Drs. Cynthia Ramsey, Nancy Poy, Sheilah Robertson, and Rodney Oakley for their assistance in compiling this chapter.

SUPPORTIVE CARE AND REHABILITATION

E.A. GORECKI

NURSING CARE FOR RECUMBENT PATIENTS

A number of conditions can cause recumbency in patients, including pelvic fractures, head trauma, and herniated intervertebral discs. A major concern in recumbent patients is formation of decubital ulcers (e.g., bed sores, pressure sores). The best treatment is prevention. Animals must be kept clean. Urine and feces should not be allowed to remain on the skin and haircoat. Poor sanitation promotes skin breakdown and formation of decubital ulcers. Frequent baths should be given, and the animal should be dried completely. Shaving the hair around the perineal region on animals that are incontinent or have diarrhea can save time in baths and drying. Sponge baths can be done instead.

Decubital ulcers develop rapidly (within 2 or 3 days) but heal slowly. Once the underlying muscle and/or bone is exposed, it can become infected. Small, superficial ulcers can be managed conservatively with doughnut bandages and topical astringents and antibiotics. Ointments with a petroleum base are not recommended, because these can harbor bacteria. Deep, extensive ulcers require surgical treatment. This may include wound debridement, placement of drains, and secondary closure. If bone is exposed, proper care is to be taken to prevent the periosteum from drying.

Prevention and treatment of infection are essential. Areas affected most are the sternum, shoulders, sides of the fifth digits, stifles, and hips.

Turning. Turning the patients every 2 to 4 hours helps prevent formation of ulcers and dependent pulmonary atelectasis. After turning, the pressure points should be checked. Redness should be only temporary. If redness persists 30 minutes or longer, decrease the time on that side. After a position change, stimulate areas over pressure points by massaging. This increases circulation to those areas.

Padding. Padding the recumbent patient is essential in preventing the formation (and treatment) of decubital ulcers. Paralyzed animals frequently thrash about; padding helps prevent animals from harming themselves. Any animal with paralysis or paresis, seizures, vestibular problems, encephalopathy resulting from neoplasia of the brain, orthopedic disease, or metabolic disease should have padding placed in the cage. Animals with vestibular disease, neoplasia of the brain, or frequent seizures should be placed in cages with padded doors and walls. Types of padding include fleece pads, sponge rubber egg crates, diapers, and waterbeds. Household items, such as blankets, sheets, and foam rubber placed in plastic bags, can be used as padding. Fleece pads are synthetic sheep skins. They are washable, absorbent, very soft, and airy. These can be combined with other forms of padding. If used alone, they are best for patients under 25 pounds.

Foam rubber egg crates are especially good for larger patients (see Fig. 26-22). A big disadvantage, however, is that they act like a sponge, absorbing urine and water. Place them in plastic bags to keep them clean and dry. Owners can purchase these crates at medical supply stores or in the bedding department of retail stores.

Waterbeds are especially good in preventing decubital ulcers (Fig. 26-38). Animal waterbeds are made in various sizes so that most standard veterinary cages will accommodate them. The bed should be placed in a cage of nearly the same area so that the patient will not fall off and become stuck between the bed and the cage wall. Animal waterbeds are thermostatically heated and provide warmth and comfort to animals placed upon them. If they become unplugged, they require about 12 hours to heat up before they can be used. Temperature can be adjusted easily on the waterbeds to prevent the animal from becoming overheated or too cold. Heat eases muscle soreness, stimulates circulation, and helps animals relax. Waterbeds should never be used without turning on the heat. A cold waterbed draws heat from the animal and produces hypothermia.

Disposable diapers or bed pads are placed on top of all padding to help keep the padding clean. Use of diapers saves valuable nursing time. Soiled diapers are simply thrown away, leaving the underlying padding reasonably clean and dry. In pet stores, they are called *puppy training pads*.

Bladder Maintenance. Every effort should be made to promote voluntary urination so that expressing the bladder and catheterization are kept to a minimum. Taking the animal outside may stimulate or promote voluntary urination. Before expressing, allow the patient to urinate. Attention should be given to bladder size, the act of urination, and the amount, color, and odor of the urine. When leg muscle function starts to return, some bladder function usually returns, also. Time should be allowed for the patient to totally evacuate its bladder.

Palpate the bladder with even, steady pressure. Sudden movement may cause the patient to tense the abdominal muscles. In toy breeds and cats, it is easiest to use one hand. Use both hands for larger breeds. Placing patients on their side is easier than trying to hold them up while expressing the bladder, especially if the patient starts to struggle. Once the bladder is palpated, apply pressure. Several seconds may be required to override the sphincter tone, especially in animals with neurologic injury.

A urinary catheter and collection set may be used in a paralyzed animal for better nursing care. The urinary catheter should be left in place only 3 to 4 days because of the risk of infection. If hematuria or some other change in urine color develops, removal of the catheter should be considered. The risk of infection can be decreased if the animal is catheterized only when necessary. The major disadvantage is the time required to catheterize the animal.

Bowel Maintenance. Keep a record of the patient's bowel movements. An enema may be required if the patient becomes constipated. This is not generally the case, however. If the patient has a flaccid anal sphincter,

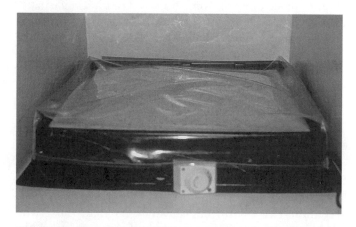

FIG. 26-38 Waterbed placed in a cage. Note that the edges of the bed meet the cage wall, so the animal cannot become wedged between the bed and cage wall.

nursing care and adequate sanitation can be especially difficult. The hindquarters of long-haired dogs and cats should be clipped closely so that feces do not smear or entangle in the haircoat. Clipping also facilitates bathing and drying if the animal becomes soiled.

NURSING CARE IN SPECIAL CIRCUMSTANCES

Head Trauma and Seizure Patients. Continuous monitoring of semicomatose or comatose patients is necessary. Monitoring includes heart rate, respiration, temperature, mucous membrane color, and neurologic function. Reevaluation is done every 15 to 60 minutes, depending upon deterioration or improvement.

Patients in status epilepticus (continuous seizures) and those that have head trauma usually have increased intracranial pressure. Cerebral edema peaks at 24 to 48 hours after trauma and can last up to 96 hours. Extending and evaluating the head and neck help cerebral venous outflow. Care should be taken not to occlude the jugular veins.

Excessive fluid therapy and hypoxia contribute to cerebral edema. Fluid therapy should be administered only to maintain hydration and normal blood pressure (after shock treatment). To combat potential hypoxia, oxygen should be given by mask, nasal catheter, or oxygen cage. If intubation is required, it should be done as quickly and smoothly as possible. Struggling and coughing increase intracranial pressure.

Caloric needs for these patients can increase as much as two and a half times. A highly caloric diet is recommended. Patients in stuporous or comatose states can receive nutrition by nasogastric tube, percutaneous enterogastric tube, or intravenously.

Spinal Trauma. Owners calling with concerns that their pets may have sustained spinal trauma should be told to place them on some form of board. They can use duct tape to help stabilize them. If the animal is brought to the clinic not on such a board, the animal should be placed on one immediately. Assessments, treatments, and diagnostics should be done with the animal on the board until the patient is stabilized. Only lateral views and across-table radiographs should be made.

REHABILITATION

Rehabilitation is an extremely important part of medical management. Patients that receive some form of rehabilitative treatment recover faster than those who do not. The type of therapy used depends upon the severity of the problem and condition of the patient. "Rehab" therapy can prevent decubital ulcers, enhance blood and lymphatic circulation, prevent muscle contracture, maintain muscle tone and joint flexibility, produce relaxation, and reduce pain.

Although some types of rehabilitation can be expensive, most are not. Many are easy to perform so that the owners can do it at home, if needed. This helps keep costs down, or, if done in the clinic, does not require much overhead. Types of rehab therapy include thermal therapy, passive exercise, and active exercise.

Local Hypothermia/Cold Therapy. Hypothermia is most effective during the first 24 to 48 hours after surgical procedures and after acute soft tissue contusions, muscle/tendon strains, and ligament sprains or lacerations. The cold decreases the tissue temperature, which decreases pain perception and reduces nerve conduction and muscle spasms. Local vasoconstriction also helps decrease edema.

Local hypothermia can be as easy as applying an ice pack to the affected area. These can be the cold packs used for shipping by drug companies, ice cubes wrapped in a towel, or continuous surface cooling blankets. Cold packs should be covered with a towel; ice should be placed in a plastic leak-proof bag wrapped in a towel. Applications should be for 5 to 10 minutes, two to four times a day. Treatment should not last longer than 30 minutes. Edema may become more severe if treatments exceed 30 minutes. Open wounds must be protected with a sterile, water-impermeable dressing to avoid contamination; use light pressure and avoid excessive cold. If the condition worsens at any point, discontinue treatment.

Local Hyperthermia/Heat Therapy. Hyperthermia is applied 48 to 72 hours after injury. Caution should be used when applying heat. Patients with sensory nerve involvement and those recovering from anesthesia could sustain thermal injuries. Before applying hot packs or a hot towel to any patient, some form of insulation, such as a towel, should be placed on the skin. The hot pack should be 104° to 113° F and applied for 10 minutes, two to four times a day. Every 1 to 2 minutes, the skin should be checked to see if it is overly hot. If so, another towel should be placed over the treatment area.

The therapeutic benefits of hyperthermia include muscle relaxation, pain relief, localized vasodilation, and localized increase in metabolic rate. This form of treatment is contraindicated for acute injuries, because it increases edema. Some of the different forms of heat treatments are radiant heat (applied with infrared lamps), ultrasound, and some forms of warm-water hydrotherapy.

Combination Therapy. Combination therapy is used in the later stages of healing and can be used with other forms of physical therapy. Heat applied before massage or exercise can improve muscle relaxation and circulation. Cold applied to the injured area after exercise helps decrease swelling and pain. If the patient has just had surgery, it is best to wait 2 to 3 days before beginning physical therapy.

Passive Exercise. No voluntary muscle activity is required by the patient in passive exercise. Two forms of passive exercise include massage and range of motion.

Massage. Massage is used to rehabilitate patients with diseases of the bone, muscle, joints, nerves, and skin, as well as patients with decubital ulcers. Massage can be administered a couple of days after surgery. The patient that is treated medically can also receive massage, but care should be taken to prevent aggravating the existing lesion. Massage can also be done after a session of active therapy is performed (combination therapy).

The primary objective of massage is to increase flow of blood and nutrients to the tissue, which in turn will provide quicker elimination of wastes. Deeper forms of massage can decrease the chances of fibrosis. Massage contraindications include acute inflammation of soft tissue, bones, and joints, recent fractures, sprains, foreign bodies under the skin, hemorrhage or lymphangitis, advanced skin diseases, fever or heat stroke, round incision sites, and torn muscles.

There are five factors to consider when administering massage: the direction of the massage (which should always be toward venous return); amount of pressure to use (start with superficial pressure and gradually work to deeper muscles); duration of massage; rate and rhythm of massage (which depends on the type used); and frequency of massage.

In *effleurage,* strokes are given with the palm and fingers, slowly and lightly, just like petting. Gradually increase the pressure of the strokes. This produces a calming effect, which allows the animal to relax. This also allows the animal to become accustomed to the therapist. With light strokes, apply fifteen per minute; with heavy strokes, apply five per minute. Give 5- to 10-minute sessions of effleurage. This type of massage enhances draining of veins and lymph channels.

With *fingertip massage,* use two or three fingers and keep them close together. Do not lose contact with the skin. Massage slowly and gently in a circular motion, increasing the pressure as the animal relaxes. This massages underlying muscles. Massage for 5 to 10 minutes.

Petrissage or deep massage is used on the back, flank, and chest. The skin is lifted, pulled, and rolled between the fingers and thumb, like rolling dough. For the shoulder, thigh, and limbs, the deeper muscles and tendons can be kneaded between the thumb and fingers of the right hand, while the left hand holds the limb and occasionally flexes and extends it. The kneading movements should be slow and rhythmic. Muscle is compressed from side to side and always in the direction of venous return. Deep massage enhances circulation, stretches muscles and tendons, and prevents adhesions and contracture.

Friction massage is fast, invigorating, circular massage given with the first two or three fingers. Massage at a rate of one circular motion every second, gradually increasing to twice that rate. This massage helps loosen superficial scar tissue and adhesions, as well as remove loose hair from the coat.

Stretch pressure massage combines pressure on a muscle with a stretching motion. This type of massage provides mechanical deformation of the skin and elongation of underlying muscle fibers and spindles. It helps maintain skin compliance and benefits muscle.

Range-of-motion therapy. Range-of-motion therapy helps maintain the proper range of motion of a limb by minimizing muscle and joint contraction from disuse. Take the affected limb and slowly move it through its normal range, making sure not to hyperextend the limb. Treatment should be for 5 or 10 minutes, two to four times a day. Range of motion can be combined with other forms of rehabilitation.

For patients with orthopedic injuries/conditions and muscle contractions, a slow controlled movement should be applied. Caution should be used not to over-stress the limb, because this may loosen fixation devices or cause muscle/tendon/ligament damage.

Active Exercise. The intent of active exercise is to stimulate as much voluntary activity as possible. Voluntary muscle contraction is the most beneficial form of therapy. Most patients must be supported with a towel/stockinette used as a sling or supporting them at the base of the tail (Figs. 26-39 and 26-40). Exercise carts and hoists can also be used to help them walk (Fig. 26-41). These exercises should be done on textured surfaces, because most patients slip or slide on tile floors. Treatment time depends on the patient. Once you notice the patient becoming tired, treatment should end. This may be as short as 1 to 2 minutes. Within the first few weeks, treatment should not extend past 20 minutes.

Standing exercises are done when the patient starts supporting weight. Allow the animal to do so for as long as possible. It may be only a second or two in the beginning. After the patient sinks back down, pick it up and repeat for as long as possible. As the patient becomes stronger and can support its total weight, gently apply downward pressure over the hips or shoulders. This helps strengthen the muscles as the animal attempts to resist.

Walking exercises are performed when patients start to regain voluntary muscle movements or with paraplegic patients. Although the patients may only have function of their forelimbs, they must start exercising them again as soon as possible. A leash should always be used to restrict their activity.

Hydrotherapy. Hydrotherapy provides passive and active therapy. Passive hydrotherapy is provided with the whirlpool, whereas active hydrotherapy is swimming (underwater exercise). Animals may be fearful of the water; time should be allowed to acclimate the animal to the water.

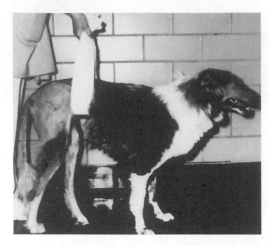

FIG. 26-39   A bath towel can be used to support the hindquarters during active exercise of animals with caudal paresis.

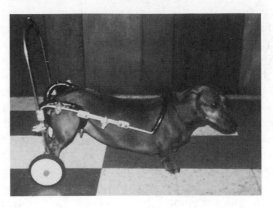

FIG. 26-41   A commercially available cart used for dogs with caudal paralysis.

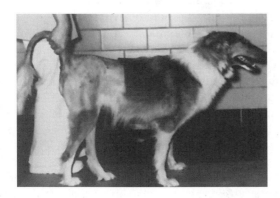

FIG. 26-40   The tail can be used to support the hindquarters during active exercise therapy of dogs with caudal paresis. Note that the tail is grasped at its base so as to avoid tail injury.

Contraindications of hydrotherapy include peripheral vascular disease, acute injury, acute inflammation, fever, recent surgery, hemorrhage, cardiac disorders, and respiratory disorders. Hydrotherapy should not commence until at least 5 days after surgery. In animals treated medically, wait 10 to 30 days. Before placing an animal in the tub, water temperature should be checked to be sure it is appropriate. The patient should never be left alone in the tub!

An animal with an elevated temperature should not be treated with warm-water therapy until its temperature has been normal for 72 hours. Animals with respiratory or cardiac insufficiency should not be treated.

Whirlpool therapy provides a vigorous hydromassage. This massaging effect helps in removing dirt, necrotic tissue, and purulent exudates, and can also help fight infection if povidone-iodine is added. It speeds wound healing, reduces hyperesthesia of the skin, and may facilitate urination and defecation.

Before putting the animal in the whirlpool, remove all bandage material. During treatment, the water surface should be skimmed to remove hair and other debris. The water temperature should be 102° to 105° F. Caution should be taken not to scald the animal. For the first treatment, the animal should just sit in the tub for 5 minutes to become accustomed to immersion. Each treatment should increase in duration, ending up with a 20-minute treatment after several days.

Swimming is an excellent form of physical therapy. Buoyancy and hydrostatic pressure in a pool provide support and allow voluntary exercise with a minimum of effort. Animals with paresis must be helped through the motions of walking or swimming. Weights can be added to the animal's legs to build strength and endurance. Water also creates resistance to movement, which helps strengthen weakened muscles as exercise sessions continue. Because a patient produces heat while exercising, the water temperature should be 80° to 90° F.

RECOMMENDED READING

Abood SK, Buffington CA: Use of nasogastric tubes: indications, technique, and complications. In Kirk RW, Bonagura JD, editors: *Kirk's current veterinary therapy XI*, Philadelphia, 1992, WB Saunders.

Donoghue S: Nutritional support of hospitalized patients, *Vet Clin North Am Sm Anim Pract* 19(3), 1989.

Lippert AC, Armstrong PJ: Parenteral nutritional support. In Kirk RW, editor: *Current veterinary therapy X*, Philadelphia, 1989, WB Saunders.

McGuire BH: Intravenous catheters. In McCurnin DM, Poffenbarger EM: *Small animal physical diagnosis and clinical procedures*, Philadelphia, 1991, WB Saunders.

Pratt PW: *Medical, surgical, and anesthetic nursing for veterinary technicians*, ed 2, St Louis, 1994, Mosby.

Stein D: *Natural healing for dogs and cats*, Freedom, Calif, 1993, Crossing Press.

Wheeler SL, McGuire BH: Enteral nutritional support. In Kirk RW, editor: *Current veterinary therapy X*, Philadelphia, 1989, WB Saunders.

CHAPTER 27

Nursing Care of Horses

T. Kemper
C. Hayes

Learning Objectives

After reviewing this chapter, the reader should understand the following:

Methods of sample collection for laboratory analysis
Routes of administration of medication
Procedure for intravenous catheterization in horses
Techniques used in general nursing care of horses

Procedures used in grooming and foot care
Principles of feeding, watering, exercising, and bedding of horses
Procedures used in caring for recumbent horses
Procedures used in caring for critically ill foals
Procedures used in caring for infected horses

GROOMING

Equine patients should be groomed daily, unless the horse has a condition whereby vigorous grooming would be painful or damaging (e.g., severe skin infections, cutaneous burns). A rubber currycomb should be used in a circular motion to remove dried sweat or mud. Next a stiff-bristled brush can be used to remove dirt and loose hair. If stiff brushes and rubber currycombs are used on the horse's face and distal limbs, they should be used gently, because overly vigorous grooming may be uncomfortable for the animal. Metal currycombs should not be used on the horse's head or distal limbs. A soft brush can be used to finish removing loose hair and dirt. If needed, a damp or dry cloth can be used to remove the remaining dust from the horse's coat. A stiff brush, hair brush, or metal mane comb should be used on the tail and mane.

HOOF PICKING

A horse's hooves should be picked clean daily. Most adult horses raise the foot when a hand is run down the caudal aspect of the distal limb and gentle pressure is exerted over the caudal aspect of the limb at the level of the distal splint bones. The hoof is then cleaned with a hoof pick by removing debris from the lateral and central sulci, starting at the heel and working toward the toe, and then from the rest of the hoof (Fig. 27-1). A degenerative condition called *thrush* is common in feet that are infrequently cleaned, or if the horse stands for long periods in damp bedding or muddy soil. Thrush may occur secondary to a bacterial infection and appears as black, malodorous material in the region of the frog. Various medications can be used topically to dry the foot and kill the bacteria. Bleach or 2% iodine can be applied to the lateral and cen-

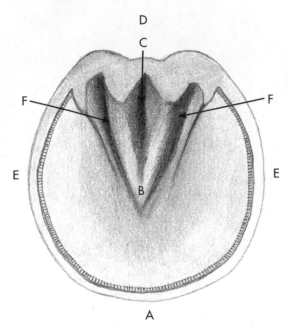

FIG. 27-1 Ventral view of the equine hoof. **A**, Toe. **B**, Frog. **C**, Central sulcus or cleft of the frog. **D**, Heel. **E**, The quarters. **F**, Lateral sulci.

tral sulci. Commercial formulations containing formalydehyde or copper can also be used. Care must always be used to avoid spilling caustic solutions on the coronary band or other parts of the horse's leg. The technician should wear gloves to protect herself/himself from the solutions. Some animals with severe thrush require foot trimming to remove diseased hoof tissue and wraps to help keep the foot clean and dry while it is being medicated.

FLY CONTROL

The best method of fly control is to maintain a clean barn with frequent manure removal. Various topical fly sprays are available. Those containing permethrins, pyrethrins, or citronella sprays are the safest for sick horses. Fly repellents containing organophosphates should not be applied to debilitated horses or foals. Overhead fly systems that release fly repellents at regular intervals can also minimize the fly population. A soft cloth can be used to apply fly repellent to the horse's face, taking care to apply the repellent around the eyes without getting any into the eyes. Fly masks are available for the face and the ears of sensitive patients. A fly sheet can also be used.

FEEDING AND WATERING

Hospitalized horses often have special dietary needs. Their diseases can often create a catabolic state. The horse may require extra calories to maintain its weight. Horses that can chew and swallow normally should be fed their usual diet if their disease permits. Good-quality alfalfa or grass hay, such as timothy hay, can be fed. Good-quality oat hay is also a suitable feed. Horses with gastrointestinal disturbances, such as colic or diarrhea, need special consideration. Horses recovering from impactions may need more laxative feeds, such as alfalfa hay, grass pasture, and even bran mashes. Horses with diarrhea or operated on for colic may benefit from a diet that is not quite so rich, such as timothy or oat hay. Hay pellets or cubes that contain alfalfa or a mixture of alfalfa and bermuda or oat hay can also be used. If added carbohydrate is needed, a pelleted feed that also contains grains may be fed.

Pelleted feed produces less dust and may be better for horses recovering from respiratory allergies or pneumonia. Horses recovering from gastrointestinal ulceration may also need to be fed a pelleted ration, because the increased fiber and stem in hay may irritate and exacerbate certain kinds of ulcers.[1] Pellets soaked to make a gruel can be fed to horses with oral lesions, facial fractures, dental problems, or recurrent episodes of choke. Feed softened in this manner is easier for the animal to chew and swallow. Horses with neuromuscular disorders, such as botulism, may be unable to chew and swallow normally. A pelleted ration that has been soaked may be the only feed the animal can eat.

Fresh water should always be available. Some horses may not know how to use an automatic waterer if it requires the horse to push on a lever to fill the water cup. Water buckets or tubs should always be provided in these cases. Salt may need to be provided topically on the feed or in the form of a salt lick during hot weather, or for horses that have diseases that create a sodium deficiency, such as colitis.

NASOGASTRIC INTUBATION

A horse that cannot chew or swallow normally, but with a functional gastrointestinal tract, can be fed and hydrated through a *nasogastric tube*. Nasogastric intubation should be done in the presence of a veterinarian until the technician has become proficient in the technique. Feeding through a nasogastric tube requires a larger-bore stomach tube than does water administration. The length of tube necessary to reach the horse's stomach should be determined before the procedure.

The tube is first lubricated with a water-soluble lubricant jelly (e.g., K-Y Jelly) or even plain water. The tube is then inserted into the nostril with one hand. The other hand is used to guide the tube through the most ventral portion of the nasal passage, the ventral meatus. Care must be taken to ensure that the tube is directed caudoventrally, because it will not easily pass into the pharynx if it is inserted into the middle or dorsal meatus. The tube should never be forced if it will not pass easily. If the tube strikes the ethmoturbinates as it is being passed through the ventral meatus to the pharynx, the nasal membranes may bleed profusely. This may happen if the horse moves at the wrong moment, or if the technician or veterinarian is not careful.

Once the tube has been inserted to the level of the pharynx, the horse's head should be lowered and the neck flexed slightly to facilitate entrance of the tube into the esophagus and not the trachea. The tube is passed into the esophagus as the horse swallows. If the horse will not swallow, the tube can be gently moved back and forth to stimulate swallowing. If the tube passes into the trachea by mistake, the horse may cough and resist. However, sedated or severely debilitated horses may not resist or cough if the tube is erroneously placed into the trachea. If the trachea is grasped in one hand and moved back and forth, the tube can be felt rattling within the cartilaginous structure. The tube will not rattle if it is in the esophagus, because this is a collapsible structure composed of striated and smooth muscle. If the tube is in the esophagus, it can often be seen on the left side of the neck near the jugular furrow as it is being passed. If the tube cannot be seen, it can be palpated as it passes through the esophagus. If the horse has an esophageal obstruction, the tube may be difficult to pass. The esophagus may be ruptured by overaggressive nasogastric intubation. The tube should be passed caudally, all the way into the stomach, but never forced.

Once the tube enters the stomach, the typical sweet and slightly fetid odor of the stomach contents may be discernible through the tube. No material should be pumped through the stomach tube unless you are absolutely certain that the tube is in the stomach and not in the trachea. Horses cannot vomit, so always check for excessive gastric contents (gastric reflux) before administration of fluid, feed, or medication. Checking for gastric reflux is done by creating a siphon effect by injecting a small amount of water into the tube with a stomach pump or dose syringes and disconnecting the pump or syringe to see if fluid or ingesta flows freely back out of the tube. If excessive fluid or ingesta is present, it may be necessary to medicate the horse at a later time, when no reflux is present. Overfilling the stomach can result in gastric rupture and death. The adult horse's stomach can hold 8 to 15 liters, but this varies between horses.[2]

Medication or fluid should be given by gravity flow through a funnel, when possible, to prevent overfilling of the stomach. If a stomach pump must be used to administer water or mineral oil, it should be periodically disconnected to check for increased pressure and backflow of fluid out of the stomach tube. Before the nasogastric tube is withdrawn, all of the fluid should be removed from the tube. This can be done by pumping a small amount of air through the tube while it is still in the stomach and then kinking the end of the tube or placing a finger over the end while it is being removed. This prevents the horse from aspirating fluid into the lungs as the tube is being removed.

Horses can be rehydrated by administering water through the nasogastric tube. If IV administration of fluids is not possible or practical, the stomach tube can be taped where it exits the nostril and then taped to the horse's halter. The tube is then wrapped around and taped in one additional site on the halter to minimize movement of the tube. A syringe can be placed in the end of the tube to prevent air from filling the stomach. Water can be given every 2 hours or as needed in this manner. Horses must not be allowed to eat or drink with a large-bore stomach tube in place, because they cannot adequately protect the airway when they swallow.

BEDDING

Horses can be bedded on a variety of materials. It is important that the bedding be clean, as dust free as possible, and relatively deep. Pine shavings are adequate for most patients, but they tend to be very dusty. This may not be acceptable for horses with open wounds or respiratory disorders. Pine shavings with minimal dust or shredded paper bedding is preferable for horses with severe respiratory problems. It is best to obtain wood shavings from a known source to prevent accidental exposure to black walnut shavings, which can cause laminitis when the horse stands in the shavings. Black walnut wood is darker than pine but can be difficult to recognize if the bedding is soiled or if multiple types of wood chips have been mixed. Straw bedding is often used for mares with newborn foals. Bedding should always be deep unless the horse has a problem that necessitates a firmer surface for standing. Regardless of the type of bedding used, it should be kept very clean by removing the urine and feces at least once daily.

Recumbent adult horses must have very deep bedding to help prevent formation of decubital ulcers (pressure sores). Alternatively, large mattresses or specially designed water beds can be used. Critically ill foals can be kept on mattresses with waterproof covers and fleece pads to keep them clean and dry. It may be necessary to clean the stall or change the bedding each time the horse or foal urinates or defecates if the animal is recumbent. Strategically placed diapers or absorbent mats may help reduce the number of bedding changes needed with a recumbent foal.

EXERCISE

Adult horses and foals should have some form of exercise daily unless their medical problem requires stall rest. Walking on soft dirt or grass surfaces is preferable to walking on concrete or asphalt. Foals may be allowed to run freely along side the mare if they do not have a condition that warrants more restricted activity, and if the area is properly fenced with no hazards, such as drains or moving vehicles. If the foal's activity must be controlled, the foal can be walked using a halter and a rope around the foal's hindquarters in the area of the semimembranosus and semitendinosus muscles. Good judgment and caution are needed to prevent the foal from rearing and flipping over backward. Neonates whose exercise must be limited can be walked by placing one arm in front of the foal's chest and one arm behind the foal to cradle it while walking. Alternatively, an adult horse halter can be used over the foal's body like a harness, with the nose piece around the foal's neck, the buckle strapped around the ventral thorax, and the rope clip located on the caudodorsal portion of the foal's back. The hind end of the foal may still need to be supported.

COLLECTING BLOOD SAMPLES

To obtain a blood sample from a horse, the animal must be properly restrained. The jugular vein is most commonly used to obtain blood samples and lies directly under the skin in the jugular furrow. The vein should be entered at the most cranial one third of the neck, where the vein is more superficial and somewhat better separated from the carotid artery. The jugular vein and carotid artery exit the thoracic inlet closely together but become more separated as the vessels course cranially toward the head.

When first learning to draw blood, you should start on the right side of the neck to prevent inadvertent puncture of the esophagus on the left side. The vein is distended by occluding it with a thumb placed proximal (ventral) to the venipuncture site. Once the vein fills, a 20-gauge or larger needle is quickly and smoothly inserted. The entire length of the needle's shaft should be well seated in the vein. Blood should become visible at the hub of the needle. The syringe is then attached and the sample is aspirated (Fig. 27-2). Alternatively, a double-ended blood collection needle (Monoject, Sherwood Medical) can be used by inserting the unsheathed longer portion into the vein and attaching the collection vials to the shorter, sheathed end. The vacuum within the collection device allows the blood to flow freely into the vial. For either method, the needle is removed after the vein is no longer occluded and distended.

In a seriously ill horse, the jugular veins may need to be preserved to allow continued venous access for delivery of medications and fluids. In this case another site should be used for routine blood collection. A venous

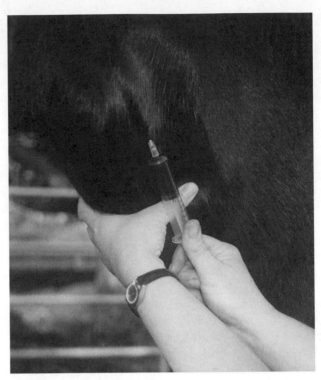

FIG. 27-2   Collecting blood from the jugular vein.

sinus ventral to the facial crest can be used for obtaining blood samples. It should be entered just caudal to its midpoint between the medial canthus of the eye and the rostral end of the facial crest, just ventral to the facial crest. This should only be attempted by experienced technicians or veterinarians because of the proximity to the horses's eye. Care must be taken to avoid inadvertently puncturing the eyeball if the horse turns its head suddenly. The cephalic vein dorsal to the carpus can also be used for venipuncture when the jugular veins are no longer patent. However, this puts you in a vulnerable position and you may be struck by the front leg of the horse while attempting to draw blood.

ADMINISTRATION OF MEDICATION
Oral Administration

Medications that are in liquid form and required in only small doses may be administered with a dose syringe or a syringe with the locking tip removed. The syringe is placed through the side of the mouth in the area of the diastema (space between the teeth). The medication is deposited on the caudal portion of the tongue if possible. Medications in pill form can be crushed with a mortar and pestle and then mixed with something sweet, such as molasses, and given in a similar manner. It is best not to mix medication with the feed, because horses often eat around the medication and do not consume the full dose. Medication that must be given in large doses requires use of a nasogastric tube for delivery into the stomach.

Parenteral Injections

Drugs and other liquids can be injected into a muscle (IM) or vein (IV), under the skin (SC), or into a layer of the skin (ID). Some medications can be given by multiple routes, either intravenously or intramuscularly. It is very important to know which routes of administration are acceptable for each drug administered, because injection by an inappropriate route can have harmful or even lethal effects on the horse. For example, procaine penicillin should be given only in the muscle (IM). If this medication is given in the vein (IV), the procaine component may cause excitation, seizures, and death. Some medications, such as phenylbutazone and tetracycline, should be administered intravenously only. These medications can be very caustic and cause tissue sloughing if administered outside the vein (perivascular) or in the muscle.

Intradermal Injections

Rarely an injection must be given in the skin. Some forms of allergy testing use intradermal injections of allergens. Lidocaine can be injected intradermally to block the skin for certain procedures. A very small amount, usually 0.1 to 1 ml, is injected using a 25-gauge, 5/8-inch needle. The skin is cleaned with alcohol if needed, and the needle is inserted into the skin (not underneath it). The plunger is withdrawn slightly to make sure a blood vessel has not been entered. If no blood is aspirated, the medication is injected. Because the medication is being injected into the skin, a small bleb becomes visible in the skin.

Subcutaneous Injections

Occasionally medications are injected subcutaneously. These medications are usually given in smaller doses, such as for allergy desensitization. A 20- or 21-gauge, 1-inch needle should be used. Any area where the skin can easily be lifted from the underlying muscle and fascia may be used; the lateral aspect of the neck where IM injections are also given is a suitable site. The skin is first cleaned with alcohol if necessary and then pulled laterally to form a "tent." The needle is then inserted under the skin. Always aspirate to make sure no blood enters the syringe and then inject.

Intramuscular Injections

Various sites can be used for IM injections. The safest muscle for technicians to use is in the neck area. The neck muscles of the horse can be used only for administering small volumes of medication. The area to be used is a triangular portion on the side of the neck formed by the ligamentum nuchae dorsally, the spine ventrally, and the shoulder caudally (Fig. 27-3). In horses, the safest muscles for IM injection are in the hind leg (semitendinosus and semimembranosus muscles). This is the preferred site for IM injections in neonates. If this site becomes infected and an abscess forms, this is the easiest area to establish adequate drainage to allow for healing.

The person administering the injection should stand on one side of the horse and inject the semitendinosus/semimembranosus muscles on the *opposite* leg (Fig. 27-4). If the horse kicks when the needle is inserted, it typically kicks with the leg on the side of the injection and not where the person is standing. This is a very vulnerable position for the technician. Horses that are known to kick should not be injected at this site. An alternative site is the gluteal (hip) muscles. This allows the person giving the

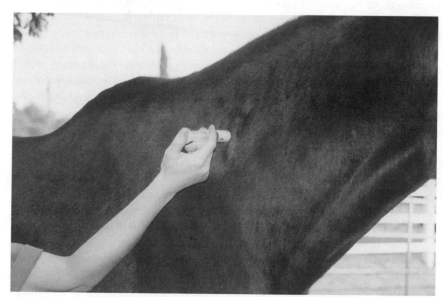

FIG. 27-3 Intramuscular injection using the brachiocephalicus muscle.

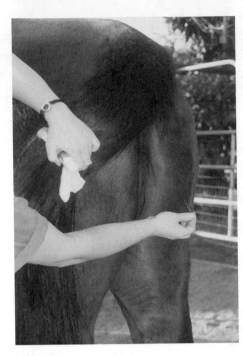

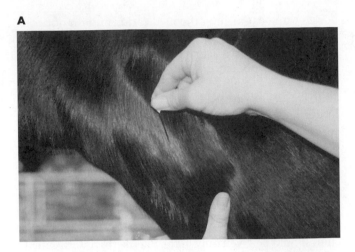

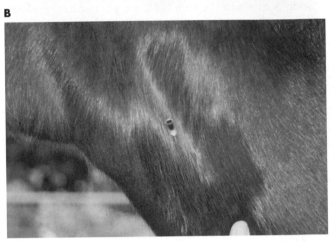

FIG. 27-4 Intramuscular injection using the semimembranosus/semitendinosus muscles. Note that the needle is inserted into the opposite leg.

injection to stand in a somewhat safer position, but if the horse develops an abscess subsequent to gluteal injection, it can be very difficult to establish adequate drainage. There should always be a handler available to restrain the horse's head when injecting the hind limb muscles of a horse.

A 16- or 18-gauge, 1.5-inch needle should be used for IM injections in adults. A 20-gauge, 1-inch needle should be used for small foals and neonates. The site is cleaned with alcohol if necessary, and the needle is inserted with a quick jab. Some people prefer to tap on the area to be injected a few times with their fist before injecting in an attempt to desensitize the area. When injecting the neck muscles, a fold of skin can be grasped and pulled slightly away from the neck to act as a skin twitch and distract the horse before inserting the needle. Always disconnect the needle from the syringe before inserting it so that if the horse kicks or jumps, the needle will remain in place and not be pulled out by the weight of the syringe. Then the syringe is attached and the plunger aspirated to make sure a blood vessel has not been entered. If no blood is visible in the syringe, the medication can be injected. The needle and syringe are then removed. No more than 20 ml of solution should be given to mature horses in one IM site.

Intravenous Injections

When administering medication IV, the blood dilutes the medication, causing it to become less caustic. The jugular vein is the only appropriate vein for IV injections in horses. The jugular vein runs caudally along the jugular

FIG. 27-5 **A,** Needle insertion for intravenous administration of medication. **B,** Blood should drip, not spurt, from the needle hub when the jugular vein is occluded before an intravenous injection.

furrow from the head and then enters the thoracic inlet on its way to the heart. The carotid artery runs deep to the jugular vein in the same vicinity, but it courses deeper into the neck and is separated from the jugular vein in the more cranial portion of the neck. This is a very important point to remember. It is safer to attempt venipuncture and IV administration of medications in the cranial one third of the neck, because you are less likely to inadvertently enter the carotid artery when aiming for the jugular vein. If a large-bore needle is used (18 gauge) and the syringe is removed before venipuncture, it should be apparent which blood vessel has been entered. Blood drips out of the hub of an 18-gauge needle if it has been placed in the jugular vein but spurts out of the needle if it is within the high-pressure carotid artery. Smaller-bore needles (20 gauge or smaller) are suitable for obtaining blood samples; however, they do not allow differentiation between arterial or venous puncture, because in both cases blood drips from the needle. Medications inadvertently injected into the carotid artery pass directly to the brain and can cause severe seizures, collapse, and even death.

When administering drugs IV, the needle is inserted in the direction of the flow of blood in the jugular vein (pointed caudally, Fig. 27-5, *A*). Some people prefer to insert the needle pointed cranially. Regardless of which direction the needle is placed, it should be well seated into the vein so that there is little chance for perivascular or intraarterial injection. The vein is distended by occluding it with the thumb of one hand and then the needle is inserted into the vein. Blood should drip from the hub of the needle while the vein remains occluded (Fig. 27-5, *B*). The syringe is attached to the needle and the plunger is gently withdrawn to produce back flow of blood. The medication is then injected slowly.

Medication should not be quickly injected as a bolus, because this could cause an adverse reaction. If the medication is given slowly, administration can be halted if a reaction occurs. Even with good technique, movement of the horse during injection can drive the needle through the jugular vein and into the carotid artery. If the horse moves after connection of the syringe to the needle, the syringe should once again be removed from the needle to check the needle's position. If all is well, the injection can be continued. Remember that arterial blood and venous blood cannot be distinguished by color when withdrawn into a syringe filled with a drug. If multiple IV injections are required daily or if large volumes of fluid must be administered, placement of an indwelling catheter is advisable.

Adverse Reactions

Adverse reactions may occur to medications given by any route. In general, these reactions occur more rapidly with intravascular injections. Reactions can range from mild sweating, urticaria, and colic, to respiratory distress, collapse, and death. With any reaction, administration of the medication should be stopped immediately and, if time allows, the veterinarian should be contacted. Epinephrine 1:1000 (American Regent Laboratories) given SC or IM at 0.5 to 1 ml/100 lb of body weight, as well as dexamethasone (Azium Schering) given IV at 0.02 to 2 mg/kg, may be needed to stop an anaphylactic reaction and save the horse's life. It is always wise to know the appropriate dosage for these drugs and to have them within reach when medication is to be given. The horse's medical record should always be tagged to indicate medications to which the animal has previously reacted.

Intravenous Catheterization

Box 27-1 details the procedure for intravenous catheterization.

Sites. In adult horses, the jugular vein is preferred for catheter placement. Alternative sites include the lateral thoracic vein, cephalic vein, and, in extreme cases when there are no remaining accessible veins, saphenous vein. In foals and neonates, the cephalic vein is the preferred site, with the jugular vein as an alternate site.

Catheterizing veins in the hind legs of adult horses can be very dangerous and should only be attempted by experienced technicians or veterinarians. The principles of venous catheterization are similar, regardless of the site.

The lateral thoracic vein lies in the ventral one quarter of the thorax on either side. It is visible coursing along the side of the thorax and runs cranially toward the axilla. This vein can be catheterized from its mid to caudal section. The catheter is directed cranially so that it runs with the flow of the blood. It can be secured by suturing in the same manner as for a jugular catheter. The cephalic vein is entered proximal to the carpus and the catheter directed proximally. The saphenous vein is entered proximal to the hock and also directed proximally. It is advisable to wrap the catheter with sterile gauze sponges and an elastic bandage (e.g., Elastikon) when using one of these alternative sites for catheterization. If long-term catheterization is anticipated, it is best to use polyurethane or Silastic catheters.

Catheter Care. If the insertion site has not been bandaged, clean the insertion site gently with povidone-iodine solution and then apply an antibacterial ointment over the insertion site at least once daily or more often if needed. Catheters that have been bandaged should have the dressing changed as needed. Foals that spend much time lying down should always have the catheter site bandaged. Bandages covering cephalic catheters usually do not need changing until it is time for the catheter to be removed. Bandages over jugular vein catheters frequently need changing because the wrap becomes loose and allows bedding material to accumulate under it.

Stent bandages can be used instead of elastic bandages to protect the catheter site (Fig. 27-9). Four sutures are placed around the insertion site to form a rectangle that is smaller than the size of a gauze roll. These sutures are placed loosely so that a loop remains, through which a piece of umbilical tape can be placed. The umbilical tape is threaded through the sutures and then tied to keep a gauze roll in place over the catheter at its insertion site. The insertion site can be cleaned daily and a new gauze roll placed over the insertion site.

Teflon catheters can be left in the vein for 3 to 5 days if the insertion site is kept clean and there is no sign of swelling or thrombophlebitis. Silastic or polyurethane catheters can be left in the vein for up to 2 weeks if adequate care is used in preserving the catheter. This type of catheter is much less thrombogenic than the Teflon type and causes less irritation to the vein.[4] The injection plug and IV tubing should be changed every 24 hours, because bacteria may proliferate within the lines. The injection plug should be cleaned with an alcohol swab before administration of medication or fluids through the port. Sterile technique must always be used when handling IV catheters or giving IV infusions, because thrombophlebitis can result from bacterial contamination.

Box 27-1 Procedure for intravenous catheterization

Materials: (Fig. 27-6)

gauze sponges, povidone-iodine scrub, povidone-iodine solution, alcohol, water, razor, 2% lidocaine

for adults, 14- to 16-gauge, 140-mm Teflon catheter or 150-mm polyurethane catheter for the jugular vein

2-0 or 0 nonabsorbable suture, such as polypropylene (Fluorofil, Pittman-Moore)

injection plug

sterile latex gloves

heparinized saline (2500 units in 250 ml saline for adults; 1000 units in 250 ml saline for neonates)

T-port (Becton-Dickinson Vascular Access) (optional)

for foals, elastic tape (Elastikon, Johnson & Johnson), sterile gauze sponges and antibacterial ointment. For adults, similar to foal or stent bandage using stretch gauze roll bandage (Conform, Kendall) and umbilical tape.

Procedure:

1. Shave and aseptically prepare the site to be catheterized.

2. Inject 0.5 to 1 ml of lidocaine intradermally to block the skin.

3. Wearing sterile gloves, take the catheter from the package and place the end of the stylet at the appropriate site. Always insert the catheter with the direction of blood flow.

4. With a sharp and quick jab, insert the catheter through the skin and into the vein. Hold the catheter at about a 90-degree angle to the skin until the vein is penetrated (Fig. 27-7, *A*). Blood should flow freely into the hub if the vein is occluded (jugular) or flows freely without holding the vein off for the other sites. If the horse is severely dehydrated or hypovolemic, backflow of blood may not

occur. For the compromised patient, it may be helpful to have the catheter filled with heparinized saline so that once the vein is penetrated, the heparinized saline starts to flow retrograde out the hub of the catheter.

5. Once the vein has been entered, orient the catheter and stylet parallel to the vein and advance the catheter ½ inch for adults and ¼ inch for foals. This ensures that both the catheter and stylet are within the lumen of the vein.

6. Hold the stylet in place and slide the catheter down the stylet and into the vein (Fig. 27-7, *B*). This should be a smooth action; the catheter should easily slide down the stylet and not feel like it is sticking. Never advance the stylet into the catheter or pull the catheter onto the stylet once the catheter has been advanced, because this could sever the tip of the catheter off within the vein. If the catheter is not correctly placed with the lumen of the vein, simply remove the entire unit and try again. Always check the tip of the catheter to make sure it has not been damaged in the attempt, because this could damage the vein. A new catheter should be used if there is any chance that the original catheter was damaged or contaminated during the procedure.

7. Once the catheter is in place, remove the stylet and place a T-port with injection plug or just an injection plug over the end of the catheter (Fig. 27-7, *C*).

8. The catheter should be sutured in place using the grooves in the hub to mark the site for the first suture, then around the narrow portion of the injection plug or T-port. If a T-port is used, another suture should be placed over the "T" to secure it. In adults, it may be advantageous to also suture the arm of the T-port loosely to add stability without creating tension at the catheter insertion site (Fig. 27-8). The arm of the T-port should slide easily through the loose loop of suture as the horse changes its neck position.

9. Flush the catheter with 3 ml of heparinized saline.

Catheter Complications. Teflon catheters can kink, obstructing the flow of IV solutions. The smaller-gauge catheters used in foals (18 gauge) have been known to break off if the catheter is placed in an area where there is much mobility, such as the jugular vein. The catheter first bends and then develops a crease. As the foal continues to move its head, the catheter may become weaker at the kinked site and can eventually break. For this reason, the cephalic vein is a better site for IV catheter placement in newborn foals.

Catheter sites should be checked frequently to avoid major complications. Local reactions at the insertion site can occur at any time. The swelling may not involve the vein itself but only the skin and subcutaneous tis-

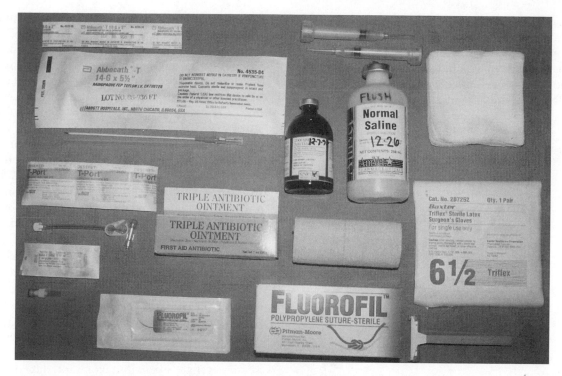

FIG. 27-6 Materials needed for intravenous catheterization.

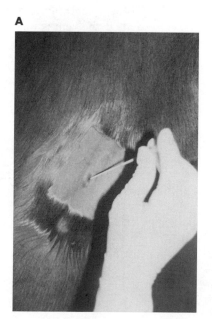
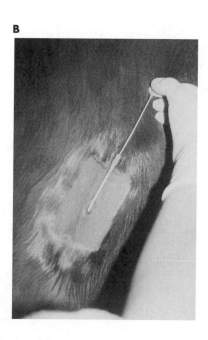
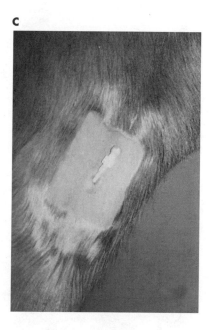

FIG. 27-7 A, Catheterization of the jugular vein. The catheter is placed at about a 90-degree angle to the vein, and the vein is entered with a sharp, quick jab. **B,** Once the vein has been entered, the catheter is oriented parallel to the vein and advanced about ½ inch to make sure the catheter and stylet are within the lumen. The catheter is then advanced while the stylet is held stationary. **C,** The stylet is removed once the catheter is in place and an injection plug is used to cap the catheter.

sues. This type of swelling may resolve with careful, gentle cleaning of the insertion site. If the swelling persists or progresses, the catheter should be removed and a new catheter inserted at a different site.

Thrombosis can develop secondary to irritation of the vessel walls, with subsequent release of thrombogenic

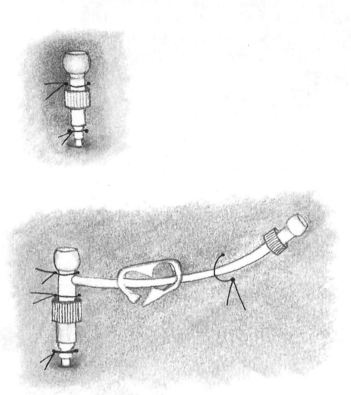

FIG. 27-8   Suture placement for the catheter, showing an injection plug *(top)* and T-port *(bottom)*.

factors that initiate the clotting cascade and platelet adherence. This occurs more frequently with severely compromised patients that may already be prone to coagulation disorders. Horses with endotoxemia, any type of gastrointestinal disorder, or gram-negative infections are at highest risk. A thrombosed vein appears corded and feels firm to the touch. It may not be painful if it is not infected. It is best to avoid use of the remaining patent jugular vein, because if the remaining jugular vein also develops thrombosis, venous return from the head is impaired, and the horse may develop severe swelling of the face and head. This may cause dyspnea (difficult breathing) and dysphagia (difficulty in eating). If jugular thrombosis develops, the horse should be fed from an elevated position to prevent dependent edema in the head. Softer feed is sometimes beneficial, such as soaked hay pellets and mashes. Thrombosed veins can be treated with application of warm compresses two or three times daily and application of dimethyl sulfoxide gel (Domoso Gel, Syntex).

Thrombophlebitis is inflammation of a vein. This can occur after administration of irritating substances, such as tetracycline, phenylbutazone, or dimethyl sulfoxide solution at concentrations greater than 10%. Thrombophlebitis can also result from bacterial colonization (infection) of the vein. This can lead to disastrous effects for the horse. The infected vein may be larger than normal size, corded, painful, and warm to the touch. The horse may resent having the vein manipulated. Ultrasound examination may show the vein to be hyperechoic, with or without fluid (blood) centrally. A hyperechoic core may also be present. If the vein is infected, an aspirate can be taken aseptically and cultured for bacterial growth. Alternatively, the catheter tip can be

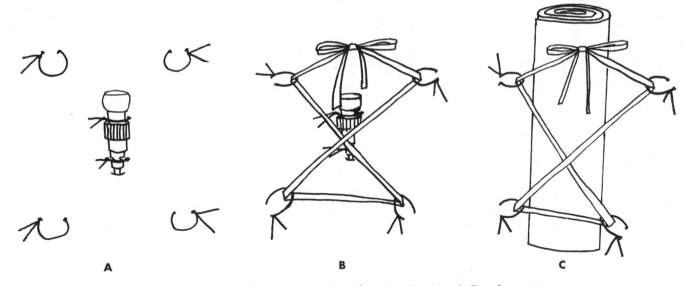

FIG. 27-9   Placement of a stent bandage to protect the catheter insertion site. **A,** Four loose sutures are placed around the insertion site. **B,** Umbilical tape is threaded through the sutures in cruciform pattern. **C,** A roll of gauze is placed over the catheter and held in place by the umbilical tape.

cultured immediately after catheter removal. Affected horses require appropriate systemic antibiotics, as well as local therapy of hot compresses.

Intravenous Infusions

Various intravenous infusions can be used to treat sick horses. Crystalloid fluids, such as lactated Ringer's solution or sodium chloride (saline), can be used to combat dehydration and hypovolemia. Colloid solutions, such as plasma or serum, can also be administered to animals requiring protein or antibody supplementation. Large volumes of fluids may be rapidly infused as a bolus in adult horses, but various fluid delivery systems are available to provide continuous fluid drip administration when needed. Care must be taken to change or remove the IV fluid bag when the fluids run out so that blood does not back up from the catheter into the IV line. If blood is allowed to fill the catheter, it may become clotted.

Commercial fluid delivery systems are available from International Win, Limited. Fluid bags can be hung from a swivel hook and line fixed at the top of the stall (Fig. 27-10). Alternatively, IV fluid administration lines and extension tubes can be attached to rubber tubing. The rubber tubing extends from the hook holding the IV fluids and is attached to the horse's halter on the same side as the catheter. The IV line is secured to the rubber tubing so that it forms loops as it travels down the rubber tubing (Fig. 27-11). This allows the horse to move freely

in the stall without pulling out the IV line. Horses must be attached so that they do not become entangled in the rubber tubing. If continuous fluid therapy is not necessary, the horse can be restrained in stocks and fluids given as a bolus infusion using a pressure bulb.

Foals require special consideration. Care must be taken not to overhydrate neonates. Special IV delivery pumps can be used to deliver fluids at the desired rate continuously. Administration systems with an in-line reservoir that holds up to 150 ml of fluid can prevent accidental delivery of excessive fluid volumes. Critically ill neonates are often hypothermic, so IV fluids should be warmed to body temperature before infusion. This can be done by heating the fluids in a bucket of warm water, or by microwaving the fluids (only if they are in plastic bags!). It is important to check the fluids to make sure they have not become too hot. Seriously compromised adult horses may also benefit from warm fluids, although this may not be practical.

Medication may be given through an injection port of the IV line if no other drugs have been added to the fluid bag. Various fluid additives are incompatible with certain medications and form a precipitate in the

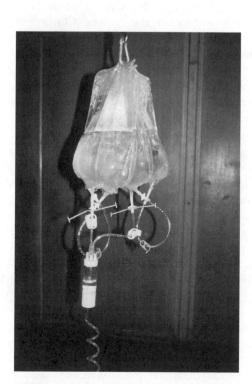

FIG. 27-10 Continuous intravenous infusion using a multiple-bag administration set.

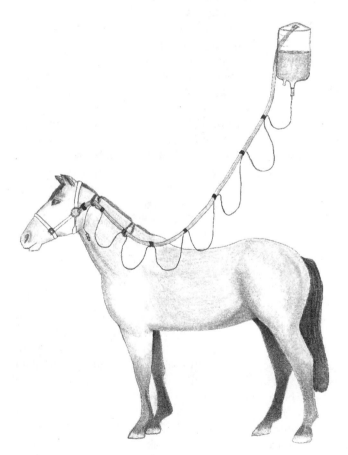

FIG. 27-11 Arrangement for continuous intravenous infusions that allows the horse to move freely in the stall.

IV line. If there is any doubt about the compatibility of the medication with the fluids, administration of the fluids should be stopped. The catheter is flushed with sterile saline and the medication is injected through the injection port. The catheter is flushed again with saline to clear the medication and fluid administration can be restarted.

The volume of saline needed to flush the catheter depends upon the catheter used; in general, 3 ml are sufficient to flush a catheter and T-port. If extension tubing is used, more flush solution may be required. If more than one type of medication is to be given, the catheter must be flushed with saline between injections of each medication. If fluids are not being infused, the final flush should be with heparinized saline to prevent clotting within the catheter. Catheters must be flushed with heparinized saline every 4 to 6 hours when fluids are not being given. Medications should not be given in IV lines delivering plasma, blood products, or parenteral nutrition.

Horses with protein-losing gastroenteropathies, such as gastric ulcers, colitis, or right dorsal colon ulcers, may require IV plasma therapy. Plasma provides for volume expansion and much-needed protein. Foals with failure of passive transfer of maternal antibodies may also require IV plasma administration to obtain protective antibodies that were not absorbed from the mare's colostrum. Plasma can be harvested directly from an appropriate donor previously screened for compatibility, or more conveniently obtained from commercial sources. Plasma is also available from donors hyperimmunized against *Rhodococcus equi, Salmonella, Clostridium botulinum,* and the J-5 endotoxin. This plasma contains antibodies directed against specific bacterial or the toxins produced by the bacteria.

Plasma is stored frozen and requires thawing in warm water, *not* in the microwave. This should be done as quickly as possible without overheating the plasma and denaturing the protein. Water that is warm to the touch, but not hot, should be added frequently to facilitate thawing. Special IV administration sets that contain a filter to catch any fibrin clots are necessary when administering plasma or blood products. Some serum products that can be stored in the refrigerator instead of the freezer are also available in concentrated form. These also require warming to body temperature.

Whole-blood transfusions may be needed in cases of severe blood loss or with such conditions as neonatal isoerythrolysis. Blood transfusions should be considered when the hematocrit falls below 12% to 15%. Horses that become anemic or lose blood gradually over a longer period can tolerate relatively lower hematocrits. If a neonate or adult rapidly loses blood to a hematocrit of 15% or less, arrangements should be made to obtain fresh, whole blood. This should be harvested from a donor that has previously been screened for compatibility or, in an emergency, from a gelding that has not received any blood or plasma transfusions. Foals with neonatal isoerythrolysis may be transfused with the dam's red blood cells after they have been separated from the plasma and washed with saline to remove the mare's antibodies that are responsible for lysis of the foal's red blood cells. The mare's washed red blood cells must then be resuspended in saline to a packed cell volume of 50% before administration.[3]

Plasma, serum, and blood should be infused slowly, giving 1 L/hr, if possible, to reduce the chance of an adverse reaction. Plasma or blood is administered very slowly at first to observe for reactions. The speed of the drip can be increased to the desired rate if the horse or foal tolerates it well. Rapid administration may be necessary if the horse is hemorrhaging. Adverse reactions range from mild tachypnea (rapid breathing), shivering, hives, or fever, to severe respiratory distress, colic, hypotension, collapse, and death.

MEDICATION OF THE EYE

Topical ointments or solutions can be applied directly to the eye. Once the horse is adequately restrained, the eye is gently pried open with clean fingers, being careful to touch only the outer lids. The medication is applied into the lower conjunctival sac. Care must be taken not to scratch the surface of the cornea. Ointments can be applied by placing a small bead of ointment in the lower conjunctival sac. Ophthalmic drops can be placed in the lower conjunctival sac using the plastic dispenser vial provided or using a sterile tuberculin syringe (no needle!) if the solution is to be used on multiple horses.

Severe corneal ulcers may require topical treatments as often as every 1 to 2 hours. For horses that become head shy and resentful with this frequent treatment schedule, alternative medication delivery systems can be used. Lavage systems can be placed in the upper eyelid (subpalpebral) or inserted into the tear duct (nasolacrimal). Liquid medications can be delivered easily through either of these systems. Severe corneal ulcers and some other abnormalities may require extra protection for the eye. A protective eye cup (Eye-Saver, Jorvet) can be used to protect the eye and keep the horse from dislodging the lavage system. The black plastic cup also protects the eye from direct sunlight that could cause pain. This may be very important, because many corneal ulcers require treatment with atropine to inhibit ciliary spasm. This makes the horse unable to constrict the pupil when exposed to direct sunlight. Netted fly masks can also be used to provide some protection for the eyes. Horses that spend a lot of time lying down may accumulate shavings or bedding in the eyes. Eye cups or netted fly masks can be used to help keep the shavings out.

BANDAGING

Materials needed to bandage the distal limbs include cotton quilts or sheet cottons (three), and track wraps, brown roll gauze, or Elastikon. Leg wraps can be used to protect a wound, to give additional support, or to apply medication. The wrap should be applied with even pressure so that the tendons running along the caudal aspect of the leg (superficial and deep digital flexor tendons) are protected and pressure is evenly applied over the entire length of the tendons.

To start, a quilt or some other thick padding is wrapped around the leg. Sheet cotton can be used; at least three sheets are needed for sufficient padding. Start the wrap at the front portion of the leg and then bring the quilt across the outside of the leg, around the back and then inside of the leg, maintaining even tension at all times (Fig. 27-12, A and B). Once the quilt is in place, a track wrap brown gauze roll or other type of outer wrap is used. The same principle is followed, with the wrap being placed from lateral toward medial across the

back of the leg. It is best to start this part of the wrap near the bottom of the leg (distally) and work up (proximally) (Fig. 27-12, C, D, and E).

The outer wrap is secured with Velcro attachments or adhesive tape. If adhesive tape is used, the ends should not overlap, because the tape is relatively inelastic and may produce uneven pressure across the tendons. If roll gauze is used, this can be secured with adhesive tape; alternatively, an additional layer can be applied using Elastikon or Vetwrap (3M Animal Products). When the wrap is finished, a small strip of padding should be visible in the innermost layer of the wrap both proximally and distally. Care must be taken to make sure that the wrap is snug but not too tight. Two fingers should be able to fit snugly between the leg and the wrap, but the wrap should feel firm and should not slip down the leg. If the wrap is applied to protect a wound, antibacterial ointment and a nonstick dressing must first be applied to the area and held in place with a layer of stretch gauze.

If the full length of the leg must be wrapped, an additional wrap can be applied so that it overlaps the lower limb wrap to some extent. This additional wrap is applied in a similar manner. The proximal wrap should overlap the distal wrap and extend to the mid-radius area. Often, a piece of the wrap is cut out over the accessory carpal bone to prevent development of pres-

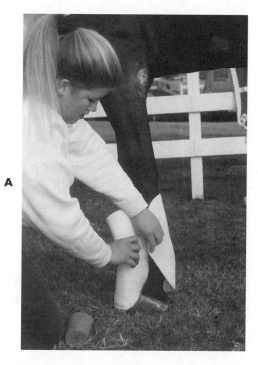 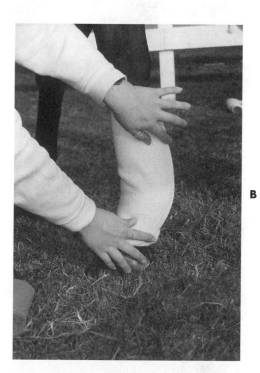

FIG. 27-12 A through E, Application of a wrap to the distal limb of a standing horse.

Continued.

sure sores over this bone. This is more difficult to do on the hind leg, because special consideration must be given to the highly movable hock joint. Often the Elastikon or Vetwrap is applied in a figure-8 around the hock so that only the sheet cotton contacts the point of the hock.

Foot Wraps

There are many different ways to wrap feet. The foot is first picked clean and then washed and dried if needed. If the foot requires medication, this can be applied and then covered with a gauze sponge secured with a layer of rolled gauze (Fig. 27-13, *A*, *B*, and *C*).

C
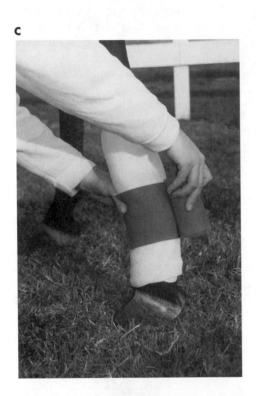

E
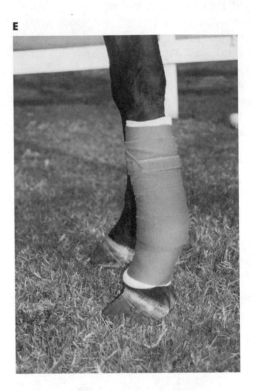

FIG. 27-12, CONT'D A through E, Application of a wrap to the distal limb of a standing horse.

D
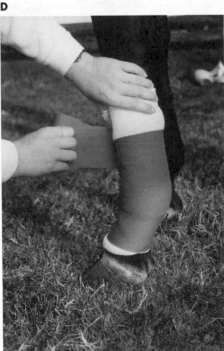

If padding is needed for protection, roll cotton or two to three sheets of cotton are used to wrap around the foot (Fig. 27-13, *D* and *E*). Next, rolled brown gauze or stretch gauze can be used to secure the sheet cotton. This is applied in figure-8 fashion to make the sheet cottons lie flat across the bottom of the foot (Fig. 27-13, *F, G,* and *H*). Finally, elastic tape, such as Elastikon or Vetwrap, or duct tape is applied to provide additional support and protection, and secure the bandage in place (Fig. 27-13, *I* and *J*). It is very important to have the ground surface of the foot wrap flat, rather than convex and bulging, so that even pressure is applied to the bottom of the foot. If no padding is

needed and the foot wrap is being used to apply medication to an area of the foot, the duct tape or Elastikon can be applied directly to the foot after a dressing, such as a Telfa pad (Kendall) or gauze sponge, is placed over the medication.

Be careful not to wrap up over the coronary band if no protective padding is in place, because excessive pressure directly on the coronary band can reduce circulation to hoof tissues and cause damage or sloughing of the hoof. If there is any question about the amount of pressure on the coronary band, one or more vertical slits can be cut in the bandage where it covers the coronary band to relieve pressure.

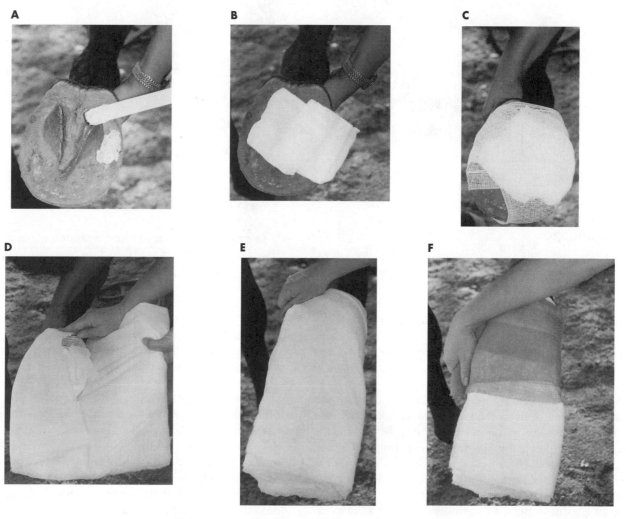

FIG. 27-13   A through **J,** Application of a foot wrap.

Continued.

G

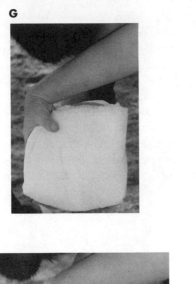

H

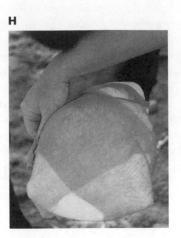

I

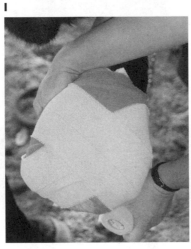

J

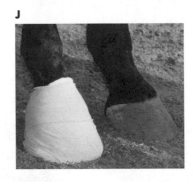

FIG. 27-13, CONT'D A through J, Application of a foot wrap.

Tail Bandages

Tail wraps can consist of Vetwrap, rolled brown gauze, or even commercial tail bags. It is important that the wrap not extend proximally to include the tail bones (coccygeal vertebrae), because the tail has little muscular padding and a tight wrap can occlude blood circulation to the tail and create a tissue slough or even loss of the entire tail. If it is necessary to wrap more proximally on the tail, a nonconstricting wrap should be loosely applied and changed daily.

At times it is necessary to wrap the tail of a horse with severe diarrhea to keep the tail clean. This can be done using a plastic rectal sleeve. Holes can be cut in the sleeve to help keep the tail from "sweating." The tail hair should first be braided and the sleeve can be tied at the most proximal part of the braid, or the sleeve can be anchored to the most proximal part of the tail with a strip of Elastikon placed lengthwise from the sleeve cranially along the midline of the back.

The tail may also need to be wrapped when a mare is about to foal or for a reproductive examination. Rolled brown gauze is applied, starting at the tail head (proximal area) and working distally, being sure to incorporate all of the tail hairs within the wrap. When the wrap reaches just distal to the last tail bone, the remaining tail hairs can be folded and incorporated within this section of the wrap. The brown gauze is then tied to itself to end and secure the wrap.

Abdominal Bandages

It may be necessary to wrap a horse's abdomen to protect a wound or an abdominal incision following colic surgery. A sterile nonstick pad is placed over the wound. Next, a dressing made from large folded sheet cotton can be placed against the sterile dressing. Elastikon is wrapped around the abdomen and over the back to hold the bandage in place. It may be necessary to use four to six rolls of Elastikon when applying a full abdominal bandage.

Padding in the form of leg rolls or quilts should be used across the horse's back to protect the skin if the backbone is prominent. Because pressure is applied with the wrap, skin necrosis can occur in this area if there is little muscle or fat across the back. The same application principles are used as for leg wraps. The Elastikon is applied evenly, starting at the cranial part of the abdomen and working caudally. The Elastikon is applied snugly to provide support, but not too tight. Each layer of Elastikon should overlap the last pass until the wrap is completed. This type of wrap is very expensive and usually does not need changing unless there is excessive drainage, or if the wound or incision must be evaluated. Thoracic wraps can be applied in a similar manner to cover a thoracic wound or protect a thoracic drain.

Chapter 23 contains detailed information on wound management and bandaging.

MONITORING PATIENTS

Hospitalized patients must be monitored regularly for changes in their condition. Horses only slightly ill can develop more severe and even life-threatening illness while receiving treatment. For instance, a horse receiving antibiotic therapy for a mild respiratory infection can develop life-threatening diarrhea from changes in bowel microflora. A horse receiving nonsteroidal antiinflammatory drugs for an orthopedic problem can develop gastrointestinal ulceration or renal dysfunction secondary to the antiinflammatory medication, particularly if the animal is not eating and drinking normally.

The heart rate, respiratory rate, rectal temperature, mucous membrane color, capillary refill time, attitude, digital pulses, urine and fecal output, gastrointestinal motility, and appetite should all be monitored at least once or twice daily. Critically ill neonates require more frequent monitoring, sometimes as often as every 2 hours, as their condition can deteriorate rapidly. Adult horses should be weighed at admission with a walk-on scale, if available, or else a weight tape can be used to estimate the horse's weight. Neonates should be weighed at admission and then daily. Most newborn foals can be weighed by picking them up and weighing the handler and foal together on a conventional scale and then subtracting the handler's weight. This may not be feasible with larger foals.

CARE OF RECUMBENT HORSES

Nursing care for recumbent animals must be meticulous. Caring for a horse that is unable to rise is tedious and often unrewarding. Horses that remain recumbent for prolonged periods eventually develop various complications, regardless of the primary disease. Because of the weight of the animal, several people are needed to frequently turn the animal from one side to the other. This is usually done with long ropes looped, not tied, around the pasterns so that the handlers can stand farther from the limbs of the horse, or by using a winch and harness, when available. When a horse is turned from one side to another, the animal often kicks, which can be very dangerous for anyone standing in the vicinity. No one should stand within striking range of the limbs of a recumbent horse. The animal must be turned as frequently as possible to prevent development of decubital ulcers on the skin and edema and congestion in the dependent portion of the lung. Helmets can be applied to horses that tend to flail about and hit their head against the wall or ground. Often the corneas become ulcerated when the animal rubs its eyes on the ground.

The primary disease must be resolved as quickly as possible so that the animal may once again stand. If the horse can stand but only with assistance, the hind limbs can be supported by suspending a rope attached to the tail from a ceiling beam. The head may also need to be supported. Commercial slings are available that provide support for horses that have some ability to support themselves but require additional help. A sling cannot be used for horses with flaccid paralysis or other conditions that make them unable to support themselves at all, because they can only slump down in the sling. Slings must be well padded to prevent development of pressure sores.

Regardless of how meticulous the nursing care, decubital ulcers (pressure sores) may develop over bony prominences, such as the tuber coxae, carpus, hock, shoulder joint, or elbow. These must be cleaned with a mild antibacterial soap. Topical antibacterial powders or sprays can also be used. A spray that creates a "breathable" bandage, such as AluSpray (Immuno Vet), may provide the best protection. Any bony protuberance that can be protected by wraps should be wrapped.

The recumbent animal may not eat or drink well. Soft, highly palatable feeds should be offered. If mashes are offered but not eaten, they must be replaced frequently to ensure palatability. Fresh, clean water should be offered to the recumbent animal every 2 hours, if possible. Feed and water may have to be given by nasogastric tube. This must be done carefully, because the animal may aspirate feed or water into the lungs when in lateral recumbency. If possible, it is preferable to feed the horse while it is in a more sternal position. Infusion of IV fluids may be required in more debilitated or dehydrated animals. It is important to keep the animal clean and dry. Frequent cleaning can help to prevent urine scalding and reduce the severity of decubital ulcers.

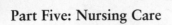

REFERENCES

1. Cohen ND et al: Medical management of right dorsal colitis in 5 horses: a retrospective study (1987-1993), *J Vet Intern Med* 9:272-276, 1995.
2. Getty R: *Sisson and Grossman's, the anatomy of the domestic animals,* ed 5, Philadelphia, 1975, WB Saunders.
3. Madigan JE: *Manual of equine neonatal medicine,* ed 2, Woodland, Calif, 1991, Live Oak Publishing.
4. Spurlock SL et al: Long-term jugular vein catheterization in horses, *J Am Vet Med Assoc* 196:425-430, 1990.

Nursing Care of Food Animals, Camelids, and Ratites

L.R. Krcatovich
S.M. Wing-Proctor
S. Mobini
M.E. Gemus
M. Levy
J.T. Blackford

Learning Objectives

After reviewing this chapter, the reader should understand the following:

Methods of sample collection for laboratory analysis
Routes of administration of medication in cattle, sheep, goats, pigs, and ratites

Procedure for intravenous catheterization
Techniques used in general nursing care of food animals and ratites
Procedures used in grooming and foot care
Procedures used in caring for ratites

CARE OF CATTLE

L.R. KRCATOVICH

INTRAVENOUS INJECTIONS

The veins most often used for IV injections in cattle are the jugular veins, coccygeal (tail) vein, and subcutaneous abdominal (milk) veins. The jugular veins are most often used for large-volume IV injections and blood collection. In addition to their accessibility, there is less chance of being kicked when using these veins. The jugular vein is always used for IV injections in calves because it is the largest accessible vessel.

The coccygeal (tail) vein is used for IV injection of small volumes (3 to 5 ml) of drugs and blood sample collection. Although most cows are more tolerant of tail venipuncture than jugular injections, there is a greater chance of being kicked. This can be minimized with proper restraint.

The subcutaneous abdominal vein, also called the "mammary" or "milk" vein, is used mainly when the jugular veins are thrombosed (occluded) or cannot be located. There are several disadvantages to milk vein injections. The technician has an increased risk of being kicked. A second person may be required to provide additional restraint. The milk vein rolls easily under the skin, making it hard to puncture the vein and thread the needle. Finally, hematomas are easily formed and may result in thrombosis of the vein.

Preparation for venipuncture is similar for all three veins. A disinfectant, such as 70% alcohol, should be applied to the injection site to remove gross contamination, provide antibacterial activity, and increase visibility of the vein. Venipunctures should not be made through dirt or fecal material, as phlebitis, septicemia, and/or contamination of medication and samples may result.

Jugular Venipuncture

Restraint. Good restraint is necessary when attempting any venipuncture. Ideally, the animal should be restrained in a head gate or stanchion. Injecting medication into the jugular vein of an animal that is not properly restrained is difficult and dangerous. Therefore, never attempt venipuncture on a free, moving large animal. A halter should be applied and the head raised and pulled to one side. A quick-release knot should be used when tying an animal to a stationary object. If the animal should fall during infusion of medication, the head can be released immediately to prevent injury to the animal. If a recumbent cow must be treated, its head can be secured by tying the free end of the halter back above the hock with a quick-release knot. Tying the head to one side secures it, making the vein accessible, but it may also make it more difficult to distend the vein.

A standing calf may be restrained by pulling it close to your body, immobilizing its head. Older calves can be restrained like adult cattle, but application of nose tongs is usually not necessary. A recumbent calf should have its head firmly held with the neck extended. If the calf moves excessively, a second person should aid in restraint.

Materials. All required materials should be assembled before attempting venipuncture. The needle selected for IV injection of large volumes of fluids varies according to personal preference and the flow rate desired. A 12- to 14-gauge, 2- to 3-inch needle is best for giving large volumes to adult cattle. Needles less than 2 inches long should not be used. A correctly threaded 3-inch needle is not likely to slip from the vein if the cow thrashes around, decreasing the chances of perivascular infiltration of irritants and hypertonic solutions. For injections of small volumes into the jugular vein, use of a 16-, 18-, or 20-gauge, 1.5-inch needle is recommended for cows and calves. These small-gauge, disposable needles are easier to insert than the reusable, large-bore needles, because disposable are used only once and are very sharp, whereas reusable needles tend to become dull.

A rubber IV line, referred to as a *simplex,* is used for IV infusions. A syringe may also be used to inject medication. Its size depends on the volume of medication to be injected.

Technique. One should never kneel or stand directly in front of the animal during jugular venipuncture. To distend the jugular vein, apply pressure at the jugular furrow, about two thirds of the way caudad on (down) the neck. Allow time for the vein to fill. Briskly stroking the vein with a finger in a downward motion (toward the heart) helps raise it for easy visualization. Unless the animal is in shock or is severely dehydrated, jugular venipuncture should not be attempted without sufficiently raising the vein. Although the jugular vein is quite large when raised, it is easily missed by the inexperienced technician.

Bovine skin is thick and difficult to penetrate with a large-gauge needle; therefore, the needle must be inserted with considerable force. Grasp the needle by the hub, using the thumb and first knuckle of the forefinger (Fig. 28-1). Warn the cow of the impending needle insertion by repeated taps on the neck, near but not over the injection site, using the back of the hand holding the needle. These warning strokes may upset the animal more than the insertion of the needle. Gradually increasing the intensity of the strokes often prevents this. After two or three warning strokes, flip the hand over and thrust the needle through the skin at a 45- to 90-degree angle to the vessel, with the needle directed toward the heart. Keeping the jugular vein occluded to observe for blood flow from the needle, indicating proper placement.

If the vein was entered on the initial attempt and a steady flow of blood exits the needle, lay the needle parallel to the skin and advance it further caudad into the vein. The needle may be directed toward the head for administration of small volumes, but larger volumes should be given with the needle directed toward the heart. If the needle slips out of the vein during insertion, retract it until blood steadily flows from it; then attempt to rethread it.

Occasionally, the needle does not enter the vein, but only penetrates the skin. When this occurs, relocate the vein and thrust the needle into it without withdrawing it from the skin. Redirection of the needle may be necessary to find the vein. Once a steady flow of blood is present, the needle should be threaded to its hub. If the needle has been inserted too deeply and has penetrated entirely through the vessel, pull the needle back slowly until the blood flows freely from the hub; at this point the needle can be threaded. Apposition of the bevel of the needle against the vessel wall may also occlude it. This may be corrected by slightly rotating the needle. Care must be

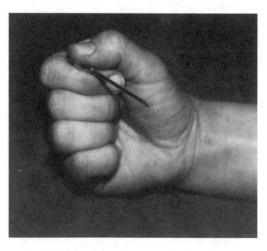

FIG. 28-1 Correct positioning of the needle for jugular venipuncture.

taken when redirecting the needle to prevent laceration of the vein and consequent hematoma formation.

Small-gauge, disposable hypodermic needles may be inserted as are large-bore needles. However, it is not necessary to use as much force to insert these needles or to strike the animal before insertion, because they are very sharp and easily penetrate the skin. The needle is introduced into the vein at a 30- to 45-degree angle, with or without a syringe attached. The needle may be correctly positioned by attaching a syringe and aspirating blood.

When the needle is correctly threaded, the syringe or simplex is attached. Aspirate (slightly withdraw the syringe barrel) and then inject the medication. If a bottle is used, it should be held in an inverted position. A steady bubbling in the bottle indicates that the medication is flowing into the vein and is being replaced by air in the bottle. If the bubbling becomes irregular or stops, the needle may be occluded or out of the vein. In such cases, lower the bottle, check the needle for correct positioning, and make the appropriate adjustments. When the inverted bottle is lowered, blood flows into the IV line. This can be used to check correct positioning of the needle.

Whether using a simplex or a syringe to administer fluid, observe the jugular furrow for gradual swelling around the needle. This may indicate that medication is flowing into the perivascular space (outside the vein). Correct the needle's position and continue. After IV injection is complete, remove the needle and apply digital (finger) pressure for 15 to 20 seconds over the venipuncture site to prevent a hematoma.

Coccygeal Venipuncture

For smaller volumes of medication, the coccygeal (tail) vein is often used rather than the jugular vein. Cattle usually become less agitated when the tail is used for venipuncture. This method also usually requires less restraint than when the jugular vein is used.

Restraint. Limited restraint is needed for coccygeal venipuncture. Dairy cattle require a halter or stanchion and a "tail jack" (see chapter 17). Beef cattle generally are more fractious and may require restraint in a chute. A tail jack must be used for coccygeal venipuncture, because it is impossible if the tail is not held in a vertical position. Holding the tail in this manner also simultaneously serves as restraint.

Materials. An 18- or 20-gauge, 1.5-inch needle attached to a 3-, 5- or 10-ml syringe is appropriate for coccygeal venipuncture. A needle larger than 18 gauge is too large for the coccygeal vein. A 20-gauge needle is most commonly used.

Technique. The first three coccygeal vertebrae (near the tail base) are the best sites for the coccygeal venipuncture. To locate the correct site, apply a tail jack and clean the ventral surface of the tail to remove gross contamination (Fig. 28-2). Palpate the tail for the bony

protrusions (hemal arches) of the vertebrae while gently aspirating, directly on the midline at a 45-degree angle to the tail. If the blood is not withdrawn into the syringe, check the needle for the correct angle and position. It may be necessary to advance or retreat the needle to locate the vein. Remove the needle and redirect it if necessary. Inject the medication when the needle is correctly positioned. Periodically aspirate blood into the syringe and reinject this to clear the needle of residual medication. Either the coccygeal artery or vein may be used for injection. After the injection is completed, remove the needle, lower the tail, and apply digital pressure for 10 to 15 seconds. Hematoma formation is usually not a problem, although digital pressure should be applied if the artery was punctured.

Subcutaneous Abdominal Venipuncture

The milk veins are used when the jugular veins cannot be raised or are inaccessible for other reasons. These veins should be used for administration of large volumes of medication only. It is too dangerous to obtain routine blood samples from them.

Restraint. The animal should be tied securely or restrained in a stanchion. Stand close to the cow's flank, facing the same direction as the cow. One should not face the cow's rear, as the cow may kick.

Materials. A 14-gauge, 2- to 3-inch needle is used for venipuncture. A syringe may be used to inject medication; however, a simplex system is frequently used. Because blood flows slowly in this vein, administration through a simplex may require more time than anticipated.

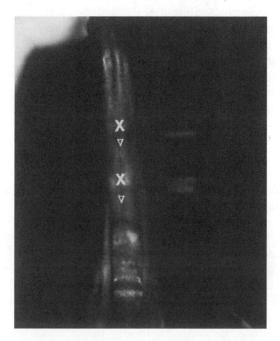

FIG. 28-2 Location of the hemal arches *(X)* and venipuncture sites *(arrowheads)* on the ventral aspect of the bovine tail.

Technique. It is not necessary to occlude the milk vein before puncturing it, because it is normally distended. The preferred venipuncture site is immediately caudal to the point where the vessel enters the abdomen; this section of the vein is the most stable. As with jugular venipuncture, it takes some force to introduce the needle through the skin. The needle should be inserted caudad and threaded into the vein. If blood does not flow freely from the needle, check the position of the needle and redirect it. Exercise caution when redirecting the needle, for it is easy to create hematomas in this area. Observe the area for perivascular infiltration during administration. When the injection has been completed, remove the needle and apply digital pressure for several minutes. Even with digital pressure, hematomas form easily.

INTRAVENOUS CATHETERIZATION

Intravenous catheterization is used primarily for prolonged fluid therapy, but it is also used for administration of injectable anesthetics or repeated IV injections. The jugular vein is most often chosen for IV catheterization in cattle. The caudal auricular vein can be catheterized in cattle, although this vein is used mainly for injection of small volumes of medication. It is difficult to secure a catheter in the ear vein for an extended period because of its location.

Restraint. Restraint required for IV catheterization is identical to that described for IV injection. Restraint needed for catheterizing the auricular vein involves securing the head and possibly use of nose tongs. It may help to cover the animal's eyes with a towel.

Materials. A 10- to 14-gauge catheter is used for adult cattle. Calves require a smaller-gauge catheter (14, 15, or 18 gauge).

To catheterize the ear vein of cattle, one can use an 18- to 20-gauge, 1.5- to 2-inch over-the-needle catheter. On large bulls, a 14-gauge, 2-inch catheter may be used if the ear vein is large enough.

Technique. The site should be clipped and surgically scrubbed. Local anesthesia is not required. An antiseptic is applied to complete skin preparation. Because of the skin's thickness, attempts to introduce a catheter through it may bend the catheter or damage the tip. To help introduce a catheter, a disposable needle of the same gauge is used to puncture the skin. This enables the catheter to pass through the skin with ease. A No. 15 surgical blade can be used for this purpose also.

For catheterization of the auricular vein, a local anesthetic is useful to decrease ear movement. Skin glue or a suture can be used to secure the catheter. The catheter site should be bandaged. To give the ear some stability, insert a 4-inch roll of gauze into the ear before bandaging the ear.

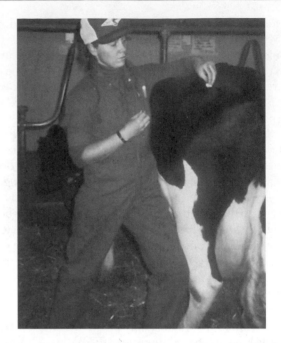

FIG. 28-3 Correct position for IM injection into the gluteal muscle mass on the cow's opposite side.

INTRAMUSCULAR INJECTIONS

Intramuscular (IM) injections are commonly used in cattle. Several large muscle masses are available, including the gluteals, semimembranosus, semitendinosus, and lateral cervical muscles. The gluteals are located on the dorsal aspect of the rear legs (Fig. 28-3). The semimembranosus and semitendinosus are located in the rear limbs, between the stifle joint and ischium. The lateral cervical muscles are cranial to the scapula, dorsal to the cervical vertebrae, and ventral to the ligamentum nuchae.

The needle selected for IM injection depends on the viscosity (thickness) of the medication to be administered and the size of the muscle mass selected. A 16-, 18- or 20-gauge, 1.5-inch needle is commonly used for adults. A smaller-gauge needle is used for calves (18, 20, or 22 gauge).

SUBCUTANEOUS INJECTIONS

Subcutaneous (SC) injections are given anywhere loose skin can be raised with one's fingers. In cattle this is easily done on the lateral aspect of the neck and thorax, the axillary region, the fold of the flank, and the brisket.

Restraint. Subcutaneous injections generally require minimal restraint. Calves can be cornered in a small area. Adult cattle should have a halter applied to be placed in a headgate or stanchion. Aggressive animals may require a chute.

Materials. An 18-, 20-, or 22-gauge, 1.5-inch needle is used for SC injections in calves. A 14-, 16-, or 18-gauge, 1.5-inch needle is used for cattle. The needle size selected depends on the viscosity of the drug and thickness of the skin. A syringe is used to inject small quantities. A simplex system may be used to administer larger quantities.

Technique. The site should be cleaned with an antiseptic, such as 70% alcohol. Pinch the skin and raise it to form a "tent," taking care not to penetrate the other side with the needle. After the needle is positioned, aspirate. If blood is not observed upon aspiration, inject the medication. If there is blood present in the needle, withdraw the needle and attempt the injection at a new site. When the injection is completed, withdraw the needle, release the skin fold, and massage the area to enhance spread of the medication and increase its absorption rate.

The volume of medication injected at each SC site varies according to personal preference and the animal's size. For cattle, 50 to 100 ml per site is the recommended maximum, although up to 250 ml may be given SC. When giving large volumes, intermittently direct the needle to prevent depositing large quantities in one site. The amount that can be injected at each SC site for calves varies from 2 to 30 ml, with a maximum volume of 50 ml.

INTRADERMAL INJECTIONS

Intradermal (ID) injection is directed into the dermis, the skin layer underlying the most superficial epidermis. Intradermal injections are used mainly to aid in diagnosis of certain diseases. Cattle are tested for tuberculosis using ID injection of bovine tuberculin. Intradermal injections are also used for allergy testing, a procedure usually limited to companion animals. Local anesthetics are injected ID to anesthetize sites for surgery or other invasive procedures.

The caudal tail fold is the site used most often for ID injections of tuberculin. They may also be given on the lateral aspect of the neck and abdomen.

Restraint. The restraint required depends on the site chosen, the number of injections to be given, and the animal's temperament. Most animals require minimal restraint. The sites must be free of hair before ID injection is attempted. If a diagnostic test is to be performed, the site should not be cleaned with antiseptics, because they might create a skin reaction and interfere with test results. Usually removal of dirt and feces is all that is required for preparation. Antiseptics can be applied to the site if local anesthetics are being deposited before surgery.

Materials. Cattle require a large needle, such as a 20- to 22-gauge, 1.5-inch needle, because of their thick skin. A tuberculin or 3-ml syringe is adequate for injecting small volumes ID.

Technique. The needle, with the syringe attached, is placed parallel to the skin. The free hand is used to pinch the skin. This pulls the skin taut and helps stabilize it. With the bevel directed up, gently insert the needle into the dermis of the skin. Aspirate if the injection is for local anesthesia over a vessel. A bleb should be visualized as the drug is deposited. If a bleb does not form, the needle is too deep; retract it a small distance and inject the drug. It is not necessary to massage the site, because the goal is to keep the drug localized.

INTRAMAMMARY INFUSION

Veterinarians and dairy farmers often employ intramammary infusions to treat mastitis or to infuse udder quarters when cows are dry (not lactating). The best time to infuse the udder is after the last milking of the day, which allows the medication to remain in the udder overnight. The udder should not be infused before milking because the beneficial effect of the medication would be lost. Because intramammary antibiotic therapy affects the results of milk culture, milk samples from mastitic quarters must be obtained before treatment.

Restraint. Minimal restraint is required for intramammary infusion. Tail restraint may be necessary for fractious cows. Care must be taken with beef cows, especially if they have been separated from their calves, because they are usually very aggressive.

Technique. Crouch beside the udder to work; never sit down or kneel. This makes it easier to avoid injury from kicking. Thoroughly clean the udder before treatment, using warm water and antiseptic soap. Use a separate cloth or paper towel to wash each teat so as to decrease the spread of microorganisms among the quarters. Dry each teat with a separate towel to remove contaminated water droplets. Wipe the teat orifice with an alcohol swab and allow to air dry. If all four quarters are to be infused, swab the far teats before swabbing the near ones, so as to prevent contamination when reaching past the near teats.

Empty the quarter by manually "stripping" out the milk before infusing medication, because residual milk mixes with the medication and dilutes it. Collect the discarded milk in a bucket to prevent contamination of the environment by the bacteria in the milk. After the teat is prepared, grasp it near the base and insert a teat cannula or sterile, disposable mammary infusion cannula into the teat orifice. More commonly, commercially prepared, disposable syringes with an attached cannula are used. Advance the cannula just through the teat sphincter a short distance and inject the medication slowly. Do not insert the cannula to the hub, because this predisposes to mastitis. As little as 10 to 20 ml or as much as 250 ml may be infused into a quarter. Remove the cannula and massage the teat and quarter to disseminate the medication. When the procedure is completed, dip the teat in teat dip to prevent invasion of microbes. If the weather is extremely cold (0° C or less), do not let the cow outside until the udder is dry, so as to prevent chapping and frostbite. Mark the cows that were treated so that their milk can be discarded.

INTRANASAL INSUFFLATION

The intranasal route is the most commonly used to administer vaccines and local anesthetics. As of this writing, intranasal vaccines have been approved only for infectious bovine rhinotracheitis (IBR) and parainfluenza-3 (PI$_3$) infection. Vaccines not designed for intranasal use are not effective when given by this route.

Intranasal anesthetics may be given before potentially painful procedures on the nasal cavity, such as nasogastric intubation, bronchoalveolar lavage, and endoscopy.

Restraint of the head is a necessity. Calves may be manually restrained, whereas adults should be secured with a halter and headgate.

Nasal secretions should be wiped from the nostril with moist cotton before medication administration. A 3- to 5-ml syringe is filled with the vaccine or local anesthetic, with a disposable, blunt tip attached to inject the drug, although the syringe alone may be used. Facing the same direction as the animal, place one hand over the animal's head, pulling it close to your body. The head must be slightly elevated to prevent the medication from running out of the nostril. The free hand is used to insert the syringe into the nostril. When the injection is completed, elevate the head for 10 to 15 seconds before releasing it.

INTRAUTERINE MEDICATION

Medication is placed in the uterus to locally treat metritis. Although this technique may be performed by veterinary technicians, they are not routinely instructed in this procedure. It is up to the veterinarian as to whether technicians should perform this procedure.

Uterine medication is available as boluses, capsules, and solutions. The form of the drug used depends on the condition of the uterus, stage of the reproductive cycle, types of drugs available, and personal preference.

Cows require minimal restraint for this procedure. The tail should be secured away from the perianal region. Feces should be "raked" (manually removed) from the rectum before the vulva is cleaned, so as to aid in palpation and prevent contamination of the area and equipment. An antiseptic soap, warm water, and cotton are used to wash the vulva and surrounding area. Wipe the vulva, starting at the dorsal commissure of the labia and progressing down to the ventral commissure. The soap should be rinsed off before treatment.

Intrauterine Infusion

A uterine pipette is used to infuse solutions into the uterus, using a syringe to inject the medication through the pipette. An equine nasogastric tube and stomach pump may be used to inject large volumes of medication into the uterus.

To aid passage of the pipette into the uterus, guide it with the opposite hand, placed into the rectum. Grasp the cervix, which lies about 3 to 4 inches cranial to the vulva, with the left hand (for a right-handed person) so that the thumb is dorsal to the cervix and the fingers are located ventrad. Insert the pipette into the vulva, exercising care to avoid touching the pipette's tip to the labia. Advance the pipette at a 30- to 40-degree angle for 3 to 4 inches. This prevents the pipette from entering the urethral opening, located on the floor of the vagina. Once the tip is past the urethral orifice, advance the pipette in a horizontal position. To aid in passage of the pipette, pull the cervix craniad to straighten the folds of the vagina. As the pipette is advanced, it may become caught in a vaginal fold. If this occurs, do not force the pipette craniad, but simply withdraw and redirect it.

Introduce the pipette's tip into the cervical opening, which is usually in the center of the cervix. Gently manipulate the cervix over the pipette. Once the pipette is through the cervix, it slides craniad easily and may be palpated rectally. Beginners commonly deposit the medication in the vagina or cervix rather than in the uterus. Always make certain the tip has passed into the uterus. Inject the medication and then flush the pipette with air to remove residual medication.

Through the entirety of this procedure, it is important never to force the pipette craniad, because this may damage vaginal or cervical tissue. Also, the vaginal and rectal walls may be penetrated if excessive force is used. This could result in such complications as peritonitis, metritis, abscesses, and reproductive disorders.

Intrauterine Boluses

A sterile sleeve should be worn to insert boluses or capsules into the uterus. Advance the hand into the animal's vulva and vagina until the cervix is located. Form your hand into a wedge, insert it into the patient's dilated os cervix (cervical orifice), and advance it into the uterus, where the medication is deposited. There are fewer complications with this method of intrauterine medication than with infusion. The primary complication is introduction of bacteria into the uterus by using poor sanitary techniques. Rough handling can damage vaginal and cervical tissue.

Many farmers medicate their animals with these methods. They should be carefully instructed in use of the proper techniques and informed of possible complications. They should also be informed of drug withdrawal times so that meat or milk from treated animals is not immediately sold.

ORAL MEDICATION
Balling Gun

Boluses, capsules, or magnets may be given per os (PO) with a balling gun (Fig. 28-4). This instrument is available in various sizes for use in different species. Cattle require a gun with a large head and long handle, with a metal or flexible plastic head. The plastic head produces less trauma to the pharyngeal tissue than a metal head but is easily damaged by teeth. Small balling guns are manufactured for use in calves.

The methods of introducing a balling gun, dose syringe, drench bottle, or Frick's speculum are similar in all species. For cattle, standing cranial to the animal's shoulder and facing the same direction as the animal, place one arm over the animal's head and caudal to the poll, with the animal's head positioned on your hip. This technique may not be possible for people with short arms. In this case, reaching across the bridge of the nose is acceptable. Insert the fingers of this hand into the mouth at the interdental space and apply pressure to the hard palate, which causes the animal to open its mouth.

Insert the balling gun or similar instrument at an upward angle at the interdental space, opposite the restraining hand. Direct the instrument caudad and advance it over the base of the tongue. Once it is over the tongue's base, advance the balling gun caudad in a horizontal position until the rings of the handle reach the buccal commissure (corner of the mouth) (Fig. 28-5). This ensures that the gun is back far enough in the

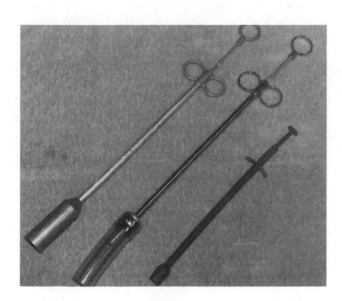

FIG. 28-4 Various sizes of balling guns are available.

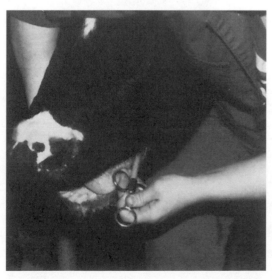

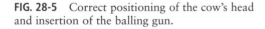
FIG. 28-5 Correct positioning of the cow's head and insertion of the balling gun.

mouth to deposit the bolus, forcing the cow to swallow and preventing expulsion of the medication. Depress the plunger to eject the bolus and remove the instrument. Observe the animal to be sure the medication was swallowed. It is not necessary to elevate the head until the bolus is swallowed if the bolus was deposited correctly.

Frick's Speculum

A Frick's speculum may be used to give two or more boluses to cattle (Fig. 28-6). Insert the speculum in the same manner as the balling gun. Once the speculum is placed over the base of the tongue, the boluses are inserted into the speculum. Allow the boluses to travel down the speculum and into the mouth. Remove the speculum and observe for swallowing. This method is used to save time but has the added danger of aspiration of medication.

Drenching

Giving small volumes of liquids PO is often referred to as "drenching." Drenching is done with a dose syringe or a drench bottle (Fig. 28-7). A 60-ml catheter-tipped syringe or a bulb syringe may be used as a dose syringe in calves. The drench bottle, commonly a wine or a soft drink bottle, should be made of strong glass and have a long, tapered neck and smooth mouth.

The technique for drenching is similar to that described for the balling gun. Be certain to insert the drench bottle at the interdental space to prevent the cow from breaking it with its molars. The head should be held slightly elevated so that the nose is level with the animal's eye. If the head is raised excessively, the animal could aspirate some of the medication. Give the medication slowly, allowing the animal to swallow at its own pace.

Dose syringes are also used to give pastes. Commercially prepared syringes containing medication are available, although these are used more often in horses.

Orogastric Intubation

"Stomach tubing" is a quick and relatively painless method to deliver large quantities of liquid medication or fluids. A stomach tube may be passed through the nasal cavity, as in horses, but this method is not commonly used in food animals. In food animals, the stomach tube is usually passed through the oral cavity, with the aid of a metal speculum.

An oral speculum is required to prevent damage to the soft stomach tube from the animal's teeth. The Frick's speculum is inserted into the mouth and held in place by an assistant.

Stomach tubes are available in different lengths and diameters. Choose an appropriately sized tube for the individual animal. A tube with an outside diameter of 5/8 to 1 inch is the average size used for adult cattle. A foal stomach tube is often used for "tubing" calves. A stomach pump or a funnel can be used to facilitate administration.

Measure the distance externally from the mouth to the rumen and insert the tube approximately this distance. The mouth-rumen distance is then easily estimated. The first 3 feet of the tube should be lubricated with water or water-soluble lubricating jelly before intubation. With an assistant holding an oral speculum in place, insert the tube into the speculum and advance it with gentle pressure. Some resistance may be felt when the tube reaches the esophagus. Observe for swallowing, then advance the tube into the esophagus. If passage is difficult, rotate the tube slightly and apply gentle pressure to advance the tube.

After inserting the tube the measured distance, check for correct placement in the rumen. If the stomach tube was inadvertently placed in the trachea, the animal may cough, although this should not be used alone to determine correct placement. If the tube has been inadvertently passed down the trachea, air may be felt exiting

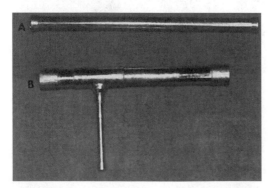

FIG. 28-6 A, Regular Frick's speculum. B, A modified Frick's speculum.

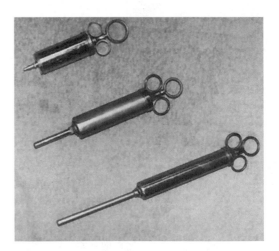

FIG. 28-7 Various sizes of dose syringes.

the tube upon exhalation. Remove the tube and reintubate. Another test used to check if the tube has been passed into the rumen is to have one person blow air into the end of the tube while another listens with a stethoscope at the rumen. A gurgling should be heard as air is blown into the tube. The smell of rumen gas may sometimes be detected exiting the tube. In some lightly muscled animals, the tube can be observed progressing caudally down the esophagus. In these animals, one may also palpate the neck for two tubular structures, i.e., the trachea and the stomach tube within the esophagus.

Once the stomach tube is correctly positioned, the medication can be given. After the medication has been infused, rinse the tube with water to flush out remaining medication. Kink the tube or occlude its end and withdraw it quickly. This prevents any fluid remaining in the tube from entering the trachea upon tube removal.

RECOMMENDED READING

Howard JL: *Current veterinary therapy 3: food animal practice,* Philadelphia, 1993, WB Saunders.
Radostits OM et al: *Herd health: food animal production medicine,* ed 2, Philadelphia, 1994, WB Saunders.
Smith BP: *Large animal internal medicine,* ed 2, St Louis, 1996, Mosby.

CARE OF SHEEP

S.M. WING-PROCTOR

ADMINISTRATION OF MEDICATION
Stomach Tubing

Placement of a stomach tube is the fast and effective method of delivering large volumes of liquid to the rumen or relieving rumen gas bloat. The tube can be passed through a mouth speculum or through the nasal cavity. When using the oral route in neonatal lambs, a mouth speculum is usually not required. Equipment should be gathered before attempting to pass a stomach tube. Required equipment includes a mouth speculum (swine mouth speculum, Frick's speculum, PVC pipe, or a roll of Elastikon) and a stomach tube of appropriate size (10- to 18-French rubber urinary catheter or 14- to 18-French infant feeding tube for lambs, small to medium foal stomach tube for sheep), and a dose syringe or funnel.

Measure from the front of the mouth to the rumen for the correct length of tube needed. Lubricate the distal one third of the tube with water, mineral oil, or water-soluble lubricating jelly. Introduce the mouth speculum into the interdental space, being careful not to

damage the animal's teeth. Pressing your thumb against the animal's tongue prompts the sheep to open its mouth. Place the tube into the speculum and advance steadily with gentle pressure; resistance might be felt at the esophagus. Correct tube placement can be determined by watching the animal swallow the tube or by blowing into the tube while someone listens for gurgling sounds in the paralumbar fossa region. Generally, rumen odor is emitted from the tube. An incorrectly placed tube stimulates a cough reflex (tube is in the trachea) and air can be felt on exhalation. Administer fluids or liquid medications through the tube using a funnel or dose syringe. When the treatment is completed, flush the tube with water until it runs clear, then kink or occlude the tube and withdraw it quickly. Failure to occlude the end of the tube can lead to aspiration of fluid into the lungs. Remove the speculum.

Dose Syringe

Dose syringes allow oral administration of liquid medications without use of a stomach tube. This technique is simple, but there is always a chance of aspiration into the lungs. Liquid medications should be limited to a volume of 30 ml. The sheep should be standing, with its head parallel to the ground or tilted slightly upward. Insert the tip of a dose syringe/backpack syringe tip into the interdental space and dispense the medication. Cup the animal's head with your hand during this procedure to keep the animal from spitting the fluid out. Withdraw the syringe and turn the sheep loose.

Bolus or Pill Administration

Boluses are large pills that require a sheep-sized balling gun, either plastic or metal, for administration. The balling gun is introduced into the sheep's mouth at the interdental space. The gun is advanced into the mouth and over the base of the tongue, being careful to avoid injury to the roof of the mouth or the teeth. Push the plunger gently to deliver the bolus. Sheep do not like this method of treatment and begin resisting the procedure if it is performed frequently. It is possible to "pill" a sheep using your fingers to introduce the pill over the base of the tongue, but you can be bitten for your efforts. Remember not to overextend the sheep's neck, because this can cause the bolus to enter the trachea instead of the esophagus.

Rumen Inoculation

It is useful to know how to inoculate the rumen of a sick sheep. Without the normal microorganisms in the gut, the sheep is unable to properly digest its food. Rumen contents can be siphoned from a healthy sheep and introduced into the rumen of the debilitated animal through a stomach tube. At least 1 quart of rumen liquid should be administered to the unhealthy animal.

Another method is to take a cud from a healthy sheep and place it into the mouth of the sick animal. This does not work well if the animal is debilitated, but the cud can be mixed with water and given via a stomach tube.

Intramuscular Injection

An intramuscular (IM) injection is best done with the animal standing (Fig. 28-8). In adult sheep, an 18-gauge, 1½-inch needle is used for IM injection; for lambs, use a 20-gauge, 1-inch needle. Only the semimembranosus, semitendinosus, and triceps muscles are substantial enough for IM injection.

Part the wool and swab the injection site with an antiseptic. Hold the needle by the hub between your thumb and forefinger, avoiding contact with the sterile shaft. Grasp the muscle near the injection site with your thumb and fingers of the opposite hand, squeeze the muscle, and quickly thrust the needle into the muscle. Attach the syringe and aspirate to check for blood; redirect the needle if necessary. Inject the medication and withdraw the needle and syringe as a unit.

Subcutaneous Injection

Subcutaneous (SC) injections can be administered with the sheep in a standing, lateral, or set up position. In adult sheep, an 18-gauge, 1-inch needle is used for SC injection; for lambs, use a 20-gauge, 1-inch needle. Any area with loose skin can be used for SC injection, although using the wool-free areas caudal to the front legs and cranial to the rear legs reduces the chance of pelt damage (see Fig. 28-8). Some caregivers prefer to use the loose skin around the neck, cranial to the scapula, or along the back for SC injections. Injections in these areas can lead to abscesses, a sore neck (which prevents the patient from eating and drinking), or pelt damage.

After wiping the area with an antiseptic, pinch the skin between the fingers to form a tent. Insert the needle into the tent, making sure the needle is under the skin. Aspirate to check for blood. If the needle is correctly positioned, inject the medication. Depending on the substance being injected, hold your finger over the puncture site as the needle is withdrawn. This prevents leaking from the injection site and helps control minor skin bleeding. It also prevents entry of air at the site, which can cause painful cysts.

Intraperitoneal Injection

The intraperitoneal (IP) route is usually used in neonates when an intravenous injection is not possible. The caudoventral abdominal wall cranial to the cranial border of the pubis is the best site for IP injections in sheep. The site is prepared by clipping the area and prepping with a surgical scrub. The animal is restrained in dorsal recumbency, with the hindquarters elevated. To avoid puncturing the bladder or injuring the penis in males, insert the needle slightly off midline. Gently insert an 18-gauge, 1- to 1½-inch needle, aspirate, and

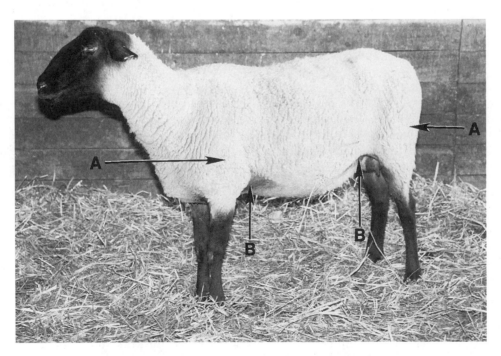

FIG. 28-8   Injection site. **A,** Intramuscular. **B,** Subcutaneous.

inject the medication. The medication should flow easily if the needle is in the peritoneal cavity. Many problems, such as peritonitis from improper site preparation or puncturing of abdominal organs, can result if improper technique is used in this procedure.

Intravenous Injection

The jugular vein is routinely used for administering medications intravenously (IV) and for drawing blood samples. It can be easily accessed in the standing sheep (Fig. 28-9). The cephalic and femoral veins may also be used, with the sheep in a standing or lateral position. Depending on the size of the sheep, an 18- or 20-gauge, 1- to 1½-inch needle is used for IV injection.

Part the wool along the jugular furrow and wipe the area with an antiseptic. Occlude the vessel at or slightly cranial to the thoracic inlet, stroking or tapping the vessel to help define the borders of the vessel. Insert the needle at a 30- to 45-degree angle, with or without the needle attached to a syringe. Thread the needle into the vessel. Aspirate and check for blood. If the needle is positioned in the vessel, inject the medication slowly. Redirect the needle if necessary. Withdraw the needle while attached to the syringe and apply pressure over the injection site to prevent formation of a hematoma. A blood sample may be obtained with a Vacutainer system using this same process. The jugular vein appears deeper in an unshorn sheep because the wool prevents the technician from resting the syringe/Vacutainer tube against the animal's skin.

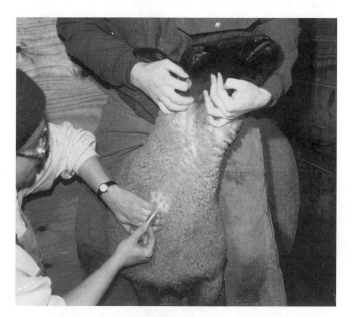

FIG. 28-9 Two-person restraint for intravenous injection or blood sampling using the jugular vein.

Intravenous Catheterization

Intravenous catheters should be placed in animals that require continuous fluid therapy, repeated IV treatments, or administration of irritating medications. The jugular vein is the vessel of choice. The cephalic or femoral veins may be used if the jugular vein is not patent. Catheter dimensions vary, depending on the size of the sheep. In adults, use 14-, 16-, or 18-gauge, 3½- to 5¼-inch catheters. In lambs, use 18-, 20-, or 22-gauge, 1½- to 3½-inch catheters.

The skin over the jugular furrow should be clipped and aseptically prepared for introduction of the catheter. Local anesthetic may be used at the catheter introduction site. An IV catheter should be placed in a sterile manner, which should include wearing sterile gloves. Occlude the vein caudal to the insertion site. Puncture the skin at the catheter site with a disposable needle the same diameter as the catheter. This prevents the catheter tip from becoming dull as it passes through the skin. Place the catheter through the needle hole at a 15- to 30-degree angle and quickly thrust the catheter into the vein and advance it toward the heart. Occlude the vessel to ensure backflow of blood through the catheter; this indicates proper placement of the catheter. Cap the catheter and flush with 10 to 15 ml of heparinized saline.

The catheter must be secured to the neck. Bandaging alone is not sufficient to keep the catheter from slipping out of place. Catheters with wings can be sutured to the skin by placing an 18-gauge, 1½-inch hypodermic needle into the skin near the wing and threading a 2/0 nonabsorbable suture material through the tip of the needle and out the needle hub. The needle is then removed and the suture is threaded into the hole of the wing and tied. The procedure is repeated on the other wing. Catheters without wings can be secured by placing the first suture caudal to the hub and a second suture cranial to the hub on the extension or IV line. At least two sutures should be placed to secure the catheter. Suturing the catheter increases the likelihood that the catheter will stay in place.

After the catheter is secured, apply an antibiotic ointment over the catheter exit with a sterile tongue depressor. Place a sterile gauze pad over the ointment and secure the setup with elastic tape (Elastikon, Johnson & Johnson) around the sheep's neck. An IV drip line should be looped into or on top of the bandage and held in place with adhesive tape. The loop in the extension line prevents direct tension on the catheter as the animal moves about the stall. The catheter and IV lines should be changed every 3 days to prevent thrombophlebitis and infection. Flushing the catheter every 4 hours with heparinized saline helps keep the catheter patent.

Intradermal Injection

Intradermal (ID) injections are used infrequently in sheep. The main use of ID injection is for tuberculosis testing. The caudal tail fold is the preferred site in sheep. A 25-gauge, 5/8-inch or 26-gauge, 3/8-inch needle is used for ID injections. The needle with the syringe attached is placed parallel to the skin. The free hand is used to pinch the skin taut and helps stabilize it for the injection. With the bevel directed up, gently insert the needle into the dermis. Aspirate if the injection is for local anesthesia over a vessel. A bleb or wheal should be visualized as the drug is deposited. Tuberculin testing uses only 0.1 ml of testing solution, so care must be taken to deposit material accurately.

Intramammary Infusion

It may be necessary to check or treat the udder for mastitis. A physical examination is best performed with the sheep in a set up position. Treatments or milk testing in the ewe are usually done with the ewe in a standing position. Thoroughly wash the teats with warm water, an antiseptic soap, and a separate cloth or paper towel. Dry each teat with an individual towel; this decreases the number of contaminating bacteria. Wipe the teat orifices with an alcohol-drenched swab, starting with the far teat and ending with the near. Allow the teats to air dry. Discard the milk in the streak canal. The teat is now prepared for collecting a milk sample for testing or for infusion of the udder.

For testing, collect a midstream squirt of milk into an appropriate container (e.g., strip cup or sterile milk culture tube). Look for flakes or blood in the milk. When treating the udder, grasp the teat near the base and insert the cannula into the teat orifice and deliver the medication into the teat. Remove the cannula, occlude the teat end, and massage the teat to disseminate the medication. Dip the teat in an approved teat dip preparation. If the ewe is to be turned outside and the weather is cold (0° C), allow the udder to dry thoroughly before turning the ewe out. Failure to do this may cause the udder to become chapped, sore, or frostbitten.

OTHER PROCEDURES
Urine Collection

Collecting urine from sheep is easier than with many other animals. Have a specimen cup ready before starting. Hold the sheep in a standing position and pinch the nostrils closed until urination occurs. Generally, the sheep will urinate within 30 seconds. The nostrils may be held off for up to 1 minute. If the sheep does not urinate in that minute, allow the animal to rest for 1 or 2 minutes. Repeat the procedure as necessary to obtain a sample.

Hoof Trimming

Sheep that are not allowed to graze or that are raised in confinement tend to develop overgrown feet. Typically the sidewalls and the toes overgrow. The hoofs should be trimmed as needed (Fig. 28-10). The sidewalls should be trimmed to keep the sole flat and the toes pointing forward. Toes are normally squared off. Trimming is done with heavy scissors, hoof rot shears, or a sharp knife (Fig. 28-11). If bleeding occurs, apply hemostatic powder or copper naphthenate (Kopertox, Fort Dodge). Severe bleeding may require bandaging.

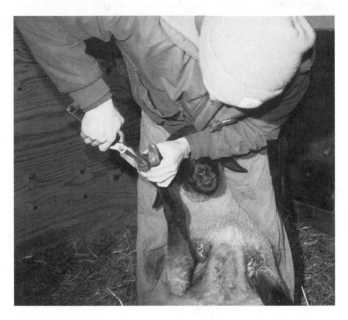

FIG. 28-10   Hoof trimming on a set-up sheep.

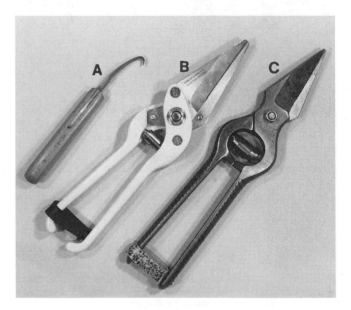

FIG. 28-11   Hoof trimming equipment. **A,** Double-sided narrow knife. **B,** Heavy-duty scissors. **C,** Hoof rot shears.

Crutching

Ewes close to parturition should be crutched. This procedure removes the wool from around the vulva and the udder. A clean vulval area facilitates passage of the lamb and allows the birthing process to proceed easily. Removing the wool from around the udder assists the lambs in finding and suckling the teats. Lambs suck on anything on the ewe's body, including wool and fecal tags. Trimming this debris from around the vulva and udder areas prevents the lambs from sucking inappropriately.

RECOMMENDED READING

Pratt PW: *Medical, surgical and anesthetic nursing for veterinary technicians,* ed 2, St Louis, 1994, Mosby.

The sheep production handbook, Englewood, Calif, 1988, American Sheep Industry Association.

The Shepherd, New Washington, Ohio, Sheep and Farm Life, Inc.

Thedford TR: *Sheep health handbook,* Morrilton, Ariz, 1983, A Winrock International Information Services Publication.

CARE OF GOATS

S. MOBINI

Goats are rising in popularity as an alternative farming enterprise and as pets. They are also used in many teaching and research institutions as models for animal or human diseases. The rise in popularity of goats has increased the need for veterinary team members to familiarize themselves with the nursing care and treatment techniques applicable to goats. Many of the techniques described below are similar to those used for other food animal species, with some adjustments for the species. The importance of the correct method of application of medications and correct dosage for the species cannot be overemphasized. The veterinary technician must be familiar with several basic principles of pharmacology to choose and consider the route of administration.

ROUTES OF DRUG ADMINISTRATION
Oral Medication

Oral administration is generally suitable for medications that act on the stomach or intestines or for systemic action after intestinal absorption. Addition of drugs to feed and water can provide therapeutic amounts of drug only if such adulterated feed or water has an acceptable smell or taste, and if the appetite of the animal is normal. Mass medication of feed and water is not reliable in goats, because sick goats are likely to have reduced feed and water intake. In addition, goats are very peculiar and may detect a change in odor or flavor and refrain from consumption.

Oral liquid medication can be administered as a drench by use of a dosing bottle, drenching gun, or dosing syringe and stomach tube. Small volumes of fluid can be given with a drenching bottle. The head of the goat should be stabilized and held horizontally at a normal to slightly raised position. With the animal's chin firmly held, the neck of the bottle is inserted into the corner of the mouth and on the back of the tongue, and the liquid medication is poured in the mouth to be swallowed by the goat. If the goat becomes restless or begins to cough, or if the fluid runs out of the mouth, treatment must be stopped and the head lowered to prevent inhalation of the fluid. A drenching gun with a short nozzle or a catheter-tip dose syringe is preferred for oral dosing of medications. The tip of the drenching gun or dose syringe is inserted at the commissure of the lips, over the tongue. The nostrils are held off while the liquid medication is quickly dispensed over the tongue.

Boluses (large tablets) can be administered to goats by use of a balling gun. A sheep and goat balling gun is available commercially, or a calf-size balling gun will work equally well. It is best to have the goat in a corner so that it cannot back up. Fit a bolus snugly into the end of the balling gun. With the goat standing, insert one hand in the interdental space at the commissure of the lips to open the mouth. Insert the balling gun at the opposite corner of the mouth and direct it carefully over the base of the tongue. Push the gun to the dorsal prominence of the tongue, being careful not to scrape the roof of the mouth. With the head lifted at about a 45-degree angle, push the plunger to "pop" the bolus down the throat. Anything deposited farther rostrally is usually chewed and rejected. Observe the goat for several seconds to be certain that it has swallowed the bolus and does not spit it out.

Orogastric Intubation

An orogastric tube (stomach tube) can be used in goats for administration of a large volume of liquid medication or fluids. A 9.54-mm-diameter foal stomach tube works well for an adult goat. The goat should be restrained appropriately. A wood block with a hole in the middle, a tape roll, or an appropriately sized syringe case with the end smoothed should be used as a mouth speculum. The speculum is placed in the mouth and the lubricated stomach tube is passed through the speculum and over the base of the tongue, into the esophagus and into the rumen. The correct location of the tube can be assessed by feeling the neck. Passage of the tube into the trachea usually elicits a pronounced cough. You can also smell the end of the tube for rumen gas, which has a characteristic smell. It is also possible to check for correct tube placement by auscultation of the left flank while air is blown into the tube in short, repeated puffs. A stomach pump or a dose syringe could be attached to the stomach tube for administration of the liquid. After fluid administration, flush the tube with some water, blow it free of fluid, kink the free end (to prevent residual fluid from falling into the pharynx or larynx), and withdraw the tube slowly.

In a goat herd, some kids are born very weak or become dehydrated after birth. A feeding probe or stomach tube can be used for administration of colostrum or oral electrolyte solution to save the kid. A commercially available baby lamb probe works very well for kids. This instrument, a stainless-steel ball probe attached to a syringe or dose gun (Fig. 28-12), is designed to prevent accidental entry into the trachea, thus protecting against fluid administration into the lungs. Place the kid on its right side with the head and neck extended. As you insert the probe in the mouth, place one hand around the kid's neck so that you can feed the instrument's end into the esophagus. Do not force the probe. Give the kid a chance to relax and swallow to ease the tube's entry. Attach the syringe and administer fluid.

The author of this section prefers to use the lamb probe for kids; however, you can give oral fluids to kids using a small flexible rubber tube (see Fig. 28-12), as in adult goats. These tubes are also available commercially. Hold the tube from the mouth to the end of the last rib (flank area) to estimate the length necessary to reach the rumen. Mark near the top as a guide. Place the kid on its right side with head and neck extended slightly. Open the mouth slightly by pressing on either side of the jaw with your fingers. Slide the tube down the kid's throat as far as the previously marked area. You should feel slight resistance as the tube passes the back of the throat and enters the esophagus. If you feel no resistance, you have probably entered the trachea. The kid may also cough if

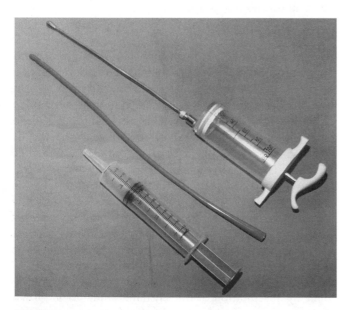

FIG. 28-12   Stainless-steel lamb probe *(top)*, flexible rubber tube *(center)*, and syringe *(bottom)*.

the tube is in the trachea. In the goat, the chance of placing the tube in the trachea is very slim because of the anatomy of their pharynx; almost always the tube passes directly into the esophagus.

Parenteral Injections

Parenteral administration techniques routinely used in goats are subcutaneous, intramuscular, and intravenous. Whenever the efficacy of treatment is not compromised, drugs and vaccines should be given subcutaneously rather than intramuscularly in goats to minimize damage to muscle tissue. It is advisable to use a separate sterile needle for each goat to prevent the spread of caprine arthritis encephalitis (CAE) virus.

Subcutaneous Injection. Subcutaneous injection in the goat is best made into the loose skin of the lateral side of the neck or on the chest wall about 5 cm caudal to the shoulder. Drug absorption is slower after subcutaneous injection than after intramuscular, but tissue tolerance is better. The skin of the injection site must be vigorously rubbed with a piece of cotton soaked with 70% alcohol to clean and disinfect the skin before injection. Repeat the swabbing process with a new cotton swab until the cotton is no longer dirty after swabbing. A fold of skin should be pinched up to form a tent. Insert a sharp needle by a sudden thrust at a 30- to 45-degree angle to the skin, with or without the syringe attached. An 18- to 20-gauge, 2- to 3-cm-long needle is used for adult goats and a 20- to 22-gauge, 2- to 3-cm-long needle for kids. Limit the volume of medication to 5 ml per site. If a large volume is to be injected, divide the dose into several portions injected at different sites. If done correctly, subcutaneous injection should leave a bleb under the skin. After withdrawal of the needle, massage the site to disperse the medication. Avoid subcutaneous injection along the back and dorsal flank if the hide is to be marketed. Vaccines should be injected subcutaneously caudal to the shoulder, because local reactions near the prescapular lymph node may be confused with caseous lymphadenitis (lymph node abscess).

Intramuscular Injection. Intramuscular injections in the goat are administered on the lateral aspect of the neck or semitendinosus/semimembranosus muscle (thigh) (Fig. 28-13). However, the preferred site for intramuscular injections is the lateral aspect of the neck, in a triangular region bounded by the vertebral column ventrally, the ligamentum nuchae dorsally, and the shoulder caudally. Injection into the thigh muscles should be avoided, because the muscle mass is small and sciatic nerve damage is a common complication. This is one of the most valuable parts of a goat carcass, and muscle damage may devalue the marketability of the meat. Gluteal muscle should not be used for injection in goats because of its small mass and the possibility of muscle damage.

The size of the needle for intramuscular injection in an adult goat is 18 to 20 gauge and 2 to 3 cm long. Use a 20- to 22-gauge, 2.5-cm-long needle for kids. The volume of injection should not be more than 5 ml per site. Use the same cleaning procedure as described for subcutaneous injection. The needle for IM injections should be inserted at a 90-degree angle (perpendicular) to the muscle. Before injecting, withdraw the syringe plunger a little to ensure that the needle is not in a blood vessel. If blood enters the syringe, withdraw the needle and reinsert in another direction or choose another site. Massage the injection site after injection and removing the needle.

Intradermal Injection. Intradermal injection is used for tuberculosis testing in goats. The injection site is the caudal tail fold. The skin is pinched and stabilized between the thumb and middle finger. A 25-gauge, 1-cm-long tuberculin needle is used. After cleaning the injection site, direct the needle bevel upward, hold the needle parallel to the skin, and gently insert it into the dermis. A small "bleb" should be visualized as the drug is deposited. If a bleb is not formed, the needle tip is too deep; retract the needle and inject again.

Intravenous Injection. The jugular vein is always used for intravenous injections and blood sampling in the goat. The goat is best restrained by an assistant's backing the animal into a corner and holding it between one's legs, with the goat's neck extended and turned slightly to one side (Fig. 28-14). The upper two thirds of the jugular furrow is cleansed with a swab soaked in 70% alcohol to remove dust and to make the hair lie flat so that the vein is easier to see. The vein is occluded about two thirds of the way down the neck, at the jugular furrow or thoracic inlet. The needle is inserted at a 45-degree angle with the tip directed cranially or caudally, with or without the syringe attached. After the needle enters the vein, thread the needle into the vein and aspirate or occlude the vein to make sure the needle is in the vein before injecting the medication. If the needle comes out of the vein because of movement of the goat, stop injection at once and reposition the needle. It

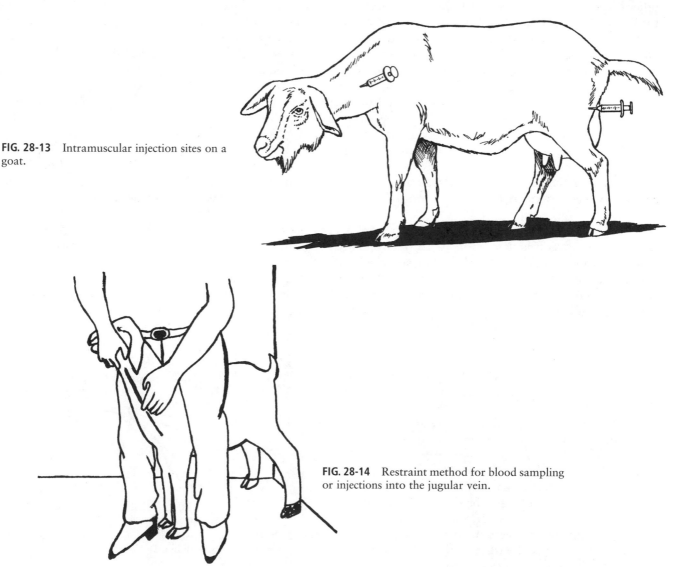

FIG. 28-13 Intramuscular injection sites on a goat.

FIG. 28-14 Restraint method for blood sampling or injections into the jugular vein.

is best to give the injection in the opposite jugular vein if you are unsuccessful in reentering the vein.

Needle size used depends on the viscosity of the drug to be administered. Use the smallest needle possible, because this reduces discomfort to the patient and minimizes trauma. An 18- to 20-gauge, 2- to 3-cm-long needle is most commonly used.

Jugular Venipuncture and Catheterization. The jugular vein is commonly used to obtain blood samples from goats for various diagnostic tests. The procedure is the same as for intravenous injection. A Vacutainer (Becton-Dickinson) needle and needle holder work well in goats for blood sampling.

Intravenous catheterization of the jugular vein is commonly performed in goats for fluid therapy. If properly maintained, an IV catheter may remain functional for several days. An 18-gauge, 5- to 6-cm-long over-the-needle catheter is most often used in goats. Shorter catheters tend to come out of the vein. The jugular vein area should be clipped and surgically scrubbed as in other species. The vein is located as previously described for IV injection. The catheter is inserted into the vein at a 45-degree angle, toward the heart. Occlude the vein to ensure a backflow of blood before threading the catheter down the vein. Advance the catheter off of the needle until the catheter's entire length is in the vein. Cap the catheter and flush with heparinized saline. Place a butterfly tape around the catheter and suture it to the skin. Securing a catheter by bandaging alone is not adequate in goats. Place a sterile gauze pad covered with an antiseptic ointment over the site where the catheter enters the skin and wrap elastic adhesive tape around the neck to secure the suture butterfly.

Intrauterine Infusion

Intrauterine infusion is done in goats to treat retained placenta or metritis. The vulva should be scrubbed and rinsed thoroughly to remove contaminants. A sterile vaginal speculum and a light source are needed. The vaginal speculum, lubricated with sterile, water-soluble jelly, is inserted into the vagina. The light source is inserted inside the speculum, and the speculum is rotated cranially until the cervix is located. A sterile bovine insemination pipette is then inserted into the cervix by applying moderate pressure to penetrate the cervix and enter the uterus. A syringe is attached to the end of the pipette, and the appropriate amount of medicated fluid is infused into the uterus.

Intramammary Infusion

Intramammary infusion is routinely used in dairy goats for treatment of mastitis and before drying off. It consists of introduction of medication through the teat canal. The tips of the teats must first be thoroughly cleaned and disinfected with alcohol swabs to prevent introduction of bacteria with the medication. Intramammary products formulated for cows are usually used in goats. These are available in special plastic syringes with a nozzle suitable for insertion into the teats. The end of the teat is held between two fingers of one hand, and the nozzle is inserted halfway into the teat canal and medication injected. Upon withdrawal of the nozzle, the teat is occluded and the teat is massaged, directing the fluid from the teat cistern into the glandular (udder) tissue. For very small teat openings, a sterile tomcat catheter can be used for teat infusion.

Urine and Milk Collection

A female goat (doe) generally urinates just after standing. However, urine samples for bacteriologic, chemical, and microscopic testing can be collected directly from the bladder by inserting a catheter using aseptic technique.

The doe should be suitably restrained and the vulva cleaned. A double-bladed small animal vaginal speculum is inserted into the vagina. Under visual control with illumination from a light, a sterile curved metal urinary catheter is inserted into the urethra. The tip of the catheter is first pushed a few millimeters into the suburethral diverticulum. Then the tip of the catheter is raised a little to pass over the fold of mucous membrane at the entrance to the urethral orifice (Fig. 28-15). From this point cranially, no resistance should be encountered. If there is any resistance, the tip of the catheter is probably still in the suburethral diverticulum.

Urethral catheterization of a male goat (buck) is very difficult. Because of the presence of a urethral diverticulum at the level of the ischial arch, it is impossible to introduce a catheter into the urinary bladder of the buck.

Milk samples are commonly collected from dairy goats for bacteriologic examination and somatic cell counts. Each teat end should be disinfected with an alcohol-soaked cotton swab. The teat on the far side of the udder is disinfected first, then the one on the near side. The sterile sample tubes are labeled as to the par-

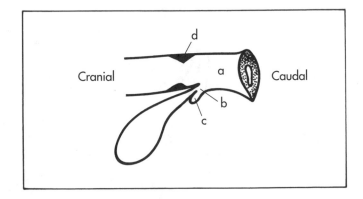

FIG. 28-15 Female goat genitalia. **A,** Vagina. **B,** Urethral orifice. **C,** Suburethral diverticulum. **D,** Cervix.

ticular quarter, the stopper is removed, and milk is directed into the tube held at a 45-degree angle, rather than held vertically. Milk samples are collected first from the near teat and then from the far one. Before a sample is collected, a small squirt of milk is discarded from each teat to flush out any bacteria present in the teat canal.

RECOMMENDED READING

Ballaglia RA, Mayrose VB: *Handbook of livestock management techniques,* Minneapolis, 1981, Burgess Publishing.

McCurnin DM: *Clinical textbook for veterinary technicians,* ed 3, Philadelphia, 1993, WB Saunders.

Pratt PW: *Medical, surgical and anesthesia nursing for veterinary technicians,* ed 2, St Louis, 1994, Mosby.

Sinn R: *Raising goats for milk and meat,* Little Rock, Ark, 1985, Heifer Project International.

Smith MC, Sherman DM: *Goat medicine,* Philadelphia, 1994, Lea & Febiger.

CARE OF SWINE

M.E. GEMUS

OVERVIEW OF SWINE PRODUCTION

The present trend in swine production is increased use of confinement rearing facilities. These facilities allow producers to raise more pigs per farm and to market pigs in 5 to 6 months. The increase in pig density raises concerns in regard to prevention of disease. If a disease occurs, the herd is affected and the economic loss can be devastating. Pigs become unhealthy because of disease transmission from adjacent pigs or infections from outside sources (e.g., trucking, feed, personnel, wind, or other species of animals).

Disease is best prevented by ensuring good health status, nutrition, housing, management, and husbandry. Diseases and production problems are primarily investigated on a herd level.

Terminology

Terms used to describe gender or stages of production within a herd follow:

Male pig, intact: *boar*
Male pig, castrated: *barrow*
Baby pig (before weaning): *piglet*
Female pig, preparturient: *gilt*
Female pig, postparturient: *sow*
Pigs less than 25 kg: *weaner pig*
Pigs 25 kg to market weight: *grower-finisher pig*

Farrowing and Piglets. Sows enter the farrowing room a few days before expected parturition. The farrowing room should be clean and disinfected with a solution containing chlorhexidine, formaldehyde solution, phenols, or a quaternary ammonium compound. The area provided for the piglets should be warm (30° to 35° C) and dry to reduce the incidence of chilling and stress in newborn piglets.

Litter sizes range from 7 to 12, and the average birth weight is approximately 1.5 kg. Maternal antibodies are transferred to piglets by ingestion of the sow's colostrum. The colostral antibodies are absorbed by the intestinal epithelial cells. Intestinal absorption of colostrum halts by about 24 hours after birth. Therefore, to ensure adequate maternal antibody transfer, it is important that piglets begin nursing within 12 hours after birth.

Hypothermia is also a problem in newborn piglets. The piglet's body temperature at birth is 39° C but decreases to 37° C within a few hours. Over the next 24 hours, the piglet's body temperature returns to 39° C. An environmental temperature of 30° to 35° C should be maintained with heat lamps and heat mats during this time of relative hypothermia.

Weaner Pigs. This stage of growth is a stressful period. It begins with weaning and placement in a nursery barn. Pigs are approximately 5 to 8 kg at weaning and remain in the nursery until they weigh 25 kg. The diet at the time of weaning changes from predominantly milk to a highly palatable, digestible dry food diet. The level of maternal antibody is declining at this time and the weaner pig is just beginning to produce its own antibodies, stimulated by natural exposure or vaccination. Feed-grade antibiotics are usually added to the diet to improve metabolism of feed. Warm (25° to 30° C), dry housing and a clean, sanitized environment are also important to this group of pigs.

Grower-Finisher Pigs. This phase includes gilts, and barrows from 25 kg up to market weight at 90 kg to 110 kg. Finisher pigs are fed a mixture of ground corn, and soybean meal, and a vitamin-mineral premix.

Breeding Stock. Breeding stock includes gilts, sows, and boars. Females are considered gilts until after they farrow their first litter; at that point they become sows. In addition to the farrowing facility, housing for this phase is provided in the breeding and gestating areas. Breeding stock also require an environment that is clean and dry, with good lighting and minimal stress.

HANDLING AND RESTRAINT

A significant animal welfare and production concern is the potential for stress from improper handling of pigs. Proper handling reduces stress during routine production practices, such as moving of hogs, blood sampling, vaccinating, clipping tails and teeth, ear notching, detusking, castration, and administration of therapeutics. Chapter 17 presents information on handling of pigs.

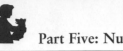
ADMINISTRATION OF MEDICATION
Oral Medication

To administer oral medication, restrain the pig as follows: Place the left thumb caudal to the pig's right ear, assuming the handler is right handed. Place the left index finger in the corner of the left side of the mouth, bringing the lips inside the pig's mouth caudal to the needle teeth to protect the handler from the sharp teeth. Placing the finger inside the mouth also encourages swallowing. Place the remaining fingers under the jaw to support the pig's weight. *Caution:* Piglets can be choked if the remaining fingers are placed around the throat instead of under the jaw.

Intramuscular Injection

Use the area of the neck muscle caudal to the ear (Fig. 28-16). Avoid injecting pharmaceuticals into the shoulder, loin, or ham so as to prevent contamination of the meat if an abscess should develop at the injection site. Pull the skin back, seat the needle into the neck muscle, inject the substance, and release the skin. Use finger pressure if the injection site is bleeding. Do not inject more than 2 ml of an injectable into one site (Table 28-1). Try to use the same injection site for each product. If a particular site shows signs of irritation, you can determine which product is causing the reaction.

Subcutaneous Injection

Some vaccines and anthelmintics are given subcutaneously (SC) (see Table 28-1). The lower vascularity of the subcutaneous layer allows for slower release of product into the system. Subcutaneous injections in pigs less than 25 kg are given primarily in the loose skin of the flank or caudal to the elbow. If injecting into the flank, inject into the folds of the skin and not into the peritoneal cavity. In larger pigs, the preferred injection site is the loose skin caudal to the ear.

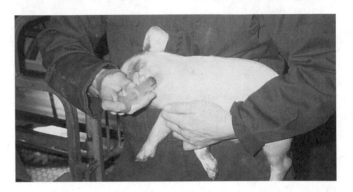

FIG. 28-16   Site for intramuscular injection.

TABLE 28-1 Recommended needle sizes, injection volumes, and blood sample volume, based on pig size

	Injections			Blood sampling					
	IM	SC	IV	Cranial vena cava	Jugular vein	Ear vein	Medial canthus	Tail vein	Cephalic vein
Piglet									
Needle	18-20 gauge, 11 mm	21 gauge, 11 mm	20 gauge, 38 mm	20 gauge, 38 mm			20 gauge, 25 mm		
Quantity	1-2 ml/site		Unlimited				5-10 ml		
Weaner									
Needle	18-20 gauge, 18 mm	21 gauge, 25 mm	20 gauge, 38 mm	20 gauge, 38 mm			20 gauge, 25 mm		20 gauge, 38 mm
Quantity	1-2 ml/site		Unlimited				5-10 ml		5-10 ml
Grower-finisher									
Needle	16 gauge, 18-25 mm	18 gauge, 25 mm	18 gauge, 65 mm	20 gauge, 38 mm		20 gauge, 25 mm	16 gauge, 38 mm		
Quantity	1-3 ml/site		Unlimited			1-2 ml	5-10 ml		
Breeding stock									
Needle	14-16 gauge, 38 mm	18 gauge, 38 mm	16 gauge, 90 mm	20 gauge, 38 mm		20 gauge, 25 mm	14 gauge, 38 mm	20 gauge, 25 mm	
Quantity	1-3 ml/site		Unlimited			1-2 ml	5-10 ml	5-10 ml	

Intranasal Injection

Pigs less than 15 kg can be held, whereas larger pigs should be snared and the head elevated. Use a syringe (without a needle) or a special adapter to dispense the medication. Direct the product into the nostril, keeping the pig's head tilted upward during and immediately following administration. To prevent the pig from ejecting the solution by sneezing, time the injection with inspiration.

Intravenous Injection

Intravenous injections are commonly given in the auricular vein (see Table 28-1). Pigs less than 15 kg can be held, whereas larger pigs should be restrained using a snare. The auricular vein, near the lateral border of the ear, is prominent when held off using a hand or a rubber band as a tourniquet at the base of the ear. After a minute the ear veins become engorged. A butterfly catheter set may be placed for administration of solutions.

BLOOD SAMPLING

Venipuncture is an integral part of blood sampling and administration of solutions. Venipuncture can be achieved using the cranial vena cava, jugular vein, auricular (ear) vein, medial canthus of the eye, or cephalic vein. Techniques for collecting blood from pigs depend on the age and weight of the pigs and restraint techniques available. Appropriate blood collection techniques and needle sizes required for various sizes of pig are given in Table 28-1.

Cranial Vena Cava and Jugular Vein

The cranial vena cava and jugular vein venipuncture techniques are most commonly used to retrieve 5 to 20 ml of blood from a large number of pigs. These techniques are cost effective and expedient; however, some skill is required by the handler and the blood collector. The methods used and anatomy of the area have been described elsewhere. The handler, restraining the pig with a snare, should ensure that the pig is aligned with the shaft of the snare, with the head raised, and neck extended to expose the jugular fossa (Fig. 28-17).

Cranial Vena Cava. To access the cranial vena cava, the collector should identify the right jugular furrow to the point just cranial to and to the right of the manubrium. The approach is made from the pig's right side because the right vagus nerve provides less innervation to the heart and diaphragm than the left vagus (accidental puncture of the vagus nerve can cause cyanosis, dyspnea, and convulsive struggling). The needle is directed toward the top of the opposite shoulder blade while a slight vacuum is maintained in the syringe. When the vena cava is entered, blood fills the test tube or syringe.

Jugular Vein. The collector identifies the deepest hollow in the jugular furrow approximately 5 to 8 cm cranial to and to the right of the manubrium. The needle, usually seated on a Vacutainer (Becton-Dickinson), is positioned perpendicular to the skin. The needle and Vacutainer are then directed toward the same shoulder blade of the pig. The advantage of jugular venipuncture is the high degree of safety for the pig. The needle length (38 mm) is unlikely to penetrate the vagus nerve and lymphatics. The jugular vein is not as large as the cranial vena cava, however, and the shorter needle makes the jugular vein more difficult to penetrate in older and overweight pigs.

Auricular Vein

This vein is generally used for collecting small samples of only 2 to 5 ml. The procedure is the same as for intravenous injection. An 18- to 20-gauge butterfly catheter can be used for collection of blood.

Medial Canthus

Blood can be collected from the venous sinus located near the medial canthus of the eye (Fig. 28-18). A small pig can be held in dorsal recumbency on a 45-degree incline, with the head down and the hind end elevated. A larger pig should be restrained with a snare. The needle, which is positioned at a 45-degree angle from both the surface of the eye and the nose, is passed into the medial canthus, just inside (deep to) the nictitating membrane. The needle is directed toward the other side of the jaw until it strikes the lacrimal bone. Rotate the needle until blood flows.

Tail Vein

Blood collection from the tail vein is limited to adult pigs without docked tails. The tail vein is found on the ventral midline of the tail at the junction of the tail with the body. The volume of blood typically obtained is approximately 2 to 5 ml.

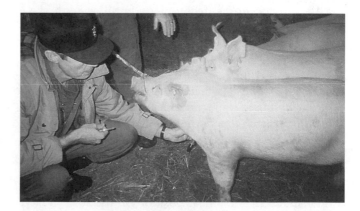

FIG. 28-17 Proper positioning of the pig for blood collection from the cranial vena cava and jugular vein. This pig is being restrained with a hog snare.

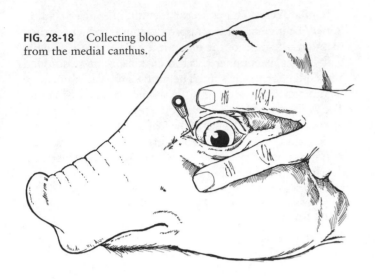

FIG. 28-18   Collecting blood from the medial canthus.

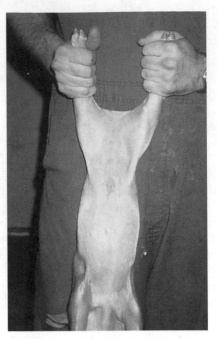

FIG. 28-19   Restraint for subcutaneous injection and castration.

Cephalic Vein

The cephalic vein is not a common site for venipuncture. It is considered inaccessible and a poor venipuncture location as compared with the other sites described. The cephalic vein is found on the medial aspect of the forelimb, between the shoulder and the elbow. The cephalic vein can be raised with digital pressure. The pig is restrained on its back, with its front legs stretched cranially and slightly laterally.

SURGICAL AND PROCESSING PROCEDURES

Veterinary technicians are often involved in processing procedures as part of the herd health program. Although most producers are quite skilled in performing these procedures, technicians familiar with these procedures can assist new producers or help train farm employees. Processing includes clipping teeth, umbilical cord clipping, tail docking, ear notching, and castration. Supplies and equipment needed for these practices are a disinfectant (chlorhexidine), tincture of iodine, side cutters, ear notching tool, and a castration knife or scalpel. Place the instruments in the disinfectant between uses.

Clipping Teeth

The newborn piglet has eight very sharp canine (wolf) teeth. These teeth arm the piglet against its littermates to establish and maintain teat position on the sow. In large litters, if the needle teeth are left intact, the piglets scratch each other, causing infection. Cutting the teeth in smaller litters may be unnecessary, but many producers clip teeth as a precaution. Using clean, sharp side cutters, position the side cutters parallel to the gum line and clip off the distal half of each tooth. Take care not to cut the pig's gum or tongue. Cutting too short may shatter the teeth, leading to gum infection.

Umbilical Cord Clipping

The umbilical cord can act as a portal of entry for bacteria. If the piglet is bleeding from the umbilical cord, tie off the cord immediately using string. Using disinfected side cutters, cut the cord 4 to 5 cm from the abdominal wall. Spray with or dip the end of the cord in 2% povidone-iodine.

Tail Docking

The tail of piglets is commonly clipped to reduce the incidence of tail biting later in the grower-finisher stage. This behavioral vice may result in stress, lameness, and paralysis. The tail is docked approximately 2 cm from the base of the tail using clean, slightly dull side cutters to crush the tail. Cauterizing clippers tend to reduce the amount of bleeding. Cutting the tail too short may result in anal prolapse.

Castration and Inguinal Hernia Repair

After puberty, male pigs may have an offensive odor or "boar taint" that is evident in pork during cooking. Therefore, marketing of intact males is not allowed in the United States or Canada. There are various techniques of castration, each determined by the age and size of the pig. The best time to castrate is before 3 weeks of age and preferably before 2 weeks.

The disadvantage to early castration is reduced detection of inguinal hernias. A knife blade can be used in boars of any size. A hooked blade (No. 12) works well with pigs weighing less than 15 kg.

Pigs castrated between 2 weeks and 16 weeks of age can be held by the back legs, with the abdomen toward the operator and the back of the pig cradled between the restrainer's legs (Fig. 28-19).

RECOMMENDED READING

Leman AD et al, editors: *Diseases of swine*, ed 7, Ames, Iowa, 1992, Iowa State University Press.

Pond WG, Houpt KA: *The biology of the pig*, London, England, 1978, Cornell University Press.

Reeves D, editor: *Guidelines for the veterinary practitioner: care and management of miniature pet pigs*, Santa Barbara, Calif, 1993, Veterinary Practice Publishing.

CARE OF CAMELIDS

M. LEVY

Llamas and alpacas are part of a larger group of South American camelids or New World camelids. In recent years, South American camelids have gained popularity and increasing numbers are now being raised in the United States. Four species of the Lamini tribe are found in South America. The llama (*Lama glama*) and the alpaca (*Lama pacos*) were domesticated about five thousand years ago, whereas the guanaco (*Lama guanicoe*) and the vicuna (*Vicugna vicugna*) are undomesticated.

ANATOMIC AND PHYSIOLOGIC CHARACTERISTICS

The *llama* is the largest of the four species. The face is usually free of wool, with a long, straight to slightly rounded nose (Fig. 28-20). The ears are also long and erect. The wool covers much of the neck and the body. The back is flat, ending in a tail that curls up and back. The colors are solid black, white, brown, or shaded, but they can also be spotted (Appaloosa), patched, or multicolored.

The *alpaca* is smaller than the llama. It has short ears, a wooly face, a rounded rump, and a straight tail (Fig. 28-21). In the United States 22 colors are recognized. The *guanaco* is slightly smaller than the llama but of similar conformation. The ears and nose are smaller than those of the llama. All guanacos have the same color pattern: soft brown to rust on the upper body and a white underbelly. Guanacos can be unpredictable and are undomesticated. The *vicuna* is the smallest and the rarest of the four species. They have a small head and a long, thin neck. Their color pattern is consistently golden brown, with a white chest. The vicuna is also undomesticated and in South America is protected from hunting.

A unique feature of camelids is that they have a stomach with three compartments, rather than four like other ruminants. For this reason, they are not considered true ruminants, although they do ruminate, chew their cud, and digest cellulose. The first compartment represents more than 80% of the total stomach in volume and is equivalent to the rumen and reticulum of true ruminants.

A split upper lip facilitates food prehension. Only three pairs of incisors are found in the lower jaw. Together with the upper dental pad, these teeth facilitate browsing and nipping. Eruption of the adult incisors starts at 2 years for the central incisors, 3 years for the middle incisors, and 4 years for the corner incisors. The upper corner incisors and upper and lower canines develop into sharp scimitar-shaped teeth that are used by males in fighting. These teeth erupt in males around 2 to 3 years and are usually removed surgically.

Llamas have two digits on each foot. The second and third phalanges are positioned horizontally and do not bear weight, whereas the first phalanx is in an upright position. The end of the foot is protected by a nail (not a hoof), and the remainder of the foot is supported by a digital cushion and a soft pad on the palmar surface. The nail may need periodic trimming.

The skin in the cranial cervical region is very thick (up to 1 cm in adult males) and the ventral projection of the transverse processes of the caudal cervical vertebrae forms an inverted U, covering the vessel of the neck. The jugular vein is deep in the neck and close to the carotid artery. The location of the jugular vein makes blood sampling and intravenous injection difficult.

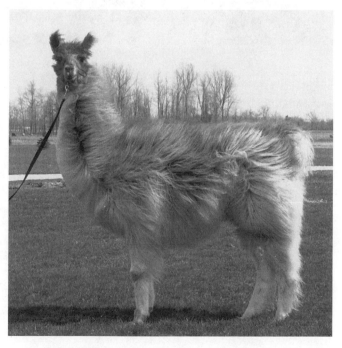

FIG. 28-20 Lateral view of an adult llama.

The uterus of the female llama is bicornuate, with a small uterine body. Most pregnancies occur in the left horn. Although pregnancies have been observed in female llamas as young as six (6) months, it is recommended to delay breeding until 12 months of age. Breeding usually takes place while the female assumes a sternal recumbent position with the male straddling her. Copulation usually lasts about 20 minutes. Ovulation is induced during copulation. Pregnancy is confirmed by rectal palpation at 35 to 40 days, ultrasound findings, or serum progesterone levels above 1 ng/ml at 21 days. The normal gestation period is 335 to 350 days. Most births occur rapidly and typically during daylight hours. Teat enlargement usually happens 1 to 3 weeks prepartum, with milk letdown 48 to 72 hours before parturition, although the teats can also enlarge after parturition.

Table 28-2 lists physical and physiologic characteristics of camelids.

Behavior, Handling, and Restraint

Llamas and alpacas are shy but curious animals that are usually easy to handle. They are social animals with a strong herd instinct. In a comfortable environment, the ears of the llama are erect and directed rostrally (forward). When a llama is upset, the ears are flattened against the head and the nose is elevated. They begin to vocalize (orgle); if the perturbation continues, the llama may spit (actually regurgitate stomach contents) and continue to vocalize. Although llamas frequently spit at each other when competing for food or to assess territoriality, they rarely spit at humans. To handle a spitting animal, a towel or other type of cloth can be placed over the muzzle.

Male llamas may bite, charge, and butt with their chest. They can also kick with their rear legs and inflict injury. Llamas rarely charge or bite humans, except for the so-called berserk male syndrome or aberrant male syndrome displayed by some bottle-raised male llamas.

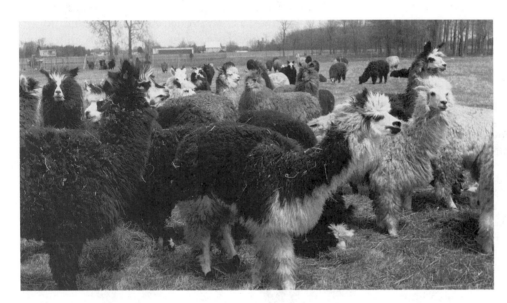

FIG. 28-21   A herd of alpacas. Note the varied coloration.

TABLE 28-2 Physical and physiologic characteristics of South American camelids				
	Llama	Alpaca	Guanaco	Vicuna
Height (cm)				
At the withers	115-130	75-95	——	90
At the poll	150-180			
Weight (kg)				
Male	132-244	60-80	100-150	40-65
Female	108-200	55	100-120	30-40
Rectal temperature (°Celsius)	37.2-38.7	37.2-38.7	37.2-38.7	37.2-38.7
Heart rate (beats/min)	60-90	60-90	60-90	60-90
Respiratory rate (resp./min.)	10-30	10-30	10-30	10-30

In most cases, a satisfactory approach to working with llamas is to have the owner catch and halter the animal before the animal is seen by a veterinarian. If it has not been caught, it is easier to move the whole herd to a smaller enclosure before trying to isolate one animal for examination. Once cornered, the animal can be approached to place a lead rope or an arm around the neck or apply a halter. The person placing the halter should avoid direct eye contact; touching the head of the llama should be minimized. Adult llamas can be easily restrained with a halter and lead rope. Crias (juvenile llamas) can be handled by placing a hand around the front of the neck and grasping around the rump or at the base of the tail. A restraining chute can be very useful for veterinary procedures. Temporary restraint can be achieved using an ear twitch. The base of the ear is encircled with the palm of the hand and squeezed. The ear should not be twisted. The owner should be consulted before using this method.

Blood Collection

Superficial veins are not readily accessible. There is no jugular groove and visualization of the jugular vein is impossible. Jugular venipuncture can be done at a cranial or caudal location on the neck. The landmark in the cranial location is ventral to a line extending from the ventral border of the mandible to the lateral surface of the neck. The tendon of the sternocephalicus muscle should be located on the neck and the vein should be penetrated just caudal to the tendon (Fig. 28-22). The site on the caudal neck is identified by palpation of the vertebral process of the fifth or sixth cervical vertebra. The needle is inserted slightly medial to the tip of the process and directed toward the center of the neck. This must be done carefully because the carotid artery is close to the jugular vein. Blood can also be collected from an ear vein near the caudal edge of the pinna. The ear is bent and a needle is inserted into the vein. Blood is collected while dripping from the hub. This method is less desirable because llamas are usually head shy. The midventral vein of the tail is located in a similar location as in cattle. The saphenous artery and vein can be used for blood collection in recumbent llamas. The artery and vein can be located on the medial aspect of the stifle. In crias, the cephalic vein can also be used. The location is similar to the position of the cephalic vein in dogs.

Urine Collection

If urine cannot be collected by free catch, bladder catheterization can be performed in female llamas. Free-catch collection of urine is better done in the morning, when llamas go to the dung pile. Bladder catheterization is virtually impossible in the male. In the female llama, catheterization is fairly easy. The external urethral orifice is easily palpated on the floor of the vulva. The ven-

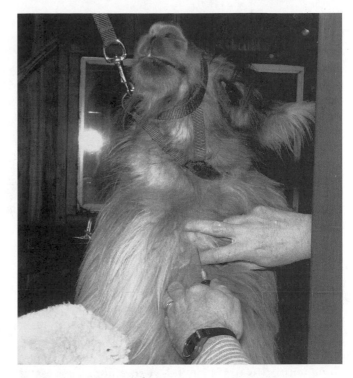

FIG. 28-22 Collecting blood from the jugular vein of an adult llama.

tral suburethral diverticulum complicates catheterization. After the vulva has been thoroughly cleaned, a sterile gloved finger is advanced in the vulva to palpate the meatus. The finger is withdrawn slightly and the catheter (No. 5 French) is advanced into the urethra above the finger to avoid the diverticulum. If the meatus is difficult to palpate, a sterile bitch speculum can be used to visualize it.

Intramuscular Injections

The general rules for giving injections are similar to those for other species, including the need for proper restraint, swabbing of the injection site, and checking for the presence of blood by pulling back on the syringe plunger before injecting the product. Intramuscular injections can be done in any large muscle mass using a 4-cm, 22- to 16-gauge needle, depending on the viscosity of the drug. The neck region should be avoided. On most llamas restrained in a chute, the hind legs are most accessible. The semimembranosus and semitendinosus muscles are the sites of choice. If frequent injections are needed, the injection sites should be rotated to avoid soreness. The area of the triceps in the angle formed by the scapula and the humerus may also be used.

Subcutaneous Injections

The technique is similar to that used in other species. The preferred sites include the skin of the thorax and caudal to the elbow, where wool is usually absent.

Intravenous Injections

The landmarks and the technique are similar to those used for blood collection. The tip of the needle is directed caudally so that the operator is warned of inadvertent carotid artery penetration by high-pressure, bright red blood exiting the hub of the needle. If intravenous catheterization is required, the same technique can be applied in the midcervical area. The right jugular is preferred to avoid the esophagus. A large area is clipped and prepared. Except in juveniles or adults with thin skin, the turgid vein is not seen but can occasionally be felt upon percussion. The skin is usually penetrated superficially with a No. 15 scalpel blade first and then a sterile 14-cm, 16- or 14-gauge catheter is inserted and secured to the skin.

Orogastric Intubation

Medication, fluids, or food can be administered with a stomach tube. The technique is fairly similar to the procedure for sheep and cattle. Adult llamas usually resist and may regurgitate, increasing the likelihood of aspiration pneumonia. Restraint is important and use of a chute with cross-ties is helpful. A speculum is necessary to protect the tube. The Frick's speculum used in cattle is usually too big, except for the largest llamas. A 20-cm-long segment of PVC pipe, slightly wider than the stomach tube, can be used. The edges must be smoothed or wrapped with adhesive tape. Once the head is secured and slightly flexed, the lubricated tip of the stomach tube is advanced caudally through the speculum to the throat. Gentle pressure and rotation of the tube encourage swallowing. A little resistance should be felt as the tube is advanced into the esophagus. The most reliable sign of correct tube placement is palpating it in the left cervical region.

Neonatal Care

At birth, crias are covered by a semitransparent epidermal membrane attached to all mucocutaneous junctions. Within an hour after birth, normal crias can stand and nurse. Average birth weight ranges from 8 to 18 kg. Llama crias weighing less than 8 kg are considered premature or dysmature and may require some special attention. Alpaca crias are somewhat smaller; crias weighing less than 5 kg are considered premature.

The first consideration is to make sure the cria can breathe by clearing the membranes and mucus away from the mouth and nostrils. A bulb syringe can be used to carefully suction mucus from the nostril. In addition, lifting and supporting the cria can help clear amniotic fluid from the respiratory tract. Respiration can be stimulated by rubbing the back or tickling the nose with a piece of straw. Artificial respiration can be done by mouth to nose resuscitation or more effectively by placing a small rubber tube (6 to 7 mm in diameter) in the cria's nostril and gently blowing intermittently at about 10 times/minute. Choanal atresia is a frequent congenital abnormality of llamas of which to be aware. Because llamas and alpacas are obligate nasal breathers, crias with these congenital abnormalities show difficulty in breathing, even when fluids have been cleared.

Postpartum care of the cria should include dipping the umbilical cord in 7% tincture of iodine or chlorhexidine (Nolvasan) diluted to a 0.5% solution. This should be done three times within the first 24 hours. Additional care includes drying and weighing the cria and watching for nursing of the colostrum. Normal crias nurse within the first hour following delivery. Crias nurse three or four times per hour, usually for less than 30 seconds each time. If the cria has not been observed nursing for 6 hours, supportive care should be given and llama colostrum should be given in feedings of about 100 to 200 ml every 2 to 3 hours. Goat or cow colostrum can be used as a substitute. Passage of meconium (first bowel movement) should occur within the first 18 to 20 hours.

For compromised crias, oxygen support is provided with a small tube inserted in one nostril and taped to the bridge of the nose. The tube is connected to humified oxygen and is advanced to the premeasured level of the eye. Initially, the oxygen flow rate is set at 5 L/minute and adjusted to the patient's needs, based on serial evaluations of arterial blood gases. Intravenous fluid is delivered via a 5-cm, 16- to 18-gauge catheter placed aseptically in the jugular vein or, alternatively, in the saphenous vein. The skin of the neonate is usually thin and may not require incision as in the adult, although this author finds it easier to make a small incision after disinfection and lidocaine desensitization. If long-term catheterization is necessary, a longer, flexible, 14-cm catheter is used. Cyanoacrylate glue is used to bond the hub of the catheter to the skin. Fluid maintenance requirements have not been established for crias. A rate of 60 to 80 ml/kg/day, plus additional fluid requirements to replace ongoing losses, is often used. The efficacy of fluid support is evaluated by frequent weight determination, urine production, and signs of overhydration.

If the cria does not or is not able to nurse, nutritional support can be provided by bottle feeding (soft plastic bottle with a lamb nipple) or orogastric tubing (Fig. 28-23). Tube feeding a cria is easy. A stallion catheter or soft rubber feeding tube is convenient for this use. Before insertion, the tube is held against the cria's side and the distance from the mouth to the base of the neck is measured. Water-soluble lubricant (K-Y Jelly) is applied to the tube, which is then slowly passed into the mouth. As the tube is swallowed and advanced to the premeasured length, it should be seen and felt on the side of the neck next to the trachea. To ensure that the tube is in the esophagus and not in the trachea, blow on the tube and watch for the stomach to expand or listen for gurgling sounds. Inject 10 to 15 ml of water into the tube before feeding. If the animal gags and/or coughs, the tube is probably in the lungs and should be withdrawn. If a substitute for the dam's milk is necessary, straight goat's milk or a 3:1 volume to volume mixture of goat milk and goat yogurt is recommended.

Herd Health

Immunization. A minimal vaccination program should include *Clostridium perfringens* C/D and tetanus. Recommendations include annual C/D and tetanus administration for all juveniles (starting at 3 months) and adults. Pregnant females should receive a C/D and tetanus booster 1 month before the anticipated parturition date. Recent information indicates that vaccination of the cria within the first week of age, followed by two monthly boosters, is effective irrespective of colostral immunity. Immunization with 7- or 8-way clostridial vaccine may cause significant injection site reactions. Other vaccinations to consider vary with the area of the country. If leptospirosis is a problem in the region, biannual vaccination of brood females should be considered. No rabies vaccine efficacy testing has been conducted in the llama, yet no adverse reaction following administration of the killed vaccine has been reported.

Parasite Control. New World camelids are susceptible to all the nematode parasites that affect ruminants. *Parelophostrongylus tenuis* is a major concern in areas inhabited by white tail deer. In enzootic liver fluke areas, llamas should be checked periodically for flukes. Coccidiosis may be a significant cause of diarrhea in young animals. Establishment of a parasite-control program depends on the geographic area, climatic conditions, number of animals, and stocking rate. Fenbendazole and ivermectin have been used successfully to control most nematodes. A minimum of two dewormings (spring and fall) is recommended. In areas with meningeal worms, monthly deworming with ivermectin or daily administration of Strongid C can be used.

Lice are the most common external parasites of llama herds. Topical treatment with organophosphate or carbamate powder is effective. Mange mite infestation is not very common, probably because of extensive use of ivermectin.

Common Procedures. Male llamas generally need to have their fighting teeth (incisors and canines) cut by 2 to 2.5 years of age. This procedure can be rapidly done in a restraining chute or under general anesthesia using a surgical wire. Castration is usually performed after 2 years of age but can be done earlier if necessary.

Acknowledgment. The author is grateful to Kesling's Llamas and Alpacas for their assistance in obtaining the photographs used in this section.

RECOMMENDED READING

Alpaca Net, Internet web site, address: http://www.alpacanet.com/
Fowler ME: *Medicine and surgery of South American camelids,* Ames, Iowa, 1989, Iowa State University Press.
Johnson LW: *Vet Clin North Am* 5(1), 1989 and 10(2), 1994.
McGee M, Tellington-Jones T: *Llama handling and training,* Dundee, New York, 1992, Zephyr Farm Press.
Llama Banner, monthly magazine, PO Box 1968, Manhattan, Kan 66502.
Llamas, bimonthly magazine, PO Box 100, Herald, Calif 85638.
Llama Web, Internet web site, address: http://www.webcom/com/degraham/

CARE OF RATITES

J.T. BLACKFORD

Ratites are a group of nonflying birds that include the ostrich (*Struthio casmelus*), the emu (*Dromaius novaehollandiae*), and the rhea (*Rhea americana*). The cassowary (*Casuarius casuarius*) is also included in this group; they are primarily concentrated on the west coast of the United States.

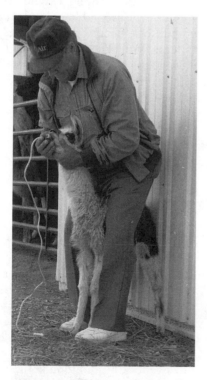

FIG. 28-23 Passing a flexible feeding tube into the nostril of a cria. Note that the cria is restrained by backing against a wall.

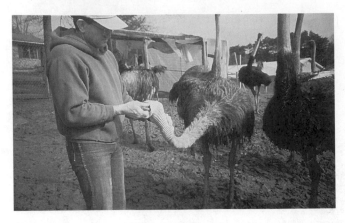

FIG. 28-24   Ostriches can be calmed by applying a cloth hood, such as a sock with the toe cut off.

RESTRAINT

Restraining is one of the most important skills to master when working with ratites. Many owners are unable to restrain their own birds and frequently their facilities are less than ideal. The birds have very powerful legs that can inflict severe trauma from kicking. The emu, rhea, and cassowary have sharp claws that can easily lacerate the handler. The danger zone when working on ratites is directly in front of the birds, because they strike forward when they kick. The emu and rhea can also kick to the side, but the most powerful segment of the kick is in front.

Chicks can easily be handled by placing a hand between their legs while cupping the sternum and picking them up, much like holding a football. While in a sitting position, the handler can treat small juvenile birds by placing the bird in the lap, with the bird's legs squeezed between the handler's knees. Larger juveniles can be held standing from the back or from the side, keeping the bird close to the handler's body. When restraining from the back, your feet should be spread apart to help maintain balance, but your knees should be held close together to prevent the bird from backing under you.

Adult birds are more difficult and risky to handle. It is frequently necessary to capture large juveniles or adult ostriches in an open pen. Applying a loose, tubular cloth hood over the head and covering the eyes commonly calms the bird so that evaluation and treatment can be carried out (Fig. 28-24). These birds are generally curious and will approach strangers. The hood is placed over the handler's forearm. When the bird is within reach, the neck is grasped and pulled down parallel to the ground with the opposite hand. Simultaneously the beak is grasped and the hood is everted over the head, leaving the nares exposed. If the bird does not approach the handler, a shepherd's hook can be used to capture the head.

The hood is then applied as described. To move the bird, a second handler grasps the tail from behind, pushing forward as gentle traction on the neck steers in the desired direction. Ostriches can also be restrained in stocks or in chutes designed for the birds. When this type of facility is not available, the birds can be restrained by squeezing the bird between a solid gate and a wall. Caution should be used when working around adult birds, especially males during the breeding season, as these birds can be aggressive.

Emus in general are not aggressive and males frequently become more docile during the breeding season. Adult emus present more difficulty in handling, because they commonly become very fractious when restrained. Their sharp claws and rough, scaly tarsometatarsus can tear clothing and severely abrade the handler's skin. Many emus do not resist mild restraint. To catch and restrain them, pass an arm around the neck near the sternum and pull the bird firmly into your upper legs and trunk, tilting the bird into an upright position. Low placement of the arm minimizes the chance of injury from kicking. The bird can be moved from this position, being careful to keep the animal in contact with your body. Sometimes moving the bird backward is easier than moving forward and it is occasionally necessary to simply pick the birds up to move them.

Male rheas are the most aggressive of the three common species. Restraint is most easily accomplished by two handlers. The first handler catches the bird as described for emus. The second handler then grasps the bird's legs and pulls the bird to the ground between the first handler's legs. With the bird's legs held, one individual straddles the recumbent bird on his or her knees, placing gentle pressure on the dorsum of the bird.

A hood can be applied to rheas, but the results are much less predictable than with ostriches. Another option that should be considered, when possible, is working on the birds in a darkened enclosure. This environment has a calming effect on the birds.

Visual Evaluation

Visual assessment of the entire flock may provide pertinent information about individual health. The birds' activity level should be noted. The initial response when a stranger approaches and enters a pen is for the birds to run from the intruder. Most will then return out of curiosity. When possible, the birds should be observed while they are eating. A food bolus can normally be observed as it passes down the cervical esophagus. Unhealthy or sick birds may go through the motions as if they are eating, pecking and throwing their head upward as if to swallow, but no food bolus is seen passing down the neck. Closer examination should be performed on birds that are inactive, that lag behind, or that are not actively eating.

Note asymmetry of the neck and dorsal spine, and deviations of the appendages. During the visual examination note condition of the integumentary system. Unthrifty plumage may indicate trauma, ectoparasites, nutritional deficiency, or feather plucking by other birds, suggesting overcrowding or boredom.

Physical Examination

The heart rate (60 to 120 beats/min) is most easily determined by auscultation laterally, between the ribs. The respiratory rate (10 to 40 breaths/min) is best determined visually in the unrestrained patient. Temperature (100° to 104° F) can be measured with a rectal or tympanic membrane thermometer. The external ear canal is a large opening caudal to the mandible at the base of the skull. Cloacal temperatures may be 1 or 2 degrees lower than tympanic membrane temperature.

The eye can be superficially examined with a good penlight. The ear canal is easily explored with an otoscope for parasites, hemorrhage, or masses. When the mouth is opened, the mucous membranes are evaluated for color (pink) and capillary refill time (< 2.5 sec). Symmetry of the choana (nasopharynx), glottis, and rostral trachea should be noted. Choanal or tracheal swabs can be made for bacterial culture and cytology when a discharge is noted. The neck is palpated for asymmetry of the trachea, right jugular vein, and vertebrae.

The thorax is auscultated and palpated. Auscultation is performed, noting abnormal respiratory sounds associated with the lungs or air sacs. Heart murmurs can also be detected by auscultation of the thorax. There is very little muscle over the thorax, making palpation easy for any signs of asymmetry associated with rib fractures or masses.

The abdomen is easily palpated in the chick. Structures that should be noted include the proventriculus and yolk sac. The proventriculus lies just to the left of the midline, caudal to the rib cage. The structure is firm to the touch and should have feed material within it that is easily compressed with gentle pressure. An empty proventriculus is firm. The yolk sac has the feel of a large bladder, decreasing in size over a 2-week period, when it should be absorbed. As the yolk sac is absorbed, the intestines become more palpable in the young chick.

These structures are not as evident in the adult bird. However, impaction associated with the proventriculus or egg retention can be recognized during careful evaluation of the adult bird's abdomen.

The cloaca should be examined for accumulation of fecal matter and urates on the feathers surrounding the opening. This commonly indicates illness or depression. Mucosal prolapse may be indicative of intestinal obstruction or local trauma. The genitalia can also be evaluated within the cloacal sphincter.

The skin and feathers are evaluated for parasites and trauma. These birds groom themselves, so the feathers should be relatively clean and well separated, unless they have recently given themselves a dust bath. Feather regrowth is a good indicator of adequate nutrition.

The wings and limbs of the birds should be examined closely, both visually and by palpation. Ostriches and rheas have well-developed wings, whereas the wing of the emu is vestigial and difficult to see when it is held close to the body. Asymmetry is noted and the structures are palpated for fractures and dislocations.

The thigh and calf regions are well muscled, making direct palpation of the femur and tibiotarsus difficult. The tarsometatarsus and phalanges are easily palpated, because there is very little tissue covering these areas. Swollen joints should be noted and the cause explored. The tendons and their sheaths should be examined for pain and swelling. Tendon luxation over the tibiotarsus and the metatarsophalangeal joint are common injuries. The foot should always be examined closely for heat, pain, and swelling. Asymmetry surrounding a phalangeal joint should be carefully explored because of the common incidence of puncture wounds involving these joints. Traumatic avulsion of the toenails may lead to localized infection.

COMMON DIAGNOSTIC AND THERAPEUTIC TECHNIQUES

Blood Sampling and Catheterization

Blood sampling and catheterization can be performed on the right jugular, cutaneous ulnar, and medial metatarsal veins. The jugular vein is easily distended and visualized in the ostrich and rhea. Watching for feather motion along the course of the distending vein on the neck helps to locate it in the emu. Feathers can be plucked to help visualize the vessel. When this vessel is catheterized, placement is in the upper (cranial) one third of the neck, to prevent the bird from pulling it out. Care is taken not to penetrate the trachea or esophagus.

In the ostrich and rhea, the cutaneous ulnar vein is located on the ventral aspect of the wing, coursing over the distal antebrachium. The vestigial wing in the emu makes this vein impractical for blood sampling and catheterization. Catheters placed in the wing vein should be protected to prevent the bird from pulling them out.

The medial metatarsal vein is located on the medial aspect of the leg, paralleling the metatarsus. Care is taken when collecting blood from this area, because the vessel is easily lacerated if the bird kicks during sampling.

Needles and catheters of 20 to 22 gauge are commonly used in these birds. Larger catheters can be placed in the jugular vein when rapid fluid volume replacement is indicated.

Heparin tubes should be used for collecting ostrich blood, because it is adversely affected by EDTA. This sample can be used for both hematologic and serum chemistry evaluations. EDTA and clot tubes are suitable for blood collection in emus and rheas.

Fluid Therapy

Fluids can be administered parenterally or enterally. Parenteral administration is performed subcutaneously or intravenously. Maintenance fluids are administered at 13 ml/kg/hr (range 5 to 28 ml/kg/hr). Enteral fluid administration is performed via an orogastric tube.

Orogastric Tube Placement

Gastric intubation is used to administer fluids, nutrients, and medication. The mouth is opened by grasping the upper beak and the tube is then directed over the glottis. Once past the glottis, the tube is easily visualized externally, passing down the cervical esophagus. Care is taken to prevent regurgitation while administering substances through the tube. Esophagostomy tube placement should be considered when long-term enteral nutrition is indicated.

Injections

Subcutaneous injections can be given over the lateral thorax caudal to the leg. The skin is lifted and the needle is inserted with care to prevent inadvertent penetration into the chest cavity. Intramuscular injections are usually given in the abaxial muscles over the rump and in the proximal thigh. Intravenous injections are administered in the same locations as described for blood sampling, although the metatarsal vein is seldom used for this purpose.

Pill Administration

Pills or boluses can be given by grasping the upper beak and gently prying the mouth open. Occasionally a finger must be inserted into the commissure to assist in opening the mouth. The pill is then placed over the glottis and a finger is used to push it into the cervical esophagus.

RECOMMENDED READING

Jensen J et al: *Husbandry and medical management of ostriches, emus and rheas,* College Station, Texas, 1996, Wildlife and Exotic Animal Consultants.

Tully TN, Shane SM: *Ratite management, medicine, and surgery,* Malabar, Fla, 1996, Krieger Publishing.

CHAPTER 29

Nursing Care of Cage Birds and Poultry

G.L. De Longe

Learning Objectives

After reviewing this chapter, the reader should understand the following:

Anatomy of birds
Behavior of birds
Capture and restraint techniques used for birds

Methods of sample collection for laboratory analysis
Routes of administration of medication
Techniques used in general nursing care of birds
Procedures used in nail, beak, and feather care
Principles of poultry health management

CAGE BIRDS

The pet birds seen in practice usually are members of the psittacine or passerine family. These are distinguished by a number of physical characteristics.

Psittacines, or parrots, make up the majority of avian patients. They are more numerous and their owners have usually invested $200 to $2500, with some of the more exotic macaws retailing for up to $15,000. Owners who have purchased a bird of this value are very willing to consult a veterinarian.

The psittacines are also known as hookbills because of their highly curved beak. Their feet are characterized by two toes pointing forward and the same number pointing backward. Many parrots use these agile feet to hold food while they eat or manipulate objects they are interested in exploring. They tend to be good climbers, often moving around their cage using a combination of beak and feet. Many parrots are well socialized and hand trained, coming out of their cage to spend a portion of their day associating directly with their human families. These birds range in weight from a few grams up to 1700 g. Many of them can become accomplished talkers. Most commonly seen in practice are the larger parrots, such as African grays, Amazons, cockatoos, Eclectus, and the large macaws. Occasionally presented for treatment are cockatiels, lovebirds, and the budgerigar, or budgie, known as the *parakeet* in the United States.

Passerines are usually small birds with a pointed or slightly curved beak. Their feet are shaped so that three toes point forward and one toe points to the rear. Many species of these birds are very active and tend to hop or fly about their cage. Most are not trained to sit on their owner's hand and remain inside their cages. Canaries and finches are the most frequently kept passerines.

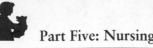

ROLE OF THE VETERINARY PRACTICE IN BIRD CARE

Many birds are seen for the first time in practice when they are exhibiting obvious signs of disease. Generally, birds mask their illness until it is far advanced. Owners who recognize a slight difference in behavior, attitude, or physical condition should be asked to bring their bird in for immediate examination.

Any new bird should be examined by a knowledgeable veterinarian within 3 days of purchase, preferably before it is taken to its new home. Many breeders and pet stores offer a limited health guarantee, and it is important for the bird to be seen before this agreement expires. Once at its new home, the new bird should be isolated from any other birds until all test results are received.

In addition to being weighed and thoroughly examined, a new bird should at a minimum be tested for common avian diseases, be swabbed for cultures and/or Gram stains of the choana and cloaca, and have a baseline set of tests including a CBC and blood chemistries performed. Some practices may elect to include a fecal examination and urinalysis. Because the sex of cage birds is impossible to determine in most species by feather coloration or physical appearance, new owners may request sexing using a blood sample.

A regular annual physical examination is very important. Because birds often cover up signs of illness and the feathers may hide weight loss, owners should bring their bird in for a physical, a CBC, basic blood chemistries, and possibly a screening culture or swab of the choana and cloaca annually. If the bird has been exposed to other birds that were or later became ill, it may be tested for other specific diseases as well. Vaccination of birds is not a routine matter as in cats or dogs, so it is important to emphasize the health value of annual checkups and testing.

A bird is often presented for routine grooming procedures, such as wing clipping, nail trimming, or beak shaping. Implantation of microchips or application of leg bands for identification are performed. Removal of the closed leg bands placed on a domestically bred, hand-raised baby bird is often requested because of safety concerns.

Specific diagnostic procedures, such as radiography, endoscopy, and ultrasound examination, are common. Surgical procedures, such as sexing, fracture repair, and removal of feather cysts, are often done in practice. Anesthesia of birds is similar to that performed in small animals but may actually be used more often for minor procedures where total restraint is required.

Avian emergencies are not unusual. Birds are curious, fragile, easily startled creatures that can readily be injured. Poisonings, reproductive disorders, gastrointestinal problems, dyspnea, seizures, and traumatic injuries are all common.

Disease related to nutritional problems is one of the primary reasons birds are brought to the veterinary hospital. Discussion of a bird's diet and eating habits is a major part of working with the bird owner. A thorough knowledge of basic bird nutrition and available commercial foods is an essential part of avian practice.

Sick birds must be medicated in the hospital or by the owner at home. The hospital staff must be experienced and competent at administering medication and instructing clients in proper techniques.

Client education is an important part of avian practice. Clients considering purchase of a pet bird sometimes consult with a veterinary practice about the characteristics of a given species. They often have questions concerning proper diets, grooming procedures, and behavior. Many practices prepare educational materials on these topics for distribution to clients.

Basic behavioral counseling should be done only by hospital personnel very familiar with the nature and needs of both hand-raised and wild-caught parrots. In difficult cases, the client can be referred to an avian behaviorist, several of whom are veterinary technicians.

Time is an important part of the bird owner–practice relationship. Pet bird appointments take longer than those for small animals, generally at least 30 minutes. Taking a complete history, discussing nutrition, observing the bird, completing a physical examination, and performing laboratory procedures are all time-consuming. Owners recognize the willingness of a practice to devote the necessary time to their birds and feel confident in the diagnosis and treatment recommended.

BASIC PET BIRD BEHAVIOR

Pet birds retain many behaviors inherent in their wild ancestors. New owners who have not thoroughly researched species characteristics before purchasing their bird may be unpleasantly surprised by some of the traits exhibited by their pet. Veterinary personnel working with birds must also understand some of the expected reactions of their patients to common procedures.

A natural behavior in psittacines is *mouthing* or using the tongue to explore surfaces. Juvenile parrots pass through an innocent "beaking" phase, in which they attempt to taste or chew almost anything, somewhat like puppies do. People unfamiliar with this behavior often feel the bird is attempting to bite, so they pull back suddenly, which encourages the bird. Most well-adapted young hand-raised birds do not bite humans unless they have been frightened or hurt.

Mature parrots are more likely to bite during handling as a defensive move. The larger psittacines, such as macaws, can exert up to 300 pounds of pressure per square inch, inflicting deep bruises and even lacerations that require suturing. Birds as small as cockatiels have the potential to draw blood. Birds may strike at any portion of the body, so handlers must be alert and cautious when working with them.

All birds commonly show fear reactions when startled. They may fling themselves about the cage, struggle violently, flap their wings, scream loudly, or take flight in response to sudden movements or unfamiliar sights. Birds may easily be injured in their efforts to get away.

Psittacines tend to vocalize in response to discomfort or restraint. Unhappy parrots can scream loudly enough to damage human hearing. Some clinics' employees routinely wear hearing protection when handling birds or working near birds in a boarding facility.

All birds defecate frequently, at least every 15 to 20 minutes, and more often when afraid or stressed. The typical behavior that indicates defecation in a calm bird is a slight wiggle of the tail, followed by a squat and an uplifted tail. Watching for this action can help prevent soiled clothing.

Other common behaviors may be disconcerting to those new to birds. Wagging of the tail back and forth usually indicates a relaxed, happy bird. Beak grinding in a bird that is sitting quietly usually signals readiness to fall asleep. Young hand-fed birds or older birds that are very bonded to their owners may regurgitate food from the crop into the mouth as a sign of affection, which owners may interpret as a sign of illness.

Care must be taken when speaking around birds at the clinic. More than one practice has been embarrassed when a talking bird repeats an unsavory word or derogatory phrase after a stay at the clinic. Birds also tend to readily imitate piercing, repetitive, or bodily function sounds.

The behavior of pet birds is very different from that of cats or dogs and techniques that work well in those species are often inappropriate for use in birds. The emotional intelligence of many of the large psittacines is on the level of a 2-year-old child. Some African grays approach the abilities of a 5-year-old human in problem-solving skills and speech patterns. This high level of intelligence results in a patient that is both entertaining and challenging.

Owners of pet birds often seek help with such problems as biting, screaming, or destructive feather picking. Many of the behaviors that owners wish to modify are the result of instinctive avian reactions or related to the stresses of captivity.

Psittacines attempt to become dominant over their flock, in this case their human family. It is important that the owner and other household members use certain techniques to maintain the dominant position in the home. Birds should be taught to consistently step up on or down from the owner's hand when asked. Clipping the bird's

wings to limit its flying ability will diminish dominance behaviors, such as flying down from a curtain rod to attack a person. When holding the bird, keep it at midchest level. Never allowing it to sit on the head or shoulders keeps it from attaining the highest perch, a position of great power. Situating the cage or perches so that the bird is below eye level also discourages dominant behavior.

Biting is a common behavior problem. Birds bite to exhibit dominance, express fear, or exhibit jealousy, or as a result of hormonal fluctuations during puberty or the breeding season. It is important for the owner to realize that the bird must not be allowed to bite as a way of controlling any situation.

Vocalization is essential to birds, but it may become a problem in some insecure or dependent birds that call constantly to their owner. Birds tend to be very noisy at dawn and dusk, around feeding time, in response to loud sounds, in an effort to locate flock members, or out of loneliness. Some species are relatively quiet, but all birds make a certain amount of noise. Owners may accidentally encourage the bird to make more noise if they respond to loud calls with anger or shouting in an effort to quiet the bird.

Feather picking, or plucking, is a well-known but poorly understood condition. The bird uses its beak to pull out any feathers that are accessible, including any that start to grow back. Some birds remove all but the feathers on their heads and some may damage skin as well as muscle. Some affected birds have an underlying physical illness that initiates plucking, but some healthy birds respond to stress, such as from separation from their owner or change in their cage location, by pulling out feathers. This is a difficult problem to solve and may become a chronic condition.

Correction of behavior problems takes time, an understanding of the underlying cause, and judicious use of behavior modification. Prolonged physical or mental isolation of the bird, withholding food or water, and physical punishment are totally unacceptable methods of dealing with these problems. All may result in permanent emotional or physical damage to the bird.

Unfortunately, many people do not know where to go to receive accurate and helpful advice, often first seeking answers from poorly informed pet store employees. In addition, readily available older books often contain advice that might apply to wild-caught parrots, but is not suitable for hand-raised birds. Many misinformed owners have worsened the very behavior they wish to eliminate by using inappropriate techniques. A veterinary clinic that treats pet birds must know the basics of bird behavior and be prepared to refer problem cases to avian behaviorists. The most current listing of behavioral consultants is found in reputable avian magazines. Practices should provide the client with several references and encourage the owner to interview the behaviorists until they find one who is compatible and whose techniques make sense.

AVIAN ANATOMY
Feathers and Skin

Feathers, which are arranged in distinct tracts over the surface of the body, provide warmth and protection. Molting occurs in all species and results in periodic replacement of old feathers. A new, growing feather has a vascular supply until it reaches full size. The shafts of these blood feathers appear dark and bleed profusely if broken, possibly leading to the death of the bird.

Birds spend several hours daily preening, or rearranging and conditioning their feathers. Almost all species have a preen gland located at the base of their tail. The oily secretion from this gland is spread over the surface of the feathers to make them more water resistant.

Birds have several types of feathers (Figs. 29-1 and 29-2). The *contour feathers* cover the body and wings and are identified as flight feathers or body feathers. The large, *primary flight feathers (remiges)* are found on the outer end of the wing. The *secondary flight feathers* are located on the wing between the body and the primaries. *Body feathers*, also known as *coverts*, provide surface coverage over most of the rest of the bird.

Down feathers insulate the bird and have a soft, fluffy appearance. Cockatoos, cockatiels, and African grays have powder down, which breaks down to produce a white dusty powder. A healthy bird of these species produces dust that is evident on dark clothing after the bird makes contact with it and the bird's beak after a grooming session.

The skin is very delicate and has a dry, slightly wrinkled appearance. Underlying muscles and blood give the skin a reddish appearance in some areas. The skin on the legs resembles the scales of reptiles. The cere, or the area around the nostrils, the beak, and the nails are all modified skin (see Fig. 29-1).

Pet birds often have spectacularly colorful plumage. However, it is important to realize that it is virtually impossible to determine the sex of cage birds by appearance, because males and females of each species look identical. The major exception to this rule is the Eclectus parrot, in which the female is a deep reddish color with a dark beak, and the male is bright green with an orange beak. Some owners attempt to sex their birds using a combination of head and beak shape or size, pelvic bone configuration, and overall size. Blood testing is available to reliably determine the sex of the bird from a small sample.

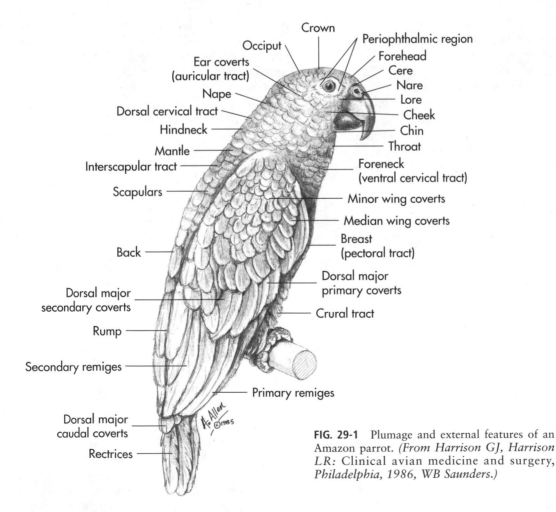

FIG. 29-1 Plumage and external features of an Amazon parrot. *(From Harrison GJ, Harrison LR: Clinical avian medicine and surgery, Philadelphia, 1986, WB Saunders.)*

Musculoskeletal System

The skeleton of birds is highly modified. Some bones are *pneumatized*, or contain air, which results in a lighter skeleton. The bones have thin walls, which makes them lighter but also more fragile. The skull bones are fused, which strengthens the beak structure. The vertebrae of the neck are shaped in such a way as to create a long, flexible neck. The large sternum, or keel, supports the pectoral muscles that are needed for flight. A large portion of the caudal vertebrae is fused to form the synsacrum, which stabilizes the back during flight.

The largest muscles in the body are the pectorals, which account for approximately 20% of the bird's weight. Because of their mass, they are used to determine the body condition of the bird and ideal for intramuscular injections.

Respiratory System

Air enters the respiratory system through the nostrils, travels through the many sinuses in the head, and then enters the oral cavity through the slit-like opening in the roof of the mouth known as the *choana*. It then travels into the opening of the trachea at the base of the tongue and through the syrinx, or vocal organ. The air continues into the small lungs, where air exchange takes place, but which do not have alveoli and therefore do not inflate. Air next flows into the *air sacs*, which are hollow membranous bags that help move air throughout the respiratory system. Birds have one single and four paired air sacs located within the body cavity. Birds lack a muscular diaphragm and depend on the movement of the rib cage to push air through the respiratory tract. Two complete breath cycles are necessary to move a breath of air completely through the respiratory system.

Digestive System

The high metabolism of birds requires ingestion of large amounts of food. The beak is used to grasp food and crush it with the aid of the tongue. Birds do not have teeth. The mouth is relatively dry, because little saliva is produced. Another avian anatomic variation is the location of the esophagus, which lies on the right side of the neck, as opposed to the left side as in mammals.

When food is swallowed, it travels through the esophagus to the crop at the base of the neck (Fig. 29-3). The crop, an enlargement of the esophagus in most birds, softens food and allows continuous passage of small amounts of food to the proventriculus, or true stomach. In young birds, the crop may become very distended after a meal. The proventriculus is very similar to the stomach of mammals, containing digestive acid and enzymes.

The food next passes into the ventriculus, or gizzard. This is a thickly muscled organ that grinds food into smaller particles. Most wild birds need grit, or small pieces of gravel, in the gizzard to break down hard foods. Pet birds may develop an impaction if given grit.

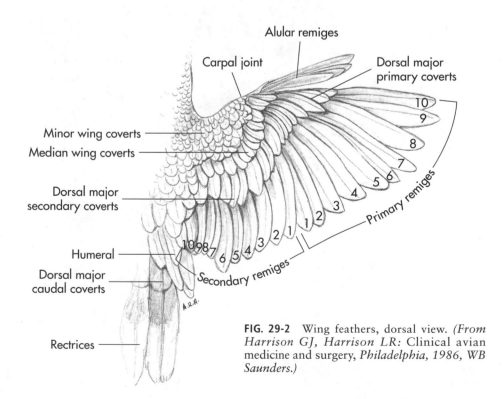

FIG. 29-2 Wing feathers, dorsal view. *(From Harrison GJ, Harrison LR: Clinical avian medicine and surgery, Philadelphia, 1986, WB Saunders.)*

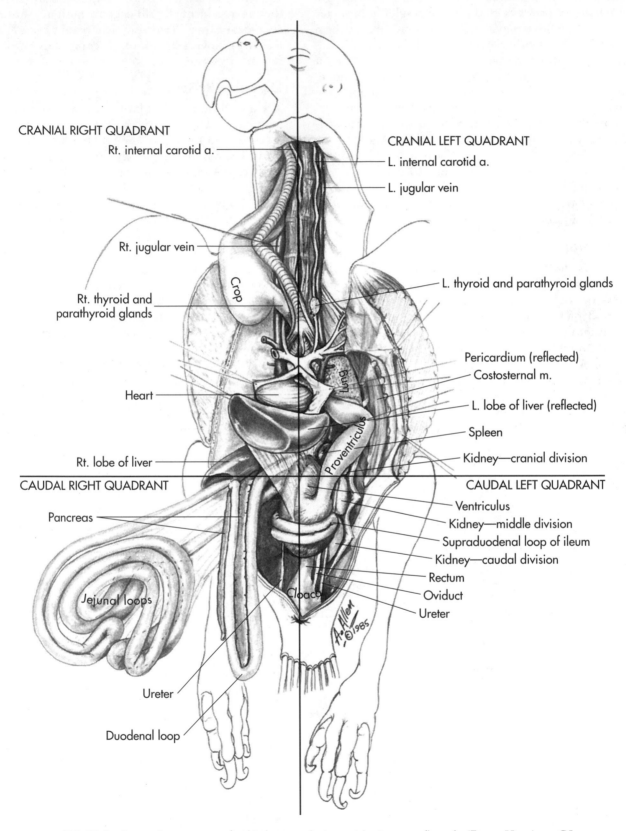

CRANIAL RIGHT QUADRANT

CRANIAL LEFT QUADRANT

Rt. internal carotid a.

L. internal carotid a.

L. jugular vein

Rt. jugular vein

Crop

L. thyroid and parathyroid glands

Rt. thyroid and parathyroid glands

Pericardium (reflected)

Costosternal m.

Lung

Heart

L. lobe of liver (reflected)

Proventriculus

Spleen

Kidney—cranial division

Rt. lobe of liver

CAUDAL RIGHT QUADRANT

CAUDAL LEFT QUADRANT

Ventriculus

Pancreas

Kidney—middle division

Supraduodenal loop of ileum

Kidney—caudal division

Jejunal loops

Rectum

Cloaca

Oviduct

Ureter

Ureter

Duodenal loop

A. Allen ©1985

FIG. 29-3 Internal structures of a bird, ventral view with viscera reflected. *(From Harrison GJ, Harrison LR: Clinical avian medicine and surgery, Philadelphia, 1986, WB Saunders.)*

The intestinal tract is very similar to that of mammals. Birds have a pancreas and bilobed liver that produce digestive enzymes and bile. The large intestine terminates at the cloaca, which is the chamber into which materials from the digestive, urinary, and reproductive systems pass before release from the body (see Fig. 29-3). The external opening of the cloaca is termed the vent, from which the droppings are passed. The droppings, which include feces, urine, and urates, vary in consistency, depending on the diet.

Urinary System

The paired kidneys of birds are closely attached to the vertebrae (see Fig. 29-3). They empty into ureters, which carry the liquid urine and semisolid urates to the cloaca. Urates, or uric acid, are the major excretion product in birds and comprise the white portion of the droppings. Birds do not have a urinary bladder.

Reproductive System

In the female bird, only the left side of the reproductive tract develops fully. As in mammals, an ovary, oviduct, and vagina are present. Various regions of the oviduct produce the egg white and eggshell. The entire process from ovulation to egg laying takes approximately 15 hours. The female lays eggs even if no male is present. If she is bred and produces fertile eggs, she is the one that determines the sex of the offspring.

The male bird has paired testes located internally near the kidneys. Sperm cells travel to the cloaca through the epididymis and then the ductus deferens. Most birds do not have a penis and mating takes place when the vents of the male and female birds come in contact.

Circulatory System

The heart of birds closely resembles that of mammals, but it is proportionally about one and one half times larger (see Fig. 29-3). Heart rates range from 150 to 300 beats per minute in large parrots, to 1400 beats per minute in the very small species. Blood pressure in birds is higher than in mammals.

The circulatory system of birds differs from that of mammals in several ways. The red blood cells of birds are oval and contain a nucleus (see Chapter 11). Birds do not have lymph nodes and the lymphatic system is less extensive.

Special Senses

The eyes of birds are relatively large. Their vision is very acute and they can perceive color. Birds often look closely at something with one eye, tilting their head for a better view. In many species, the color of the iris is often darker in young birds. Birds also have voluntary control of the muscles of the iris and often rapidly change the size of the circular pupil when excited or intrigued. Blinking is done using the almost transparent nictitating membrane, or third eyelid. Most birds close their eyes only when they sleep.

The ears of birds are hidden from view by feathers, which have a slightly different appearance and sometimes are a different color. The external opening is located caudal and ventral to the eye (see Fig. 29-1). The auditory range is similar to that of humans.

Taste and smell are difficult senses to evaluate. Birds have fewer taste buds than humans, and these taste buds are located on the roof of the mouth, not on the tongue. Birds can taste, but it is unknown how well. Smell appears to be poorly developed.

RESTRAINT

A cornerstone of avian practice is proper restraint. Restraint is often required to ensure the safety of the avian patient and the personnel handling the bird during diagnostic and therapeutic procedures. Effective restraint often requires two or more people, so good planning and communication between those involved are vital. This section details many of the techniques commonly used in practice for capture, restraint, and release of pet birds.

Typical reactions to restraint include struggling, vocalizing loudly, flapping of the wings, attempting to bite, and grasping with the feet. Individual birds react differently to being restrained. Their actions depend on their species, previous experiences with restraint, and types of contact with people. Young, hand-fed parrots are often very accepting of human handling, whereas wild-caught birds used for breeding may be extremely difficult to capture and restrain. The speed and agility of small species, such as finches, which are never handled by the owner because of their temperament and size, make them challenging to catch and hold.

Restraint Techniques

A terry cloth towel is often useful when capturing and restraining birds ranging in size from the cockatiels or conures to the largest parrots (Fig. 29-4). Paper towels are sometimes used when restraining budgies, cockatiels, or conures. The towel, which is often draped over the hand during capture, is arranged during restraint so that the bird's nares are exposed without uncovering the eyes. The bird should be allowed to chew on the towel if it wishes, which keeps its beak busy and makes it less likely for the holder to be bitten. The smallest birds, such as finches, canaries, and budgerigars, are usually captured using a bare hand. The nails or wings of the very small birds may become entangled in a towel, leading to traumatic fractures or other related problems. It is also difficult to evaluate very small patients held in a towel.

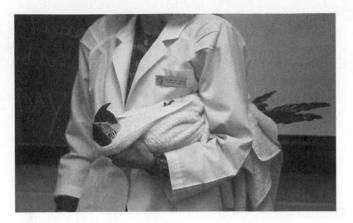

FIG. 29-4   Blue and gold macaw wrapped in a towel and restrained by one person for treatment.

The technician should approach any size bird with confidence so that capture is prompt. Once the capture process is initiated, the technician must remain in control of the situation and persist until the bird is well secured. Birds are often captured from the back in order to avoid the beak, but some birds are less frightened if approached from the front.

Once the patient is caught, the basic towel-wrapping technique is similar for all sizes of birds. The head is firmly gripped from the rear without putting pressure on the eyes. In the larger birds, the ear openings are convenient positioning areas that are easily felt through the towel. Next, the body is grasped and the wings are quickly folded close to the body in their natural position. This protects the wings from damage and prevents trauma to the holder from flapping wings. The towel is then tucked around the bird, which is positioned so that its chest is exposed. The feet must next be restrained so that the holder is not hurt by the sharp nails as the bird uses its legs and feet to grasp anything in an effort to free itself. A firm grip of the body is necessary, but it is easy to suffocate the bird by squeezing it too tightly.

Correct placement of the technician's hands is essential for proper positioning. When working with the smallest birds, grip the bird's head between your thumb and index finger. The little finger of the same hand restrains the bird's legs, while the remaining fingers circle the bird's trunk. This technique works well in both quiet and struggling birds.

In larger birds, such as cockatiels and conures, the head, neck, and trunk are grasped with one hand. The other hand is used to secure the feet or perform techniques, such as administration of medication. Larger birds sometimes require a two-handed restraint method, in which the head is held in one hand and the feet are gripped in the other hand. This allows the bird to be stretched and held very securely so that procedures can be readily performed by another person.

One person can single-handedly restrain most birds for a majority of procedures. Once the bird is caught and securely wrapped, the handler can control both the head and feet. The bird can be wrapped in such a way that the feet are immobilized, allowing the technician to administer medications and vaccinations (see Fig. 29-4).

Capture Techniques

Small pet birds, such as canaries, budgerigars, and conures, are usually transported to the veterinarian in their own cage. They must be safely and gently removed for a hands-on physical examination. Slow and deliberate movements minimize stress to the bird, accompanied by a quiet tone of voice for reassurance. It may be helpful to dim the room lights before proceeding, because this calms some birds.

Large pet birds are generally brought to the clinic in a carrier, because their cages are usually too large to transport. Allowing the bird to ride freely on the owner's hand or shoulder should be discouraged, because the bird may escape after a frightening incident even if its wings have been trimmed to prevent flight.

Larger parrots may be caught in the cage, in the carrier, on the floor, or from a table top. As with small birds, a slow and deliberate approach works best. A quiet, soothing tone of voice should be used when relating to the bird. In most cases a towel is used during capture to avoid injury to the bird or technician. It is extremely important to exhibit confidence in the approach to large birds, because they may become aggressive when they detect uncertainty. Birds that are easily removed from the cage may be placed on the floor by the owner or technician. Once on the floor, the bird feels vulnerable, is less likely to fight, and is unable to move very quickly. The towel is thrown over the bird and it is picked up. This technique is often used with Amazons and macaws. Birds that are accustomed to being handled with a towel by the owner may sometimes be caught by approaching from the front while on the floor or a table top and gently wrapping the towel from front to back.

A larger bird that was caught on the floor or countertop is usually released onto the floor. The holder positions the wrapped patient so that it will be standing when the towel is removed. Keeping a good grip on the head and body, place the bird feet down on the floor. The towel is then smoothly removed from the body, the head is released, and the restrainer steps back to avoid a strike by the bird.

If a bird is to be released into a cage or carrier, care must be taken to avoid injury by placing it onto the floor of the container, never on a perch. Hands should be quickly withdrawn after release to avoid being bitten by an angry bird.

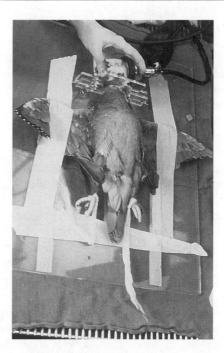

FIG. 29-5 Anesthetized double yellow-head Amazon parrot taped to a restraint board in dorsal recumbency. Note the mask in place over the face to maintain anesthesia.

Restraint Board. The restraint board is used for procedures that require the awake (not anesthetized) bird to remain completely still, such as for radiographs or implantation of microchips for identification. In other situations, both hands may be needed to perform complicated tasks. Anesthetized birds can be positioned on the restraint board for surgery (Fig. 29-5). The patient is usually secured on the board in dorsal recumbency or in a lateral position.

Two persons are necessary to place an awake bird on the restraint board. The person restraining the bird positions the head and neck as the second person fastens the neck restraint. The legs are then immobilized by looping gauze strips on the legs, proximal to the feet, and taping these strips tautly to the board. The wings, which have been held close to the body as the neck and legs are fastened, are restrained by taping them to the board surface using masking tape. Cloth tape should not be used, because it may pull or damage feathers.

Use of Gloves. Some practices and textbooks suggest the routine use of leather gloves to protect the handler when catching and restraining large pet birds. Unfortunately, birds may respond to gloves as if they are hands and subsequently become afraid of being handled in any situation. For this reason, use of towels is strongly recommended. Gloves should be avoided if possible.

PHYSICAL EXAMINATION

A physical examination in birds is very similar to that performed in other animals. Because of the unique anatomy of the avian patient, the exam is modified somewhat. The technician must be aware of the anatomic features and differences found in birds.

Physical examination is divided into three parts. A thorough history is first obtained from the client, followed by careful observation of the bird for signs of health and disease. Finally, the bird is captured and examined.

Ask the client the age of the bird, the sex of the bird, how long the owner has had the bird, where it was obtained, exposure to new or visiting birds, a description of the diet and any supplements fed, any signs of illness observed, current or past medications used to treat the bird, and the possibility of exposure to toxic plants or poisons.

If the bird is transported in its cage, the cage itself can offer insight into the type of care the bird receives. Close attention should be paid to whether the size of the cage is appropriate for the species of bird. The condition of the cage, the number and type of toys, and the presence of adequate food bowls should be noted. The cage bedding should be inspected. If paper is used, the condition of the droppings should be evaluated.

A small bird should be evaluated in its cage, whereas a large bird should be observed in the carrier if practical or out of the carrier in a nonthreatening location. The bird should exhibit normal posture and movement. It should be active, bright, alert, and responsive. Any obvious indications of illness, such as difficulty breathing or sitting fluffed up on the bottom of the cage, signal that the bird is extremely sick and is to be considered an emergency case.

Special equipment needed for the avian physical examination includes a pediatric stethoscope and several sizes of metal oral specula used to keep the mouth open for examination. Some practices purchase a trans-illumination device that can be used to backlight air-filled structures, such as the beak and sinuses.

Weighing the bird is generally the first step of the hands-on examination. Avian scales, which are available in a variety of configurations, must be accurate to a gram. It is important to weigh the bird each time it visits the clinic, because owners often do not notice fluctuations in weight. However, most very small birds are not weighed because of the stress associated with handling.

Small birds, such as budgerigars and cockatiels, are often caught by hand and placed in a cloth or paper bag, which is then laid on the scale platform. Some birds weigh only a few grams and the bag may weigh as much as the bird. To offset the weight of the bag, the scale must first be adjusted to zero with the empty bag on it.

Large birds, such as Amazons and cockatoos, often stand or perch on the scale long enough to be weighed. These birds may also be placed in a pillowcase or other large bag for weighing. The scale must be zeroed with the bag before the weight is taken.

Physical examination of larger birds requires two people, one to restrain the bird and the other to examine it. Small birds that can be grasped in one hand may be restrained and evaluated by a single person. The bird is usually wrapped in a cloth or paper towel but may be held in the bare hand if the bird is very small. Care must be taken to avoid restricting chest movement, because the lack of a muscular diaphragm limits the bird's ability to breathe.

Physical examinations generally start with the head. External structures that should be identified and evaluated include the cere, nostrils, beak, ear openings, eyes, and feathers. Evidence of discharge, irritation, or matting of feathers should be noted. The eyes should be clear and bright. The beak should be properly shaped for the species and free of obvious damage. There should be no discharge or odor from the ears. Larger parrots can be checked for dehydration by gently lifting the skin above the eyelid and watching to see how long it takes for the skin to return to its normal position.

The mouth must be held open using either a metal speculum or gauze strips that are looped over the upper and lower beaks (Fig. 29-6). The mouth should be fairly dry, with no lesions, discharges, blood, or odors present. The choana should have obvious papillae, or finger-like projections. The tongue shape and coloration should be normal for the species.

Moving down the neck, palpate the crop. This structure may be very obvious in young birds, birds who have eaten recently, or those with digestive problems. It may be impossible to detect a crop in older or very small birds. Some species do not have a crop.

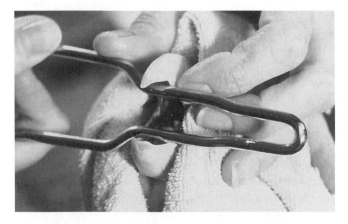

FIG. 29-6 A metal speculum holds the beak open to allow examination of the mouth.

The breast of the bird should be evaluated for good muscling. The keel, or breastbone, should be palpable as a low ridge surrounded by muscle on about the same level on either side. Birds in poor condition have a very prominent keel, with low, receding muscles. Overweight birds have a keel buried in a valley between the pectoral muscles.

Evaluation of the abdomen is very limited or impossible in small birds. In larger birds, abdominal palpation should be used to detect organs that feel hard or unusually shaped. In all birds, the vent should be clean and covered by dry feathers.

A pediatric stethoscope is useful for assessing the heart and respiratory system. The heart rate and respiratory rate should be within normal limits for the species, but stress may result in unreliable numbers.

The feathers should be clean, symmetric, smooth, and structurally sound. Evidence of blood feathers (i.e., growing feathers) should be noted. The presence of the powder down, which is produced by cockatoos, cockatiels, and African grays, should be evaluated. The delicate skin is usually white and underlying structures, such as muscle or blood vessels, are somewhat visible. The nails and skin on the legs should be inspected for condition and any abnormal growth. The preen gland, located at the base of the tail in most species, may not be easily found. Swelling or any discharge indicates a problem.

Both wings should be gently examined, with care taken to curve the wing in the direction of the body at all times. Some birds are very sensitive and struggle when their wings are manipulated. Any of the rest of the musculoskeletal system that was not palpated should be checked at this time.

Several procedures typically performed in the examination of domestic animals are omitted in birds. First, the temperature of birds, which ranges from 40° to 44° C, is not measured. There is wide variation between individual birds and the stress associated with the procedure would raise the temperature, resulting in an inaccurate number. Second, the capillary refill time cannot be evaluated using the oral mucosa. Third, birds have no external lymph nodes to palpate.

The hands-on examination should be completed quickly to minimize stress on the patient. A thorough examination should take no longer than 15 minutes. If the patient appears extremely distressed during the examination, it must be released and placed in a quiet location until it has recovered enough to continue.

GROOMING

The health of a bird can depend on several grooming procedures that are routinely performed at the veterinary clinic. Veterinary technicians must be familiar with and competent in these techniques. Effective restraint is often a vital part of these procedures.

Bathing

A very basic technique that many birds enjoy is a bath. Of the several ways to do this, gently misting the bird with a spray bottle filled with warm water is most common. The warm mist should be directed so that it falls from above the bird, not sprayed directly toward it. The bird may be bathed in this manner either inside or out of the cage, depending on its temperament. Some birds readily bathe in a shallow pan of water. Others like to clean themselves by rolling in wet vegetation, such as lettuce or nonpoisonous house plants. Soap should not be used, because it has a drying effect on the feathers and any residue could be toxic.

Nail Trimming

A regularly requested service is trimming of long or sharp nails. The size and temperament of the bird determines the number of people required to perform the trim. Towel restraint is commonly used.

Birds with light-colored nails have easily visible blood vessels, improving the chances of a nail trim without any bleeding. In birds with black nails, an understanding of structure of the nail is important. However, even with extreme care it is not unusual to cut the quick of at least one nail, causing bleeding. Owners should be warned that this may happen.

The most common tools used for nail trims include Resco trimmers, the Dremel (motorized) tool, files, nail scissors, fingernail trimmers, and cautery instruments. These should be disinfected or sterilized after using to help prevent the spread of disease between birds. Each clinic and veterinarian prefers certain instruments for nail trims. The typical small animal practice could easily trim bird nails without purchase of additional equipment.

Resco guillotine clippers are commonly used on birds the size of conures and larger. A pair should be reserved for use in birds only.

The Dremel tool, typically used on large birds, uses a grinding tip to blunt the tips of the nails. This handheld motorized tool is noisy, can overheat nail tissues if applied too long, and may carry contaminants to other birds on which it is used if the grinding head is improperly cleaned.

Flat or rounded fine tooth files are preferred by some for nail trims of birds of any size. This method slowly blunts the nail tips, causing some birds to become impatient.

The scissor trimmers used on cat nails work well in birds up to Amazon size. Human fingernail clippers may be used in small birds.

Some veterinarians use electrocautery instruments to trim nails and prevent bleeding at the same time. Many birds exhibit pain reactions, presumably related to the high heat of the instrument.

Small birds, such as budgerigars or finches, can be held in one hand and the nails trimmed with the other. Trimming the nails of Amazons and larger birds generally involves two people, one to restrain the bird and the other to trim the nails. Birds generally grasp at anything that touches their feet, so the toes not being trimmed must be held out of the way of the trimmers.

Each nail is closely examined before proceeding. If there is any doubt about how much to remove, only a short tip should be clipped off. More can be removed if necessary.

Any blood loss in birds should be considered serious. In very small birds, loss of what appears to be a minute amount of blood is potentially fatal. When bleeding is noticed, a hemostatic powder must be pressed immediately onto the nail.

Wing Clipping

Most pet bird owners have their bird's wings clipped to limit its flying ability. This helps prevent the bird from escaping through an open window or door or injuring itself by flying through the house. Wing trimming also inhibits development of many dominance behaviors and makes taming and training easier. The wing trim should allow the bird to glide to the floor a short distance from where it began flapping its wings.

Bandage scissors are most often used because of the protected tip. However, any type of scissors can be used if handled carefully. The scissors selected should be suitably sized for the bird to be trimmed.

One person may easily position and trim the smaller species of birds. Two or more handlers are required to trim larger birds. The person performing the wing trim must have a thorough knowledge of wing anatomy and double-check before cutting any feathers. Incorrect trimming procedures may result in accidental wing tip amputation. The wings must be handled carefully to minimize bruising and prevent fractures. They must always be curved toward the body in a natural position, never bent backward. Personnel working with the bird must also be aware that flapping wings can cause bruising and abrasions to human handlers.

Many birds have one or more immature, growing feathers concealed by their mature feathers. These blood feathers can be difficult to locate and identify without inspecting the underside of the wing. When a blood feather is accidentally cut, the hollow shaft bleeds profusely. The bleeding feather must be pulled out immediately using hemostats or a pair of pliers. Without intervention, the bird may die of blood loss.

There are several types of wing trims. The standard wing clip, where all primary feathers are trimmed, is most common (Fig. 29-7). Cockatoos and other heavy birds that fly slowly may need trimming of only the tips of the primaries. Cockatiels fly so well that their feathers must be trimmed to the level of the covert feathers. Other clips involve trimming only a few primaries on each wing to give the bird a more natural look. Some birds still fly quite well after these trims.

A newly trimmed bird should be placed on the floor and gently encouraged to fly. In this way, the bird becomes aware of its limited abilities in a safe location. This also reveals whether further trimming is necessary before the bird leaves the clinic.

Beak Trimming

All pet birds, most commonly parrots, may be presented with overgrown, damaged, poorly aligned, or sharply pointed beaks. Usually only the upper beak needs attention. Most healthy birds provided with plenty of toys to chew on and play with never need a beak trim.

The Dremel tool or files are used to shape and modify the beak. Flaky material on the sides of the beak is care-

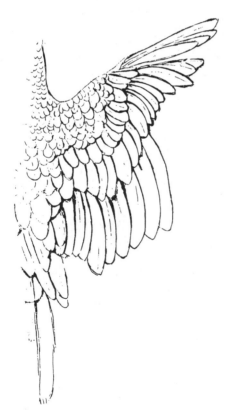

FIG. 29-7 Trimming the primary feathers at the level of the coverts on both wings is not attractive but may be necessary to restrict flight in some species (*dorsal view*). *(From Harrison GJ, Harrison LR: Clinical avian medicine and surgery, Philadelphia, 1986, WB Saunders.)*

fully ground away. If the upper beak is badly overgrown, the tip of the beak may be clipped using nail trimming instruments, such as Resco clippers. Because the beak has a central blood supply, trimming the tip too short may cause bleeding. A hemostatic powder should be ready. After the beak trim is finished, some practices apply mineral oil to provide an attractive gloss.

One or two people are needed for a beak trim, depending on the size of the bird. A small bird may be managed by one person; a larger bird must be restrained by one person while the other does the trim. It is important to keep the bird from mouthing or biting the tools, because they may damage sensitive soft tissue.

ADMINISTERING MEDICATION

The avian patient may need to be tube fed because it has a digestive disorder, nebulized to treat a pulmonary disease, vaccinated against any of several diseases, given fluid therapy, or medicated topically for an infection. The techniques used in small animals are not always directly applicable to birds.

Parenteral Injection

A bird with a life-threatening disease often refuses to eat and may regurgitate oral medication. Parenteral treatments, or medication by injection, can often be quickly administered without undue stress to the patient. Needles suitable for injecting birds range from 22 to 26 gauge. Tuberculin or insulin syringes are used most often, although larger syringes may be needed to administer larger volumes.

Intramuscular Injection

The intramuscular (IM) route is most commonly used. The large, well-developed pectoral muscles are the site of choice. The bird must be restrained well to prevent struggling during IM injection, because muscle may be damaged if the needle is not held steady. Two people should work together to inject birds of cockatiel size or larger (Fig. 29-8). However, one person with good restraint skills can single-handedly inject IM medications in almost any bird.

Intramuscular injections should be given into the thickest part of the breast muscle. The feathers may be wet down with water before inserting the needle. Once the needle is in place, the syringe plunger is pulled back to see if any blood is aspirated into the hub. If blood is present, the needle should be pulled out and placed in a new site. Once a satisfactory location is determined, the syringe is held steady while the plunger is quickly depressed. The needle is then removed and pressure applied to the puncture site for several seconds. If relatively large amounts of medication must be given, it

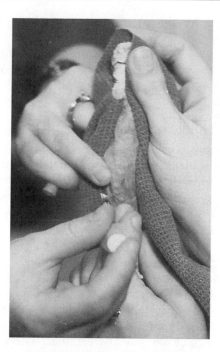

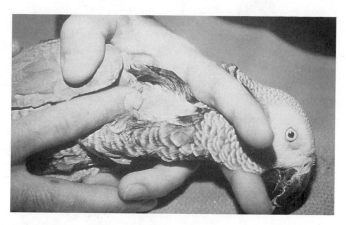

FIG. 29-9 Location of the right jugular vein in an African gray parrot. The feathers over the area have been plucked. The technician is restraining the head and occluding the vein. *(Courtesy of Dr. Heidi Hoefer, Animal Medical Center, New York, New York.)*

FIG. 29-8 Cockatiel restrained for IM injection into the pectoral muscles. Note the hand placement used to restrain the bird. The injection site is indicated by the pointed finger.

should be distributed over several sites. It is important to determine that no surface blood is visible before the bird is released.

Intravenous Injection and Blood Collection

The sites for IV injections include the wing (cutaneous ulnar) vein, the medial metatarsal vein, the brachial vein, and the right jugular vein (Fig. 29-9). Simple restraint is usually adequate for administration of small volumes of a drug, but a bird requiring a large volume of fluids may be anesthetized to keep it completely still.

Blood is usually collected using a 23- or 25-gauge needle. A venous sample may be aspirated into a heparinized syringe and transferred to a microhematocrit tube. The sample can be collected directly into a heparinized microhematocrit tube by holding the tube to the hub of a needle in place in a vein. An alternate method is to clip a toenail short enough to induce bleeding and collect the blood into the microhematocrit tube. If the toenail technique is used, the nail should be thoroughly cleaned with alcohol to prevent contaminating the sample with urates from the stool.

Avian veins are extremely delicate and hematoma formation is common. Use of small-bore, 25- or 26-gauge needles causes the least damage to the vein and minimizes hematomas. The jugular vein is especially fragile and some practices use it as the last choice, because any hematoma is very visible.

The person restraining the bird is also responsible for occluding the selected vein and releasing the pressure after the needle is successfully inserted. The injection should be smooth and fast, unless the medication must be given slowly. Once the needle is removed, direct pressure is applied to the site for 30 to 60 seconds. A cottonball soaked in cold water may be used to apply pressure and cause the vessel to constrict somewhat in response to the chilly temperature. The injection site must be evaluated closely for bleeding before releasing the bird.

Intravenous Fluid Administration

When a volume of IV fluids must be supplied to a bird, they may be infused using a needle, a butterfly catheter, or a flexible indwelling catheter. A 23- to 25-gauge needle is suitable for large parrots and a 27- to 30-gauge needle is best for the smallest birds, such as budgies. Most birds toy with and destroy IV tubing connected to their catheter, so fluids are often given as a single large-volume injection. A bird in stable condition may be anesthetized to give IV fluids over a more prolonged period.

Before placing a catheter or administering fluids, pluck and surgically prepare the injection site. The fluid usually selected is lactated Ringer's solution, which should be warmed before infusion. Typical replacement fluid volumes for a 10% dehydrated bird are 0.5 ml for a finch, 2 ml for a cockatiel, 8 ml for an Amazon, and 14 ml for a macaw.

Intraosseous Injection

When large volumes of fluids must be given to a bird, especially one in shock with collapsed veins, the intraosseous route is preferred. A needle is inserted directly into the lumen of a long bone that contains marrow, because using one of the pneumatic bones, such as the humerus or femur, directs fluids into the respiratory system and can drown the bird. The principal sites are the distal end of the ulna and the proximal end of the tibia. The feathers over the site must be plucked and the skin surgically prepared before the needle is inserted.

Subcutaneous Injection

The subcutaneous (SC) route is not often used, because injected liquid tends to leak readily from the site. However, if necessary, the dorsal scapular area and the ventrolateral abdomen are used. Replacement fluids are the most commonly used SC medications.

Oral Medication

Most birds reject drugs placed in the mouth, and there are no pilling instruments appropriate for birds. However, certain infections of the intestinal tract must be treated with oral drugs. In some exceptional cases, young hand-fed birds may consume medicated food from a syringe or spoon.

One method of treating birds per os (PO) is administering the medication in the food or water. Medicated food or water may have a different taste and not be consumed or therapeutic levels may never be achieved in the bloodstream. Medicated food allows treatment of large numbers of birds or birds that are impossible to treat in any other manner. Specialized coated feeds and medicated pellets are available commercially. Medicated water is generally used in flock situations.

Tube Feeding

The best way to administer oral medication is the technique known as *gavage*, in which a feeding tube is passed directly into the crop and the medication is injected with a syringe. This is a dangerous and stressful procedure for both patient and technician, because misdirected medication enters the respiratory system or tube insertion may rupture the esophagus or crop.

A metal feeding tube or red rubber tube may be used. The metal tube is preferable because it is easily palpated to determine correct placement and can be passed without a mouth speculum (Fig. 29-10).

The bird is restrained in a towel in an upright position facing the person passing the tube and held as still as possible. Cockatiels and smaller birds may be handled by one skilled person, but larger birds usually require two experienced people. The tube is inserted between the beaks on the bird's left side and is directed over the tongue and into the esophagus, which lies on the right side of the bird's neck. Placement into the crop is slow and gentle, with palpation of its progress until the crop is reached. Once the medication is infused, the tube is slowly withdrawn in the same manner. The bird must be observed for several minutes for adverse reactions.

Budgies can receive up to approximately 1 ml of medication, cockatiels up to 8 ml, Amazons and cockatoos 15 ml, and the large macaws no more than 30 ml. The proper amount is injected slowly until the crop is full, because excess medication may be regurgitated and aspirated.

Topical Medication

Skin conditions and eye disorders are sometimes treated with topical medication. Feathers that come in contact with topical medications may have to be cleaned with a mild detergent. Birds sometimes ingest any medication applied to the skin and may need to be fitted with an Elizabethan collar.

Sinus Flushes

A common problem in pet birds is sinusitis, which may cause signs ranging from sneezing to regional swelling of the head and nasal discharge. Flushing of the sinuses with sterile saline or dilute antibiotic or disinfectant solutions is one method of treatment. The solution is injected directly into the sinus using a needle and syringe or flushed into the sinus through a nostril using a syringe without a needle.

Nebulization Therapy

In birds with severe or unresponsive respiratory tract infections, nebulization is an effective method of deliv-

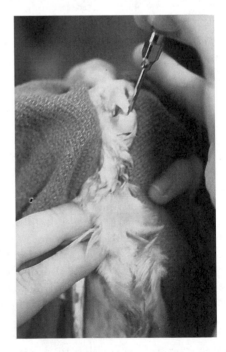

FIG. 29-10 Using a metal feeding tube to administer oral medication to a cockatiel. The tube has been passed into the mouth from the bird's left to the right, and then into the esophagus. The technician is palpating the location of the tube as it is passed. The bird is restrained by a second person.

ering medication directly to the lungs and air sacs. A nebulizer, a machine that creates particles of water minute enough to reach deep into the lung tissue, is required. Nebulization therapy may be done with the bird in a closed chamber or through an anesthetic face mask. A typical treatment regimen is 15 to 30 minutes every 6 to 8 hours using an antimicrobial solution.

POULTRY

Avian medicine also includes domestic poultry, most commonly chickens and turkeys. The birds seen in clinical practice are often members of a backyard flock, ranging in size from a few birds up to several hundred. Private practices rarely are involved with commercial poultry medicine, because the large corporations producing poultry for consumers employ their own veterinary personnel.

GENERAL INFORMATION

Unlike pet birds, most poultry show sexual dimorphism at maturity. The sex of young chicks is often impossible to determine by appearance. At commercial hatcheries chicks are sexed at 1 day of age by examining their vents. Accuracy rates can approach 95%.

Roosters can be very aggressive and attack people with their beak, wings, and leg spurs. Hens are pursued by the cock until he is able to catch and mount her for breeding. Females may be injured if there is too little space for her to escape. A hen is typically docile but will peck at anyone attempting to remove the eggs on which she is sitting.

Poultry Health Management

Poultry present many different challenges than cage birds. First, the birds are housed together, complicating diagnosis and treatment of disease. If one bird becomes ill, the entire flock may be exposed. It is important for the owner to obtain a rapid, accurate diagnosis if there is an outbreak of illness in the flock in order to prevent spread to other birds. Second, owners have access to over-the-counter medications and may have treated their birds before contacting a veterinarian. This may limit the usefulness of diagnostic tests, such as microbial culture and sensitivity tests. Third, the meat and eggs of poultry are often intended for human consumption and this limits the selection of medications that can be used. Withdrawal times must be considered when the veterinarian decides on treatment. Fourth, the conditions under which poultry are kept often promote growth and spread of potentially pathogenic organisms. Wet or dirty bedding, dusty conditions, overcrowding, poor ventilation, high ambient temperatures, and poor nutrition all are contributing factors in disease outbreaks.

Examination Techniques. Physical examination of poultry is very similar to that of cage birds. Restraint techniques are very different from those used with pet birds and depend on the species and size of the bird. In general, poultry are docile and more easily handled than pet birds, once they are caught.

Poultry are often presented for necropsy. A dead bird may be submitted or a sick bird may be euthanized for diagnostic purposes. Samples collected for submission to the diagnostic laboratory must be properly collected, labeled, and packaged. A complete history, including the flock and individual bird's presenting signs, must accompany the samples (see Chapter 12).

Examination of birds for external parasites is part of the physical examination. Mites and lice are generally easily visible to the naked eye, whereas a skin scraping is needed to confirm scaly leg mite infestation. Internal parasites, such as roundworms and coccidia, are diagnosed with a fecal flotation.

Medication Techniques. In a flock situation, individual birds may be medicated or the entire flock is treated by placing medication in the water or feed. Some drugs must be injected, whereas others are given orally.

Vaccinations are often used only by owners raising poultry for sale. The typical backyard flock owner may purchase mail-order day-old birds that have been vaccinated and come from immunized stock. Poultry vaccines can be administered by injection to individual birds when necessary. If large numbers are to be immunized, the vaccination method may be through drinking water, intranasal administration, or the intraocular route.

Blood collection sites include the jugular and wing veins. IV injections can be made at the same locations.

Husbandry. Backyard poultry are most often kept in flocks in common housing that combines indoor and outdoor facilities. It is important for the owner to minimize the chances of infection by using proper bedding, periodic cleaning, practicing biosecurity, and careful flock management.

The indoor area must be well ventilated and well insulated in colder climates, because the bird's comb is susceptible to frostbite. Bedding such as pine shavings must be regularly cleaned. Cobwebs and dust often contribute to respiratory infections, so overall cleanliness of the house is important. Chickens prefer to roost on perches at least 18 inches above the floor at night.

The outdoor area should be as large as possible and enclosed with wire mesh that is small enough to keep the birds from sticking their head through. Some owners also cover the top with mesh to prevent the birds from flying out and predators from coming in.

Most poultry are fed commercially available diets suitable for their stage of life or stage of production.

This diet may be supplemented with fresh green plants, garden waste, or household scraps. Nutritional imbalances are rare unless owners are attempting to feed a totally homemade diet without knowledge of poultry requirements.

RECOMMENDED READING

Beynon PH: *Manual of psittacine birds*, Ames, Iowa, 1996, Iowa State University Press.

Calnek BW et al: *Disease of poultry*, ed 9, Ames, Iowa, 1991, Iowa State University Press.

Gallerstein GA: *The complete bird owner's handbook*, New York, 1994, Macmillan.

Pet bird report. Published bimonthly, 2236 Mariner Square Dr, #35, Alameda, Calif, 94501.

Ritchie BW et al: *Avian medicine: principles and application*, Lake Worth, Fla, 1994, Wingers Publishing.

CHAPTER 30

Nursing Care of Small Mammals

S.P. Messonnier

Learning Objectives

After reviewing this chapter, the reader should understand the following:

Methods of sample collection for laboratory analysis
Routes of administration of medication
Techniques used in general nursing care of rabbits, rodents, and ferrets

Principles of feeding, watering, exercising, and bedding of small mammals
Procedures used in forced feeding of small mammals
Techniques used for diagnosing disease in small mammals

Small mammals are popular pets. These include ferrets, rabbits, mice, rats, gerbils, guinea pigs, and hamsters. The term *pocket pets* should probably be abandoned, because owners should not be encouraged to carry these pets around in their pockets. Although small mammals are easy to care for, they require care different from that of dogs and cats.

Small mammals do not currently require annual vaccinations. However, an annual examination and fecal analysis is recommended to ensure good health and husbandry. At the very least, a "new pet" visit, which includes an examination and microscopic fecal analysis, is necessary to ensure health, maintain the "health guarantee" that might accompany the purchase, and allow the technician and doctor to educate the owner on proper feeding, housing, and handling for the species (Fig. 30-1).

Small mammals are often purchased as first pets for children. Small mammals can make acceptable pets for children, but children should always be supervised when handling these delicate creatures. Small mammals can bite; children should be made aware of this and told that these pets are "real live creatures" and not stuffed animals. All pets should be handled with care. Small mammals should not be allowed free run of the house, because this can prove fatal to these small pets. Finally, because the average life span of most small mammals is only 2 to 3 years, children should be counseled so that an "early" death is not unexpected.

HOUSING

It is most convenient to house small rodents in a glass aquarium, although cages are available specifically for these pets. Ferrets and rabbits can be housed in a large cat or dog carrier; some owners build rather elaborate "condos" for their pet rabbits and ferrets. Wooden cages are not suitable; small mammals, particularly rodents, love to chew and can destroy their homes. Wire rabbit cages are also fine, but to decrease foot trauma (which results in "sore hocks"), at least half of the wire

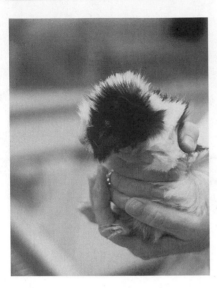

FIG. 30-1   Clients should be instructed on the proper way to handle small mammals. This illustration shows the correct way to carry a guinea pig, with the body supported by one hand.

floor should be covered with toweling, plexiglass, or wood. Place the litterbox and ceramic or steel food and water bowls in the carrier for rabbits and ferrets. Rodents can have their food placed in the cage in bowls and usually drink out of sipper bottles, which must be inspected daily for clogging of the dispenser tip. Rodent cages can be left open at the top, as long as the pet cannot escape and other pets (such as the family dog or cat) cannot get to the pet. Cages must be escape-proof to prevent injury or fatality.

The environmental temperature should be kept between 65° and 80° F; fatal heat stroke is not uncommon. Because rodents and ferrets like to burrow, some type of hiding place should be provided for them in the cage. Tubular, hollow objects can be purchased at pet stores, or cleaned empty cans (such as an orange juice can), terry cloth towels, or paper towel cardboard rolls can be provided. If using a can, be sure there are no exposed sharp metal edges that can cause injury. Small mammals often chew paper towel or toilet paper cardboard rolls rather quickly, so these need to be replaced fairly often.

Rabbits can be housed outdoors, but care must be taken to prevent heat stroke, myiasis (fly strike), and dog and cat attacks. Rabbits housed outdoors should be provided shelter from direct sunlight, rain, or snow, and wind.

Wood shavings, such as pine or cedar, are usually provided for bedding material for rabbits and rodents. However, the aromatic oils from these shavings, particularly cedar, may induce liver changes. Shredded paper or paper towels are also fine and may be preferred. Avoid using sawdust, sand, or dirt as bedding.

The cage should be cleaned and the bedding changed as often as it gets dirty, but at least weekly. A major cause of respiratory disease in pet rodents is poor environmental ventilation, which allows ammonia from accumulation of urine to irritate the pet's airways. A frequently cleaned, well-ventilated environment is important in controlling respiratory infections. Any toys should be cleaned weekly as well.

FEEDING

Pet rodents can be fed commercial rodent chows or pellets. The "party mix" diets containing seeds and nuts are not recommended. These are high in fat, and many rodents prefer these to the formulated pellets. Seeds and nuts can be offered as an occasional treat (less than 10% of the daily diet). Fresh, well-cleaned vegetables and occasionally a small amount of fruit can be offered as well. Leafy green vegetables (not lettuce or celery) can be offered, as well as yellow and orange vegetables. The total daily amount of these "people foods" should not make up more than 10% of the diet. The pets should eat mainly a commercial pelleted diet (90% of the diet), 5% to 10% vegetables and fruits, and occasionally a few seeds or nuts as treats. Hay (alfalfa or clover), a source of fiber, can be offered free-choice as a source of fiber.

Unlike most other pets, guinea pigs require a dietary source of vitamin C. They should be fed guinea pig chow (pellets), which is supplemented with vitamin C. However, the shelf-life of vitamin C is about 90 days from the time of milling, not from the time of purchase. Therefore, vitamin C should also be supplied in the drinking water. A simple way to do this is to crush a 200-mg vitamin C tablet into powder. Mix the powder in 1 liter of water. This solution should be made fresh *daily* and used as the pet's drinking water. Fresh green vegetables (broccoli, cabbage, bok choy) can also be used to supply vitamin C.

Rabbits should be fed mainly free-choice hay. Alfalfa hay can be offered in small amounts, but it is too rich to be the sole source of fiber. Timothy, grass, or clover hay are better choices. Commercial pelleted feed should be offered at no more than 1/4 cup per 5 pounds of body weight each day. The increased fiber helps prevent diarrhea and formation of trichobezoars (hairballs).

Ferrets can be fed commercial kitten food or cat food, or specially formulated ferret diets. As with dogs and cats, periodontal disease is common in ferrets. A dry diet can help reduce tartar accumulation.

CAGE TOYS

Cage toys can provide psychological stimulation as well as exercise for small mammals. Tubes and mazes are popular, as are exercise wheels. "Open-track" (wire mesh) exercise wheels are not recommended, because rodents, especially hamsters, can be injured by catching a foot in the wheel while exercising. Hamsters with severe foot and leg injuries are either euthanized or require a leg amputation. Although not every animal with an open-track exercise wheel will be injured, it is best to avoid this type of wheel. The safest exercise wheel is composed of plastic and has no openings in the track ("solid track") where a foot can get caught.

GENERAL NURSING CARE

Because of the cost involved in hospitalization and intensive care, most pet rodents are treated on an outpatient basis, whereas rabbits and ferrets are often hospitalized. As with any other sick pet, proper nursing care is vital to maximize the pet's chances for full recovery.

Pet rodents that must be hospitalized are usually critically ill. Fluid therapy, antibiotics, forced feeding, and proper environment are important. These patients should be handled as little as possible. The proper ambient temperature must be maintained; human pediatric incubators serve this function well. Many can be purchased as used units rather inexpensively through medical suppliers or directly from human hospitals. Because of the sensitivity of all small exotic mammals to extremes in heat, the ambient temperature should be kept no warmer than 80° F. Temperatures above this often result in death from heat stroke.

When necessary, oxygen can be supplemented through a port on most pediatric incubators.

Food and water should be offered even if forced feeding is needed. Overfeeding is rarely a problem. Rabbits that refuse to eat often resume eating if offered hay, carrot tops, cilantro, parsley, or other green vegetable matter.

When possible, small mammals should be isolated from other hospitalized animals. This is due to not only the risk of disease spread (e.g., *Bordetella* passed from rabbits or dogs to guinea pigs) but also the fact that these sick pets are extremely stressed. Remember that most small mammals are prey in the wild. Housing them near a natural predator (dog or cat) may increase their stress.

DIAGNOSTIC AND TREATMENT TECHNIQUES

Diagnostic testing is important in small mammals. Many of these pets are presented because of vague complaints, such as lethargy and lack of appetite. Although certain syndromes are more common in certain species, diagnostic testing can help determine a definitive diagnosis and proper treatment plan.

Unfortunately, many owners of some less expensive small mammals, particularly rodents, may not allow diagnostic testing because of the expense involved. Regardless, the veterinary technician must have a working knowledge of the various diagnostic tests available.

Venipuncture

Venipuncture is commonly used in ferrets and rabbits, and infrequently used in diagnosing diseases of pet rodents. Venipuncture is used for withdrawing blood for hematologic and biochemical analysis, administration of certain medications, and catheterization for administration of fluids. Anesthesia may be required when performing venipuncture on small mammals; the technician must be thoroughly acquainted with delivery of anesthetic agents and monitoring of anesthesia in small mammals. Additionally, technicians should check with the veterinary supervisor to make sure that technician-induced anesthesia of these pets is allowed under the state veterinary practice act. Except under certain specific circumstances, anesthesia may not be required once the technician has developed proficiency at venipuncture.

Although each diagnostic laboratory has specific requirements, for the volume of blood required for various tests, most laboratories can perform a mini-battery of tests on 0.5 ml of blood collected in a green-top (lithium heparin) tube. To prevent volume depletion in pet rodents, some clinicians replace the volume of blood withdrawn with an equal volume of balanced electrolyte solution, given intravenously or subcutaneously.

Rabbits. The following sites can be used for blood collection in rabbits: cephalic vein, lateral saphenous vein, jugular vein, marginal ear vein, and the central ear artery. For collection of small volumes of blood, the author of this chapter routinely uses a marginal vein or central artery of the ear (Fig. 30-2). Cannulate the vein with a 27- or 28-gauge needle and collect the blood in a blood tube or heparinized microhematocrit tube as it drips freely from the cannulated vessel. Alternatively, blood can be collected using a 27- or 28-gauge needle attached to a tuberculin syringe. For tuberculin syringes with non-removable needles, after blood collection the needle can be clipped off the end with nail clippers and the blood emptied from the syringe into the appropriate tube.

Jugular venipuncture is also fairly easy in rabbits. After hair on the neck is clipped, the rabbit is restrained in ventral recumbency as for jugular venipuncture on a dog or cat. The forelegs can be extended, but rabbits may resist this. The skin over the vein is disinfected with alcohol and pressure applied at the jugular furrow to make the vein stand out. Blood is then collected using a 23-gauge or larger needle; a sample of 1 to 2 ml is adequate for most assays.

Cephalic venipuncture may be difficult in rabbits except in those with heat stroke, in which case the increased body temperature allows the vein to maximally

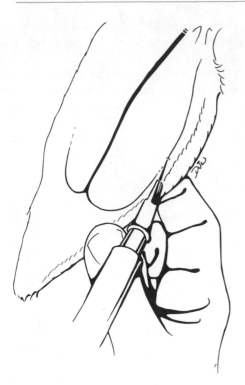

FIG. 30-2 The marginal ear vein can be used for blood collection or small-volume intravenous injections in rabbits. *(From Harkness JE, Wagner JE: The biology and medicine of rabbits and rodents, Baltimore, 1995, Williams & Wilkins.)*

dilate. In rabbits with heat stroke use the cephalic vein for catheterization, blood collection, and fluid therapy.

Ferrets. The following sites can be used for blood collection and venipuncture in ferrets: cephalic vein, jugular vein, cranial vena cava, lateral saphenous vein, and the ventral artery of the tail. The author routinely uses the jugular vein or cranial vena cava for blood collection. Venipuncture is most easily performed under isoflurane anesthesia maintained by face mask, although jugular venipuncture can also be done in unanesthetized ferrets. Obtaining small volumes of blood from larger ferrets is possible using the central artery of the tail.

Place the anesthetized ferret in dorsal recumbency. For jugular venipuncture, clip the hair and clean the skin with an alcohol swab. The legs are pulled caudally while the head and neck are extended dorsally. Applying digital pressure in the jugular furrow allows visualization of the jugular vein. A 23-gauge or larger needle is used to collect 1 to 2 ml of blood.

For venipuncture of the cranial vena cava, anesthesia must be used.[2] The anesthetized ferret is placed in dorsal recumbency and the front limbs are pulled caudally and the head held steady. A 25-gauge needle attached to a 3-ml syringe is inserted at the palpable notch between the manubrium of the sternum and the first rib. The needle is held at a 45-degree angle to the skin and is directed toward the opposite hip. The nee-

---

Box 30-1 Venipuncture technique

Materials:

appropriately sized needle and syringe or microhematocrit tubes

collection vial

alcohol swab

IV catheter, 24 gauge (if catheterization will be performed)

Procedure:

1. Gently restrain the animal. If anesthesia is used, another person must monitor the anesthetized animal.

2. Identify the venipuncture site. Warming of the area (e.g., a tail vein with warm water, an ear vein with warm water, or a focal heat light) may improve visualization.

3. Clean the area with an alcohol swab; for catheterization, prepare the area as for surgery.

4. For some peripheral vessels (jugular, cephalic), entering the skin just lateral to the vessel and then penetrating the vessel may improve the chance for successful venipuncture. For other vessels (rabbit ear vessels, ferret cranial vena cava), directly enter the vessel through the skin.

5. Withdraw the amount of blood needed (generally 1 to 2 ml in rabbits and ferrets) no more than 25% of the total blood volume in pet rodents (blood volume is approximately 6% of body weight) in a 2-week period.

6. Withdraw the needle and apply pressure for 30 to 60 seconds.

---

dle is inserted almost to the hub and blood is gently aspirated into the syringe as the needle is slowly withdrawn. Once blood begins entering the syringe, the needle and syringe are held in place and the appropriate volume of blood (usually 1 to 2 ml) is removed. The needle is then withdrawn and pressure applied over the venipuncture site.

Rodents. The following sites can be used for blood collection and venipuncture in pet rodents: lateral saphenous vein, cephalic vein, jugular vein, orbital sinus, and the ventral tail artery (Box 30-1). The central vena cava of anesthetized guinea pigs is easily accessed for blood collection.

Parenteral Injection

Injectable medications are usually preferred over oral medications in hospitalized small mammals. Medications that cannot be safely given orally (penicillin in rabbits) must be given by injection. With the exception of ferrets, small mammals are difficult to medicate with pills. Extremely ill pets may have reduced intestinal function, making absorption of oral medication erratic and unpredictable. You may want to instruct owners on how to give injectable medication. When this is not possible, prescribe oral liquid medication for the pet.

Injections are usually given subcutaneously or intramuscularly, although when a catheter is in place, intravenous or intraosseous administration may be preferred. The most common sites used for subcutaneous administration of medications in small mammals are over the dorsal neck, back, and flank. Intramuscular injections are commonly given in the muscles of the caudal thigh. In small rodents, intraperitoneal injections can be given in the caudal left quadrant of the abdomen. The choice of fluids follows the same guidelines as in dogs and cats; lactated Ringer's solution is commonly used.

Intraosseous Catheterization[1]

Because of the difficulty in venous catheterization in small mammals, some doctors and technicians prefer intraosseous catheterization. This is the author's method of choice for delivering fluids to critically ill exotic pets. Some pets require general anesthesia for placement of the catheter; those that are gravely ill often require only local anesthesia. An intraosseous catheter is ideal for delivering fluids and most medications that can be safely given intravenously.

The rate of absorption of a substance injected into the bone marrow is equal to that after injection into a peripheral vein. Intraosseous catheterization is preferred in patients with complete circulatory collapse. With respect to the rate of fluid uptake, the intraosseous route is second only to a central venous route, with the tip of the catheter residing in the cranial vena cava.

Intraosseous catheterization is not without risks, however. Contraindications include sepsis, skeletal abnormalities, skin and wound infections, abscesses over the bone, and recent fracture of that bone. With regard to sepsis, the risk of causing osteomyelitis must be weighed against the risk of mortality if insufficient fluids are delivered.

Supplies needed include a local anesthetic (1% or 2% lidocaine), suture material, bandaging material, triple antibiotic ointment, and an appropriate needle (Box 30-2). Depending upon the size of the pet, a 20-gauge spinal needle or 18- to 25-gauge hypodermic needle may be used. Several sites are available for intraosseous catheterization; the author's preferred site is the trochanteric fossa of either femur.

Box 30-2 Intraosseous catheterization

Materials:

1% to 2% lidocaine

suture material

adhesive tape

20-gauge spinal needle or 18- to 25-gauge hypodermic needle

bandaging dressing material

antibiotic ointment

Procedure:

1. Gently restrain the animal. If anesthesia is necessary, another person must monitor the anesthetized animal.

2. Identify the catheterization site; prepare the area as for surgery.

3. Infiltrate the area with lidocaine (not needed if general anesthesia is used but may provide some analgesia when the pet awakens).

4. Use a twisting motion while advancing the needle into the bone.

5. Aspirate to check for needle position. Any marrow that is aspirated can be saved for analysis, if indicated. Injection of a small amount of electrolyte solution (or heparinized saline) can also be used to check for proper positioning of the needle (extravasation of fluid indicates accidental penetration of bone cortex; the needle must be removed).

6. Apply antibiotic ointment and a light dressing to the site.

7. Apply a tape butterfly using adhesive tape around the hub of the needle. Suture the tape to the skin.

8. Bandage the catheter to the limb; flush with heparinized saline and apply a cap to the needle when fluids are not being administered. To make a cap for the needle, cut off the end of a 1-ml syringe (including the stopper) with nail clippers.

After the site is aseptically prepared, the skin, subcutis, and periosteum are infiltrated with lidocaine (if needed). The needle is inserted through the skin (a small stab incision can be made through the skin if needed before needle insertion) and advanced until bone is met.

To avoid penetrating the sciatic nerve, walk the needle off the medial aspect of the greater trochanter into the trochanteric fossa. The hip joint should remain in a neutral position during needle advancement. Internally rotating the hip and adducting it also helps to protect the nerve. While applying firm and steady pressure, rotate the needle in 30-degree turns until it penetrates into the bone. Once the cortex has been penetrated, resistance to needle passage is reduced. The needle is flushed with a small amount of heparinized saline, which should flow freely.

If resistance to fluid flow is encountered, a bone or marrow plug might be obstructing the needle. This can be prevented by using sterilized stainless-steel wire as a stylet during introduction of the needle or removing the needle and reinserting another one (preferably the next larger size) into the same hole. Observe the subcutaneous tissue for leakage of fluid. If this occurs, the needle must be removed and placed into another bone. A bone should not be catheterized again for 24 hours after previous attempts at catheterization.

Once the needle is seated firmly in place, a tape butterfly is placed around the hub of the needle and sutured to the skin. The area is covered with antibiotic ointment and bandaged securely.

Fluids can be given at a maximum rate of 11 ml/min by gravity flow and 24 ml/min using 300 mm Hg pressure. The catheter should be flushed every 6 hours with heparinized saline and removed after 48 to 72 hours. Most drugs suited for intravenous routes can be safely infused into the marrow. Check with the drug manufacturer if there are any questions.

Oral Drug Administration

Because of the difficulty in giving tablets and capsules to small mammals (except possibly ferrets), most oral medications are given in a liquid form. When possible, injectable medications are preferred to decrease the possibility of gastrointestinal problems and increase the chance of successful treatment (GI absorption of drugs may be erratic in sick pets, especially if they are anorectic).

Safe antibacterials for use in rabbits and rodents include chloramphenicol, trimethoprim-sulfas, enrofloxacin, amikacin, gentamicin, and tetracyclines (although tetracyclines have been implicated in guinea pig deaths). If diarrhea develops during use of any antibacterial, drug administration should be stopped, the diarrhea treated, and another antibacterial used if needed (preferably given parenterally). Rabbits can be treated short term with injectable penicillin or amoxicillin if these drugs are indicated. If diarrhea develops, drug administration should be stopped immediately and the rabbit examined. Ferrets can safely be treated with most antibacterials used in cats.

Fecal Analysis

Microscopic fecal analysis is used to evaluate animals with diarrhea and any nonspecific complaint (anorexia, lethargy). The method is similar to that used in dogs and cats. For cases of diarrhea, a fecal smear of *fresh* feces mixed with a small amount of warm tap water and a flotation (using zinc sulfate or sodium nitrate solution) should be performed. A parasitology text should be consulted for details on identifying the ova.

Forced Feeding

Many exotic mammals are presented for veterinary care because of anorexia and lethargy. In addition to the need for rehydration, nutritional supplementation is often required (and often overlooked). Animals that are not eating are in a *catabolic state*. Decreased food intake results in breakdown of protein and fat for energy. This can contribute to hepatic lipidosis (especially in rabbits), acidosis, azotemia, muscle wasting, impaired gastrointestinal function, and decreased immunity. To prevent these complications (or correct them, because many are probably in existence when the pet is initially examined), supplementation with food is important. This can be done in the hospital or by the owner at home if the pet will be treated on an outpatient basis.

Rabbits. Sick rabbits often eat hay or greens (e.g., carrot tops, parsley, cilantro) even if they refuse pellets. These greens and hay can be offered free choice. Rabbits with intestinal hypomotility or suspected "hairballs" can be fed a 1:1:1 mix of strained baby food vegetables, powdered pellets, and water, lactated Ringer's solution, or pineapple juice (from fresh pineapples, not canned) at 10 ml/lb two to three times/day. If needed, a nasogastric tube (5 to 8 French) can be passed (after instilling topical anesthetic in the nostrils) for feeding. Rabbits may not cough if the tube is erroneously passed into the trachea, even if water is injected to check for correct positioning. For this reason, a radiograph should be made before tube feeding.

Rodents. Most rodents are treated on an outpatient basis, and forced feeding is done by the owner. Recommend supplementation with fluids, such as water or preferably lactated Ringer's solution, Pedialyte, or even Gatorade. The normal daily maintenance requirement for fluids is 10 ml/100 g; more will be needed, because these anorectic pets are invariably dehydrated. Also, 200 to 1000 mg of vitamin C must be added to the fluids for guinea pigs. For feeding, a mixture of powdered pellets, water (or lactated Ringer's solution), strained baby food vegetables, and/or a soy-based enteral feeding product, using an equal amount of all ingredients, can be infused through a syringe.

Ferrets. Hospitalized ferrets can be force-fed any of the diets suitable for cats, including a/d (Hill's), strained meat baby food, Deliver 2.0, "duck soup" (Box 30-3),

Box 30-3 Recipe for "Duck Soup"

1 can Sustacal (8 oz)
1 can water (8 oz)
2 scoops KMR kitten weaning formula (optional)
4 oz ProPlan Kitten Growth Formula (dry) soaked
   in water to soften
Mix thoroughly and gently warm.

CliniCare, or RenalCare. The food can be offered to the ferret to eat voluntarily (slight warming may increase appetite, especially of the a/d), or given with a syringe or through a tube. In extreme cases, the doctor may wish to place an esophagostomy tube for feeding. Give 10 ml/lb for each meal three to four times a day.

Fluorescein Staining of the Cornea

Rabbits, ferrets, and rodents may be presented for evaluation of ocular irritation or discharge. The source of this discomfort is often a corneal ulcer. In rabbits, corneal ulcers often appear as a white, opaque film that can mimic hypopyon. Before any ophthalmic medication is applied, the cornea should be evaluated by fluorescein staining. The procedure is the same as in dogs and cats. Briefly, a drop of water is placed on the end of the fluorescein strip. The moistened strip is gently touched to the sclera or palpebral conjunctiva and the eyelids closed to allow distribution of the stain. Areas of ulceration retain the fluorescent dye, whereas intact corneal epithelium does not. If the eye contains a large amount of mucus, this can be removed by gentle flushing with water after the stain is applied. Often the eye may be painful, especially if ulceration is present. In this case, one to two drops of topical ocular anesthetic can be applied to minimize blepharospasm before stain is applied.

Cytologic Examination

Small mammals are sometimes presented for evaluation of cutaneous masses. These may represent tumors or abscesses. These masses should be initially evaluated by needle aspiration of their contents. All masses should be aspirated so that the doctor can formulate the proper diagnosis and treatment plan. A 22- to 25-gauge needle and 3- to 12-ml syringe are used for aspirating the mass. After material has been aspirated from the mass, the needle is removed from the syringe, air is aspirated into the syringe, and the needle is replaced on the air-filled syringe. A clean glass slide is readied. The air is then pushed through the needle, which causes the small amount of aspirated material trapped in the needle to be deposited on the slide.

To prepare the slide for staining, use a squash technique, in which a clean slide is gently placed at right angles on top of the slide containing the aspirated material. The two slides are gently "squashed" together, and the top slide is pulled away. The material can be stained with Diff-Quik and examined for evidence of inflammation, infection, or neoplasia.

Skin Scrapings and Fungal Culture

The skin of small mammals may become infested with parasitic mites (*mange*) or infected with fungi called dermatophytes (*dermatophytosis* or *ringworm*) (see Chapter 11). Depending upon the practice area, the prevalence of mange and ringworm in small mammals can be quite high. As with dogs and cats, skin scrapings and fungal cultures on areas of alopecia and crusting are often indicated. This can be challenging in rodents because these pets are often very mobile and difficult to restrain. A brief period of isoflurane anesthesia may be required to collect skin scrapings using a scalpel blade. In addition to (or in place of) a skin scraping, a cellophane-tape preparation can be made by applying cellophane tape onto an area of affected skin. The tape is then placed on a slide and examined microscopically for parasites.

Some doctors choose to forgo a skin scraping and fungal culture in pet rodents and recommend a skin biopsy or a trial dose of ivermectin, especially if anesthesia would be required to obtain the necessary samples for skin scraping or fungal culture.

REFERENCES

1. Otto C et al: Intraosseous infusion of fluids and therapeutics, *Compend Cont Educ Pract Vet* 2:421-430, 1989.
2. Rosenthal K: Ferrets, *Vet Clin No Am* 24:1-24, 1994.

CHAPTER 31

Nursing Care of Reptiles, Amphibians, and Aquarium Fish

S.P. Messonnier
R. Francis-Floyd

Learning Objectives

After reviewing this chapter, the reader should understand the following:

Methods of sample collection for laboratory analysis
Routes of administration of medication to reptiles and aquarium fish
Techniques used in general nursing care of reptiles and fish

Principles of feeding, watering, exercising, and bedding of reptiles
Procedures used in forced feeding of reptiles
Techniques used for diagnosing disease in reptiles and fish
Techniques used to ensure good water quality for aquarium fish

CARE OF REPTILE AND AMPHIBIAN PETS

S.P. MESSONNIER

Reptiles are often kept as pets; amphibians are rarely kept as pets except by experienced hobbyists. When a reptile or amphibian becomes ill, many owners turn to the veterinarian only after consulting with the "local expert" at the pet store. Additionally, because of the preservation response (discussed below), reptiles are usually critically ill by the time they are examined by the veterinarian. Because few veterinarians have the expertise to properly diagnose and treat these exotic species, another less-qualified veterinarian may have given inappropriate treatment before the animal was presented to your clinic. All of these factors contribute to a severely compromised patient and worsened prognosis.

Although kept as pets, reptiles and amphibians still retain many wild animal characteristics. One is called the *preservation response*. In the wild, an animal cannot have the luxury of acting "sick" when it is ill. If it did, it would risk being killed by others of its species or by predators. Therefore, a wild animal must give the appearance of being healthy so as to preserve itself even when it is ill. There comes a time, however, when the animal becomes so ill that it can no longer pretend to be healthy. At this point, usually when the illness is well advanced, the animal begins showing signs of illness. If the animal has been sick for some time, its condition deteriorates quickly after illness becomes apparent. Owners often state that the pet was "fine yesterday and now it's dying." Understanding and explaining the preservation response to owners will help them appreciate the severity of their pets' illnesses.

Reptiles and amphibians do not require vaccinations; however, they should receive an annual physical examination and fecal test for parasites. All new pets should receive the examination and fecal analysis within 48 hours of purchase. Ideally, prophylactic dewormings for various internal parasites can also be given at this time.

Owners should be counseled about the likely possibility that their reptile pet may serve as an asymptomatic carrier of *Salmonella* bacteria.[6] Culturing the feces in an attempt to detect *Salmonella* can also be done during this initial visit.

HOUSING
Reptiles

Reptiles can be housed in a simple aquarium with appropriate substrate or in something more elaborate. As a rule, the simpler the housing setup, the easier it is to observe the pet and clean the environment.

An aquarium of appropriate size can easily accommodate most pet reptiles.[1] There are many choices of substrates (bedding material). Artificial turf is most commonly used. It is easy to clean and is attractive. Care should be taken to make sure the edges do not become frayed; reptiles may chew on and subsequently ingest this frayed material, which may cause an impaction.

Other suitable substrates include terry cloth towels, newspaper, and butcher paper. Unacceptable substrates include dirt, sand, cat litter, crushed corn cobs, and crushed peanut shells. These substrates are difficult to keep clean, retain moisture that favors the growth of microorganisms, and may be ingested (causing an obstruction).

Lighting is important for reptile pets. Although species requirements may vary, as a general rule reptiles need approximately 12 hours of light and 12 hours of darkness. The light can be room light or preferably a full-spectrum light.

Heat is critical for reptiles. These pets are cold-blooded (ectotherms) and cannot regulate body temperature as mammals do. Owners must maintain the ambient temperature in the *thermoneutral zone* for that species (between a minimum and maximum temperature needed to preserve life). Iguanas require ambient temperatures between 75° and 100° F, box turtles 75° to 85° F, and most pythons and boa constrictors 75° to 90° F (Fig. 31-1). Species requirements vary and appropriate texts should be consulted as to each species' thermoneutral zone. Failure to provide the correct environmental temperature may contribute to anorexia, failure to breed, failure to gain weight, failure to thrive, and a host of medical problems. An important part of treating reptile diseases is to supply heat, because this allows the pet's immune system to function at its maximum capability.

Unfortunately, many owners take the advice of pet store employees when purchasing products for heating the reptile's environment. "Hot rocks" are often used as the pet's sole supply of heat. This practice should be discouraged for several reasons. First, although these artificially heated rocks may heat the pet's abdomen, they

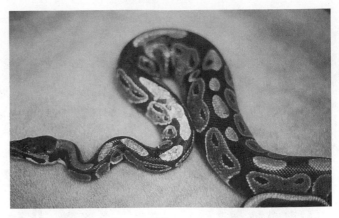

FIG. 31-1 Most pythons and boa constrictors require ambient temperatures between 75° and 90° F.

do not supply necessary environmental heat. Second, if the pet is weak, it may not have the energy to climb onto the hot rock and receive any heat. Third, these rocks may become too hot, causing severe burns. Their use should be discouraged.

Acceptable sources of heat include heating pads placed beneath the cage, or hot lights hung above or placed within the cage. Hot lights (basking lights) can often be purchased from pet stores; they are supplied as bulbs or ceramic heating elements. Owners can construct their own hot light using a 100-watt bulb with a reflector hood. Whichever method of heating is used, the owner should place two aquarium thermometers in the cage, one at the cool end and one at the end containing the heat source. This allows owners to know the range of temperatures in the pet's cage. Owners should also protect the pet from direct contact with the heat source, because severe burns can result from contact between the pet and the hot light. If heat is to be supplied at night, an infrared bulb or ceramic heating element can be used.

Amphibians

Most amphibians are kept at cooler temperatures and in a more humid environment than used for reptile pets. Although species differences occur, most amphibians do well at an ambient temperature of 70° to 85° F and humidity of 75% to 95%. Hiding places and full-spectrum and ultraviolet lighting should be provided. Terrestrial amphibians can be maintained on 1 to 4 inches of treated topsoil substrate covered with leaves or sphagnum moss and variously sized pieces of bark. The cage can be misted regularly to keep the soil moist. Aquatic amphibians, such as frogs, are housed in a typical aquarium with underwater filter. Obviously, the environment of pet amphibians must be kept clean. Hyperthermia and dehydration are common problems seen in amphibians housed in improper environments.

FEEDING

The subject of feeding reptiles and amphibians is vast and beyond the scope of this chapter. However, it is important to understand the dietary needs of reptiles, especially because improper diet is a common cause of many diseases in pet reptiles. This section discusses the general dietary needs of common pet reptiles and amphibians.

Iguanas[3]

Regardless of what pet store clerks tell owners, iguanas (Fig. 31-2) are *herbivorous*. This means that a major portion of the diet must be plant material. There is some controversy among veterinarians as to whether it is acceptable to feed iguanas small amounts of animal protein, such as crickets, moths, or worms. Most veterinarians would probably agree that limiting these animal protein sources to no more than 10% of the diet is safe, although the iguana may not even require these foods (and some iguanas will not eat them).

Most of an iguana's diet should consist of flowers (and leaves), such as roses, hibiscus, carnations, and mums, and green leafy vegetables (not celery and iceberg lettuce, which are low in nutritional value). A small amount of fruits can also be offered. Commercial dog and cat foods are too high in protein and vitamin D and are not recommended. The vegetable and flower "salad" should be chopped into pieces of a size suitable for the iguana's size and offered fresh daily or every other day. A *light* dusting of calcium powder (daily) and vitamin powder (weekly) is often recommended. Fresh water should be available at all times. Metabolic bone disease is common in green iguanas and results from a deficiency of dietary calcium, such as when only lettuce and fruit or lettuce and crickets are fed.

Snakes

Most species of snakes are carnivorous and eat whole prey. Suitable prey items include rats, mice, hamsters, and gerbils. Some species prefer one type of rodent, so it is wise to check reference texts regarding the snake species in question. To prevent injury or death of the snake, it is best to feed killed prey, either freshly killed (or stunned) or thawed, frozen prey. If the snake will eat only live prey, the owner *must* observe the snake after feeding it the prey. If the snake has not killed and eaten the prey within 15 minutes, the prey should be removed and the snake fed at a later time.

Box Turtles[2]

Like iguanas, box turtles eat a large amount of plant material; like snakes, they also eat animal protein. As a rule, the diet of box turtles should consist of about 50% plant material (similar to that for the iguana; hay can

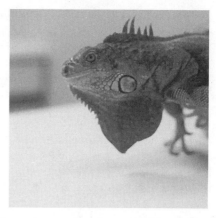

FIG. 31-2 Green iguana. Iguanas are herbivorous and should not be fed excessive amounts of animal protein.

also be offered) and 50% animal protein. This can include commercial turtle pellets, tofu, sardines, crickets, or worms. Vitamin A deficiency commonly results when turtles are offered only lettuce and fruit or lettuce and crickets. A proper diet helps prevent this common disorder. As with iguanas, a *light* daily sprinkling of calcium and weekly sprinkling of vitamins can help supplement the diet of box turtles.

Amphibians

Most amphibians are carnivorous as adults. Improper diet, such as a diet consisting of only crickets, can cause nutritional problems, such as metabolic bone disease. An improper diet, such as one consisting entirely of dog or cat food, may cause the opposite problem and lead to hypervitaminosis D or gout. Reference texts should be consulted regarding the proper diet for the species of amphibian in question.

GENERAL NURSING CARE

Although some sick reptiles and amphibians can be treated on an outpatient basis, many must be hospitalized for intensive care to maximize the chances for successful recovery.

Pet reptiles and amphibians that must be hospitalized are usually critically ill.[4] Fluid therapy, antibiotics, forced feeding, and proper environment are important. These sick pets should be handled as little as possible. The proper ambient temperature must be maintained; human pediatric incubators serve this function well. Incubators can be purchased as used units rather inexpensively through medical suppliers or directly from human hospitals. Most hospitalized reptiles must be maintained at ambient temperatures above 90° F while hospitalized, although the preferred optimum temperatures vary between species. Reference texts should be consulted regarding this temperature. Amphibians have a lower preferred temperature of approximately 70° to 75° F. If the need for hospitalization arises, sick amphibians do better when kept at this lower temperature and in an environment with approximately 75% to 95% humidity. When necessary, oxygen can be supplemented through a port on most pediatric incubators.

When possible, sick reptiles and amphibians should be isolated from other hospitalized animals. This is not only because of the risk of disease spread but also because these sick pets are extremely stressed. Many reptiles and amphibians are prey in the wild. Housing them near a natural predator (dog or cat) may serve to increase their stress.

DIAGNOSTIC AND TREATMENT TECHNIQUES

Diagnostic testing is routinely used in reptiles and amphibians. Commonly, such vague complaints as lack of appetite and lethargy are the only clues to illness. Although certain syndromes are more common in certain species, diagnostic testing helps the practitioner formulate a definitive diagnosis and proper treatment plan.

Unfortunately, many owners of some of the less expensive pets, particularly small iguanas and turtles, may not allow diagnostic testing because of the expense involved. Regardless, the veterinary technician must have a working knowledge of the various diagnostic tests available.

Venipuncture[8]

Venipuncture is commonly used in reptile patients and is less commonly used in amphibian pets. Venipuncture is used for withdrawing blood for hematologic and biochemical analysis, administration of certain medications, and intravenous catheterization for administration of fluids. Larger pets, such as large iguanas, usually present little difficulty for venipuncture, other than the need for adequate restraint. Venipuncture is challenging and at times impossible in the smaller reptiles and amphibians.

Anesthesia may be required when performing venipuncture on pets that are difficult to manually restrain; the technician must be thoroughly acquainted with delivery of anesthetic agents and monitoring of anesthesia in reptiles and amphibians. Additionally, technicians should check with the veterinary supervisor to make sure that technician-induced anesthesia of these pets is allowed under the state veterinary practice act. Except under certain specific circumstances, anesthesia may not be required once the technician has developed proficiency at venipuncture.

Although each diagnostic laboratory has specific requirements for the volume of blood required for vari-

ous tests, most laboratories can perform a mini-battery of tests on 0.5 ml of blood collected into a green-top (lithium heparin) tube. To prevent volume depletion in the smaller pets, some clinicians replace the volume of blood withdrawn with an equal volume of balanced electrolyte solution, given intravenously or subcutaneously.

Iguanas. The ventral coccygeal vein (tail vein) and ventral abdominal vein can be used for venipuncture in iguanas. The author prefers the ventral coccygeal vein and uses a 23- or 25-gauge needle (depending upon the size of the iguana) attached to a small syringe. The pet can be restrained on its back with the ventral aspect of the tail facing upward (dorsally), or the patient can be gently restrained in ventral recumbency on the table, with the tail hanging off of the table, and the vessel approached ventrally in this fashion. The needle is usually held vertical to the tail and vessel, although rarely the needle can be angled to allow cannulation of the vessel. The vessel lies on the midline; the needle is inserted to the depth of the bone, the syringe plunger is withdrawn slightly, and the needle is withdrawn away from the bone until blood appears in the syringe.

For puncture of the ventral abdominal vein, the patient is restrained in dorsal recumbency or supported in the axillary region and held vertically off of the table. The vein lies on the ventral midline just under the skin. Aspiration of blood is usually easier in the cranial half of the abdomen. Because it is easy to miss this vessel or actually pass the needle through the vessel, you may want to use the tail vein.

Snakes. The heart, ventral coccygeal vein, and palatine veins can be used for blood collection in snakes. For withdrawing blood from the ventral coccygeal vein, the same procedure used in iguanas is used in snakes. A point caudal to the vent or hemipenes is chosen for the venipuncture.

The palatine veins in the roof of the mouth can also be used, although these present some difficulty, especially in smaller snakes. Using a 25- or 27-gauge needle to cannulate the vein, you can collect blood that flows into the hub of the needle in heparinized microhematocrit tubes.

Cardiac puncture is most commonly used in snakes for blood collection. The heart is located by palpation or observing individual beats; this is not always as easy as it sounds. Once identified, the heart is stabilized between the thumb and index finger placed cranial and caudal to the heart. Blood is collected with a 23- to 27-gauge needle attached to a syringe. The needle is advanced between scales (scutes) and into the heart, and blood is withdrawn slowly.

Turtles. The following sites can be used for blood collection in pet turtles: jugular vein, dorsal coccygeal vein, clipped nail, brachial vein, and the postoccipital vein/venous plexus. Most clinicians prefer the right jugular vein for blood collection (the right vein is often larger than the left one). The most difficult part is in restraining the head; this is usually no problem in debilitated pets but is quite challenging in stronger, healthier specimens. The needle is introduced most easily in a cranial to caudal direction in the vein (which is superficial and located just beneath the skin). Depending upon the size of the patient, a 23- to 27-gauge needle attached to a syringe can be used.

The dorsal tail vein is commonly used in large tortoises. The tail is extended and a 25-gauge needle is placed into the vessel at the dorsal midline close to the base of the tail; a small volume of blood can be collected from this vessel.

A nail can be clipped as a last resort. Make sure to thoroughly clean the nail so as not to contaminate the blood specimen (falsely elevated uric acid levels are often reported if the specimen is contaminated with urates from droppings on the nail). The blood is collected into microhematocrit tubes by capillary action after the nail is clipped. Avoid "milking" the nail; simply allow the blood to flow freely.

Blood can be collected from the brachial vein or postoccipital vein; however, these samples are often contaminated with lymph from vessels in the area. For this reason, techniques for venipuncture from these sites are not discussed here.

Amphibians.[5] The lingual venous plexus, ventral abdominal vein, ventral caudal vein, and heart can be used for blood collection in amphibians. The lingual venous plexus, located on the ventral surface of the tongue and floor of the mouth, is often used even in small amphibians. After withdrawing the tongue with a cotton-tipped applicator, nick the vessels with a 25- to 28-gauge needle and collect blood in heparinized microhematocrit tubes. Releasing the tongue when finished usually causes the vessels to cease bleeding, although direct pressure can also be applied with the applicator. The area under the tongue should be swabbed to remove mucus and saliva before blood collection to minimize contamination.

The ventral abdominal vein, which courses just over the linea alba, can be cannulated with a 26- or 27-gauge needle in larger amphibians. A point midway between the pelvis and sternum is often chosen for venipuncture.

The ventral caudal (tail) vein is useful in collecting blood from species with a tail (salamanders). A 25- to 28-gauge needle is used for the technique. In species with tail autotomy (ability to regrow the tail), this site should not be used, because the tail may become separated during the procedure.

Cardiac puncture with a 25- to 28-gauge needle can be used for blood collection. The apex of the ventricle is entered after the cardiac impulse is identified visually by placing the pet on its back; sedation may be necessary (Box 31-1).

Box 31-1 Venipuncture technique

Materials:

appropriately sized needle and syringe or microhematocrit tubes

blood tube

alcohol swab

Procedure:

1. Gently restrain the pet. If anesthesia is used, another person must monitor the anesthetized animal.

2. Identify the venipuncture site. Warming of the area (e.g., with warm water on the jugular vein in turtles) may improve visualization.

3. Clean the area with an alcohol swab.

4. Withdraw the required amount of blood (limited to no more than 5% to 10% of body weight in a 2-week period).

5. Withdraw the needle; apply pressure for 30 to 60 seconds.

Parenteral Injection

Injectable medications are usually preferred over oral medications in hospitalized reptiles and amphibians. Medications that cannot be given orally (aminoglycosides) must be given by injection. Reptiles are difficult to medicate with pills. Extremely ill reptiles may have reduced intestinal function, making absorption of oral medication erratic and unpredictable. Most owners can be taught to give injections to their pets. Because most injections need to be given only once daily (and some just once every 48 to 72 hours), the task is not as difficult as it sounds.

Injections can be given subcutaneously, although the intramuscular route is often preferred. Because of the renal portal system in reptiles and amphibians, intramuscular injections should be given in the cranial half (forelimbs) of the body when possible. Injection of some medications may sting, and injection of some medications given subcutaneously may cause discoloration of the scales. Medications can also be given intravenously or via intraosseous catheterization. Intraperitoneal injection is another common route of drug administration in reptiles and amphibians. In turtles, the intracoelomic or epicoelomic routes are also used.

Amphibians can often be treated topically by dripping the solution onto the pet or by immersing it in a bath of solution. Amphibians can be injected subcutaneously (i.e., over the dorsum, pelvis, or shoulder) or intramuscularly (i.e., in the cranial half of the body in the epaxial musculature or front legs). Fluids are best given intracoelomically.

Hydration fluids may also be given to reptiles and amphibians. Although many clinicians used lactated Ringer's solution, a more appropriate solution is made by combining equal parts of lactated Ringer's solution with 2.5% dextrose or 2 parts of 2.5% dextrose in 0.45% saline with 1 part of lactated Ringer's solution.

Intraosseous Catheterization[7]

Because of the difficulty in venous catheterization in reptiles and amphibians, some doctors and technicians prefer intraosseous catheterization. Some pets require general anesthesia for placement of the catheter; those that are gravely ill often require only local anesthesia. An intraosseous catheter is ideal for delivering fluids and most medications that can be safely given intravenously. With regard to reptiles and amphibians, an intraosseous catheter is most easily placed in iguanas. The following discussion refers to intraosseous catheterization of iguanas.

The rate of absorption of a substance injected into the bone marrow is equal to that after injection into a peripheral vein. Intraosseous catheterization is preferred in patients with complete circulatory collapse. With respect to the rate of fluid uptake, the intraosseous route is second only to a central venous route, with the tip of the catheter residing in the cranial vena cava.

Intraosseous catheterization is not without risks, however. Contraindications include sepsis, skeletal abnormalities, skin and wound infections, abscesses over the bone, and recent fracture of that bone. With regard to sepsis, the risk of causing osteomyelitis must be weighed against the risk of mortality if insufficient fluids are delivered.

Supplies needed include a local anesthetic (1% or 2% lidocaine), suture material, bandaging material, triple antibiotic ointment, and an appropriate needle. Depending upon the size of the pet, a 20-gauge spinal needle or 18- to 25-gauge hypodermic needle may be used. The areas most commonly catheterized are the femur and fibial crest.

After the site is aseptically prepared, the skin, subcutis, and periosteum are infiltrated with lidocaine (if needed). The needle is inserted through the skin (a small stab incision can be made through the skin if needed before needle insertion) and advanced until bone is met. To avoid penetrating the sciatic nerve, walk the needle off the medial aspect of the greater trochanter into the trochanteric fossa. The hip joint should remain in a neutral position during needle advancement. Internally rotating the hip and adducting it also helps to protect the nerve. While applying firm and steady pressure, rotate the needle in 30-degree turns until it penetrates into the bone. Once the cortex has been penetrated, resistance to needle passage is reduced. The needle is flushed with a small amount of heparinized saline, which should flow freely. If resistance to fluid flow is encountered, a bone or marrow plug might be obstructing the needle. This can be prevented by using sterilized stainless-steel wire as a stylet during introduction of the needle or removing the needle and reinserting another one (preferably the next larger size) into the same hole. Observe the subcutaneous tissue for leakage of fluid. If this occurs, the needle must be removed and placed into another bone. A bone should not be catheterized again for 24 hours after previous attempts at catheterization.

Once the needle is seated firmly in place, a tape butterfly is placed around the hub of the needle and sutured to the skin. The area is covered with antibiotic ointment and bandaged securely.

Fluids can be given at a maximum rate of 11 ml/minute by gravity flow and 24 ml/minute using 300 mm Hg pressure. The catheter should be flushed every 6 hours with heparinized saline and removed after 48 to 72 hours. Most drugs suited for intravenous routes can be safely infused into the marrow. Check with the drug manufacturer if there are any questions (Box 31-2).

Water Soaks

An often neglected but important part of rehydration therapy in reptiles involves soaking the pet in warm water for 5 to 10 minutes several times a day. This can be done in the hospital and by owners when the pet is treated at home. The water baths often stimulate elimination, seem to be psychologically beneficial for the pet, and may allow for per-cloacal fluid absorption. The author recommends three to four baths each day. Place water in a sink. The water should be as warm as your hand will comfortably tolerate. The depth of the water should allow the pet to submerge most of its body, but let its head remain out of the water. The animal must be monitored at all times while it is immersed in the bath so as to prevent drowning.

Forced Feeding

Many pet reptiles and amphibians are presented for veterinary care because of anorexia and lethargy. In addition to the need for rehydration, nutritional supplementation is often required (and often overlooked). Animals that are not eating are in a *catabolic state*. Decreased food intake results in breakdown of protein and fat for energy. This can contribute to hepatic lipidosis, acidosis, azotemia, muscle wasting, impaired gastrointestinal function, and decreased immunity. To prevent these complications (or correct them, because

Box 31-2 Intraosseous catheterization

Materials:

1% to 2% lidocaine

suture material

adhesive tape

20-gauge spinal needle or 18- to 25-gauge hypodermic needle bandaging/dressing material

antibiotic ointment

Procedure:

1. Gently restrain the pet. If anesthesia is necessary, another person must monitor the anesthetized animal.

2. Identify the catheterization site; prepare the area as for surgery.

3. Infiltrate the area with lidocaine (not needed if general anesthesia is used but may provide some analgesia when the pet awakens).

4. Use a twisting motion while advancing the needle into the bone.

5. Aspirate to check for needle position. Any marrow that is aspirated can be saved for analysis, if indicated. Injection of a small amount of electrolyte solution (or heparinized saline) can also be used to check for proper positioning of the needle (extravasation of fluid indicates accidental penetration of bone cortex; the needle must be removed).

6. Apply antibiotic ointment and a light dressing to the site.

7. Apply a tape butterfly using adhesive tape around the hub of the needle. Suture the tape to the skin.

8. Bandage the catheter to the limb; flush with heparinized saline and apply a cap to the needle when fluids are not being administered. To make a cap for the needle, cut off the end of a 1-ml syringe (including the stopper) with nail clippers.

tube is passed into the esophagus and into the stomach (on longer snakes, it may not be possible for the tube to reach the stomach). The slurry is given down the tube, and the tube is withdrawn. Because reptiles have a cranially located glottis (often at the base of the tongue) that is easily visualized upon opening the mouth, it is difficult (if not impossible) to accidentally intubate the trachea.

Amphibians. A slurry of Emeraid II (Lafeber) and Repto-Min can be used (not to exceed 2% of the pet's body weight every 24 hours) or a slurry of pinkie mice supplemented with vitamins and crickets.

Iguanas/Turtles. Diluted Emeraid II can be used for forced feeding. Alternatively, a slurry of ground alfalfa mixed with water or an electrolyte replacement solution could be used.

Snakes. Snakes can be force-fed well-lubricated whole prey (mice). You may use a slurry of turkey baby food mixed with diluted Emeraid II and give this by stomach tube.

Fecal Analysis

Microscopic analysis of fecal samples is used to evaluate animals with diarrhea and any nonspecific complaint (anorexia, lethargy). The method is similar to that used in dogs and cats. For cases of diarrhea, a fecal smear of *fresh* feces mixed with a small amount of (warm) tap water and a flotation (using zinc sulfate or sodium nitrate solution) should be performed. Gram stains may be helpful as well, especially if a yeast infection is suspected. A parasitology text should be consulted for details on identifying the ova. Fecal cultures can also be used, especially when *Salmonella* or *Campylobacter* infection is suspected. A reference laboratory should be consulted regarding specific requirements for fecal cultures.

Fluorescein Staining of the Cornea

When ocular disease is suspected, fluorescein staining of the cornea is indicated. The procedure is the same as in dogs and cats. Briefly, a drop of water is placed on the end of the fluorescein strip. The moistened strip is gently touched to the sclera or palpebral conjunctiva and the eyelids closed to allow distribution of the stain. Areas of ulceration retain the fluorescent dye, whereas intact corneal epithelium does not. If the eye contains a large amount of mucus, this can be removed by gentle flushing with water after the stain is applied. Often the eye may be in pain, especially if ulceration is present. In this case, one to two drops of topical ocular anesthetic can be applied to minimize blepharospasm before stain is applied.

Cytologic Examination

Reptiles are sometimes presented for evaluation of cutaneous masses. These may represent tumors, abscesses,

many are probably in existence when the pet is initially examined), supplementation with food is important. This can be done in the hospital or by the owner at home if the pet will be treated on an outpatient basis.

The force-feeding procedure is relatively straightforward. An appropriately sized red rubber feeding granulomas, or parasites. These masses should be initially evaluated by needle aspiration of their contents. All masses should be aspirated so that the doctor can formulate the proper diagnosis and treatment plan. A 22- to 25-gauge needle and 3- to 12-ml syringe are used for aspirating the mass. After material has been aspirated from the mass, the needle is removed from the syringe, air is aspirated into the syringe, and the needle is replaced on the air-filled syringe. A clean glass slide is readied. The air is then pushed through the needle, which causes the small amount of aspirated material trapped in the needle to be deposited on the slide.

To prepare the slide for staining, use a squash technique, in which a clean slide is gently placed at right angles on top of the aspirated material. The two slides are gently "squashed" together, and the top slide is pulled away. The material can be stained with Diff-Quik and examined for evidence of inflammation, infection, or neoplasia.

REFERENCES

1. de Vosjoli P: *The general care and maintenance of ball pythons*, Lakeside, Calif, 1990, Advanced Vivarium Systems.
2. de Vosjoli P: *The general care and maintenance of box turtles*, Lakeside, Calif, 1991, Advanced Vivarium Systems.
3. de Vosjoli P: *The general care and maintenance of the green iguana*, Lakeside, Calif, 1990, Advanced Vivarium Systems.
4. Frye F: *Reptile care: an atlas of diseases and treatments*, Neptune City, NJ, 1991, TFH.
5. Mader D: *Reptile medicine and surgery*, Philadelphia, 1996, WB Saunders.
6. Messonnier SP: *Exotic pets: a veterinary guide for owners*, Plano, Tex, 1995, Wordware Publishing.
7. Otto C et al: Intraosseous infusion of fluids and therapeutics, *Compend Contin Educ Pract Vet* 4:421-430, 1989.
8. Messonnier SP: *Common reptile diseases and treatment*, Cambridge, Mass, 1996, Blackwell Science.

CARE OF AQUARIUM FISH

R. FRANCIS-FLOYD

HOUSING SICK FISH

For small fish ($\leq$ 10 cm), a 38-L aquarium with a sponge filter and air stone is adequate for a hospital tank. Fish should be housed in a tank where they can be readily observed and isolated from other fish, easily caught and handled for diagnostic evaluations or treatment, and given medication safely and accurately.

Care of hospitalized fish must include cleaning and disinfecting equipment, maintaining appropriate water quality, and feeding. An easy and effective method of removing debris from a tank is to siphon it from the bottom with a hose. Daily cleaning is probably not necessary unless excessive debris accumulates (usually caused by overfeeding); however, tanks should be thoroughly cleaned once or twice a week. Because of concerns about transmission of infectious disease, each tank should have its own siphon hose, net, etc., or each piece of equipment must be disinfected (and thoroughly rinsed) between uses. Ideally, a dilute chlorine or quaternary ammonium solution should be circulated through the tank (not containing fish), and all filters used for at least an hour, followed by thorough rinsing. If chlorine is used, a standard colorimetric chlorine test kit can be used to ensure that no residual chlorine remains. Chlorine bleach should not be used as a disinfectant in the immediate vicinity of live fish, because it is very volatile and a small amount (0.02 mg/L) can kill fish.

WATER QUALITY MANAGEMENT

Water quality should be monitored daily and results entered into the medical record of all hospitalized fish. Various water quality test kits available are easy to use, inexpensive, and reasonably accurate. No ammonia, nitrite, or nitrate should be present in freshwater or saltwater systems at any time. Of these, ammonia is most likely to be of concern because of the lack of established biologic filtration in a hospital setting. Nitrogenous wastes are removed primarily by regular water changes. Never use distilled or deionized water to fill fish tanks, because these lack essential minerals.

Saltwater systems should be maintained at a pH of 8.2 to 8.3 and a salinity approaching 33 ppt (parts per thousand), or a specific gravity of 1.023 at 25° C, unless there is a medical order to the contrary.[3] Freshwater systems should be maintained with a pH of 6.5 to 9.0, with the understanding that ammonia toxicity increases substantially when pH is above 8.0.[2,5] Total alkalinity (carbonate) and total hardness (mineral cations, usually predominantly calcium) should be greater than 50 mg/L in freshwater systems, and should exceed several hundred mg/L in saltwater systems. If city water is used, water must be dechlorinated by an activated carbon filter or by adding sodium thiosulfate at 6.99 mg/L to remove each 1 mg of chlorine from 1 L of solution.[2] If well water is used, vigorous aeration should be used to eliminate potential problems caused by gas supersaturation. Overviews of water quality management for freshwater and saltwater systems are available in other references.[2,3,5]

FEEDING SICK FISH

Hospitalized fish are likely to have a poor appetite, although many species of pet fish begin to eat as soon as they feel better. Improvement in feeding activity is an excellent gauge of response to therapy for many species. Wild-caught fish (e.g., reef fish) are less likely to eat, especially if recently captured. For most fish, a maximum feeding rate of 0.5% to 1% body weight per day provides plenty of food for body maintenance while in the clinic.

A standard flake or pelleted food may be all that is required for feeding most fish. Fish foods should be stored in a cool, dry place and discarded after 1 to 3 months. Herbivorous species often thrive on fresh vegetables, including romaine lettuce, fresh broccoli, spinach, or bok choy. Diced zucchini, an excellent source of B and C vitamins, is usually acceptable to many carnivorous fish. If it is necessary to soften fresh vegetables, they may be briefly parboiled or blanched in a microwave oven; however, even brief exposure to heat destroys some vitamins.

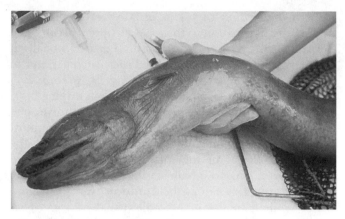

FIG. 31-3 This moray eel has been anesthetized in preparation for aspiration biopsy.

HANDLING FISH

Most species of pet fish tolerate a considerable amount of handling if it is done carefully. First, never move an animal until a plan is in place as to where it is being moved, the purpose of the move, and assignment of responsibility so that all involved are aware of their role and equipment is ready to accomplish their task. From a practical perspective, if a fish is to be moved to another container filled with water, such as an anesthetic solution, be sure that the two solutions are the same temperature. It is easy to accidentally kill a fish by moving it from warm water to cool water or vice versa. Sudden changes in temperature greater than 4° C should be avoided. If city water is being used, be sure to dechlorinate receiving water. If well water is being used, be sure it is well aerated and degassed.

If fish must be netted, a small-mesh net should be used and great care should be taken to minimize scale damage. If fish can be collected with something less damaging than a net (wet hand or plastic barrier), this is preferable. When fish are removed from water, they should be placed on a wet, slippery surface rather than a dry counter or table top. It is usually advisable to place freshwater fish in weak salt solution (1 to 10 ppt, depending on species and exposure time) following handling. A similar decrease in salinity may benefit saltwater species, although less data are available to confirm this.

RESTRAINT OF AQUARIUM FISH

In many instances it may be easiest to restrain fish chemically before beginning a procedure (Fig. 31-3).

Methane tricaine sulfonate or MS-222 (Finquel, Argent Chemical) is a safe and effective anesthetic that can be used for freshwater or saltwater fish. Concentrations of 50 to 100 mg/L are generally safe and effective for most species.[1] During induction of anesthesia, fish go through a brief excitement phase characterized by rapid swimming, followed by loss of equilibrium and nonresponsiveness to stimuli.[1] Monitoring the respiratory rate is essential for safe anesthesia of fish. If opercular movements cease at any time, the fish should be moved to clean water immediately.

Manual restraint is possible if fish are too sick to tolerate anesthesia or if the procedure is of very short duration (≤ 1 to 2 min). An unanesthetized fish can be restrained by holding the fish's head while covering the eyes, and applying gentle but firm pressure to the peduncle. If the animal objects strenuously, use of anesthesia is recommended.

ADMINISTERING MEDICATION TO FISH

Bath treatments are ideal for eliminating external parasites, fungi, or bacteria, and may be somewhat analogous to dipping a dog. A few antibiotics and anthelmintics can be administered through a bath treatment, but these are limited. When administering a bath treatment, it is important to understand that the concentration used is inversely proportional to the time that the fish should be left in the medicated water. Therefore, if a fish is to be in contact with the medication for a very short time, the concentration of chemical is likely to be quite high. On the other hand, if the medication is to be placed in the water as a permanent treatment, such as when adding salt to a recirculating system, the concentration of chemical should be very low.

Oral medication of fish is usually accomplished by adding the medication to their food. A premix can often be added directly to the usual food, but occasionally it is necessary to make a specialized diet. Medication can be added to pelleted food by adding the premix to a small amount of vegetable or cod liver oil, mixing thoroughly, and drizzling the resulting suspension over pellets as they are vigorously stirred or shaken. The most common site for intramuscular (IM) injection is the epaxial muscles along the dorsal body wall, just caudal to the dorsal fin. To administer an intraperitoneal (IP) injection, the fish can be held in dorsoventral recumbency while a small-gauge needle (usually 25 gauge) is inserted in a dorsocranial direction just cranial to the pelvic bone and pelvic fin. To avoid damaging internal organs, the needle should be lifted so that it lies just within the peritoneal space. Irritating substances should be given IM rather than IP.

Topical medication, usually in ointment form, is easily administered by gently removing the fish from the water, applying ointment to the desired site, and holding the fish out of water for about 30 seconds, then releasing it. Topical medication is usually limited to small, localized injuries.

REFERENCES

1. Brown LA: *Anesthesia and restraint.* In Stoskopf MK: *Fish medicine*, Philadelphia, 1993, WB Saunders.
2. Boyd CE: *Water quality in ponds for aquaculture*, Alabama Agricultural Experiment Station, Auburn, Ala, 1990, Auburn University.
3. Spotte S: *Captive seawater fishes*, New York, 1992, John Wiley & Sons.
4. Stoskopf MK: *Fish medicine*, Philadelphia, 1993, WB Saunders.
5. Tucker CS: *Water analyses.* In Stoskopf MK: *Fish medicine*, Philadelphia, 1993, WB Saunders.

CHAPTER 32

Nursing Care of Orphaned and Injured Wild Animals

S.L. Porter
L.J. Gage

Learning Objectives

After reviewing this chapter, the reader should understand the following:

Assessing the condition of orphaned wild animals
Methods of sample collection for laboratory analysis
Routes of administration of medication

Principles of rehabilitating orphaned wild animals and marine mammals in captivity
Procedures used in forced feeding of marine mammals
Techniques used for diagnosing disease in wild animals and marine mammals

RABBITS, BIRDS, AND RAPTORS

S.L. PORTER

GENERAL CONSIDERATIONS

Native wild animals that become injured or orphaned are commonly found by well-meaning individuals. If the veterinary hospital does not accept wild animals as patients, callers should be referred to licensed wildlife rehabilitators, wildlife centers, zoos, or other veterinary hospitals that do accept such cases. If only giving advice, the professional staff must provide advice that is medically sound and legal. Because many of these "rescued" animals have no true owners, the practice is often not paid for services rendered. Potential professional liability issues, such as possible zoonoses and staff injuries, must be considered.

PHYSICAL EXAMINATION OF WILDLIFE

Physical examination may be done by the technician and/or the veterinarian. Most of the commonly seen wild animals are easily handled if one pays attention to their offensive and defensive weapons, such as teeth, beaks, claws, antlers, and hooves. These weapons must be neutralized to prevent injury to personnel (Fig. 32-1). Gloves, towels, snares, nets, shields, and other restraint aids may be necessary. These animals are often severely compromised and are poor candidates for general anesthesia. Only vicious animals, such as carnivores, bears, and some rodents, must be anesthetized for this initial examination. Because most of these animals are trauma victims, multiple injuries are very common. Do not stop the examination after finding one lesion.

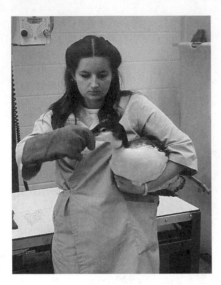

FIG. 32-1 Technician restraining a loon, which is a heavy-bodied bird with a thick, pointed beak. Note that the technician wears heavy gloves and holds the beak while pressing the bird's wings to its body. When working with birds with a pointed beak, grasp the beak first to prevent injury, and do not release your grip until the bird is placed back in its enclosure.

RELEASABILITY

The concept of *releasability* must be considered. The goal of wildlife rehabilitation is to release the animal back to the wild so that it may survive. A wild bird with one functional wing, or one leg, or any totally blind animal should not be released. Part of the hospital plan should consider the factors that determine whether an animal can be successfully returned to the wild. Unless the nonreleasable animal is a threatened or endangered species, it should be humanely euthanized if it cannot be released. Euthanasia may be performed by the same methods used in small animal practice. Birds are readily euthanized by injecting a small amount (0.1 to 0.3 ml) of barbiturate euthanasia solution into the suboccipital sinus at the base of the skull. Small wild animals may be humanely euthanized by placing them in a small, glass chamber containing halothane.

Legal placement of unreleasable animals is difficult and time consuming. Government agencies will not grant permits for individuals to keep nonreleasable wildlife, including hand-raised orphans, in their homes. Placement can be arranged through professional wildlife rehabilitation organizations and via the Internet, but these are often overwhelmed with too few legal outlets for these animals. Avian species, except house sparrows, English starlings, and pigeons, are all protected by the Fish and Wildlife Service of the U.S. Department of Interior; nonendangered or nonthreatened mammals and reptiles are protected by state

wildlife agencies. When endangered species are presented, the nearest FWS office should be notified. Unless the veterinarian is working with licensed rehabilitators, the veterinarian should have permits from the state wildlife agency and the Fish and Wildlife Service of the Department of Interior. State wildlife laws vary, and veterinarians should contact their local game wardens for specific information.

DIAGNOSTIC TESTING

After the physical examination, such diagnostic tests as complete blood counts, blood chemistries, radiographs, fecal examination, and toxicologic tests may be required to further evaluate the patient. These procedures are similar to those done on domestic animals.

CARE OF ORPHANED WILDLIFE

During the spring, citizens find many young wild animals. These young animals have fallen from nests, have had their nests destroyed, or are just found on the ground. Many times these people call the hospital for information about what to do. If at all possible, the young animal should be placed back in the nest or the nest should be rebuilt or replaced. Fledgling birds may be placed in a bush so that they can still be fed by their parents.

If these "orphans" are brought to the veterinary practice, they should be handled like other wild animals. They often are hypothermic and/or dehydrated. Any other medical problems, such as wounds, parasite infestation, and fractures, must be addressed. The diet used varies with the species. There are many milk substitutes on the market, including Esbilac (Pet-Ag, Elgin, Ill), Unilac (Upjohn, Kalamazoo, Mich), KMR (Pet-Ag), Zoologic (Pet-Ag), Nurturall (Vet Products Labs, Phoenix, Ariz), and Just Born (Farnham Pet Products, Phoenix, Ariz). These can be used to feed baby squirrels, opossums, foxes, raccoons, and other small mammals. Baby rabbits require more fat in their diets, so whipping cream is often added to the commercial preparations or Lamb Milk Replacer (Land O Lakes, Fort Dodge, Iowa) is used. Goat milk or Lamb Milk Replacer is also used for the fawns of white-tailed deer. These formulas may be administered by a variety of means, including dosing needles, eyedroppers, pet nursers, baby bottles, or lamb nipples attached to soda bottles. The amount fed and frequency of administration vary with the size of the animal, but usually 10% to 20% of the body weight is given in divided doses two to four times a day. After the baby mammal opens its eyes, the feeding frequency is decreased, the formula is thickened, and weaning begins.

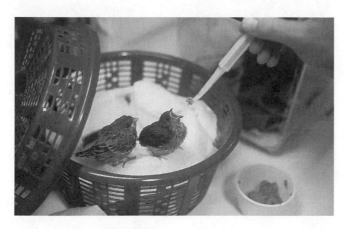

FIG. 32-2 The baby songbird on the right gapes as a food dropper approaches its mouth. These young birds are kept in a simple basket but will be moved to a proper enclosure as they learn to fly.

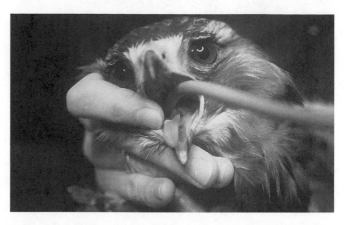

FIG. 32-3 A rubber feeding tube is used to provide fluids and nutrients to this red-tailed hawk. The glottis is visible ventral to the tube.

Bird diets also vary with the species. Commercial diets, such as Nutristart (Lafeber, Odell, Ill) and Lake's Hand Rearing Formula (Lakes Unlimited) are available. For songbirds, a nonoily canned dog food is mixed 2:1 with chick starter and fed whenever the baby bird gapes for food (Fig. 32-2), or about every 15 to 60 minutes, depending on age of the bird. Insects, such as mealworms, waxworms, and crickets, may be added to the diet at weaning. Young waterfowl and quail may be fed chick or turkey starter. Baby doves and pigeons must be tube fed formula until weaning. Raptors or birds of prey should be hand fed chopped rodents or another balanced diet for the first two weeks of life, before they begin eating on their own. Hamburger and organ meat should not be fed, because it causes severe bone abnormalities in all young animals. The young of some species, such as wood ducks, killdeer, and chimney swifts, are difficult and time consuming to raise. Proper training is essential to success with these species.

Before they are released, wild animals must be introduced to natural foods. Predatory species must be given the opportunity to practice killing live prey before release. Various behavioral abnormalities, especially taming, may develop in hand-raised wildlife, so experienced wildlife rehabilitators should be consulted. Imprinting, or species identification, occurs at birth or hatching in precocious species, such as deer, ducks, and quail, and later in development in altricial species, such as raptors.

CARE OF INJURED ADULT WILDLIFE

The most common reason adult wild animals are presented to veterinarians is vehicular trauma. These animals suffer the same types of injuries as seen in dogs and cats. Therapy for shock includes fluids and glucocorti-coids. Intravenous fluids are best, but intraperitoneal fluids work well in small mammals; intraosseous fluids are commonly used in birds and mammals. In birds, intraosseous fluids may be administered into the distal ulna or the proximal tibiotarsus. The intraosseous route may also be used in small mammals by placing an 18-gauge needle through the trochanteric fossa into the proximal femur. If the animal is conscious, oral fluids may be administered via a stomach tube (Fig. 32-3).

Because many injured wild animals are hypothermic, warming is an essential part of the treatment. These animals may be placed in an infant incubator, on a warm-water circulating pad, or carefully on a towel-covered heating pad or under a heat lamp. It is important to carefully monitor and frequently move animals placed on electric heating pads or under heat lamps.

Open wounds require attention, especially in birds in which there is little soft tissue under the skin and the exposed bone or connective tissue may become dry or infected. Wounds should be flushed, debrided, and protected by suturing or bandaging. It is important not to damage a bird's feathers by smearing them with oily topicals or covering them with sticky tape. Masking tape works well to hold bandaging material or immobilize extremities in small animals. Nonstick elastic tape (VetWrap, 3-M Animal Care, St. Paul, Minn) can be used over or under masking tape.

Traumatized wild animals often exhibit neurologic signs because of brain injury. Signs include ataxia, depression, head tilt, torticollis, or blindness. These animals require supportive therapy to see if they improve. Corticosteroids may be used for several days. The condition of these animals may improve within days to weeks, may worsen, or may improve to some extent and then remain static. Euthanasia is indicated if the animal's condition worsens or ceases to improve. Those

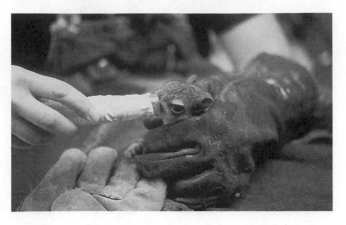

FIG. 32-4 A plastic syringe casing has been modified to serve as a mask for induction of anesthesia in an immature gray squirrel.

that appear normal must be permitted to demonstrate the ability to find food and perches and move normally in an enclosure larger than a dog kennel.

Eye problems also commonly result from collisions with vehicles. These injuries may be obvious, involving the globe, cornea, iris, or lens, or they may be obscure, involving the posterior segment. A complete eye examination should include observing if the animal can visually follow a finger moved near its face, pupillary light reflex, and ophthalmoscopy. An animal that is totally blind should never be released back into the wild. Most animals with vision in only one eye, however, can survive in the wild and may be released once they have demonstrated that they have otherwise recovered.

Fractures are common in traumatized wild animals and require at least stabilization initially. Many fractures in smaller animals can be treated only with external immobilization by taping the extremity to the body, or splinting it in extension using aluminum rods, tongue depressors, syringe casings, finger splints, or casting material. Some fractures may require surgery, but surgery should be performed after the animal's condition has stabilized. It is wise to combine internal fixation with external fixation to provide additional support. Because contracture of connective tissue is a common problem in birds, extremities should not be immobilized longer than 3 to 4 weeks. Physical therapy involving joint massage, flexing and extending joints, and exercise in a flight pen is essential for birds that have had their wings immobilized.

CHEMICAL RESTRAINT AND ANESTHESIA

General anesthesia is most rapidly and safely induced with isoflurane (Aerrane, Anaquest, Madison, Wisc).

Other inhalation agents may be used, but they are generally not as safe as isoflurane (see Chapter 20). If the animal can be physically restrained, induction by mask works well (Fig. 32-4). Endotracheal intubation is usually performed except for quick procedures or in species that are difficult to intubate, such as rodents, rabbits, and deer.

It is important to allow the animal to recover from general anesthesia in a dark, quiet, warm space to prevent its injuring itself. With isoflurane anesthesia, the animals are physically restrained until they are standing, usually within 5 to 10 minutes.

CARE OF POISONED WILDLIFE

Although trauma is the most common cause of neurologic signs, poisonings also commonly affect the nervous system. The poisonings may be intentional or accidental. Birds are most commonly involved. Nonspecific clinical signs include convulsions, ataxia, depression, diarrhea, salivation, nystagmus, and opisthotonos. Usually one patient is presented at a time, but if many animals are affected, the state or federal wildlife officials should be contacted immediately.

The two most common types of poisonings seen are lead toxicity and organophosphate/carbamate toxicity. Lead toxicity may be diagnosed by radiographic evidence of lead shot in the gastrointestinal tract or by elevated lead levels in the blood. The most common treatment for lead toxicity is calcium disodium edentate (Calcium Disodium Versenate, Riker Labs, St. Paul, Minn) IM at 35 mg/kg BID for 5 days.

Organophosphate or carbamate toxicity is diagnosed by finding depressed levels of cholinesterase in the blood or by identifying the chemical in the crop or stomach contents. The treatment for organophosphate poisoning is atropine at 0.5 mg/kg IV or IM. Atropine only alleviates clinical signs and does not affect cholinesterase levels. Affected birds require several weeks to fully recover.

Botulism, also called *limberneck*, is a major cause of death in wild birds. It is frequently seen in waterfowl; many birds may be affected at one time. Affected birds exhibit an inability to control their neck or wings and a prolapsed nictitans (third eyelid). Treatment is primarily supportive, although neostigmine (Prostigmin, Roche, Nutley, NJ) may increase neuromuscular function.

CARE OF WILDLIFE IN CAPTIVITY

Diagnosis and treatment of injury or illness in wildlife can be relatively easy, but coaxing the patient to eat while in captivity may be more of a challenge. It is not unusual for a wild animal to become debilitated or even to starve to death while in captivity. Providing a proper diet is essential for maintaining wild animals in captivity. Canned dog food is used as a base diet for a variety of species, including song birds, opossums, raccoons, skunks, foxes, and bears. Commercial diets are also available. The diet can be made more appealing by adding mealworms for insectivores, honey for bears, and banana for other species. Rabbits, squirrels, and other rodents are fed sweet feed, sweet potato, dark green leafy vegetables, and rodent or rabbit pellets. Owls, hawks, vultures, and eagles may be fed laboratory rodents, chopped chicken, carrion, or prepared, supplemented horse meat (Bird of Prey Diet, Animal Spectrum, North Platte, Neb).

Some species will not eat in a small cage but readily accept the same food in a quiet, larger pen. If the animal will not eat on its own, then nourishment must be provided to it. Various hyperalimentation formulas, such as Isocal (Mead Johnson, Evansville, Ind), Emeraid II (Lafeber, Odell, Ill), and Clinical Care (Pet-Ag, Elgin, Ill), are administered by stomach tube. Nutrical (Evsco, Buena, NJ) works well when force fed to mammals.

In addition to an adequate diet, proper management of captive wild animals also includes housing so that the animal does not injure its feathers, wings, legs, or head. Birds often destroy feathers or break their legs when kept in wire cages. Excessive noise and activity often excite the animal, causing it to bang its head or wings against the sides of the enclosure. Birds of prey in particular are subject to infections on the bottoms of their feet from inadequate perches. The veterinary hospital is not the ideal place to house wild animals unless they can be kept in an isolated, quiet area.

RETURN TO THE WILD

A major consideration in wildlife rehabilitation is determination of when the patient is ready for release. Criteria used must be aimed at ensuring the survival of the animal in the wild. These may include healed injuries, normal blood values, ability to fly or run, and ability to obtain food.

Once the animal has been judged ready for release, then thought must be given to proper release sites. It is not acceptable to just open the door and toss out the animal. In some cases it is best to release the animal where it was found; however, this may be contraindicated, such as if the animal was found near a busy highway. Some animals, such as groundhogs, deer, and beavers, are considered pests, and should be released only where permission has been granted by the landowner. The animal should be released in suitable habitat, away from people, pets, and motor vehicles. It is not uncommon for a family to work hard to raise a songbird, release it in their back yard, and then watch in horror as it is killed by their cat. Some captive raised orphans, such as Canada geese and wood ducks, imprint on their release site and return there to nest. Consideration should also be given to the weather and time of year. Animals should not be turned out during or just preceding inclement weather. Releasing reptiles and adolescent mammals in winter is also not a good idea. Migrating birds should not be released after the migration has finished. Some birds have been transported to Florida for release during the winter.

RECOMMENDED READING

Davidson WR, Nettles VF: *Field manual of wildlife diseases in the southeast United States*, Athens, Ga, 1988, Southeast Cooperative Wildlife Disease Study.

Fowler M, editor: *Zoo and wild animal medicine: current therapy 3*, Philadelphia, 1993, WB Saunders.

Friend M, editor: *Field guide to wildlife diseases*, Washington, DC, 1987, USDI, FWS (Resource Publication #167).

McKeever K: *Care and rehabilitation of injured owls*, Vineland, Ontario, Can, 1987, WF Rannie.

Moore AT and Joosten S: *NWRA principles of wildlife rehabilitation*, St. Cloud, Minn, 1997, National Wildlife Rehabilitators' Association.

Redig PT et al, editors: *Raptor biomedicine*, Minneapolis, 1993, University of Minnesota Press.

Ritchie BW, Harrison GJ, Harrison LR; *Avian medicine: principles and application*, Lake Worth, Fla, 1994, Wingers Publishing.

Wildlife rehabilitation listserver: LISTSERV@VM1.NODAK.EDU

Wildlife health listserver: WildlifeHealth@relay.doit.wisc.edu

Wildlife Rehabilitation Today Magazine, Coconut Creek Publishing, 2201 NW 40th Terrace, Coconut Creek, FL 33060-2032.

WILDLIFE REHABILITATION ORGANIZATIONS

National Wildlife Rehabilitators Association (NWRA)
14 North 7th Avenue
St. Cloud, MN 56303-4766

International Wildlife Rehabilitation Council
4437 Central Place, B-4
Suisun, CA 94585

MARINE MAMMALS

L.J. GAGE

Marine mammals are mammals that have adapted to living in a marine environment. Cetaceans and sirenians are "true" marine mammals, spending their lives in water. Pinnipeds, polar bears, and sea otters are also considered to be marine mammals, because they have adapted to and depend on the marine environment for survival.

REHABILITATION OF PINNIPEDS

The order Pinnipedia includes the families Phocidae (true seals), Otariidae (eared seals, such as sea lions and fur seals), and Odobenidae (walruses). Representatives of all of these families are found in captive situations. Phocids and otariids are the most common marine mammals found in rehabilitation centers worldwide.

Wild, stranded pinnipeds often require intensive nursing care. When possible, the animal should be sent in a timely manner to the closest rehabilitation center. The only time an individual should try rehabilitation of marine mammals is if there is no marine mammal rehabilitation center in the state or country where the animal is stranded.

Pinnipeds become stranded because they are ill, injured, or orphaned. They can be transported to a rehabilitation center via truck or airplane. One should ensure they are kept cool during their trip, because they are prone to overheating. Once they arrive at a rehabilitation center, a physical examination should be performed. Blood can be collected for a complete blood count and serum biochemical analysis (Fig. 32-5). The lungs and heart should be auscultated and all information entered into an individual record. Fecal analysis is done to detect parasite eggs. Feces can be cultured for the more common pathogens, such as *Salmonella* or *Plesiomonas* (typically a human pathogen). An individual treatment regimen is prescribed for each animal, based on laboratory and clinical findings.

Most sick, injured, or orphaned pinnipeds are dehydrated when they are rescued and require fluid replacement therapy. Some will drink fresh water, but the most reliable way to rehydrate them is to administer subcutaneous fluids. This is achieved by swift placement of a l-inch, 18-gauge needle subcutaneously between the shoulders or over the hips. Lactated Ringer's solution is a good choice of fluids initially. Fluids can be given at a rate of 50 ml/kg/day. Depressed animals tolerate subcutaneous fluid administration from a 1-L bag with a drip set hung above the animal. Small pinnipeds can be restrained and given subcutaneous fluids in a single dose at several sites. Intravenous fluids are nearly impossible to administer to otariids because of the difficulty of catheterizing a vein. Intravenous fluids can be given easily to phocids that are depressed and stationary through the extradural intravertebral sinus. Always remember that restraint for treatment is very stressful to wild animals and the stress of restraint may outweigh the benefits of giving the fluids.

California sea lions are the most common otariid found in rehabilitation centers on the west coast of the United States. The most prevalent findings in these animals are heavy parasite infections, respiratory problems, and renal disease. Northern fur seals and Steller's sea lions are infrequently rescued and usually are presented to rehabilitation centers as emaciated pups.

Northern elephant seals and harbor seals are the most common phocids found in rehabilitation centers. Most elephant seals are found stranded as orphan pups or yearlings with skin problems. Most harbor seals admitted to rehabilitation centers are orphaned pups.

Rehabilitation of harbor seal pups involves diagnosis and treatment of illness or injury and day-to-day hand-rearing of all pups. A formula for hand-rearing most otariids and phocids is Borden's Multimilk, which is available in powdered form and is mixed with equal parts of water (Fig. 32-6). Feedings of formula should

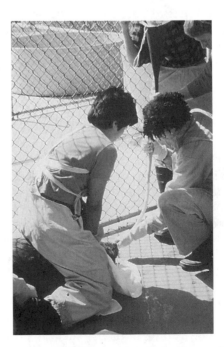

FIG. 32-6   Tube feeding an orphaned elephant seal pup.

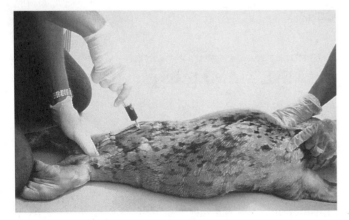

FIG. 32-5   Obtaining a blood sample from the extradural intravertebral vein of a harbor seal.

be gradually brought up to 100 ml/kg/day, divided into five feedings. If the pup vomits during or shortly after tube feeding, decrease the feeding amount.

MEDICAL CONSIDERATIONS

Premature harbor seal pups are characterized by a long, silky lanugo coat, normally shed *in utero*, and low body weight. These pups are often jaundiced and have bilirubin levels measuring as high as 17 mg/dl. Their immune system is often depressed, as evidenced by low globulin levels. They can become hypoglycemic and care should be taken to monitor their blood glucose levels. If their blood glucose levels fall below 80 mg/dl, 5 to 10 ml of 50% dextrose should be added to each tube feeding. Pups with a blood glucose level under 40 mg/dl usually have tremors or seizures. These pups should be given 10 to 20 ml of 20% dextrose IV and then maintained on an IV drip of 5% dextrose solution.

Pups often have respiratory problems and are best treated by placing them in an oxygen cage for several days. Many do quite well in a clean environment with good husbandry. Some of the more common medical problems seen in harbor seal pups are enteritis, pneumonia, omphalitis, and parasitic infections.

Common medical problems seen in elephant seal pups are *Otostrongylus* infections, pneumonia, and enteritis. Many yearling elephant seals that are rescued have had an abnormal molt. These animals lose all of their hair and outer layers of skin during the molt and are quite susceptible to a variety of pathogens at this time. If the animal is immunocompromised, pathogens can infect the skin and the infection can spread to internal tissues. They are treated with broad-spectrum antibiotics and the skin lesions are cleaned daily with jets of water from a hose. These animals also often have roundworm and/or tapeworm infections.

RESCUE AND REHABILITATION OF SMALL STRANDED CETACEANS

The order Cetacea has two suborders: Mysticeti (baleen whales) and Odontoceti (toothed whales, dolphins, and porpoises). Cetaceans become stranded singularly or in groups. Single stranded Odontocetes are the most successfully rehabilitated. Large baleen whales are difficult to rescue and rehabilitate and most often cannot be treated, or can be treated only at the stranding site. Smaller cetaceans can be taken off the beach by cradling them in a heavy flexible material or, ideally, by the use of a canvas stretcher designed for cetaceans.

Much of the success of rehabilitating cetaceans depends on the speed of the rescue and early treatment.

The rescue vehicle should be equipped with foam pads, towels, a stretcher to carry the animal, buckets, water sprayers, zinc oxide, or anhydrous lanolin ointment and, when possible, plenty of ice for the larger species. The animal should be removed from the beach as quickly and quietly as possible. Wet towels should be used to cover the body, and anhydrous lanolin or zinc oxide ointment should be placed around the blowhole and on the areas not covered by towels to prevent windburn or sunburn of the skin. The animal should be kept cool and moist for the duration of the trip to the rehabilitation center. A saltwater tank filled with water at a level of 3 to 4 feet should be made available.

The initial physical examination is extremely important and should be done as soon as the animal arrives at the rehabilitation facility. Rescue personnel should note the respiratory pattern of the animal as it travels. Respiratory rates above 6 breaths per minute indicate a compromised animal. Respiratory rates higher than 10 breaths per minute indicate extreme stress and warrant a poor prognosis.

The animal should be examined for external lesions. During this examination the sex of the animal can be determined. The genital slit in females includes, at its distal end, the anal orifice. In males there is noticeable space between the genital slit and the anal orifice.

The mouth should be examined for ulcers or lacerations. The teeth should be examined. Worn teeth usually indicate that the animal is aged. Feces can be collected from the stretcher for parasitic ova examination. Because beached cetaceans are often extremely debilitated, giving them broad-spectrum antibiotics, oral fluids, vitamins, and IV corticosteroids before transferring them to a saltwater tank can improve their chances of survival.

When the initial examination has been completed, the animal should be introduced to a saltwater pool and given assistance if necessary. Many stranded animals are in shock when they arrive at the facility and need aid in swimming. This usually entails lightly supporting the animal while walking it around the pool. One method of support for small cetaceans involves rigging floats on either side of the animal. The float arrangement can be adjusted so that the animal can easily float, breathe, and swim at the surface. This provides stability without human contact. Another method of support involves placing a towel under the jaw, with rehabilitation personnel on either side of the animal to support it and guide it around the pool. It is best to keep the water level waist deep until the animal shows signs that it can swim on its own. Once the animal is swimming, a 24-hour watch should be started, with personnel ready to assist the animal should it falter.

Stranded cetaceans do not readily eat, and must be force fed or given food by stomach tube. Most stranded small cetaceans are dehydrated. Giving 1 or 2 L of water via stomach tube to larger species, such as *Tursiops*, or 0.5 to 1 L to smaller species, such as *Delphinus*, with a vitamin supplement often improves their clinical appearance.

Rolled towels are worked between the jaws and the mouth opened just enough to pass a large equine stomach tube. The esophagus is large and the tube can be easily passed past the blowhole apparatus and into the stomach. Tube feedings can include a fish slurry, antibiotics, and an anti-ulcer drug. Passing a stomach tube can be very stressful to the animal, and it may be wise to do this only once a day. The tubing effort should be well organized so that it takes as little time as possible. While the animal is being tube fed, a physical examination can be done. Injections or blood sampling should be done before the tube feeding. These animals often start to eat fish voluntarily after one or two tube feedings.

Forced feeding is done with whole fish and is necessary if the animal does not eat voluntarily for more than 2 days. The animal is restrained and two rolled towels are worked between the jaws. The mouth is opened just enough to introduce a medium-size, firm fish to the back of the mouth. Be careful not to twist or torque the lower jaw when opening the mouth, because it is fragile in the smaller species and could be dislocated or broken. Once the fish is in the back of the mouth, the animal will swallow it. The animal should be allowed to relax briefly between each fish to encourage it to swallow completely. At the end of each forced-feeding session, a fish can be placed between the animal's jaws just before it is released. Occasionally the animal swallows this fish and subsequently accepts fish.

Vitamin supplements should include 500 to 1000 mg of vitamin B_1 (thiamin), 400 to 1000 IU of vitamin E, and multiple vitamins. These can be put into the daily tube feedings or fed in fish each day.

The amounts of fish fed to stranded cetaceans varies with the species. Most animals can be maintained on 6% to 10% of their body weight in fish per day. Smaller species, such as *Delphinus* or *Lagenorhynchus*, need up to 20% of their body weight in fish each day. When an animal is first admitted, assume it has not eaten for some time. Feed only 1 to 3 kg of fish the first day, working up gradually to its maintenance amount.

Water quality for cetaceans is even more important than for pinnipeds. They cannot be maintained for any prolonged time in fresh water. Water salinity should exceed 25 parts per thousand. The water should be filtered and free of bacteria.

RECOMMENDED READING

Dierauf LA: CRC *handbook of marine mammal medicine*, Boca Raton, Fla, 1990, CRC Press.

Fowler ME: *Zoo & wild animal medicine, current therapy 3*, Philadelphia, 1993, WB Saunders.

Nursing Care of Laboratory Animals

K. Hrapkiewicz

Learning Objectives

After reviewing this chapter, the reader should understand the following:

Methods of sample collection for laboratory analysis
Routes of administration of medication
Techniques used in general nursing care of mice, rats, hamsters, gerbils, guinea pigs, and rabbits

Principles of feeding, watering, and housing of laboratory animals
Principles of sanitation of the laboratory animal environment
Techniques used for diagnosing disease in laboratory animals

HUSBANDRY
Housing

Most animals used in research are reared in special environments to reduce disease potential. Animals in the pet trade are not raised under as stringent conditions and are frequently exposed to more disease-causing agents. In a research setting, different species are housed in separate rooms to meet experimental requirements, prevent interspecies disease transmission, and reduce anxiety because of interspecies conflict.

Rodents used in research or as pets are usually housed in plastic or metal cages with slotted bar or wire mesh lids. Shoebox-type cages made of plastic materials are popular for housing rodents (Fig. 33-1, *A*). Cages hung from a supporting frame are frequently seen in research settings (Fig. 33-1, *B*). Several individual cages can be placed on a shelving unit called a *rack* (Fig. 33-1, *C*). Cage flooring can be either a solid bottom or wire mesh. Solid flooring with bedding material is generally preferred. If mesh flooring is used, care must be taken to prevent foot injury and loss of neonates through the flooring.

Special housing may be required in research settings. Immunocompromised rodents are housed in microisolator cages or other protective cages to reduce their exposure to viruses or bacteria. Metabolism cages allow for collection of urine and feces, and inhalation chambers provide a way to expose an animal to various agents.

Glass terraria are adequate to house pet rodents. When terraria are used for housing, care should be taken to ensure that rodents have access to food and water. Rabbits can be housed in wire or front-opening cages with catch pans to collect urine and feces (Fig. 33-1, *D*).

Animals should be housed in caging that is appropriate for the animal's size and weight and in accordance with current regulations or guidelines. Cage height should allow an animal to make normal postural adjustments. For example, gerbils frequently sit upright, so the height of their caging should allow them to do so. The cage should be located in an area protected from climatic extremes. Changes in temperature and humid-

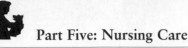

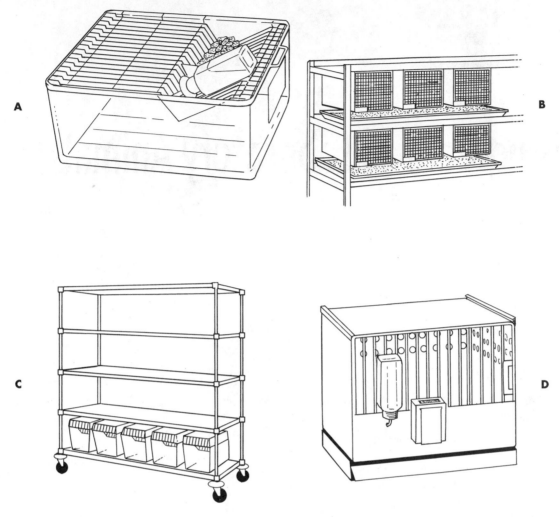

FIG. 33-1   Caging used for rodents and rabbits. **A,** Shoebox cage. **B,** Suspended cages. **C,** Rack holding shoebox cages. **D,** Rabbit cage with J feeder. *(From McBride DF:* Learning veterinary terminology, *St Louis, 1996, Mosby.)*

ity and/or drafty conditions should be avoided, because they can be stressful and predispose the animal to disease. The recommended housing temperature for mice, rats, hamsters, gerbils, and guinea pigs is 18° to 26° C and for rabbits is 16° to 22° C. The acceptable range of relative humidity is 30% to 70%. The guideline for ventilation in an animal housing room is 10 to 15 air changes per hour. A light cycle of 12 hours of light to 12 hours of darkness is most commonly used in animal housing rooms. Albino rodents are susceptible to phototoxicity, so care should be taken to ensure safe illumination levels in their housing area. Noise should be minimized in animal housing areas, because excessive sound exposure can be stressful and produce untoward effects. It is important to remember that many species can hear frequencies of sound that are inaudible to humans. Some rodents, such as gerbils, are prone to sound-induced seizures.

Bedding used for solid-bottom caging should be absorbent, comfortable, nonnutritive, nontoxic, and disposable. A variety of bedding material can be used,

including paper, sawdust, and soft pine, aspen, cedar, corncob, or hardwood chips. Cedar and soft pine shavings are frequently used for pet rodent bedding because of their pleasant aroma. These should be avoided in a research setting, however, because they emit aromatic hydrocarbons that induce liver changes and cytotoxicity.

Diet

Animals should be fed a clean, wholesome, and nutritious diet *ad libitum*. It is important to feed a balanced diet, freshly milled, formulated for that particular species. In most instances, the food should be placed in a feeder hung in the animal's cage. This prevents soiling of the food with urine and feces, keeping it dry and clean. If vegetables or fruit are offered to supplement the diet, they should be fresh and washed before feeding them. Any uneaten vegetables or fruits should be removed daily. Animals should have access to fresh water via an automatic watering system or water bottles with sipper tubes.

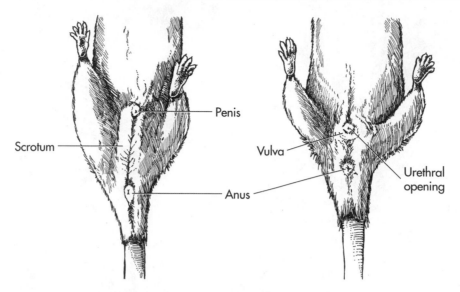

FIG. 33-2 The sex of most rodents can be determined by the distance between the anus and urogenital opening. This anogenital distance is greater in males (*left*) than in females (*right*). (*Adapted from the* American Association for Laboratory Animal Science training manual series, vol 1: assistant laboratory animal technician, *Cordova, Tenn, AALAS.*)

SANITATION

Sanitation involves bedding changes, cleaning to remove dirt and debris, and disinfection to reduce or eliminate microorganisms. All animal caging and bedding must be cleaned or changed as often as necessary to prevent accumulation of odor and waste, and to keep the animals clean and dry. Caging is usually cleaned once or twice a week. After removal of gross dirt, urine, and feces, cages should be disinfected by washing all surfaces with hot water (82° C) or by applying a disinfectant solution. A good, safe, readily available disinfectant for animal cages is laundry bleach (5% sodium hypochlorite), prepared by mixing 30 ml in 1 L of water. A fresh mixture should be prepared daily, because it deteriorates upon standing. Rabbit, guinea pig, and hamster urine is alkaline and contains crystals. When accumulated on caging, the crystals form a scale that can be difficult to remove. Acidic products available commercially or white vinegar can be used to remove the scale. It is important to thoroughly rinse detergents and disinfectants from cleaned cages and feeders, because residues may cause health problems. Deodorizers should not be used to mask animal odors, because they can be toxic to the animal or add a variable to a research study.

CARE OF RODENTS AND RABBITS

Mice, rats, hamsters, gerbils, and guinea pigs characteristically have long, chisel-shaped incisors that grow continuously and must be worn down by abrasion. Rodents are for the most part nocturnal. The sex of most rodents can be determined by anogenital distance, the distance being longer in males and shorter in females (Fig. 33-2).

Mice

The mouse (*Mus musculus*) is a small rodent, easily housed and handled, and relatively inexpensive to purchase and maintain as a pet. It is the most commonly used laboratory animal. Balb/ (albino), C57BL (black), and C3H (agouti) are common inbred strains of mice. Swiss and ICR are outbred strains of mice.

Mice may live up to 3 years. They weigh 20 to 40 g and have a rapid heart rate (approximately 500 to 600 beats/min) and a body temperature of 36.5° to 38° C.

The mammary glands reach from the ventral midline to the back and neck. Mice are sexed by anogenital distance. Mice are continuously polyestrous, with an estrous cycle lasting only 4 days. Mating can be confirmed by the presence of a vaginal plug, a white, waxy copulatory plug located in the vagina. The gestation length is 21 days, with pups born hairless and helpless. Young mice are weaned at 21 days of age.

Mice can be caught and safely picked up by grasping the scruff of the neck with forceps or by grasping the base of the tail with the fingers (Fig. 33-3, *A*). For manipulation or examination, the animal is caught by the base of the tail and placed on a surface it can grasp, such as the cage lid. The scruff of the neck is then grasped by the thumb and forefinger (Fig. 33-3, *B*), and the mouse is inverted to lie on its back with the tail positioned between the palm of the hand and the little finger. Clear plastic restraint devices can also be used for restraint and manipulation.

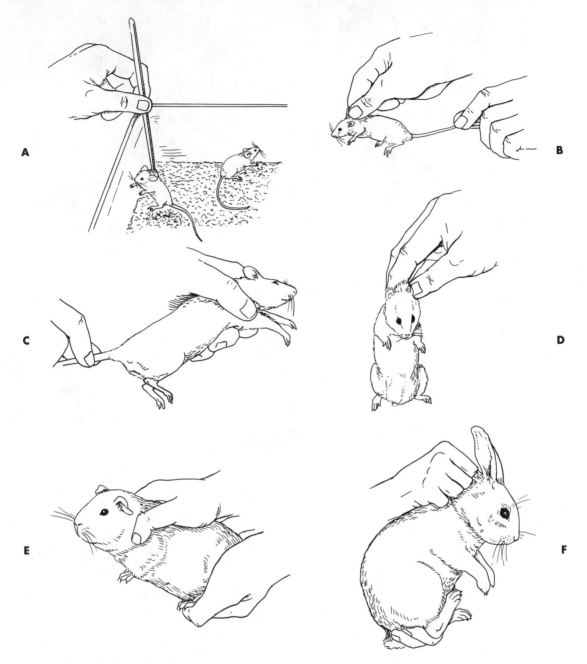

FIG. 33-3 Handling laboratory animals. **A,** Picking up a mouse with forceps. **B,** Restraining a mouse by the scruff. **C,** Restraining a rat. **D,** Picking up a hamster by the scruff. **E,** Restraining a guinea pig. **F,** Lifting a rabbit by the scruff while supporting the hindquarters. *(From McBride DF: Learning veterinary terminology, St Louis, 1996, Mosby.)*

Rats

The common rat (*Rattus norvegicus*), found in pet stores or in research laboratories, was developed from the wild brown Norway rat. Rats are easily maintained and make excellent pets if handled gently. They are the second most commonly used laboratory animal. Hooded or Long-Evans rats have pigmented eyes and are white, with a black hood over the head and shoulders. They tend to be smaller than albino rats, such as Sprague-Dawley and Wistar.

The life span of the rat is 2½ to 3½ years. Rats weigh 250 to 500 g, with females being smaller than males. Their body temperature is 36° to 37.5° C. The Harderian gland, a lacrimal gland located caudal to the eyeball, secretes a red porphyrin-rich secretion that lubricates the eye. In times of stress or illness, red tears overflow and stain the face and nose. Rats are susceptible to respiratory disease caused by *Mycoplasma pulmonis* and cilia-associated respiratory bacillus.

Rats are continuously polyestrous, with an estrous cycle length of 4 to 5 days. Mating can be confirmed by the presence of a plug in the vagina. The vaginal plug can also be discharged in the cage or litter pan. Females are usually separated from the male before parturition. Gestation is 21 days in length, with pups born hairless and helpless. Young rat pups are weaned at 21 days of age.

Rats can be caught and safely picked up by grasping the base of the tail to transport them a short distance, such as when changing cages. When rats are held upside down, they are more interested in righting themselves rather than in biting the handler. To restrain for manipulation or examination, pick up the rat by placing the hand firmly over the back and rib cage and restraining the rat's head and shoulders with one's thumb and forefinger. If additional control is needed, the base of the tail may be restrained with the other hand (Fig. 33-3, C). An alternative method is to pin the rat with your free hand while pulling on the base of the tail. Position your index and third fingers to firmly grasp either side of the rat's neck caudal to the mandible; the thumb and other fingers are used to gently restrain the chest.

Hamsters

The Syrian or golden hamster (*Mesocricetus auratus*) originated in the Middle East. It is the most common hamster in the pet trade and in research. It is noted for its ease of taming, low waste production, and lack of odor. The golden hamster is stocky and short-tailed, weighs approximately 120 g, and has a reddish-golden brown body color with a gray ventrum. Other color varieties, such as cinnamon, cream, white, piebald, albino, and the long-haired teddy bears, are popular as pets. The Chinese or striped hamster (*Cricetulus griseus*) is a gray-brown with a dark strip down its back and is smaller than the golden, weighing 35 g. They tend to be more difficult to handle and thus are not as popular as pets. Female Chinese hamsters are belligerent and must be housed individually.

Hamsters usually have a life span of 1½ to 2 years. They have cheek pouches that can transport an amazing amount of food and bedding. A female hamster sometimes packs her whole newborn litter in her pouches to move them to another location. Hamsters have extremely loose skin. Marking glands, called *flank* or *hip glands*, are located in the skin of both flanks and are more prominent in males. At temperatures below 8° C, some hamsters become inactive for periods of 2 to 3 days. During this transient state of hibernation, they have a reduced body temperature and reduced heart and respiratory rates.

Hamsters are sexed by anogenital distance. Females have an estrous cycle length of 4 days. They are commonly belligerent toward the male unless sexually receptive. During the winter, hamsters have a normal seasonal breeding quiescence. Hamsters have a gestation length of 16 days, the shortest of the laboratory animals. Cannibalism is common during the first pregnancy and in the first week postpartum. Care should be taken not to disturb a new litter during this period. Hamster urine is normally turbid and milky, because it contains a large amount of crystals.

An important point to remember when handling a hamster is to avoid surprising it. Hamsters are sound sleepers, so make sure the hamster is awake and knows the handler intends to pick it up. Startled or awakened hamsters often bite, so use caution. Hamsters are most easily moved by grasping the loose skin across the shoulders or by using the hands as a scoop to transfer the hamster from one cage to another. They can also be picked up in a small can or cup. To restrain a hamster, gently grasp the loose skin across the back by curling the fingers and thumb around opposite sides of the animal to gather in as much loose skin as possible. Grasp the *skin*, not the body, of the hamster (Fig. 33-3, D). An alternative method is to reverse your hand so that your thumb and forefinger hold the skin at the base of the tail.

Proliferative ileitis, or wet tail, is caused by a bacterial infection and is the most common spontaneous disease of hamsters. Young animals are affected most often. Affected hamsters produce foul-smelling, watery diarrhea, hence the term *wet tail*.

Gerbils

The Mongolian gerbil (*Meriones unguiculatus*) is a native to desert regions of Mongolia and northeastern China. It is an active, burrowing, social animal. The gerbil is clean and produces little waste, making it one of the simplest laboratory animals to maintain. It is relatively odorless, unaggressive, and easy to handle, making it a good pet. The agouti or mixed-brown gerbil is the color variety most commonly seen, but black and other colors, such as piebald, white, and cinnamon, are available.

The gerbil, or jird, as it is sometimes referred to, has an average life span of 3 years and weighs less than 100 g when mature. It has long hind limbs adapted for leaping and, unlike most other rodents, has a hair-covered tail. Both sexes have a distinct dark orange midventral sebaceous gland, which is used for territorial marking. Gerbils form stable lifelong monogamous arrangements and breed throughout the year. The female is polyestrous and has an estrous cycle of 4 to 6 days in length. Gestation normally lasts 24 days but can be as long as 48 days. The male can be left in the cage, because it participates in care of the young. Gerbils are weaned at 21 days of age.

A gerbil can be safely picked up by cupping both hands under it or by grasping the base of the tail to lift it from its cage. To restrain the gerbil for examination or injection, the loose skin at the nape of the neck is grasped with one hand and the base of the tail is grasped with the other hand. Extreme care must be taken not to grasp the tip of the tail because the skin may tear and slip off, exposing the underlying muscle and vertebrae. Alternatively, an over-the-back grip can be used. Gerbils resist being placed on their back.

Spontaneous seizures frequently occur when gerbils are stimulated by loud noises, rough handling, or a novel environment. The seizure is usually short, lasting from a few seconds to more than a minute. During a seizure, the gerbil freezes and holds its legs stiffly extended, while the body trembles. No treatment is necessary. Sorenose, or rednose, is common in gerbils. This nasal dermatitis is associated with excessive porphyrin secretion and staphylococcal infection.

Guinea Pigs

The guinea pig (*Cavia porcellus*) is tailless, with a compact, stocky body and short legs. It originated in South America and is a hystricomorph, or hedgehog-like rodent, related to chinchillas and porcupines. The guinea pig makes a nice children's pet because it is docile and seldom bites or scratches. It has been associated with research for so long that a human volunteer for an experiment is often called a "guinea pig." Guinea pigs can be monocolored, bicolored, or tricolored. The most common pet and laboratory variety is the English, American, or short-haired guinea pig. The Abyssinian has short, rough hair arranged in whorls or rosettes; the Peruvian or "rag mop" variety has long, silky hair.

The guinea pig, or *cavy* as it is commonly called, weighs 700 to 1200 g as an adult. It has a normal body temperature of 37.2° to 39.5° C and a life span of 4 to 5 years. Guinea pigs have four digits on their front limbs and three digits on their hind limbs. Their urine is normally opaque and creamy yellow, and contains crystals. Both male and female guinea pigs have inguinal nipples. Sexing is difficult because, unlike other rodents, there is little difference in the anogenital distance in males and females. The female has a Y-shaped anogenital opening and vaginal membrane that remains intact and closed except during the few days of estrus and at parturition. Males have scrotal pouches lateral to the anogenital line and a penis that can be protruded by manual pressure.

Female guinea pigs are called *sows*, males are called *boars*, and the act of giving birth is called *farrowing*. The sow is polyestrous throughout the year and has an estrous cycle of 15 to 17 days. A sow should be bred for the first time before 7 months of age, before fusion of the pubic bones, to prevent dystocia. The gestation period is lengthy, averaging 68 days. Neonates are precocious and nearly self-sufficient. They are born fully furred, with eyes and ears open and teeth erupted. Young guinea pigs eat solid food within the first few days postpartum and can be weaned at 14 to 21 days.

To restrain a guinea pig, lift the animal by grasping under the trunk with one hand while supporting the rear quarters with the other hand (Fig. 33-3, *E*). It is especially important to use a two-hand support method with adult and pregnant animals. An alternative method is to place one hand over the shoulder area, with the thumb and forefingers just caudal to the front legs, while the other hand supports the rear quarters. Use care not to overly compress the chest with this method.

Dietary vitamin C must be provided to guinea pigs because, like primates, they cannot synthesize their own vitamin C. Even under ideal storage conditions, the vitamin C content of food deteriorates rapidly, so it is important to use freshly milled food. Commercial rabbit and guinea pig foods look alike; both are small pelleted chows, but they differ in vitamin C content. Citrus fruits, cabbage, peppers, and kale can be fed to supplement vitamin C. Penicillin should not be used in guinea pigs, because it often induces fatal reactions in this species.

Rabbits

The domestic rabbit (*Oryctolagus cuniculus*) is a descendant of the wild rabbits of Europe. The Flemish Giant is a large breed weighing 6 to 7 kg, the New Zealand and Californian are medium-size breeds weighing 2 to 5 kg, and the Dutch and Polish are small breeds weighing 1 to 2 kg. The albino New Zealand is popularly used for meat production and research. The smaller breeds are used as pets and in research. Rabbits make good pets; they are mild tempered, seldom bite, and can be housetrained.

Rabbits are lagomorphs, differentiated from rodents by the presence of two upper pairs of incisors that continuously grow. The rabbit has a life span of 5 to 6 years or more, body temperature of 38.5° to 40° C, heart rate 130 to 325 beats per minute, and respiratory rate of 30 to 60 breaths per minute. They have a wide field of vision, can readily detect motion, and see well in dim light. Their ears are highly vascular and function in heat regulation. They have a small skeletal mass as compared with similar-sized animals and large hindquarter muscles that make them prone to back fractures.

Rabbits have several unusual features to their intestinal tract, including a sacculus rotundus located at the terminal end of the ileum, a large cecum that terminates in a vermiform process or appendix, and a colon with regular sacculations called *haustra*. Rabbits are coprophagic and pass two types of feces. Soft, moist "night feces" are rich in vitamins and protein and are eaten directly from the anus. Firm, dry pellets are passed during the daytime. The color of rabbit urine varies from orange-red to brown.

Male rabbits are called *bucks* and female rabbits are called *does*. Sexing can be accomplished by gently pressing the skin back from the genital opening. Females have an elongated vulva, with a slit opening; males have a rounded, protruding penile sheath. The dewlap, a heavy fold of skin at the throat, is more prominent in females. Rabbits do not have a true estrous cycle but have periods of sexual receptivity. They are induced ovulators. Because the doe is territorial, she is taken to the buck's cage for mating, which usually occurs within minutes. Gestation is approximately 31 days. Parturition in the rabbit is called *kindling* and the young are called *kits* or, more commonly, *bunnies*. Young rabbits are born naked and helpless, yet they require little maternal care. Does nurse young rabbits only for a few minutes once or twice daily. Weaning occurs at 6 to 8 weeks of age.

To remove a rabbit from a cage or to carry it a short distance, grasp the scruff of the rabbit's neck with one hand and support the hindquarters and back with the other (Fig. 33-3, *F*). When carrying a rabbit longer distances, its head should be tucked into the crook of the arm that is supporting the hindquarters (Fig. 33-4, *A*). Rabbits that are incorrectly handled can injure either themselves by struggling and fracturing their back or their handler by scratching him or her. A towel wrapped around the rabbit works well for restraint, especially if the eyes are covered. Mechanical devices made of plastic or metal are frequently used for restraint during minor procedures, such as blood collection from an ear vein, IV injections, or treatments. The restraining device holds the head in place and has a sliding partition that fits snugly against the rabbit's rump (Fig. 33-4, *B*). Rabbits should never be lifted or restrained by grabbing their ears, because the ears are sensitive and fragile. When returning a rabbit to its cage, place it in the cage rump first to prevent injury to the rabbit or handler. A rabbit has a tendency to leap toward the cage if allowed to enter the cage head first.

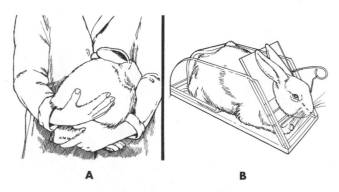

A   **B**

FIG. 33-4 **A,** Rabbits can be carried by supporting the body while directing the head into the crook of the elbow. **B,** Device to restrain rabbits. *(Adapted from the* American Association for Laboratory Animal Science training manual series, vol 2: laboratory animal technician, *Cordova, Tenn, 1991, AALAS.)*

Malocclusion can result in overgrown incisors that may need to be trimmed every 2 to 3 weeks. Ear mite infections with *Psoroptes* are common in pet rabbits. The mites characteristically cause a dry, brown, crusty material to accumulate on the inner surface of the ears. Pododermatitis, a pressure necrosis of the plantar surface of the metatarsal area, commonly called *sore hocks*, is seen in heavy, obese rabbits. Rabbits are susceptible to infection with *Pasteurella multocida*. Several clinical forms of the disease occur; the most common are rhinitis ("snuffles") and pneumonia.

TECHNIQUES AND TREATMENTS

Medication can be administered orally by mixing the medication in the water or feed, and by gavage needle or eye dropper.

The standard routes of injection (IV, IM, SC, ID, IP) are used in laboratory animals. Rodents have few readily accessible veins, making it difficult to administer drugs IV. Tail veins can be used in the mouse and rat. The margin ear veins, located on the lateral sides of the pinna in the rabbit, are accessible and can be used for IV injections. The small muscle mass of rodents makes it difficult to inject drugs IM. For this reason the IP (intraperitoneal) route is more commonly used in rodents. When giving IP injections, it is best to use the caudal left abdominal quadrant and tilt the animal's head and forequarters ventrally. This helps to avoid accidental puncture of the large cecum in these animals.

Small blood samples can be collected from rodents and rabbits by toenail clip or superficial venipuncture. The orbital sinus is frequently used to collect blood from rodents, but they must first be anesthetized. Cardiac puncture can also be used in an anesthetized rodent or rabbit, but it is not recommended except for collection before euthanasia. The margin ear veins and artery of the rabbit are easily visualized and can be used to collect blood (see Chapter 30). The jugular vein can also be used in rabbits.

Urine samples can be obtained by gentle digital pressure or cystocentesis. Rodents can be placed on a cold surface or in a cooled plastic bag until urine is voided.

Identification of individual animals is important in a research setting. Rodents are identified by ear tag or by an ear notch or punch pattern. Ear tags or ear tattoos are used in rabbits. A microchip can be implanted subcutaneously in laboratory animals for quick electronic identification.

Many factors, such as species, strain, ingesta content, weight, and nutritional and health status, affect the response of rabbits and rodents to anesthesia. Small rodents are not fasted before inducing anesthesia. Food, but not water, should be withheld for 3 to 6 hours from guinea pigs and rabbits before inducing anesthesia. A small scale should be used to obtain an accurate weight of the animal to calculate the dose when using injectable anesthetic agents. Inhalation agents, such as isoflurane and halothane, can also be used; however, they should be delivered using a calibrated vaporizer to prevent anesthetic overdose. Inhalation agents are commonly administered via chamber, face mask, or nose cone because it is difficult to intubate these species. It is essential to monitor the animal closely and keep it warm to prevent hypothermia. Hydration and nutritional support are important postoperative considerations.

Techniques used to diagnose disease in companion and food animals are used in laboratory animals. The small size of laboratory animals makes it more difficult to obtain adequate laboratory samples. In the research setting, the health status of the rodent colony is often more important than the health status of an individual animal. Health status is frequently monitored by serologic testing of sentinel animals that are placed in the colony.

RECOMMENDED READING

American Association for Laboratory Animal Science training manual series, volume I, assistant laboratory animal technician, Cordova, Tenn, 1991, AALAS.

American Association for Laboratory Animal Science training manual series, volume II, assistant laboratory animal technician, Cordova, Tenn, 1991, AALAS.

Harkness JE, Wagner JE: *The biology and medicine of rabbits and rodents*, ed 4, Media, Penn, 1995, Williams & Wilkins.

CHAPTER 34

Nursing Care of Pediatric and Geriatric Patients

A.P. Davidson
W.E. Vaala
F.B. Garry
B.J. Deeb

Learning Objectives

After reviewing this chapter, the reader should understand the following:

Procedures used for examining, resuscitating, and caring for neonatal puppies, foals, and calves
Complications commonly affecting neonates and how to combat them

Methods used to provide nutritional support of neonates
Effects of aging
Procedures used for maintaining the health of aged animals
Special anesthetic considerations for aged animals

CARE OF NEONATAL PUPPIES AND KITTENS

A.P. DAVIDSON

EXAMINATION

Signs of distress or disease in neonates are usually nonspecific, most commonly including continuous vocalization, ineffective nursing, and restlessness. Careful examination of the neonate and its environment can yield specific clues. The normal neonate is warm to the touch and is vigorous and vocal in its objection to handling. Body temperature ranges from 35.5° to 36.5° C. The mucous membranes are pink to red and moist. Capillary refill time is less than 2 seconds. Respiration is regular (15 to 35 breaths per minute), and no fluid is auscultated over the lung fields. Minimal clear nasal discharge may be evident. The heart rate is rapid, usually 180 to 250 beats per minute. Normal hydration is evidenced by normal skin turgor. Urination and defecation are easily elicited by gentle stimulation of the anogenital area with a moistened cotton ball. The umbilical area is normally not inflamed, and the anus and genitalia are clean. The limbs and paws, including nails (claws), should be well developed and properly oriented. The haircoat is full, shiny, and free of parasites or fecal contamination. The bedding of the nest box should not show evidence of diarrhea.

RESUSCITATION

Resuscitation of the neonate is necessary when the bitch or queen fails or is unable to perform this (such as after cesarean section or with maternal behavioral problems), or when a puppy or kitten does not respond to typical maternal manipulation (licking and nuzzling by the bitch or queen). An airway free of amniotic fluid, placental membranes, and meconium (first neonatal feces) should be established within 3 to 5 minutes after birth.

The placental membranes, if present, are removed first, by tearing from the neonate's face. The oral cavity and trachea are cleared by swabbing with cotton-tipped applicators or gentle suction with a bulb syringe. Carefully swinging the neonate headfirst in a downward arc, while supporting the head and trunk in a towel, assists removal of airway fluids by centrifugal force (Fig. 34-1). Clearing the airway prevents aspiration of potentially damaging meconium-containing fluids.

Respiration can be stimulated by thoracic and facial massage with a dry, warm towel. Oxygen can be supplied by a small face mask if cyanosis persists. The size of most canine and feline neonates precludes nasal oxygen insufflation and intubation, but positive-pressure ventilation can be achieved with a properly fitted face mask. Care should be taken not to overinflate the neonatal lungs. External cardiac massage is performed if the heart rate is very low (less than 80 to 100 beats per minute) or not detectable. The umbilical cord should be clamped and ligated if bleeding and coated with tincture of iodine (Fig. 34-2). Tincture of iodine is preferable to povidone-iodine because it is more astringent (drying) because of its alcohol content. Gut suture material (2-0 or 3-0) is ideal for ligation of the umbilical cord.

The neonate should be completely dried and warmed. Immediate suckling is encouraged, because it provides colostrum (first milk), calories, and glucose, sparing the neonate's limited glycogen stores. If nursing is not immediately available, glucose should be provided via oral administration of one or two drops of Karo (corn) syrup. Subcutaneous administration of 5% dextrose (2 to 4 ml/kg) is possible, but this runs the risk of abscessation.

The subcutaneous route is convenient for delivery of balanced, preservative-free electrolyte solutions to mildly dehydrated puppies and kittens, but it is not adequate for dehydrated individuals. Intravenous catheterization of the jugular vein in kittens and small-breed puppies or the cephalic vein in larger neonatal puppies is possible. The intraosseous route of fluid administration is optimal in very small neonates; it permits rapid administration of large volumes of fluids to the venous system via the bone marrow sinusoids and medullary venous channels. The trochanteric fossa of the femur and the greater tubercle of the humerus are preferred sites. An 18- to 20-gauge spinal needle is advanced into the marrow cavity and secured to the skin. Oral administration of fluids is useful for neonates without gastric disorders (not vomiting), but it is also not adequate for dehydrated individuals. Fluids administered by any route should be first warmed to body temperature.

Poorly responsive neonates can benefit from drug therapy. For the purposes of drug dosing, normal puppies weigh 100 to 700 g (0.1 to 0.7 kg) at birth, whereas normal kittens weigh approximately 100 g (0.1 kg). Reversal of the effects of any narcotic or barbiturate anesthetic agent used during anesthesia of the dam can improve the status of neonates born by cesarean section. Naloxone, a narcotic antagonist, and doxapram, a respiratory stimulant, can be administered (0.1 to 0.2 ml) into the tongue (or other muscle) or umbilical vein of the neonate.

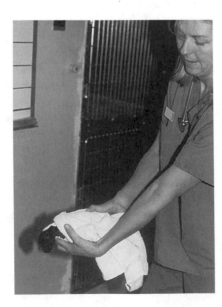

FIG. 34-1 Proper positioning of a neonate for swinging to expel fluid from the lungs.

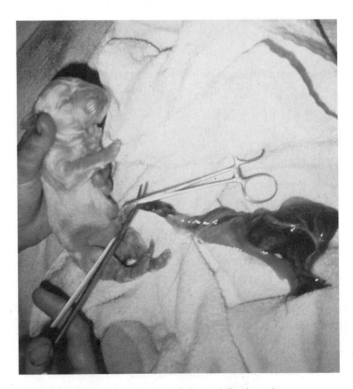

FIG. 34-2 Ligation of the umbilical cord.

Apnea (lack of breathing) lasting longer than 5 minutes can warrant therapeutic intervention to correct acidemia and provide substrate for myocardial metabolism. Sodium bicarbonate, diluted 1:1 with 5% dextrose (0.5 mEq/ml), can be administered at 0.5 to 1 mEq/kg via the umbilical vein, over 2 to 4 minutes. Prolonged bradycardia or cardiac standstill can be treated with epinephrine (1:10,000 solution given IV at 0.1 ml/kg) and atropine (0.03 mg/kg IM or IV).

The ambient temperature of neonates during the first few weeks of life (30° to 32° C) can be maintained with an infrared lamp, positioned 6 feet above the draft-free nest box, illuminating half of the area available to the dam and neonates. Heating pads can cause thermal burns and their use is discouraged. The temperature within the nest box should be monitored with a thermometer. Hypothermia of neonates predisposes to hypoglycemia, hypoxemia, and poor digestive function. Nest box surfaces should be lined with smooth, nonporous materials to facilitate cleaning and avoid abrading the neonates.

Disinfectants used on nest box surfaces must not leave caustic or toxic residues. Bedding material should not impair respiration or obscure neonates from the dam's view, but it should provide good footing and absorb wastes. Shredded, unprinted newspaper and washable terry cloth toweling are superior.

Acquired disorders of the postpartum period include immunodeficiencies, malnutrition, and infectious disease. Orphaned neonates are at increased risk. Neonatal congenital immunodeficiencies associated with thymus dysfunction have been proposed. Acquired immunodeficiencies result from failure of passive transfer of maternally derived antibodies, acquired primarily by ingestion of colostrum during the first 24 hours of life. Acquired immunodeficiencies also occur secondary to distemper and parvoviral infections and dietary zinc deficiencies.

Neonatal malnutrition can result from poor milk production or quality, crowding, and ineffectual nursing. Malnutrition is evidenced by failure to gain weight steadily. The birth weight should double by 12 days of age. Rotating neonates in the whelping box gives smaller, weaker individuals first access to the teats. Supplemental feeding with commercially available artificial bitch and queen milk is often indicated. Approximately 22 to 26 kcal per 100 g of body weight should be fed daily. Commercial milk replacers generally provide 1 to 1.24 kcal/ml of formula. The neonate should receive 13 to 22 ml of formula per 100 g of body weight, divided into four meals daily, over the first 4 weeks of life.

Neonates rarely nurse effectively from artificial nipples and bottles because of problems with equipment size and shape, as well as milk flow and variable suckling reflexes. Gastric intubation is preferred. Large-bore, soft, red rubber catheters, cut to proper length

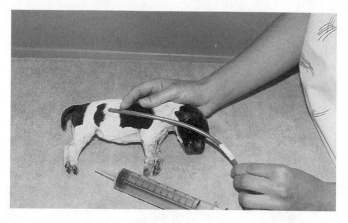

FIG. 34-3 Proper measurement of feeding tube length for an orphan puppy.

(from mouth to stomach), minimize inadvertent tracheal intubation (Fig. 34-3). Frequent small-volume feedings reduce the risk of regurgitation and aspiration. Commercial milk substitutes are closer to bitch or queen milk than most homemade recipes. Milk should be warmed to body temperature just before administration. Hand-fed neonates should be weighed daily.

RECOMMENDED READING

Hoskins JD: *A practitioner's guide to puppy and kitten care*, The American Animal Hospital Association Professional Library Series, Denver, 1995, American Animal Hospital Association.

Hoskins JD: *Veterinary pediatrics: dogs and cats from birth to six months*, ed 2, Philadelphia, 1995, WB Saunders.

Wallace MS, Davidson AP: *Abnormalities in pregnancy, parturition, and the periparturient period*. In Ettinger SJ, Feldman EC, editors: *Textbook of veterinary internal medicine*, ed 4, Philadelphia, 1995, WB Saunders.

CARE OF NEONATAL FOALS

W.E. VAALA

Healthy, full-term foals are precocious neonates that can sit sternal within 10 minutes of birth, develop a suckle reflex within 20 minutes of delivery, and can stand and nurse from the udder by 2 hours of age. Any foal that is not standing and nursing from the dam within 3 hours of birth should receive a thorough medical examination. A healthy foal has a regular heart rate between 70 and 100 beats per minute, a regular respiratory rate between 25 and 40 breaths per minute and a temperature between 37.2° and 38.6° C. Newborn foals have a bright, inquisitive attitude and an erect, angular body posture. Foals nurse several times an hour, consume between 15% and 30% of their body weight per day in milk, and gain an average of 0.5 to 1 kg/day.

Because there is no transfer of antibodies across the equine placenta before birth, foals depend on ingestion of good-quality colostrum during the first 18 hours after birth to absorb sufficient antibodies to provide protection against infection during the first few weeks of life. After consuming 1 to 1.5 L of colostrum, healthy foals should have a serum concentration of IgG, the primary immunoglobulin in colostrum, above 800 mg/dl. An IgG level below 200 to 400 mg/dl is considered failure of passive transfer (FPT) of immunoglobulins. A foal with FPT requires antibody supplementation in the form of colostrum or plasma, depending on the foal's age.

UMBILICAL CORD CARE AND COMPLICATIONS

Following delivery the umbilical cord usually ruptures naturally 3 to 4 cm from the foal's body wall. The umbilical stump contains the remnants of the umbilical vein, two umbilical arteries, and the urachus. It represents a potential portal of entry for environmental bacteria. Therefore, the umbilical cord should be disinfected promptly after birth with 2% iodine. Ideally, the stump is submersed in iodine solution using a 20-ml sterile syringe case or other narrow container. Avoid splashing iodine on the prepuce or groin area. Disinfect the umbilical cord twice daily for 2 days or until the stump remains dry.

The urachus, which is the fetal conduit for urine *in utero*, should close spontaneously at birth or shortly thereafter. The urachus may fail to close (congenital patent urachus) or may reopen postpartum (acquired patent urachus). Most cases of urachal patency are acquired and are associated with inflammation of the umbilical remnants. Conditions favoring reopening of the urachus include prolonged recumbency associated with urine scalding and bladder overdistention, exposure to excessively dirty or damp bedding, ligation or cutting of the umbilical cord, and any condition that produces increased intraabdominal pressure, such as straining to defecate because of constipation or straining to urinate because of cystitis or bladder rupture.

A foal with a patent urachus dribbles urine from the urachus during micturition, resulting in a persistently moist umbilicus. Initial treatment focuses on again disinfecting the umbilicus, keeping the surrounding area as dry as possible, maintaining the foal on clean, absorbent bedding, and encouraging the foal to spend increasing amounts of time standing. If urachal patency persists, systemic antibiotics should be given to reduce the risk of ascending bacterial infection. The urachus can also be cauterized using a silver nitrate applicator stick inserted gently into the end of the urachus and twirled slowly.

The applicator should not be inserted any deeper than 1 cm into the distal urachus.

During the first few weeks of the foal's life, the umbilical stump should be examined daily for signs of infection, characterized by swelling, heat, pain, or purulent discharge. Abscessation of the internal umbilical remnants within the abdominal cavity is best detected by using transabdominal ultrasonography.[1] Most umbilical stump infections respond to medical management using systemic, broad-spectrum, bactericidal antibiotics. Refractory infections or large internal abscesses require excision of the internal umbilical remnants.

MECONIUM PASSAGE

Meconium is the first manure passed and is composed of swallowed amniotic fluid, cellular debris, and intestinal secretions. It is dark black or brown in color, and pelleted or firm in consistency. Because of the tenacious nature of meconium, foals usually strain a little to pass their first manure. Meconium should be eliminated within 24 hours of birth, followed by passage of soft, yellow or tan milk feces.

Meconium impaction is the most common cause of colic in newborn foals, especially colts because of their narrow pelvic canal. Therefore, it is a sound management practice to administer an enema prophylactically to foals soon after birth to facilitate meconium passage (Fig. 34-4).

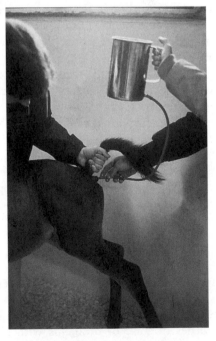

FIG. 34-4 Gravity enema administration using a stainless-steel enema bucket and red rubber stallion urinary catheter.

CARING FOR SICK FOALS
Weakness and Recumbency

Generalized weakness and prolonged recumbency predispose to pressure sores, poor umbilical hygiene, and urachal patency; interfere with lung function; contribute to collapse of the dependent lung; increase the risk of pneumonia; exacerbate preexisting musculoskeletal weakness; compromise gastrointestinal function; and increase the likelihood of constipation. Weak foals should be kept on soft absorbent bedding. Mattresses covered with sheets and absorbent synthetic fleece pads are ideal. Pillows can be used to prop foals into sternal recumbency. Recumbent foals must be turned every 2 hours and encouraged to stand. Cornstarch powder can be used to help keep foals clean and dry.

Hypothermia

Sick foals become hypothermic very quickly from heat loss to the environment and inability to regulate body temperature. Warmth can be provided by insulating foals from the cold ground and drafty environment using mattresses, closed-cell camping pads, sleeping bags, and blankets. Additional warmth can be provided using intravenous fluids warmed in the microwave or heated in a fluid jacket containing a chemical heat pack, and by placement of hot-water bottles close to highly vascular areas, such as the axilla and groin. Circulating hot-water pads (Aquamatic K pads and K-module, Baxter Hospital Supply Division, Chicago, Ill), circulating hot-air blankets, and radiant heat lamps (suspended a minimum of 52 cm above the foal) can be used to provide additional heat. Cold, dehydrated foals require concurrent volume expansion with intravenous fluid in addition to external heat.

Dehydration and Hypotension

Foals become dehydrated from decreased fluid intake from poor nursing or fluid loss from diarrhea. Ideally, intravenous fluids should be administered continuously using infusion pumps or controlled drip chambers, such as Buretrol (Microdrip Infusion, Travenol Labs, Deerfield, Ill) or dial-a-flow regulator IV extension sets (Abbot Labs, Chicago, Ill). For maintenance, fluids should be infused at 4 to 6 ml/kg/hr (e.g., 200 to 300 ml/hr for a 50-kg foal). Replacement fluid needs are calculated using the following formula:

Fluid deficit (L) = % dehydration × body weight (kg)

For example, a 50-kg foal that is 5% dehydrated would require 0.05 × 50 = 2.5 L of fluid to correct the existing deficit. This fluid deficit is in addition to the foal's maintenance fluid requirements.

Many sick foals become hypotensive from dehydration, hypovolemia, and poor control of blood pressure associated with severe bacterial infections. Weak, thready peripheral pulses are indicative of low blood pressure. Blood pressure can be measured indirectly and noninvasively using one of a variety of oscillometric blood pressure monitors (e.g., Dinamap Monitor, Critikon, Tampa, Fla). The coccygeal artery at the base of the tail is the preferred site to measure blood pressure.[2]

Inability to Nurse

Never feed a cold, shocky foal, because the gastrointestinal tract is poorly perfused and not functioning normally. If the foal cannot be fed orally, intravenous nutrition must be initiated using a continuous infusion of a hypertonic solution containing dextrose, lipids, amino acids, and vitamins administered through a long, indwelling jugular catheter (Arro Cath, Arro International, Reading, Pa).

If the foal can be fed orally and has a strong suckle reflex and can swallow well, you can attempt bottle feeding. Keep the foal's head and neck flexed, and encourage udder-seeking behavior by offering the foal the bottle under your armpit (Fig. 34-5). Auscultate the trachea immediately after nursing to be certain the foal is not aspirating milk into the lungs. Aspiration is characterized by a loud fluid rattle heard over the trachea.

If the foal cannot suckle and/or swallow effectively, milk must be fed via a small-diameter nasogastric tube

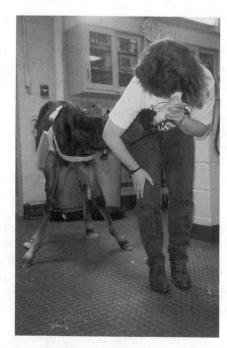

FIG. 34-5 Bottle feeding a foal from under the handler's armpit to encourage udder-seeking and udder-bumping behavior.

(silicone nasogastric tube 91 cm long, 5 mm ID, Cook Veterinary Products, Bloomington, Ind; indwelling Kangaroo feeding tubes, 190 cm long, Sherwood Medical, St. Louis, Mo). If the nasogastric tube is left in place between feedings, the end should be capped and firmly secured to the foal's halter. Always confirm proper placement of the nasogastric tube by feeling the end of the tube pass down the esophagus, sucking on the end of the tube to confirm negative pressure, and blowing on the end of the tube while simultaneously auscultating over the stomach to ensure the end of the tube is unkinked and in the stomach.

Ideally, a foal should consume 20% to 30% of its body weight in milk per day. However, it is reasonable to begin feeding a sick foal 10% of its body weight per day. If the foal tolerates this volume, the amount of milk can be increased gradually. Small feedings should be given every 1 to 2 hours to newborn foals. "On-demand" feeding is ideal, but it is often too labor intensive to be practical. Mare's milk or an artificial, commercially available mare milk replacer can be used. Small amounts of active culture yogurt or commercially available intestinal inocula can be given to stimulate normal enzyme production and improve digestion.

Newborn orphan foals are best fed by bottle initially. Once they have received adequate colostrum and are consuming 20% to 25% of their body weight in milk daily, these foals can be trained to drink from a bucket or bowl. The feeding container should be clean and shallow. Placing the nipple in the bowl as a "straw" helps some foals learn to drink more readily from the bowl. Milk should be room temperature or slightly warmer. Make any changes in formula composition of volume slowly. After the first week of life, the frequency of feedings can be reduced to every 3 hours. A foal that is consuming adequate nutrition should gain 0.5 to 1.0 kg/day. An alternative to bucket raising orphans is to rent a foster "nurse mare" to raise the foal. If a foal is to be bucket raised, a "four-legged" companion is essential to help the orphan learn to socialize and to teach the foal such basic skills as grazing and eating solid foods.

Breathing Difficulties

Clinical signs of respiratory distress include nostril flare, increased abdominal component to breathing, rib retractions, grunting on expiration, paradoxic respiration (e.g., chest wall collapses inward during inspiration), and cyanotic mucous membranes. The most accurate way to assess lung function is to obtain an arterial blood gas measurement. The preferred site for arterial puncture is the great metatarsal artery. If the foal shows signs of respiratory distress or if hypoxemia is documented on analysis of an arterial blood gas sample, intranasal oxygen therapy is indicated.

Seizures

Convulsing foals can injure themselves. Head trauma and corneal abrasions are the most common self-inflicted wounds. Convulsing foals require rapid sedation initially with 5 to 10 mg of diazepam (Valium, Roche) administered intravenously. If seizures persist or recur, additional Valium may be given, followed by a slow infusion of phenobarbital (3 to 10 mg/kg administered as a slow intravenous infusion over 15 to 20 minutes). Affected foals should have their head protected with a soft helmet (High Horse, Reno, Nev.), and their legs and hooves wrapped with soft bandages. Continuous supervision is required until neurologic signs have subsided.

Infection and Failure of Passive Transfer

Foals showing signs compatible with septicemia should be treated with broad-spectrum, bactericidal antibiotics. A popular drug combination is intravenous penicillin and amikacin. Amikacin can be nephrotoxic. Therefore, renal function and hydration status should be monitored before and during this drug treatment. Foals with a serum IgG level below 800 mg/dl should receive immunoglobulin supplementation. Colostrum is the richest and cheapest source of antibodies. Unfortunately, the foal intestine absorbs large immunoglobulin molecules most efficiently only during the first 10 to 12 hours of life. Negligible antibody absorption occurs after 24 hours of age.

Good-quality colostrum can be administered to foals less than 12 to 18 hours of age that have no evidence of gastrointestinal dysfunction. Ideally, colostrum supplementation should begin within 1 to 2 hours of birth. Administration of at least 1 L of colostrum with a specific gravity above 1.060 is recommended. The specific gravity of colostrum can be measured using an Equine Colostrometer (Jorgenson Laboratories, Loveland, Colo).

If the foal with FPT is older than 18 to 24 hours of age or has signs of gastrointestinal disease, a plasma transfusion is the preferred route of antibody supplementation. The volume of plasma given depends on the serum IgG level, the IgG concentration in the donor plasma, the foal's body weight and general health status, and the final desired serum IgG concentrations. Most foals require 1 to 2 L of plasma to increase their serum IgG concentration above 800 mg/dl. Commercially available plasma with high levels of IgG is available (HiGamm Equi, Lake Immunogenetics, Ontario, NY; Polymune Plus, Veterinary Dynamics Inc., Chino, Calif). Plasma donors should be negative for A and Q blood groups, which are the two blood types responsible for the most serious hemolytic reactions in horses.

Plasma should be administered at an average rate of 10 ml/kg/hr using an in-line filter. It is advisable to give the first 50 ml of the transfusion slowly over 15 to 20 minutes while monitoring the foal's heart rate, respiratory rate, and general attitude for any adverse reactions. Serum IgG concentration should be measured after the plasma transfusion is complete. Foals catabolize protein rapidly and may require additional plasma transfusions during their illness.

While treating the sick neonate, it is important to keep the mare within sight of her foal to remind her of her maternal responsibilities. Until the foal is ready to nurse again from the mare, the mare's udder should be stripped of milk every 2 to 3 hours. To enhance milk letdown in the mare, 10 to 15 units of oxytocin can be administered intramuscularly 5 to 10 minutes before milking the mare.

REFERENCES

1. Reef V: *Abnormalities of a neonatal umbilicus detected by diagnostic ultrasound.* In the *Proceedings of the 32nd annual meeting of American Association of Equine Practitioners,* 32:157, 1986.
2. Vaala WE, Webb AI: *Cardiovascular monitoring of the critically ill foal.* In Koterba AM, editors: *Equine clinical neonatology,* Philadelphia, 1990, Lea & Febiger.

CARE OF NEONATAL CALVES

F.B. GARRY

The most common problems in neonatal calves are prematurity, metabolic problems that may result from dystocia or illness of the dam, neonatal calf enteritis, and neonatal septicemia. As in other species, septicemia in neonatal calves can be a life-threatening problem before it is recognized. The prognosis for an affected calf is guarded or poor. Calves affected by the other three general neonatal problems, however, can look every bit as bad as the septicemic calf but survive if appropriate care is provided.

Dairy calves are usually orphaned at birth; therefore, sick dairy calves are treated as individuals without major concern about "bonding" with the dam. For beef calves, however, a major consideration is development of a maternal-neonatal bond. This determines the manner in which supportive care is provided to the calf. For example, with a beef calf born to a first-calf heifer, special care must be taken early in the calf's life to make sure the dam will recognize and care for the calf. In some cases, if the calf is separated at birth following a dystocia, the dam may either reject the calf by ignoring it or may traumatize the calf when it is returned to her. For these reasons, try to establish contact between the dam and beef calf as early as possible and devise means for caring for the calf in the close presence of the cow.

RESUSCITATION

Calves born during dystocia, whether delivered via cesarean section or per vagina, may require resuscitation. Resuscitation procedures are similar for calves as for other species. If assisted ventilation is required, intubate calves via the oropharynx (7 to 9 mm ID endotracheal tube). The anatomy of the bovine pharynx and larynx makes intubation by feel very difficult. In most cases, the larynx must be visualized using a mouth speculum and in some cases it is very useful to employ an aluminum stylet threaded through the endotracheal tube, which can be inserted through the larynx and the tube advanced thereafter.

Once the trachea is intubated or if the calf did not require assisted ventilation, the calf is laid in sternal recumbency to allow for better ventilation. Keeping the calf sternal is easier if the hind limbs are stretched cranially along either side, similar to a dog-sitting position. The calf's initial respiratory efforts are shallow and erratic, but a rhythmic pattern should be established within a couple of minutes. Placement of a piece of straw, a flexible tube, or a finger into the nares and ears stimulates the calf to take deeper breaths and/or to cough and clear the airways.

Amniotic fluid and debris should be cleared from the oropharynx and nasal passages. This is most effectively done with suction. Hanging and/or swinging the calf does not effectively clear the fluid from the lower airways as is commonly thought, but it does stimulate the calf's respiration and heart rate. Fluid in the lungs is then absorbed more quickly.

Supplemental oxygen can be via nasal insufflation (Fig. 34-6). If nasal oxygen is provided, it is important to measure the length of the intranasal tube before its introduction. A length of tube that stretches from the calf's naris to eye is sufficient. If the tube is advanced too far caudally (a surprisingly easy error to make as a stimulated calf jerks its head vigorously about), the tube most commonly passes into the esophagus, inflating the calf's stomach with gas. Because the rumen is very small in the ruminant neonate, some of this gas advances into the abomasum, making it difficult or impossible to remove the gas via intubation.

Preventing Hypothermia

For any newborn calf, drying the amniotic fluid off the haircoat is very important. Evaporative heat loss is a major contributor to neonatal hypothermia. One of the most important functions of a dam with good mothering ability is to lick the calf dry. If the calf is separated from the dam immediately after birth, the calf should be rubbed dry with towels. Use of a hair dryer can be very helpful.

In addition to drying the calf, provision of additional warmth is very important to survival of the compro-

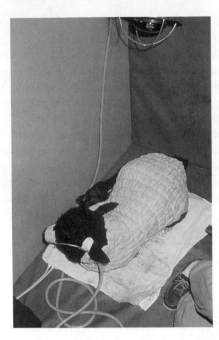

FIG. 34-6 This calf was born weak and is being treated with nasal insufflation of oxygen, with the tube taped to the ear and muzzle. The calf has been covered with a blanket and is under a heat lamp.

mised neonate. Shivering and the metabolic heat produced by attempts to stand and walk provide heat production. Calves suffering from hypoxemia, hypoglycemia, acidosis, or dehydration show little or no shivering and generally remain inactive. Therefore, calves with these problems can very rapidly become hypothermic.

At birth the average calf has a rectal temperature of about 103.5° F, which is about 1° to 1.5° higher than the body temperature of the dam. Within the first half hour of life, body temperature drops rapidly and, in normal calves, usually stabilizes around 101° to 102° F. In compromised calves it is quite common for the body temperature to continue to drop to levels below 100° F within the first hour of life. Drying the calf and providing a heat lamp, a water blanket, or some kind of protective covering are very important. Body temperature should be very carefully monitored through the first several hours of life because development of hypothermia, which may occur even when additional warmth is provided, is an important clue to concurrent problems. Most calves stand and suck the dam within about 1 hour after delivery.

Feeding Colostrum

Because calves are born essentially agammaglobulinemic (without immunoglobulins), provision of colostrum shortly after birth is critically important for the calf to obtain passive maternal antibodies. As a rule of thumb, beef calves should be fed all of the dam's first-milking colostrum as soon as they develop a suckle reflex. If dairy cow colostrum is used, make sure that the colostrum is of sufficient quality. The "quality" of colostrum is a rough measure of the concentration of immunoglobulin. This is most easily determined by use of a colostrometer, a simple tool that measures the specific gravity of the colostrum.

Dairy cows produce much more colostrum than do beef cows, but generally the quality is lower and also the concentration of immunoglobulin. As a rule of thumb, if calves are provided with dairy cow colostrum, it can be administered orally at 10% of body weight over the first 24 hours of life. Absorption of maternal colostral immunoglobulin by the calf's intestine usually begins to decrease after the first feeding of colostrum or at about 8 hours of age. Therefore, it is important that the first feeding of colostrum is usually of fairly large magnitude. If the calf has a vigorous suckle reflex, allow the calf to nurse all of the dam's colostrum that it will consume. If more colostrum is available, continue to feed it throughout the first 24 hours, offering it at 2-hour intervals and allowing the calf to suckle. If the calf does not have a suckle reflex, continue to offer the colostrum frequently, looking for development of a suckle reflex up to about 6 hours of age. If at that time the calf has not developed a suckle response, intubate the calf and give all of the dam's colostrum if it is out of a beef heifer or give 5% of the calf's body weight in colostrum if dairy cow colostrum is available.

Allowing the calf to suckle versus orogastric intubation for administration of colostrum or milk is an important question. If the calf has already been nursing the dam and is presented for treatment beyond the first several days of age, it is common for the calf to refuse a rubber nipple feeder. It may be worthwhile to reintroduce the calf to the dam because it may then suckle the dam quite readily. On the other hand, if this is a newborn calf that has not yet suckled the dam, it will usually suckle from a nipple feeder as readily as from the dam's teats.

Development of a suckle reflex is a very important indicator of the calf's status. Calves with a variety of problems, including hypoxemia, hypoglycemia, hypothermia, or acidosis resulting from dystocia, frequently do not develop the reflex until these problems are corrected. Therefore, lack of a suckle reflex is a good indicator of one or more of these problems. In some cases, if these problems are present, the calf may not absorb immunoglobulin, even if colostrum is provided via intubation.

For these reasons, allow the calf to suckle because development of a suckle reflex usually suggests some improvement in the underlying condition. Further, when other problems are present, the calf's gastrointestinal tract may not be fully functional. Therefore, repeated intubation of newborn calves or calves of older ages suffering from similar problems may result in large accumulations of fluid in the forestomachs or abomasum. If you resort to intubation to supply the calf with oral fluids or milk, carefully monitor the calf for fecal production and palpate its abdomen, looking for evidence that the fluid administered is sequestering in the gastrointestinal tract, rather than proceeding on through and being absorbed. If the calf will not suckle and there is evidence that fluid has accumulated in the gastrointestinal tract, continue to offer fluids frequently via nipple feeder but discontinue orogastric intubation.

Stimulation of the calf to develop a suckle reflex is another important function of the dam. Most calves are very responsive to stroking or rubbing along the back, especially near the tailhead. If the calf is not suckling well, such rubbing stimulation can often provide very rewarding results. If the calf has been sleeping or is compromised by one of the aforementioned problems, it may require several minutes before the calf begins to suckle. Therefore, it is worthwhile to repeatedly introduce the nipple into the calf's mouth and try to deliver a small amount of milk in the calf's mouth before giving up and assuming the calf does not have a suckle reflex.

Feeding Milk

Beyond colostral feeding, provision of milk as nutrition is obviously of critical importance. Although dairy calves are often raised with the provision of only 10% of body weight per day as fluid milk, this practice should not be mistakenly construed as providing optimal nutrition. The strategy of providing 10% of body weight per day is geared to enhancing intake of solid feeds so that dairy calves can be weaned at an early age. Most calves, if given the opportunity, freely consume between 20% and 30% of their body weight in milk per day. Although sick calves may not have a very hearty appetite, a recovering calf or premature calf commonly has an exaggerated appetite. For these reasons, provide a calf with up to 3% of its body weight per feeding and offer milk feedings at approximately 2-hour intervals. With this regimen, some calves consume over 30% of their body weight in milk per day.

Feeding Electrolytes

For calves with fluid loss because of neonatal enteritis, oral electrolyte solutions are commonly offered as a means to provide additional fluid therapy. Calves with mild to moderate dehydration may respond adequately with only oral fluid supplementation, whereas calves with severe dehydration require intravenous fluid support. It has been a common practice to withhold milk from calves with enteritis. You do not have to hold to that practice, but rather offer milk via nipple feeder if the calf will accept it. Because milk alone will not provide the electrolytes that have been lost through the gastrointestinal tract, provide oral electrolyte solutions at alternate feedings with the milk. The electrolyte fluids and milk or milk replacer should not be mixed, because this adversely influences normal milk digestion. Offer milk at 2% to 3% of body weight maximum, alternating with oral fluid feedings offered at 5% of body weight per feeding, with the alternate feedings at 2-hour intervals. Many calves refuse the milk feedings but eagerly suckle the electrolyte. With this regimen, even when calves do refuse the milk, they can be provided as much as 30% of body weight per day in additional oral electrolyte fluids.

RECOMMENDED READING

Aldridge B et al: Role of colostral transfer in neonatal calf management; failure of acquisition of passive immunity, *Compend Contin Educ Pract Vet* 14:265-270, 1992.

Howard JL: *Current therapy 3: food animal practice*, Philadelphia, 1993, WB Saunders.

Smith BP: *Large animal internal medicine*, ed 2, St Louis, 1996, Mosby.

CARE OF GERIATRIC PATIENTS

B.J. DEEB

Humans and their animal companions are living longer than ever before. The expectation of societies in most developed countries is that advances in health care and life quality are applicable to animal companions as well as humans. Nursing care of geriatric patients requires special considerations.

THE EFFECTS OF AGING

Old age brings about numerous gradual degenerative changes. Body weight increases, the skin loses elasticity and becomes dry and scaly, and the haircoat becomes dull and sparse. The footpads become hyperkeratinized and the nails become brittle. In carnivores, dental calculus increases; in older rabbits or rodents, dental malocclusion becomes more common. Digestion is less efficient and reduced colonic motility leads to constipation.

Cardiac output decreases with age, usually as a result of mitral valve insufficiency. The lungs lose elasticity, and increased susceptibility to respiratory infection can lead to chronic obstructive pulmonary disease, chronic bronchitis, bronchiectasis, and emphysema. Diminished kidney function leads to polydipsia, polyuria, urinary incontinence, anemia, and wasting.

TABLE 34-1 Recommendations for common age-related health problems	
Problem or disease	**Treatment**
Dry skin and haircoat	Use oil-free humectants, bathe with oil-based conditioners
Thickened footpads	Apply keratolytic gel
Dental tartar and gingivitis	Brush teeth, massage gums twice a week, routine scaling of dental calculus
Malocclusion (rabbits/rodents)	Routine trimming of maloccluded teeth, check for points on premolars and molars
Decreased gastrointestinal function	Add pancreatic enzymes to food, increase dietary fiber, reduce dietary fat
Constipation	Add psyllium hydrophilic mucilloid (Metamucil) to food
Fecal incontinence	Low-fiber diet
Congestive heart failure	Low-sodium diet, restrict activity, cardiac drugs
Chronic lung disease	Restrict activity, mucolytic expectorants, bronchodilators
Renal failure	Restrict dietary protein and phosphate, fluid therapy, supplement diet with vitamins
Degenerative joint disease	Reduce activity, reduce body fat, increase muscle mass, gentle massage, acupuncture, polysulfated glycosaminoglycan, control pain with nonsteroidal antiinflammatory drugs
Behavior problems	Behavior modification, anxiolytic drugs

In addition, muscle and bone atrophy. Degenerative joint disease and vertebral spondylosis are common in older animals. Changes in the nervous system lead to loss of short-term memory, changes in sleep patterns, and incontinence. Hearing, vision, and taste decrease; the sense of smell is preserved to some extent in most aged companion animals. Altered immune function leads to reduced antibody response to antigens, autoimmune diseases, and a higher incidence of neoplasia.

Geriatric pets are less able to adjust to stressful conditions and some react with stereotypic, destructive, or aggressive behaviors or depression and anorexia. Separation anxiety or excessive vocalization is certainly a consideration whenever the geriatric patient is hospitalized. An animal with failing vision or hearing is more apt to be startled and overreact aggressively. Housesoiling is another common geriatric problem. Musculoskeletal disease may make movement to the appropriate place for elimination difficult or painful. Inappropriate elimination caused by medical problems must be differentiated from that related to behavior.

Table 34-1 summarizes some of the changes seen in geriatric animals, and ways in which owners can accommodate the needs of geriatric patients.

Geriatric Criteria

When the changes described above have taken a toll on the animal's well being, that animal can be considered *geriatric*. The age at which this occurs depends on the expected life span of the species, as well as various individual factors. In general, species that grow to large size live longer than smaller mammals. If there is wide vari-ation in size within a species, such as with the many dog breeds, the smaller breeds tend to live longer than the largest breeds (Table 34-2).

NURSING CONSIDERATIONS FOR GERIATRIC PATIENTS

Handling

When providing nursing care for a geriatric companion animal, assume that the effects of aging are affecting the health and behavior of that animal. Old pets brought to the veterinary hospital may be overly anxious and have any number of problems, such as impaired vision and hearing; painful joints; thin bones; weak muscles; poor kidney function; congestive heart failure; chronic bronchitis; decreased liver, pancreatic, and gastrointestinal function; periodontal disease; malodorous breath; flaky skin; and a sparse haircoat.

Schedule office visits for geriatric patients during less busy times of the day and week. Never rush examinations or sample collection. Take time for discussion with the owner. Handle the geriatric animal gently and deliberately. Avoid sudden movements. Let the animal know where you are at all times; this is especially important with old horses, because they may be more prone to kick or bolt. Keep your hands on the animal and gently stroke it. Be careful moving or manipulating the limbs. If the animal is to be left at the hospital, expect separation anxiety. Placing the pet's blanket or food dish or a piece of the owners' clothing in the cage

TABLE 34-2 Approximate life span of companion animals

	Approximate life span	Age when considered geriatric
Dogs		
Small (less than 20 lb)	15 years	12 years
Medium (21 to 50 lb)	13 years	10 years
Large (51 to 90 lb)	11 years	8 years
Giant (more than 90 lb)	9 years	6 years
Cats	15 years	10 years
Ferrets	8 years	5.5 years
Rabbits	10 years	7 years
Guinea pigs	8 years	5.5 years
Rats	3 years	2.5 years
Hamsters	2 years	1.5 years
Horses	24 years	18 years

or run may help reduce stress. Polydipsia and polyuria necessitate attention to the water supply and may require more frequent cleaning of the enclosure. If possible, do not leave a geriatric patient overnight unattended in the hospital.

Body Condition and Diet

A rule of thumb for body condition is that the animal's ribs should be easily felt but not seen. In carnivores, a waist should be obvious caudal to the ribs. Older animals tend to become less active, especially if musculoskeletal problems have made exercise difficult, and they require fewer calories for maintenance. If owners cannot resist giving treats, recommend use of low-calorie treats (see Chapter 14). The diet of overweight carnivores should provide less than 20% of total daily calories as fat and at least 20% as protein.

Because of changes in the digestive system, the diet should be supplemented with vitamins, unsaturated fatty acids, and zinc. Increased fiber content aids intestinal mobility as well as calorie restriction. Feeding small portions three to four times daily reduces begging for food and improves digestion. Commercial "senior" diets provide the right balance for older dogs and cats. For geriatric rabbits and rodents, the typical high-protein, high-calorie, high-calcium alfalfa/seed diets should be replaced with low-protein, low-calorie, low-calcium grass hay and vegetables.

Older horses may require chopped, wafered, or moistened pelleted feed. Hay should be of high quality and leafy. Older horses tend to require a diet with more protein and phosphorus than younger horses. Aged horses should be observed while eating in an effort to detect problems related to chewing, as from dental disease. Older horses may have to be fed individually so as to prevent injury or food theft by aggressive, younger horses.

Exercise is essential in maintaining a desirable body weight and good muscle tone, as well as providing periods of interest and interaction with human companions. Walks or games with the pet make life more enjoyable for all.

Weight loss is usually an indication of organ dysfunction and requires diagnosis and dietary adjustment as dictated by the problem. Whatever the cause of anorexia, sometimes the patient can be encouraged to eat when given human attention, stroking, and hand feeding. One should vary the choices of food, offering fresh choices frequently. Syringe or tube feeding of a balanced semiliquid diet is a short-term alternative.

Drug Therapy

Drug absorption, disposition, and excretion are affected by age-related organ and metabolic changes. These alterations should be considered to ensure efficacy and avoid toxicity during drug therapy. Absorption of orally administered drugs is affected by an increase in gastric pH, loss of intestinal absorptive surface area, prolonged intestinal transit time, and decreased blood flow to the liver and gastrointestinal tract. Absorption of parenterally administered drugs is affected by increased fat deposits and decreased vascularity.

While body fat increases, muscle and body fluid decrease in many older patients. Lipophilic drugs, such as some anesthetics, will be distributed more to body fat and less to the plasma, altering their effects and rate of elimination. Hydrophilic drugs, such as aminoglycosides, accumulate less in fat-containing tissues and more in plasma. Renal excretion of drugs may be reduced; the likelihood of nephrotoxicity can be reduced by reducing the frequency of dosing or reducing the drug dose.

Anesthesia

Any geriatric pet requiring anesthesia should be thoroughly examined and have a panel of laboratory tests performed (e.g., CBC, blood chemistry panel) to obtain baseline blood values. The doses of preanesthetics and anesthetics may need to be altered and usually reduced. Small doses of neuroleptic-analgesic combinations work well for geriatric patients. Drugs with profound effects on the cardiovascular system should be avoided. Of the inhalant anesthetics, isoflurane is preferred. It has minimal effects on cardiac, renal, and hepatic function, and it provides rapid induction and recovery. Chapter 20 contains detailed information on anesthetic agents available for geriatric patients.

Client Education

Aging affects all animals, but the effects of aging on each individual varies. Serious problems can be prevented by knowing the history of the geriatric patient and scheduling regular physical examinations, with appropriate laboratory tests. Veterinary technicians should educate the client on the effects of aging and the special requirements of geriatric animals. Discussions should include diet, body condition, grooming, dental problems, vaccinations, internal parasites, and the value of regular examinations. Solicit questions from the client during office visits or field calls and periodically contact the client to inquire about the patient's well-being. A health care program for the geriatric patient is more apt to be implemented by animal owners if they are convinced of the benefits.

RECOMMENDED READING

Deeb BJ, Wolf NS: Studying longevity and morbidity in giant and small breeds of dogs, *Vet Med* 89 (suppl 7):702-713, 1994.
Goldston RT: Geriatrics and gerontology, *Vet Clin North Am Small Anim Pract* 19:1, 1989.
Goldston RT, Hoskins JD: *Geriatrics and gerontology of the dog and cat*, Philadelphia, 1995, WB Saunders.
Hunthausen W: Identifying and treating behavior problems in geriatric dogs, *Vet Med* 89 (suppl 7):688-694, 1994.

APPENDIX A

Review Questions

CHAPTER 2: OCCUPATIONAL HAZARDS

1. The primary and most effective method of preventing disease transmission is:

   a. Vaccination for possible diseases
   b. Proper personal hygiene
   c. Routine use of protective equipment
   d. Quarantine of suspect animals

2. According to the National Institutes of Occupational Safety & Health (NIOSH), up to 90% of health care workers' exposure to waste anesthetic gases can be attributed to:

   a. Inaccurate vaporizers
   b. Leaks in anesthetic machine connections
   c. Excess flow in relation to the size of the patient
   d. Refilling the vaporizer

3. Infection of a human with the common canine roundworm (Toxocara canis) causes a condition known as:

   a. Cutaneous larva migrans
   b. Visceral larva migrans

   c. Ringworm
   d. Toxoplasmosis

4. The most serious hazard from sharps (e.g., needles, scalpel blades) in a veterinary hospital is:

   a. Tetanus
   b. Hepatitis
   c. Physical trauma
   d. Infection with human immunodeficiency virus

5. In most instances, when a chemical is transferred from the original bottle to another bottle for use within the hospital, the secondary bottle must be labeled with:

   a. The name of the chemical and the appropriate warnings
   b. The chemical name, any appropriate warning, and the name and address of the manufacturer
   c. A proper prescription label
   d. The chemical's name and concentration

627

CHAPTER 3: ETHICS, ANIMAL WELFARE, AND LAW

6. Which of the following does *not* represent a major ethical influence on veterinarians?

   a. Obligations to peers
   b. Obligations to animals
   c. Obligations to clients
   d. Obligations to the news media

7. The new consensus ethic for animals in society is best characterized as:

   a. An ethic of anticruelty
   b. Dealing with animal suffering that is not the result of cruelty
   c. Freeing animals from all human use
   d. Aimed at ferreting out sadists and psychopaths

8. A client may sue and recover from a veterinarian for malpractice:

   a. Any time the veterinarian fails to perform in accordance with professional standards
   b. If the veterinarian's negligence is the cause of injury to the client's animal
   c. If the veterinarian fails to adhere to the requirements of the governing state's practice act
   d. If the veterinarian uses an unapproved drug to treat the client's animal, and the drug causes adverse effects

9. The veterinarian is required to perform in accordance with standards of the veterinary profession:

   a. As defined in each individual state's practice act
   b. Which standard does not depend on the specialized training of the veterinarian
   c. As is determined by a judge or jury after hearing expert testimony on the matter
   d. Only if the veterinarian has a written contract with the client to do so

10. As an employer, a veterinarian can be sued for the negligent actions of assistants:

    a. Under the doctrine *respondeat superior*
    b. Only if the veterinarian instructed the assistant to take such negligent action
    c. Only if the veterinarian was on site
    d. Even if the assistant performed actions outside of his or her scope of employment

CHAPTER 4: VETERINARY MEDICAL TERMINOLOGY

For questions 11 through 15, select the correct answer from the following five choices:

   a. An-
   b. Brady-
   c. Contra-
   d. Hypo-
   e. Pyo-

11. Prefix meaning "against" or "opposed"

12. Prefix meaning "insufficient" or "abnormally low"

13. Prefix meaning "without" or "not having"

14. Prefix meaning "abnormally slow"

15. Prefix meaning "pus-related"

For questions 16 through 20, select the correct terms from the following five choices:

   a. Mesial
   b. Ventral
   c. Supine
   d. Proximal
   e. Superficial

16. What is the correct term for "in dorsal recumbency"?

17. What is the correct term for "situated nearer to the central axis of the body, relative to another body part"?

18. What is the correct term for "contact surface of a tooth, closest to the midline of the dental arcade"?

19. What is the correct term for "pertaining to the underside of a quadruped, or denoting a position more toward the abdomen"?

20. What is the correct term for "situated near the surface of the body or a structure"?

CHAPTER 5: RECORDKEEPING, BUSINESS TRANSACTIONS, AND CLINIC ADMINISTRATION

21. When hiring an applicant for a veterinary staff position, it is best to hire the applicant:

    a. With the highest level of education and then provide training on working as a team member
    b. With the most animal-related experience and then provide training on working as a team member
    c. With experience in working as a team member and then provide training in the required job skills
    d. Willing to work for the least pay

22. Extending credit to a few qualified clients can benefit the practice because:

    a. These desirable clients are likely to refer other, similarly qualified clients to the practice
    b. The clinic can provide services to clients who otherwise might be turned away and the interest on the unpaid balance adds to practice revenues
    c. Collecting part of the fees in the initial payments is better than losing the entire amount through nonpayment
    d. It is always best to recruit as many new clients as possible, regardless of their ability to pay

23. Which statement concerning medical records is most accurate?

    a. By law, medical record forms must measure 8½ x 11 inches.
    b. Any errors in transcribing medical information should be masked with typing correction fluid ("white out").
    c. By law, clients are not entitled access to their animal's medical record.
    d. Information must be entered accurately and at the time service is provided.

24. The most economical amount of a particular product to order, calculated by factoring in fixed costs, carrying cost, and purchase price, is known as the:

    a. Restocking cost
    b. Economic order quantity

    c. Rollover quantity
    d. Cost-reversal quotient

25. Dividing the total annual purchases of an item by the average value of that item on hand yields that item's:

    a. Rolling average inventory value
    b. Inventory turnover
    c. Return on investment
    d. Profit ratio

CHAPTER 6: HUMAN INTERACTIONS IN THE VETERINARY WORKPLACE

26. Most employers consider all of the following as desirable traits in employees *except*:

    a. A positive attitude
    b. Versatility and adaptability to change
    c. Ability to both lead and follow
    d. Extensive experience in only a single field or area

27. Concerning sexual harassment on the job, which statement is most accurate?

    a. If your supervisor asks you to become romantically involved, it is best to do so without question.
    b. If other employees routinely use sexually explicit language in the workplace, it is appropriate for you to do so also.
    c. The employer is ultimately responsible for providing employees with a workplace free from sexual harassment.
    d. In the eyes of the law, employees must fend for themselves in the work environment.

28. Animal owners become clients that patronize veterinary practices because they:

    a. Have a relationship with their animal and wish to preserve that relationship
    b. Believe it is socially acceptable to take their animal to a veterinarian
    c. Are required by law to have their animal cared for by a veterinarian
    d. Want to avoid feeling guilty if their animal becomes ill and dies without veterinary care

29.   When making appointments for clients, it is best to offer:

a. Two choices of appointment times
b. At least three choices of appointment times
c. An appointment at any time they consider convenient
d. One specific appointment time, with no alternative times

30.   Concerning the doctor's punctuality in seeing clients during office visits, which statement is most accurate?

a. Staying on schedule is unimportant, because most clients expect to wait to see the doctor.
b. Staying on schedule is very important, because it shows respect for the client and keeps the clinic running smoothly.
c. The doctor's punctuality is unimportant, because a client's time is not as important as the doctor's time.
d. The doctor's punctuality is important only for desirable, "grade A" clients.

31.   When presenting a client with the bill for veterinary services, it is best to:

a. Explain the fees in a quiet, businesslike manner, with a minimum of conversation
b. Apologize for the high fees and explain that these fees are lower than those of other practices
c. Hand the client the bill and ask by what method the client wishes to pay
d. Apologize to the client and offer to extend credit under generous terms

32.   When your verbal response summarizes what the client is verbally expressing, this is called:

a. Validation
b. Effective listening
c. Reflection
d. Attending

33.   Of the stages of grieving, which is recognized as the first to occur?

a. Denial
b. Anger
c. Resolution
d. Guilt

CHAPTER 7: ANATOMY AND PHYSIOLOGY

34.   Which of the following is *not* one of the basic tissues of an animal's body?

a. Connective tissue
b. Endocrine tissue
c. Muscle tissue
d. Nervous tissue

35.   Which group of bones of the pelvic limb is listed in the correct order from proximal to distal?

a. Femur, tibia, tarsals, metatarsals
b. Humerus, radius, carpals, metacarpals
c. Metatarsals, carpals, ulna, femur
d. Phalanges, metatarsals, fibula, femur

36.   Where does external respiration take place?

a. At the nostrils
b. In the lungs
c. In the upper respiratory tract
d. Throughout the body tissues

37.   Severe damage to which part of the central nervous system is likely to cause rapid death of an animal?

a. Brainstem
b. Cerebellum
c. Cerebrum
d. Spinal cord

38.   Which endocrine gland is often called the "master endocrine gland" because many of the hormones it produces direct the activity of other endocrine glands?

a. Adrenal gland
b. Parathyroid gland
c. Pituitary gland
d. Thyroid gland

39.   Where are ova usually fertilized by spermatozoa?

a. Cervix
b. Oviduct
c. Uterus
d. Vagina

CHAPTER 8: PATHOLOGY AND RESPONSE TO DISEASE

40. Which of the following is *not* a cardinal sign of inflammation?

    a. Heat
    b. Cold
    c. Swelling
    d. Redness

41. Which of the following is considered to be a pyogenic bacterium?

    a. *Mycobacterium*
    b. *Mycoplasma*
    c. *Streptococcus*
    d. *Clostridium*

42. Which components of the immune system are involved in cell-mediated immunity?

    a. B-lymphocytes
    b. T-lymphocytes
    c. Immunoglobulins
    d. Plasma cells

43. What is the predominant cell type in a suppurative exudate?

    a. Histiocytes
    b. Red blood cells
    c. Neutrophils
    d. Lymphocytes

44. What is the initiating factor that results in traumatic reticulopericarditis?

    a. Ulceration of the reticulum caused by bovine virus diarrhea virus
    b. Liver abscessation caused by *Corynebacterium*
    c. Excessive grain intake and rumenal atony
    d. Ingestion of a metallic foreign body that penetrates the reticulum

CHAPTER 9: PREVENTIVE MEDICINE

45. All of the following are aspects of appropriate animal housing *except*:

    a. Pleasing to the owner
    b. Prevents escape

    c. Provides shelter from the elements
    d. Appropriate for the species

46. Against which disease are dogs or cats *not* routinely vaccinated?

    a. Panleukopenia
    b. Rabies
    c. Parvovirus infection
    d. Tetanus

47. Against which disease are cattle *not* vaccinated?

    a. Rhinopneumonitis
    b. Leptospirosis
    c. Parainfluenza-3
    d. Vibriosis

48. Which agent is *least* appropriate for cleaning or disinfecting water containers for animals?

    a. Phenols
    b. Hypochlorites
    c. Quaternary ammonium compounds
    d. Dishwashing detergent

49. What is a very common, controllable factor predisposing to disease in companion animals?

    a. Genetic mutations
    b. Extremes of weather
    c. Obesity
    d. Old age

CHAPTER 10: ANIMAL DISEASE AND PEOPLE

50. Zoonoses are defined as diseases that:

    a. Are transmitted between animals and people
    b. Commonly occur in animals and people
    c. Occur only in zoo animals
    d. Occur in animals and people that are exposed to the same source of infection

51. A disease can be indirectly transmitted in all of the following ways *except*:

    a. Inhalation of infectious droplets
    b. Bite of an arthropod vector
    c. Contact with infectious blood
    d. Ingestion of contaminated food

52. All of the following diseases are transmitted by ingestion of unpasteurized milk *except*:

   a. Listeriosis
   b. Q fever
   c. Brucellosis
   d. Giardiasis

53. All of the following are control or prevention programs for zoonoses *except*:

   a. Flea and tick dip for hunting dogs
   b. Deworming of 6-week-old puppies
   c. Testing of cattle and then vaccination against brucellosis
   d. Rectal examination of horses

54. The role of the veterinary technician in preventing and controlling zoonotic diseases includes all of the following *except*:

   a. Noticing the first signs of a zoonotic disease
   b. Educating clients, especially those most susceptible, about the risk of zoonoses
   c. Treating clients and their pets for certain common zoonoses
   d. Participating in disease control and prevention programs

CHAPTER 11: LABORATORY PROCEDURES

55. Which anticoagulant is preferred for routine hematologic studies because it preserves cell morphology?

   a. Heparin
   b. Sodium citrate
   c. EDTA
   d. Ammonium oxalate

56. What effect does an icteric sample have on total plasma protein determination by refractometry?

   a. No effect
   b. Slightly increased value
   c. Decreased value
   d. Markedly increased value

57. Reticulocytes are found in all of the following species *except*:

   a. Cats
   b. Dogs
   c. Pigs
   d. Horses

58. Which of the following is a toxic change observed in neutrophils?

   a. Döhle bodies
   b. Howell-Jolly bodies
   c. Heinz bodies
   d. Nuclear hypersegmentation

59. Which test of the coagulation system requires a blood tube containing diatomaceous earth?

   a. Activated clotting time
   b. Bleeding time
   c. Whole blood clotting time
   d. One-stage prothrombin time

60. Trematodes and cestodes are similar because they:

   a. Are dorsoventrally flattened and have muscular suckers for attachment
   b. Lack a digestive tract
   c. Have direct life cycles
   d. Have separate sexes

61. Samples collected for parasitologic examinations should be:

   a. Examined grossly for consistency, color, odor, blood, mucus, and foreign bodies
   b. Examined 48 hours after collection
   c. Collected off the ground to include grass and soil from the environment
   d. Conducted using a direct smear only

62. Lungworm infections are best diagnosed using:

   a. Sedimentation of feces
   b. Fecal flotation using saturated sodium chloride flotation solution
   c. The Baermann technique
   d. Modified McMaster egg count

63. The recommended flotation solution for recovery of *Giardia* oocysts is:

   a. Sheather's sugar
   b. Zinc sulfate
   c. Magnesium sulfate
   d. Potassium dichromate

64. In an emergency situation, when results are needed as soon as possible, in what type of tube should blood be collected for a blood chemistry profile, and what sample is tested?

   a. EDTA tube, plasma
   b. Heparin tube, plasma
   c. Serum tube, serum
   d. Citrate tube, whole blood

65. Which of the following describes the correct sample-handling technique when submitting a serum sample to the laboratory?

   a. Collect the blood in a serum tube and send the tube to the laboratory.
   b. Collect the blood in a serum separator tube. Allow the blood to clot at room temperature. Centrifuge and send the tube to the laboratory.
   c. Collect the blood in a serum tube. Allow the blood to clot at room temperature. Centrifuge, harvest the serum, transfer the serum to a second tube, and send this tube to the laboratory.
   d. Collect the blood in a tube containing EDTA as an anticoagulant. Send this tube along with a cold pack to the laboratory.

66. Assay for which of the following is used to assess carbohydrate metabolism?

   a. Fibrogen
   b. GGT
   c. Bile acids
   d. Glucose

67. What is the preferred sample for assay of fibrogen?

   a. Serum
   b. EDTA plasma
   c. Sodium heparin plasma
   d. Potassium heparin plasma

68. In cases of leptospirosis, the sample of choice for dark-field examination is a:

   a. Midstream urine sample
   b. Sample of kidney tissue
   c. Blood sample
   d. Fecal sample

69. To confirm the diagnosis of ringworm (dermatophytosis), which type of specimen should you collect and submit to the diagnostic laboratory?

   a. Feces
   b. Stomach contents
   c. Blood sample
   d. Skin scapings

70. Specimens for bacteriologic examination should be submitted:

   a. On dry ice in a well-sealed container for both aerobic or anaerobic cultures
   b. On dry ice in an unsealed container, because aerobic bacteria cannot thrive in sealed environments because of lack of oxygen
   c. At room temperature (20° C)
   d. At body temperature (37° C) because organisms thrive best at this temperature

71. Concerning collection and handling of specimens for virologic examination, which statement is most accurate?

   a. Leave the specimens at room temperature, because viruses do not deteriorate at this temperature.
   b. Do not leave virologic specimens at room temperature, because viral titers decrease rapidly as temperature increases.
   c. Ship virologic specimens on dry ice only if the ambient temperature is high.
   d. Never ship virologic specimens on dry ice.

72. Compared with a 50× oil-immersion lens with an N.A. of 0.85, a 40× lens with an N.A. of 0.66 has resolving power and magnification that are:

   a. Increased and higher, respectively
   b. Increased and lower, respectively
   c. Decreased and higher, respectively
   d. Decreased and lower, respectively

73. For which fluid is a complete fluid analysis *least* appropriate?

    a. Thoracic fluid
    b. Cerebrospinal fluid
    c. Synovial fluid
    d. Hematoma

74. If a urine sample is left standing for some time, which of the following changes is *least* likely to occur?

    a. Precipitation of crystals
    b. Bacterial overgrowth
    c. Decrease in pH
    d. Rupture of cellular elements (e.g., RBCs, WBCs)

75. In which condition are large numbers of white blood cells *least* likely to be observed in the urine sediment?

    a. Infection of the urinary bladder
    b. Infection of the kidneys
    c. Inflammation of the urinary bladder secondary to uroliths
    d. Rhabdomyolysis

76. The instructions included with a test kit explicitly state that hemolyzed samples should not be tested. When preparing to perform the test, you notice the serum sample is slightly red. Most appropriately you should:

    a. Run the test anyway
    b. Refrigerate the sample to see if the discoloration disappears
    c. Collect another blood sample to obtain clear serum
    d. Centrifuge the sample until the color is gone

77. Which item is *not* an essential part of a page in a maintenance notebook for laboratory instruments?

    a. Components to be checked
    b. Instrument serial number
    c. Manufacturer's address and telephone number
    d. Interval of checks

CHAPTER 12: EUTHANASIA METHODS, SPECIMEN COLLECTION, AND NECROPSY TECHNIQUES

78. The technique often used for euthanizing very small, immature animals, such as young mice and rats, and small birds is:

    a. Electrocution
    b. Injectable anesthetics
    c. Inhalant anesthetics
    d. Cervical dislocation

79. Which type of laboratory test requires the greatest amount of tissues for examination?

    a. Bacteriologic
    b. Virologic
    c. Parasitologic
    d. Toxicologic

80. Sections of tissues collected for histopathologic examination should be no thicker than:

    a. 10 mm
    b. 5 mm
    c. 1 mm
    d. 15 mm

81. Which species does *not* have a gallbladder?

    a. Cats
    b. Mice
    c. Horses
    d. Rabbits

82. Specimens for virologic testing are most likely to be diagnostic if collected from:

    a. Animals that have been chronically sick
    b. Animals that are in the acute stages of illness
    c. Animals that have been ill for only a few days
    d. Dead animals

CHAPTER 13: PHARMACOLOGY AND PHARMACY PRACTICES

83. The doctor asks you to dispense drug tablets for a 22-lb dog, to be given at 5 mg/kg TID for 5 days. How many 25-mg tablets should you dispense?

a. 5
b. 10
c. 20
d. 30

84. Which type of insulin is most appropriate for IV infusion in animals with diabetic ketoacidosis?

a. NPH insulin
b. Regular insulin
c. Lente insulin
d. Ultralente insulin

85. Which drug is most likely to cause nephrotoxicosis?

a. Penicillin G
b. Gentamicin
c. Oxytetracycline
d. Ampicillin

86. Which compound is a biguanide antiseptic that binds to the outer surface of the skin, producing some residual activity?

a. Povidone-iodine
b. Benzalkonium chloride
c. Hexachlorophene
d. Chlorhexidine

87. Which drug is most likely to be effective against adult heartworms?

a. Thiabendazole
b. Melarsomine dihydrochloride
c. Pyrantel pamoate
d. Diethylcarbamazine

CHAPTER 14: NUTRITION

88. The daily weight gain of an average growing puppy is approximately:

a. 2 to 4 g/kg of anticipated adult weight
b. 1 to 2 g/kg of anticipated adult weight
c. 5 to 7 g/kg of anticipated adult weight
d. 0.25 to 0.5 g/kg of anticipated adult weight

89. A pet's diet should be changed:

a. Periodically to maintain interest and stimulate appetite

b. Frequently to avoid problems associated with poor diet quality
c. Only when necessary and after careful consideration of nutritional requirements
d. Abruptly, with no transitional period

90. Which cat has the highest daily energy requirement?

a. 12-year-old, 3-kg, castrated male
b. 2-year-old, 3-kg queen nursing 3-week-old kittens
c. 4-year-old, 9-kg, intact male
d. 5-year-old, 4-kg, pregnant queen

91. Which species ferments predigested feed material?

a. Cattle
b. Sheep
c. Goats
d. Horses

92. An animal that is consuming much more feed than it requires for maintenance is likely to have a body condition score of:

a. 1
b. 5
c. 9
d. 12

CHAPTER 15: REPRODUCTION

93. The correct order of stages in the estrous cycle is:

a. Anestrus, proestrus, diestrus, estrus
b. Anestrus, diestrus, proestrus, estrus
c. Anestrus, estrus, diestrus, proestrus
d. Anestrus, proestrus, estrus, diestrus

94. Concerning use of equine chorionic gonadotropin (ECG) as a blood test for pregnancy in the mare, which statement is *least* accurate?

    a. The ECG test can give a false positive ("pregnant" when really not pregnant) if the fetus dies after 35 days of gestation.
    b. The ECG tests can give a false negative ("not pregnant" when really pregnant) if done too early or too late in pregnancy.
    c. The ECG test must be done between 120 and 250 days of gestation, when estrogen levels are high in the mare.
    d. The ECG test is the basis of the MIP test.

95. Concerning B-mode, real-time ultrasonography, which statement is *least* accurate?

    a. It allows us to see movement of the fetus.
    b. It can detect a foal's heartbeat as early as 25 days of pregnancy.
    c. It can be used to determine the sex of embryos.
    d. It must be used transabdominally in mares.

96. When dealing with a live neonate, the most important immediate consideration is to:

    a. Clear the airway and establish respiration
    b. Dip the umbilical cord end in disinfectant
    c. Ensure that it received colostrum
    d. Check for congenital defects

97. The male breeding soundness examination should include all of the following *except:*

    a. A good physical examination, including the reproductive organs
    b. Evaluation of the quantity of sperm in the ejaculate
    c. Estimation of the percentage of normally shaped and motile sperm
    d. Evaluation of the bull's genetic potential

CHAPTER 16: BEHAVIOR

98. It is reasonable to confine a puppy in a crate as part of a house training program for:

    a. An entire 8-hour workday
    b. All of the time, except when the puppy is taken outside to eliminate

    c. Only for as long as the puppy can be expected to control its bladder and bowels, based on its age
    d. Never more than an hour at a time

99. The best way to establish good litterbox habits in a kitten is to:

    a. Take the kitten to the box whenever it needs to eliminate, grasp its paws, and make scratching motions
    b. Be sure the kitten observes the queen eliminating in a litterbox
    c. Confine the kitten in a small room with a litterbox
    d. Provide a clean, accessible litterbox with fine-grained litter material at a moderate depth

100. The *best way* to prevent or resolve normal "puppy destructive behavior" is to:

    a. Show the dog the object it has previously chewed and verbally scold it
    b. Provide appropriate chew toys
    c. Provide a variety of toys and make household objects less appealing
    d. Put the dog on a "time out" whenever it is caught chewing

101. Concerning behavior in dogs and cats, which statement is *least* accurate?

    a. Puppy testing is an accurate way of predicting a dog's adult personality
    b. Aggressive behavior is normal behavior for all animals
    c. Providing puppies and kittens with many pleasant socialization opportunities may prevent fear-motivated aggression problems later in life
    d. Intact males are more likely to display aggressive problems than are females or castrated males

102. It has been scientifically proven that:

    a. Allowing a dog to sleep on the owner's bed creates aggressive behavior problems
    b. Playing tug-of-war games with a dog creates aggressive behavior problems
    c. Cats generally do not form linear dominance hierarchies as do dogs
    d. Forcing puppies to assume submissive positions prevents aggressive behavior problems

103. Punishment:

    a. Is relatively easy to administer correctly

    b. Is the application of any aversive stimulus that results in reduced frequency of a behavior

    c. Is the best method to resolve most behavior problems

    d. Can be administered appropriately if the animal is shown the results of its misbehavior, even if the misbehavior is not observed

CHAPTER 17: PHYSICAL RESTRAINT

104. For veterinary treatment, friendly cats are best restrained by:

    a. The owner

    b. Pressing onto the examination table

    c. Petting and minimal physical restraint

    d. A sharp tone of voice

105. Solid wooden panels are best used as a herding device for:

    a. Llamas

    b. Cats

    c. Miniature horses

    d. Pigs

106. Which species should *never* be restrained by the scruff?

    a. Hamster

    b. Guinea pig

    c. Gerbil

    d. Mouse

107. Concerning restraint of pet birds, which statement is *least* accurate?

    a. One hand should be used to compress the trachea and thorax.

    b. Birds are not susceptible to hyperthermia and can be safely restrained in a towel for long periods.

    c. When experienced, one person can restrain a small bird for jugular venipuncture.

    d. It is preferable to have the owner remove the bird from its cage.

108. *Before* attempting to remove an animal from its cage, the first consideration is to:

    a. Talk to it in a loud, commanding voice

    b. Find an escape route for yourself

    c. Have a sedative injection ready for administration

    d. Close all escape routes

CHAPTER 18: PATIENT HISTORY AND PHYSICAL EXAMINATION

109. Concerning history taking, which statement is *least* accurate?

    a. The information gathered from the history can direct attention to potential problems or affected body areas.

    b. One must be careful not to jump to conclusions about the diagnosis.

    c. Information about the animal's environment or activity is rarely relevant.

    d. The nature and dates of past illnesses may aid diagnosis of the current problem.

110. Possible causes of an animal's illness are termed:

    a. Definitive possibilities

    b. Differential diagnoses

    c. Circumstantial presumptions

    d. Tentative conclusions

111. A musical or drumlike sound elicited by percussion over an air-filled organ is termed:

    a. Tympany

    b. Dullness

    c. Sibilance

    d. Emphysema

112. Which sign indicates upper airway disease?

    a. Tenesmus

    b. Stridor

    c. Strabismus

    d. Opisthotonos

113. In horses and cattle, rhythmic pressing of a fist into an abdominal area is termed:

    a. Ballottement

    b. Palpation

    c. Abdominocentesis

    d. Decoupage

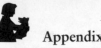

CHAPTER 19: DIAGNOSTIC IMAGING

114.   Which substance absorbs the most x-rays?

    a. Bone
    b. Fat
    c. Water
    d. Metal

115.   Which of the following controls the degree of contrast on a radiograph?

    a. Focal spot size
    b. Focal-film distance
    c. kVp
    d. mAs

116.   Which type of x-ray machine allows for higher output and faster exposure times?

    a. Full-wave rectified, single phase
    b. Full-wave rectified, three phase
    c. Self-rectified
    d. Half-wave rectified, single phase

117.   Which term best describes an area with the same echotexture as surrounding tissues?

    a. Hyperechoic
    b. Hypoechoic
    c. Anechoic
    d. Isoechoic

118.   If resistance is encountered when passing the biopsy forceps through the endoscope to collect a biopsy specimen:

    a. Try to open the forceps while in the channel to unlock the jaws
    b. Straighten out the distal end of the endoscope until passage is possible
    c. Force the forceps through the channel
    d. Abandon the procedure because difficult passage indicates a large neoplasm

119.   Which statement concerning video endoscopes is most accurate?

    a. They use glass fiber bundles for transmission of the image.
    b. Broken fibers show up on the monitor screen as black dots.
    c. They are composed of a metal tube, lenses, and glass rods.
    d. A microchip records and transmits the image.

CHAPTER 20: PRINCIPLES OF ANESTHESIA, ANALGESIA, AND ANESTHETIC NURSING

120.   Monitoring the perfusion of body tissues during anesthesia refers to:

    a. Maintaining normal blood pressure
    b. Administering adequate fluid volume during anesthesia
    c. Administration of oxygen during anesthesia
    d. Ensuring the flow of oxygenated blood to tissues

121.   The best indication of hypoventilation in an anesthetized patient is:

    a. Cyanotic (blue) mucous membranes
    b. Pale mucous membranes
    c. Abnormal arterial blood gas results
    d. Respiratory rate

122.   If the heart rate should increase dramatically during anesthesia, the anesthetist's initial response should be to:

    a. Turn up the anesthetic concentration on the vaporizer
    b. Inject additional anesthetic
    c. Evaluate the patient's overall status to determine cause
    d. Turn down the anesthetic concentration on the vaporizer

123.   The most frequent complication associated with phenothiazine administration is:

    a. Hypertension
    b. Hypotension
    c. Cardiac arrhythmia
    d. Excitement upon recovery

124.   When comparing the heart rate and peripheral pulse rate, the heart rate:

    a. Should equal the pulse rate
    b. Should be more rapid than the pulse rate
    c. Should be lower than the pulse rate
    d. Is not exactly correlated with the pulse rate

125.   The recommended rate of intravenous fluid infusion during anesthesia in small animals is:

    a. 5 to 10 mg/kg/hr
    b. 10 to 20 ml/kg/hr

c. 20 to 30 ml/kg/hr

d. 30 to 40 ml/kg/hr

126. Moderate acute hemorrhage during surgery can be compensated for by infusing standard replacement fluids at the rate of:

a. 1 ml of fluid/ml of blood lost

b. 2 ml of fluid/ml of blood lost

c. 3 ml of fluid/ml of blood lost

d. 90 ml of fluid/kg/hr

127. Which of the following is a neuroleptanalgesic combination?

a. Xylazine and ketamine

b. Ketamine and acepromazine

c. Fentanyl and droperidol

d. Oxymorphone and atropine

CHAPTER 21: PRINCIPLES OF SURGICAL NURSING

128. Which abdominal incision is made parallel to the long axis of the body and lateral to the ventral midline?

a. Paracostal

b. Flank

c. Paramedian

d. Ventral midline

129. An accumulation of serous fluid in dead space in the region of an incision is called a:

a. Hematoma

b. Keratoma

c. Seroma

d. Subcutoma

130. Which of the following is *not* a general rule of aseptic technique?

a. Only sterile items should touch other sterile items.

b. Any sterile item touching another sterile item becomes nonsterile.

c. If the sterility of an item is in question, it should be considered nonsterile.

d. Nonscrubbed personnel should not reach over sterile fields.

131. Which wrapper has the longest sterile shelf-life for a sterilized pack?

a. Heat-sealed plastic pouch

b. Double-wrapping with two-layer muslin

c. Double-wrapping with paper

d. Double-wrapping with two-layer muslin, heat-sealed in a dust cover

132. Which item *cannot* be safely sterilized using steam sterilization?

a. Rubber catheter

b. Stainless-steel suture wire

c. Gauze sponges

d. Fiberoptic endoscope

133. Concerning preoperative scrubbing of the hands and arms, which statement is most accurate?

a. For the first case of the day, a 2-minute scrub is adequate.

b. During and after scrubbing, the hands should be kept higher than the elbows.

c. A separate scrub brush must be used for each hand and for each arm.

d. The objective of preoperative scrubbing is to sterilize the skin.

134. Which antimicrobial soap is a good virucide and has good residual activity because it binds with the keratin of skin?

a. Hexachlorophene

b. Triclosan

c. Chlorhexidine

d. Povidone-iodine

135. Concerning the counted brush stroke method of preoperative scrubbing of the hands and arms, which statement is *least* accurate?

a. The counted brush stroke method provides much better disinfection than the anatomic timed method.

b. The tips of the fingers and thumbs should each receive 30 strokes.

c. Each of the four surfaces of each part of each finger and thumb should receive 20 strokes.

d. Each of the four surfaces of each arm should receive 20 strokes.

136. Which suture material has the largest diameter and is most coarse?

a. 9-O monofilament nylon
b. 2-O chromic surgical gut
c. 20-gauge stainless-steel wire
d. #1 polypropylene

137. Which suture material is nonabsorbable?

a. Polyester
b. Polyglycolic acid
c. Polyglactin 910
d. Polyglyconate

CHAPTER 22: EMERGENCY AND CRITICAL CARE

138. Diminished or absent breath and heart sounds are most compatible with:

a. Laryngeal paralysis
b. Pulmonary edema
c. Pneumothorax
d. Asthma

139. Prolonged capillary refill time is an indicator of:

a. Increased blood pressure
b. Poor peripheral perfusion
c. Increased cardiac output
d. Poor pulse pressure

140. All of the following are crystalloid solutions *except*:

a. Hetastarch
b. Normal saline
c. Lactated Ringer's
d. Plasmalyte 148

141. The cornerstone of shock therapy is:

a. Fluid therapy
b. Antibiotic therapy
c. Corticosteroid administration
d. Sympathomimetic administration

142. In cases of suspected toxin ingestion, clinical signs of nervousness, apprehension, and seizures most likely suggest toxicity caused by:

a. Organophosphate
b. Ethylene glycol

c. Metaldehyde
d. Anticoagulant rodenticide

CHAPTER 23: MANAGEMENT OF WOUNDS, FRACTURES, AND OTHER INJURIES

143. In which category is an abdominal surgical wound that has minor contamination, but not with organ contents?

a. Clean
b. Clean-contaminated
c. Contaminated
d. Dirty

144. Which of the following is *not* a characteristic of wound infection?

a. Fewer than 100,000 microorganisms per gram of tissue
b. Pus
c. Elevated white blood cell count
d. Erythema

145. A length of gauze or tape placed in a wound to prolong drainage and to keep the wound from closing prematurely is called a:

a. Seton
b. Penrose drain
c. Scranton loop
d. Robert Jones bandage

146. Which type of wound closure is recommended 3 to 5 days after cleaning and debridement, and *after* granulation tissue forms?

a. Primary closure
b. Delayed primary closure
c. Secondary closure
d. Nonclosure

147. Which orthopedic device is most suitable for temporary immobilization of fractures on the distal limb?

a. Robert Jones bandage
b. Spica splint
c. Ehmer sling
d. Velpeau sling

148. Concerning various types of wounds, which statement is most accurate?

a. High-velocity gunshot wounds tend to create little tissue destruction and no exit wound.
b. The owner should be encouraged to pull a protruding arrow out of the animal's body.
c. Horses and cattle almost always die after a venomous snakebite.
d. First-degree burns destroy the full thickness of the skin.

CHAPTER 24: FLUID THERAPY AND BLOOD TRANSFUSIONS

149. Which of the following represents a high concentration of hydrogen ions?

    a. Alkalosis
    b. pH 7.6
    c. pH 8.0
    d. Acidosis

150. Which solution is most appropriate for maintenance of fluids and electrolyte balance?

    a. Lactated Ringer's
    b. Normosol-M
    c. 0.9% Saline
    d. 5% Dextrose in water

151. After a dog's nail (cuticle) is clipped to induce bleeding, the normal bleeding time is less than:

    a. 5 minutes
    b. 2 minutes
    c. 1 minute
    d. 6 minutes

152. What is the "universal donor" blood group of dogs?

    a. DEA 7 positive
    b. DEA 1.1 negative
    c. DEA 9 negative
    d. DEA 4.3 positive

153. Which substance should *not* be used to anticoagulate and preserve blood to be collected and stored for transfusion?

    a. Citrate-phosphate-dextrose-adenine
    b. Citrate-phosphate-dextrose
    c. Acid-citrate-dextrose
    d. Heparin

CHAPTER 25: DENTISTRY

154. How much attachment loss can be expected in an area with stage-2 periodontal disease?

    a. Up to 10%
    b. Up to 25%
    c. Up to 50%
    d. More than 50%

155. Which of the following is *not* a typical characteristic of bacteria found in periodontal pockets in advanced (stage-4) periodontal disease?

    a. Spirochetes
    b. Gram negative
    c. Motile
    d. Anaerobic

156. Which of the following is *not* an advantage of intraoral films in dental radiography?

    a. Double emulsion provides good detail
    b. Flexible for easy positioning
    c. Can pass through automatic processor by itself
    d. Inexpensive

157. Which permanent teeth are deflected rostrally (mesially) if their deciduous counterparts are not exfoliated at the appropriate time (retained)?

    a. Lower canines
    b. Upper canines
    c. Lower incisors
    d. Upper incisors

158. Which term accurately describes a forming tooth that attempts to duplicate but does not completely split?

    a. Dens-in-dente
    b. Fusion tooth
    c. Germination tooth
    d. Twinning

159. Which teeth are considered the carnassial teeth of dogs and cats?

    a. The four canines
    b. The upper first molars and lower fourth premolars
    c. The upper first molars and lower first molars
    d. The upper fourth premolars and lower first molars

160. Which of the following is *not* an appropriate treatment for a fractured tooth with an open canal?

    a. Endodontics (root canal therapy)
    b. Extraction
    c. Vital endodontics (vital pulpotomy/pulp capping on recently exposed canal)
    d. Wait to see if it causes problems

CHAPTER 26: NURSING CARE OF DOGS AND CATS

161. Concerning venipuncture and blood collection, which statement is *least* accurate?

    a. The vessels of cats are usually very deep and thick-walled.
    b. The jugular vein runs in a line from the point of the mandibular ramus to the thoracic inlet.
    c. The jugular vein of short-nosed dog breeds tends to be more lateral than that of other breeds.
    d. Animals with endocrine disorders tend to have thin skin and friable vessels.

162. For which assay should a vacuum-filled collection tube (e.g., Vacutainer) *not* be used for blood collection?

    a. Potassium
    b. Blood gases
    c. Creatine phosphokinase
    d. Complete blood count

163. Which site is most commonly used for subcutaneous injection of small volumes of medication or fluid?

    a. Between the scapulae, at the back of the neck
    b. Lateral aspect of the thigh
    c. Lateral aspect of the proximal foreleg
    d. Ventral abdomen

164. Concerning use of catheters, which statement is *least* accurate?

    a. The shorter the catheter, the less likely it is to cause phlebitis and complications.
    b. A jugular catheter is less likely to cause phlebitis with injection of irritating solutions.
    c. Butterfly catheters are not appropriate for long-term IV infusions.
    d. Catheters should not be inserted into vessels near areas of infection, scars, wounds, or fractures.

165. Which catheterization site is most appropriate for long-term infusion of fluids and nutrients?

    a. Medial auricular (ear) vein
    b. Femoral artery
    c. Saphenous vein
    d. Jugular vein

166. Which of the following is *not* recommended to maintain body temperature in hospitalized animals?

    a. Circulating warm-water blanket
    b. Incubator
    c. Warm-water bottles
    d. Electric heating pad

167. Blowing or administration of a powder, vapor, or gas into a body cavity or airway is termed:

    a. Auscultation
    b. Insufflation
    c. Aspiration
    d. Intussusception

168. Concerning enteral feeding by nasogastric tube, which statement is *least* accurate?

    a. Hyperosmolar diets may cause diarrhea.
    b. Accidental tracheal intubation can lead to aspiration pneumonia.
    c. A nasogastric tube should remain in place for no longer than 48 hours.
    d. Before each feeding, the tube should be aspirated and sterile water injected.

CHAPTER 27: NURSING CARE OF HORSES

169. Which type of wood shavings contains a toxin that can cause laminitis?

    a. White pine shavings
    b. Yellow pine shavings
    c. Cedar shavings
    d. Black walnut shavings

170. If a horse has gastric reflux, the animal:

    a. Is likely to vomit
    b. Can be rehydrated with fluids administered by nasogastric tube
    c. Can be fed a bran mash and allowed free access to water
    d. Is at risk of gastric rupture if the reflux is excessive and pressure is not relieved by passing a nasogastric tube

171. Concerning infectious diseases, which statement is most accurate?

    a. Always disinfect equipment before cleaning the dirt, debris, or manure off of it.
    b. Always handle infected horses before handling other horses in the barn.
    c. Horses can spread diseases only by coughing.
    d. Coveralls, plastic bottles, and gloves should be worn when working with horses with contagious disease.

172. Concerning intravenous infusions, which statement is most accurate?

    a. Large volumes of fluid can be rapidly infused as a bolus in neonatal foals.
    b. Care must be taken to prevent the fluid in an IV bag from completely running out, allowing blood to flow back into the IV line.
    c. Medication may be injected through the IV line injection port while parenteral nutrition is being administered to foals.
    d. Frozen plasma should be thawed quickly by microwaving on a high setting for 20 minutes.

173. Concerning leg wraps, which statement is most accurate?

    a. Leg wraps should be applied using even distribution of tension so that they are snug, but not so tight as to damage the tendons.
    b. Leg wraps should be applied to produce more pressure over the front of the leg and no pressure over the tendons.
    c. The point of the hock should be double-wrapped with elastic bandage material to decrease joint motion.
    d. Leg wraps should always be applied to the leg as tightly as possible to prevent slippage.

174. Concerning recumbent horses, which statement is *least* accurate?

    a. Three people can easily turn an adult horse with two grasping the distal legs at the pastern while the third person lifts the head.
    b. The horse should be turned as frequently as possible.
    c. Recumbent animals must be kept on thick padding or deep bedding.
    d. Slings should not be used to support horses with flaccid paralysis.

175. What is the most effective and most desirable way to control flies in a stable with a sick horse?

    a. Organophosphate sprays
    b. Pyrethrin sprays
    c. Frequent stall cleaning and manure removal
    d. Overhead fly spray systems

CHAPTER 28: NURSING CARE OF FOOD ANIMALS, CAMELIDS, AND RATITES

176. Concerning venipuncture and blood collection in cattle, which statement is *least* accurate?

    a. The subcutaneous abdominal vein is preferred for routine collection of blood samples.
    b. The jugular vein is often used for infusion of large volumes of fluid.
    c. The coccygeal vein can be used for injection of small volumes of drugs.
    d. Bovine skin is thick and difficult to penetrate with large-bore needles.

177. Which vein should be used for intravenous injections in calves?

    a. Subcutaneous abdominal vein
    b. Coccygeal vein
    c. Jugular vein
    d. Saphenous vein

178. Concerning milk sampling and intramammary infusions, which statement is most accurate?

    a. Milk samples from mastitic quarters should be obtained after a week of antibiotic treatment.
    b. The quarter should be stripped of milk before infusing medication.
    c. The cannula should be inserted into the teat full length, up to the hub, when infusing medication.
    d. Intramammary infusions should be performed 10 to 15 minutes before each milking.

179. Effective ways to move sheep include all of the following *except*:

    a. Moving sheep along slight curves where they cannot see ahead
    b. Keeping noise at a quiet-soft tone
    c. Taking into account a sheep's flight zone
    d. Providing bright or shadowy lighting

180. Which sign indicates incorrect placement of a stomach tube in the trachea instead of in the rumen?

    a. A cough reflex
    b. Swallowing as the tube is advanced
    c. Rumen odor exiting the tube
    d. Gurgling sounds in the paralumbar fossa

181. When therapeutic efficacy would not be compromised, drugs and vaccines in the goat should be given:

    a. Subcutaneously
    b. Intravenously
    c. Intramuscularly
    d. Orally

182. Subcutaneous injections in the goat are best administered at the:

    a. Top of the neck
    b. Upper flank
    c. Lateral aspect of the neck
    d. Dorsal aspect of the back

183. In adult goats, what is the largest volume of solution that can be safely injected intramuscularly at any single site?

    a. 5 ml
    b. 10 ml
    c. 15 ml
    d. 20 ml

184. What is the most appropriate needle size for injections in adult goats?

    a. 14 gauge, 2 to 3 cm
    b. 16 gauge, 2 cm
    c. 18 to 20 gauge, 2 to 3 cm
    d. 21 to 22 gauge, 2 to 3 cm

185. In chronologic order, the stages of pig production are:

    a. Piglet, grower, boar, sow, weaner
    b. Piglet, weaner, grower-finisher
    c. Piglet, boar, gilt, sow, weaner
    d. Piglet, weaner, sow, grower-finisher

186. Piglets acquire most of their material antibodies from:

    a. Placental transfer of antibodies
    b. Colostral antibodies in the first 24 hours of life
    c. Milk in the first 24 hours of life
    d. Colostrum and milk in the first week of life

187. Llamas differ from other ruminants because they have:

    a. Three digits on each foot, rather than two
    b. Only an upper dental pad, with no upper incisors
    c. A stomach with three compartments instead of four
    d. An esophagus on the right side of the neck, rather than on the left

188. Which species has vestigial wings?

    a. *Rhea americanus*
    b. *Struthio camelus*
    c. *Casuarius casuarius*
    d. *Dromaius novaehollandiae*

CHAPTER 29: NURSING CARE OF CAGE BIRDS AND POULTRY

189. The anesthetic agent of choice in cage birds is:

    a. Sodium thiopental
    b. Isoflurane
    c. Ketamine
    d. Acepromazine

190. Which muscle area is the preferred site of IM injection?

    a. Gluteal
    b. Biceps
    c. Triceps
    d. Pectoral

191. Which feathers are clipped in a wing trim?

    a. Primary flight
    b. Covert
    c. Down
    d. Contour

192. What is the best way to give a bird oral medication?

    a. By gavage
    b. With a pilling device
    c. Squirt the liquid drug into the mouth using a syringe
    d. In the feed or water

193. Concerning cage birds, which statement is *least* accurate?

    a. Behavior problems constitute the primary reason owners sell their pet birds.
    b. Psittacines are also known as parrots or hookbills.
    c. Owners of birds requiring behavior counseling should be referred to local pet stores for authoritative advice on correcting the problem.
    d. Appointments for examination and treatment of pet birds generally take longer than appointments for dogs and cats.

194. Concerning poultry management, which statement is *least* accurate?

    a. Young, commercially raised birds are commonly vaccinated.
    b. Withdrawal times must be considered when prescribing medication.

    c. The sex of adult poultry is easy to determine from their appearance.
    d. Birds are housed individually to prevent disease transmission and fighting.

CHAPTER 30: NURSING CARE OF SMALL MAMMALS

195. Which species requires vitamin C in the diet?

    a. Mouse
    b. Guinea pig
    c. Ferret
    d. Gerbil

196. To decrease the chance of hairball formation, rabbits should be fed a large amount of:

    a. Hay
    b. Vegetables
    c. Pellets
    d. Fruit

197. All of the following are recommended sites for blood collection in ferrets *except* the:

    a. Cranial vena cava
    b. Heart
    c. Jugular vein
    d. Cephalic vein

198. Which of the following is *not* a reason why parenteral injection is the preferred route of drug administration in small mammals?

    a. Decreased gastrointestinal problems
    b. Increased chance of successful treatment
    c. More choices of injectable medications
    d. More accurate dose delivery

CHAPTER 31: NURSING CARE OF REPTILES, AMPHIBIANS, AND AQUARIUM FISH

199. As compared with the environment of reptiles, the environment of amphibians should be:

    a. Warmer and more humid
    b. Warmer and less humid
    c. Cooler and more humid
    d. Cooler and less humid

200. The site most commonly used to collect blood from snakes is the:

    a. Tail vein
    b. Palatine vein
    c. Cephalic vein
    d. Heart

201. The site most commonly used to collect blood from turtles is the:

    a. Jugular vein
    b. Axillary vein
    c. Dorsal coccygeal vein
    d. Toenail

202. Decreased food intake results in all of the following *except*:

    a. Protein and fat anabolism
    b. Hepatic lipidosis
    c. Acidosis
    d. Impaired gastrointestinal function

203. The best indicator that a fish is being maintained in a safe plane of anesthesia is:

    a. Respiratory movement
    b. Response to stimuli
    c. Loss of equilibrium
    d. Eye movement

CHAPTER 32: NURSING CARE OF ORPHANED AND INJURED WILD ANIMALS

204. Which animal is most likely to survive if released from captivity?

    a. Songbird with a missing toe
    b. Blind rabbit
    c. Hawk with a broken wing
    d. Duck with a missing leg

205. What approximate amount should be fed to a captive baby animal?

    a. 3% to 5% of body weight divided three times daily
    b. 1% to 2% of body weight divided two times daily
    c. 10% to 20% of body weight divided two to four times daily
    d. 7.5% of body weight once daily

206. What is a common cause of mass death in wild avian species?

    a. Salmonellosis
    b. Botulism
    c. Vehicular trauma
    d. Heat stroke

207. Which parasite affects the esophagus and crop of pigeons and doves?

    a. *Leukocytozoon*
    b. *Sarcoptes*
    c. *Toxoplasma*
    d. *Trichomonas*

208. What two dietary supplements are essential to pinnipeds housed in fresh water?

    a. Vitamin E and sodium chloride
    b. Vitamin A and vitamin E
    c. Vitamin B_1 and sodium chloride
    d. Vitamin B_1 and vitamin E

CHAPTER 33: NURSING CARE OF LABORATORY ANIMALS

209. The species with the shortest gestation period is the:

    a. Gerbil
    b. Hamster
    c. Rabbit
    d. Mouse

210. All of the following species are rodents *except*:

    a. *Oryctolagus cuniculus*
    b. *Mus musculus*
    c. *Cavia porcellus*
    d. *Mesocricetus auratus*

211. Penicillin can cause a fatal reaction in:

    a. Guinea pigs
    b. Rats
    c. Hamsters
    d. Rabbits

212. Which rodent is most prone to seizures?

    a. Rabbit
    b. Guinea pig
    c. Hamster
    d. Gerbil

213. Which bedding material should *not* be used in a research setting?

   a. Aspen chips
   b. Paper
   c. Cedar chips
   d. Corncob chips

CHAPTER 34: NURSING CARE OF PEDIATRIC AND GERIATRIC PATIENTS

214. The optimal chronology of resuscitation events for the neonate after cesarean section includes:

   a. Clearing the airway, initiating respiration, and stimulating cardiac function, followed by attention to the umbilical cord and drying
   b. Drying the neonate, stimulating cardiac function, and initiating respiration, followed by administration of glucose and care of the umbilical cord
   c. Ligation and cauterization of the umbilical cord, followed by clearing the airways, stimulating respiration and cardiovascular function, and drying the neonate
   d. Rubbing the neonate to stimulate respiration, drying to stimulate cardiovascular function, and swinging to clear the airways, followed by umbilical care

215. Fluid administration to a dehydrated, volume-depleted neonate is best achieved via:

   a. Intraosseous or intravenous catheterization for administration of a balanced electrolyte solution
   b. Subcutaneous administration of balanced electrolyte solution at several sites
   c. Oral administration of a balanced electrolyte solution via stomach tube
   d. Oral administration of an artificial milk product as per the manufacturer's recommendation

216. As compared with the body temperature of the dam, the body temperature of normal neonatal calves is approximately:

   a. 2° cooler
   b. Equal
   c. 1° warmer
   d. 3° warmer

217. A common cause of aggressive behavior in geriatric animals is:

   a. Pain from degenerative joint disease
   b. Congestive heart failure
   c. Incontinence
   d. Unfulfilled hunger

218. Which change is recommended for an overweight geriatric dog?

   a. Feed a reduced amount of maintenance diet and institute vigorous exercise
   b. Feed a low-fat, high-fiber diet and gradually increase periods of gentle exercise
   c. Feed one large meal of the maintenance diet once daily and institute moderate exercise
   d. Feed a diet with 30% of the total daily calories from fat and 15% from protein, and institute 30 to 60 minutes of vigorous exercise daily

Answers

CHAPTER 2: OCCUPATIONAL HAZARDS

1. b. Personal hygiene is the first line of defense in preventing transmission of disease from patient to patient or from the patient to the worker. Hand washing is the most common form of personal hygiene, but other practices, such as eating and drinking only in areas free from chemical or biologic hazards, are also included.

2. b. According to NIOSH studies, leaks in connections and cracked or worn hoses are the most likely source of exposure when a proper machine and scavenging unit are used. The anesthetic system should be checked for leaks daily or before each use.

3. b. Migration of roundworm larvae causes visceral larva migrans.

4. c. The most serious risk is from puncture or laceration and the possibility of subsequent bacterial infection associated with the trauma. Although tetanus is a possibility in some situations, the likelihood of needle contamination with a tetanus organism is remote. There is no evidence that HIV or hepatitis virus can be transmitted from animals to people.

5. a. OSHA Standard 1910.1200 requires the label of secondary chemical containers for in-house use to specify the identity of the chemical contents and the appropriate hazard warnings. The manufacturer's name and address are not required for containers used in the clinic.

CHAPTER 3: ETHICS, ANIMAL WELFARE, AND LAW

6. d. Veterinarians have no ethical obligations to the news media.

7. b. Society is becoming more concerned with animal suffering from any cause.

8. b. Malpractice is one type of negligence. For negligence to be a basis for a lawsuit brought by the client, the negligence must cause damage to the client, in this case, injury to the client's animal.

9. c. The standards of professional practice and whether the veterinarian performed in accordance with these standards are presented by expert testimony during trial. The judge or jury decides if the veterinarian performed in accordance with these standards. Practice acts dictate whom and under what conditions a person may practice veterinary medicine, but they do not define the standards of professional practice.

10. a. A veterinarian is liable for the actions of employed assistants under the doctrine *respondeat superior*. The assistant, however, must be acting within the scope of employment.

CHAPTER 4: VETERINARY MEDICAL TERMINOLOGY

11. c.

12. d.

13. a.

14. b.

15. e.

16. c.

17. d.

18. a.

19. b.

20. e.

CHAPTER 5: RECORDKEEPING, BUSINESS TRANSACTIONS, AND CLINIC ADMINISTRATION

21. c. The ability to work as a team member indicates character traits that are desirable in the veterinary workplace. Skills related to a specific position can be learned on the job.

22. b. Extending credit to certain qualified clients is advantageous to the client and the clinic.

23. d. The size of medical record forms varies. Information should never be "whited-out."

Clients legally are allowed access to their animal's records.

24. b. The economic order quantity is calculated to determine the most appropriate amount of a product to order at one time.

25. b. A high inventory turnover is more desirable than low inventory turnover (in stock for long periods).

CHAPTER 6: HUMAN INTERACTIONS IN THE VETERINARY WORKPLACE

26. d. Many employers consider broad, diversified work experience more desirable than a highly focused background.

27. c. It is the employer's responsibility to create an environment free of harassment of any kind.

28. a. Clients present their animal for veterinary care because they want to preserve their relationship with the animal.

29. a. Clients should be given a choice of two appointment times. A single specified time, without any other choices, might be inconvenient. Offering more than two choices tends to confuse clients.

30. b. The doctor should be encouraged to stay on schedule so as to show clients respect for their time and to keep the clinic running smoothly.

31. a. Present the bill without apology and explain the fees in quiet, businesslike manner.

32. c. With the technique of reflection, you restate what the client has already expressed.

33. a. Denial is typically the first stage of the grieving process.

CHAPTER 7: ANATOMY AND PHYSIOLOGY

34. b. The four basic types of tissues in an animal's body are connective tissue, epithelial tissue, muscle tissue, and nervous tissue.

35. a. The pelvic limb is the hind limb. Listing the bones from proximal to distal means starting close to the body and working down the limb.

36. b. External respiration is the exchange of oxygen and carbon dioxide between air in the lungs and blood in the pulmonary capillaries.

37. a. The brainstem contains centers that control many vital functions of the body. Severe damage to it can cause immediate failure of circulation and respiration, resulting in rapid death.

38. c. Many pituitary hormones stimulate production and release of hormones from other endocrine glands.

39. b. Spermatozoa usually arrive at the oviduct before the ovum. They undergo the process of capacitation there to improve their chances of fertilizing the ovum once it arrives.

CHAPTER 8: PATHOLOGY AND RESPONSE TO DISEASE

40. b. Cold is not a cardinal sign of inflammation.

41. c. Of the bacteria listed, *Streptococcus* is the only one considered pyogenic. It can produce a purulent exudate at the site of infection.

42. b. Of the choices listed, T-lymphocytes are the only component of cell-mediated immunity. All of the other answer choices are involved in humoral immunity.

43. c. A suppurative exudate is characterized by a predominance of neutrophils. A histiocytic or granulomatous inflammatory response is composed primarily of histiocytes. A hemorrhagic exudate is characterized primarily by extravasation of erythrocytes (red blood cells). A lymphoplasmacytic (or lymphocytic/plasmacytic) exudate is characterized by a predominance of lymphocytes and plasma cells.

44. d. The initiating event of traumatic reticulopericarditis involves penetration of a metallic foreign body (nail or wire) through the wall of the reticulum, with subsequent penetration of the diaphragm and pericardium. The foreign body is commonly ingested along with forage. Use of baling string (rather than wire), oral administration or rumen magnets, and application of good management procedures have greatly decreased the incidence of this disease.

CHAPTER 9: PREVENTIVE MEDICINE

45. a. Animal housing should be designed for the comfort and safety of the animals, without regard to the owner's sense of aesthetics.

46. d. Dogs and cats are unlikely to contract tetanus.

47. a. This disease affects horses.

48. a. Phenols can be toxic to some species and should not be used to sanitize water containers.

49. c. Obesity is very common and can be prevented by proper feeding and sufficient exercise.

CHAPTER 10: ANIMAL DISEASE AND PEOPLE

50. a. Some diseases are common to people and animals but are not considered true zoonoses. Only diseases that are transmitted between animals and people are considered zoonoses.

51. a. Inhalation of infectious droplets is considered transmission by direct means because the droplets only travel a few feet and are inhaled directly.

52. d. Giardiasis is transmitted by ingestion of water that is contaminated by animals in the reservoir population.

53. d. Rectal palpation is used to diagnose pregnancy and detect some types of abdominal disorders but is not used to control or prevent zoonotic disease.

54. c. It is illegal for veterinary professionals to prescribe drugs for or treat humans.

CHAPTER 11: LABORATORY PROCEDURES

55. c. EDTA is preferred for routine hematologic studies.

56. a. Icteric serum has no effect on plasma protein determination.

57. d. Reticulocytes are not found in equine blood.

58. a. Döhle bodies are a mild toxic change seen in neutrophils.

59. a. Diatomaceous earth tubes are required to determine activated clotting time (ACT).

60. a. Trematodes and cestodes are similar because they are dorsoventrally flattened and have muscular attachment structures. Trematodes have a digestive tract, whereas cestodes lack a digestive tract. Both trematodes and cestodes have indirect life cycles requiring intermediate hosts, and both male and female reproductive organs are found in the same individual, with the exception of schistosomes.

61. a. Fecal samples should be examined for consistency, color, odor, blood, mucus, and foreign bodies. They should be examined ideally within the first hour after elimination with a direct smear and fecal flotation. A direct smear facilitates detection of motile protozoan trophozoites that do not survive in the environment for more than 24 hours. Fecal flotation detects protozoan cysts and helminth eggs in the sample. Samples collected rectally or off of clean surfaces are better than samples collected with grass and dirt because of contamination of the samples with stages of free-living nematodes in the environment.

62. c. When lungworm infections are suspected, fecal samples should be examined by a Baermann test. Fecal flotation solutions, such as sodium chloride solution, distort the larvae and make identification difficult. Flotation with zinc sulfate solution is recommended for recovery of some lungworms. Larvae can be recovered by sedimentation, but this technique concentrates fecal debris as well as larvae and is not as efficient. The modified McMaster egg counting technique uses flotation solutions that crenate larvae and it is not as sensitive.

63. b. The recommended flotation solution for recovery of *Giardia* oocysts is zinc sulfate. This solution has a lower specific gravity and floats less fecal debris. It also does not distort oocysts as much as other salt solutions.

64. b. For a blood chemistry profile, blood should be collected in a heparin tube, and plasma is submitted for assay.

65. c. None of the other sample handling methods described is appropriate.

66. d. The blood glucose level is used to assess carbohydrate metabolism.

67. b. Serum contains no fibrinogen. Heparinized plasma should not be used.

68. a. Urine is the sample of choice for dark-field, morphologic examination of leptospires.

69. d. Ringworm is a skin infection.

70. b. CO_2 from dry ice can escape into the container and kill pH-sensitive microorganisms by lowering the pH of fluids.

71. b. Virologic specimens should be immediately placed on dry ice.

72. d. Magnification of an object is determined by the power of the ocular lens × the power of the objective lens. A 50× lens produces higher magnification. The N.A. is directly proportional to the resolving power of the lens; the higher the N.A., the greater the resolution.

73. d. Complete analysis of fluid (blood) from a hematoma is not necessary. An aspirate from a hematoma should be handled in the same manner as an aspirate from a fluid-filled mass.

74. c. The pH usually increases if urine is left standing for some time.

75. d. Rhabdomyolysis, a condition characterized by muscle damage and release of myoglobin, does not cause increased WBC numbers in the urine.

76. c. For reliable results, kit instructions should be followed exactly. Refrigeration or centrifugation does not clear hemolysis.

77. c. Although it may be convenient to list the instrument manufacturer's address and telephone number, this information is not necessary on the maintenance log.

CHAPTER 12: EUTHANASIA METHODS, SPECIMEN COLLECTION, AND NECROPSY TECHNIQUES

78. d. Cervical dislocation is used for poultry, other small birds, and other small animals, such as mice and immature rats.

79. d. Unlike other laboratory tests, toxicologic testing requires large quantities of tissue or specimen.

80. b. Specimen sections thicker than 5 mm are not adequately penetrated by fixative. Thicker unfixed sections allow autolysis to progress.

81. c. Horses do not have a gallbladder.

82. b. Many viruses are successfully isolated from animals in the acute stages of a viral illness, as opposed to animals that have been sick for many days, or dead.

CHAPTER 13: PHARMACOLOGY AND PHARMACY PRACTICES

83. d. 22 lb = 10 kg × 5 mg/kg = 50 mg per dose = 2 tablets × 3 doses daily = 6 tablets daily × 5 days = 30 tablets

84. b. This is the only type of insulin that can be safely given IV.

85. b. Gentamicin is an aminoglycoside, which can produce nephrotoxicity.

86. d. Chlorhexidine is a biguanide and is the active ingredient in Nolvasan.

87. b. Melarsomine may eventually displace thiacetarsamide as the most widely used heartworm adulticide.

CHAPTER 14: NUTRITION

88. a. Each day, an average growing puppy gains about 2 to 4 g/kg of anticipated adult weight.

89. c. Abrupt or frequent diet changes are not recommended.

90. b. A queen nursing a litter or growing kittens has a very high daily energy requirement.

91. d. The other species digest prefermented feed material.

92. c. The highest rating on the scale is 9, or grossly obese.

CHAPTER 15: REPRODUCTION

93. d. Anestrus is followed by proestrus, then estrus, and finally diestrus.

94. c. ECG levels tend to be highest between 35 and 120 days of gestation.

95. d. Mares can be examined with use of a transrectal probe.

96. a. The other items listed can be attended to after adequate respiration is ensured.

97. d. Genetic potential is evaluated by breeding trials rather than by a breeding soundness examination.

CHAPTER 16: BEHAVIOR

98. c. A crate should not be used to the detriment of the puppy's socialization needs or for such long periods that the puppy is forced to eliminate in it. A crate is only a tool to supervise a puppy during housetraining; it does not constitute the complete housetraining process.

99. d. Eliminating in loose, particulate substrates is a normal developmental process that does not require observational learning or owner assistance.

100. c. It is not realistic to attempt to eliminate chewing behavior through punishment. The goal is to redirect the behavior to appropriate objects.

101. a. Scientific studies have shown that puppy tests do not predict adult behavior.

102. c. Several studies on cat behavior have shown this to be true. The other statements are hypotheses and/or opinions not substantiated by scientific behavioral research.

103. b. This is the technical, precise definition of punishment. All of the other choices listed are incorrect.

CHAPTER 17: PHYSICAL RESTRAINT

104. c. Most friendly cats can be restrained with minimal handling.

105. d. Pigs are best driven with a solid panel, because they naturally back away from it.

106. b. Guinea pigs have no loose skin on the nape of their necks.

107. b. Care should be used to prevent hyperthermia when restraining birds with a cloth or towel.

108. d. All escape routes should be closed before the cage door is opened.

CHAPTER 18: PATIENT HISTORY AND EXAMINATION

109. c. Such information may aid diagnosis.

110. b. Differential diagnoses comprise the possible causes of illness in a specific case.

111. a. Tympany describes the drumlike sound produced by percussion of a gas-filled organ.

112. b. Stridor is loud breathing that can be heard without the aid of a stethoscope.

113. a. The fist is rhythmically pressed in an effort to bump underlying masses or organs.

CHAPTER 19: DIAGNOSTIC IMAGING

114. d. Metal is the most dense and has a higher atomic number; therefore, it absorbs more x-rays.

115. c. kVp controls contrast. A higher kVp produces a radiograph with a long scale of contrast or more grays.

116. b. With full-wave rectified, three phase, a constant positive electrical potential is applied from the cathode to the anode, allowing faster times to be used.

117. d. *Isoechoic* is used to describe tissues with the same echotexture as surrounding tissues.

118. b. Straightening the distal end of the endoscope facilitates passage of the biopsy forceps.

119. d. Microchips are used in video endoscopes.

CHAPTER 20: PRINCIPLES OF ANESTHESIA, ANALGESIA, AND ANESTHETIC NURSING

120. d. Although the other answer choices help maintain perfusion, perfusion involves flow of oxygenated blood to tissues.

121. c. Answers *a*, *b*, and *d* may indicate other conditions in addition to hypoventilation. Abnormal blood gas results provide specific indications of inadequate gas exchange.

122. c. It is always wise to evaluate the patient's overall condition before making decisions.

123. b. Phenothiazines are alpha-blocking agents that may cause significant vasodilation and hypotension.

124. a. Only answer *a* describes a normal situation in which there is a pulse for each beat of the heart. Answer *b* describes an abnormal condition called *pulse deficit*. Answer *c* is physiologically impossible. Answer *d* is incorrect.

125. b. This infusion rate replaces fluids lost because of inhalation of dry gases and supplements the fluid volume to offset the hypotensive effects of anesthesia. A given patient may need more or less fluids at various stages of the procedure, however.

126. c. Standard replacement fluids containing sodium are distributed one third in the intravascular space and two thirds in the extravascular space. For adequate volume replacement, one must administer three times the blood volume lost. Answer *d* is the maximum fluid delivery rate used in shock patients.

127. c. This combination is commercially available as Innovar-Vet.

CHAPTER 21: PRINCIPLES OF SURGICAL NURSING

128. c. A paramedian incision is made on either side of and parallel to the ventral midline.

129. c. Such accumulations of fluid are called *seromas*.

130. b. Sterile items can safely come in contact with other sterile items.

131. a. An intact, heat-sealed plastic pouch generally ensures sterility for a year.

132. d. This delicate instrument would be damaged by steam sterilization

133. b. This prevents water from running down the arms and contaminating the hands.

134. c. Chlorhexidine binds with keratin.

135. a. Both methods provide about the same degree of disinfection.

136. c. Wire of this size is thicker than the other materials listed.

137. a. The other materials listed are absorbable.

CHAPTER 22: EMERGENCY AND CRITICAL CARE

138. c. Laryngeal paralysis is associated with loud, sonorous sounds; pulmonary edema has a crackling sound; a wheezing sound is associated with asthma.

139. b. Capillary refill time is only an indicator of peripheral perfusion.

140. a. All of the other fluids listed contain electrolytes and are similar to plasma.

141. a. Antibiotics do not help the clinical signs of shock. Corticosteroids may or may not be beneficial. Sympathomimetics are used when the patient is unresponsive to fluid therapy.

142. c. Organophosphate poisoning is associated with salivation, lacrimation, miosis, and muscle tremors. Signs of ethylene glycol toxicity include depression and acute renal failure. Anticoagulant rodenticide toxicity is associated with anemia and signs of hemorrhage.

CHAPTER 23: MANAGEMENT OF WOUNDS, FRACTURES, AND OTHER INJURIES

143. b. This is considered a clean-contaminated wound.

144. a. A wound is considered infected when the microbial count exceeds this level.

145. a. Setons are less useful once they have become saturated with exudates.

146. c. This is also a form of third-intention healing.

147. a. The Robert Jones bandage provides compression and immobilization of the distal limb until definitive treatment is available.

148. c. Protruding arrows are best removed by a veterinarian.

CHAPTER 24: FLUID THERAPY AND BLOOD TRANSFUSIONS

149. d. Acidosis is a high concentration of hydrogen ions, with corresponding low pH.

150. b. The other solutions listed are most appropriate for replacement therapy.

151. a. Normal cuticle bleeding time in dogs is less than 5 minutes.

152. b. Blood of DEA 1.1 negative type can be safely infused into recipients.

153. d. Heparin has no preservative properties and is not recommended for transfusion purposes.

CHAPTER 25: DENTISTRY

154. b. Stage 3 involves up to 50%; stage 4 involves greater than 50%.

155. a. Typical bacteria in pockets are anaerobic, gram-negative motile bacilli.

156. c. An intraoral film must be taped to a standard film before putting it through the processor and even then it can still get lost. They are inexpensive and flexible and have a double emulsion.

157. b. The upper canines are deflected rostally (mesially) by retained deciduous teeth; the other teeth listed are deflected lingually.

158. c. Fusion refers to two separate teeth that fuse together; twinning is the complete duplication and split.

159. d. The carnassial teeth are the upper front premolars and lower front molars.

160. d. Teeth with open canals should *NEVER* be ignored because of the great potential for infection and bacteremia spreading to the rest of the body.

CHAPTER 26: NURSING CARE OF DOGS AND CATS

161. a. The vessels of cats tend to be superficial and fragile.

162. b. Samples for blood gas assays should be collected in a syringe or in special arterial blood samplers.

163. a. None of the other sites is commonly used for SC administration.

164. a. Longer catheters are more stable and less likely to irritate the vein.

165. d. None of the other sites is appropriate for long-term use.

166. d. Heating pads can easily cause thermal burns if not used carefully.

167. b. This most commonly involves administration of oxygen via mask or nasal tube.

168. c. A nasogastric tube can safely remain in place for at least a week.

CHAPTER 27: NURSING CARE OF HORSES

169. d. Black walnut shavings contain a substance that can be toxic.

170. d. Horses usually cannot vomit. If a horse has gastric reflux, it should not be given anything by nasogastric tube, nor should it be allowed to eat or drink.

171. d. Disinfection is ineffective if organic material is present. Infected horses should be handled last, if possible. Diseases can also be spread through secretions, feces, and via people and objects, not just by coughing.

172. b. Care must be taken not to overhydrate foals with large boluses of IV fluids. Nothing should be injected into an IV line containing par-

enteral nutrition solution, because it is easily contaminated. The proteins in plasma become denatured if the plasma is thawed too quickly or if it is "cooked" in a microwave.

173. a. Leg wraps should be snug but not too tight and applied to distribute pressure uniformly. The point of the hock is often left unwrapped to prevent development of pressure sores.

174. a. To turn a recumbent horse, long ropes should be looped around the pasterns and pulled to flip the horse, making sure that there is plenty of room to get out of the way once the horse starts to turn over. One should always stay out of range of the limbs of a recumbent horse.

175. c. Organophosphate sprays may be dangerous to sick horses. The other methods of fly control can be helpful, but frequent manure removal and keeping stalls clean provide the *best* fly control.

CHAPTER 28: NURSING CARE OF FOOD ANIMALS, CAMELIDS, AND RATITES

176. a. This vein is not routinely used for blood collection because of the danger of being kicked.

177. c. The jugular vein is the largest accessible vein in calves.

178. b. Milk in the gland tends to dilute the infused medication.

179. d. Bright, glaring, or shadowy lighting makes sheep uneasy.

180. a. A cough reflex indicates the tube is in the trachea and not in the esophagus. Air may be felt exiting the tube on exhalation.

181. a. Subcutaneous injection prevents muscle damage, which would diminish the value of the carcass.

182. c. Injections along the back and dorsal flank damage the hide. There is no loose skin at the dorsal aspect of the neck, as in dogs and cats.

183. a. Intramuscular injections should be limited to 5 ml per site.

184. c. A needle of this size minimizes patient discomfort while allowing for injection of fairly viscous medications.

185. b. Sows, gilts, and boars denote reproductive stages and not a stage of production.

186. c. Absorption of colostrum halts by 24 hours after birth.

187. c. The stomach of llamas has three compartments rather than four.

188. d. Emus have vestigial wings; the other species have relatively well-developed wings.

CHAPTER 29: NURSING CARE OF CAGE BIRDS AND POULTRY

189. b. Isoflurane gas is safe and provides extremely fast induction and recovery.

190. d. The pectoral muscles are the largest in the body.

191. a. The primary flight feathers provide the lift required for flying.

192. a. Gavage, or tube feeding, places medication directly into the crop.

193. c. Behavior counseling should be performed by a person with a strong background in pet birds and who is familiar with current behavior theory.

194. d. Poultry are housed in a flock situation, not individually.

CHAPTER 30: NURSING CARE OF SMALL MAMMALS

195. b. Guinea pigs require a dietary source of vitamin C.

196. a. Feeding roughage in the form of hay helps prevent hairball formation.

197. b. Cardiac puncture is not recommended in ferrets.

198. c. The number of injectable drugs available is irrelevant. The other reasons listed constitute the advantages of parenteral injection.

CHAPTER 31: NURSING CARE OF REPTILES, AMPHIBIANS, AND AQUARIUM FISH

199. c. Amphibians require a cooler and more humid environment than do reptiles.

200. d. Blood is often collected from the heart of snakes.

201. a. Blood is usually collected from the jugular vein of turtles.

202. a. Anabolism is the process of tissue generation. Reduced food intake leads to catabolism, or tissue degeneration.

203. a. Respiratory rate is the most important sign to monitor when a fish is anesthetized. If opercular movement ceases at any time, the fish should be removed from the anesthetic solution at once.

CHAPTER 32: NURSING CARE OF ORPHANED AND INJURED WILD ANIMALS

204. a. The other injuries listed are likely to lead to that animal's death after release.

205. c. The other amounts listed are insufficient.

206. b. Botulism commonly causes death of large numbers of aquatic birds at one time.

207. d. *Trichomonas* affects the esophagus and crop of pigeons and doves.

208. c. Pinnipeds housed in fresh water require supplemental salt (sodium chloride) and thiamin (B_1). Because pinnipeds are marine mammals, they require extra salt in their diet when housed in fresh water. They can become hyponatremic (sodium deficient) if they do not receive the supplement. This can lead to neurologic problems and death. Thiamin is destroyed over time by the action of thiaminase present in the tissues of frozen fish. Thiamin deficiency can lead to neurologic problems progressing to death.

CHAPTER 33: NURSING CARE
OF LABORATORY ANIMALS

209. b. The hamster has a gestation period of 16 days; mouse, 21 days; gerbil, 24 days; and rabbit, 31 days.

210. a. The rabbit has two pairs of upper incisors that distinguish them as lagomorphs.

211. a. Penicillin can induce fatal enterotoxemia in guinea pigs.

212. d. Spontaneous seizures occur when gerbils are stimulated by loud noises, rough handling, or a new environment.

213. c. Cedar should be avoided because it emits aromatic hydrocarbons that induce liver changes.

CHAPTER 34: NURSING CARE
OF PEDIATRIC AND GERIATRIC
PATIENTS

214. a. Only this answer lists the procedures according to appropriate priority.

215. a. Intraosseous or intravenous administration is most appropriate for administration of fluids to volume-depleted neonates.

216. c. A neonatal calf's body temperature is normally about 1° to 1.5° warmer than the dam's.

217. a. Aggression may be a result of pain or fear. Pain is associated with degenerative joint disease. Fear is associated with failing eyesight and hearing or anxiety but usually not the other ailments listed.

218. b. Weight reduction in an overweight geriatric pet can be achieved by feeding a diet low in fat and high in fiber, feeding small meals more frequently, and gradually increasing gentle exercise. Because of possible cardiovascular, respiratory, and joint disease, sudden vigorous exercise should be avoided.

Index

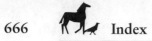

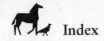

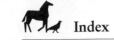

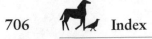